PEDIATRIC PARAMETERS AND EQUIPMENT

Age	Pre-term	Newborn	3 Mo	6 Mo	1 Yr	2 Yr	3 Yr	4 Yr	6 Yr	8 Yr	12 Yr	Adolescent
Wt (kg)	1.5	3.5	6	8	10	12	15	17	20	25	40	50
HR	160	130	140	130	120	115	100	100	100	90	85	85
RR	40	40	30	30	26	26	24	24	20	20	20	20
SBP	60	70	80	80	90	90	95	95	95	95	105	110
Cuff	Preemie	Newborn	Infant	Small child	Small child	Child	Child	Child	Child/small adult	Small adult	Adult	Adult
BVM	Newborn	Infant	Infant	Child	Child	Child	Child	Child	Child	Child/adult	Adult	Adult
Oral Airway	Newborn 40 mm	Infant 50 mm	Small 60 mm	Small 60 mm	Small 60 mm	Small 70 mm	Small 70 mm	Med 80 mm	Med 90 mm	Med 90 mm	Large 100 mm	Large 100 mm
ETT Blade	#0	#0–1	#1	#1	#1	#2	#2	#2	#2	#2–3	#3	#3
ETT Size	2.5–3.0	2.5–3.5	3.5–4.0	3.5–4.0	4.0–4.5	4.0–4.5	4.5–5.0	4.5–5.0	5.0–5.5	5.5–6.5*	6.0*–7.0*	7.0*–8.0*
Sx Cath	5Fr	6Fr	8Fr–10Fr	8Fr–10Fr	8Fr–10Fr	10Fr	10Fr	10Fr	10Fr	10Fr	12Fr	14Fr
NGT	5Fr	5Fr–8Fr	5Fr–8Fr	8Fr–10Fr	10Fr	10Fr	10Fr	10Fr–12Fr	12Fr–14Fr	14Fr	14Fr–18Fr	14Fr–18Fr
IV Cath	24G	22–24G	22–24G	20–24G	20–24G	18–22G	18–22G	18–22G	18–20G	18–20G	16–20G	16–20G
Chest Tube	8Fr–10 Fr	12Fr	16Fr	16Fr	16Fr	16Fr	16Fr	16Fr	20Fr	24Fr	28Fr	30Fr
Urine Cath	5Fr	6Fr	8Fr	8Fr	8Fr	8Fr	8Fr	8Fr	10Fr	12Fr	14Fr	14Fr

*8 yr and greater: Should have cuffed ETT.

ETT Size = (Age [years] + 16)/4.

Avg. tube depth from lip/teeth = 3 × ETT size (i.e., 3.0 × 3 = 9 cm@lip).

Hypotension = SBP ≤70 mmHg + (2 × age in years over 1 yr).

<1 mo SBP ≤60, 1 mo–1 yr SBP ≤70.

From The Johns Hopkins Children's Center Kids Kard, 2007.

IV INFUSIONS* $$6 \times \frac{\text{Desired dose (mcg/kg/min)}}{\text{Desired rate (mL/hr)}} \times \text{Wt (kg)} = \frac{\text{mg drug}}{\text{100 mL fluid}}$$

Medication	Dose (mcg/kg/min)	Dilution in 100 mL D_5W	IV Infusion Rate
Alprostadil (Prostaglandin E_1)	0.05–0.1	0.3 mg/kg	1 mL/hr = 0.05 mcg/kg/min
Amiodarone	5–15	6 mg/kg	1 mL/hr = 1 mcg/kg/min
DOPamine	2–20	6 mg/kg	1 mL/hr = 1 mcg/kg/min
DOBUTamine	2–20	6 mg/kg	1 mL/hr = 1 mcg/kg/min
EPINEPHrine	0.1–1	0.6 mg/kg	1 mL/hr = 0.1 mcg/kg/min
Lidocaine	20–50	6 mg/kg	1 mL/hr = 1 mcg/kg/min
Phenylephrine	0.05–2	0.3 mg/kg	1 mL/hr = 0.05 mcg/kg/min
Terbutaline	0.1–10	0.6 mg/kg	1 mL/hr = 0.1 mcg/kg/min
Vasopressin (pressor)	0.5–2 milliunits/kg/min	6 milliunits/kg	1 mL/hr = 1 milliunit/kg/min

*Standardized concentrations are recommended when available.

RESUSCITATION MEDICATIONS

Adenosine • Supraventricular tachycardia	**0.1 mg/kg IV/IO RAPID BOLUS** May repeat at 0.2 mg/kg IV/IO after 2 min Max first dose 6 mg, max subsequent dose 12 mg
Amiodarone • Ventricular tachycardia • Ventricular fibrillation	**5 mg/kg IV/IO** Push if no pulse Give over 20–60 min if pulse Monitor for hypotension
Atropine • Bradycardia (increased vagal tone) • Primary AV block	**0.02 mg/kg IV/IO, 0.04–0.06 mg/kg ETT** Min dose 0.1 mg Max single dose 0.5 mg Repeat once if needed
Calcium chloride (10%) • Hypocalcemia	**20 mg/kg IV/IO (0.2 mL/kg)** Max dose 2 grams
Dextrose	**<5 kg 10% dextrose 10 mL/kg** **5 to <45 kg 25% dextrose 4 mL/kg** **≥45 kg 50% dextrose 2 mL/kg**
EPINEPHrine • Pulseless arrest • Bradycardia (symptomatic)	**0.01 mg/kg (0.1 mL/kg) 1 : 10,000 IV/IO every 3–5 min (max 1 mg)** **0.1 mg/kg (0.1 mL/kg) 1 : 1,000 ETT every 3–5 min (max 2.5 mg)**
Insulin • Hyperkalemia	**0.1 units/kg IV/IO with 1 g/kg of dextrose**
Magnesium sulfate • Torsades de pointes • Hypomagnesemia	**50 mg/kg IV/IO** Push if no pulse Give over 15–20 min if pulse Max dose 2 grams Monitor for hypotension/bradycardia
Naloxone • Opioid overdose • Coma	**First dose: 0.001–0.005 mg/kg to reverse respiratory depression associated with opioid overdose** **High dose: <5 yr or <20 kg: 0.1 mg/kg IV/IO/IM/SubQ** **>5 yr or >20 kg: 2 mg IV/IO/IM/SubQ** ETT dose 2–3 times IV dose. May give every 2 min prn
Sodium bicarbonate • Metabolic acidosis • Hyperkalemia • Tricyclic antidepressant overdose	**1 mEq/kg IV/IO** Dilute 1 : 1 with sterile water for <10 kg
Vasopressin	**0.5 units/kg/dose IV/IO**

ETT Meds (NAVEL: naloxone, atropine, vasopressin, epinephrine, lidocaine)—dilute meds to 5 mL with NS, follow with positive-pressure ventilation.

Adapted from the Johns Hopkins Children's Center Kids Kard, 2007, and the American Heart Association, PALS Pocket Card, 2007.

Special thanks to LeAnn McNamara and Angela Martinez, Clinical Pharmacy Specialists for their expert guidance with IV infusion and resuscitation medications guidelines.

GLASGOW COMA SCALE

Activity	Score	Child/Adult	Score	Infant
Eye Opening	4	Spontaneous	4	Spontaneous
	3	To speech	3	To speech/sound
	2	To pain	2	To pain
	1	None	1	None
Verbal	5	Oriented	5	Coos/babbles
	4	Confused	4	Irritable cry
	3	Inappropriate	3	Cries to pain
	2	Incomprehensible	2	Moans to pain
	1	None	1	None
Motor	6	Obeys commands	6	Normal spontaneous
	5	Localizes to pain	5	Withdraws to touch
	4	Withdraws to pain	4	Withdraws to pain
	3	Abnormal flexion	3	Abnormal flexion (decorticate)
	2	Abnormal extension	2	Abnormal extension (decerebrate)
	1	None	1	None

From The Johns Hopkins Children's Center Kids Kard, 2007.

nineteenth
EDITION

THE HARRIET LANE HANDBOOK

A Manual for Pediatric House Officers

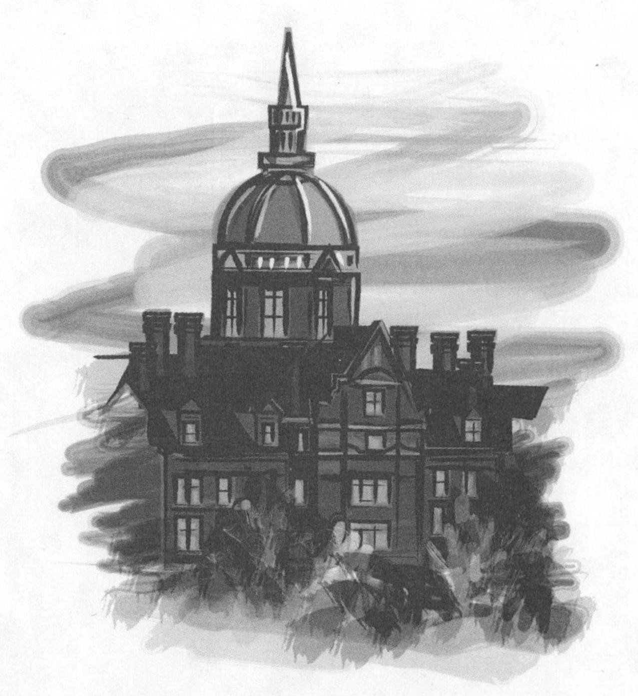

nineteenth
EDITION

THE HARRIET LANE HANDBOOK

A Manual for Pediatric House Officers

The Harriet Lane Service
Children's Medical and Surgical Center of
The Johns Hopkins Hospital

EDITORS
Megan M. Tschudy, MD
Kristin M. Arcara, MD

with more than 110 illustrations and over 55 color plates

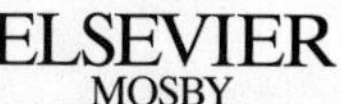

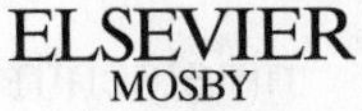

1600 John F. Kennedy Blvd.
Suite 1800
Philadelphia, PA 19103-2899

THE HARRIET LANE HANDBOOK, NINETEENTH EDITION ISBN: 978-0-323-07942-6
International Edition: 978-0-8089-2435-7

Notices

Knowledge and best practice in this field are constantly changing. As new research and experience broaden our understanding, changes in research methods, professional practices, or medical treatment may become necessary.

Practitioners and researchers must always rely on their own experience and knowledge in evaluating and using any information, methods, compounds, or experiments described herein. In using such information or methods they should be mindful of their own safety and the safety of others, including parties for whom they have a professional responsibility.

With respect to any drug or pharmaceutical products identified, readers are advised to check the most current information provided (i) on procedures featured or (ii) by the manufacturer of each product to be administered, to verify the recommended dose or formula, the method and duration of administration, and contraindications. It is the responsibility of practitioners, relying on their own experience and knowledge of their patients, to make diagnoses, to determine dosages and the best treatment for each individual patient, and to take all appropriate safety precautions.

To the fullest extent of the law, neither the Publisher nor the authors, contributors, or editors, assume any liability for any injury and/or damage to persons or property as a matter of products liability, negligence or otherwise, or from any use or operation of any methods, products, instructions, or ideas contained in the material herein.

Library of Congress Cataloging-in-Publication Data
The Harriet Lane handbook : a manual for pediatric house officers / the Harriet Lane Service, Children's Medical and Surgical Center of the Johns Hopkins Hospital.—19th ed. / editors, Megan M. Tschudy, Kristin M. Arcara.
p. ; cm.
Includes bibliographical references and index.
ISBN 978-0-323-07942-6 (pbk. : alk. paper)—ISBN 978-0-8089-2435-7 (international ed. : pbk. : alk. paper)
1. Pediatrics—Handbooks, manuals, etc. I. Tschudy, Megan M. II. Arcara, Kristin M. III. Johns Hopkins Hospital. Children's Medical and Surgical Center.
[DNLM: 1. Pediatrics—Handbooks. WS 29]
RJ48.H35 2012
618.92—dc22

2011005581

Acquisitions Editor: James Merritt
Developmental Editor: Barbara Cicalese
Publishing Services Manager: Pat Joiner-Myers
Senior Project Manager: Joy Moore
Designer: Steve Stave
Marketing Manager: Helena Mutak

Printed in the United States of America

Last digit is the print number: 9 8 7 6 5 4 3 2

To our loving families:

Diane and Donald Arcara,
whose love and unending sacrifice have given me
wings to fly and roots to
keep me grounded, without which I wouldn't be where I am today.

To Kenneth Aiello, my family and friends,
every step of the way you have been there to support,
listen to, and love me; I don't know
what I would do without each of you.

Mary and Ted Tschudy,
for loving me selflessly and supporting me unconditionally,
you laid the strong foundation for all I am today and will become.

To my family and friends who have become my family,
thank you for teaching me by loving example,
wholeheartedly believing in me,
and always walking by my side.

To our patients and their families,

You constantly challenge us to improve ourselves as clinicians,
communicators, and educators, inspire us with your courage,
and enrich our lives.

To our role model, teacher, and friend

Julia McMillan

And to

George Dover,
Chairman of Pediatrics
The Johns Hopkins Hospital,
Devoted advocate for residents, children, and their families

Preface

"The good physician treats the disease; the great physician treats the patient who has the disease."

—*Sir William Osler*

The Harriet Lane Handbook was first developed in 1953 after Harrison Spencer (Chief Resident in 1950–1951) suggested that residents should write a pocket-sized "pearl book." As recounted by Henry Seidel, the first editor of *The Harriet Lane Handbook,* "Six of us began without funds and without [the] supervision of our elders, meeting sporadically around a table in the library of the Harriet Lane Home." The product of their efforts was a concise yet comprehensive handbook that became an indispensable tool for the residents of the Harriet Lane Home. Ultimately, Robert Cooke (Department Chief, 1956–1974) realized the potential of the handbook, and, with his backing, the fifth edition was published for widespread distribution by Year Book. Since that time, the handbook has been regularly updated and rigorously revised to reflect the most up-to-date information and clinical guidelines available. It has grown from a humble Hopkins resident "pearl book" to become a nationally and internationally respected clinical resource. Now translated into many languages, the handbook is still intended as an easy-to-use manual to help pediatricians provide current and comprehensive pediatric care.

Today *The Harriet Lane Handbook* continues to be updated and revised *by* house officers *for* house officers, with each edition improving in content from the previous edition. Recognizing that including all of the information we would like to present would push the book past the size of a useful pocket book and that many physicians have access to online references, for the first time the nineteenth edition includes online-only content. This symbol throughout the chapters denotes online content in Expert Consult. This content is meant to provide in-depth information that might be beyond the scope of a pocket-sized, printed resource. The online-only content includes expanded text, tables, additional images, and other references. The nineteenth edition also provides a number of pertinent websites at the beginning of many chapters.

Notable changes to this edition include a significant reorganization of text and figures to improve flow and ease of use. In addition to including the most up-to-date guidelines, practice parameters, and references, we will highlight some of the most important improvements in the nineteenth edition of *The Harriet Lane Handbook.*

- Reflecting the importance of mental health care in pediatrics, the Behavior and Development chapter has been significantly expanded to include information about pediatric psychiatry and renamed, **"Development, Behavior, and Mental Health"** to reflect the enhanced content. This chapter reviews the identification and management of basic mental health disorders, including pharmacologic management of attention deficit/hyperactivity disorder (ADHD) and depression.

- The **Microbiology and Infectious Disease** chapter has been completely reorganized to improve organization and ease of use. We have also included guidelines for the management of newborns with in utero HIV exposure.
- The **Hematology** chapter includes significantly revised guidelines for monitoring unfractionated heparin and Coumadin.
- The **Genetics** chapter has been expanded to include a hypoglycemia decision tree algorithm and information on mitochondrial disorders.
- The **Immunoprophylaxis** chapter has also been completely updated with the most current immunization guidelines, including human papillomavirus (HPV) for females and males, revised respiratory syncytial virus (RSV) prophylaxis, and PCV13 guidelines.
- The **Poisonings** chapter has been expanded to include information on lead poisoning as well as envenomation management.
- Given the delicate nature and paramount importance of fluid and electrolyte management in pediatrics, the **Fluid and Electrolytes** chapter has been broken down to separate these two aspects of management and then recombined with an easy-to-follow set of equations for various clinical scenarios.
- The chapter on **Gastroenterology** has been reorganized and now includes information on inflammatory bowel disease as well as antibody production in response to hepatitis B infection.
- The **Rheumatology** chapter features a new easy-to-use table providing an overview of vasculitides, a new section on treatment of systemic lupus erythematosus, and a table detailing the differences and similarities among the juvenile rheumatoid/idiopathic arthritis classifications.

Designed for pediatric house staff, *The Harriet Lane Handbook* would not have been possible without the substantial efforts of this year's senior resident class, the members of which balanced their busy resident schedules with authoring the chapters that follow. They truly are the heart and soul of this handbook. Watching their growth in clinical skill and character since their internship and their dedication to patients gives us the utmost confidence in the bright future of pediatrics. Each of these residents worked with a faculty advisor, who selflessly dedicated his or her time and expertise to improve the quality and content of this publication. We are indebted to both of these groups for their tireless work.

Chapter Title	Resident	Faculty Advisor
1. Emergency Management	Christopher Valente, MD	Allen Walker, MD
2. Poisonings	Tina Rezaiyan, MD	Mitchell Goldstein, MD
3. Procedures	Laura J. Sigman, MD, JD	Jason Custer, MD
4. Trauma, Burns, and Common Critical Care Emergencies	Katherine M. Steffen, MD	Allen Walker, MD
5. Adolescent Medicine	Nicole Brown, MD, MPH	Hoover Adger, MD, PhD Arik Marcell, MD, MPH
6. Analgesia and Sedation	Kristin M. Arcara, MD	Jennifer Anders, MD
7. Cardiology	Elaine Giannakos Lennox, MD	Jane Crosson, MD William Ravekes, MD W. Reid Thompson, MD
8. Dermatology	Nisha Kapadia, MD	Bernard Cohen, MD
9. Development, Behavior, and Mental Health	Jessica Perniciaro, MD	Mary Leppert, MB, BCh, BAO
10. Endocrinology	Lauren Cohee, MD	David Cooke, MD
11. Fluids and Electrolytes	Elizabeth Quaal Hines, MD	Michael Barone, MD
12. Gastroenterology	Rebecca F. Rabin, MD, MHS	Maria Oliva-Hemker, MD
13. Genetics	Emily Spengler, MD	Ronald Cohn, MD
14. Hematology	Sama Ahsan, MD Julia Noether, MD	James Casella, MD Clifford Takemoto, MD
15. Immunology and Allergy	Wonha Kim, MD	Howard Lederman, MD, PhD Robert Wood, MD
16. Immunoprophylaxis	Kristin Santini Casasanta, MD	Ravit Boger, MD
17. Microbiology and Infectious Disease	Benjamin Lee, MD Tracy McCallin, MD	Aaron Milstone, MD
18. Neonatology	Matthew H. Merves, MD	Sue Aucott, MD
19. Nephrology	Stacy Cooper, MD	Susan Furth, MD
20. Neurology	Delphine Robotham, MD	Thomas Crawford, MD
21. Nutrition and Growth	Brandi Kaye Freeman, MD Jenifer Hampsey, MS, RD, CSP	Maria Oliva-Hemker, MD
22. Oncology	Catherine M. Albert, MD	Kenneth Cohen, MD Patrick Brown, MD
23. Palliative Care	Judson Heugel, MD	Nancy Hutton, MD
24. Pulmonology	Allison Kirk, MD	Laura Sterni, MD
25. Radiology	Judson Heugel, MD	Jane Benson, MD
26. Rheumatology	Marc A. Callender, MD	Sangeeta Sule, MD, PhD Edward Sills, MD
27. Blood Chemistries and Body Fluids	Kristin M. Arcara, MD	
28. Biostatistics and Evidence-Based Medicine	Karsten Lunze, MD, MPH	Leon Gordis, MD, MPH, DrPH
29. Drug Doses	Carlton K. K. Lee, PharmD, MPH Megan M. Tschudy, MD Kristin M. Arcara, MD	
30. Formulary Adjunct	Kristin M. Arcara, MD	
31. Drugs in Renal Failure	Megan M. Tschudy, MD	

The Formulary, which is undoubtedly one of the most referred to handbook sections, is complete, concise, and up-to-date thanks to the efforts of Carlton K. K. Lee, PharmD, MPH. With each edition, he carefully updates, revises, and improves the section. His herculean efforts make the Formulary one of the most useful and cited pediatric drug reference texts available.

Generations of Johns Hopkins residents have met for teaching conferences in the Frank Oski Conference Room. On a centrally located bookshelf stand all of the previous editions of *The Harriet Lane Handbook*. They remind us daily of the remarkable legacy of leadership left by the previous authors and editors whose work is the foundation of this book. We truly are humbled to have the opportunity to build on the great work of the preceding editors: Drs. Harrison Spencer, Henry Seidel, Herbert Swick, William Friedman, Robert Haslam, Jerry Winkelstein, Dennis Headings, Kenneth Schuberth, Basil Zitelli, Jeffery Biller, Andrew Yeager, Cynthia Cole, Mary Greene, Peter Rowe, Kevin Johnson, Michael Barone, George Siberry, Rob Iannone, Christian Nechyba, Veronica Gunn, Jason Robertson, Nicole Shilkofski, Jason Custer, and Rachel Rau. Many of these previous editors continue to contribute to the learning and maturation of the Harriet Lane house staff. They all are true examples of outstanding clinicians, educators, and mentors.

An undertaking of this magnitude could not have been accomplished without the support and dedication of some extraordinary people. Special thanks to Megan Brown and Kathy Miller for providing tremendous support and counsel. They are the backbone that holds together our program. We truly appreciate their friendship. We also offer our deepest gratitude to George Dover, whose constant desire for change and improvement and whose tireless service continues to push the Johns Hopkins Children's Center, pediatric resident education, and each of us further toward excellence. We who are fortunate enough to work with him are better equipped to care for our patients and contribute to advancement in the field of pediatrics because of his inspiring leadership. A heartfelt "thank you" goes to Drs. Henry Seidel, Barton Childs, and Fred Heldrich, whose professionalism and commitment to pediatrics we can only hope to emulate. Their legacy lives on in the generations of pediatricians trained under their steady guiding hands who now teach new generations. They will be missed. Our special thanks go to our friend and mentor Janet Serwint, whose leadership continues to deeply enrich our lives. She is the consummate example of unwavering commitment to excellence in patient care, research scholarship, and teaching. Finally, none of this would have been possible without Julia McMillan. She is a true leader in every sense of the word with her reach extending well past our institution. Her commitment to the care of all children and her passion for medical education has nurtured a love of pediatrics and learning in all of us. We are forever indebted to her.

Residents

Lubna Abdullah
Breanna Barger-Kamate
Katherine Beckwith-Fickas
Challice Bonifant
Rebecca Carlin
Susan Davidson
Marissa DeFreitas
Neal deJong
Branden Engorn
Alisa Khan
Jessica Komlos
Jamie Laubisch
Hanna Lemerman
Monica Lemmon
Jean Limpert
Melissa Long
Nicole Marsh
Courtney McGuire
Anna Minta
Jana Mohassel
Tamar Rubinstein
Jane Park Sando
Laura Tochen
Elizabeth Tucker
Darcy Weidemann
Karen Zimowski

Interns

Sean Barnes
Tal Berkowitz
Meghan Bernier
Jason Cervenka
Gordon Cohen
Paul Doherty
Cullen Dutmer
Erica Elzey
Oluwatosin Fatusin
Marie Fiero
Michael Goldsmith
Abha Gupta
Christa Habela
Julia Johnson
Kristen Johnson
Sarah Kachan-Liu
Julie King
Jessica Klein
Erin Mack
Crystal Malvoisin
Sara Mixter
Monica Mix
Jonathan Mullin
David Myles
Chinedu Onyedike
Robin Punsalan
Siddharth Srivastava
Christina Ulen
Caleb Ward
Deanna Wilson

Megan M. Tschudy

Kristin M. Arcara

Contents

Part I Pediatric Acute Care

1 Emergency Management 3
Christopher Valente, MD

2 Poisonings 19
Tina Rezaiyan, MD

3 Procedures 57
Laura J. Sigman, MD, JD

4 Trauma, Burns, and Common Critical Care Emergencies 89
Katherine M. Steffen, MD

Part II Diagnostic and Therapeutic Information

5 Adolescent Medicine 117
Nicole Brown, MD, MPH

6 Analgesia and Sedation 137
Kristin M. Arcara, MD

7 Cardiology 154
Elaine Giannakos Lennox, MD

8 Dermatology 201
Nisha Kapadia, MD

9 Development, Behavior, and Mental Health 226
Jessica Perniciaro, MD

10 Endocrinology 243
Lauren Cohee, MD

11 Fluids and Electrolytes 271
Elizabeth Quaal Hines, MD

12 Gastroenterology 293
Rebecca F. Rabin, MD, MHS

13 Genetics 309
Emily Spengler, MD

14 Hematology 322
Sama Ahsan, MD, and Julia Noether, MD

15 Immunology and Allergy 354
Wonha Kim, MD

16 Immunoprophylaxis 370
Kristin Santini Casasanta, MD

17 Microbiology and Infectious Disease 405
Benjamin Lee, MD, and Tracy McCallin, MD

18 Neonatology 455
Matthew H. Merves, MD

19 Nephrology 476
Stacy Cooper, MD

20 Neurology 504
Delphine Robotham, MD

21 Nutrition and Growth 524
Brandi Kaye Freeman, MD, and Jenifer Hampsey, MS, RD, CSP

22 Oncology 564
Catherine M. Albert, MD

23 Palliative Care 577
Judson Heugel, MD

24 Pulmonology 584
Allison Kirk, MD

25 Radiology 606
Judson Heugel, MD

26 Rheumatology 620
Marc A. Callender, MD

Part III Reference

27 Blood Chemistries and Body Fluids 639
Kristin M. Arcara, MD

28 Biostatistics and Evidence-Based Medicine 651
Karsten Lunze, MD, MPH

Part IV Formulary

29 Drug Doses 661
Carlton K. K. Lee, PharmD, MPH; Megan M. Tschudy, MD; and Kristin M. Arcara, MD

30 Formulary Adjunct 989
Kristin M. Arcara, MD

31 Drugs in Renal Failure 1012
Megan M. Tschudy, MD

Index 1037

PART I

PEDIATRIC ACUTE CARE

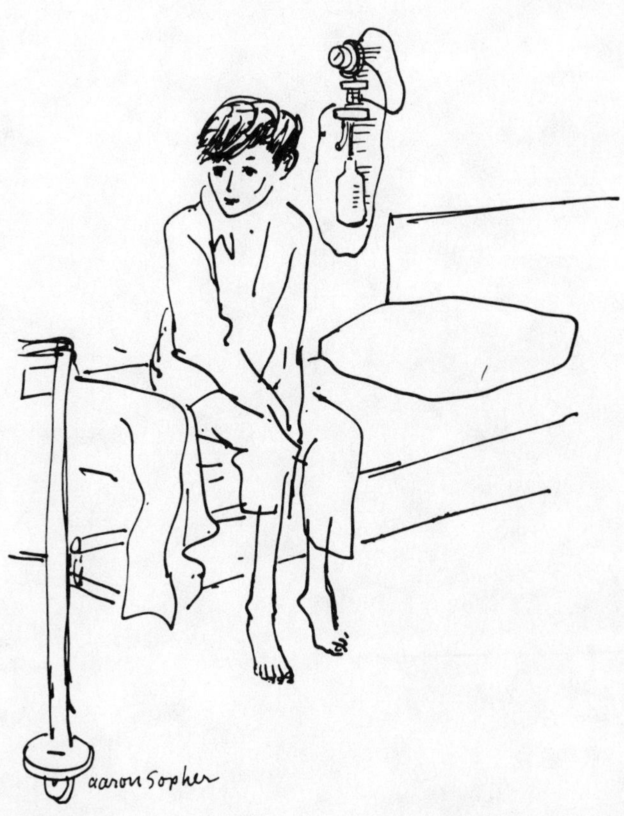

Chapter 1

Emergency Management

Christopher Valente, MD

When approaching a patient in cardiopulmonary arrest, one must first and foremost focus on A, B, C, D, and Es. The history, physical exam, and laboratory studies should closely follow a rapid primary assessment. **NOTE:** The 2010 American Heart Association Guidelines for Cardiopulmonary Resuscitation and Emergency Cardiovascular Care updates the 2005 guidelines by recommending that immediate chest compressions should be the first step in reviving **victims of sudden cardiac arrest,** thus the new acronym C-A-B has been put forth. The original A-B-C pathway is presented in this section as it remains the accepted way in which to rapidly assess and manage any critically ill patient.[1]

I. AIRWAY[2–5]

A. Assessment

1. Is airway patent?
   Think about obstruction: Head tilt/chin lift (or jaw thrust if injury suspected) to open airway
2. Is the child breathing spontaneously?
   If not, must immediately begin ventilating via rescue breaths, bag-mask, or endotracheal tube
3. Are respirations adequate?
   a. Look for chest rise
   b. Recognize signs of distress (stridor, tachypnea, flaring, retractions, accessory muscle use, wheezes)

B. Management[2–10]

1. **Equipment**
   a. Use oral or nasopharyngeal airway in patients with altered mental status
      (1) Oral: Unconscious patients—measure with flange at teeth and tip at mandibular angle
      (2) Nasal: Conscious patients—measure tip of nose to tragus of ear
   b. Laryngeal mask airway (LMA): Simple way to secure an airway (no laryngoscopy needed), especially in difficult airways; does not prevent aspiration
   c. Bag and mask ventilation with cricoid pressure may be used indefinitely if ventilating effectively (look at chest rise)
2. **Intubation:** Indicated for (impending) respiratory failure, obstruction, airway protection, pharmacotherapy, or need for likely prolonged support

a. Equipment (see page i): **SOAP** (**S**uction, **O**xygen, **A**irway Supplies, **P**harmacology)
   (1) Laryngoscope blade: Straight (or Miller) blade typically used in children
      (a) Size: #00-1 for premie–2 month, #1 for 3 month–1 year, #2 for >2 years, #3 for >8 years
      (b) Curved (or Mac) blade may be helpful in patients >2 years
   (2) Endotracheal tube (ETT):
      (a) Size determination: Internal diameter of ETT (mm) = (Age/4) + 4, or use length-based resuscitation tape to estimate
      (b) Approximate depth of insertion in cm = ETT size × 3
      (c) Uncuffed ETT for patients <9 years of age
      (d) Mind the stylet; it should not extend beyond the distal end of the ETT
      (e) Attach end-tidal CO_2 monitor as confirmation of placement and effectiveness of chest compressions if applicable
   (3) Nasogastric tube (NGT): To decompress the stomach; measure from nose to angle of jaw to xiphoid for depth of insertion
b. Rapid sequence intubation (RSI) recommended unless patient is newborn or unconscious, and results in higher success rates with lower aspiration risk
   (1) Preoxygenate with non-rebreather at 100% O_2 for minimum of 3 minutes
      (a) Do not use positive pressure ventilation (PPV) unless patient effort is inadequate
      (b) Children have less oxygen/respiratory reserve than adults due to higher oxygen consumption and lower functional residual capacity
   (2) See Figure 1-1 and Table 1-1 for drugs used for RSI: (Adjunct, sedative, paralytic) important considerations in choosing appropriate agents include clinical scenario (e.g., bronchospasm, increased intracranial pressure, neurologic status, hyperkalemia), allergies, presence of neuromuscular disease or anatomic abnormalities, hemodynamic status
   (3) For patients difficult to bag or with difficult airways, may consider sedation without paralysis and the assistance of subspecialists (anesthesia and otolaryngology)
c. Procedure: Attempts should not exceed 30 seconds
   (1) Preoxygenate with 100% O_2 as above
   (2) Administer intubation medications (Fig. 1-1 and Table 1-1)
   (3) Apply cricoid pressure to prevent aspiration (Sellick maneuver) during bag-valve-mask ventilation and intubation
   (4) Use scissoring technique to open mouth
   (5) Hold laryngoscope blade in left hand. Insert blade into right side of mouth, sweeping tongue to the left out of line of vision

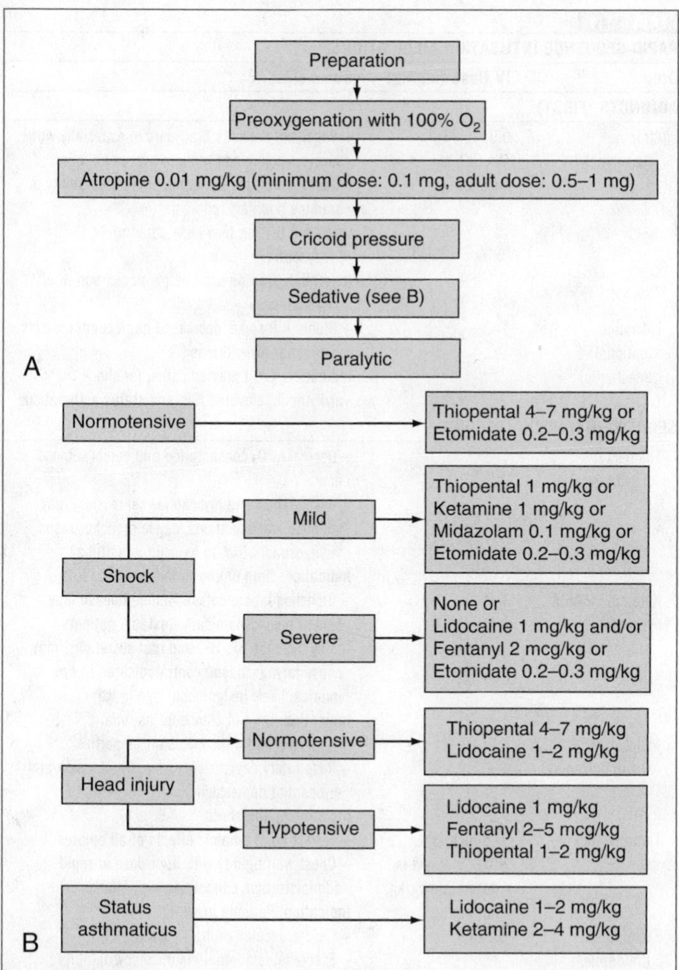

FIGURE 1-1

A, Treatment algorithm for intubation. **B,** Sedation options. *(Modified from Nichols DG, Yaster M, Lappe DG, et al [eds]: Golden hour: The handbook of advanced pediatric life support. St. Louis, Mosby, 1996, p. 29.)*

TABLE 1-1

RAPID-SEQUENCE INTUBATION MEDICATIONS

Drug	IV Dose (mg/kg)	Comments
ADJUNCTS (FIRST)		
Atropine (vagolytic)	0.01–0.02 Min: 0.1 mg Max: 1 mg	+ Vagolytic; prevents bradycardia, especially with succinylcholine and reduces oral secretions – Tachycardia, pupil dilation eliminates ability to examine pupillary reflexes Less than 0.1 mg may case paradoxical bradycardia **Indication:** Can be used as premedication in all circumstances
Lidocaine (optional anesthetic)	1–2	+ Blunts ICP spike, decreased gag/cough; controls ventricular arrhythmias **Indication:** Good premedication for shock, arrhythmia, elevated ICP, and status asthmaticus
SEDATIVE-HYPNOTIC (SECOND)		
Thiopental (barbiturate)	1–5	+ Decreases O_2 consumption and cerebral blood flow – Vasodilation and myocardial depression; may increase oral secretions, cause bronchospasm/laryngospasm (Not to be used in asthma) **Indication:** Drug of choice for increased ICP
Ketamine (NMDA receptor antagonist)	1–4	+ Bronchodilation; catecholamine release may benefit hemodynamically unstable patients – May increase BP, HR, and oral secretions; may cause laryngospasm; contraindicated in eye injuries; likely insignificant rise in ICP **Indication:** Drug of choice for asthma
Midazolam (benzodiazepine)	0.05–0.1	+ Amnestic and anticonvulsant properties – Respiratory depression/apnea, hypotension and myocardial depression **Indication:** Mild shock
Fentanyl (opiate)	1–5 mcg/kg **NOTE:** fentanyl is dosed in mcg/kg, not mg/kg	+ Fewest hemodynamic effects of all opiates – Chest wall rigidity with high-dose or rapid administration; cannot use with MAOIs **Indication:** Patients in shock
Etomidate (imidazole/hypnotic)	0.2–0.3	+ Cardiovascular neutral; decreases ICP – Exacerbates adrenal insufficiency (inhibits 11-beta hydroxylase) so consider administration of steroids in patients with shock **Indication:** Patients with severe shock, especially cardiac patients
Propofol (sedative-hypnotic)	1.5–3	+ Extremely quick onset and short duration; blood pressure lowering; good anti-emetic – Hypotension and profound myocardial depression; contraindicated in patients with egg allergy **Indication:** Induction agent for general anesthesia

TABLE 1-1

RAPID-SEQUENCE INTUBATION MEDICATIONS (Continued)

Drug	IV Dose (mg/kg)	Comments
PARALYTICS (NEUROMUSCULAR BLOCKERS) (THIRD)		
Succinylcholine (depolarizing)	1–2	+ Quick onset (30–60 sec), short duration (3–6 min) make it an ideal paralytic – Irreversible; bradycardia in <5 year old or with rapid doses; increased risk of malignant hyperthermia; contraindicated in burns, massive trauma/muscle injury, neuromuscular disease, myopathies, eye injuries, renal insufficiency
Vecuronium (non-depolarizing)	0.1–0.2	+ Onset 70–120 sec; cardiovascular neutral – Duration 30–90 minutes; Must wait 30–45 min to reverse with atropine and neostigmine **Indication:** When succinylcholine contraindicated or when longer term paralysis desired
Rocuronium (non-depolarizing)	0.6–1.2	+ Quicker onset 30–60 sec, shorter acting than vecuronium; cardiovascular neutral – Duration 30–60 min; may reverse in 30 min with atropine and neostigmine

+, Potential advantages; –, potential disadvantages or cautions; BP, blood pressure; HR, heart rate; ICP, intracranial pressure; MAOI, monoamine oxidase inhibitor.

(6) Advance blade to epiglottis. With straight blade, lift laryngoscope straight up, directly lifting the epiglottis to view cords. With curved blade, place tip in vallecula and lift straight up to elevate the epiglottis and visualize the vocal cords

(7) If possible, have another person hand over the tube, maintaining direct visualization, and pass through cords until black marker reaches the level of the cords

(8) Hold firmly against the lip until tube is securely taped

(9) Verify ETT placement: observe chest wall movement, auscultation in both axillae and epigastrium, end-tidal CO_2 detection (there will be a false-negative response if there is no effective pulmonary circulation), improvement in oxygen saturation, chest radiograph, repeat direct laryngoscopy to visualize ETT

II. BREATHING[2,3,11,12]

A. Assessment

Once airway is secured, continually reevaluate ETT positioning (listen for breath sounds). Acute respiratory failure may signify **D**isplacement of the ETT, **O**bstruction, **P**neumothorax, or **E**quipment failure (DOPE)

B. Management

1. **Mouth-to-mouth or mouth-to-nose breathing:** Provide two slow breaths (1 sec/breath) initially. For newborns, apply one breath for every three chest compressions. In infants and children, apply two breaths after

30 compressions (one rescuer) or two breaths after 15 compressions (two rescuers). Breaths should have adequate volume to cause chest rise

2. **Bag-mask ventilation** is used at a rate of 20 breaths/min (30 breaths/min in infants) using the E-C technique
   a. Use non-dominant hand to create a C with thumb and index finger over the top of the mask. Ensure a good seal but do not push down on the mask. Hook the remaining fingers around the mandible (not the soft tissues of the neck!) with the fifth finger on the angle creating an E, and lift the mandible up toward the mask
   b. Assess chest expansion and breath sounds
   c. Decompress stomach with orogastric or nasogastric tube with prolonged bag-mask ventilation
3. **Endotracheal intubation:** See prior section

III. CIRCULATION[2–4,11]

A. Assessment

1. **Rate/rhythm:** Assess for bradycardia, tachycardia, abnormal rhythm or asystole. Generally, bradycardia requiring chest compressions is <60 beats/min; tachycardia of >240 beats/min suggests tachyarrhythmia rather than sinus tachycardia
2. **Perfusion:**
   a. Assess pulses, capillary refill (<2 sec = normal, 2–5 sec = delayed, >5 sec suggests shock), mentation, and urine output (if Foley in place)
   b. If one cannot identify a pulse within 10 seconds, initiate cardiopulmonary resuscitation (CPR)
3. **Blood pressure (BP):** Hypotension is a late manifestation of circulatory compromise;

$$\text{Hypotension} = \text{systolic BP} < [70 + (2 \times \text{age in years})]$$

B. Management (Table 1-2)[13]

1. **Chest compressions**
   a. Press hard (⅓ to ½ anteroposterior [AP] diameter of chest) and fast (at least 100/minute) on backboard base with full recoil and minimal interruption

TABLE 1-2

MANAGEMENT OF CIRCULATION

	Location*	Rate (per min)	Compressions:Ventilation
Infants	1 fingerbreadth below intermammary line	>100	15:2 (2 rescuers) 30:2 (1 rescuer)
Pre-pubertal children	2 fingerbreadths below intermammary line	≥100	15:2 (2 rescuers) 30:2 (1 rescuer)
Adolescents/adults	Lower half of sternum	100	30:2 (1 or 2 rescuers)

*Depth of compressions should be one third to one half anteroposterior diameter of the chest.

b. Use end-tidal CO_2 to estimate effectiveness (<10–12 mmHg indicates inadequate compressions)
c. If single rescuer in infant, use two finger technique; otherwise two thumbs with hands encircling chest technique is preferable
2. **Use of automated external defibrillator (AED):** For children >1 year, use an AED/defibrillator after sudden, witnessed arrest or after 5 cycles of cardiopulmonary resuscitation if arrest is unwitnessed
3. **Resuscitation with poor perfusion and shock:**
a. Optimize oxygen delivery with supplemental O_2
b. Support respirations to reduce work of patient
c. Place intraosseous (IO) immediately if intravenous (IV) access not obtained in 90 sec or if patient is in cardiac arrest
d. Resuscitation fluids are lactated Ringer's or normal saline
  (1) Give up to four 20 mL/kg boluses each over ≤5 min for a total of 80 mL/kg in the first 20 min after presentation, feeling for hepatomegaly after each one
  (2) 5–10 mL/kg bolus in patient with cardiac insufficiency
  (3) Consider colloid such as albumin, plasma, packed red blood cells (PRBCs) if poor response to crystalloids
e. Identify type of shock: Hypovolemia, cardiogenic (congenital heart disease, myocarditis, cardiomyopathy, arrhythmia), distributive (sepsis, anaphylaxis, neurogenic), obstructive (pulmonary embolus [PE], cardiac tamponade, tension pneumothorax)
f. Pharmacotherapy (see inside front cover and consider stress dose corticosteroids and/or antibiotics if applicable)

IV. ALLERGIC EMERGENCIES (ANAPHYLAXIS)[14,15]

A. Definition

1. A rapid-onset IgE-mediated systemic allergic reaction involving multiple organ systems, including two or more of the following:
a. **Cutaneous/mucosal** (flushing, urticaria, pruritus, angioedema); seen in 90%
b. **Respiratory** (laryngeal edema, bronchospasm, dyspnea, wheezing, stridor, hypoxemia); seen in ~70%
c. **Gastrointestinal (GI)** (vomiting, diarrhea, crampy abdominal pain); seen in ~40%–50%
d. **Circulatory** (tachycardia, hypotension, syncope); seen in ~30%–40%
2. Initial reaction may be delayed for several hours AND symptoms may recur up to 72 hours after initial recovery. Patients should therefore be observed for a minimum of 6–24 hours for late-phase symptoms

B. Initial Management

1. Remove/stop exposure to precipitating antigen
2. Give epinephrine intramuscular (IM) immediately while performing ABCs. Delayed administration is associated with increased mortality

a. Establish airway and give O_2 and PPV as needed.
b. Obtain IV access, Trendelenburg position with head 30 degrees below feet, fluid boluses followed by pressors as needed
3. **Epinephrine** = Mainstay of therapy. Immediately give epinephrine, 0.01 mL/kg (1 : 1000) IM, maximum dose 0.5 mL. Repeat every 5 min as needed. The site of choice is the lateral aspect of the thigh due to its vascularity
4. **Histamine-1 receptor antagonist** such as diphenhydramine, 1 to 2 mg/kg through IM, IV, or oral (PO) route (maximum dose, 50 mg). Also, consider a histamine-2 receptor antagonist (e.g., ranitidine)
5. **Corticosteroids** help prevent the late phase of the allergic response. Administer methylprednisolone in a 2 mg/kg IV bolus, followed by 2 mg/kg per day IV or IM divided every 6 hours, or prednisone, 2 mg/kg PO once daily
6. **Albuterol** 2.5 mg for <30 kg, 5 mg for >30 kg for bronchospasm or wheezing repeated every 15 min as needed
7. **Racemic epinephrine** 0.5 mL inhaled for signs of upper airway obstruction
8. Patient should be discharged with an **Epi-Pen** (>30 kg), Epi-Pen Junior (<30 kg), or comparable injectable epinephrine product with specific instructions on appropriate use as well as an anaphylaxis action plan

V. RESPIRATORY EMERGENCIES[16]

The hallmark of upper airway obstruction is inspiratory stridor, whereas lower airway obstruction is characterized by cough, wheeze, and a prolonged expiratory phase

A. Asthma[17,18]

Lower airway obstruction resulting from triad of inflammation, bronchospasm, and increased secretions

1. **Assessment:** Assess respiratory rate (RR), work of breathing, O_2 saturation, heart rate (HR), peak expiratory flow, alertness, color
2. **Initial management**

a. Give O_2 to keep saturation >95%
b. Administer inhaled β-agonists: Nebulized albuterol, 0.05 to 0.15 mg/kg/dose as often as needed
c. Ipratropium bromide, 0.25 to 0.5 mg, nebulized with albuterol acts to decrease airway secretions. Benefit has been demonstrated only for moderate to severe exacerbations and its effect is not titratable (give early, but no benefit has been shown from repeated doses)
d. Steroids: Methylprednisolone, 2 mg/kg IV/IM bolus, then 2 mg/kg/day divided every 6 hr or prednisone/prednisolone, 2 mg/kg PO every 24 hr; requires minimum of 3 hours to take effect
e. If air movement is still poor despite maximizing above therapy
   (1) Epinephrine: 0.01 mL/kg SC or IM (1 : 1000; maximum dose, 0.5 mL) every 15 min up to three doses

(a) bronchodilator, vasopressor and inotropic effects
(b) short acting (~15 min) and should be used as temporizing rather than definitive therapy

(2) Magnesium sulfate: 25–75 mg/kg/dose IV or IM (maximum 2 g) infused over 20 min every 4 to 6 hr up to three to four doses
(a) Smooth muscle relaxant; relieves bronchospasm
(b) Many clinicians advise giving a saline bolus prior to administration as hypotension may result
(c) Contraindicated if patient already has significant hypotension or with renal insufficiency

(3) Terbutaline: 0.01 mg/kg SC (maximum dose, 0.4 mg) every 15 min up to two doses
(a) Systemic beta-2 agonist limited by cardiac intolerance
(b) Monitor continuous 12-lead electrocardiogram (ECG), cardiac enzymes, urinalysis (UA), and electrolytes
(c) IV route is preferred when available (see below)

3. **Further management** if incomplete or poor response: Consider obtaining an arterial blood gas value if breath sounds are minimal.

NOTE: A normalizing Pco_2 is often a sign of impending respiratory failure

a. Maximize and continue initial treatments
b. Terbutaline 2 to 10 mcg/kg IV load, followed by continuous infusion at 0.1 to 1.0 mcg/kg/min titrated to effect with appropriate cardiac monitoring in intensive care unit as above
c. A helium (≥70%) and oxygen mixture may be of some benefit in the critically ill patient but is more useful in upper airway edema. Avoid use in the hypoxic patient
d. Methylxanthines, such as aminophylline, may be considered in the intensive care unit (ICU) setting, but have not been shown to affect intubation rates or length of hospital stay and have significant side effects
e. Noninvasive positive pressure ventilation (i.e., BiPAP) may be used in patients with impending respiratory failure both as temporizing measure and to avoid intubation, but requires a cooperative patient with spontaneous respirations

4. **Intubation** of those with acute asthma is dangerous and should be reserved for impending respiratory arrest

a. Indications for endotracheal intubation include deteriorating mental status, severe hypoxemia, and respiratory or cardiac arrest
b. Premedicate with ketamine, lidocaine, or midazolam (see Fig. 1-1 and Table 1-1)
c. Consider using an inhaled anesthetic, such as isoflurane

5. **Hypotension:** The result of air trapping, hyperinflation, and therefore decreased pulmonary venous return. See Section III.B.3 for management. Definitive treatment is reducing lower airway obstruction

B. Upper Airway Obstruction[19–22]

Upper airway obstruction is most commonly caused by foreign-body aspiration or infection

1. **Epiglottitis:** Most often affects children between 2 and 7 years, though may occur at any age. It is a true emergency involving cellulitis and edema of the epiglottis, aryepiglottic folds, and hypopharynx
   a. Patient is usually febrile, anxious, and toxic appearing with sore throat, drooling, respiratory distress, stridor, tachypnea and *tripod* positioning (sitting forward supported by both arms with neck extended and chin thrust out). Any agitation of the child may cause complete obstruction so avoid invasive procedures/evaluation until airway is secured
   b. Unobtrusively give O_2 (blow-by). NPO, pulse ox, and allow parent to hold patient
   c. Summon epiglottitis team (most senior pediatrician, anesthesiologist, intensive care physician, and otolaryngologist in hospital)
   d. Management options
      (1) If unstable (unresponsive, cyanotic, bradycardic) → emergently intubate
      (2) If stable with high suspicion → take patient to operating room for laryngoscopy and intubation under general anesthesia
      (3) If stable with moderate or low suspicion → obtain lateral neck radiographs to confirm
   e. After airway is secure, obtain cultures of blood and epiglottic surface. Begin antibiotics to cover *Haemophilus influenzae* type B, *Streptococcus pneumoniae,* group A streptococci, *Staphylococcus aureus*
   f. Epiglottitis may also be caused by thermal injury, caustic ingestion, or foreign body
2. **Croup (laryngotracheobronchitis):** Most common in infants 6 to 36 months. It is a common syndrome involving inflammation of the subglottic area, presenting with fever, barking cough, and stridor. Patients rarely appear toxic as in epiglottitis
   a. Mild (no stridor at rest): Treat with minimal disturbance, cool mist, hydration, antipyretics and consider steroids
   b. Moderate to severe
      (1) The efficacy of mist therapy is not established
      (2) Racemic epinephrine (2.25%), 0.05 mL/kg/dose (maximum dose, 0.5 mL) in 3 mL normal saline (NS) over 15 min every 1 to 2 hr, or nebulized epinephrine, 0.5 mL/kg of 1 : 1000 (1 mg/mL) in 3 mL NS (max dose, 2.5 mL for <4 years old, 5 mL for >4 years old). Observe for a minimum of 2 to 4 hr after administering nebulized epinephrine due to potential for rebound obstruction. Hospitalize if more than one nebulization is required
      (3) Dexamethasone, 0.3 to 0.6 mg/kg IV, IM, or PO once. Effect lasts 2–3 days. Alternatively, nebulized budesonide (2 mg) may be

used, though little data exist to support its use and some studies find it to be inferior to dexamethasone

(4) A helium-oxygen mixture may decrease resistance to turbulent gas flow through a narrowed airway

c. If a child fails to respond as expected to therapy, consider other etiologies (e.g. retropharyngeal abscess, bacterial tracheitis, subglottic stenosis, epiglottitis, or foreign body). Obtain airway radiography, computed tomography (CT), and evaluation by otolaryngology or anesthesiology

3. **Foreign-body aspiration:** Occurs most often in children 6 months to 3 years old. It frequently involves hot dogs, candy, peanuts, grapes, or balloons. Most events unwitnessed, so suspect this in children with sudden-onset choking, stridor, or wheezing

a. If the patient is stable (i.e., forcefully coughing, well oxygenated), removal of the foreign body by bronchoscopy or laryngoscopy should be attempted in a controlled environment

b. If the patient is unable to speak, moves air poorly, or is cyanotic

(1) Infant: Place infant over arm or rest on lap. Give five back blows between the scapulae. If unsuccessful, turn infant over and give five chest thrusts (not abdominal thrusts)

(2) Child: Perform five abdominal thrusts (Heimlich maneuver) from behind a sitting or standing child

(3) After back, chest, and/or abdominal thrusts, open mouth using tongue-jaw lift and remove foreign body if visualized. Do not attempt blind finger sweeps. Magill forceps may be used to retrieve objects in the posterior pharynx. Ventilate if unconscious and repeat sequence as needed

(4) If there is complete airway obstruction and the patient cannot be ventilated by bag-valve mask or ETT, consider percutaneous (needle) cricothyrotomy (Fig. 1-2)[3]

VI. NEUROLOGIC EMERGENCIES

A. Altered States of Consciousness[23]

1. **Assessment:** Range of mental status includes alert, confused, disoriented, delirious, lethargic, stuporous, and comatose

a. History: Consider structural versus medical causes (Box 1-1). Obtain history of trauma, ingestion, infection, fasting, drug use, diabetes, seizure, or other neurologic disorder

b. Examination: Assess HR, BP, respiratory pattern, Glasgow Coma Scale (Table 1-3), temperature, pupillary response, funduscopy (a late finding, absence of papilledema does not rule out increased intracranial pressure [ICP]), rash, abnormal posturing, and focal neurologic signs

2. **Management of coma**

a. **A**irway (with C-spine immobilization), **B**reathing, **C**irculation, **D**-stick, **O**xygen, **N**aloxone, **T**hiamine (ABC DON'T)

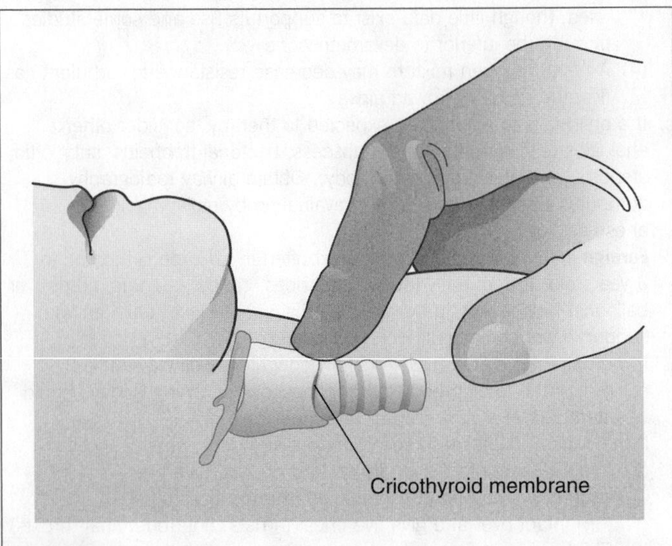

FIGURE 1-2

Percutaneous (needle) cricothyrotomy. Extend neck, attach a 3-mL syringe to a 14- to 18-gauge intravenous (IV) catheter, and introduce catheter through the cricothyroid membrane (inferior to the thyroid cartilage, superior to the cricoid cartilage). Aspirate air to confirm position. Remove the syringe and needle, attach the catheter to an adaptor from a 3.0-mm endotracheal tube, which can then be used for positive-pressure oxygenation. *(Modified from Dieckmann RA, Fiser DH, Selbst SM: Illustrated textbook of pediatric emergency and critical care procedures. St. Louis, Mosby, 1997, p. 118.)*

(1) Naloxone, 0.1 mg/kg IV, IM, subcutaneous (SC), or ETT (maximum dose, 2 mg). Repeat as necessary given short half-life (in case of opiate intoxication)
(2) Thiamine, 100 mg IV (before starting glucose in adolescents, in case of alcoholism or eating disorder)
(3) $D_{25}W$, 2 to 4 mL/kg IV bolus if hypoglycemia is present

b. Laboratory tests: Consider complete blood count, electrolytes, liver function tests, NH_3, lactate, toxicology screen (serum and urine; always include salicylate and acetaminophen levels), blood gas, serum osmolality, prothrombin time (PT)/partial thromboplastin time (PTT), and blood/urine culture. If patient is an infant or toddler, consider assessment of plasma amino acids, urine organic acids, and other appropriate metabolic workup

c. If meningitis or encephalitis is suspected, consider lumbar puncture (LP) and start antibiotics and acyclovir

BOX 1-1

DIFFERENTIAL DIAGNOSIS OF ALTERED LEVEL OF CONSCIOUSNESS

STRUCTURAL CAUSES

Vascular—e.g., cerebrovascular accident, cerebral vein thrombosis

Increased intracranial pressure—e.g., hydrocephalus, tumor, abscess, cyst, subdural empyema, pseudotumor cerebri

Trauma (intracranial hemorrhage, diffuse cerebral swelling, shaken baby syndrome)

MEDICAL CAUSES

Anoxia

Hypothermia/hyperthermia

Metabolic—e.g., inborn errors of metabolism, diabetic ketoacidosis, hyperammonemia, uremia, hypoglycemia, electrolyte abnormality

Infection—e.g., sepsis, meningitis, encephalitis, subdural empyema

Seizure/post-ictal state

Toxins/ingestions

Psychiatric/psychogenic

Modified from Avner J: Altered states of consciousness. Pediatr Rev 2006;27(9):331–337.

TABLE 1-3

COMA SCALES

Glasgow Coma Scale		Modified Coma Scale for Infants	
Activity	**Best Response**	**Activity**	**Best Response**
EYE OPENING			
Spontaneous	4	Spontaneous	4
To speech	3	To speech	3
To pain	2	To pain	2
None	1	None	1
VERBAL			
Oriented	5	Coo/babbles	5
Confused	4	Irritable	4
Inappropriate words	3	Cries to pain	3
Nonspecific sounds	2	Moans to pain	2
None	1	None	1
MOTOR			
Follows commands	6	Normal spontaneous movements	6
Localizes pain	5	Withdraws to touch	5
Withdraws to pain	4	Withdraws to pain	4
Abnormal flexion	3	Abnormal flexion	3
Abnormal extension	2	Abnormal extension	2
None	1	None	1

Data from Jennet B, Teasdale G: Aspects of coma after severe head injury. Lancet 1977;1:878, and James HE: Neurologic evaluation and support in the child with an acute brain insult. Pediatr Ann 1986;15:16.

d. Request emergent head CT after ABCs are stabilized; consider neurosurgical consultation and electroencephalogram (EEG) if indicated
e. If ingestion is suspected, airway must be protected before GI decontamination (see Chapter 2)
f. Monitor Glasgow Coma Scale and reassess frequently (Table 1-3)

TABLE 1-4

ACUTE MANAGEMENT OF SEIZURES

Time (min)	Intervention
0–5	Stabilize the patient
	Assess airway, breathing, circulation, and vital signs
	Administer oxygen
	Obtain intravenous or intraosseous access
	Consider hypoglycemia, thiamine deficiency, intoxication (dextrose, thiamine, naloxone may be given immediately if suspected)
	Obtain laboratory studies: Consider glucose, electrolytes, calcium, magnesium, blood gas, CBC, BUN, creatinine, and LFTs, toxicology screen, anticonvulsant levels, blood culture (if infection is suspected)
	Initial screening history and physical examination
5–15	Begin pharmacotherapy
	Lorazepam (Ativan), 0.05–0.1 mg/kg IV, up to 4–6 mg
	Or
	Diazepam (Valium), 0.2–0.5 mg/kg IV (0.5 mg/kg rectally) up to 6–10 mg
	May repeat lorazepam or diazepam 5–10 min after initial dose
15–25	If seizure persists, load with one of the following:
	1. Fosphenytoin† 15–20 mg PE/kg IV/IM at 3 mg PE/kg/min via peripheral IV live (maximum 150 mg PE/min). If given IM, may require multiple dosing sites
	2. Phenytoin* 15–20 mg/kg IV at rate not to exceed 1 mg/kg/min via central line
	3. Phenobarbital 15–20 mg/kg IV at rate not to exceed 1 mg/kg/min
25–40	If seizure persists:
	Levetiracetam 20–30 mg/kg IV at 5 mg/kg/min or valproate 20 mg/kg IV at 5 mg/kg/min
	May give phenobarbital at this time if still seizing at 5 minutes and (fos) phenytoin previously used
	Additional phenytoin or fosphenytoin 5 mg/kg over 12 hr for goal serum level of 10 mg/L
	Additional phenobarbital 5 mg/kg/dose every 15–30 min (maximum total dose of 30 mg/kg; be prepared to support respirations)
40–60	If seizure persists,‡ consider pentobarbital, midazolam, or general anesthesia in intensive care unit. Avoid paralytics

*Phenytoin may be contraindicated for seizures secondary to alcohol withdrawal or most ingestions (see Chapter 2).

†Fosphenytoin dosed as phenytoin equivalent (PE).

‡Pyridoxine 100 mg IV in infant with persistent initial seizure.

BUN, Blood urea nitrogen; CBC, complete blood count; CT, computed tomography; EEG, electroencephalogram; LFTs, liver function tests; IM, intramuscular; IV, intravenous.

Modified from Abend, NS, Dlugos, DJ: Treatment of refractory status epilepticus: literature review and a proposed protocol. Pediatr Neurol 2008;38:377.

B. Status Epilepticus[24,25]

See Chapter 20 for non-acute evaluation and management of seizures

1. **Assessment:** Common causes of childhood seizures include electrolyte abnormalities, hypoglycemia, fever, subtherapeutic anticonvulsant levels, central nervous system (CNS) infections, trauma, toxic ingestion, and metabolic abnormalities. Consider specific patient history such as shunt malfunction in patient with ventriculoperitoneal shunt. Less common causes include vascular, neoplastic, and endocrine diseases
2. **Acute management of seizures** (Table 1-4): If CNS infection is suspected, give antibiotics and/or acyclovir early
3. **Diagnostic workup:** When stable, workup may include CT or magnetic resonance imaging, EEG, and lumbar puncture (LP)

REFERENCES

1. Field JM, Hazinski MF, Sayre MR, et al. 2010 American Heart Association Guidelines for Cardiopulmonary Resuscitation and Emergency Cardiovascular Care. *Circulation.* 2010:Nov 2;122(18 Suppl 3):S640–656.
2. American Heart Association. Pediatric advanced life support. *Pediatrics.* 2006;117(5):e1005–e1028.
3. Nichols DG, Yaster M, Lappe DG, et al. eds. *Golden hour: the handbook of advanced pediatric life support.* St. Louis: Mosby; 1996.
4. Ralston M, Hazinski MF, Zaritsky AL, et al. eds. *Pediatric advanced life support provider manual.* Dallas: American Heart Association, Subcommittee on Pediatric Resuscitation; 2006.
5. Sagarin MJ, Barton ED, Chng YM, et al. Airway management by US and Canadian emergency medicine residents: a multicenter analysis of more than 6,000 endotracheal intubation attempts. *Ann Emerg Med.* 2005;46:328–336.
6. American Heart Association. Pharmacology. In: *Pediatric advanced life support provider manual.* Dallas: American Heart Association, Subcommittee on Pediatric Resuscitation; 2006:228.
7. Sagarin MJ, Chiang V, Sakles JC, et al. Rapid sequence intubation for pediatric emergency airway management. *Pediatr Emerg Care.* 2002;18:417.
8. Zelicof-Paul A, Smith-Lockridge A, Schnadower D, et al. Controversies in rapid sequence intubation in children. *Curr Opin Pediatr.* 2005;17:355.
9. Sivilotti ML, Filbin MR, Murray HE, et al. Does the sedative agent facilitate emergency rapid sequence intubation? *Acad Emerg Med.* 2003;10:612.
10. Perry J, Lee J, Wells G. Rocuronium versus succinylcholine for rapid sequence induction intubation. *Cochrane Database Syst Rev.* 2003;CD002788.
11. Pediatric basic life support. *Circulation.* 2005;112:IV156.
12. Berg RA, Sanders AB, Kern KB, et al. Adverse hemodynamic effects of interrupting chest compressions for rescue breathing during cardiopulmonary resuscitation for ventricular fibrillation cardiac arrest. *Circulation.* 2001;104:2465.
13. Stevenson AG, McGowan J, Evans AL, et al. CPR for children: one hand or two? *Resuscitation.* 2005;64:205.
14. Sampson HA, Munoz-Furlong A. Second symposium on the definition and management of anaphylaxis: summary report—Second National Institute of Allergy and Infectious Disease/Food Allergy and Anaphylaxis Network symposium. *J Allergy Clin Immunol.* 2006;117(2):391–397.

15. Lee JM, Greenes DS. Biphasic anaphylactic reactions in pediatrics. *Pediatrics.* 2000;106:762.
16. Luten RC, Kissoon N. The difficult pediatric airway. In: Walls RM, ed. *Manual of emergency management.* 2nd ed. Philadelphia: Williams and Wilkins; 2004:236.
17. National Asthma Education and Prevention Program. *Expert panel report III: Guidelines for the diagnosis and management of asthma.* Bethesda, MD: National Heart, Lung and Blood Institute; 2007.
18. Carroll CL, Schramm CM. Noninvasive positive pressure ventilation for the treatment of status asthmaticus in children. *Ann Allergy Asthma Immunol.* 2006;96:454.
19. Cherry JD. Croup (laryngitis, laryngotracheitis, spasmodic croup, laryngotracheobronchitis, bacterial tracheitis, and laryngotracheobronchopneumonitis). In: Feigin RD, Cherry JD, Demmler H, et al. eds. *Textbook of pediatric infectious diseases.* 6th ed. Philadelphia: Saunders; 2009:254.
20. Alberta Medical Association. Guideline for the diagnosis and management of croup. Alberta Clinical Practice Guidelines 2008. Published on the Alberta Medical Association Practice Guideline Website.
21. McMillan JA, Feigin RD, DeAngelis C, et al. *Epiglottitis. Oski's pediatrics: principles and practice.* 4th ed. Philadelphia: Lippincott, Williams and Wilkins; 2006:695.
22. Beharloo F, Veyckemans F, Francis C, et al. Tracheobronchial foreign bodies. Presentation and management in children and adults. *Chest.* 1999;115:1357.
23. Avner J. Altered states of consciousness. *Pediatr Rev.* 2006;27(9):331–337.
24. Abend NS, Dlugos DJ. Treatment of refractory status epilepticus: literature review and a proposed protocol. *Pediatr Neurol.* 2008;38:377.
25. Wheless JW. Treatment of status epilepticus in children. *Pediatr Ann.* 2004;33:377–383.

Chapter 2

Poisonings

Tina Rezaiyan, MD

2

See additional content on Expert Consult

I. WEBSITES

American Association of Poison Control Centers: http://www.aapcc.org/dnn/Home.aspx

American Academy of Clinical Toxicology: http://www.clintox.org/index.cfm

Centers for Disease Control and Prevention, Section on Environmental health: http://www.cdc.gov/Environmental/

II. INITIAL EVALUATION

A. History

1. **Exposure history**
   a. Obtain history from family members and/or friends
   b. Route, timing and number of exposures (acute, chronic, or repeated ingestion), prior treatments or decontamination efforts[1,2]
2. **Substance identification**
   a. Attempt to identify exact name of substance ingested and constituents, including product name, active ingredients, possible contaminants, expiration date, concentration, and dose
   b. Consult local poison control for pill identification
3. **Quantity of substance ingested:** Attempt to estimate a missing volume of liquid or the number of missing pills from a container
4. **Environmental information:** Accessible items in the house or garage; open containers; spilled tablets; household members taking medications, herbs, or other complementary medicines[2]

B. Laboratory Findings

1. **Toxicology screens:** Screens include analgesics, amphetamines, antidepressants, barbiturates, cocaine, ethanol, and opiates. If a particular type of ingestion is suspected, verify that the agent is included in the toxicology test[2]
2. When obtaining a blood or urine toxicology test, consider measuring both aspirin and acetaminophen levels because these are common analgesic ingredients in many medications (Section IV)[2]
3. Gas chromatography or gas mass spectroscopy can distinguish medications that may cause a false-positive toxicology screen for tricyclic antidepressants, such as antihistamines, antipsychotics, and cyclobenzaprine[3]
4. Recognize drugs not detected by routine toxicology screens[4]

C. Clinical diagnostic aids (Table 2-1)

D. Toxidromes (Table 2-2)

III. ACUTE MANAGEMENT

A. Airway, Breathing, Circulation

Establish intravenous (IV) access, contact local poison control center

B. General Decontamination

1. **Skin:** Indicated if patient was exposed to concentrated lipid-soluble toxins. Avoid secondary exposure by wearing protective clothing.

TABLE 2-1

CLINICAL DIAGNOSTIC AIDS

Clinical Sign	Intoxicant
VITAL SIGNS	
Hypothermia	Alcohols, antidepressants, barbiturates, carbamazepine, carbon monoxide, clonidine, ethanol, hypoglycemics, opioids, phenothiazines, sedative-hypnotics
Hyperpyrexia	Amphetamines, anticholinergics, antihistamines, atropinics, β-blockers, cocaine, iron, isoniazid, monoamine oxidase inhibitors (MAOIs), phencyclidine, phenothiazines, quinine, salicylates, sympathomimetics, selective serotonin reuptake inhibitors, theophylline, thyroxine, tricyclic antidepressants (TCAs)
Bradypnea	Acetone, alcohol, barbiturates, botulinum toxin, clonidine, ethanol, ibuprofen, narcotics, nicotine, sedative-hypnotics
Tachypnea	Amphetamines, barbiturates, carbon monoxide, cyanide, ethylene glycol, isopropanol, methanol, salicylates *Direct pulmonary insult:* hydrocarbons, organophosphates, salicylates
Bradycardia	α-Agonists, alcohols, β-blockers, calcium channel blockers, central α_2-agonist, clonidine, cyanide, digoxin, narcotics, organophosphates, plants (lily of the valley, foxglove, oleander), sedative-hypnotics
Tachycardia	Alcohol, amphetamines, anticholinergics, antihistamines, atropine, cocaine, cyclic antidepressants, cyanide, iron, phencyclidine, salicylates, sympathomimetics, theophylline, TCAs, thyroxine
Hypotension	α-Antagonists, angiotensin-converting enzyme (ACE) inhibitors, barbiturates, carbon monoxide, cyanide, iron, methemoglobinemia, opioids, phenothiazine, sedative-hypnotics, TCAs *Profound hypotension:* β-blockers, calcium channel blockers, clonidine, cyclic antidepressants, digoxin, imidazolines, nitrites, quinidine, propoxyphene, theophylline
Hypertension	Amphetamines, anticholinergics, antihistamines, atropinics, clonidine, cocaine, cyclic antidepressants (early after ingestion), diet pills, ephedrine, MAOIs, nicotine, over-the-counter cold remedies, phencyclidine, phenylpropanolamine, pressors, sympathomimetics, TCAs *Delayed hypertension:* thyroxine
Hypoxia	Oxidizing agents

2

TABLE 2-1

CLINICAL DIAGNOSTIC AIDS (Continued)

Clinical Sign	Intoxicant
NEUROMUSCULAR	
Nervous system instability	*Insidious onset:* acetaminophen, benzocaine, opioids *Abrupt onset:* lidocaine, monocyclic or tricyclic antidepressants, phenothiazines, theophylline *Delayed onset:* atropine, diphenoxylate *Transient instability:* hydrocarbons
Depression and excitation	Clonidine, imidazolines, phencyclidine
Ataxia	Alcohol, anticonvulsants, barbiturates, carbon monoxide, heavy metals, hydrocarbons, solvents, sedative-hypnotics
Chvostek/Trousseau signs	Ethylene glycol, hydrofluoric acid-induced hypocalcemia, phosphate-induced hypocalcemia from Fleets enema
Coma	Alcohols, anesthetics, anticholinergics (antihistamines, antidepressants, phenothiazines, atropinics, over-the-counter sleep preparations), anticonvulsants, baclofen, barbiturates, benzodiazepines, bromide, carbon monoxide, chloral hydrate, clonidine, cyanide, cyclic antidepressants, γ-hydroxybutyrate (GHB), hydrocarbons, hypoglycemics, inhalants, insulin, lithium, opioids, organophosphate insecticides, phenothiazines, salicylates, sedative-hypnotics, tetrahydrozoline, theophylline
Delirium, psychosis	Alcohol, anticholinergics (including cold remedies), cocaine, heavy metals, heroin, LSD, marijuana, mescaline, methaqualone, peyote, phencyclidine, phenothiazines, steroids, sympathomimetics
Miosis	Barbiturates, clonidine, ethanol, opioids, organophosphates, phencyclidine, phenothiazines, muscarinic mushrooms
Mydriasis	Amphetamines, antidepressants, antihistamines, atropinics, barbiturates (if comatose), botulism, cocaine, glutethimide, LSD, marijuana, methanol, phencyclidine
Nystagmus	Barbiturates, carbamazepine, diphenylhydantoin, ethanol, glutethimide, MAOIs, phencyclidine (both vertical and horizontal), sedative-hypnotics
Paralysis	Botulism, heavy metals, paralytic shellfish poisoning, plants (poison hemlock)
Seizures	Alcohol, ammonium fluoride, amphetamines, anticholinergics, antidepressants, antihistamines, atropine, β-blockers, boric acid, bupropion, caffeine, camphor, carbamates, carbamazepine, carbon monoxide, chlorinated insecticides, cocaine, cyclic antidepressants, diethyltoluamide, ergotamine, ethanol, GHB, *Gyromitra* mushrooms, hydrocarbons, hypoglycemics, ibuprofen, imidazolines, isoniazid, lead, lidocaine, lindane, lithium, LSD, meperidine, nicotine, opioids, organophosphate insecticides, phencyclidine, phenothiazines, phenylpropanolamine, phenytoin physostigmine, plants (water hemlock), propoxyphene, salicylates, strychnine, theophylline

Continued

TABLE 2-1

CLINICAL DIAGNOSTIC AIDS (Continued)

Clinical Sign	Intoxicant
CARDIOVASCULAR	
Hypoperfusion	Calcium channel blockers, iron
Wide QRS complex	TCAs
ELECTROLYTES	
Anion gap metabolic acidosis	Acetaminophen, carbon monoxide, chronic toluene, cyanide, ethanol, ethylene glycol, ibuprofen, iron, isoniazid, lactate, methanol, metformin, paraldehyde, phenformin, salicylates
Electrolyte disturbances	Salicylates, theophylline
Hypoglycemia	Alcohols, β-blockers, hypoglycemics, salicylates
Serum osmolar gap	Acetone, ethanol, ethylene glycol, isopropyl alcohol, methanol, propylene glycol Calculated osmolarity = (2 × serum Na) + BUN/2.8 + glucose/18. Normal osmolarity is 290 mOsm/kg
SKIN	
Asymptomatic cyanosis	Methemoglobinemia
Cyanosis unresponsive to oxygen	Aniline dyes, benzocaine, nitrites, nitrobenzene, phenazopyridine, phenacetin
Flushing	Alcohols, antihistamines, atropinics, boric acid, carbon monoxide, cyanide, disulfiram
Jaundice	Acetaminophen, carbon tetrachloride, heavy metals (iron, phosphorus, arsenic), naphthalene, phenothiazines, plants (mushrooms, fava beans)
ODORS	
Acetone	Acetone, isopropyl alcohol, phenol, salicylates
Alcohol	Ethanol
Bitter almond	Cyanide
Garlic	Heavy metal (arsenic, phosphorus, thallium), organophosphates
Hydrocarbons	Hydrocarbons (gasoline, turpentine, etc.)
Oil of wintergreen	Salicylates
Pear	Chloral hydrate
Violets	Turpentine
RADIOLOGY	
Small opacities on radiograph	Halogenated toxins, heavy metals, iron, lithium, densely packaged products

Remove contaminated clothing and seal in plastic bag. Wash the patient with soap and water[1]

2. **Eye flushing:** Remove contact lenses. Irrigate with lukewarm water for at least 20 min or at least 1 liter normal saline per eye with lids fully retracted before re-evaluating

C. Gastrointestinal (GI) Decontamination

1. **Airway protection:** Extremely important when attempting GI decontamination because of the risk for aspiration. If no gag reflex

TABLE 2-2
TOXIDROMES

Drug Class	Vital Signs	Neurologic	Skin, Mucous Membranes	GI	GU	Other
ADRENERGIC/SYMPATHOMIMETIC						
Amphetamines, cocaine, epinephrine, albuterol, ephedrine	↑ or ↔ RR ↑ HR ↑ T ↑ BP	Alert, agitation, dilated and reactive pupils, hyperreflexia, tremor, delirium, psychosis, seizures	Diaphoresis	Hyperactive bowel sounds, emesis, abdominal pain		
ANTICHOLINERGIC						
Antihistamines, atropine, belladonna alkaloids, jimsonweed, some mushrooms, phenothiazines, scopolamine, tricyclic antidepressants **"Mad as a hatter, red as a beet, blind as a bat, hot as a hare, dry as a bone."**	↔ RR ↑ HR ↑ T ↔ or ↑ BP	Depressed mental status, confusion, psychosis, paranoid ideation, delirium, ataxia, agitation, seizures, coma, extrapyramidal symptoms, dilated and sluggish pupils, normal DTRs	Dry skin, flushing, dry mucous membranes, decreased sweating	Hypoactive bowel sounds, ileus	Urine retention	Respiratory failure

Continued

TABLE 2-2

TOXIDROMES (Continued)

Drug Class	Vital Signs	Neurologic	Skin, Mucous Membranes	GI	GU	Other
ANTICHOLINESTERASE (CHOLINERGIC)						
Black widow spider bites, some mushrooms, organophosphate nerve agents, organophosphate and carbamate pesticides, tobacco **SLUDGE:** ***s***alivation, ***l***acrimation, ***u***rination, ***d***efecation, ***g***astric cramping, ***e***mesis **DUMBELS:** ***d***iarrhea, ***u***rination, ***m***iosis, ***b***ronchospasm, ***e***mesis, ***l***acrimation, ***s***alivation	↑ or ↔ RR ↓ or ↑ HR ↔ T ↔ BP	Confusion, depressed mental status, coma, pupillary constriction, normal DTRs or hyporeflexia, seizures, muscle fasciculations, weakness, paralysis	Diaphoresis, wet mucous membranes, salivation, lacrimation	Hyperactive bowel sounds, diarrhea, cramping, emesis	Increased urination	Respiratory failure
EXTRAPYRAMIDAL						
Haloperidol, metoclopramide, phenothiazines		Tremor, rigidity, opisthotonos, torticollis, dysphonia, oculogyric crisis				

Fentanyl, meperidine, heroin, hydrocodone, oxycodone, propoxyphene, morphine, clonidine	↓ RR ↔ or ↓ HR ↔ or ↓ T ↔ or ↓ BP	Confusion, lethargy, euphoria, somnolence, seizures, ataxia, coma, pupillary constriction, normal DTRs or hyporeflexia	Normal skin and mucous membranes	Decreased bowel sounds, constipation	Urine retention	Pulmonary edema
SEDATIVE-HYPNOTIC						
Benzodiazepines, barbiturates	↓ RR ↔ or ↓ HR ↑ or ↓ T ↓ BP	Depressed mental status, CNS depression, normal pupils, normal DTRs or hyporeflexia	Normal	Normal	Normal	
WITHDRAWAL						
Cessation of alcohol, barbiturates, benzodiazepines, γ-hydroxybutyrate	↑ HR ↑ RR ↑ BP ↑ T	Restlessness, hallucinations, anxiety, hyperalgesia, mydriasis	Lacrimation, "goose bumps," sweating	Abdominal cramps, diarrhea		Yawning, rhinorrhea

BP, Blood pressure; DTR, deep tendon reflex; HR, heart rate; GI, gastrointestinal; GU, genitourinary; RR, respiratory rate; T, temperature.
Data from references 1 and 2.

2

exists or the patient has altered mental status, intubation is necessary before decontamination efforts

2. **Syrup of ipecac**[4,5]: Not recommended for routine management of poisonings
3. **Cathartics**[4,5]: Not recommended for routine management of poisonings
4. **Activated charcoal**[1,6]

a. Indications: Carbamazepine, barbiturates, dapsone, quinine, and theophylline ingestions. Some evidence for use with digoxin and phenytoin ingestions. Little evidence for use with salicylates
b. Risks: Bowel obstruction, bowel perforation, pulmonary aspiration, hypernatremia, hypermagnesemia
c. Contraindications: Ileus, mechanical bowel obstruction, altered mental status with unprotected airway, caustic ingestion, hydrocarbon ingestion, ingestion of foreign body
d. Most effective if given within 1 hour of ingestion
e. Procedure/dosage: Activated charcoal 1 g/kg oral (PO) or via nasogastric (NG) tube every 1–6 hr. For adolescents or adults, give 50–100 g
f. Activated charcoal poorly adsorbs most electrolytes, iron, lithium, mineral acids, mineral bases, alcohols, cyanides, most solvents, and most water-soluble compounds (hydrocarbons)

5. **Nasogastric/orogastric lavage**[1,6,7]

a. Indications: Tricyclic antidepressants (TCAs), calcium channel blockers, iron, lithium, alcohols, substances that delay gastric emptying
b. Risks: Mechanical trauma to oropharynx or esophagus, aspiration
c. Contraindications: Ingestion of corrosive substances or hydrocarbons, altered mental status, unprotected airway
d. Most effective within 1 hour of ingestion
e. Procedure/dosage: Place patient in Trendelenburg or left lateral decubitus position, and pass the largest-bore NG tube. Confirm tube placement by aspiration of gastric contents. Administer normal saline solution, 50–100 mL in young children or 150–200 mL in adolescents. Withdraw the fluid by aspiration and repeat until lavaged fluid is clear

6. **Whole-bowel irrigation**[5,7,8]

a. Indications: Sustained-release or enteric-coated preparations, heavy metals, or illegal drug packets
b. Contraindications: Altered mental status with unprotected airway, caustic ingestion, hydrocarbon ingestion, ingestion of foreign body, ileus, bowel perforation
c. Procedure/dosage
   (1) Administer 30 mL/kg/hr of osmotically balanced polyethylene glycol electrolyte solution to induce liquid stool. Alternatively, can give up to 500 mL/hr in children or 2 L/hr in adults
   (2) Continue until rectal effluent is clear. Slow administration and antiemetic medications may be necessary to reduce bloating, nausea, and emesis

D. Enhanced Elimination

1. **Urinary alkalinization with forced diuresis**[1,4]
a. Indications: Salicylates, isoniazid, dichlorophenoxyacetic acid, phenobarbital, chlorpropamide, chlorophenoxy herbicides
b. Procedure/dosage
   (1) Use this equation to determine dosage

$$0.6 \times \text{weight (kg)} \times 5\,\text{mEq} = \text{mEq of sodium bicarbonate to be given over 4 hr}$$

   (2) Administer the sodium bicarbonate in intravenous fluid drip containing glucose and KCl
c. Alternate dosing: Sodium bicarbonate, 1–2 mEq/kg IV over 1–2 hr
d. Monitor: Maintain urine pH 7.5–7.8; correct hypokalemia (hypokalemia reduces the ability to alkalinize the urine)
2. **Urinary acidification:** Not recommended secondary to exacerbation of metabolic acidosis and myoglobin deposition

E. Active Removal

Hemodialysis and hemofiltration: Consult local poison control center and a pediatric nephrologist

F. Antidotes (See Formulary for Specific Antidotes)

G. Inhalation Injuries[9]

1. **Physical examination:** Symptoms may be delayed after the inhalational injury occurs. Symptoms that may predict acute inhalational injury include cough, facial burns, inflamed nares, stridor, sputum production, wheezing, and altered mental status
2. **Management**
a. Assess stability of the airway and intubate if there are signs of airway edema

NOTE: Upper airway obstruction progresses rapidly with thermal or chemical burns to the face, nares, or oropharynx

b. Administer supplemental oxygen through a non-rebreather mask. Give aerosolized bronchodilators as needed with or without corticosteroids to decrease airway edema
c. Check chest radiograph, arterial blood gases (ABGs) with co-oximetry, and bedside spirometry

NOTE: Use co-oximetry instead of pulse oximetry to measure oxyhemoglobin.

d. Obtain 12-lead electrocardiogram (ECG) to evaluate for myocardial ischemia or infarction
e. Observe for at least 24 hr

IV. INGESTIONS (TABLE 2-3, BOX 2-1)

In general, there are a few principles for management of ingestions. The half-life of the drug will effect management and appropriate length

Text continued on page 48

TABLE 2-3

MEDICATION INGESTIONS

Ingestion	Signs and Symptoms	Management
Acetaminophen[5,10,11,12] paracetamol, APAP	**Phase 1 (first 24 hr):** Anorexia, nausea, malaise, pallor, vomiting, diaphoresis, or may be asymptomatic. **NOTE:** Initial manifestations do not predict subsequent hepatotoxicity **Phase 2 (24–72 hr):** Hepatomegaly, right upper quadrant (RUQ) pain, hyperbilirubinemia, elevated liver enzymes, elevated prothrombin time, oliguria **Phase 3 (72–96 hr):** Liver enzymes peak, encephalopathy, cardiomyopathy, hepatic failure and necrosis, coagulopathy, renal failure, emesis, malaise **Phase 4 (4 days–2 weeks):** Recovery or fatal hepatic failure. The end point of liver damage is reached during this phase	**1. Initial Considerations:** a. Hepatotoxicity with >150 mg/kg ingested or >7.5 g in adults b. Alanine aminotransferase (ALT) >1000 IU/L is a marker of severe liver injury, but not prognostic c. High-risk groups for hepatotoxicity: concurrent use of cytochrome P-450 enhancing drugs, current viral illness, diabetes mellitus, or malnourished d. *Start treatment immediately if* (1) Single ingestion >150 mg/kg or 7.5 g by history (2) Unknown time of ingestion and acetaminophen level >10 mcg/mL (3) Severe clinical symptoms and abnormal liver function (4) Chronic or subacute overdose with risk (5) Acetaminophen level above "possible hepatic toxicity" on nomogram **2. Monitoring:** a. Obtain baseline electrolytes, liver function, coagulation factors, and urinalysis. **NOTE:** Recheck labs every 12–24 hr until normal b. Acetaminophen level 4–24 hr after ingestion best predicts hepatotoxicity. **NOTE:** Levels <4 hr postingestion are unreliable due to drug absorption c. Recheck levels 8 hr postingestion if extended release ingested d. Compare measured level with the nomogram (Fig. 2-1)

3. **Supportive Care/Decontamination:**
   a. *Activated charcoal:* Most useful within 1–2 hr of ingestion and improves outcome if used concurrently with antidote
   b. Hemodialysis and hemoperfusion are NOT recommended
4. **Antidote:** *N*-acetylcysteine (NAC)
   a. *Drug information:* Increases glutathione stores and conjugates toxic metabolites
   b. See Formulary for complete dosing instructions
   c. *PO/nasogastric dosing:* Most effective if administered within 8 to 10 hours of ingestion. Contraindicated with corrosive ingestions, gastrointestinal (GI) bleed, or bowel obstruction
   d. *IV dosing:* IV NAC should be administered only if there are contraindications to PO dosing or when patients are treated more than 10 hours postingestion. Anaphylactoid reactions, bronchospasm, and angioedema occur more frequently in patients treated with the IV preparation
5. **Adjunct:** Use antiemetics (metoclopramide, ondansetron) as needed

Continued

TABLE 2-3

MEDICATION INGESTIONS (Continued)

Ingestion	Signs and Symptoms	Management
Alcohols[1,8] a. Ethanol (see Box 2-1, Drugs of Abuse) b. Ethylene Glycol c. Methanol d. Isopropanol	*Ethylene Glycol:* **Early (<12 hr):** central nervous system (CNS) depression similar to ethanol ingestion, nausea, vomiting, seizures. Hypoglycemia, elevated osmolar gap, anion gap metabolic acidosis **Late (12–24 hr):** cardiopulmonary effects: tachycardia, hypertension, heart failure, respiratory distress **Delayed (24–72hr):** Toxic-metabolite mediated nephrotoxicity. Calcium oxalate crystals, hypocalcemia, tetany, prolonged QT. Elevated lactate *Methanol:* **Early (<12 hr):** CNS depression similar to ethanol ingestion, nausea, vomiting. Hypoglycemia, elevated osmolar gap, anion gap metabolic acidosis **Late (12–72 hr):** Blindness, changes in visual acuity or color vision, basal ganglia lesions	1. **Initial Considerations:** a. Ethylene glycol and methanol toxicity may be delayed with co-ingestion of ethanol b. GI decontamination is rarely indicated because of rapid absorption and limited binding to activated charcoal 2. **Monitoring:** a. Electrocardiogram b. Chest radiograph should be obtained if there is concern for aspiration c. Lab evaluation: ethylene glycol and methanol levels, serum ethanol level, arterial blood gas, electrolytes, lactate, urinalysis d. Urine may fluoresce with ingestion of ethylene glycol-containing products containing fluorescein **NOTE:** Most routine alcohol screens do not include ethylene glycol 3. **Supportive Care:** a. Fluids. Glucose, and bicarbonate as needed b. Calcium gluconate should be given only for symptomatic hypocalcemia; it may increase the formation of calcium oxalate crystals with ethylene glycol ingestions 4. **Antidote:** a. Fomepizole (See Formulary for dosing instructions) b. Ethanol: indicated only if unable to give fomepizole Loading dose: 1 mL/kg (95% ethanol) diluted in D_5W to make a 10% IV solution given over 1 hr. Maintenance dose: 0.8–1.5 mL/kg/hr (80–150 mg/kg/hr) IV to target blood ethanol levels to 100–150 mg/dL 5. **Cofactors:** used to optimize nontoxic pathways a. *Ethylene glycol:* Pyridoxine and thiamine b. *Methanol:* Leucovorin and folic acid

	Isopropanol: (rubbing alcohol, disinfectants) Similar to ethanol ingestion. Hemorrhagic gastritis and hematemesis. Respiratory depression, coma, and hypotension with large ingestions. Ketonemia and ketonuria without glycosuria or hyperglycemia. Elevated osmolar gap. Isopropanol does NOT cause an anion gap acidosis	1. **Initial Considerations:** a. The irritant effects usually deter children from ingesting large amounts b. If large ingestion does occur, maintain a low threshold for intubation and ventilation 2. **Monitoring:** a. Close cardiorespiratory monitoring b. Chest radiograph if concerned for aspiration c. Electrolytes and urinalysis 3. **Supportive Care:** a. Fluids for hypotension b. Protect and maintain airway c. Patients who remain asymptomatic for 6 to 8 hours may be discharged home
Anticholinergics[1] (antidepressants, antihistamines, antispasmodics, phenothiazines)	See Table 2-2 Symptoms may develop 12–24 hr after ingestion secondary to decreased GI motility and delayed absorption Elimination half-life is 8–55 hr	1. **Supportive Care/Decontamination:** a. If <8 hr of ingestion, give activated charcoal b. Consider a cathartic, because drug-charcoal complex is excreted in feces 2. **Antidote:** Physostigmine—See Formulary for dosing a. Administer physostigmine only if electrocardiogram (ECG) is normal b. *Risks:* Seizures, bradycardia, hypotension, bronchospasm. Risks increase when physostigmine is given rapidly or in large doses c. *Contraindication:* Ingestion of drug affecting cardiac conduction (tricyclic antidepressant [TCA]) d. Treat muscarinic side effects of physostigmine with atropine IV at one half of the dose of physostigmine

Continued

TABLE 2-3

MEDICATION INGESTIONS (Continued)

Ingestion	Signs and Symptoms	Management
Antidepressants[13,14,15] a. *Tricyclic antidepressants (TCAs):* amitriptyline, clomipramine, desipramine, doxepin, imipramine, nortriptyline, protriptyline, trimipramine b. *Selective serotonin reuptake inhibitors (SSRIs):* amoxapine, citalopram, clomipramine, fluoxetine, fluvoxamine, nefazodone, paroxetine, sertraline, venlafaxine c. *Monoamine oxidase inhibitors (MAOIs):* phenelzine, tranylcypromine, isocarboxazid, moclobemide, pargyline, procarbazine, selegiline d. *Serotonin syndrome:* Occurs with co-ingestion of MAOIs with sympathomimetic or serotonergic drugs. e. Bupropion	See Table 2-2, Anticholinergic *TCAs:* seizures, delirium, arrhythmias (ventricular tachycardia, ventricular fibrillation), hypotension, significantly decreased GI motility *SSRIs:* CNS depression, seizures, coma, agitation, tremor, drowsiness, nystagmus, delirium, arrhythmias, hypertension, emesis, hepatotoxicity *MAOIs:* CNS hyperstimulation, seizures, muscle rigidity, hyperpyrexia, blood pressure instability (rapid hemodynamic changes), rhabdomyolysis *Co-ingestion of MAOIs and food or drugs with biogenic amines (wine, cheese, soy sauce, decongestants):* stroke, seizures, severe hypertension *Serotonin syndrome:* autonomic dysfunction, seizures, muscle rigidity, myoclonus, hyperpyrexia, circulatory collapse, rhabdomyolysis, flushing *Bupropion:* An atypical antidepressant. Lowers seizure threshold and has a narrow therapeutic window	1. **Initial Considerations:** a. Ingestions > 20–35 mg/kg of TCA are typically fatal. Doses as low as 15 mg/kg can be fatal in toddler-aged children b. TCAs significantly decrease GI motility c. TCAs have long half-life and slow elimination rates, necessitating prolonged treatment and decontamination 2. **Monitoring:** a. Check 12-lead ECG and continuous cardiac monitoring b. Monitor potassium levels if administering sodium bicarbonate 3. **Supportive Care/Decontamination:** a. Activated charcoal 1 g/kg b. Consider gastric lavage even in delayed presentations c. If cardiac arrhythmias or widened QRS, administer sodium bicarbonate 1–2 mEq/kg bolus followed by continuous infusion; goal serum pH 7.45–7.55 **NOTE:** Use lidocaine, atenolol, propranolol, or magnesium for arrhythmias. Class Ia (quinidine and procainamide) and Ic antiarrhythmics are contraindicated 4. **MAOI Overdose: Key Points** a. 24-hr observation is recommended due to possible delayed side effects b. Treat hypertension with short-acting antihypertensive (nitroprusside) c. Treat severe muscle rigidity and hyperthermia with benzodiazepines and neuromuscular blockade d. Monitor creatine kinase, electrolytes, and urine myoglobin for rhabdomyolysis

Antihistamines[16] a. *Second/third generation:* Azelastine, brompheniramine, doxylamine, ebastine, fexofenadine, loratadine, mizolastine, cetirizine b. *First generation:* Diphenhydramine, chlorpheniramine, hydroxyzine	See Table 2-2, *Anticholinergic* Paradoxical CNS stimulation, hyperactivity, tremors, dizziness, coma, hypotension, arrhythmias, cardiorespiratory arrest, muscle weakness, seizures, hyperpyrexia	1. **Initial Considerations:** a. Antihistamines may be in cough syrups, sedatives, antiemetics, drugs to prevent motion sickness, cold preparations, and sleep aids b. Second-generation antihistamines cause prolonged QT and arrhythmias c. Observe patient for at least 4 hr postingestion. If ingestion of second generation or slow-release form, admit and observe regardless of symptoms d. Obtain acetaminophen level in antihistamine ingestions due to its presence in cough/cold remedies 2. **Monitoring:** a. 12-lead ECG; continuous cardiac monitoring b. **NOTE:** May cause false-positive TCA test 3. **Supportive Care/Decontamination:** a. Give activated charcoal if <4 hr postingestion b. Hemodialysis is NOT indicated 4. **Antidote:** Physostigmine (See Formulary for dosing information) 5. First-line treatment for arrhythmia: sodium bicarbonate; then consider magnesium, propranolol

Continued

TABLE 2-3

MEDICATION INGESTIONS (Continued)

Ingestion	Signs and Symptoms	Management
Barbiturates Amobarbital, butalbital, pentobarbital, phenobarbital, secobarbital	Slurred speech, ataxia, lethargy, nystagmus, confusion, coma, cutaneous bullae, respiratory depression, flaccid, hyporeflexia, hypotension, hypothermia; "absent EEG activity" See Box 2-1, Sedative-Hypnotics	1. **Initial Considerations:** a. Phenobarbital levels are most useful within 1–2 hr postingestion b. Ingestion of >6 mg/kg long-acting or >3 mg/kg short-acting barbiturate is usually toxic 2. **Supportive Care/Decontamination:** a. One or more doses activated charcoal for phenobarbital b. Hemodialysis if large doses of phenobarbital ingested 3. **Adjunct:** Sodium bicarbonate to keep urine pH >7.5, which increases phenobarbital elimination
Benzodiazepines[17,18] a. Sedatives, anxiolytics, muscle relaxants, hypnotics b. Alprazolam, clorazepate, chlordiazepoxide, clonazepam, diazepam, flurazepam, lorazepam, midazolam, oxazepam, temazepam, triazolam	Coma, dysarthria, ataxia, drowsiness, hallucinations, confusion, agitation, bradycardia, hypotension, respiratory depression	1. **Initial Considerations:** Half-life can be 2–48 hr 2. **Monitoring:** Can be detected by urine and serum toxicology tests 3. **Supportive Care/Decontamination:** Administer activated charcoal if within 1 hr of ingestion and consciousness is not impaired 4. **Antidote:** Flumazenil (See Formulary for dosing) a. May precipitate seizures; therefore, it is only indicated in cases of respiratory distress or circulatory compromise

β-Blockers[19,20,21] a. β_1 *selective:* Atenolol, esmolol, metoprolol b. β_1 and β_2 *selective:* Labetalol, nadolol, pindolol, timolol	Coma, seizures, altered mental status, hallucinations, cardiac arrhythmia (atrioventricular [AV] node blockade, accelerated junctional rhythms), bradycardia, congestive heart failure (CHF), hypotension, respiratory depression, bronchospasm, hypoglycemia	1. **Monitoring:** a. Serial 12-lead ECG for conduction delays every 1–2 hr b. Observe regular-release preparation for 6-hr postingestion and sustained release for 24 hr c. Observe ingestions with timolol eye drops for 24 hr d. Echocardiogram to evaluate myocardial function e. Measure serum glucose, renal function and acid base status 2. **Supportive Care/Decontamination:** a. Activated charcoal recommended if <1 hr postingestion b. Pretreat bradycardia with atropine before gastric lavage. **NOTE:** Lavage can cause vagal response and worsen bradycardia c. Whole bowel irrigation for sustained-release preparations d. Hemodialysis and hemoperfusion not indicated 3. **Antidote:** Glucagon. See Formulary for side effects and dosing a. Glucagon infusion should be started at the response dose per hour (e.g., if patient receives 7 mg glucagon before response occurs, then start infusion at 7 mg/hr) b. Glucagon has inotropic and vasopressor effects; administer normal saline during glucagon treatment 4. **Adjuncts:** a. Atropine, IV fluids, vasopressors for hypotension or myocardial depression b. Insulin—to facilitate myocardial utilization of glucose and increase contractility. Recommended rate of up to 0.5–1 Units/kg/hr

Continued

TABLE 2-3
MEDICATION INGESTIONS (Continued)

Ingestion	Signs and Symptoms	Management
Calcium Channel Blockers[20–21] Amlodipine, bepridil, diltiazem, isradipine, nicardipine, nifedipine, verapamil	Seizures, coma, dysarthria, lethargy, confusion, decreased myocardial contractility, cardiac arrhythmia, profound hypotension, peripheral vasodilation, apnea, pulmonary edema, bowel infarction, lactic acidosis, hyperglycemia, mild hyperkalemia, flushing, peripheral cyanosis	1. **Initial Considerations:** Small ingestions may cause significant toxicity. Onset of symptoms usually occur within 1–2 hours, but may develop 24 hours after ingestion with sustained-release preparation 2. **Monitoring:** a. Serial 12-lead ECG to evaluate conduction delays b. Observe regular-release preparation for 6 hr postingestion and sustained-release for 24 hr 3. **Supportive Care/Decontamination:** a. Gastric lavage if <1 hr postingestion and life-threatening ingestion b. Activated charcoal recommended c. Whole-bowel irrigation for sustained-release preparations d. Hemodialysis and hemoperfusion not indicated 4. **Antidote:** Calcium salts (see Formulary for calcium chloride dosing) **NOTE:** if digoxin toxicity is being considered, avoid treatment with calcium salts 5. **Adjunct:** a. Atropine, IV fluids, and vasopressors for hypotension or myocardial depression b. Consider insulin therapy to increase myocardial glucose utilization and contractility
Clonidine[21]	Symptoms resemble an opioid toxidrome CNS depression, coma, lethargy, hypothermia, miosis, bradycardia, profound hypotension, respiratory depression	1. **Initial Considerations:** a. Small ingestions cause significant toxicity in children b. Symptoms occur within 1 hr postingestion and last up to 24 hr **NOTE:** 10–20 mcg/kg = cardiovascular compromise; >20 mcg/kg = respiratory depression 2. **Monitoring:** 12-lead ECG to evaluate for heart block and continuous cardiorespiratory monitoring

		3. Supportive Care/Decontamination: a. Single dose of activated charcoal if <1 hr postingestion b. Whole-bowel irrigation is effective for clonidine patch ingestions **NOTE:** Rapid drug absorption makes decontamination ineffective after 2 hr postingestion **4. Antidote:** Naloxone—See Formulary a. Treat for neurologic, cardiovascular, or respiratory symptoms b. Give 1–2 mg initially. Large doses (up to 10 mg) may be necessary. If the patient responds to naloxone, continue to give boluses, or start an infusion **5.** Give atropine if bradycardia does not respond to naloxone
Hypoglycemics[8] a. *Sulfonylureas:* Glipizide, glyburide, glimepiride, chlorpropamide b. *Biguanides:* Metformin	Status epilepticus, fatigue, dizziness, agitation, confusion, tachycardia, cardiovascular compromise, poor feeding, diaphoresis. **Metformin may cause metabolic acidosis**	**1. Initial Considerations:** Small ingestions can cause significant clinical toxicity **NOTE:** Hypoglycemia can be delayed 16–24 hr postingestion **2. Monitoring:** Hourly glucose checks **3. Supportive Care/Decontamination:** a. Single dose of activated charcoal b. Hemodialysis and hemoperfusion may be necessary in severe ingestions **4. Adjunct:** a. Hypertonic glucose ($D_{10}W$, neonates; $D_{25}W$, children; $D_{50}W$, adults) boluses as needed to treat hypoglycemia. Glucose infusion is necessary for several days b. Octreotide 1–2 mcg/kg subcutaneously to treat refractory hypoglycemia c. Glucagon 0.025 to 0.1 mg/kg (max 1mg per dose). Repeat dosing every 20 minutes as required. Only a temporary measure, hypoglycemia may persist

Continued

TABLE 2-3

MEDICATION INGESTIONS (Continued)

Ingestion	Signs and Symptoms	Management
Iron[22,23]	**Stage 1:** (0–6 hr postingestion): Abdominal pain, emesis, GI hemorrhage, diarrhea, dehydration. **Stage 2:** (6–24 hr postingestion): Latent phase. Patients are often asymptomatic. However, patients with large ingestions may progress directly from stage 1 without a latent period to stage 3 **Stage 3:** (6–48 hr postingestion): Coma, seizures, shock, cyanosis, hepatic dysfunction and necrosis, metabolic acidosis, coagulopathy, hypoglycemia **Stage 4:** (2–3 days postingestion): Hepatic failure **Stage 5:** (4–6 wk after ingestion): GI tract strictures, pyloric stenosis, acute bowel obstruction	**1. Initial Considerations:** a. Specific preparation of iron ingested will guide management. Ingestions of children's chewable multivitamin with iron, carbonyl iron preparations, and polysaccharide iron preparations are no longer referred to the emergency room b. If asymptomatic and <40 mg/kg of elemental iron consumed, no treatment necessary beyond observation c. *Toxic reference ranges:* Serum iron 350 mcg/dL = minimal toxicity Serum iron 500 mcg/dL = moderate toxicity Serum iron 1000 mcg/dL = severe life-threatening toxicity **2. Monitoring:** a. Serum iron levels after 6 hr are misleading because liver has cleared free iron b. Sustained-release preparations: check level 8 hr postingestion c. Follow abdominal radiograph d. Monitor electrolytes, anion gap acidosis, complete blood count (leukocytosis often seen) **3. Supportive Care/Decontamination:** a. Consider gastric decontamination. **NOTE:** Activated charcoal is not indicated b. Whole-bowel irrigation if iron tablets are visible on radiograph **4. Antidote:** Deferoxamine (See Formulary) a. Consider for patients who have severe symptoms, anion gap acidosis, serum iron concentrations >500 mcg/dL, or a significant number of pills visible on abdominal radiography. b. Start immediately if there are signs of organ failure **5. Adjunct:** Vigorous hydration

Nonsteroidal antiinflammatory drugs (NSAIDs) a. *COX-1 and COX-2 Inhibitors:* Salicylates, phenylbutazone, mefenamic acid, meclofenamate, ketorolac, indomethacin, ibuprofen, naproxen b. *COX-2 Inhibitors:* Celecoxib, rofecoxib	Nausea, vomiting, epigastric pain, GI hemorrhage, renal failure, hepatotoxicity, headache, behavior changes, aseptic meningitis, bronchospasm, myocardial infarction, platelet inhibition, bone marrow suppression, photosensitivity reactions	**1. Initial Considerations:** a. Ingestions >400 mg/kg can lead to significant toxicity b. If mefenamic acid or sustained-release NSAID ingested, observe for 12 hr **2. Monitoring:** Serum electrolytes, lactic acid, blood urea nitrogen (BUN), creatinine, and liver function enzymes **3. Supportive Care/Decontamination:** a. Activated charcoal b. Hemodialysis and hemoperfusion are ineffective
Phenothiazines, Butyrophenone[24] a. Tranquilizers b. Chlorpromazine, fluphenazine, haloperidol, perphenazine, prochlorperazine, promethazine, thioridazine, trifluoperazine	Orthostatic hypotension, akathisia, dystonia, hyperthermia, parkinsonism, tardive dyskinesia, decreased sweating, decreased GI motility, urine retention, miosis, mydriasis	**1. Initial Considerations:** a. Symptoms may occur 6–24 hr after ingestion b. Risk of neuroleptic malignant syndrome **2. Monitoring:** 12-lead ECG to evaluate for prolonged QT, ST changes; continuous cardiac monitoring **3. Supportive Care/Decontamination:** a. Activated charcoal if within 4–6 hr of ingestion b. Hemodialysis and hemoperfusion not indicated **4. Antidote:** Benztropine. Diphenhydramine. See Formulary for dosing. **NOTE:** Use benztropine with caution in patients with dysrhythmia **5.** Adjunct: Sodium bicarbonate can be used to treat dysrhythmias. Lidocaine is second line therapy for dysrhythmia

Continued

TABLE 2-3

MEDICATION INGESTIONS (Continued)

Ingestion	Signs and Symptoms	Management
Salicylates[8] a. Aspirin, methylsalicylate, nonaspirin salicylate b. Salicylates are also present in cough and cold preparations, topical preparations (oil of wintergreen) and creams, Pepto Bismol, wart and callus treatments	GI upset, vomiting, hyperpyrexia, dizziness, lethargy, dysarthria, seizure, respiratory depression, coma, cerebral edema, hepatic dysfunction, dehydration, electrolyte disturbances, tachypnea, respiratory alkalosis, metabolic acidosis, coagulopathy Tinnitus, impaired hearing with chronic abuse	**1. Initial Considerations:** a. Ingestions >150 mg/kg are referred to the emergency room b. Mild symptoms (GI upset, tachypnea, tinnitus) with ingestions of 150–300 mg/kg c. Moderate toxicity (agitation, fever, diaphoresis) with ingestions of 300–500 mg/kg d. Severe toxicity (seizure, coma, dysarthria, pulmonary edema, cardiorespiratory arrest) with ingestions >500 mg/kg e. *Chronic salicylism:* Symptoms of severe toxicity may occur at lower ingestion and serum salicylate levels **2. Rapid Confirmation of Salicylate Use:** a. *Ferric chloride test ($FeCl_3$):* Several drops of 10% $FeCl_3$ mixed with 1 mL urine turns purple if salicylates are in urine (extremely sensitive test) b. *Trinder Spot Test:* 1 mL Trinder reagent mixed with 1 mL urine will turn violet if salicylates are in urine

3. **Monitoring:**
   a. Check plasma salicylate level on arrival and every 2 hr until levels decline
   b. Monitor levels 6–12 hr postingestion of sustained-released formulation, and every 2 hr until levels begin to decline

   NOTE: The Done nomogram is no longer used. Plasma levels may not correlate with clinical toxicity

   c. Monitor complete metabolic panel, coagulation markers, anion gap, lactic acid
   d. Monitor urine pH and specific gravity
   e. 12-lead ECG and continuous cardiac monitoring
4. **Supportive Care/Decontamination:**
   a. Gastric lavage indicated up to 4 hr postingestion for large overdoses
   b. Activated charcoal for presentations 6–8 hr postingestion
   c. Whole-bowel irrigation for enteric-coated ingestions
   d. Hemodialysis indicated for unresponsive acidosis, seizures, coma, renal failure, CHF, hepatic compromise with coagulopathy, progressive deterioration, or salicylate level >100 mg/dL after acute ingestion
5. **Adjunct:**
   a. *Fluid resuscitation:* Give IV fluids with 5% dextrose, potassium, and 50–100 mEq/L sodium bicarbonate at twice maintenance
      Goal serum pH 7.5 to 7.55 to increase excretion and decrease CNS entry
   b. Goal urine pH >7.5. Goal urine output is 2 mL/kg/hr

   NOTE: Monitor for hypokalemia secondary to alkalinization

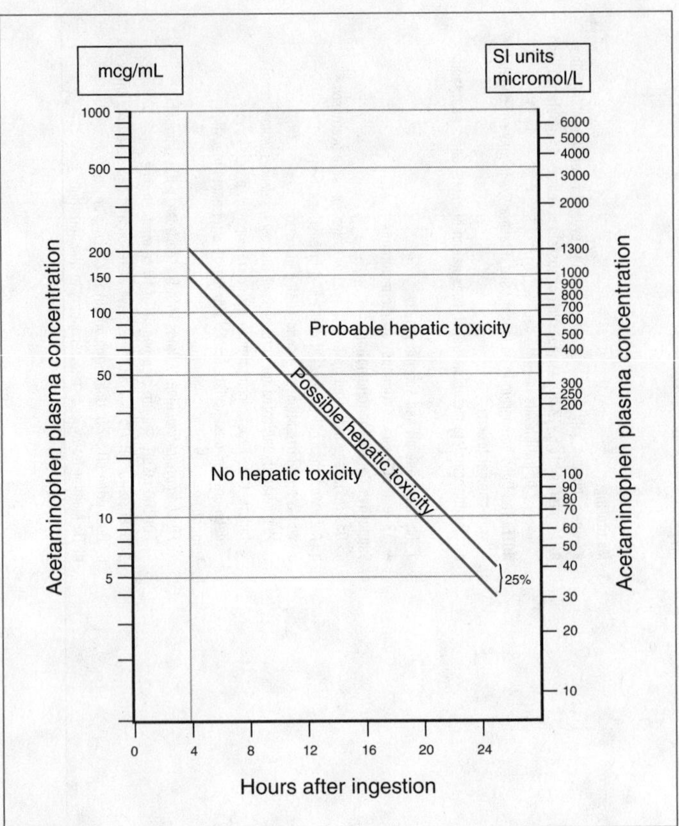

FIGURE 2-1

Semilogarithmic plot of plasma acetaminophen levels versus time. **NOTE:** This nomogram is valid for use after acute ingestions of acetaminophen. The need for treatment cannot be extrapolated based on a level before 4 hours. In chronic overdose, toxicity can be seen with much lower plasma levels. *(From Jones AL: Mechanism of action and value of N-acetylcysteine in the treatment of early and late acetaminophen poisoning: a critical review. J Toxicol Clin Toxicol 1998;36:277–285.)*

BOX 2-1

DRUGS OF ABUSE[25–28]

General management principles. Determine which drugs are included in your institution's routine urine toxicology screen. Check an abdominal radiograph if body packing or stuffing is suspected. Treat hyperpyrexia with external cooling measures. Treat agitation or seizures with benzodiazepines unless otherwise specified. Consider hemodialysis for acute renal failure.

AMPHETAMINE (STIMULANT)

1. Names: Amphetamine ("bennies, uppers"), methamphetamine ("ice, crank, crystal meth, glass"), dextromethamphetamine ("dexies"), ephedrine methylphenidate (Ritalin), phenylpropanolamine pseudoephedrine
2. Routes: enteral, intravenous, intranasal, and smoked
3. Acute intoxication: dilated pupils, euphoria, hyperactivity, hyperthermia, flushing, diaphoresis, hypertension, tachycardia, angina, arrhythmias, tremor, ataxia, dry mouth, diarrhea, insomnia, suicidal and homicidal ideations
   Toxic ingestion: coma, circulatory collapse, hypertensive crisis, cerebral hemorrhage, seizure, psychosis, rhabdomyolysis, violent behaviors
   Chronic abuse: cardiomyopathy, pulmonary hypertension, vasculitis
4. Monitoring: easily detected in urine drug screens.
   NOTE: Isomers of nasal inhalants/cold preparations cause false positives
   NOTE: Amphetamines are detectable in the urine up to 48 hr after last use
5. Supportive care/decontamination
   a. 12-lead electrocardiogram (ECG) and continuous cardiorespiratory monitoring
   b. Consider activated charcoal for recent ingestions
6. Adjunct: treat hypertensive crisis with benzodiazepines, hydralazine, nitroprusside, or phentolamine
7. Withdrawal: generalized fatigue, myalgias, poor concentration, confusion, anxiety, depression, insomnia for 1–2 days after use

COCAINE (STIMULANT)

1. Names: cocaine ("coke, crack, and freebase")
2. Routes: intranasal, intravenous, and smoked
3. Acute intoxication: dilated pupils, dry mouth, increased energy, anxiety, insomnia, paranoia, tremors, muscle rigidity, hyperpyrexia, bradycardia (low doses), tachycardia, hypertension, arrhythmia
   Acute intoxication in infants: dystonic posturing, seizure, hyperactivity, altered mental status
   Toxic ingestion: psychosis, seizures, hypertensive crisis, cerebrovascular event, myocardial infarction, rhabdomyolysis, pneumothorax, pneumomediastinum
   Chronic abuse: nasal septum ulcers, dilated cardiomyopathy, endocarditis, aortic dissection
4. Monitoring
   a. Urine toxicology: metabolites are detected in urine 2–3 days after last use
   b. Serial 12-lead ECG and cardiorespiratory monitoring
   c. Check cardiac enzymes, creatine kinase (CK), electrolytes, blood urea nitrogen (BUN), creatinine
   d. Consider head computed tomography (CT) to evaluate for acute cerebrovascular accident
   e. Consider lumbar puncture if subarachnoid hemorrhage suspected and patient has normal head CT

Continued

BOX 2-1

DRUGS OF ABUSE (Continued)

5. Supportive care/decontamination
   a. Consider multiple doses of activated charcoal or whole-bowel irrigation for body packing or body stuffing
   b. If body packer or stuffer is symptomatic, immediate surgical removal of foreign bodies is indicated
6. Adjunct
   a. Benzodiazepines are indicated for seizures, agitation, hypertension, and tachycardia. Benzodiazepines are associated with decreased mortality from cocaine use
   b. Treat hypertensive crisis with nitroprusside and benzodiazepines

   NOTE: β-Blockers are contraindicated due to risk of unopposed α-induced hypertension
   c. Treat arrhythmias according to Pediatric Advanced Life Support (PALS) protocol
   d. Treat rhabdomyolysis with aggressive hydration
7. Withdrawal: drug cravings, depression, dysphoria, irritability, lethargy, and tremors. Symptoms peak 2–3 days after last use

ECSTASY (STIMULANT)

1. Names: 3,4-methylenedioxymethamphetamine (MDMA) ("Adam, X, XTC, Love Drug")
2. Route: enteral
3. Acute intoxication: euphoria, increased psychomotor drive, tachycardia, hypertension, difficulty concentrating, headaches, palpitations, flushing, hyperthermia, nystagmus, suicidal and homicidal ideations

   Toxic ingestion: psychosis, coma, seizures, intracranial hemorrhage, cerebral infarction, asystole, pulmonary edema, multiorgan system failure, renal or hepatic failure, adult respiratory distress syndrome (ARDS), disseminated intravascular coagulation (DIC), syndrome of inappropriate antidiuretic hormone secretion (SIADH), death

   Chronic abuse: paranoid psychosis
4. Monitoring
   a. Detectable in routine urine toxicology screens
   b. 12-lead ECG and continuous cardiorespiratory monitoring
5. Supportive care/decontamination: consider activated charcoal for recent ingestions
6. Adjunct
   a. Treat hypertension with nitroprusside, phentolamine, or benzodiazepines. β-Blockers are contraindicated due to risk of unopposed α-induced hypertension
   b. Treat agitation, seizures, and delirium with abnormal vital signs with benzodiazepines
   c. Alkalinization or acidification of urine are not indicated
7. Withdrawal: generalized fatigue, myalgias, poor concentration, confusion, anxiety, depression, insomnia for 1–2 days after use

BOX 2-1

DRUGS OF ABUSE (Continued)

ETHANOL (DEPRESSANT)

1. Route: enteral
2. Legal intoxication: 50–80 mg/dL (varies by state)
3. Mild/moderate intoxication: <100–200 mg/dL; disinhibition, euphoria, impaired coordination, impaired judgment, slurred speech, sedation
4. Severe intoxication: >300 mg/dL; confusion, stupor, coma, respiratory depression, loss of protective reflexes, death
5. Chronic abuse: "wet" beriberi, "dry" beriberi, cirrhosis, pancreatitis, hepatitis, Mallory-Weiss tear
6. Initial considerations
   a. 12 oz beer, 4 oz wine, and 1.5 oz liquor increase blood ethanol levels by approximately 0.025 g/dL (varies by weight)
   b. Blood alcohol >500 mg/dL in teens may be fatal
   c. Blood alcohol >100 mg/dL in infants may cause coma and hypoglycemia
7. Monitoring
   a. Serum ethanol level and urine toxicology screen
   b. Monitor electrolytes, glucose, bicarbonate, magnesium, and phosphorus
8. Supportive care/decontamination
   a. Gastric lavage is not indicated due to quick absorption
   b. If congestion suspected, consider gastric emptying and activated charcoal
   c. Consider hemodialysis for hemodynamic instability, impaired hepatic function, or severe symptoms
9. Adjunct
   a. Hypoglycemic seizures can be treated with glucose
   b. Intravenous (IV) fluids: D_5W NS + supplements (100 mg thiamine, 2 g folate, magnesium, and possibly potassium if indicated)

γ-HYDROXYBUTYRATE (GHB) (DEPRESSANT), γ-HYDROXYBUTYROLACTONE (GBL)

1. Names: GHB ("liquid ecstasy, date rape drug")
2. Route: enteral
3. Acute intoxication: 10 mg/kg: sleep, 30 mg/kg: memory loss, 50 mg/kg: general anesthesia/coma; nystagmus, miosis, ataxia, hypothermia
   Toxic ingestion: central nervous system (CNS) and respiratory depression, agitation, seizures, bradycardia, agitation
4. Initial considerations: effects typically last 6–8 hr; toxicity prolonged with ethanol ingestion
5. Monitoring
   a. Not detectable in urine screens
   b. Detectable via gas chromatography or mass spectrometry
6. Adjunct: treat bradycardia with atropine
7. Withdrawal: feelings of doom, anxiety, insomnia, disorientation, visual and auditory hallucinations

HALLUCINOGENS

1. Names: mescaline ("cactus"), psilocybin ("mushrooms"), LSD ("acid"), phencyclidine ("PCP, angel dust"), dimethyltryptamine, diethyltryptamine
2. Routes: enteral, inhaled, intravenous

Continued

BOX 2-1

DRUGS OF ABUSE (Continued)

3. Acute intoxication: psychosis, paranoia, time and visual distortions, depersonalization, hyperreflexia, hyperthermia, dilated pupils, tachycardia, hypertension, facial flushing
   LSD intoxication: flashbacks, psychosis, delusions, grandiosity, paresthesias, weakness, drowsiness and dizziness, hyperthermia, tachycardia, hypertension
   PCP intoxication: possible bradycardia and hypotension, panic, aggression, violence, seizures, cyclic coma, nystagmus, dyskinesia, dystonia, bronchospasm, hypersalivation
   Toxic exposure: rhabdomyolysis
4. Initial consideration: half-life ranges from 1–3 days
5. Monitoring: PCP is detected by most urine screens
6. Adjunct: treat seizures, anxiety, and agitation with benzodiazepines

KETAMINE

1. Names: Ketalar ("K, Special K")
2. Routes: enteral, inhaled
3. Acute intoxication: nystagmus, analgesia, anxiety, sedation, amnesia, hallucination, hypersalivation, tachycardia, hypertension, emesis
   Toxic exposure: rhabdomyolysis, delirium, respiratory depression, respiratory arrest
4. Monitoring: not detectable in routine toxicology screens; however, detectable by high-performance liquid chromatography
5. Adjunct: treat emergence reactions or agitation with benzodiazepines

MARIJUANA

1. Names: marijuana ("pot, reefer, weed, herbs, bud"), hashish (" hash, hemp")
2. Routes: enteral, smoked
3. Acute intoxication: euphoria, relaxation, confusion, increased appetite, impaired motor skills, tachycardia, anxiety, panic attacks, conjunctival injection, depersonalization, mood change, pneumomediastinum, pneumothorax
   Toxic exposure: delusion, panic, paranoia, and psychosis
   Chronic abuse: cough, frequent respiratory infection, gynecomastia, infertility
4. Initial considerations
   Smoking is three times more potent than enteral ingestion
5. Monitoring
   a. Detected in urine toxicology screens for 3 days after single use and up to 10 days after weekly use
   b. Consider chest radiograph if low oxygen saturation, chest pain, or unequal breath sounds
6. Adjunct: treat toxic delirium and psychosis with benzodiazepines
7. Withdrawal: flulike illness, disturbed sleep, tremor, anorexia. Symptoms peak 4–5 days after last use and slowly resolve over 2 weeks

OPIOIDS (DEPRESSANT)

1. Names: buprenorphine, codeine, fentanyl, heroin, hydrocodone, hydromorphone, meperidine, morphine methadone, opium, oxycodone, pentazocine, propoxyphene
2. Routes: enteral, intranasal, intravenous, intramuscular, subcutaneous, and smoked

BOX 2-1

DRUGS OF ABUSE (Continued)

3. Acute intoxication: pinpoint pupils, euphoria, sedation, impaired thought, hypothermia, clammy skin, urine retention, constipation, increased anal tone
   Toxic exposure: hypotension, arrhythmia, respiratory depression, coma, seizure, death
   Chronic IV abuse: cellulitis, septic emboli, endocarditis, abscesses
4. Monitoring
   a. Not all opioids are detected by urine screens
   b. Thin-layer chromatography and radioimmunoassay detect opiate metabolites up to 3 days from last use
   c. 12-lead ECG and cardiorespiratory monitoring
5. Antidote: naloxone. See Formulary
6. Adjunct: consider methadone or buprenorphine to prevent withdrawal
7. Withdrawal: drug cravings, depression, irritability, anxiety, tremors, rhinorrhea, muscle aches, diarrhea, insomnia, piloerection

SEDATIVE-HYPNOTICS (DEPRESSANT)

1. Names: barbiturates (Amytal, Nembutal, Seconal, Phenobarbital), meprobamate, methaqualone, methyprylon, flunitrazepam (Rohypnol: "roofies, roofinol, date pill"), benzodiazepines (Ativan, Halcion, Librium, Valium, Xanax)
2. Routes: enteral, intranasal, intravenous
3. Acute intoxication: reduced anxiety, lowered inhibitions, shallow breathing, poor concentration, impaired coordination, impaired memory, impaired judgment, sluggish pupillary response
   Toxic exposure: hypotension, bradycardia, pulmonary edema, respiratory depression
4. Monitoring: not all barbiturates or benzodiazepines are detected on urine screens
5. Supportive care/decontamination
   a. Consider multiple doses of activated charcoal
   b. Hemodialysis or hemoperfusion in severe overdoses
6. Antidote: flumazenil. See Formulary for dosing and precautions
7. Adjunct: consider methadone to prevent withdrawal
8. Withdrawal: seizures, increased rapid eye movement sleep, tremors, insomnia, apathy, weakness, agitation, anxiety, cravings, and flulike illness. Symptoms peak 5 days after last use

INHALANTS[1,28]

1. Types: volatile hydrocarbons (lighter fluid, paint thinner, hair spray, gasoline), nitrous oxide (laughing gas), paints and varnishes containing akyl nitrates ("poppers, amys")
2. Signs and symptoms
   a. Perioral or perinasal dermatitis. Paint, other stains, or frostbite around nose or mouth. Oral or nasal ulcerations. Chemical odors on breath or clothing
   b. Sneezing, coughing, or tearing from mucosal irritation, gastrointestinal (GI) upset, palpitations
   c. Initial period of euphoria may be followed by dizziness or headache

Continued

BOX 2-1

DRUGS OF ABUSE (Continued)

3. Toxic exposure
   a. CNS depression, slurred speech, hallucinations, lethargy, seizures, coma, respiratory depression
   b. Chemical pneumonitis, hepatotoxicity, methemoglobinemia, and carbon monoxide poisoning may occur depending on the inhaled agent
   c. The most common cause of fatality related to inhalant use is sudden cardiac arrhythmia
4. Monitoring: gas chromatography may be used for diagnosis. Consider chest x-ray (CXR), 12-lead ECG, and a comprehensive metabolic panel
5. Supportive care: basic life support. Use of oxygen and albuterol as needed. Correction of electrolyte abnormalities as needed

of observation. Special attention should be paid to whether it is an immediate or sustained-release preparation. For hypotension, patients often require aggressive fluid resuscitation or vasopressors. For ingestions that cause seizure, treat with benzodiazepines unless otherwise specified. Treat hyperpyrexia with cooling measures. Hemodialysis may be indicated in cases of renal impairment.

NOTE: See Expert Consult, Chapter 2, for these drugs

A. Carbamazepine

B. Digoxin

C. Phenytoin, Fosphenytoin[25]

D. Valproate (VPA), Divalproex, Depakote

V. OTHER CAUSES OF POISONINGS

A. Carbon Monoxide (CO)[29]

1. A colorless, odorless, nonirritating, tasteless gas
2. **Environmental exposures:** House fires, automobile exhaust, gas furnaces/heaters/ovens/dryers, wood and coal heating, fireplaces, charcoal grills, generators, lawn mowers, snow and leaf blowers, paint remover or aerosol propellants containing methylene chloride
3. **Mechanism of injury:** CO has 240-fold greater affinity for hemoglobin than oxygen, leading to decreased oxygen delivery to tissues, cardiac ischemia, and neurologic injury
4. **Clinical presentation**

a. Mild poisoning: Headache, nausea, vomiting, dizziness, blurred vision
b. Moderate poisoning: Confusion, syncope, chest pain, dyspnea, weakness, tachycardia, tachypnea, rhabdomyolysis
c. Severe poisoning: Palpitations, arrhythmias, respiratory arrest, noncardiogenic pulmonary edema, seizures, coma
d. End organ damage: Cerebral edema, permanent ocular toxicity, cardiac ischemia, muscle necrosis, myoglobinuria, renal failure

NOTE: Cherry-red mucosal membranes and retinal hemorrhages are late and rare findings

5. **Management**

a. Secure the airway and avoid hypercapnia

b. Administer 100% O_2 via non-rebreather face mask until carboxyhemoglobin (COHb) is less than 10% and symptoms resolve

c. If severe respiratory compromise, cardiovascular instability, altered alertness, nervous system dysfunction, or coma is present, intubate and mechanically hyperventilate using 100% O_2

d. Consider hyperbaric oxygen therapy in cases of altered mental status, coma, seizures, loss of consciousness, cardiac dysfunction, or pregnancy with >15% COHb, although specific indications are controversial

e. Measure serum COHb levels, ABG, complete metabolic panel, cardiac enzymes, creatine kinase, and lactate

NOTE: General guidelines for COHb levels: Symptomatic at >15%, toxicity at >20%, severe neurologic effects at >40%, and irreversible central nervous system (CNS) damage at >50%. Symptoms may not correlate with COHb levels in the blood

f. Obtain ECG and chest radiograph to evaluate for myocardial ischemia and noncardiogenic pulmonary edema

g. Head computed tomography scan may show infarction and bilateral globus pallidus lesions

h. Perform neuropsychometric testing if clinically indicated or treating with hyperbaric oxygen

B. Cyanide[1,30]

(See Expert Consult, Chapter 2)

C. Lead[31,32]

1. **Etiologies:** Paint, dust, soil, drinking water, cosmetics, cookware, parental occupations, imported toys
2. Children from 1 to 5 years are at greatest risk
3. **Manifestations**

a. Centers for Disease Control and Prevention (CDC) defines toxicity as blood lead level (BLL) >10 mcg/dL

NOTE: There is good evidence to suggest that neurocognitive sequelae are likely to occur at BLL <10 mcg/dL

b. Subclinical disease with BLL <45 mcg/dL

c. Acute symptoms with BLL >45 mcg/dL: Lethargy, anorexia, decreased activity, sporadic vomiting, intermittent abdominal pain and constipation

d. Acute encephalopathy with BLL >70 mcg/dL: Coma, seizures, bizarre behavior, ataxia, apathy, incoordination, vomiting, altered state of consciousness, and loss of recently acquired skills

NOTE: It is possible for children to have lead levels >100 mcg/dL acutely and be initially asymptomatic. Elevated lead levels should never be ignored because of lack of symptoms

4. **Management** (Table 2-4)
a. BLL >10 mcg/dL: lead education. Follow-up
b. BLL >20 mcg/dL (also if BLL is rising or if blood lead level is between 15–19 mcg/dL persistently, i.e. >3 months duration): As for BLL >10 mcg/dL. Environmental investigation. In addition, complete blood count, iron level, abdominal radiography (if ingestion is suspected) with bowel decontamination if indicated and neurodevelopmental monitoring
c. BLL >45 mcg/dL: As for BLL >20 mcg/dL. In addition, check zinc protoporphyrin level and administer chelation therapy (Table 2-5)

TABLE 2-4

REPEAT BLOOD LEAD TESTING GUIDELINES

If Screening BLL Is:	Repeat BLL Within:
10–14 mcg/dL	1 month (then within 3 months)
15–19 mcg/dL	1 week–1 month (then within 2 months)
20–44 mcg/dL	1 week
45–69 mcg/dL	48 hours
>70 mcg/dL	Immediately

BLL, Blood lead level.
From American Academy of Pediatrics. Committee on Environmental health. Screening for elevated blood lead levels. Pediatrics 1998;101:1072–1078.

TABLE 2-5

CHELATION THERAPY[1]*

Chelation Agent* (See Formulary for Dosage Information)	Indication	Comments
Dimercaprol (BAL)	BLL >70 mcg/dL Encephalopathy Severe symptoms	Contraindicated in hepatic disease and peanut allergy May cause hemolysis in G6PD deficiency May also cause renal dysfunction
Calcium disodium ethylene-diamine tetraacetic acid (EDTA)	BLL >70 mcg/dL	May cause renal dysfunction Use in conjunction with BAL for BLL >70—must be given 4 hours after BAL Second line agent for BLL 45–70
Succimer (DMSA)	Preferred agent for patients with BLL >45 mcg/dL who are asymptomatic at presentation	May cause transient LFT abnormalities and reversible neutropenia

*Chelation therapy should only be given in consult with a toxicologist due to the potentially toxic effects.
BLL, Blood lead level; CBC, complete blood count; LFT, liver function test.

d. Caution should be used when prescribing chelation therapy due to the potentially toxic effects. Should only be given in consult with a toxicologist

D. Methemoglobinemia[1]

1. **Etiologies**
a. Congenital hemoglobinopathy: Genetic deficiency of enzymes that reduce methemoglobin
b. Oxidative hemoglobin injury in ill infants, i.e., diarrheal illness, poisoning, drugs, or environmental exposure
c. Agents of injury: Aniline dyes, chloroquine, dapsone, fertilizers containing nitrogens, local anesthetics, high doses of methylene blue, metoclopramide, naphthalene, nitrates, nitrites, rifampin, toluidine, contaminated well water
2. **Clinical presentation**
a. Acute-onset methemoglobinemia: CNS depression, cardiac instability, hemolysis, tissue ischemia
b. Cyanosis unresponsive to oxygen therapy but with normal Pao_2 on ABG
c. Arterial blood has chocolate-brown color and does not turn red on exposure to air

NOTE: Cyanosis occurs with 1.5 g/dL methemoglobin level or when 10% or more of the hemoglobin is methemoglobin

3. **Management**
a. Remove the offending agent
b. Administer 100% O_2. Note that pulse oximetry is not accurate
c. Perform skin decontamination if indicated
d. Give activated charcoal if suspect oxidant ingestion
e. Perform co-oximetry analysis of the blood to confirm and quantify methemoglobinemia. Estimate the oxygen-carrying capacity based on the percentage of methemoglobin and the total amount of hemoglobin
f. Serial ECGs to monitor for myocardial ischemia
g. Obtain electrolytes, creatinine, ABG, complete blood count, blood smear to evaluate for hemolysis, and urinalysis
h. Methylene blue: See Formulary for dosing instructions
 (1) Indicated for severe tissue hypoxia (beyond cyanotic discoloration), CNS depression, cardiovascular instability, coexisting medical condition that decreases tolerance for low oxygen delivery to tissues, and methemoglobin level greater than 30%
 (2) Administration causes a transient decrease in the pulse oximetry reading
 (3) Clinical improvement should be noted within one hour of administration
 (4) Contraindicated in patients with glucose-6-phosphate dehydrogenase (G6PD) deficiency
i. Consider hyperbaric oxygen therapy or exchange transfusions if methylene blue is ineffective or contraindicated

j. Cimetidine may be useful in treating dapsone-induced methemoglobinemia

E. Pesticides (Organic Phosphorus Compounds and Carbamates)[1]

1. Produces a cholinergic toxidrome (see Table 2-1)
2. **Diagnostic tests**
   a. Measure butyrylcholinesterase activity and red blood cell cholinesterase activity
   b. Persistence of cholinergic symptoms after an atropine challenge suggests organic phosphorus or carbamate poisoning
   c. Electromyogram (EMG) studies may be used to quantify acetylcholinesterase inhibition at the neuromuscular junction
3. **Initial management**
   a. Decontamination. Remove all clothing, triple-wash skin and hair. Medical personnel should wear protective gloves and clothing
   b. Orogastric lavage for acute ingestions
   c. Ensure adequate airway and ventilation

NOTE: Only a non-depolarizing neuromuscular blocking agent should be used to induce pharmacologic paralysis

4. **Antidote:** (See Formulary for dosing)
   a. Atropine. Competitively antagonizes acetylcholine at muscarinic receptors. Is not effective for reversing excessive nicotinic effects
   b. Pralidoxime. Enhances hydrolytic regeneration of acetylcholinesterase and exhibits an antimuscarinic effect on nervous tissue

NOTE: Pralidoxime is not recommended if the poisoning is from a carbamate pesticide

F. Rodenticides (Superwarfarins)[1,33]

1. Superwarfarins are long-acting, potent anticoagulants that inhibit the carboxylation of vitamin K-dependent factors
2. **Initial considerations**
   a. No intervention is needed for healthy, young children with acute unintentional exposures of small amounts. They do not develop significant laboratory or clinical evidence of anticoagulation[34]
   b. Intentional ingestions, repeated ingestions, or ingestions involving suspected child abuse warrant close follow-up
3. **Laboratory evaluation:** Serial international normalized ratios (INRs) at 24 and 48 hours post exposure. If normal, no further intervention is needed. If INR is abnormal, patients should be followed until their coagulation studies are normal while off therapy for several days
4. **Management**
   a. Orogastric lavage for patients with potentially life-threatening ingestions if presenting within 1 to 2 hours
   b. At least a single dose of activated charcoal, unless contraindicated
   c. Send blood type and cross match and establish venous access
   d. Packed red blood cells to correct anemia associated with bleeding

e. Fresh frozen plasma (FFP): 10–25 mL/kg to replace vitamin K–dependent clotting factors and reverse any coagulopathy. Multiple FFP transfusions may be required
5. **Antidote:** phytonadione/vitamin K (See Formulary for dosing)

G. Venomous Snakes[1,34]

1. Crotalids are responsible for most snake envenomations in North America. Rattlesnakes (timber, Eastern, Western diamondback, and Mojave), copperhead, and water moccasin (cottonmouth)
2. Appearance: Triangular shaped head, elliptical pupils, hollow retractable fangs
3. **Clinical findings**
a. Local: Fang marks, local tissue damage, pain, swelling
b. Systemic: Nausea, abdominal pain, coagulopathy, rhabdomyolysis, nephrotoxicity, increased vascular permeability and hypotension, neurotoxicity (with the Mojave)
4. **Laboratory evaluation:** Electrolytes, fibrinogen, partial thromboplastin time (PTT), INR, fibrin degradation products, complete blood count, creatine phosphokinase
5. **Management**
a. Cleanse wound. Minimize activity. Immobilize affected extremity with a padded splint and gently wrapped elastic bandage. Do **NOT** use a tourniquet. Elevate the extremity to a level above the heart
b. Obtain serial neurovascular checks and circumferential measurements of affected limb until progression has ceased
c. Fluid replacement, blood products, and analgesia as needed
d. Prophylactic antibiotics are **NOT** recommended
e. Consider tetanus prophylaxis
f. Patients who remain asymptomatic for 6 hours and have normal coagulation studies may be released
g. Envenomation may mimic a compartment syndrome; however, fasciotomy is rarely indicated or beneficial
6. **Antivenom (CroFab)**
a. Indications include rapid progression of swelling, significant coagulation defect, neuromuscular paralysis, or cardiovascular collapse
b. Patients who are asymptomatic or have minimal symptoms should not be treated with antivenom
c. Consult poison control center for guidelines
d. Monitor for immediate hypersensitivity reactions

H. Poisonous Spiders[1,34]

1. **Brown recluse** *(Loxosceles recluse)*
a. Habitat: Found in the midwest and southeast United States. Prefer warm, dry areas such as cupboards, attics, and basements
b. Appearance: Gray or tan with a brown violin-shaped pattern on its cephalothorax. Three pairs of eyes. On average 9 mm long with a leg span of approximately 25 mm

c. Local symptoms: Initial bite is usually painless. Within 6 hours patients may develop pain, erythema, and pruritus at the site of the bite. A small blister with a blue discoloration may develop surrounded by a ring of erythema. Most plaques resolve, some develop central necrosis, eschar, and ulceration over the next few days
d. Systemic symptoms: Typically begin 2 to 3 days after the bite, including flulike symptoms, arthralgias, convulsions, and rash. Rarely, patients develop hemolytic anemia, disseminated intravascular coagulation (DIC), thrombocytopenia, rhabdomyolysis, and kidney failure
e. Management
   (1) Cleanse wound and elevate affected extremity
   (2) Analgesics for pain relief
   (3) Tetanus prophylaxis if needed
   (4) Consider brown recluse antivenom for patients with significant toxicity (call poison control center for guidelines)

2. **Black widow** *(Latrodectus mactans)*
a. Habitat: Present throughout North America. Typically live outdoors around homes in woodpiles, garages, and gardens
b. Appearance: Shiny black with a red hourglass marking on its ventral abdomen
c. Local symptoms: Typical bite causes a pinprick sensation. A small circle of erythema or induration may be seen at the bite site
d. Systemic symptoms: Significant envenomation may cause muscle cramps and diaphoresis that remain localized to the site or spread diffusely and become severe. Abdominal or back pain, nausea, vomiting, facial edema, headache, anxiety, renal failure, and priapism may occur
e. Management
   (1) Cleanse wound
   (2) Consider benzodiazepines for muscle spasm and analgesics for pain relief
   (3) Tetanus prophylaxis if needed
   (4) Consider black widow antivenom for patients with significant toxicity (call poison control center for guidelines)

REFERENCES

1. Flomenbaum M, Goldfrank LR, Hoffman R, et al. *Toxicologic emergencies*, 8th ed. New York, McGraw-Hill; 2006.
2. Dart RC, Rumack BH. Poisoning. In: Hay WW, Levin MJ, Sondheimer JM, et al, eds: *Current pediatric diagnosis and treatment*. 19th ed. New York: McGraw-Hill; 2009:313–338.
3. Hoppe-Roberts JM. Poisoning mortality in United States: comparison of national mortality statistics and poison control center reports. *Ann Emerg Med*. 2000;35(5):440–448.
4. Bryant S, Singer J. Management of toxic exposure in children. *Emerg Med Clin North Am*. 2003;21(1):101–119.

5. Hanhan UA. The poisoned child in the pediatric intensive care unit. *Pediatr Clin North Am.* 2008;55:669–686.
6. Osterhoudt KC, Alpern ER, Durbin D, et al. Activated charcoal administration in pediatric emergency department. *Pediatr Emerg Care.* 2004;20(8):493–498.
7. Michael JB, Sztajnkrycer MD. Deadly pediatric poisonings: nine common agents that kill at low doses. *Emerg Med Clin North Am.* 2004;22(4):1019–1050.
8. Henry K, Harris CR. Deadly ingestions. *Pediatr Clin North Am.* 2006;53(2): 293–315.
9. Mlcak RP, Suman OE, Herndon DN. Respiratory management of inhalation injury. *Burns.* 2007;33(1):2–13.
10. White M, Liebelt EL. Update on antidotes for pediatric poisonings. *Pediatr Emerg Care.* 2006;22(11):740–749.
11. Calello D, Osterhoudt KC, Henretig FM. New and novel antidotes in pediatrics. *Pediatr Emerg Care.* 2006;22(7):523–530.
12. Kanter MZ. Comparison of oral and IV acetylcysteine in the treatment of acetaminophen poisoning. *Am J Health-Syst Pharm.* 2006;63:1821–1827.
13. Miller J. Managing antidepression overdoses. *Emerg Med Serv.* 2004;33(10): 113–119.
14. Rosenbaum TG, Kou M. Are one or two dangerous? Tricyclic antidepressant exposure in toddlers. *J Emerg Med.* 2005;29(2):169–174.
15. Isbister GK, Bowe SJ, Dawson A, et al. Relative toxicity of selective serotonin reuptake inhibitors (SSRIs) in overdose. *J Toxicol Clin.* 2004;24(3):277–285.
16. Scharman EJ, Erdman AR, Wax PM, et al. Diphenhydramine and dimenhydrinate poisoning: An evidence-based consensus guideline for out-of-hospital management. *Clin Toxicol (Phila).* 2006;44(3):205–223.
17. Isbister GK, O'Regan L, Sibbritt D, et al. Alprazolam is relatively more toxic than other benzodiazepines in overdose. *Br J Clin Pharmacol.* 2004;58(1): 88–95.
18. Thomson JS. Use of flumazenil in benzodiazepine overdose. *Emerg Med J.* 2006;23(2):162.
19. Love JN, Howell JM, Klein-Schwartz W, et al. Lack of toxicity from pediatric beta-blocker exposure. *Hum Exp Toxicol.* 2006;25(6):341–346.
20. Shepard G. Treatment of poisoning caused by beta-adrenergic and calcium-channel blockers. *Am J Health-Syst Pharm.* 2006;63(19):1828–1835.
21. DeWitt CR, Waksman JC. Pharmacology, pathophysiology and management of calcium channel blocker and beta-blocker toxicity. *Toxicol Rev.* 2004;23(4): 223–238.
22. Aldridge MD. Acute iron poisoning: What every pediatric intensive care unit nurse should know. *Dimen Crit Care Nurs.* 2007;26(2):43–48.
23. Manoguerra AS, Erdman AR, Booze LL, et al. Iron ingestion: an evidence-based consensus guideline for out-of-hospital management. *Clin Toxicol (Phila).* 2005;43(6):553–570.
24. Love JN, Smith JA, Simmons R. Are one or two dangerous? Phenothiazine exposure in toddlers. *J Emerg Med.* 2006;31(1):53–59.
25. Craig S. Phenytoin poisoning. *Neurocrit Care.* 2005;3(2):161–170.
26. Kuhen BM. Many teens abusing medications. *JAMA.* 2007;297(6):578–580.
27. Ruha AM, Yarema MC. Pharmacologic treatment of acute pediatric methamphetamine toxicity. *Pediatr Emerg Care.* 2006;22(12):782–785.
28. Kaul P. Substance abuse. In Hay WW, Levin MJ, Sondheimer JM, et al, eds: *Current pediatric diagnosis and treatment,* 19th ed. New York: McGraw-Hill; 2009:137–151.

29. Williams JF, Storck M, American Academy of Pediatrics Committee on Substance Abuse, et al. Inhalant abuse. *Pediatrics*. 2007;119:1009–1017.
30. Kao L, Nanagas K. Carbon monoxide poisoning. *Med Clin North Am*. 2005;89(6):1161–1194.
31. Geller RJ, Barthold C, Saiers JA, et al. Pediatric cyanide poisoning: causes, manifestations, management, and unmet needs. *Pediatrics*. 2006;118: 2146–2158.
32. American Academy of Pediatrics, Committee on Environmental Health. Lead exposure in children: prevention, detection, and management. *Pediatrics*. 2005;116:1036–1046.
33. Davoli CT, Serwint JR, Chisolm JJ. Asymptomatic children with venous lead levels > 100 mcg/dL. *Pediatrics*. 1996;98(5):965–968.
34. Mullins ME, Brands CL, Daya MR, et al. Unintentional pediatric superwarfarin exposures: do we really need a prothrombin time? *Pediatrics*. 2000;105: 402–404.
35. Singletary EM, Rochman AS, Bodmer JC, et al. Envenomations. *Med Clin North Am*. 2005;89:1195–1224.

Chapter 3
Procedures

Laura J. Sigman, MD, JD

3

I. GENERAL GUIDELINES

A. Consent

It is crucial to obtain informed consent from the parent or guardian before performing any procedure by explaining the procedure, the indications, any risks involved, and any alternatives. Obtaining consent for life-saving emergency procedures is unnecessary.

B. Risks

1. All invasive procedures involve pain and risk for infection and bleeding. Specific complications are listed by procedure
2. Sedation and analgesia should be planned in advance, and the risks of such explained to the parent and/or patient as applicable. In general, 1% lidocaine buffered with sodium bicarbonate is adequate for local analgesia. See Chapter 6 for Analgesia and Sedation guidelines. Also see the "AAP Guidelines for Monitoring and Management of Pediatric Patients During and After Sedation for Diagnostic and Therapeutic Procedures"[1]
3. Universal precautions should be followed for all patient contact that exposes the health care provider to blood, amniotic fluid, pericardial fluid, pleural fluid, synovial fluid, cerebrospinal fluid (CSF), semen, or vaginal secretions
4. Proper sterile technique is crucial to achieve good wound closure, decrease transmittable diseases, and prevent wound contamination

II. BLOOD SAMPLING

A. Heelstick and Fingerstick[2]

1. Indications: Blood sampling in infants for laboratory studies unaffected by hemolysis
2. Complications: Infection, bleeding, osteomyelitis
3. Procedure:

a. Warm heel or finger

b. Clean with alcohol

   (1) Puncture heel using a lancet on the lateral part of the heel, avoiding the posterior area

   (2) Puncture finger using a lancet on the palmar lateral surface of the finger near the tip

c. Wipe away the first drop of blood, and then collect the sample using a capillary tube or container

d. Alternate between squeezing blood from the leg toward the heel (or from the hand toward the finger) and then releasing the pressure for several seconds

B. External Jugular Puncture[3]

1. Indications: Blood sampling in patients with inadequate peripheral vascular access or during resuscitation
2. Complications: Infection, bleeding, pneumothorax
3. Procedure (Fig. 3-1):

a. Restrain infant securely. Place infant with head turned away from side of blood sampling. Position with towel roll under shoulders or with head over side of bed to extend neck and accentuate the posterior margin of the sternocleidomastoid muscle on the side of the venipuncture
b. Prepare area in a sterile fashion
c. The external jugular vein will distend if its most proximal segment is occluded or if the child cries. The vein runs from the angle of the mandible to the posterior border of the lower third of the sternocleidomastoid muscle

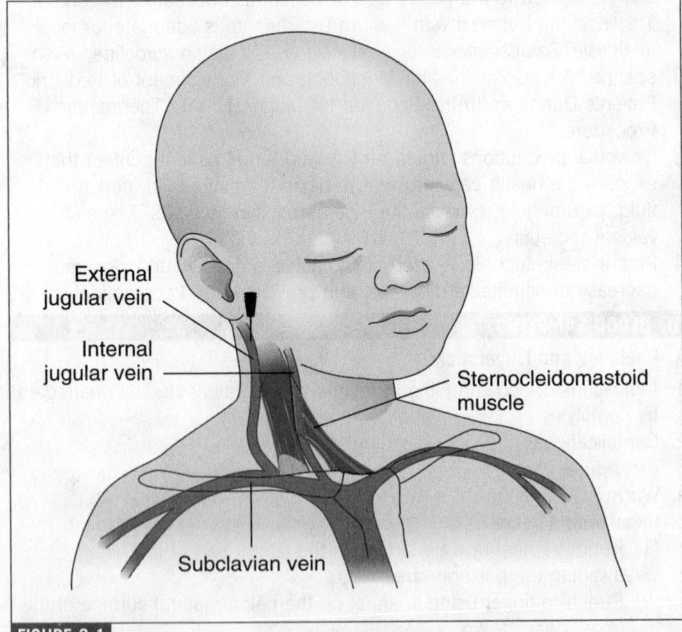

FIGURE 3-1

External jugular cannulation. *(From Dieckmann R, Fiser D, Selbst S: Pediatric emergency and critical care procedures. St. Louis, Mosby, 1997.)*

d. With continuous negative suction on the syringe, insert the needle at about a 30-degree angle to the skin. Continue as with any peripheral venipuncture
e. Apply a sterile dressing, and put pressure on the puncture site for 5 minutes

C. Femoral Artery and Femoral Vein Puncture[3,4]

1. Indications: Venous or arterial blood sampling in patients with inadequate vascular access or during resuscitation
2. Contraindications: Femoral puncture is particularly hazardous in neonates and is not recommended in this age group. There is also a risk in children for trauma to the femoral head and joint capsule. Avoid femoral punctures in children who have thrombocytopenia or coagulation disorders and in those who are scheduled for cardiac catheterization
3. Complications: Infection, bleeding, hematoma of femoral triangle, thrombosis of vessel, osteomyelitis, septic arthritis of hip
4. Procedure (Fig. 3-2):

a. Hold child securely in frog-leg position with the hips flexed and abducted. It may help to place a roll under the hips
b. Prepare area in sterile fashion
c. Locate femoral pulse just distal to the inguinal crease (note that vein is medial to pulse). Insert needle 2 cm distal to the inguinal ligament and 0.5 to 0.75 cm into the groin. Aspirate while maneuvering the needle until blood is obtained

NOTE: The right femoral vein is easier to cannulate than left owing to straighter path to inferior vena cava.

d. Apply direct pressure for minimum of 5 minutes

D. Radial Artery Puncture and Catheterization[3,4]

1. Indications: Arterial blood sampling or frequent blood gases and continuous blood pressure monitoring in an intensive care setting
2. Complications: Infection, bleeding, occlusion of artery by hematoma or thrombosis, ischemia if ulnar circulation is inadequate
3. Procedure:

a. Before procedure, test adequacy of ulnar blood flow with the Allen test. Clench the hand while simultaneously compressing ulnar and radial arteries. The hand will blanch. Release pressure from the ulnar artery, and observe the flushing response. Procedure is safe to perform if entire hand flushes
b. Locate the radial pulse. It is optional to infiltrate the area over the point of maximal impulse with lidocaine. Avoid infusion into the vessel by aspirating before infusing. Prepare the site in sterile fashion
   (1) Puncture: Insert butterfly needle attached to a syringe at a 30- to 60-degree angle over the point of maximal impulse. Blood should

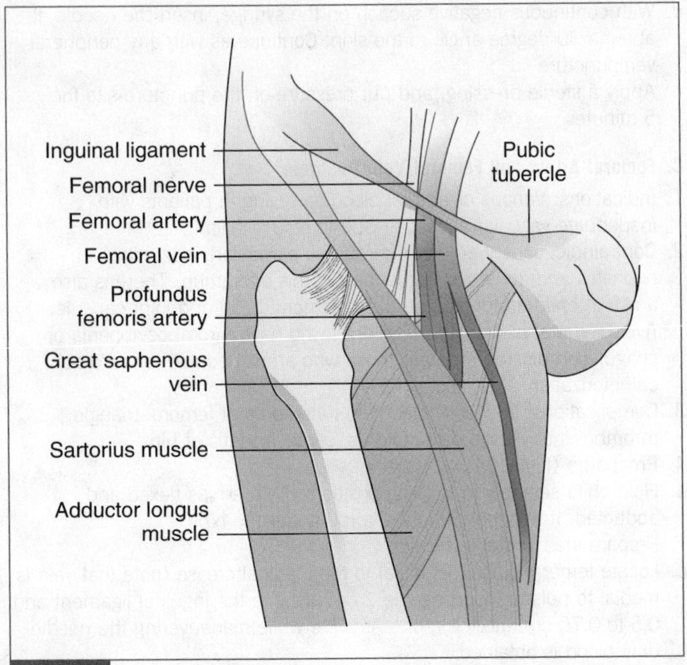

FIGURE 3-2
Femoral artery and vein anatomy. *(From Dieckmann R, Fiser D, Selbst S: Pediatric emergency and critical care procedures. St. Louis, Mosby, 1997.)*

flow freely into the syringe in a pulsatile fashion. Suction may be required for plastic tubes. Once the sample is obtained, apply firm, constant pressure for 5 minutes and then place a pressure dressing on the puncture site

(2) Catheter placement: Secure the patient's hand to an arm board. Leave the fingers exposed to observe any color changes. Prepare the wrist with sterile technique and infiltrate over the point of maximal impulse with 1% lidocaine. Make a small skin puncture over the point of maximal impulse with a needle, then discard the needle. Insert an intravenous (IV) catheter with its needle through the puncture site at a 30-degree angle to the horizontal; pass the needle and catheter through the artery to transfix it, then withdraw the needle. Very slowly, withdraw the catheter until free flow of blood is noted. Then advance the catheter and secure in place using sutures or tape. Seldinger technique using a guidewire can also be used. Apply a sterile dressing. Infuse heparinized isotonic

fluid (per protocol) at 1 mL/hr. A pressure transducer may be attached to monitor blood pressure

NOTE: Do not infuse any medications, blood products, or hypotonic or hypertonic solutions through an arterial line.

E. Posterior Tibial and Dorsalis Pedis Artery Puncture[4]

1. Indications: Arterial blood sampling when radial artery puncture is unsuccessful or inaccessible
2. Complications: Infection, bleeding, ischemia if circulation is inadequate
3. Procedure (see section II.D for technique):
a. Posterior tibial artery: Puncture the artery posterior to the medial malleolus while holding the foot in dorsiflexion
b. Dorsalis pedis artery: Puncture the artery at the dorsal midfoot between the first and second toes while holding the foot in plantar flexion

III. VASCULAR ACCESS

A. Peripheral Intravenous Placement

1. Indications: To obtain access to peripheral venous circulation to deliver fluid, medications, or blood products
2. Complications: Thrombosis, infection
3. Procedure:
a. Choose IV placement site and prepare with alcohol
b. Apply tourniquet and then insert IV catheter, bevel up, at angle almost parallel to the skin, advancing until a *flash* of blood is seen in the catheter hub. Advance the plastic catheter only, remove the needle, and secure the catheter
c. After removing tourniquet, attach T connector filled with saline to the catheter, flush with several mL of normal saline (NS) to ensure patency of the IV line

B. Central Venous Catheter Placement[3,5,6]

1. Indications: To obtain emergency access to central venous circulation, monitor central venous pressure, deliver high-concentration parenteral nutrition or prolonged IV therapy, or infuse blood products or large volumes of fluid
2. Complications: Infection, bleeding, arterial or venous perforation, pneumothorax, hemothorax, thrombosis, catheter fragment in circulation, air embolism
3. Access sites:
a. External jugular vein
b. Subclavian vein: Least common site in children due to increased complications
c. Internal jugular vein: Contraindicated with elevated intracranial pressure
d. Femoral vein: Contraindicated with severe abdominal trauma

4. Procedure: Seldinger technique
a. Secure patient, prepare site, and drape according to the following guidelines for sterile technique[6]:
 (1) Wash hands
 (2) Wear hat, mask, eye shield, sterile gloves, and sterile gown
 (3) Prep procedure site for 30 seconds (chlorhexidine), allow to dry for an additional 30 seconds (groin: Scrub for 2 minutes and allow to dry for 1 minute)
 (4) Use sterile technique to drape the site
b. Insert needle, applying negative pressure to locate vessel
c. When there is blood return, insert a guidewire through the needle into the vein. Watch cardiac monitor for ectopy
d. Remove the needle, holding the guidewire firmly
e. Slip a catheter that has been preflushed with sterile saline over the wire into the vein in a twisting motion. The entry site may be enlarged with a small skin incision or dilator. Pass the entire catheter over the wire until the hub is at the skin surface. Slowly remove the wire, secure the catheter by suture, and attach IV infusion
f. Apply a sterile dressing over the site
g. For neck vessels, obtain a chest radiograph to rule out pneumothorax

5. Approach:
a. External jugular (Fig. 3-1): Place patient in 15- to 20-degree Trendelenburg position. Turn the head 45 degrees to the contralateral side. Enter the vein at the point where it crosses the sternocleidomastoid muscle
b. Internal jugular: Place patient in 15- to 20-degree Trendelenburg position. Hyperextend the neck to tense the sternocleidomastoid muscle and turn head away from the site of line placement. Palpate the sternal and clavicular heads of the muscle and enter at the apex of the triangle formed. An alternative landmark for puncture is halfway between the sternal notch and tip of the mastoid process. Insert the needle at a 30-degree angle to the skin and aim toward the ipsilateral nipple. When blood flow is obtained, continue with Seldinger technique. Right side is preferable because of straight course to right atrium, absence of thoracic duct, and lower pleural dome on right side. The internal jugular vein runs lateral to the carotid artery
c. Subclavian vein (Fig. 3-3): Position the child in the Trendelenburg position with a towel roll under the thoracic spine to hyperextend the back. Aim the needle under the distal third of the clavicle toward the sternal notch. When blood flow is obtained, continue with Seldinger technique
d. Femoral vein (Fig. 3-4): Hold the child securely with the hip flexed and abducted. Locate the femoral pulse just distal to the inguinal crease. In infants, vein is 5 to 6 mm *medial* to arterial pulse. In adolescents, vein is usually 10 to 15 mm *medial* to the pulse. Place the thumb of the nondominant hand on the femoral artery. Insert the needle medial to

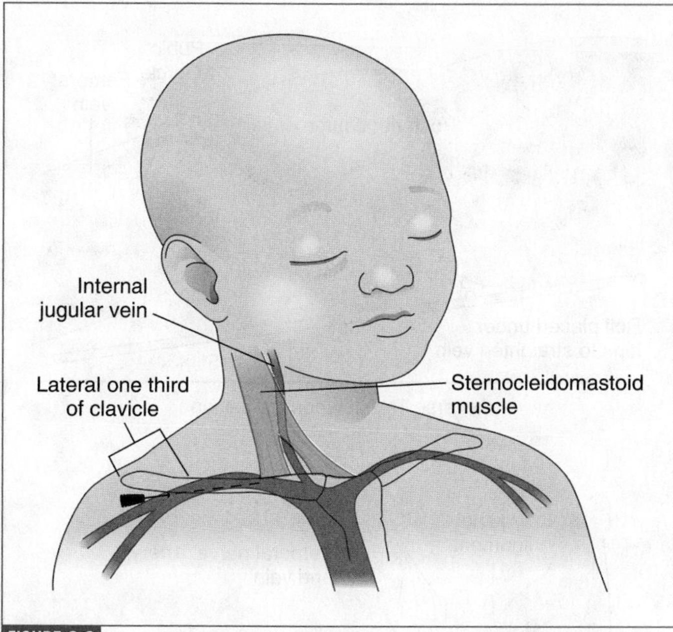

FIGURE 3-3
Subclavian vein cannulation. *(From Dieckmann R, Fiser D, Selbst S: Pediatric emergency and critical care procedures. St. Louis, Mosby, 1997.)*

the thumb. The needle should enter the skin 2 to 3 cm distal to the inguinal ligament at a 30-degree angle to avoid entering the abdomen. When blood flow is obtained, continue with Seldinger technique

C. Intraosseous (IO) Infusion[3,4] (Fig. 3-5)

1. Indications: Obtain emergency access in children during life-threatening situations. This is very useful during cardiopulmonary arrest, shock, burns, and life-threatening status epilepticus. IO line can be used to infuse medications, blood products, or fluids. The IO needle should be removed once adequate vascular access has been established
2. Complications:
   a. Complications are rare, particularly with correct technique. Frequency of complications increases with prolonged infusions
   b. Extravasation of fluid from incomplete cortex penetration, infection, bleeding, osteomyelitis, compartment syndrome, fat embolism, fracture, epiphyseal injury
3. Sites of entry (in order of preference):
   a. Anteromedial surface of the proximal tibia, 2 cm below and 1 to 2 cm medial to the tibial tuberosity on the flat part of the bone (see Fig. 3-5)

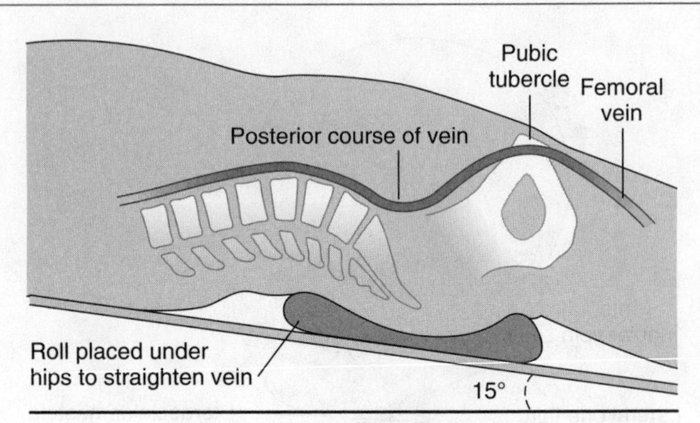

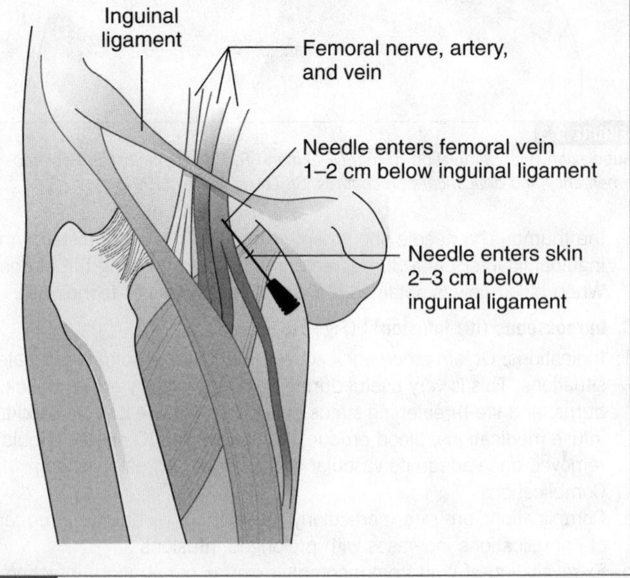

FIGURE 3-4

Femoral vein cannulation. *(From Dieckmann R, Fiser D, Selbst S: Pediatric emergency and critical care procedures. St. Louis, Mosby, 1997.)*

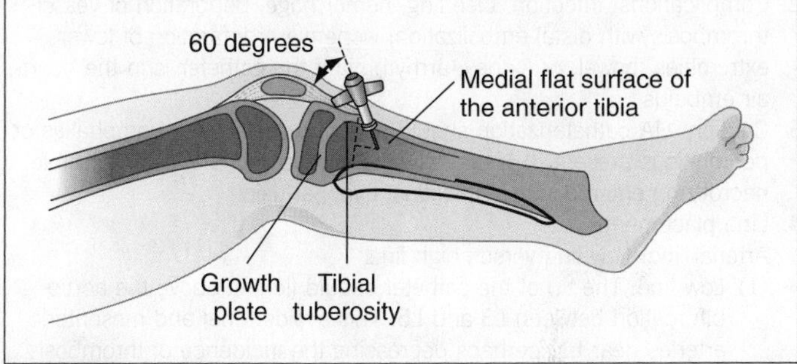

FIGURE 3-5

Intraosseous needle placement using standard anterior tibial approach. The insertion point is in the midline on the medial flat surface of the anterior tibia, 1 to 3 cm (2 fingerbreadths) below the tibial tuberosity. *(From Dieckmann R, Fiser D, Selbst S: Pediatric emergency and critical care procedures. St. Louis, Mosby, 1997.)*

b. Distal femur 3 cm above the lateral condyle in the midline
c. Medial surface of the distal tibia 1 to 2 cm above the medial malleolus (may be a more effective site in older children)
d. Anterosuperior iliac spine at an angle of 90 degrees to the long axis of the body

4. Procedure:
a. Prepare the selected site in sterile fashion if situation allows
b. If the child is conscious, anesthetize the puncture site down to the periosteum with 1% lidocaine (optional in emergency situations)
c. Insert a 15- to 18-gauge IO needle perpendicular to the skin at angle away from epiphyseal plate and advance to the periosteum. With a boring rotary motion, penetrate through the cortex until there is a decrease in resistance, indicating that you have reached the marrow. The needle should stand firmly without support. Secure the needle carefully
d. Remove the stylet and attempt to aspirate marrow. (Note that it is not necessary to aspirate marrow.) Flush with 10 to 20 mL heparinized NS. Observe for fluid extravasation. Marrow can be sent for determination of glucose levels, chemistries, blood type and cross-match, hemoglobin, blood gas analysis, and cultures
e. Attach standard IV tubing. Any crystalloid, blood product, or drug that may be infused into a peripheral vein may also be infused into the IO space, but an increased pressure (through pressure bag or push) is needed for infusion. There is a high risk for obstruction if continuous high-pressure fluids are not flushed through the IO needle

D. Umbilical Artery (UA) and Umbilical Vein (UV) Catheterization[3]

1. Indications: Vascular access (via UV), blood pressure (via UA), and blood gas (via UA) monitoring in critically ill neonates

2. Complications: Infection, bleeding, hemorrhage, perforation of vessel; thrombosis with distal embolization; ischemia or infarction of lower extremities, bowel, or kidney; arrhythmia if the catheter is in the heart; air embolus
3. Caution: UA catheterization should never be performed if omphalitis or peritonitis is present. It is contraindicated in the presence of possible necrotizing enterocolitis or intestinal hypoperfusion
4. Line placement:

a. Arterial line: Low line versus high line
   (1) Low line: The tip of the catheter should lie just above the aortic bifurcation between L3 and L5. This avoids renal and mesenteric arteries near L1, perhaps decreasing the incidence of thrombosis or ischemia
   (2) High line: The tip of the catheter should be above the diaphragm between T6 and T9. A high line may be recommended in infants weighing less than 750 g, in whom a low line could easily slip out

b. UV catheters should be placed in the inferior vena cava above the level of the ductus venosus and the hepatic veins and below the level of the right atrium

c. Catheter length: Determine the length of catheter required using either a standardized graph or the regression formula. Add length for the height of the umbilical stump
   (1) Standardized graph: Determine the shoulder-umbilical length by measuring the perpendicular line dropped from the tip of the shoulder to the level of the umbilicus. Use the graph in Figure 3-6 to determine the arterial catheter length, and the graph in Figure 3-7 to determine venous catheter length
   (2) Birth weight (BW) regression formula:

$$\text{Low line: UA catheter length (cm)} = \text{BW (kg)} + 7$$

$$\text{High line: UA catheter length (cm)} = [3 \times \text{BW (kg)}] + 9$$

$$\text{UV catheter length (cm)} = [0.5 \times \text{high line UA (cm)}] + 1$$

NOTE: Formula may not be appropriate for small-for-gestational-age (SGA) or large-for-gestational-age (LGA) infants.

5. Procedure for UA line (Fig. 3-8):

a. Determine the length of the catheter to be inserted for either high (T6 to T9) or low (L3 to L5) position

b. Restrain the infant. Maintain the infant's temperature during the procedure. Prepare and drape the umbilical cord and adjacent skin using sterile technique

c. Flush the catheter with a sterile saline solution before insertion. Ensure that there are no air bubbles in the catheter or attached syringe

d. Place sterile umbilical tape around the base of the cord. Cut through the cord horizontally about 1.5 to 2.0 cm from the skin; tighten the umbilical tape to prevent bleeding

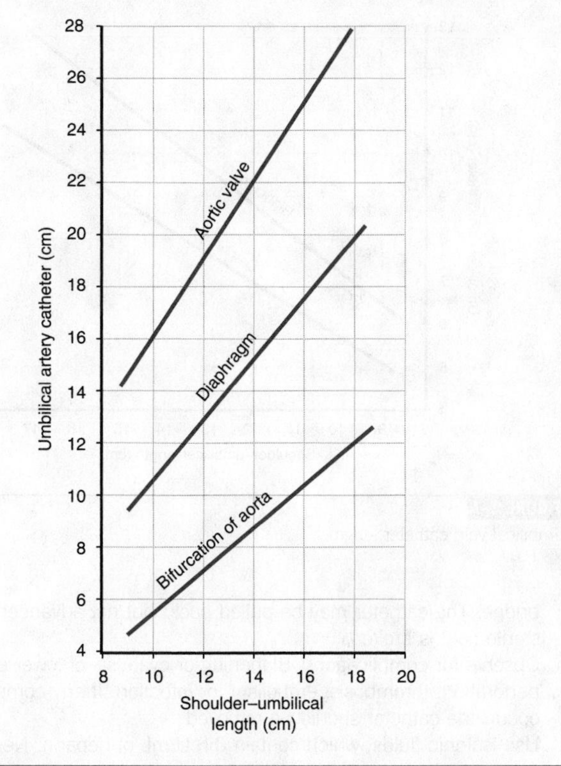

FIGURE 3-6
Umbilical artery catheter length.

e. Identify the one large, thin-walled umbilical vein and two smaller, thick-walled arteries. Use one tip of open, curved forceps to probe and dilate one artery gently; use both points of closed forceps, and dilate artery by allowing forceps to open gently
f. Grasp the catheter 1 cm from its tip with toothless forceps, and insert the catheter into the lumen of the artery. Aim the tip toward the feet, and gently advance the catheter to the desired distance. Do not force. If resistance is encountered, try loosening umbilical tape, applying steady and gentle pressure, or manipulating the angle of the umbilical cord to skin. Often the catheter cannot be advanced because of creation of a "false luminal tract." There should be good blood return when the catheter enters the iliac artery
g. Confirm the position of the catheter tip radiographically. Secure the catheter with a suture through the cord, a marker tape, and a tape

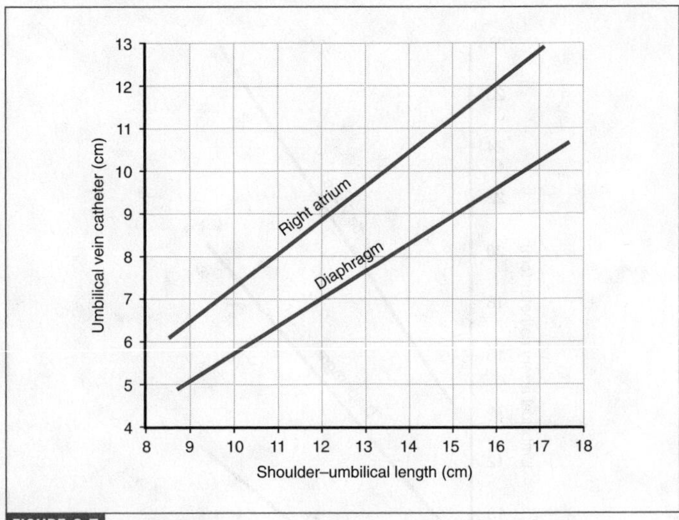

FIGURE 3-7

Umbilical vein catheter length.

bridge. The catheter may be pulled back, but not advanced once the sterile field is broken

h. Observe for complications: Blanching or cyanosis of lower extremities, perforation, thrombosis, embolism, or infection. If any complications occur, the catheter should be removed
i. Use isotonic fluids, which contain 0.5 U/mL of heparin. Never use hypo-osmolar fluids in the UA

NOTE: There are no definitive guidelines on feeding with a UA catheter in place. There is concern (up to 24 hours after removal) that the UA catheter or thrombus may interfere with intestinal perfusion. A risk-to-benefit assessment should be individualized.

6. Procedure for UV line (Fig. 3-8):
   a. Follow steps a through d for UA catheter placement. However, determine catheter length using Fig. 3-7
   b. Isolate the thin-walled umbilical vein, clear thrombi with forceps, and insert catheter, aiming the tip toward the right shoulder. Gently advance the catheter to the desired distance. Do not force. If resistance is encountered, try loosening the umbilical tape, applying steady and gentle pressure, or manipulating the angle of the umbilical cord to skin. Resistance is commonly met at the abdominal wall and again at the portal system. Do not infuse anything into liver
   c. Confirm position of the catheter tip radiographically. Secure catheter as described in step g for UA placement

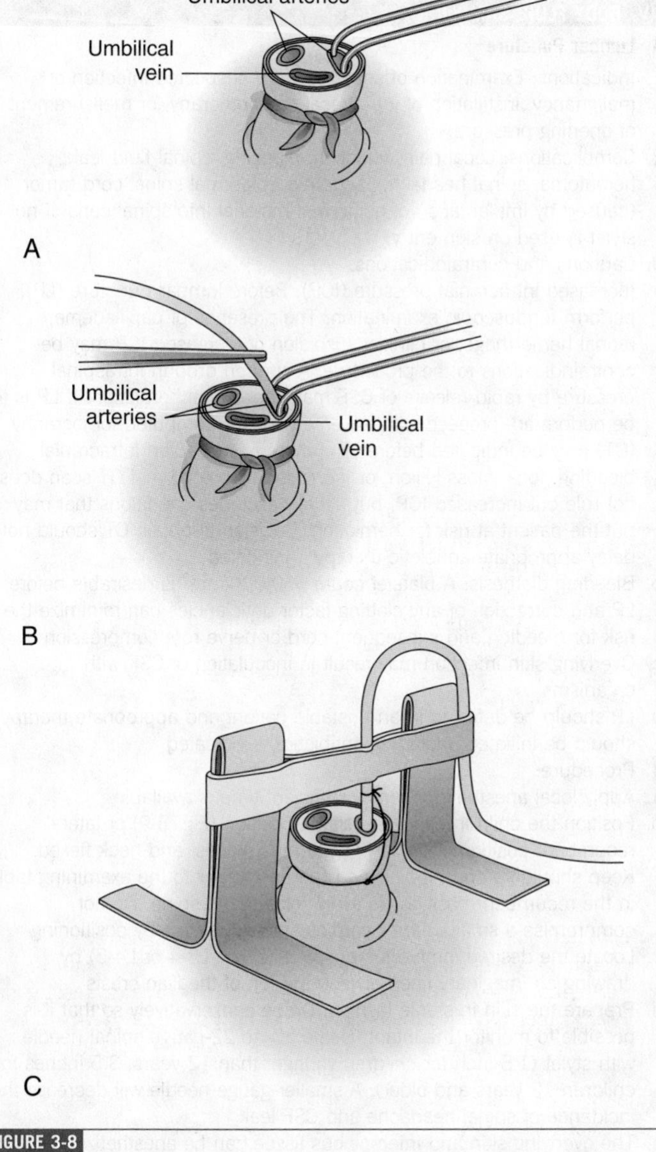

FIGURE 3-8

Placement of umbilical arterial catheter. **A,** Dilating the lumen of umbilical artery. **B,** Insertion of umbilical artery catheter. **C,** Securing the catheter to the abdominal wall using a *bridge* method of taping. *(From Dieckmann R, Fiser D, Selbst S: Pediatric emergency and critical care procedures. St. Louis, Mosby, 1997.)*

IV. BODY FLUID SAMPLING

A. Lumbar Puncture[3,4]

1. Indications: Examination of spinal fluid for suspected infection or malignancy, instillation of intrathecal chemotherapy, or measurement of opening pressure
2. Complications: Local pain, infection, bleeding, spinal fluid leak, hematoma, spinal headache, acquired epidermal spinal cord tumor (caused by implantation of epidermal material into spinal canal if no stylet is used on skin entry)
3. Cautions and contraindications:
   a. Increased intracranial pressure (ICP): Before lumbar puncture (LP), perform funduscopic examination. The presence of papilledema, retinal hemorrhage, or clinical suspicion of increased ICP may be contraindications to the procedure. A sudden drop in intraspinal pressure by rapid release of CSF may cause fatal herniation. If LP is to be performed, proceed with extreme caution. Computed tomography (CT) may be indicated before LP if there is suspected intracranial bleeding, focal mass lesion, or increased ICP. A normal CT scan does not rule out increased ICP, but usually excludes conditions that may put the patient at risk for herniation. Decision to obtain CT should not delay appropriate antibiotic therapy if indicated
   b. Bleeding diathesis: A platelet count >50,000/mm^3 is desirable before LP and correction of any clotting factor deficiencies can minimize the risk for bleeding and subsequent cord or nerve root compression
   c. Overlying skin infection may result in inoculation of CSF with organisms
   d. LP should be deferred in an unstable patient and appropriate therapy should be initiated, including antibiotics if indicated
4. Procedure:
   a. Apply local anesthetic cream if sufficient time is available
   b. Position the child in either the sitting position (Fig. 3-9) or lateral recumbent position (Fig. 3-10), with hips, knees, and neck flexed. Keep shoulders and hips aligned (perpendicular to the examining table in the recumbent position) to avoid rotating the spine. Do not compromise a small infant's cardiorespiratory status by positioning
   c. Locate the desired intervertebral space (either L3-4 or L4-5) by drawing an imaginary line between the top of the iliac crests
   d. Prepare the skin in sterile fashion. Drape conservatively so that it is possible to monitor the infant. Use a 20- to 22-gauge spinal needle with stylet (1.5-inch for children younger than 12 years, 3.5 inches for children 12 years and older). A smaller-gauge needle will decrease the incidence of spinal headache and CSF leak
   e. The overlying skin and interspinous tissue can be anesthetized with 1% lidocaine using a 25-gauge needle
   f. Puncture the skin in the midline just caudad to the palpated spinous process, angling slightly cephalad toward the umbilicus.

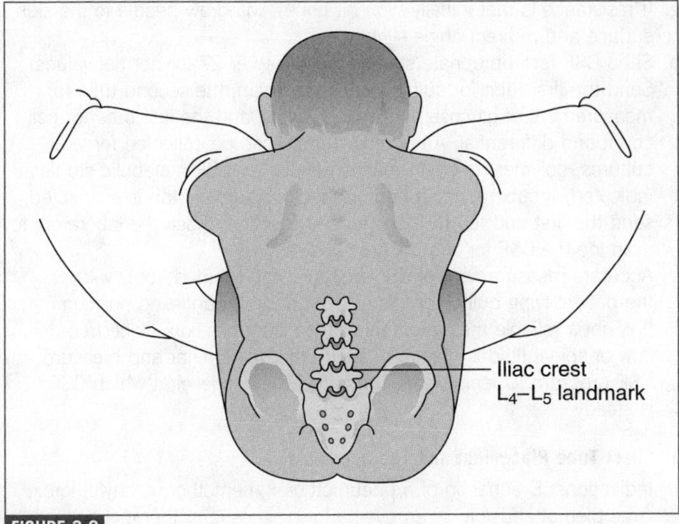

FIGURE 3-9
Lumbar puncture site in the sitting position. *(From Dieckmann R, Fiser D, Selbst S: Pediatric emergency and critical care procedures. St. Louis, Mosby, 1997.)*

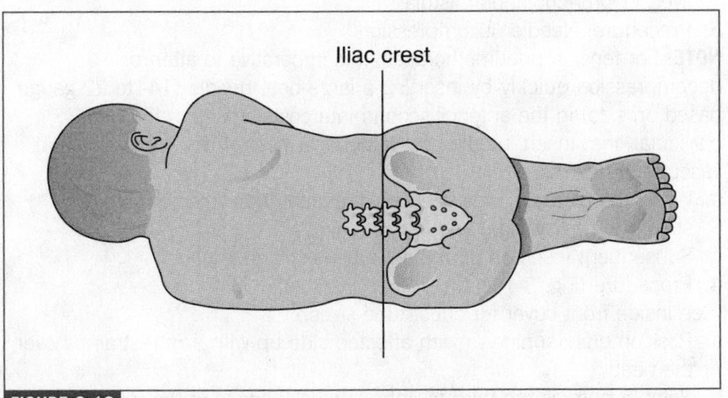

FIGURE 3-10
Lumbar puncture site in lateral (recumbent) position. *(From Dieckmann R, Fiser D, Selbst S: Pediatric emergency and critical care procedures. St. Louis, Mosby, 1997.)*

Advance several millimeters at a time and withdraw the stylet frequently to check for CSF flow. The needle may be advanced without the stylet once it is completely through the skin. In small infants, one may *not* feel a change in resistance or "pop" as the dura is penetrated

g. If resistance is met initially (you hit bone), withdraw needle to the skin surface and redirect angle slightly
h. Send CSF for appropriate studies (see Chapter 27 for normal values). Send the first tube for culture and Gram stain, the second tube for measurement of glucose and protein levels, and the last tube for cell count and differential. An additional tube can be collected for viral cultures, polymerase chain reaction (PCR), or CSF metabolic studies if indicated. If subarachnoid hemorrhage or traumatic tap is suspected, send the first and fourth tubes for cell count, and ask the laboratory to examine the CSF for xanthochromia
i. Accurate measurement of CSF pressure can be made only with the patient lying quietly on his or her side in an unflexed position. It is not a reliable measurement in the sitting position. Once free flow of spinal fluid is obtained, attach the manometer and measure CSF pressure. Opening pressure is recorded as level at which CSF is steady

B. Chest Tube Placement and Thoracentesis[3,5]

1. Indications: Evacuation of a pneumothorax, hemothorax, chylothorax, large pleural effusion, or empyema for diagnostic or therapeutic purposes
2. Complications: Infection, bleeding, pneumothorax, hemothorax, pulmonary contusion or laceration, puncture of diaphragm, spleen, or liver, or bronchopleural fistula
3. Procedure: Needle decompression

NOTE: For tension pneumothoraces, it is imperative to attempt decompression quickly by inserting a large-bore needle (14- to 22-gauge, based on size) in the anterior second intercostal space in the mid-clavicular line. Insert needle over superior aspect of rib margin to avoid vascular structures.

a. When the pleural space is entered, attach catheter to a three-way stopcock and syringe, and aspirate air
b. Subsequent insertion of a chest tube is still necessary

4. Procedure (Fig. 3-11): Chest tube insertion

(See inside front cover for chest tube sizes.)

a. Position child supine or with affected side up with arm restrained over the head
b. Point of entry is the third to fifth intercostal space in the mid to anterior axillary line, usually at the level of the nipple (avoid breast tissue)
c. Prepare and drape in sterile fashion
d. Patient may require sedation (see Chapter 6). Locally anesthetize skin, subcutaneous tissue, periosteum of rib, chest wall muscles, and pleura with 1% lidocaine
e. Make sterile 1- to 3-cm incision one intercostal space below desired insertion point, and bluntly dissect with a hemostat through tissue

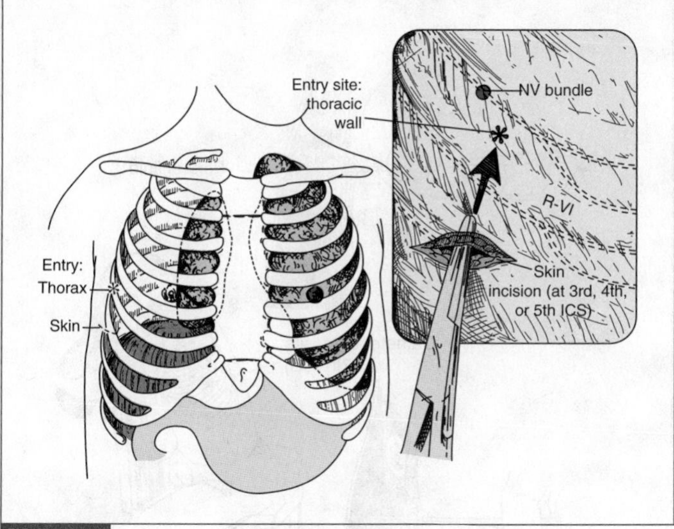

FIGURE 3-11

Technique for insertion of chest tube. ICS, intercostal space; NV neurovascular; R-VI, sixth rib. *(Modified from Fleisher G, Ludwig S: Pediatric emergency medicine, 3rd ed. Baltimore, Williams & Wilkins, 2000.)*

layers until the superior portion of the rib is reached, avoiding the neurovascular bundle on the inferior portion of the rib

f. Push the hemostat over the top of the rib, through the pleura, and into the pleural space. Enter the pleural space cautiously and not deeper than 1 cm. Spread hemostat to open, place chest tube in clamp, and guide through entry site to desired distance
g. For a pneumothorax, insert the tube anteriorly toward the apex. For a pleural effusion, direct the tube inferiorly and posteriorly
h. Secure the tube with purse-string sutures in which the suture is first tied at the skin, then wrapped around the tube once and tied at the tube
i. Attach to a drainage system with 20 to 30 cm H_2O pressure
j. Apply a sterile occlusive dressing
k. Confirm position and function with chest radiograph

5. Procedure: Thoracentesis (Fig. 3-12)

a. Confirm fluid in pleural space by clinical examination and radiographs or ultrasonography
b. If possible, place child in sitting position leaning over table; otherwise place supine
c. Point of entry is usually in the seventh intercostal space and posterior axillary line

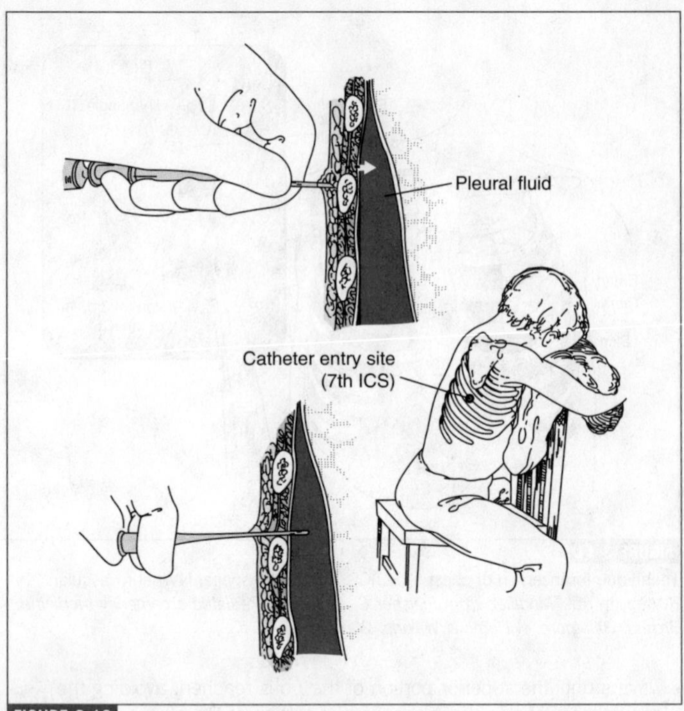

FIGURE 3-12

Thoracentesis. ICS, intercostal space. *(Modified from Fleisher G, Ludwig S: Pediatric emergency medicine, 3rd ed. Baltimore, Williams & Wilkins, 2000.)*

d. Prepare and drape area in sterile fashion
e. Anesthetize skin, subcutaneous tissue, rib periosteum, chest wall, and pleura with 1% lidocaine
f. Advance an 18- to 22-gauge IV catheter or large-bore needle attached to a syringe onto the rib, and then "walk" over the superior aspect into the pleural space, while providing steady negative pressure; often a popping sensation is generated. Be careful not to advance too far into the pleural cavity. If an IV or pigtail catheter (with guidewire) is used, the soft catheter may be advanced into the pleural space aiming downward
g. Attach syringe and stopcock device to remove fluid for diagnostic studies and symptomatic relief (see Chapter 27 for evaluation of pleural fluid)
h. After removing needle or catheter, place an occlusive dressing over the site and obtain a chest radiograph to rule out pneumothorax

C. Pericardiocentesis[3,5]

1. Indications: To obtain pericardial fluid in cardiac tamponade emergently or nonemergently for diagnostic or therapeutic purposes
2. Complications: Bleeding, infection, puncture of cardiac chamber, cardiac dysrhythmia, hemopericardium or pneumopericardium, pneumothorax, hemothorax, cardiac arrest, death
3. Procedure (Fig. 3-13):

a. Unless contraindicated, provide sedation and/or analgesia for the patient. Monitor electrocardiogram (ECG)
b. Place patient at a 30-degree angle (reverse Trendelenburg). Have patient secured
c. Prepare and drape puncture site in a sterile fashion. A drape across the upper chest is unnecessary and may obscure important landmarks
d. Anesthetize the puncture site with 1% lidocaine
e. Insert an 18- or 20-gauge needle just to the left of the xiphoid process, 1 cm inferior to the bottom rib at about a 45-degree angle to the skin
f. While gently aspirating, advance needle toward the patient's left shoulder until pericardial fluid is obtained
g. Upon entering the pericardial space, clamp the needle at the skin edge with hemostat to prevent further penetration. Attach a 30-mL syringe with a stopcock
h. Gently and slowly remove the fluid. Rapid withdrawal of the pericardial fluid can result in shock or myocardial insufficiency
i. Send fluid for appropriate laboratory studies (see Chapter 27)
j. In nonemergent conditions, this is best performed under two-dimensional echocardiographic guidance

D. Paracentesis[4]

1. Indications: Percutaneous removal of intraperitoneal fluid for diagnostic or therapeutic purposes
2. Complications: Bleeding, infection, puncture of viscera
3. Cautions:

a. Do not remove a large amount of fluid too rapidly because hypovolemia and hypotension may result from rapid fluid shifts
b. Avoid scars from previous surgery; localized bowel adhesions increase the chances of entering a viscus in these areas
c. The bladder should be empty to avoid perforation
d. Never perform paracentesis through an area of cellulitis

4. Procedure:

a. Prepare and drape the abdomen as for a surgical procedure. Anesthetize the puncture site
b. With the patient in semisupine, sitting, or lateral decubitus position, insert a 16- to 22-gauge IV catheter attached to a syringe in midline 2 cm below the umbilicus. In neonates, insert just lateral to the rectus muscle in the right or left lower quadrants, a few centimeters above the inguinal ligament

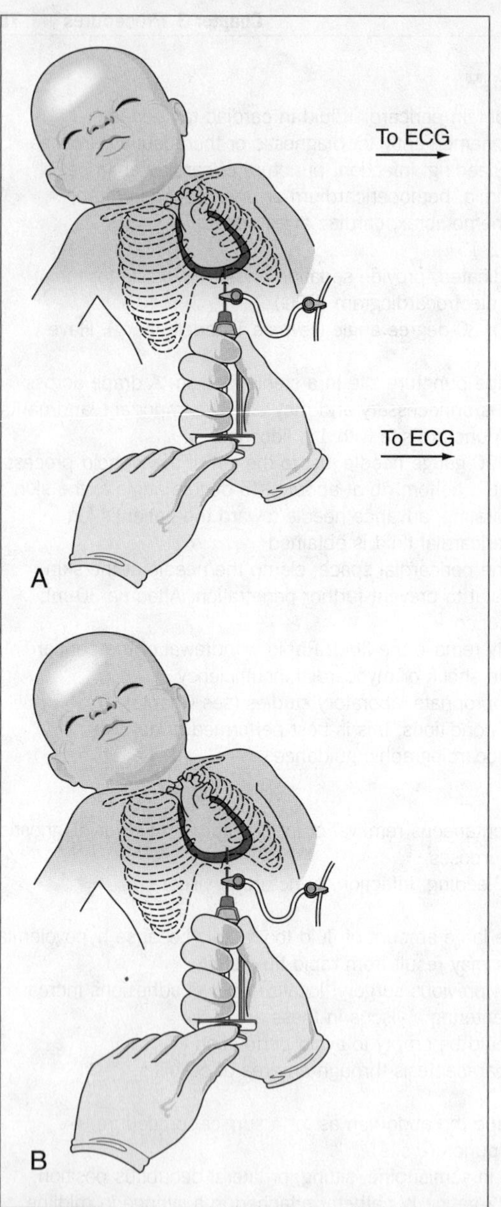

FIGURE 3-13

Subxiphoid approach for pericardiocentesis. **A,** Needle in pericardial sac with normal electrocardiogram (ECG). **B,** Needle in heart with current of injury pattern on ECG. *(From Dieckmann R, Fiser D, Selbst S: Pediatric emergency and critical care procedures. St. Louis, Mosby, 1997.)*

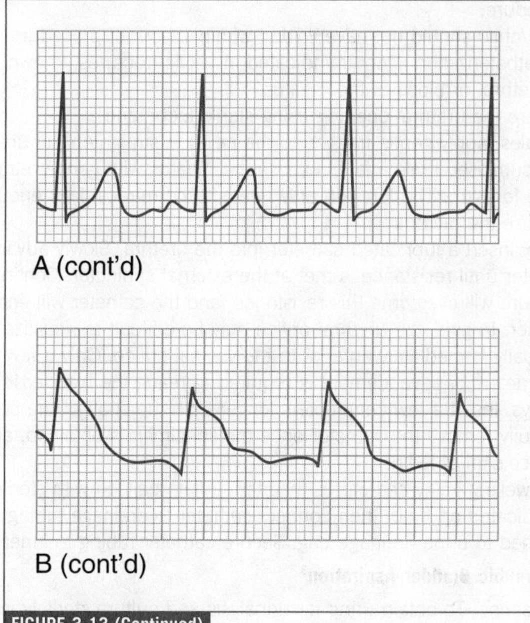

FIGURE 3-13 (Continued)

c. Aiming cephalad, insert the needle at a 45-degree angle while one hand pulls the skin caudally until entering the peritoneal cavity. This creates a Z tract when the skin is released and the needle removed. Apply continuous negative pressure
d. Once fluid appears in the syringe, remove introducer needle and leave catheter in place. Attach a stopcock and aspirate slowly until an adequate amount of fluid has been obtained for studies or symptomatic relief
e. If, on entering the peritoneal cavity, air is aspirated, withdraw the needle immediately. Aspirated air indicates entrance into a hollow viscus. (In general, penetration of a hollow viscus during paracentesis does not lead to complications.) Repeat paracentesis with sterile equipment
f. Send fluid for appropriate laboratory studies (see Chapter 27)

E. Urinary Bladder Catheterization[4]

1. Indications: To obtain urine for urinalysis and culture sterilely and to accurately monitor hydration status
2. Complications: Hematuria, infection, trauma to urethra or bladder, intravesical knot of catheter (rarely occurs)

3. Procedure:
a. Infant/child should not have voided within 1 hour of procedure

NOTE: Catheterization is contraindicated in pelvic fractures, known trauma to the urethra, or blood at the meatus.

b. Prepare the urethral opening using sterile technique
c. In males, apply gentle traction to the penis to straighten the urethra. In uncircumcised male infants expose the meatus with gentle retraction of the foreskin. The foreskin only needs to be retracted far enough to visualize the meatus
d. Gently insert a lubricated catheter into the urethra. Slowly advance the catheter until resistance is met at the external sphincter. Continued pressure will overcome this resistance, and the catheter will enter the bladder. In girls, the urethral orifice may be difficult to visualize, but it is usually immediately anterior to the vaginal orifice. Only a few centimeters of advancement is required to reach the bladder in girls. In boys, insert a few centimeters longer than the shaft of the penis
e. Carefully remove the catheter once the specimen is obtained, and cleanse skin of iodine
f. If indwelling Foley catheter is inserted, inflate balloon with sterile water as indicated on bulb, then connect catheter to drainage tubing attached to urine drainage bag. Secure catheter tubing to inner thigh

F. Suprapubic Bladder Aspiration[3]

1. Indications: To obtain urine for urinalysis and culture sterilely in children younger than 2 years (avoid in children with genitourinary tract anomalies, coagulopathy, or intestinal obstruction). Bypasses distal urethra, thereby minimizing risk for contamination
2. Complications: Infection (cellulitis), hematuria (usually microscopic), intestinal perforation
3. Procedure (Fig. 3-14):
a. Anterior rectal pressure in girls or gentle penile pressure in boys may be used to prevent urination during the procedure. Child should not have voided within 1 hour of procedure
b. Restrain the infant in the supine, frog-leg position. Prepare suprapubic area in sterile fashion
c. The site for puncture is 1 to 2 cm above the symphysis pubis in the midline. Use a syringe with a 22-gauge, 1-inch needle, and puncture at a 10- to 20-degree angle to the perpendicular, aiming slightly caudad
d. Exert suction gently as the needle is advanced until urine enters syringe. The needle should not be advanced more than 1 inch. Aspirate the urine with gentle suction
e. Cleanse skin of iodine

G. Soft Tissue Aspiration[7]

1. Indications: Cellulitis that is unresponsive to initial standard therapy, recurrent cellulitis or abscesses, immunocompromised patients in

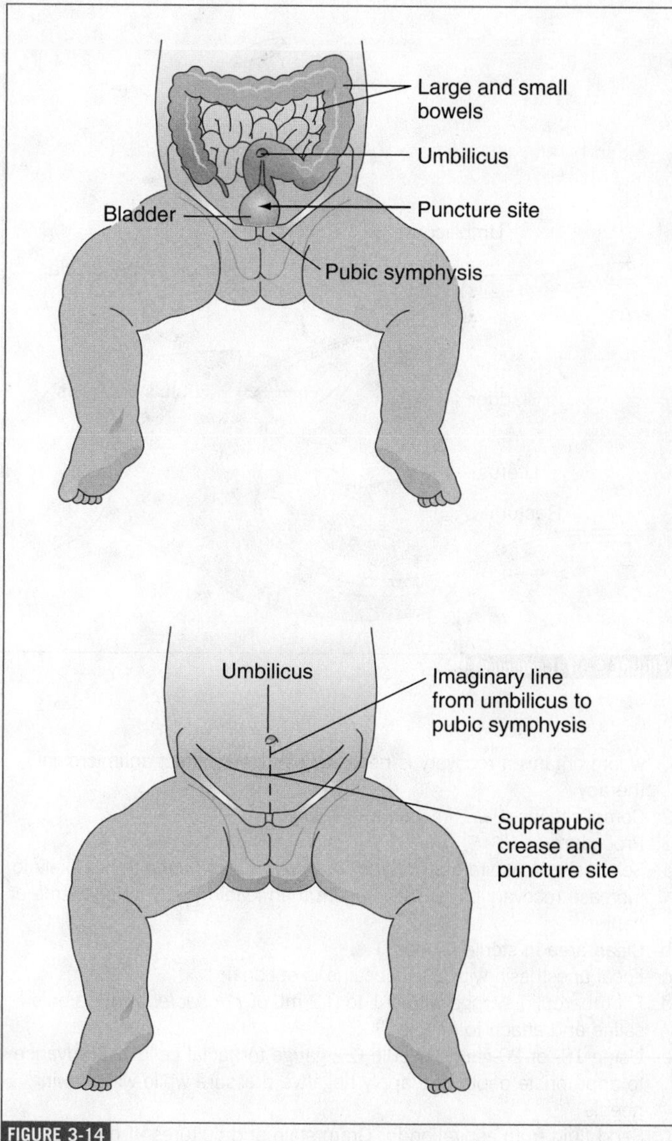

FIGURE 3-14

Landmarks for suprapubic bladder aspiration. *(From Dieckmann R, Fiser D, Selbst S: Pediatric emergency and critical care procedures. St. Louis, Mosby, 1997.)*

Continued

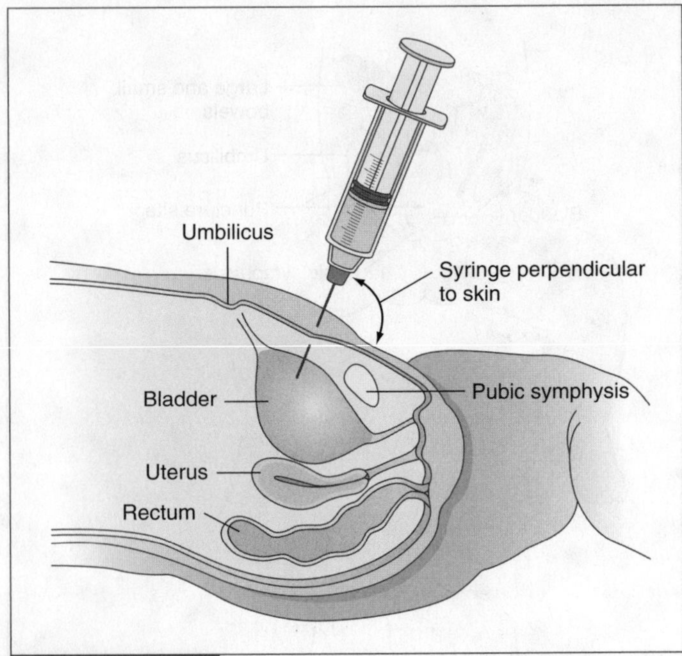

FIGURE 3-14 (Continued)

whom organism recovery is necessary and may affect antimicrobial therapy

2. Complications: Pain, infection, bleeding
3. Procedure:

a. Select site to aspirate at *point of maximal inflammation* (more likely to increase recovery of causative agent than leading edge of erythema or center)[7]
b. Clean area in sterile fashion
c. Local anesthesia with 1% lidocaine is optional
d. Fill tuberculin syringe with 0.1 to 0.2 mL of *nonbacteriostatic* sterile saline and attach to needle
e. Using 18- or 20-gauge needle (22-gauge for facial cellulitis), advance to appropriate depth and apply negative pressure while withdrawing needle
f. Send fluid from aspiration for Gram stain and cultures. If no fluid is obtained, you can streak needle on agar plate. Consider acid-fast bacillus (AFB) and fungal stains in immunocompromised patients

V. IMMUNIZATION AND MEDICATION ADMINISTRATION[4]

A. Subcutaneous Injections

1. Indications: Immunizations and other medications
2. Complications: Bleeding, infection, allergic reaction, lipohypertrophy or lipoatrophy after repeated injections
3. Procedure:
a. Locate injection site: Upper outer arm or outer aspect of upper thigh
b. Clean skin with alcohol
c. Insert 0.5-inch, 25- or 27-gauge needle into the subcutaneous layer at a 45-degree angle to the skin. Aspirate for blood, then inject medication

B. Intramuscular Injections

1. Indications: Immunizations and other medications
2. Complications: Bleeding, infection, allergic reaction, nerve injury
3. Cautions:
a. Avoid intramuscular (IM) injections in a child with a bleeding disorder or thrombocytopenia
b. Maximum volume to be injected is 0.5 mL in a small infant, 1 mL in an older infant, 2 mL in a school-aged child, and 3 mL in an adolescent
4. Procedure:
a. Locate injection site: Anterolateral upper thigh (vastus lateralis muscle) in smaller child, or outer aspect of upper arm (deltoid) in older one. The dorsal gluteal region is less commonly used because of risk for nerve or vascular injury. To find the ventral gluteal site, form a triangle by placing your index finger on the anterior iliac spine and your middle finger on the most superior aspect of the iliac crest. The injection should occur in the middle of the triangle formed by the two fingers and the iliac crest
b. Clean skin with alcohol
c. Pinch muscle with free hand and insert 1-inch, 23- or 25-gauge needle until the hub is flush with the skin surface. For deltoid and ventral gluteal muscles, the needle should be perpendicular to the skin. For the anterolateral thigh, the needle should be 45 degrees to the long axis of the thigh. Aspirate for blood, then inject medication

VI. BASIC LACERATION REPAIR[3]

A. Suturing

1. Techniques (Fig. 3-15):
a. Simple interrupted
b. Horizontal mattress: Provides eversion of wound edges
c. Vertical mattress: For added strength in areas of thick skin or areas of skin movement; provides eversion of wound edges
d. Running intradermal: For cosmetic closures

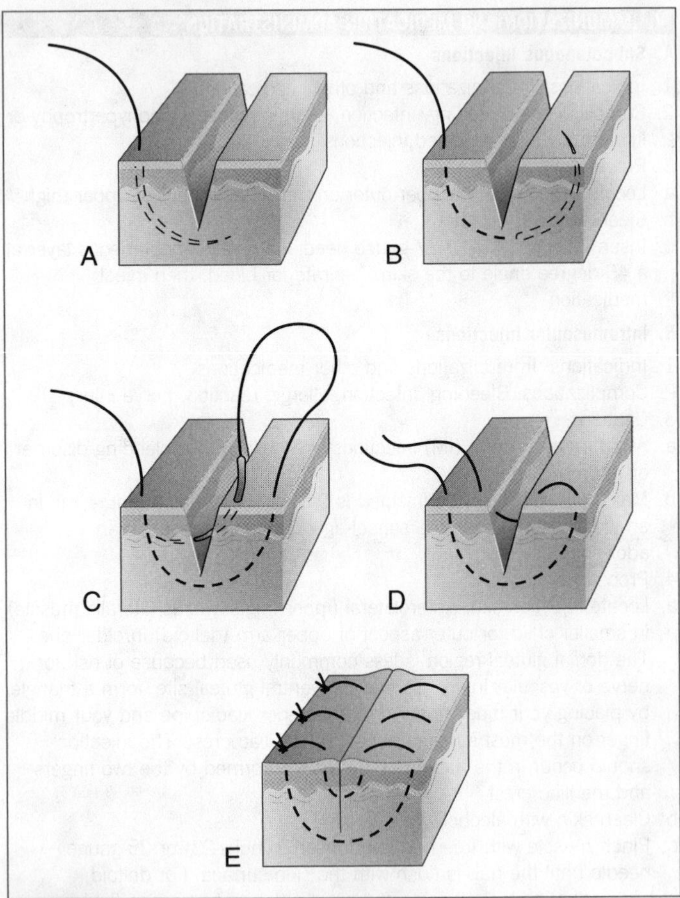

FIGURE 3-15

A–E, The vertical mattress suture. After initial placement of a simple interrupted stitch with a larger bite, make a backhand pass across the wound, taking small, superficial bites. When the knot is tied, the edges of the laceration should evert slightly. *(From Dieckmann R, Fiser D, Selbst S: Pediatric emergency and critical care procedures. St. Louis, Mosby, 1997.)*

2. Procedure:

NOTE: Lacerations of the face, lips, hands, genitalia, mouth, or periorbital area may require consultation with a specialist. Ideally, lacerations at increased risk for infection (areas with poor blood supply, contaminated/crush injury) should be sutured within 6 hours of injury. Clean wounds in cosmetically important areas may be closed up to

TABLE 3-1

GUIDELINES FOR SUTURE MATERIAL, SIZE, AND REMOVAL

Body Region	Monofilament* (for Superficial Lacerations)	Absorbable† (for Deep Lacerations)	Duration (days)
Scalp	5–0 or 4–0	4–0	5–7
Face	6–0	5–0	3–5
Eyelid	7–0 or 6–0	—	3–5
Eyebrow	6–0 or 5–0	5–0	3–5
Trunk	5–0 or 4–0	3–0	5–7
Extremities	5–0 or 4–0	4–0	7–10
Joint surface	4–0	—	10–14
Hand	5–0	5–0	7
Foot sole	4–0 or 3–0	4–0	7–10

*Examples of monofilament nonabsorbable sutures: nylon, polypropylene. Good for the outermost layer of skin. Use 4–5 throws per knot. Polypropylene is good for scalp, eyebrows.

†Examples of absorbable sutures: polyglycolic acid and polyglactin 910 (Vicryl). Good for deeper, subcuticular layers.

24 hours after injury in the absence of significant contamination or devitalization. In general, bite wounds should not be sutured except in areas of high cosmetic importance (face). The longer sutures are left in place, the greater the scarring and potential for infection. Sutures in cosmetically sensitive areas should be removed as soon as possible. Sutures in high-tension areas, such as extensor surfaces, should stay in longer (Table 3-1)

a. Prepare child for procedure with appropriate sedation, analgesia, and restraint
b. Anesthetize the wound with topical anesthetic or with lidocaine-bicarbonate by injecting the anesthetic into the subcutaneous tissues (see Formulary)
c. Forcefully irrigate the wound with copious amounts of sterile NS. Use at least 250 mL for smaller, superficial wounds and more for larger wounds. This is the most important step in preventing infection. Avoid high-pressure irrigation of deep puncture wounds
d. Prepare and drape the patient for a sterile procedure
e. Débride the wound when indicated. Probe for foreign bodies as indicated. Consider obtaining a radiograph if a radiopaque foreign body was involved in the injury
f. Select suture type for percutaneous closure (see Table 3-1)
g. Match layers of injured tissues. Carefully match the depth of the bite taken on each side of the wound when suturing. Take equal bites from both wound edges. Apply slight thumb pressure on the wound edge as the needle is entering the opposite side. Pull the sutures to approximate wound edges, but not too tightly to avoid tissue necrosis. In delicate areas, sutures should be approximately 2 mm apart and 2 mm from the wound edge. Larger bites are acceptable where cosmesis is less important[3]

h. When suturing is complete, apply topical antibiotic and sterile dressing. If laceration is in proximity of a joint, splinting of the affected area to limit mobility often speeds healing and prevents wound separation
i. Check wounds at 48 to 72 hours in cases in which wounds are of questionable viability, if wound was packed, or for patients prescribed prophylactic antibiotics. Change dressing at check
j. For hand lacerations, close skin only; do not use subcutaneous stitches. Elevate and immobilize the hand. Consider consulting a hand or plastics specialist
k. Consider the child's need for tetanus prophylaxis (see Chapter 16, Table 16-6, for guidelines)

B. Skin Staples

1. Indications
a. Best for scalp, trunk, extremities
b. More rapid application than sutures, but can be more painful to remove
c. Lower rates of wound infection
2. Contraindications
a. Not for areas that require meticulous cosmesis
b. Avoid in patients who require magnetic resonance imaging (MRI) or CT
3. Procedure
a. Appose wound edges and staple
b. Left in place for the same length of time as sutures (Table 3-1)
c. To remove, use staple remover

C. Tissue Adhesives

1. Indications
a. For use with superficial lacerations with clean edges
b. Excellent cosmetic results, ease of application, and reduced patient anxiety
c. Lower rates of wound infection
2. Contraindications
a. Not for use in areas under large amounts of tension (e.g., hands, joints)
b. Use caution with areas near the eye
3. Procedure:
a. Use pressure to achieve hemostasis and clean the wound as explained previously
b. Hold together wound edges
c. Apply adhesive dropwise along the wound surface, avoiding applying adhesive to the inside of the wound. Hold in place for 20–30 seconds
d. If the wound is malaligned, remove the adhesive with forceps and reapply
e. Adhesive will slough off after 7–10 days

VII. MUSCULOSKELETAL PROCEDURES

A. Basic Splinting[3]

1. Indications: To provide short-term stabilization of limb injuries
2. Complications: Pressure sores, dermatitis, neurovascular impairment
3. Procedure:

a. Determine style of splint needed
b. Measure and cut fiberglass or plaster to appropriate length. If using plaster, upper-extremity splints require 8 to 10 layers, and lower-extremity splints require 12 to 14 layers
c. Pad extremity with cotton Webril, taking care to overlap each turn by 50%. In prepackaged fiberglass splints, additional padding is not generally required. Bony prominences may require additional padding. Place cotton between digits if they are in a splint
d. Immerse plaster slabs into room-temperature water until bubbling stops. Smooth out wet plaster slab, avoiding any wrinkles
   Warning: Plaster becomes hot after drying.
e. Position splint over extremity and wrap externally with gauze. When dry, an elastic wrap can be added
f. Alternatively, wet one side of fiberglass until saturated. Roll or fold to remove excess water. Mold splint as indicated

NOTE: Using warm water will decrease drying time. This may result in inadequate time to mold splint. Turn edge of the splint back on itself to produce a smooth surface. Take care to cover the sharp edges of fiberglass. When dry, wrap with elastic bandage.

g. Use crutches or slings as indicated
h. The need for orthopedic referral should be individually assessed

B. Long Arm Posterior Splint (Fig. 3-16)

1. Indications: Immobilization of elbow and forearm injuries

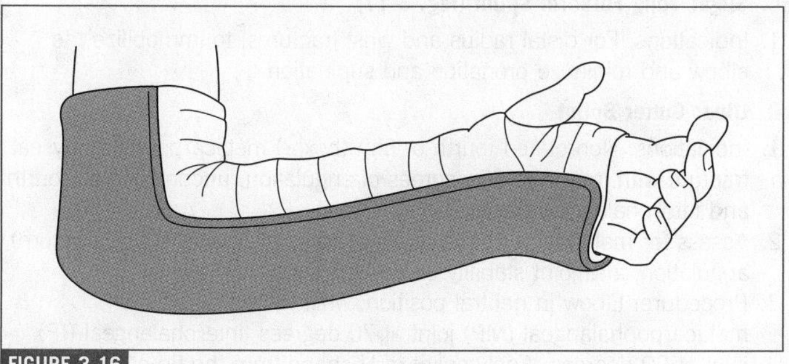

FIGURE 3-16
Long arm posterior splint.

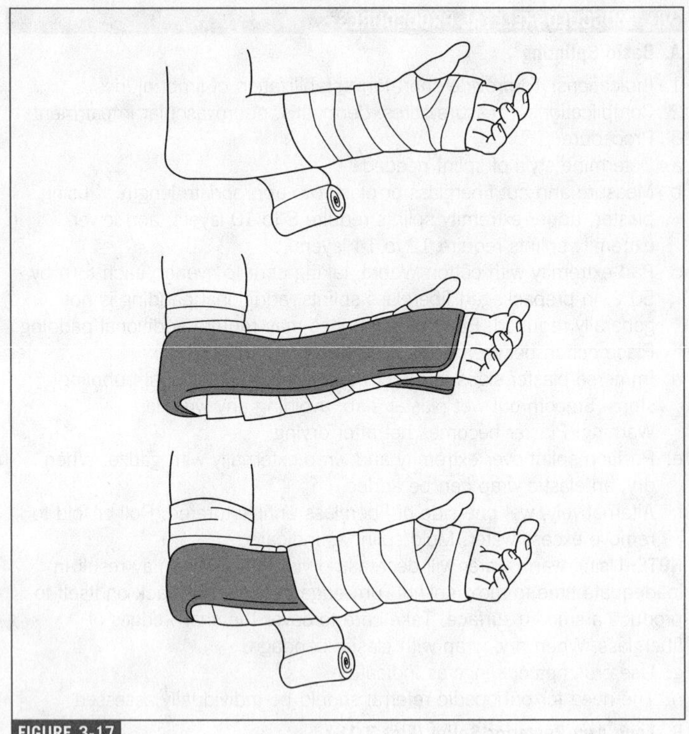

FIGURE 3-17
Sugar tong forearm splint.

C. Sugar Tong Forearm Splint (Fig. 3-17)

1. Indications: For distal radius and wrist fractures, to immobilize the elbow and minimize pronation and supination

D. Ulnar Gutter Splint

1. Indications: Nonrotated fourth or fifth (boxer) metacarpal metaphyseal fracture with less than 20 degrees of angulation, uncomplicated fourth and fifth phalangeal fracture
2. Assess for malrotation, displacement (especially Salter I–type fracture), angulation, and joint stability before splinting
3. Procedure: Elbow in neutral position, wrist in neutral position, metacarpophalangeal (MP) joint at 70 degrees, interphalangeal (IP) joint at 20 degrees. Apply splint in U shape from the tip of the fifth digit to 3 cm distal to the volar crease of the elbow. The splint should be wide enough to enclose the fourth and fifth digits

E. Thumb Spica Splint

1. Indications: Nonrotated, nonangulated, nonarticular fractures of the thumb metacarpal or phalanx, ulnar collateral ligament injury (gamekeeper's or skier's thumb), scaphoid fracture or suspected scaphoid fracture (pain in anatomic snuff box)
2. Procedure: Wrist in slight dorsiflexion, thumb in some flexion and abduction, IP joint in slight flexion. Apply splint in U shape from tip of thumb to mid-forearm. Mold the splint along the long axis of the thumb so that thumb position is maintained. This will result in a spiral configuration along the forearm

F. Volar Splint

1. Indications: Wrist immobilization
2. Procedure: Wrist in slight dorsiflexion. Apply splint on palmar surface from the MP joint to 2 to 3 cm distal to the volar crease of the elbow. It is useful to curve the splint to allow the MP joint to rest at an 80- to 90-degree angle

G. Posterior Ankle Splint

1. Indications: Immobilization of ankle sprains and fractures of the foot, ankle, and distal fibula
2. Procedure: Measure leg for appropriate length of plaster. The splint should extend to base of toes and the upper portion of the calf. A sugar tong (stirrup) splint can be added to increase stability for ankle fractures

H. Radial Head Subluxation Reduction (Nursemaid's Elbow)

1. Presentation: Commonly occurs in children ages 1 to 4 years with a history of inability to use an arm after it was pulled. The child presents with the affected arm held at the side in pronation with elbow slightly flexed
2. Caution: Rule out a fracture clinically before doing procedure. Consider radiograph if mechanism of injury or history is atypical
3. Procedure:

a. Support the elbow with one hand, and place your thumb laterally over the radial head at the elbow. With your other hand, grasp the child's hand in a handshake position
b. Quickly and deliberately supinate and externally rotate the forearm, and simultaneously flex the elbow. Alternatively, hyperpronation alone may be used. You may feel a click as reduction occurs
c. Most children will begin to use the arm within 15 minutes, some immediately after reduction. If reduction occurs after a prolonged period of subluxation, it may take the child longer to recover use of the arm. In this case, the arm should be immobilized with a posterior splint
d. If procedure is unsuccessful, consider obtaining a radiograph. Maneuver may be repeated if needed

REFERENCES

1. AAP guidelines for monitoring and management of pediatric patients during and after sedation for diagnostic and therapeutic procedures: an update. *Pediatrics.* 2006;118(6):2587–2602.
2. Barone MA. Pediatric procedures. In: *Oski's Pediatrics: Principles and Practice.* 4th ed. Philadelphia. Lippincott Williams & Wilkins; 2006:2671–2687.
3. Fleisher G, Ludwig S. *Textbook of pediatric emergency medicine.* 6th ed. Baltimore: Williams & Wilkins; 2010.
4. Dieckmann R, Fiser D, Selbst S. *Illustrated textbook of pediatric emergency and critical care procedures.* St. Louis: Mosby; 1997.
5. Nichols DG, Yaster M, Lappe DG, et al. *Golden hour: the handbook of advanced pediatric life support.* 2nd ed. St. Louis: Mosby; 1996.
6. Berenholtz SM, Pronovost PJ, Lipsett PA, et al. Eliminating catheter-related bloodstream infections in the intensive care unit. *Crit Care Med.* 2004;32(10): 2014–2020.
7. Howe PM, Eduardo Fajardo J, Orcutt MA. Etiologic diagnosis of cellulitis: comparison of aspirates obtained from the leading edge and the point of maximal inflammation. *Pediatr Infect Dis J.* 1987;6(7):685.

Chapter 4

Trauma, Burns, and Common Critical Care Emergencies

Katherine M. Steffen, MD

4

See additional content on Expert Consult

I. TRAUMA: OVERVIEW[1]

A. Primary Survey

The primary survey includes assessment of the **ABC**s: **A**irway, **B**reathing, and **C**irculation. See Chapter 1 for a complete algorithm.

B. Secondary Survey

Procedures included in a secondary survey are listed in Table 4-1. Includes assessment of neurologic status using quick screen: **AVPU** (**A**lert, **V**ocal stimulation response, **P**ainful stimulation response, **U**nresponsive) or Glasgow Coma Scale.

C. AMPLE History

Obtain an AMPLE history: **A**llergies, **M**edications, **P**ast illnesses, **L**ast meal, **E**vents preceding injury.

II. SPECIFIC TRAUMATIC INJURIES

A. Minor Closed Head Trauma (CHT)[2]

1. Introduction: Head injury can be caused by penetrating trauma, blunt force, rotational acceleration, or acceleration-deceleration injury. CHT can lead to depressed or nondepressed skull fracture, epidural or subdural hematoma, cerebral contusion, brain edema, increased intracranial pressure (ICP), brain herniation, concussion (mild to moderate diffuse brain injury), and/or coma (diffuse axonal injury [DAI]). See Section VI.B for treatment of elevated ICP associated with severe CHT
2. Evaluation:
   a. Physical examination (after ABCs and cervical spine [c-spine] immobilization):
      (1) Assign Glasgow Coma Scale (GCS) score (see Chapter 1)
      (2) Obtain vital signs, with special attention paid to Cushing's triad—hypertension, bradycardia, and irregular respiratory pattern
      (3) Perform careful neurologic examination as part of secondary survey (see Table 4-1)
      (4) If severe symptoms are present, or if major CHT, follow procedures for emergency management of increased ICP and coma (see Section VI.B)

TABLE 4-1

SECONDARY SURVEY*

Organ System	Secondary Survey
Head	Scalp/skull injury Raccoon eyes: periorbital ecchymoses; suggests orbital roof fracture Battle's sign: ecchymoses behind pinna; suggests mastoid fracture Cerebrospinal fluid (CSF) leak from ears/nose or hemotympanum suggests basilar skull fracture Pupil size, symmetry, and reactivity: unilateral dilation of one pupil suggests compression of cranial nerve III (CNIII) and possible impending herniation; bilateral dilation of pupils is ominous and suggests bilateral CNIII compression or severe anoxia and ischemia Corneal reflex Funduscopic examination for papilledema as evidence of increased intracranial pressure Hyphema
Neck	Cervical spine tenderness, deformity, injury Trachea midline Subcutaneous emphysema
Chest	Clavicle deformity, tenderness Breath sounds, heart sounds Chest wall symmetry, paradoxical movement, rib deformity/fracture Petechiae over chest/head suggest traumatic asphyxia
Abdomen	Serial examinations to evaluate tenderness, distention, ecchymosis Shoulder pain suggests referred subdiaphragmatic process Orogastric aspirates with blood or bile suggest intra-abdominal injury Splenic laceration suggested by left upper quadrant rib tenderness, flank pain, and/or flank ecchymoses
Pelvis	Tenderness, symmetry, deformity, stability
Genitourinary	Laceration, ecchymoses, hematoma, bleeding Rectal tone, blood, displaced prostate Blood at urinary meatus suggests urethral injury; do not catheterize
Back	Log-roll patient to evaluate spine for step-off along spinal column Tenderness Open or penetrating wound
Extremities	Neurovascular status: Pulse, perfusion, pallor, paresthesias, paralysis, pain Deformity, crepitus, pain Motor/sensory examination Compartment syndrome: Pain out of proportion to expected; distal pallor/pulselessness
Neurologic	Quick screen: **A**lert, **V**ocal stimulation response, **P**ainful stimulation response, **U**nresponsive (AVPU) or Glasgow Coma Scale
Skin	Capillary refill, perfusion Lacerations, abrasions, contusion

*Remove all of patient's clothing, and perform a thorough head-to-toe examination. Remember to keep the child warm during exam.

(5) Rule out possible drug or alcohol ingestion/use as etiology of altered mental status

b. Associated symptoms: Altered level or loss of consciousness (LOC), amnesia (before, during, or after the event), mental status change, behavior change, seizure activity, vomiting, headache, gait disturbance, visual change, or lethargy since event

c. Mechanism of injury:
   (1) Linear forces: Less likely to cause LOC; more commonly lead to skull fractures, intracranial hematoma, or cerebral contusion
   (2) Rotational forces: Commonly cause LOC; occasionally associated with DAI
   (3) Suspect abuse if mechanism of injury is not consistent with sustained injuries

3. Management:

a. Evaluate c-spine

b. Obtain noncontrast computed tomography (CT) scan of head (Box 4-1)
   (1) In absence of LOC, use clinical judgment based on mechanism of injury, severity of known injuries, and deficits on examination

c. Observe patient:
   (1) Monitor for 4–6 hours to detect delayed signs or symptoms of intracranial injury. A symptom-free lucid period can precede variable degrees of acute-onset mental status change with epidural bleeds
   (2) Recommend continued observation at home, or in hospital if clinically unstable, or if there are concerns about home environment (caregiver reliability, follow-up, etc.). Counsel parents on indications to have patient re-evaluated

d. Consider patients with the following symptoms for hospitalization:
   (1) Depressed or declining level of consciousness or prolonged unconsciousness (GCS 8–12)
   (2) Focal neurologic deficit
   (3) Increasing headache, persistent vomiting, or seizures
   (4) Cerebrospinal fluid otorrhea or rhinorrhea, hemotympanum, Battle's sign, or raccoon eyes
   (5) Linear skull fracture crossing the groove of the middle meningeal artery, a venous sinus of the dura, or the foramen magnum
   (6) Depressed or compound skull fracture or fracture into the frontal sinus
   (7) Bleeding disorder or patient on anticoagulation therapy
   (8) Intoxication, illness, or injury obscuring neurologic state
   (9) Suspected nonaccidental trauma
   (10) Patient is unable to return to emergency department (ED) for reassessment

e. Concussions in sports-related injuries:[3]
   (1) Definition: Trauma-induced alteration of consciousness that may or may not cause LOC

BOX 4-1

INDICATIONS FOR IMAGING IN MINOR CLOSED HEAD TRAUMA

Age <2 years	GCS ≤14 OR altered mental status OR palpable skull fracture	→ Obtain Head CT
	Occipital, parietal, or temporal scalp hematoma OR history of LOC >5 seconds OR severe mechanism of injury OR not acting normally per parent	→ Observation vs. Head CT based on other clinical factors: physician experience, multiple vs. isolated findings, worsening of signs or symptoms after ED observation, age <3 months, parental preference
	None of signs or symptoms listed above	→ No Head CT
Age ≥2 years	GCS ≤14 OR altered mental status OR signs of basilar skull fracture	→ Obtain Head CT
	History of LOC OR history of vomiting, or severe mechanism of injury or severe headache	→ Observation vs. Head CT based on other clinical factors: physician experience, multiple vs. isolated findings, worsening of signs or symptoms after ED observation, parental preference
	None of signs or symptoms listed above	→ No Head CT

LOC = Loss of consciousness
ED = Emergency Department
Modified from Kuppermann J, Holmes J, Dayan P, et al. Identification of children at very low risk of clinically-important brain injuries after head trauma: a prospective cohort study. Lancet 2009: 374:1160–70.

(2) Immediate signs: Change in playing ability, confusion, slowing, memory disturbance, incoordination, headache, dizziness, nausea, vomiting, and LOC

(3) Postconcussive symptoms: Headaches, fatigue, sleep disturbance, nausea, vision changes, tinnitus, balance problems, emotional/behavioral changes, and cognitive changes

(4) Management: Evaluate Airway, Breathing, Circulation (ABC); perform mental status assessment
   (a) Grade of concussion less important than tracking recovery course carefully over time
   (b) Return to play only if: No signs or symptoms during rest or exertion, normal neurologic exam, neuroimaging normal (if obtained)
   (c) Consider neuropsychologic testing if history of multiple injuries, recovery not progressing as expected

(5) Refer to Centers for Disease Control and Prevention Guidelines: Concussion in Youth Sports: http://www.cdc.gov/concussion/HeadsUp/youth.html

B. Neck Injuries[2]

See Chapter 25 (Radiology) for in-depth evaluation of cervical trauma and reading c-spine films

1. Immobilize c-spine prior to history and physical examination. Due to large occiput in infants, use support under neck/shoulders to maintain neutral position and avoid neck flexion
2. Radiographic studies:
   a. Posteroanterior (PA), lateral views (including C7), and odontoid view
   b. Flexion and extension views of c-spine, if:
      (1) Unstable c-spine injury not suspected
      (2) Bony point tenderness
      (3) Symptoms on palpation
      (4) Suspicion of abnormality on PA or lateral views
   c. Magnetic resonance imaging (MRI) indicated to rule out direct spinal cord damage if neurologic symptoms persist and plain films are negative
3. Clinically clear the c-spine:
   a. Patient must be awake and alert, without a distracting injury or intoxication
   b. Palpate posterior neck for localized tenderness. If there is pain, maintain c-spine collar for immobilization until further evaluation can definitively rule out injury. If there is no pain, assess active and passive range of motion

C. Blunt Thoracic and Abdominal Trauma[4]

1. Anatomic considerations in children: Pliable rib cage, solid organs proportionally larger than those of adults, underdeveloped abdominal musculature
2. Common injuries:
   a. Thoracic: Pneumothorax, hemothorax, pulmonary contusion, fractures; damage to major blood vessels, heart, diaphragm
   b. Abdominal: Hematomas within gastrointestinal (GI) tract; damage to spleen, liver, pancreas, kidneys, genitourinary (GU) system, or major blood vessels
3. Evaluation:
   a. Careful history and physical examination
   b. Laboratory studies:
      (1) Type and cross-match
      (2) Thoracic injury: Complete blood count (CBC), pulse oximetry; consider arterial blood gas (ABG)
      (3) Abdominal injury: CBC (follow serial hemoglobin values), electrolytes, liver function tests, amylase, lipase, urinalysis

c. Radiologic evaluation:
   (1) Chest radiograph with or without chest CT with IV contrast, if patient is stable
   (2) Abdominal CT with IV contrast (routine oral contrast is not indicated, secondary to high false-negative rate for hollow viscus injury)
   (3) Consider focused abdominal ultrasound when coexisting injuries (e.g., neurologic or significant orthopedic) prevent CT scan

4. Emergent treatment:
a. If significant trauma is suspected or diagnosed, consult a pediatric surgeon
b. Tension pneumothorax:
   (1) Signs: Marked respiratory distress, distended neck veins, contralateral tracheal deviation, diminished breath sounds, compromised systemic perfusion, or trauma arrest
   (2) Treatment: Needle decompression, then chest tube placement directed toward lung apex (see Chapter 3)
c. Open pneumothorax (a.k.a. sucking chest wound): Allows free flow of air between atmosphere and hemithorax. Cover defect with an occlusive dressing (i.e., petroleum jelly gauze), give positive-pressure ventilation, and insert chest tube (see Chapter 3)
d. Hemothorax: Provide fluid resuscitation followed by placement of a chest tube directed posteriorly and inferiorly
e. Abdominal trauma: Penetrating trauma requires surgical evaluation. Nonoperative management may be possible in blunt trauma, even in the presence of intra-abdominal bleeding. Bleeding from injured spleen, kidneys, or liver is often self-limited. The decision to pursue operative vs. nonoperative management should be made by a surgeon

D. Orthopedic/Long Bone Trauma[5,6]

1. Fractures: Some fracture patterns are unique to children (Fig. 4-1); growth-plate injuries are classified by the Salter-Harris classification (Table 4-2). Ligaments are stronger than bones or growth plates in children; thus, dislocations and sprains are relatively uncommon, whereas growth-plate disruption and bone avulsion are more common. For basic splinting techniques, see Chapter 3
2. Compartment syndrome[1,6]: Elevated muscle compartment pressure (enclosed by surrounding fascia) impairs blood flow, resulting in nerve and muscle damage
a. May be secondary to crush injury, fractures (most common: tibia), burns, infections (necrotizing fasciitis), or hemorrhage
b. Marked by **6 P**s: **P**ain (earliest symptom), **P**aresthesias, **P**allor, **P**oikilothermia, **P**aralysis, **P**ulselessness
   (1) Unremitting pain, even after appropriate analgesia is most sensitive sign
   (2) Pain with passive muscle stretch is a strong indicator

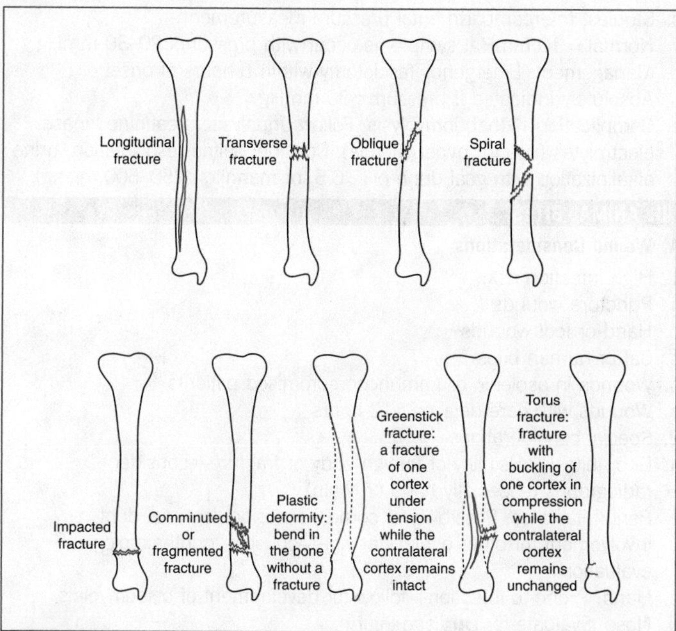

FIGURE 4-1

Fracture patterns unique to children. *(Modified from Ogden JA: Skeletal injury in the child, 3rd ed. Philadelphia, WB Saunders, 2000.)*

TABLE 4-2

SALTER-HARRIS CLASSIFICATION OF GROWTH-PLATE INJURY

Class I	Class II	Class III	Class IV	Class V
Fracture along growth plate	Fracture along growth plate with metaphyseal extension	Fracture along growth plate with epiphyseal extension	Fracture across growth plate, including metaphysis and epiphysis	Crush injury to growth plate without obvious fracture
I	II	III	IV	V

c. Studies: Intercompartmental pressure measurement. Normal = 10 mmHg; symptoms occur with pressures 20–30 mmHg
d. Management: Emergency fasciotomy within 6 hours of onset. Absolutely indicated if pressure >30 mmHg
e. Complications: Rhabdomyolysis. Follow urinalysis, creatinine kinase, electrolytes (risk for hyperkalemia). Consider saline resuscitation, urine alkalinization with goal urine pH >6.5, or mannitol (250–500 mg/kg)

III. ANIMAL BITES[2]

A. Wound Considerations

1. High infection risk:
a. Puncture wounds
b. Hand or foot wounds
c. Cat or human bites
d. Wounds in asplenic or immunocompromised patients
e. Wounds with care delayed >12 hours
2. Special considerations:
a. Deep bites: Possibility of foreign body or fracture—consider radiographs (especially hand or scalp)
b. Periorbital bites: Possibility of corneal abrasion, lacrimal duct involvement, or other ocular damage—consider ophthalmologic evaluation
c. Hand: Prone to infection—follow for development of osteomyelitis
d. Nose: Evaluate for cartilage injury
3. Animal species (Table 4-3)

B. Management

1. Wound hygiene:
a. Irrigate with copious amounts (at least 100 mL/cm of laceration) of sterile saline using high-pressure syringe irrigation. Do not irrigate puncture wounds

TABLE 4-3
ANIMAL BITES

Animal	Common Organism(s)	Special Considerations
Dog	*Staphylococcus aureus* *Pasteurella multocida*	Crush injury
Cat	*Pasteurella multocida*	Deep puncture wound Often associated with fulminant infection Slow to respond to treatment
Human	*Streptococcus viridans* *Staphylococcus aureus* Anaerobes *Eikenella corrodens*	Consider child abuse
Rodent	*Streptobacillus moniliformis* *Spirillum minus*	Low incidence of secondary infection Rat-bite fever—occurs rarely

b. Débride devitalized tissue and evaluate for foreign bodies
c. Consider surgical debridement/exploration for extensive wounds, wounds involving metacarpophalangeal joint, and cranial bites by a large animal
d. Culture only if evidence of infection is present

2. Closure:

a. Avoid closing wounds of high infection risk (see list III.A)
b. Wounds that involve tendons, joints, deep fascia, or major vasculature should be evaluated by a plastic or hand surgeon and, if indicated, closed in the operating room
c. Suturing: When indicated, closure should be done with minimal simple, interrupted, nylon sutures. Approximate wound edges loosely. Avoid deep sutures
   (1) Head and neck: Can usually be safely sutured (with the exceptions noted) after copious irrigation and wound debridement if within 6 to 8 hr of injury and no signs of infection. Facial wounds often require primary closure for cosmetic reasons; infection risk is lower due to good vascular supply
   (2) Hands: In large wounds, subcutaneous dead space should be closed with minimal absorbable sutures, with delayed cutaneous closure in 3 to 5 days if there is no evidence of infection

3. Antibiotics: Prophylactic antibiotics are only indicated in cases of high infection risk, as listed in III.A. See Chapter 17 for appropriate antibiotic therapies
4. Rabies and tetanus prophylaxis: See Chapter 16
5. Disposition:

a. Outpatient care: Obtain careful follow-up of all bite wounds within 24–48 hours, especially those requiring surgical closure. Extremity wounds, especially of the hands, should be immobilized in position of function and kept elevated. Wounds should be kept clean and dry
b. Inpatient care: Consider hospitalization for observation and parenteral antibiotics for significant human bites, immunocompromised or asplenic hosts, deep or severe infections, bites associated with systemic complaints, bites with significant functional or cosmetic morbidity, and/or unreliable follow-up or care by the parent/guardian

6. The infected wound: Wounds that subsequently become infected may require drainage and debridement, possibly under anesthesia. Adjust antibiotic therapy according to Gram stain and culture results

IV. BURNS[1,2,7]

Section edited with assistance from Susan Ziegfeld, MSN, CRNP

A. Evaluation of Pediatric Burns (Tables 4-4 and 4-5)

NOTE: Depending on the extent and type of burn, the severity may progress over the first few days after injury; complete daily assessment until burn has declared itself.

TABLE 4-4

THERMAL INJURY

Type of Burn	Description/Comment
Flame	Most common type of burn; when clothing burns, the heat exposure is prolonged, and the severity increased.
Scald/contact	Mortality is similar to that in flame burns when total body surface area involved is equivalent; see Figure 4-2.
Chemical	Tissue damaged by protein coagulation or liquefaction rather than hyperthermic activity.
Electrical	Injury is often extensive, involving skeletal muscle and other tissues in addition to the skin damage. Extent of damage may not be initially apparent. The tissues with the least resistance are most heat sensitive; bone with most resistance, nerve tissue with least. Cardiac arrest may occur from passage of the current through the heart.
Inhalation	Present in 30% of victims of major flame burns and increases mortality. Consider when there is evidence of fire in enclosed space. Signs include: singed nares, facial burns, charred lips, carbonaceous secretions, posterior pharynx edema, hoarseness, cough, or wheezing.
Cold injury/frostbite	Freezing results in direct tissue injury. Toes, fingers, ears, and nose are commonly involved. Initial treatment includes rewarming in tepid (105°–110°F) water for 20–40 min. Excision of tissue should not be done until complete demarcation of nonviable tissue has occurred.

TABLE 4-5

BURN CLASSIFICATION

Superficial	Injury to epidermis only Characterized by erythema, pain, includes sunburn or minor scalds Patients with superficial burns only usually do not require IV fluid replacement Not included in estimate of surface area burned Generally heals on its own without scarring in 3–5 days
Superficial partial thickness	Damages, but does not destroy epidermis and dermis Characterized by intense pain, blisters, pink to cherry red skin, moist and weepy Nails, hair, sebaceous glands, and nerves intact Can progress to deep partial or full thickness burn Spontaneous re-epithelialization in 2–3 weeks
Deep partial thickness	Injury to epidermis and dermis Characterized by intense pain, dry and white in color Can result in disruption of nails, hair, sebaceous glands May cause scarring: skin grafting usually required
Full thickness	Injury involves all layers of skin, characterized by charred black color, ± areas dry or white Pain may be intense or absent depending on nerve ending involvement Causes scarring; skin grafting required

B. Burn Mapping

Calculate total body surface area (TBSA) burned (Fig. 4-2): Based only on percentage of second- and third-degree burns

C. Emergent Management of Pediatric Burns

1. Acute stabilization:

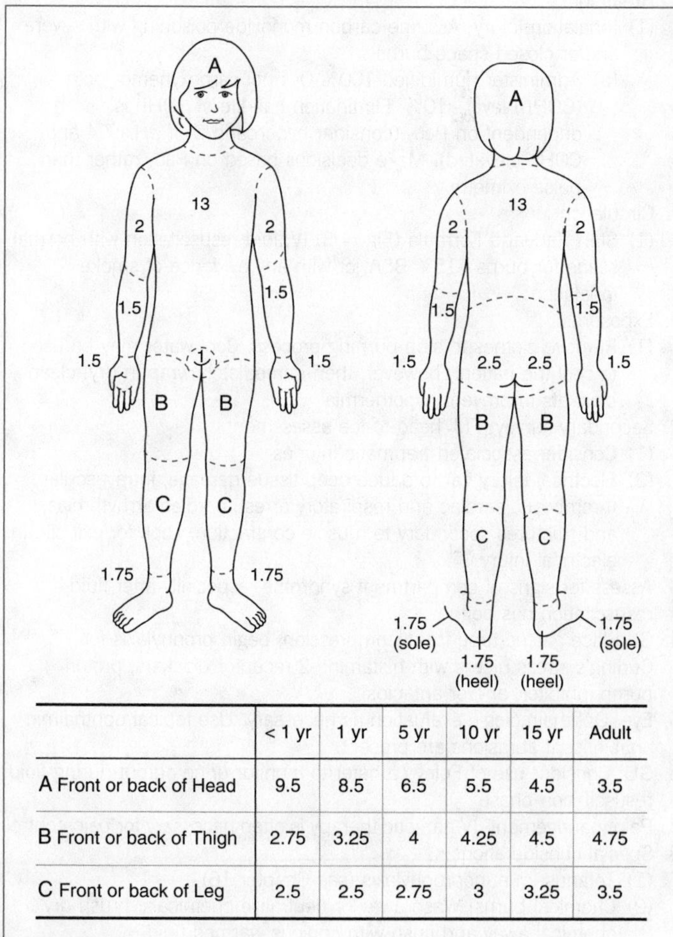

	< 1 yr	1 yr	5 yr	10 yr	15 yr	Adult
A Front or back of Head	9.5	8.5	6.5	5.5	4.5	3.5
B Front or back of Thigh	2.75	3.25	4	4.25	4.5	4.75
C Front or back of Leg	2.5	2.5	2.75	3	3.25	3.5

FIGURE 4-2

Burn assessment chart. All numbers are percentages. *(From Barkin RM, Rosen P: Emergency pediatrics: a guide to ambulatory care, 6th ed. St. Louis, Mosby, 2003.)*

a. Airway with cervical spine stabilization
  (1) Assess airway for signs of inhalation injury or respiratory distress: Soot in nares, carbonaceous sputum, stridor
  (2) Establish definitive airway early: Consider intubation for >20% TBSA burned

NOTE: Avoid late use of succinylcholine, due to increased risk of hyperkalemia (see Chapter 1).

b. Breathing:
  (1) Inhalation injury: Assume carbon monoxide poisoning with severe and/or closed-space burns
    (a) Administer humidified 100% O_2 until carboxyhemoglobin (COHb) level <10%. Elimination half-life of COHb is dependent on Pao_2 (consider hyperbaric O_2 if pH <7.4 and COHb elevated). Make decisions based on Pao_2 rather than pulse oximetry

c. Circulation:
  (1) Start Parkland Formula (Fig. 4-3) IV fluid resuscitation with normal saline for burns >15% BSA, or with any evidence of smoke inhalation

d. Exposure:
  (1) Remove clothes to stop burning process. Cool water may be used to cool the patient, however, then immediately wrap in dry, clean blankets to prevent hypothermia

2. Secondary survey: Full head-to-toe assessment
  (1) Consider associated traumatic injuries
  (2) Electrical injury can produce deep tissue damage, intravascular thrombosis, cardiac and respiratory arrest, cardiac arrhythmias, and fractures secondary to muscle contraction. Look for exit site in electrical injury
3. Assess for signs of compartment syndrome, especially after fluid resuscitation has begun
4. GI: Place gastric tube for decompression; begin prophylaxis for Curling's stress ulcers with histamine-2 receptor blockers, proton pump inhibitor, and/or antacids
5. Eye: Ophthalmologic evaluation as necessary. Use topical ophthalmic antibiotics if abrasions are present
6. GU: Consider use of Foley catheter to monitor urine output during fluid resuscitation phase
7. Pain management: IV narcotic therapy is often necessary for pain control
8. Special considerations:
  (1) Tetanus immunoprophylaxis (see Chapter 16)
  (2) Chemical burns: Wash away or neutralize chemicals: brush dry chemical away and flush with copious warmed fluid

D. Further Management of Pediatric Burns

1. Inpatient management:

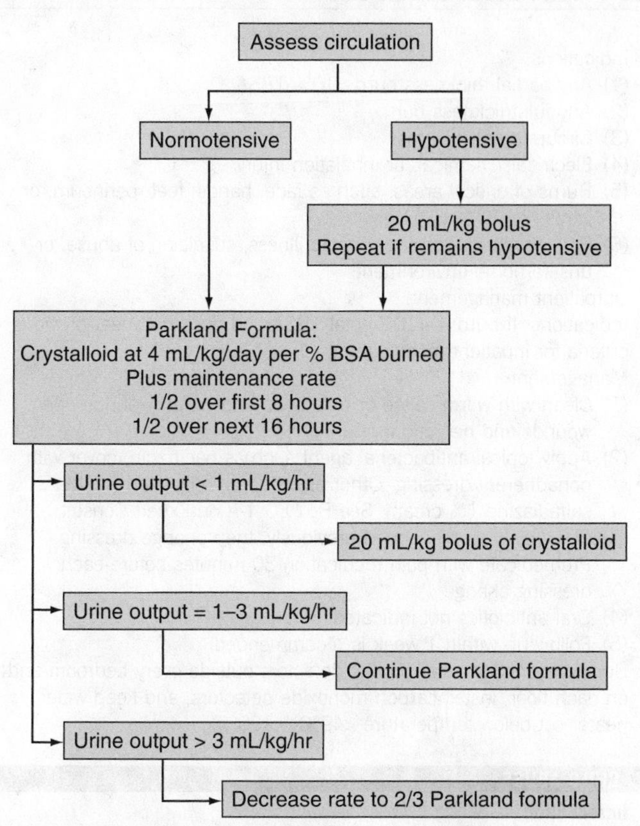

1) Consider central venous access for burns >25% BSA.

2) Use the Parkland formula as a guideline to estimate fluid need. Requirements decrease by 25% to 50% after first 24 hr. Monitor weight, serum electrolytes, urine output, nasogastric losses to determine concentrations and rates.

3) Consider adding colloid after 18–24 hr. (albumin, 1 g/kg/day) to maintain serum albumin >2 g/dL.

4) Withhold potassium generally for the first 48 hr. because of a large release of potassium from damaged tissues. To manage electrolytes most effectively, monitor urine electrolytes twice weekly and replace urine losses accordingly.

FIGURE 4-3

Fluid management of life-threatening burns. *(Modified from Nichols DG, Yaster M, Lappe DG, et al: Golden hour: the handbook of pediatric advanced life support. St. Louis, Mosby, 1996, p. 460.)*

a. Indications:
   (1) Any partial-thickness burn >10% TBSA
   (2) Any full-thickness burn
   (3) Circumferential burns
   (4) Electrical, chemical, or inhalation injury
   (5) Burns of critical areas, such as face, hands, feet, perineum, or joints
   (6) Patient with underlying chronic illness, suspicion of abuse, or unsafe home environment
2. Outpatient management:
a. Indications: If burn is <10% total TBSA and does not meet previous criteria for inpatient management
b. Management:
   (1) Clean with warm saline or mild soap and water. Débride open wounds and necrotic tissue
   (2) Apply topical antibacterial agent such as bacitracin, cover with nonadherent dressing. Other agent commonly used is silver sulfadiazine 1% cream. See Box EC 4-A on Expert Consult
   (3) Clean daily as mentioned previously, then change dressing. Premedicate with pain medication 30 minutes before each dressing change
   (4) Oral antibiotics not indicated
   (5) Follow-up within 1 week is recommended
3. Burn prevention: Install smoke detectors outside every bedroom and on each floor, install carbon monoxide detectors, and keep water heater set below temperature <49°C (<120°F)

V. CHILD ABUSE

A. Introduction

Approach should be multidisciplinary: medical professionals, social worker, and community agencies such as emergency medical service providers, police, social services, and prosecutors.

B. Management[2,8,9]

The medical professional should suspect, diagnose, treat, report, and document all cases of child abuse, neglect, or maltreatment.

1. Suspect: Increase suspicion if there is inappropriate parental response, delay in seeking medical attention, inadequate history of injury, a mechanism inconsistent with physical findings, evidence of neglect or failure to thrive, evidence of disturbed emotions or expressions in a child, prior history of suspicious events, or parental substance abuse
2. Diagnose: Concerning injuries. Attempt to correlate all physical findings with history, photodocument if possible. See Chapter 4 Plates 1–6.
a. Bruises: Shape of bruises is important. Be suspicious of bruises in protected areas (chest, abdomen, back, buttocks)

TABLE 4-6

SKELETAL INJURY IN NONACCIDENTAL TRAUMA

Skeletal injury	Correlate mechanism of injury with physical finding; rule out any underlying bony pathology.
Long bones	Classic fracture is the epiphyseal/metaphyseal fracture, seen as a "bucket handle" or "corner" fracture at the end of long bones, secondary to jerking/shaking of a child's limb. Spiral fractures may be suspicious of abuse, but can be seen with rotational forces, such as the "toddler's fracture" of the tibia.
Ribs	Posterior nondisplaced rib fractures are usually due to severe squeezing of the rib cage. May not be visible on plain film until callus formation. Chest compressions from cardiopulmonary resuscitation do not appear to cause rib fractures in children.
Skull	Fractures >3 mm wide, complex fractures, bilateral fractures, and nonparietal fractures suggest forces greater than those sustained from minor household trauma.

b. Bites: Shape, size, and location are important. Inter-canine distance of >3 cm are suggestive of human bites, which generally crush more than lacerate
c. Burns: Absence of splash marks, well-demarcated edges, stocking glove patterns, symmetrically burned buttocks and/or lower legs, spared inguinal creases, and symmetrical involvement of palms or soles are all suggestive of nonaccidental injury
d. Bleeding:
   (1) Retinal hemorrhages are virtually pathognomonic of abusive head trauma (AHT)/shaken-baby syndrome
   (2) Duodenal hematomas are suspicious for nonaccidental blunt trauma; may lead to upper GI obstruction
e. Fractures: certain fracture types are suspicious for non-accidental trauma (see Table 4-6)
f. Abusive Head Trauma (AHT)/Shaken-baby syndrome: Findings may include: retinal hemorrhages, subdural hematomas, long bone or rib fractures, and central nervous system (CNS) dysfunction such as seizure, apnea, or lethargy secondary to intracranial injury
g. Sexual abuse:
   (1) If abuse is suspected to have occurred within 72 hours, defer interview and GU exam to multidisciplinary team with expertise in evaluation of sexual abuse if available. Avoid collection of lab specimens without input from this team
   (2) Genital examination should be performed by trained forensic specialist due to anatomic variability (especially of hymen)
   (3) Normal genital exam does not rule out abuse
   (4) Document vaginal bleeding in the prepubertal female: Injury to external genitalia (especially the posterior region), bruising, or discharge can be suspicious for abuse

(5) Evaluate anus for bruising, laceration, hemorrhoids, scars that extend beyond the anal verge, absence of anal wink, or evidence of infection, such as genital warts. Circumferential hematoma of the anal sphincter is associated with forced penetration

3. Useful studies:
a. Skeletal survey is suggested to evaluate suspicious bony trauma in any child; these studies are mandatory for children <2 years of age (see Chapter 25 for components)
b. Bone scan may be indicated to identify early or difficult to detect fractures
c. Noncontrast head CT scan is useful for visualizing intracranial hemorrhage, but unreliable for detection of skull fractures
d. Magnetic resonance imaging (MRI) may identify lesions not detected by CT scan (e.g., posterior fossa injury and diffuse axonal injury)
e. Dilated, indirect ophthalmoscopy by an ophthalmologist is important for accurate detection of retinal hemorrhages in suspected AHT/ shaken-baby syndrome.
4. Treat: Medical stabilization is primary goal. Prevention of further injuries is the long-term goal
5. Report: All health care providers are required by law to report suspected child maltreatment to the local police and/or child welfare agency. Suspicion, supported by objective evidence, is criterion for reporting and should first be discussed with not only the entire medical team but also the family. The professional who makes such reports is immune from any civil or criminal liability
6. Document: Write legibly, carefully documenting the following: reported and suspected history and mechanisms of injury; any history given by the victim in his or her own words (use quotation marks); information provided by other providers or services; and physical examination findings, including drawings of injuries and details of dimensions, color, shape, and texture. Always consider early use of police crime laboratory photography to document injuries

VI. COMMON CRITICAL CARE EMERGENCIES

A. Acute Hypertension[10]

1. Assessment:
a. Use appropriate cuff size for blood pressure (BP) measurement. Correlate with BP tables for age, height, and weight (Table 7-1, 7-2, Figure 7-3, 7-4)
b. Hypertensive *urgency:* Significant elevation in BP *without* accompanying end-organ damage; more common in children. Symptoms include headache, blurred vision, and nausea
c. Hypertensive *emergency:* Elevation of both systolic and diastolic BP *with* acute end-organ damage (e.g., cerebral infarction or hemorrhage, pulmonary edema, renal failure, hypertensive encephalopathy, or seizures)

d. Possible etiologies: Cardiovascular, renovascular, renal parenchymal, endocrine, CNS, medication or ingestion

NOTE: Rule out hypertension secondary to elevated ICP before lowering BP.

e. Physical examination: Four-extremity BP, funduscopy (papilledema, hemorrhage, exudate), visual acuity, thyroid examination, evidence for congestive heart failure (tachycardia, gallop rhythm, hepatomegaly, edema), abdominal examination (mass, bruit), thorough neurologic examination, evidence of virilization, cushingoid effect
f. Initial diagnostic evaluation: Urinalysis, blood urea nitrogen, creatinine, electrolytes, chest radiograph, and electrocardiogram
g. Consider renin level, toxicology screen, thyroid and adrenal testing, urine catecholamines, abdominal ultrasound, renal Doppler ultrasound, head CT

2. Management:

a. Hypertensive emergency:
   (1) Goal: Lower BP promptly but gradually to preserve cerebral autoregulation (Table 4-7)
      (a) Mean arterial pressure (MAP) = 1/3 systolic + 2/3 diastolic BP
      (b) Lower by 1/3 of planned MAP reduction over first 6 hours, then
      (c) Lower by additional 1/3 over next 24–36 hours, then
      (d) Lower final 1/3 over next 48 hours

TABLE 4-7

MEDICATIONS FOR HYPERTENSIVE EMERGENCY*

Drug	Onset (Route)	Duration	Interval to Repeat/ ↑ Dose	Comments
Diazoxide (arteriole vasodilator)	1–5 min (IV)	Variable (2–12 hr)	15–30 min	May cause edema, hyperglycemia
Hydralazine (arteriole vasodilator)	5–20 min (IV)	2–6 hr	4–6 hr	May cause reflex tachycardia, prolonged hypotension, nausea
INFUSIONS				
Nitroprusside (arteriole and venous vasodilator)	<30 sec (IV)	Very short	30–60 min	Requires ICU setting; follow thiocyanate level
Labetalol (α-, β-blocker)	1–5 min (IV)	Variable (~6 hr)	10 min	May require ICU setting
Nicardipine (calcium channel blocker)	1 min (IV)	3 hr	15 min	May cause edema, headache, nausea, vomiting

*See Formulary for dosing.

ICU, Intensive care unit.

TABLE 4-8

MEDICATIONS FOR HYPERTENSIVE URGENCY*

Drug	Onset (Route)	Duration	Interval to Repeat	Comments
Enalapril	15 min (IV)	12–24 hr	8–24 hr	May cause hyperkalemia, hypoglycemia
Minoxidil	30 min (PO)	2–5 days	4–8 hr	Contraindicated in pheochromocytoma

*See Formulary for dosing.
PO, Per os.

(2) Consult nephrologist and/or cardiologist
(3) After elevated ICP is ruled out, do not delay treatment because of further diagnostic workup

b. Hypertensive urgency:
(1) Goal: To lower MAP by 20% over 1 hour and return to baseline levels over 24 to 48 hours (Table 4-8)
(2) An oral route may be adequate. (Use of sublingual nifedipine is not recommended, as a precipitous, uncontrolled fall in BP may result.)

B. Increased Intracranial Pressure (ICP)[11,12]

See Chapter 20 for evaluation and management of hydrocephalus

1. Assessment:

a. History: Obtain history regarding trauma, vomiting, fever, headache, neck pain, unsteadiness, seizure, vision change, gaze preference, and change in mental status. In infants, look for irritability, vomiting, poor feeding, lethargy, and bulging fontanel

b. Physical examination:
(1) Evaluate vital signs for Cushing's triad (hypertension, bradycardia, irregular respiratory pattern)
(2) Thorough neurologic examination: Attention to photophobia, pupillary response, papilledema, cranial nerve dysfunction (especially paralysis of upward gaze or abduction), neck stiffness, neurologic deficit, abnormal posturing, altered mental status, or evidence of trauma

c. Laboratory studies: CBC, electrolytes, glucose, toxicology screen, blood culture. Lumbar puncture (LP) contraindicated due to herniation risk

2. Management: Elevate head of bed 30 degrees. Obtain emergent neurosurgical consult and head CT. Do not lower BP if elevated ICP is suspected. Immobilize c-spine if trauma is suspected

a. Stable patient (responsive, stable vital signs, no focal findings): Apply cardiorespiratory monitor

b. Unstable patient:
(1) Give normal saline or hyperosmolar solutions for maintenance fluids

(2) Give 3% NaCl, 2–5 mL/kg, or mannitol, 0.25 g/kg IV, for temporary reduction of ICP. May increase mannitol gradually to 1 g/kg/dose if needed, although high-dose mannitol can produce significant hypotension from osmotic diuresis

(3) Reserve hyperventilation for acute management; keep P_{CO_2} at 30 to 35 mmHg. Provide controlled neuroprotective intubation, as outlined in Table 1-1

(4) In traumatic brain injury, consider controlled hypothermia

c. Do not delay antibiotics if meningitis suspected

d. In space-occupying lesions (tumors, abscesses), consider dexamethasone to reduce cerebral edema in consultation with a neurosurgeon

e. Consider epinephrine or phenylephrine infusion to maintain and keep systemic pressure above ICP

Cerebral perfusion pressure (CPP) = MAP − ICP

f. Prevent hyperthermia: Goal is body temperature <37.5°C

g. Avoid hypotension, hypoxia, hypercarbia, and hypovolemia

C. Shock[13]

1. Definition: Physiologic state characterized by inadequate oxygen and nutrient delivery to meet tissue demands

a. Compensated shock: Body maintains perfusion to vital organs; may be hard to detect; tachycardia may be present

b. Decompensated shock: Poor perfusion, tachycardia, hypotension

c. See Table 4-9 for categorization

2. Causes (See Table 4-10):

a. Hypovolemic shock

b. Distributive shock: Including septic, anaphylactic, and neurogenic shock

c. Cardiogenic shock

d. Obstructive shock: Including cardiac tamponade, tension pneumothorax, massive pulmonary embolism

3. Management (See Table 4-10)

D. Respiratory Failure[13]

1. Definition: Failure of the lungs to exchange oxygen and/or carbon dioxide

2. Causes:

a. Neurologic: Muscle weakness, altered sensorium

b. Obstruction: Foreign body, inflammation

c. Parenchymal disease: Pneumonia, pulmonary edema, acute respiratory distress syndrome (ARDS), asthma

d. Mechanical: Abnormal chest wall, trauma

3. Management:

a. Noninvasive positive-pressure ventilation

TABLE 4-9

CATEGORIZATION OF HEMORRHAGE AND SHOCK IN PEDIATRIC TRAUMA PATIENTS

System	Compensated Shock, Mild Hemorrhage, Simple Hypovolemia (<30% blood volume loss)	Decompensated Shock, Moderate Hemorrhage, Marked Hypovolemia (30%–45% blood volume loss)	Cardiopulmonary Failure, Severe Hemorrhage, Profound Hypovolemia (>45% blood volume loss)
Cardiovascular	Mild tachycardia	Moderate tachycardia	Severe tachycardia
	Weak peripheral pulses	Thready peripheral pulses	Absent peripheral pulses
	Strong central pulses	Weak central pulses	Thready central pulses
	Low-normal blood pressure (SBP >70 mmHg + [2× age in years])	Frank hypotension (SBP <70 mmHg + [2× age in years])	Profound hypotension (SBP <50 mmHg)
	Mild acidosis	Moderate acidosis	Severe acidosis
Respiratory	Mild tachypnea	Moderate tachypnea	Severe tachypnea
Neurologic	Irritable, confused	Agitated, lethargic	Obtunded, comatose
Integumentary	Cool extremities, mottling	Cool extremities, pallor	Cold extremities, cyanosis
	Poor capillary refill (>2 sec)	Delayed capillary refill (>3 sec)	Prolonged capillary refill (>5 sec)
Excretory	Mild oliguria, increased specific gravity	Marked oliguria, increased blood urea nitrogen	Anuria

SBP, Systolic blood pressure.
Adapted from Advanced Trauma Life Support Course. Chicago, American College of Surgeons.

b. Intubation and mechanical ventilation (see Chapter 1 for discussion of intubation)
4. Types of ventilatory support:
a. Volume limited:
   (1) Delivers a preset tidal volume to a patient regardless of pressure required
   (2) Risk for barotrauma reduced by pressure alarms and pressure pop-off valves that limit peak inspiratory pressure (PIP)
b. Pressure limited:
   (1) Gas flow is delivered to the patient until a preset pressure is reached and then held for the set inspiratory time (reduces the risk for barotrauma)
   (2) Useful for neonatal and infant ventilatory support (<10 kg), in which the volume of gas being delivered is small in relation to the volume of compressible air in the ventilator circuit, which makes reliable delivery of a set tidal volume difficult

TABLE 4-10

TYPES OF SHOCK, PHYSIOLOGIC RESPONSE, AND BASIC TREATMENT

Type of Shock	HR	Preload	Contractility	SVR	Treatment
Hypovolemic	↑	↓↓	+/–	↑	• High flow oxygen • Fluid resuscitation: evaluate perfusion after 60 mL/kg total volume bolused, then consider pressors
Septic (early, warm)	↑	↓↓	+/–	↓	• High flow oxygen • Fluid resuscitation • Antibiotics • Pressors (dopamine, norepinephrine, phenylephrine)
Septic (late, cold)	↑	↓↓	↓	↑	• High flow oxygen • Fluid resuscitation • Antibiotics • Pressors (dopamine, epinephrine, phenylephrine)
Anaphylactic	↑	↓↓	↓	↓	• High flow oxygen • Epinephrine (IM) • Fluid resuscitation
Neurogenic	↑	↓↓	+/–	↓↓	• Fluid resuscitation • Pressors (norepinephrine)
Cardiogenic	↑	↑	↓↓	↑	• High flow oxygen • Fluid resuscitation (5–10 mL/kg) • CHF management (CPAP/BiPAP, diuretics, ACE inhibitors) • Inotropes (milrinone, dobutamine)
Obstructive	Cause dependent	Cause dependent	Cause dependent	Cause dependent	• Therapy directed at primary etiology of shock

ACE, Angiotensin-converting enzyme; BiPAP, bilevel positive airway pressure; CHF, congestive heart failure; CPAP, continuous positive airway pressure; HR, heart rate; IM, intramuscular; SVR, systemic vascular resistance.

4

c. High-frequency ventilation[14]:
   (1) High-frequency oscillatory ventilation (HFOV):
      (a) High-amplitude and high-frequency pressure waveform generated in the ventilator circuit. Tidal volumes are less than dead space. Bias gas flow provides fresh gas at ventilator and maintains airway pressure
      (b) Minimizes barotrauma and oxygen toxicities
      (c) Patient must be euvolemic secondary to risk for decreased venous return
   (2) High-frequency jet ventilation:
      (a) Used simultaneously with a conventional ventilator
      (b) A jet injector port delivers short bursts of inspiratory gas
      (c) Adequate gas exchange can be achieved at low airway pressures, providing maintenance of lung volume and minimal risk for barotrauma
5. Ventilator parameters:
a. PIP: Peak pressure attained during the respiratory cycle
b. Positive end-expiratory pressure (PEEP): Airway pressure maintained between inspiratory and expiratory phases; prevents alveolar collapse during expiration, decreases work of reinflation, and improves gas exchange
c. Rate (intermittent mandatory ventilation) or frequency (Hz): Number of mechanical breaths delivered per minute or rate of oscillations in HFOV
d. Inspired oxygen concentration (Fio_2): Fraction of oxygen present in inspired gas
e. Inspiratory time (Ti): Length of time spent in the inspiratory phase of the respiratory cycle
f. Tidal volume (V_T): Volume of gas delivered during inspiration
g. Power (ΔP): Amplitude of the pressure waveform in HFOV
h. Mean airway pressure ($\overline{PAW}$): Average pressure over entire respiratory cycle
6. Modes of operation:
a. Intermittent mandatory ventilation (IMV): A preset number of breaths are delivered each minute. The patient can take breaths on his or her own, but the ventilator may cycle on during a patient breath
b. Synchronized IMV (SIMV): Similar to IMV, but the ventilator synchronizes delivered breaths with inspiratory effort and allows the patient to finish expiration before cycling on. More comfortable for patient than IMV
c. Assist control ventilation (AC): Every inspiratory effort by the patient triggers a ventilator-delivered breath at the set V_T. Ventilator-initiated breaths are delivered when the spontaneous rate falls below the backup rate
d. Pressure support ventilation (PSV): Inspiratory effort opens a valve, allowing airflow at a preset positive pressure. Patient determines rate

and inspiratory time. May be used in combination with other modes of operation. Determine effectiveness of ventilation by monitoring tidal volumes

e. Noninvasive positive-pressure ventilation (NIPPV): Respiratory support provided through face mask
   (1) Continuous positive airway pressure (CPAP): Delivers airflow (with set FiO_2) to maintain a set airway pressure
   (2) Bilevel positive airway pressure (BiPAP): Delivers airflow to maintain set pressures for inspiration and expiration

7. Initial ventilator settings:

a. Volume limited:
   (1) Rate: Approximately normal range for age (see Table 24-1)
   (2) V_T: Approximately 8–10 mL/kg
   (3) Ti: Generally use inspiration-to-expiration (I/E) ratio of 1:2. More prolonged expiratory phases are required for obstructive diseases to avoid air trapping
   (4) FiO_2: Selected to maintain targeted oxygen saturation and PaO_2

b. Pressure limited:
   (1) Rate: Approximately normal range for age (see Table 24-1)
   (2) PEEP: Start with 3–5 cm H_2O and increase as clinically indicated. Monitor for decreases in cardiac output with increasing PEEP
   (3) PIP: Set at pressure required to produce adequate chest wall movement (approximate this using hand-bagging and manometer)
   (4) FiO_2: Selected to maintain targeted oxygen saturation and PaO_2

c. HFOV:
   (1) Frequency: 10–15 Hz for neonates, 5–8 Hz for children
   (2) Power: Select to achieve adequate chest wall movement
   (3) MAP: 1–4 cm H_2O higher than settings on a conventional ventilator
   (4) FiO_2: Selected to maintain targeted oxygen saturation and PaO_2

d. High-frequency jet ventilator:
   (1) PIP: Increase 2 cm H_2O over conventional ventilator setting
   (2) Ti: Set at 0.02 sec
   (3) Frequency: In neonates, set at 420 cycles/sec

8. Further ventilator management:

a. Follow patient closely with pulse oximetry, end-tidal carbon dioxide measurements, and clinical assessment. Confirm findings with ABGs, and adjust ventilator parameters as indicated (Table 4-11)

b. In cases of ARDS or other condition of poor compliance or air leaks, permissive hypercapnia, and V_T of 5 mL/kg should be used to avoid barotrauma

c. Parameters for initiating high-frequency ventilation:
   (1) Oxygenation index (OI) >40 (See Section VI.G for calculation of OI)
   (2) Inability to provide adequate oxygenation or ventilation with conventional ventilator

TABLE 4-11

EFFECTS OF VENTILATOR SETTING CHANGES

Ventilator Setting Changes	Typical Effects on Blood Gases	
	$Paco_2$	**Pao_2**
↑PIP	↓	↑
↑PEEP	↑	↑
↑Rate (IMV)	↓	Minimal ↑
↑I:E ratio	No change	↑
↑Fio_2	No change	↑
↑Flow	Minimal ↓	Minimal ↑
↑Power (in HFOV)	↓	No change
↑$\overline{PAW}$ (in HFOV)	Minimal ↓	↑

Fio_2, fraction of inspired oxygen; HFOV, high-frequency oscillatory ventilation; I:E, inspiratory/expiratory ratio; IMV, intermittent mechanical ventilation; $\overline{PAW}$, mean airway pressure; PEEP, positive end-expiratory pressure; PIP, peak inspiratory pressure.

d. Parameters predictive of successful extubation:
  (1) $Paco_2$ appropriate for patient
  (2) PIP generally 14–16 cm H_2O
  (3) PEEP 2–3 cm H_2O (infants) or 5 cm H_2O (children)
  (4) IMV 2–4 breaths/min (infants); children may wean to CPAP or pressure support
  (5) Fio_2 <40% (maintaining Pao_2 >70)
  (6) Adequate air leak around endotracheal tube in cases of airway edema or stenosis.
  (7) Maximum negative inspiratory pressure (NIF) >20–25 cm H_2O
  (8) Minimal secretions

E. Status Epilepticus (See Chapter 1)

F. Status Asthmaticus (See Chapter 1)

G. Critical Care Reference Data

1. **Minute ventilation (V_E):**

$$V_E = \text{Respiratory rate} \times \text{tidal volume } (V_T)$$

a. $V_E \times Paco_2$ = constant (for volume-limited ventilation)
b. Normal V_T = 10–15 mL/kg

2. **Alveolar gas equation:**

$$P_{AO_2} = Pio_2 - (P_{ACO_2}/R)$$
$$Pio_2 = Fio_2 \times (P_B - 47 \text{ mmHg})$$

a. Pio_2 = Partial pressure of inspired O_2 minus 150 mmHg at sea level on room air
b. R = Respiratory exchange quotient (CO_2 produced/O_2 consumed) = 0.8
c. P_{ACO_2} = Partial pressure of alveolar CO_2 minus partial pressure of arterial CO_2 ($Paco_2$)
d. P_B = Atmospheric pressure = 760 mmHg at sea level. Adjust for high-altitude environment

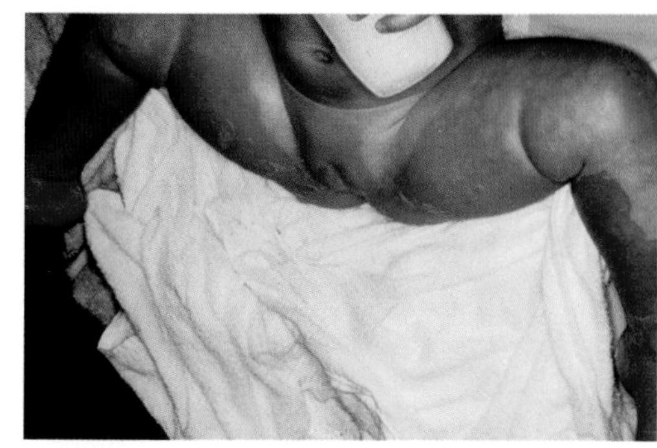

PLATE 1
Infant that has been burned when immersed in hot water, lower extremities and buttocks. *(From Zitelli B, Davis H: Atlas of pediatric physical diagnosis, 5th ed. St. Louis, Mosby, 2008.)*

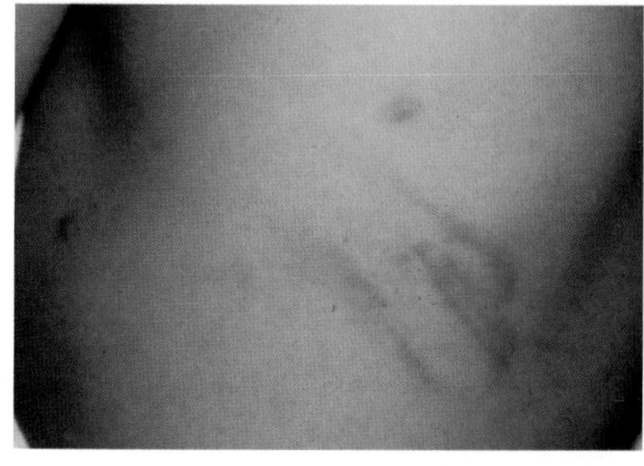

PLATE 2
Child who has been beaten with a looped cord. *(From Zitelli B, Davis H: Atlas of pediatric physical diagnosis, 5th ed. St. Louis, Mosby, 2008.)*

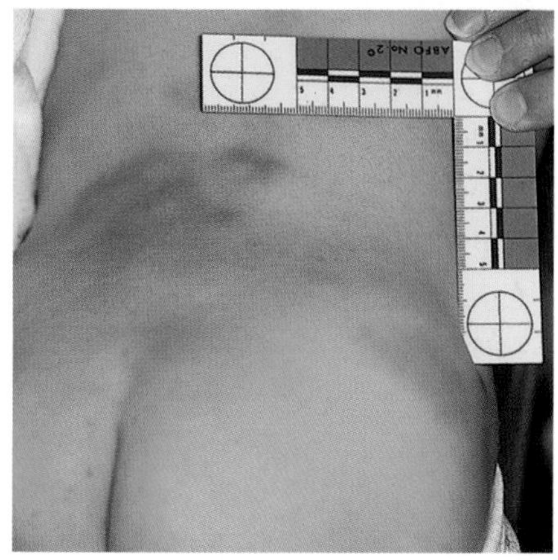

PLATE 3
Child with suspicious bruising on lower back. *(From Zitelli B, Davis H: Atlas of pediatric physical diagnosis, 5th ed. St. Louis, Mosby, 2008.)*

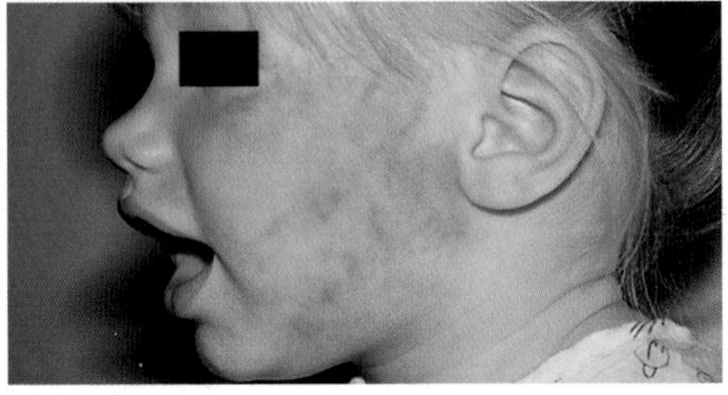

PLATE 4
Toddler slapped in the face with linear hand marks visible. *(From Zitelli B, Davis H: Atlas of pediatric physical diagnosis, 5th ed. St. Louis, Mosby, 2008.)*

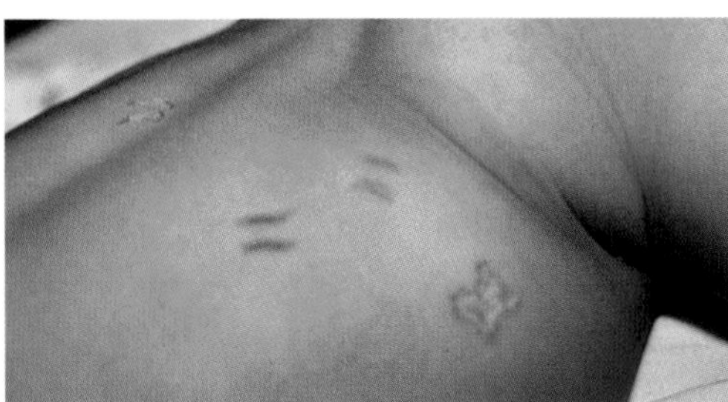

PLATE 5
Skin burned with hot cigarette lighter. *(From Zitelli B, Davis H: Atlas of pediatric physical diagnosis, 5th ed. St. Louis, Mosby, 2008.)*

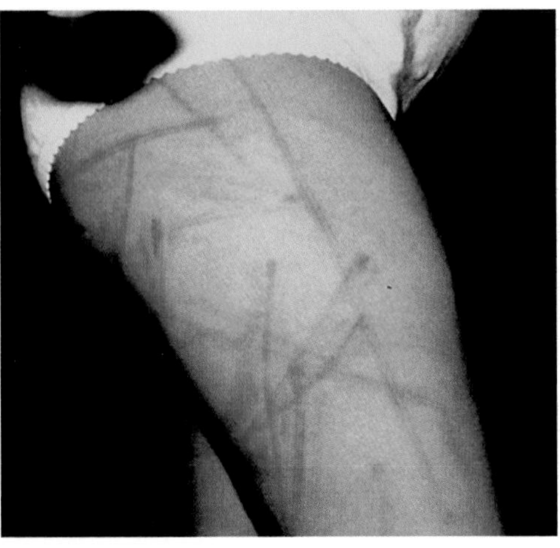

PLATE 6
Child beaten with a switch. *(From Zitelli B, Davis H: Atlas of pediatric physical diagnosis, 5th ed. St. Louis, Mosby, 2008.)*

e. Water vapor pressure = 47 mmHg
f. P_{AO_2} = Partial pressure of O_2 in the alveoli

3. **Alveolar-arterial oxygen gradient (A-a gradient):**

$$\text{A-a gradient} = P_{AO_2} - Pa_{O_2}$$

a. Obtain ABG, measuring P_{AO_2} and P_{ACO_2} with patient on 100% Fi_{O_2} for at least 15 min
b. Calculate the P_{AO_2} and then the A-a gradient
c. The larger the gradient, the more serious the respiratory compromise. A normal gradient is 20–65 mmHg on 100% O_2 or 5–20 mmHg on room air

4. **Oxygenation Index (OI):**

$$OI = \frac{\text{mean airway pressure (cm } H_2O) \times FiO_2 \times 100}{Pa_{O_2}}$$

OI >35 for 5 to 6 hours is one criterion for ECMO (extracorporeal membrane oxygen) support.

See more Critical Care Reference Data on Expert Consult, Chapter 4.

REFERENCES

1. Marx J, Hockberger R, Walls R. *Rosen's emergency medicine: concepts and clinical practice.* 7th ed. St. Louis: Mosby; 2009.
2. Fleisher GR, Ludwig S, eds. *Textbook of pediatric emergency medicine.* 5th ed. Philadelphia: Lippincott Williams & Wilkins; 2006.
3. Kirkwood MW, Yeates KO, Wilson PE. Pediatric sport-related concussion: a review of the clinical management of an oft-neglected population. *Pediatrics.* 2006;117:1359–1371.
4. Sanchez J, Paidas C. Childhood trauma: now and in the new millennium. *Surg Clin North Am.* 1999;79(6):1503–1535.
5. Green NE. *Skeletal trauma in children.* 3rd ed. Philadelphia: WB Saunders; 2003.
6. Canale ST. *Campbell's operative orthopedics.* 10th ed. St. Louis: Mosby; 2003.
7. Barkin RM, Rosen P. *Emergency pediatrics: a guide to ambulatory care.* 6th ed. St. Louis: Mosby; 2003.
8. Kellogg N. The evaluation of sexual abuse in children. *Pediatrics.* 2005;116(2): 506–512.
9. Sato Y. Imaging of nonaccidental head injury. *Pediatr Radiol.* 2009;39(Suppl 2): S230–S235.
10. Offiah A, van Rijn RR, Perez-Rossello JM, et al. Skeletal imaging of child abuse (non-accidental injury). *Pediatr Radiol.* 2009;39(5):461–470.
11. Nichols DG, Yaster M, Lappe DG, et al. *Golden hour: the handbook of advanced pediatric life support.* 2nd ed. St. Louis: Mosby; 1996.
12. Walker PA, Harting MT, Baumgartner JE, et al. Modern approaches to pediatric brain injury therapy. *J Trauma.* 2009;67(2 Suppl):S120–S712.
13. Rogers M. *Textbook of Pediatric Intensive Care.* 4th ed. Baltimore: Williams & Wilkins; 2008.
14. Mesiano G, Davis GM. Ventilatory strategies in the neonatal and paediatric intensive care units. *Paediatr Respir Rev.* 2008;9(4):281–288.

PART II

DIAGNOSTIC AND THERAPEUTIC INFORMATION

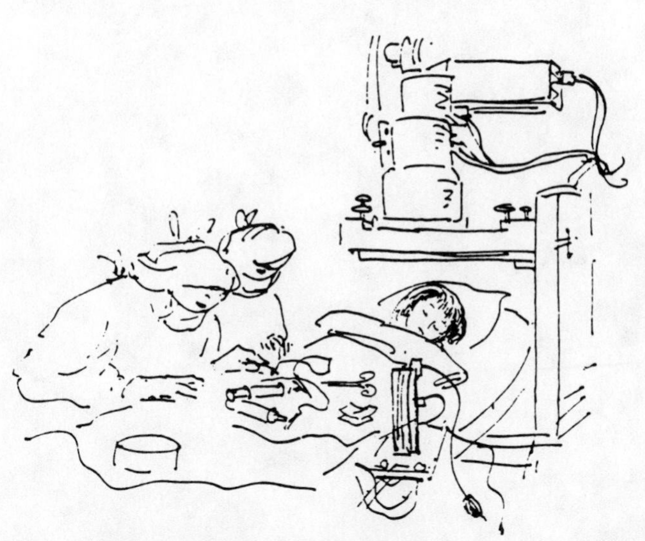

Chapter 5

Adolescent Medicine

Nicole Brown, MD, MPH

5

See additional content on Expert Consult

I. WEBSITES

Sexual health: http://www.ashastd.org
Drug abuse: http://teens.drugabuse.gov
Adolescent development: http://www.aacap.org
http://www.aap.org/sections/adolescenthealth
www.guttmacher.org/sections/adolescents.php

II. INTRODUCTION TO ADOLESCENT HEALTH

A. Pubertal Development[1–5]

1. **Pubic hair** (for males and females); see Box 5-1
2. **Female breast development** (Fig. 5-1)
3. **Male genital development** (Table 5-1). Also see Chapter 10 for testicular volumes
4. **Gynecomastia in males**
   a. Generally occurs in middle–late stages of puberty
   b. Etiology: Breast growth stimulated by estradiol
   c. Prevalence: Occurs in 50% of boys (50% unilateral, 50% bilateral)
   d. Clinical course: Regression usually occurs over 2-year period
   e. Treatment: Often no treatment necessary. Severe or nonregressing cases may warrant referral to surgeon
5. **Precocious puberty:** The onset of secondary sexual characteristics before age 8 years in girls and 9 years in boys
6. **Delayed puberty:** The lack of secondary sexual development by age 14 years (See Chapter 10 for more information)

B. Psychosocial Development (Table 5-2)

C. Psychosocial and Medicosocial History (Table 5-2)[6,7]

HEADSS[3,4,6]: Brief instrument that screens for psychosocial factors that impact adolescent mental and physical health

1. **Home:** Household composition, family dynamics and relationships, living and sleeping arrangements, guns in the home, recent changes
2. **Education/Eating:** School attendance, suspensions, grade failure; grades as compared with previous years; attitude toward school; favorite, most difficult, best subjects; special educational needs; goals for the future (See Section III B—ROS for Eating/Nutrition questions)

BOX 5-1

PUBIC HAIR TANNER STAGING

Tanner Stage	Appearance
1	No hair
2	Sparse, downy hair at base of symphysis pubis
3	Sparse, coarse hair across symphysis pubis
4	Adult hair quality, fills in pubic triangle, no spread to thighs
5	Adult quality and distribution including spread to medial thighs

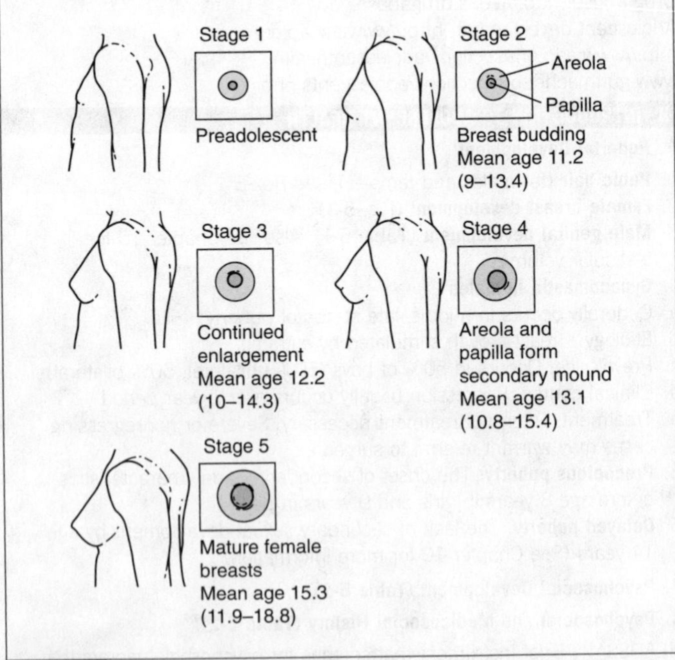

FIGURE 5-1

Tanner stages of breast development in females. *(Modified from Johnson TR et al: Children are different: developmental physiology, 2nd ed. Columbus, Ohio, Ross Laboratories, 1978. Mean age and range [2 standard deviations around mean] from Joffe A: Introduction to adolescent medicine. In McMillan JA et al [eds]: Oski's pediatrics: principles and practice, 4th ed. Philadelphia, Lippincott Williams & Wilkins, 2006, pp. 549–550.)*

TABLE 5-1

GENITAL DEVELOPMENT (MALE)

Stage	Comment (±2 standard deviation around mean age)
1	Prepubertal
2	Enlargement of scrotum and testes; skin of scrotum reddens and changes in texture; little or no enlargement of penis; mean age 11.4 yr (9.5–13.8 yr)
3	Enlargement of penis, first mainly in length; further growth of testes and scrotum; mean age 12.9 yr (10.8–14.9 yr)
4	Increased size of penis with growth in breadth and development of glans; further enlargement of testes and scrotum and increased darkening of scrotal skin; mean age 13.77 yr (11.7–15.8 yr)
5	Genitalia adult in size and shape; mean age 14.9 yr (13–17.3 yr)

Data from Joffe A: Introduction to adolescent medicine. In McMillan JA, DeAngelis CD, Feigan RD, et al (eds): Oski's pediatrics: principles and practice, 4th ed. Philadelphia, Lippincott Williams & Wilkins, 2006, pp 546–557.

TABLE 5-2

PSYCHOSOCIAL DEVELOPMENT OF ADOLESCENTS

Task	Early Adolescence (10–13 yr)	Middle Adolescence (14–16 yr)	Late Adolescence (>17 yr)
Independence	Less interest in parental activities Wide mood swings	Peak of parental conflicts	Reacceptance of parental advice and values
Body image	Preoccupation with self and pubertal changes Uncertainty about appearance	General acceptance of body Concern over making body more attractive	Acceptance of pubertal changes
Peers	Intense relationships with same-sex friend	Peak of peer involvement Conformity with peer values Increased sexual activity and experimentation	Peer group less important More time spent in sharing intimate relationships
Identity	Increased cognition Increased fantasy world Idealistic vocational goals Increased need for privacy Lack of impulse control	Increased scope of feelings Increased intellectual ability Feeling of omnipotence Risk-taking behavior	Practical, realistic vocational goals Refinement of moral, religious, and sexual values Ability to compromise and to set limits

Joffe A: Introduction to Adolescent Medicine. In McMillan JA, DeAngelis CD, Feigan RD, Warshaw J (eds): Oski's pediatrics principles and practice, 4th ed. Philadelphia, Lippincott Williams, & Wilkins, 2006.

3. **Activities:** Friendships with same or opposite sex, ages of friends, best friend, dating, recreational activities, physical activity, sports participation, hobbies and interests, job, weapon carrying, fighting
4. **Drugs:** Personal use of tobacco, alcohol, illicit drugs, anabolic steroids; peer substance use; family substance use and attitudes. If personal use, determine if ever used, frequency, quantity, binge, injury with use and administer **CAGE** questionnaire:

C—Have you ever felt the need to **C**UT down?
A—Have others **A**NNOYED you by commenting on your use?
G—Have you ever felt **G**UILTY about your use or about something you said or did while using?
E—Have you ever needed an **E**YE-OPENER (alcohol/drug use first thing in the morning or before noon)?

NOTE: Any affirmative answer on **CAGE** indicates high risk for alcoholism or dependence and requires further assessment

Also helpful in this age group is the **CRAFFT** questionnaire:

C—Have you ever ridden in a **C**AR driven by someone (or yourself) who was "high" or had been using alcohol or drugs?
R—Do you ever use alcohol or drugs to **R**ELAX, feel better about yourself, or fit in?
A—Do you ever use alcohol/drugs while you are **A**LONE?
F—Do your family or **F**RIENDS ever tell you that you should cut down on your drinking or drug use?
F—Do you ever **F**ORGET things you did while using alcohol or drugs?
T—Have you gotten into **T**ROUBLE while you were using alcohol or drugs?

NOTE: Two or more affirmative answers suggest a significant problem

5. **Sexuality:** Sexual feelings toward opposite or same sex; sexual behavior (i.e. vaginal/oral/anal sex)—age at first sex, number of lifetime and current partners, ages of partners, recent change in partners; use of condoms, hormonal contraception, dual contraception, knowledge of emergency contraception and sexually transmitted infection (STI/HIV) prevention; history of STI/HIV or testing for STI/HIV, prior pregnancies, abortions; ever fathered a child; history of nonconsensual intimate physical contact or sex; ever exchange sex for money or drugs
6. **Suicide/depression:** Feelings about self, both positive and negative; history of depression or other mental health problems; sleep problems: difficulty getting to sleep, early waking; changes in appetite or weight; anhedonia; irritability; anxiety; current or prior suicidal thoughts; prior suicide attempts

III. ADOLESCENT HEALTH MAINTENANCE

Bright Futures Guidelines for Health Supervision of Adolescents[8]
(See Box EC 5-A on Expert Consult)

A. Chief Complaint

Hidden agenda: Adolescents may present with chief complaints that are not the true concern for the visit. Gentle but persistent questioning ("Is there anything else?") often leads to the actual reason for the visit.

B. Review of Systems (Areas of Emphasis with an Adolescent)

1. Nutrition: Dietary habits, including skipped meals, special diets, purging methods, recent weight gain or loss
2. Skin: Acne, moles, rashes, warts
3. Genitourinary: Dysuria, urgency, frequency, discharge, bleeding
4. Menstrual: Menarche, frequency, duration, pain, menometrorrhagia

C. Family History[3,4]

Including psychiatric disorders, suicide, alcoholism or substance abuse, and chronic medical conditions or familial risk factors (hypertension, diabetes, cholesterol, blood clot, heart attack, stroke, cancer, asthma, tuberculosis, human immunodeficiency virus [HIV]).

D. Confidentiality

Laws governing the provision of confidential health care to adolescents vary by state. Be familiar with State Laws for consent for care of minors regarding issues of STIs, pregnancy, mental health, and substance abuse.

E. Physical Examination (Most Pertinent Aspects)[3,4,8]

Whenever possible, examine patient in a gown to ensure complete and thorough exam

1. Height, weight (calculate body mass index [BMI]), and blood pressure with percentiles
2. Dentition and gums (smokeless tobacco use, enamel erosion from induced vomiting)
3. Skin: Acne (type and distribution of lesions), scars, piercings, tattoos
4. Thyroid
5. Spine: Scoliosis (see Section V)
6. Breasts: Tanner stage (Fig. 5-1), masses (females); gynecomastia (males)
7. External genitalia:
   a. Visual inspection (human papillomavirus, ulcers, rashes, pubic lice, trauma, discharge)
   b. Pubic hair distribution: Tanner stage Box 5-1
   c. Genital examination: Tanner stage (Table 5-1, Table 10-16), masses (hydrocele, varicocele, hernia), anal inspection for patients engaging in anal sex
8. Pelvic examination: Perform in any age female who is sexually active or has a gynecologic complaint

F. Laboratory Tests and Procedures[8–14]

1. **Purified protein derivative (PPD):** If high risk for tuberculosis (see Chapter 17 for screening recommendations)

2. **Hemoglobin and hematocrit:** Recommended for females once after menarche
3. **Sexually active adolescents:**
a. Serologic tests: HIV testing is recommended for all persons 13 years and older with subsequent test at least annually for all persons at high risk.[11] Syphilis testing is recommended annually for persons at risk. Rescreening for syphilis and HIV is recommended 3 to 4 months after documented sexually transmitted infection (STI), and/or after new sexual partner in persons at high risk
b. Males: Noninvasive tests such as urine-based nucleic acid amplification tests or (NAATs) are the preferred method to screen for chlamydia and gonorrhea. These tests have high sensitivities and specificities (>90%) as well as high patient acceptability. Sexually active adolescent males are considered among the high-risk groups for STIs and should be screened even if asymptomatic. Rescreening after positive test/treatment should occur 3 months later[12]
c. Females: Detection tests for gonorrhea and *Chlamydia* (urine-based NAAT or vaginal swab)[13], wet mount saline and potassium hydroxide (KOH) preparations, mid-vaginal pH, cervical Gram stain, Pap smear (as appropriate per age and immunocompetency status (e.g. HIV, chronic immunosuppressive therapy)[10]
4. **Cholesterol:** Once during puberty or if personal or familial risk factors (refer to Chapter 7 for more information)
5. **Diabetes:** Consider fasting glucose or hemoglobin A1c in patients at risk
6. **Papanicolaou (Pap smear):**
a. Initial test: Any immunocompetent female ≥21 years
b. Subsequent tests: Annually through age 30 years. Frequency also depends on prior Pap test results
c. Treatment: See Table 5-3

G. Immunizations

Refer to Chapter 16 for dosing, route, formulation, and schedules.

IV. SEXUAL HEALTH

A. Vaginal Infections, Genital Ulcers, and Warts[14]

See Chapter 17 for discussion of infection with chlamydia, gonorrhea, pelvic inflammatory disease, and HIV and for further discussion of syphilis. See Formulary for dosage information. After diagnosis of STI, encourage the patient to refrain from intercourse until full therapy is complete, the partner is treated, and all visible lesions are resolved.

1. Diagnostic features of vaginal infections (Table 5-4)
2. Refer to Table 5-5 for diagnostic features and management of genital ulcers and warts

TABLE 5-3

SUMMARY OF TREATMENT RECOMMENDATIONS FOR CYTOLOGIC AND HISTOLOGIC ABNORMALITIES IN ADOLESCENTS

Diagnosis	ACOG Recommendation for Adolescents
ASC-US	Repeat Pap test in 12 mo
LSIL	Repeat Pap test in 12 mo
HSIL	Colposcopy
AGC	Colposcopy, endocervical assessment, possible endometrial evaluation
Cancer	Colposcopy with endocervical assessment
CIN 1	Repeat cytology at 12 mo intervals for 2 years
CIN 2	Close follow-up at 6 mo intervals (cytology or colposcopy) for up to 24 months, or treatment with either ablation or excision
CIN 3	Ablative or excision therapy

ACOG, American College of Obstetricians and Gynecologists; AGC, atypical glandular cells; ASC-US, atypical squamous cells—undetermined significance; CIN, cervical intraepithelial neoplasia; HSIL, high-grade SIL; LSIL, low-grade squamous intraepithelial lesion.

From Wright TC, Jr., Massad LS, Dunton CJ, et al. 2006 consensus guidelines for the management of women with abnormal cervical screening tests. *Am J Obstet Gynecol* 2007 Oct;197(4):346.

B. Methods of Contraception (see Table 5-6)

A more complete listing of contraceptive methods is available in expanded Table EC 5-A on Expert Consult

C. Combined Hormonal Contraceptives (Estrogen and Progesterone)[15–17]

1. Contraindications

a. Do not use (Center for Disease Control [CDC] category 4): History of deep vein thrombosis (DVT), known thrombophilia including antiphospholipid syndrome, stroke, current and history of ischemic (coronary) heart disease, complicated valvular heart disease, moderate or severely impaired cardiac function, vascular disease, lupus with positive (or unknown) antiphospholipid antibody, active cancer (metastatic, on therapy, or within 6 months of clinical remission), complicated solid organ transplantation; estrogen-dependent neoplasia; pregnancy; lactation for <6 weeks; liver disease (including liver cancer, benign hepatic adenoma, active viral hepatitis, severe cirrhosis); diabetes with vascular complications; migraine with aura (at any age); major surgery with prolonged immobilization; any surgery on the legs; hypertension with pressures higher than 160/100 mmHg or with vascular disease; thrombogenic mutation (including factor V Leiden, prothrombin mutation); protein C, S, or antithrombin deficiencies

Text continued on page 127

TABLE 5-4

DIAGNOSTIC FEATURES AND MANAGEMENT OF VAGINAL INFECTIONS

	No Infection	Yeast Vaginitis	Trichomoniasis	Bacterial Vaginosis
Etiology	—	*Candida albicans* and other yeasts	*Trichomonas vaginalis*	*Gardnerella vaginalis*, anaerobic bacteria, mycoplasma
Typical symptoms	None	Vulvar itching, irritation, ↑ discharge	Malodorous frothy discharge, vulvar itching	Malodorous, slightly ↑ discharge
Discharge				
• Amount	Variable; usually scant	Scant to moderate	Profuse	Moderate
• Color*	Clear or white	White	Yellow-green	Usually white or gray
• Consistency	Nonhomogeneous, floccular	Clumped; adherent plaques	Homogeneous	Homogeneous, low viscosity; smoothly coats vaginal walls
Vulvar/vaginal inflammation	No	Yes	Yes	No
pH of vaginal fluid†	Usually <4.5	Usually <4.5	Usually >5.0	Usually >4.5
Amine ("fishy") odor with 10% potassium hydroxide (KOH)	None	None	May be present	Present
Microscopy‡	Normal epithelial cells; *Lactobacillus* predominates	Leukocytes, epithelial cells, yeast, mycelia, or pseudomycelia in 40%–80% of cases	Leukocytes; motile trichomonads seen in 50%–70% of symptomatic patients, less often if asymptomatic	Clue cells, few leukocytes; *Lactobacillus* outnumbered by profuse mixed flora (nearly always including *G. vaginalis* plus anaerobes)
Usual treatment (See Formulary)	None	Oral fluconazole; Intravaginal azoles	Metronidazole or tinidazole	Oral/intravaginal metronidazole or clindamycin
Management of sex partners	None	None	Treatment recommended	None

NOTE: Refer to Formulary for dosing information.

*Color of discharge is determined by examining vaginal discharge against the white background of a swab.

†pH determination is not useful if blood is present.

‡To detect fungal elements, vaginal fluid is digested with 10% KOH before microscopic examination; to examine for other features, fluid is mixed (1 : 1) with physiologic saline.

From Workowski KA, Berman S. Sexually transmitted diseases treatment guidelines, 2010. *MMWR Recomm Rep.* Dec 17 2010;59(RR-12):1–110.

TABLE 5-5

DIAGNOSTIC FEATURES AND MANAGEMENT OF GENITAL ULCERS AND WARTS

Infection	Clinical Presentation	Presumptive Diagnosis	Definitive Diagnosis	Treatment/Management of Sex Partners
Genital herpes	Grouped vesicles, painful shallow ulcers	Tzanck preparation with multinucleated giant cells	HSV PCR	No known cure. Prompt initiation of therapy shortens duration of first episode. For severe, recurrent disease, initiate therapy at the start of prodrome or within 1 day Transmission can occur during asymptomatic periods. See Formulary for dosing of acyclovir, famciclovir, or valacyclovir
Chancroid	Etiology: *Haemophilus ducreyi* Painful genital ulcer; tender, suppurative inguinal adenopathy	No evidence of treponema pallidum (syphilis) on darkfield microscopy or serologic testing; negative HSV	Use of special media (not widely available in United States); sensitivity <80%	Azithromycin 1 g orally in single dose OR Ceftriaxone IM (single dose); Ciprofloxacin orally × 3 days; Erythromycin orally × 3 days Partners should be examined and treated, regardless of whether symptoms are present, or if they have had sex within 10 days preceding onset of patient's symptoms

Continued

TABLE 5-5

DIAGNOSTIC FEATURES AND MANAGEMENT OF GENITAL ULCERS AND WARTS (Continued)

Infection	Clinical Presentation	Presumptive Diagnosis	Definitive Diagnosis	Treatment/Management of Sex Partners
Primary syphilis	Indurated, well-defined, usually single painless ulcer or chancre; nontender inguinal adenopathy	Nontreponemal serologic test: VDRL, RPR, or STS	Treponemal serologic test: FTA-ABS or MHA-TP; darkfield microscopy or direct fluorescent antibody tests of lesion exudates or tissue	Parenteral penicillin G (See Chapter 17 for preparation(s), dosage, and length of treatment.) Treat presumptively for persons exposed within 3 months preceding the diagnosis of primary syphilis in a sex partner or who were exposed > 90 days preceding the diagnosis and in whom serologic tests may not be immediately available or follow up is uncertain
HPV infection (genital warts)	Single or multiple soft, fleshy, papillary or sessile, painless growths around the anus, vulvovaginal area, penis, urethra, or perineum; no inguinal adenopathy	Typical clinical presentation	Papanicolaou smear revealing typical cytologic changes	Treatment does not eradicate infection. Goal: Removal of exophytic warts. Exclude cervical dysplasia before treatment. Patient-administered therapies include podofilox and imiquimod cream. Clinician-applied therapies include podophyllin 10%–25% in compound tincture of benzoin, bichloracetic or trichloroacetic acid, surgical removal, and cryotherapy with liquid nitrogen or cryoprobe. Podofilox, imiquimod, and podophyllin are contraindicated in pregnancy. Period of communicability is unknown

NOTE: Chancroid, lymphogranuloma venereum (LGV), and granuloma inguinale should be considered in the differential diagnosis of genital ulcers if the clinical presentation is atypical and tests for herpes and syphilis are negative.

FTA-ABS, Fluorescent treponemal antibody absorbed; HPV, human papilloma virus; HSV, herpes simplex virus; MHA-TP, microhemagglutination assay for antibody to T. pallidum; RPR, rapid plasma reagin; STS, serologic test for syphilis; VDRL, Venereal Disease Research Laboratory.

Modified from Workowski KA, Berman S. Sexually transmitted diseases treatment guidelines, 2010. *MMWR Recomm Rep.* Dec 17 2010;59(RR-12):1–110.

TABLE 5-6

COMMON METHODS OF CONTRACEPTION AND FAILURE RATE (%)[17]
(See expanded Table EC 5-A on Expert Consult)

Method	Typical Use	Perfect Use	Benefits	Risks/Disadvantages
COMBINED HORMONAL				
Oral Transdermal Vaginal Ring	8 8 8	0.3 0.3 0.3	Intercourse-independent; rapid reversibility; daily, weekly, or monthly dosing options; decreased risk for dysmenorrhea, rheumatoid arthritis, iron-deficiency anemia, ovarian and uterine cancers, ovarian cysts, acne, ectopic pregnancy, benign breast disorders	Thromboembolic phenomena, cerebrovascular accident, hypertension, worsening migraines, nausea, weight gain, breast tenderness, breakthrough bleeding, amenorrhea, depression; not a barrier to STI
PROGESTIN ONLY				
DMPA Progestin pill Implant	3 8 0.05	0.3 0.03 0.05	Intercourse-independent; can be used while breast-feeding; no estrogen; decreased risk for ovarian/endometrial cancer; no drug interactions; pill and implant have rapid reversibility	Menstrual irregularity/ amenorrhea, weight gain, reversible osteopenia, mood changes, breast tenderness, headaches; not a barrier to STI; DMPA delays return to fertility
BARRIER				
Male condom	15	2	No major risks; low cost, nonprescription; male involved; protects against STI and cervical cancer	Decreased sensation; use with each act of coitus; requires male cooperation
NO METHOD	**85**			

DMPA, Depomedroxyprogesterone acetate; STI, sexually transmitted infection.
Centers for Disease Control and Prevention: Division of Reproductive Health, National Center for Chronic Disease Prevention and Health Promotion. US Medical Eligibility Criteria for Contraceptive Use, 2010, 4th ed. May 2010; 89.

b. Exercise caution (CDC category 3): Postpartum and not breastfeeding for <21 days, history of bariatric/malabsorptive procedure, diabetic nephropathy/retinopathy/neuropathy or other vascular disease, use of drugs that affect liver enzymes (e.g., rifampin, lamotrigine, anticonvulsants), medically treated or current gallbladder disease, hypertension with pressures 140–159/90–99 mmHg, or history of adequately controlled hypertension

c. Advantages generally outweigh disadvantages (CDC category 2): Major surgery without prolonged immobilization, sickle cell disease, unexplained vaginal bleeding, undiagnosed breast mass, headaches without aura and age <35 years, superficial thrombophlebitis, uncomplicated valvular heart disease, lupus with severe thrombocytopenia or on immunosuppressive treatment, cervical cancer or lesions, non-insulin and insulin dependent diabetes without complications, family history of hyperlipidemia or myocardial infarction before age 50 years

2. Serious complications (ACHES)[15]:

a. **A**bdominal pain (pelvic vein or mesenteric vein thrombosis, pancreatitis)
b. **C**hest pain (pulmonary embolism)
c. **H**eadaches (thrombotic or hemorrhagic stroke, retinal vein thrombosis)
d. **E**ye symptoms (thrombotic or hemorrhagic stroke, retinal vein thrombosis)
e. **S**evere leg pain (thrombophlebitis of the lower extremity)

NOTE: See Expert Consult, Chapter 5, for oral contraceptive pill (OCP), transdermal patch, and vaginal ring instructions.

D. Long-Acting Progestin Methods[17]

1. Do not use (Center for Disease Control Category 4): Unexplained vaginal bleeding, pregnancy, acute liver disease, lupus with positive or unknown antiphospholipid antibodies or severe thrombocytopenia, past breast cancer with no evidence of disease, hypertension with pressures greater than 160/100 mmHg, diabetes with vascular disease, ischemic heart disease, stroke
2. Not contraindicated: Breast-feeding, history of thrombosis, hypertriglyceridemia, tobacco abuse, migraine, systemic lupus, hepatic disease, sickle cell (evidence suggests reduced frequency/severity of painful crises), seizure disorder
3. Depomedroxyprogesterone acetate (DMPA) injection instructions:

a. Initial injection first 5 days after onset of menses
b. Reinjection every 11 to 13 weeks
c. Reinjection after 13 weeks or initial injection after first 5 days of cycle (Fig. 5-2)

4. No STI protection; therefore, a barrier method should be used in addition to the pill or DMPA

E. Emergency Contraceptive Pill (ECP)[17]

1. **Contraindications:**

a. For estrogen-containing regimens—same as those for OCPs (see Section IV.C.1), but use over time has shown that such stringent

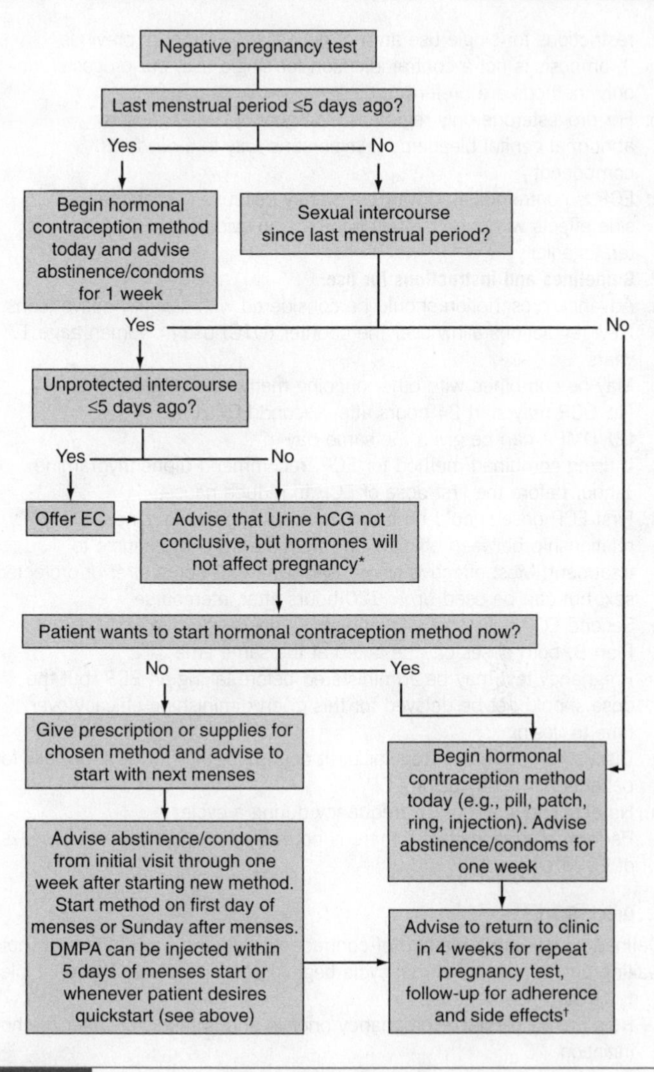

FIGURE 5-2

*Pregnancy tests may take 2–3 weeks after sex to be accurate.

†Consider pregnancy test at 2nd DMPA if QuickStart was used and patient failed 4-week follow-up visit.

Quick-start hormonal contraception algorithm including Depomedroxyprogesterone acetate (DMPA) initial and late injection. Adapted from Zieman M, Hatcher RA, Cwiak C, et al. *A pocket guide to managing contraception*. Tiger, Georgia: Bridging the Gap Foundation, 2010:142.

restrictions for single use are not necessary. History of previous thrombosis is not a contraindication for single use, but progesterone-only methods are preferred

b. For progesterone-only regimens—pregnancy, undiagnosed abnormal genital bleeding, or hypersensitivity to a product component
c. ECP is contraindicated with pregnancy because of maternal side effects without offsetting benefits; no evidence of teratogenicity

2. **Guidelines and instructions for use:**

a. Advance prescription should be considered with sexually active teens. New regulations allow over the counter (OTC) use in women ≥age 17 years
b. May be combined with other ongoing methods of birth control
   (1) OCP may start 24 hours after second ECP dose
   (2) DMPA can be given the same day
c. If using combined method for ECP, recommend diphenhydramine 1 hour before the first dose of ECP to reduce nausea
d. First ECP dose should be taken as soon as possible. Linear relationship between efficacy and the time from intercourse to treatment. Most effective when used within 72 hours after unprotected sex, but can be used up to 120 hours after intercourse
e. Second ECP dose should be taken 12 hours after the first dose. With Plan B, both doses can be taken at the same time
f. Pregnancy test may be administered before taking an ECP, but the dose should not be delayed for this given diminishing efficacy over time to dosing
g. Discuss proper use of regular birth control for the future, especially for patients frequently using ECP
h. No absolute limit of ECP frequency during a cycle
i. Perform pregnancy test if there is no menstrual period within 3 weeks of ECP treatment

F. Quick Start[18]

Defined as starting a method of contraception on the day of the visit (not waiting until a new menstrual cycle begins) see Figure 5-2. The principles of quick start regimens are to:

1. Rule out a detectable pregnancy prior to and immediately after method initiation
2. Provide emergency contraception if indicated
3. Initiate the method immediately
4. Counsel youth to use condoms for one week and obtain a follow-up pregnancy test in 4 weeks if the method was initiated after day 6 of the menstrual cycle
5. Advise that a pregnancy test at Quick Start initiation is not conclusive, but hormones will not affect pregnancy

6. Quick Start Depo Provera can be initiated if menstrual period began in the last 5 days, and initial pregnancy test is negative. Patients should be counseled that there is a small chance they could be pregnant if they have had sex within the last two weeks. Urine pregnancy test should be repeated in 4 weeks and patients should be counseled to avoid sex or use condoms for the first two weeks after getting the injection to decrease the chance of pregnancy

G. Follow-Up Recommendations[8]

Two or three follow-up visits per year to monitor patient compliance, blood pressure, and side effects

V. SCOLIOSIS[19,20]

A. Assessment

1. Routine screening for idiopathic scoliosis is no longer recommended
   a. The potential harms of screening and treating adolescents for idiopathic scoliosis include unnecessary follow-up visits and evaluations due to false positive test results and psychological adverse effects, especially related to brace wear
   b. Clinicians should be prepared to evaluate idiopathic scoliosis when it is discovered incidentally or when the adolescent or parent expresses concern about scoliosis
2. *Adams forward bend test:* Ask patient to bend forward at the hips, with knees straight and arms hanging forward. Spine is inspected from behind for symmetry. Emphasizes any asymmetry of the paraspinous muscles and rib cage (Fig. 5-3)
3. *Scoliometer:* Place midline over spot of maximum rotation during Adams forward bend test. Threshold of 5 to 7 degrees of rotation roughly correlates to 20 degree Cobb angle, and is often used as cutoff for orthopedic referral
4. Radiographic determination of the Cobb angle (Fig. 5-4): If there is clinical suspicion of significant scoliosis on screening, obtain erect thoracoabdominal spinal view
5. Bone scan with or without magnetic resonance imaging (MRI): If pain is worse at night, progressive, well localized, or otherwise suspicious, obtain bone scan or MRI to look for tumor, infection, or fracture
6. MRI: Obtain if patient is younger than 10 years or if *opposite* curves are present (i.e., left-sided thoracic and right-sided lumbar)

B. Treatment

Treatment plan determined according to the Cobb angle and skeletal maturity, which is assessed by grading the ossification of the iliac crest. It can be estimated in females; skeletal maturity is reached 18 months after menarche

1. Skeletally immature:
   a. <10 degrees: Obtain a single follow-up radiograph in 4 to 6 months to ensure there has been no significant progression of the scoliosis

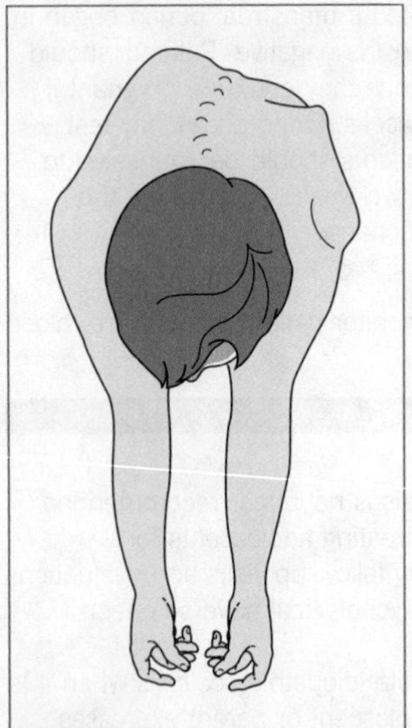

FIGURE 5-3

Forward bending test. This emphasizes any asymmetry of the paraspinous muscles and rib cage.

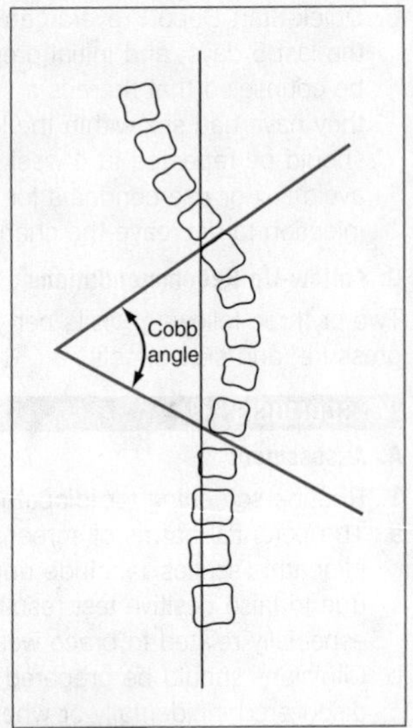

FIGURE 5-4

Cobb angle. This is measured using the superior and inferior end plates of the most tilted vertebrae at the end of each curve.

b. 10 to 20 degrees: Obtain follow-up radiographs every 4 to 6 months while still growing
c. 20 to 40 degrees: Bracing is required
d. >40 degrees: Surgical correction is necessary
2. Skeletally mature:
a. <40 degrees: No further evaluation or intervention is indicated
b. >40 degrees: Surgical correction is required
3. Orthopedic referral: Indicated if the patient is skeletally immature with a curve >20 degrees or skeletally mature with a curve >40 degrees, or in the presence of suspicious pain or neurologic symptoms

VI. PREPARTICIPATION PHYSICAL EVALUATION (PPE)[21,22]

PPE is opportunity to screen for risks related to participation in sports, but is also an opportunity to deliver adolescent clinical preventive services since this may be the only visit a young person has during adolescence. (Refer to Sections II–IV)

A. Medical History

Includes information about chronic conditions/medications (including performance-enhancing agents), hospitalizations/surgeries, use of protective equipment during sports participation, allergies (especially those associated with anaphylaxis, respiratory compromise or exercise-induced), immunizations (hepatitis B virus [HBV], measles, mumps, rubella [MMR], tetanus, varicella).

NOTE: See Chapter 7, Table 7-14, and Table EC 7-D for further information about PPE screening and exercise restrictions with cardiac disease.

B. Review of Systems and Physical Examination Items

Examination items are in italics.

1. Height and weight
2. Vision: Visual problems, corrective lenses; visual acuity, pupil equality
3. Cardiac: History of congenital heart disease; syncope, dizziness, or chest pain during exercise; history of high blood pressure or heart murmurs; family history of heart disease; history of disqualification or limited participation in sports because of a cardiac problem; *blood pressure, heart rate and rhythm, pulses (including radial/femoral lag), auscultation for heart sounds, murmurs—both standing and supine*
4. Respiratory: Asthma, coughing, wheezing, or dyspnea during exercise
5. Abdomen: Organomegaly and single kidney are contraindications for contact sports
6. Genitourinary: Age at menarche, last menstrual period, regularity of menstrual periods, number of periods in the last year, longest interval between periods, dysmenorrhea; *palpation of the abdomen, palpation of the testicles, examination of the inguinal canals*
7. Orthopedic: Previous injuries that have limited sports participation or required medical intervention; screening orthopedic examination (Fig. 5-5)
8. Neurology: History of a significant head injury/concussion; numbness or tingling in the extremities; severe headaches; seizure disorder (seizure disorder is not a direct contraindication to contact sports if seizures are well-controlled; history of seizure within the past 6 months should raise concern prior to clearance, particularly those engaged in water sports)
9. Skin: Rashes; evidence of contagious infections (e.g., varicella or impetigo)
10. Psychosocial: Weight control and body image; stresses at home or in school; use or abuse of drugs and alcohol; attention to signs of eating disorders, including oral ulcerations, eroded tooth enamel, edema, lanugo hair, calluses or ulcerations on knuckles

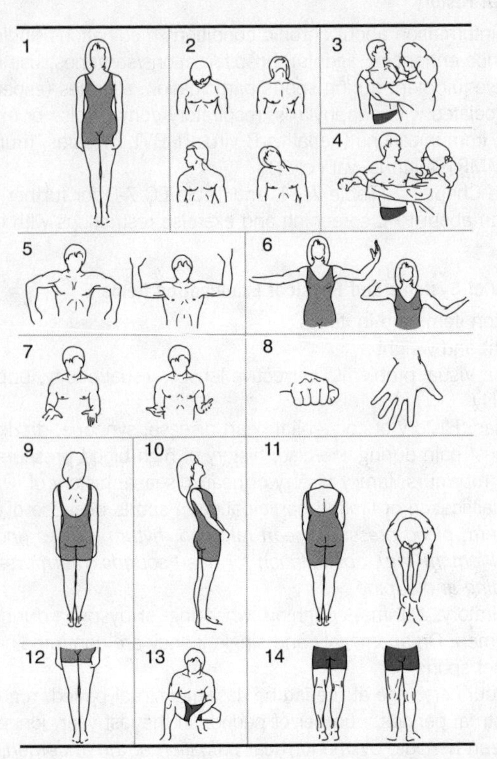

FIGURE 5-5

Screening orthopedic examination. The general musculoskeletal screening examination consists of the following: *1,* inspection, athlete standing, facing examiner (symmetry of trunk, upper extremities); *2,* forward flexion, extension, rotation, lateral flexion of neck (range of motion, cervical spine); *3,* resisted shoulder shrug (strength, trapezius); *4,* resisted shoulder abduction (strength, deltoid); *5,* internal and external rotation of shoulder (range of motion, glenohumeral joint); *6,* extension and flexion of elbow (range of motion, elbow); *7,* pronation and supination of elbow (range of motion, elbow and wrist); *8,* clenching of fist, then spreading of fingers (range of motion, hand and fingers); *9,* inspection, athlete facing away from examiner (symmetry of trunk, upper extremities); *10,* back extension, knees straight (spondylolysis and spondylolisthesis); *11,* back flexion with knees straight, facing toward and away from examiner (range of motion, thoracic and lumbosacral spine; spine curvature; hamstring flexibility); *12,* inspection of lower extremities, contraction of quadriceps muscles (alignment symmetry); *13,* "duck walk" four steps (motion of hips, knees, and ankles; strength; balance); *14,* standing on toes, then on heels (symmetry, calf; strength; balance). *(Modified from American Academy of Family Physicians: Preparticipation physical examination, 2nd ed. Kansas City, MO, American Academy of Family Physicians, 1997.)*

REFERENCES

1. Kulin H, Muller J. The biological aspects of puberty. *Pediatr Rev* 1996;17:75–86.
2. Muir A. Precocious puberty. *Pediatr Rev* 2006;27(10):373–381.
3. Joffe A. Introduction to adolescent medicine. In: McMillan JA, DeAngelis CD, Feigan RD, et al, eds. *Oski's pediatrics principles and practice.* 4th ed. Philadelphia: Lippincott Williams & Wilkins; 2006:546–557.
4. Rosen DS, Neinstein LS. Preventive healthcare for adolescents. In: Neinstein LS, ed. *Adolescent healthcare: a practical guide.* 4th ed. Philadelphia: Lippincott Williams & Wilkins, 2002:82–117.
5. Rosen D. Physiologic growth and development during adolescence. *Pediatr Rev* 2004;25:194–200.
6. Fishman M, Bruner A, Adger H. Substance abuse among children and adolescents. *Pediatr Rev* 1997;18:397–398.
7. Gutgesell M, Payne N. Issues of adolescent psychological development in the 21st century. *Pediatr Rev* 2004;25:79–85.
8. *Bright Futures Guidelines for Health Supervision of Infants, Children, and Adolescents.* 3rd ed. Elk Grove, Village, IL: American Academy of Pediatrics; 2008:515–574.
9. Greydanus D, Omar H, Patel D. What's new: cervical cancer screening in adolescents. *Pediatr Rev* 2009;30:23–25.
10. Wright TC, Jr., Massad LS, Dunton CJ, et al. 2006 consensus guidelines for the management of women with abnormal cervical screening tests. *Am J Obstet Gynecol* 2007 Oct;197(4):346–355.
11. Branson, BM, Handsfield H., et al. Revised Recommendations for HIV testing of Adults, Adolescents, and Pregnant Women in Health Care Settings. *MMWR* 2006;55:1–12.
12. Gaydos CA. Nucleic Acid Amplification Tests for Gonorrhea and Chlamydia: Practice and Applications. *Infect Dis Clin North Am* 2005 Jun;19(2): 367–386.
13. Expert Consultation Meeting Summary Report, APHL. Laboratory Diagnostic Testing for Chlamydia Trachomatis and Neiserria Gonorrhoeae. 2009;(no volume):1–6.
14. Workowski KA, Berman S. Sexually transmitted diseases treatment guidelines, 2010. *MMWR Recomm Rep.* Dec 17 2010;59(RR-12):1–110.
15. Calderoni ME, Coupey SM. Combined hormonal contraception. *Adolesc Med* 2005;16:517–537.
16. Burkett AM. Progestin only contraceptives and their use in adolescents: clinical options and medical indications. *Adolesc Med Clin* 2005;16: 553–567.
17. Center for Disease Control and Prevention: Division of Reproductive Health, National Center for Chronic Disease Prevention and Health Promotion: US medical eligibility criteria for contraceptive use, 2010. *MMWR* 2010;59: 1–84.
18. Zurawin RK, Ayensu-Coker L. Innovations in contraception: a review. *Clin Obstet Gynecol* June 2007;50(2):425–439.
19. Weinstein S, Dolan L, Cheng J. Adolescent idiopathic scoliosis. *Lancet* 2008;371:1527–1534.
20. Stewart D, Skaggs D. Consultation with the specialist: adolescent idiopathic scoliosis. *Pediatr Rev* 2006;27:299–306.

21. US Preventive Task Force: Screening for Idiopathic Scoliosis in Adolescents. http://www.uspreventiveservicestaskforce.org/uspstf/uspsaisc.htm 2004; 1–3.
22. Andrews JS. Making the most of the sports physical. *Contemp Pediatr* 1997;14:188.

Chapter 6

Analgesia and Sedation

Kristin M. Arcara, MD

See additional content on Expert Consult

I. WEB RESOURCES

International Association for the Study of Pain: http://childpain.org/
American Pain Society: http://www.ampainsoc.org/
Society for Pediatric Sedation: http://www.pedsedation.org/
American Society of Anesthesiologists: http://www.asahq.org/

II. PAIN ASSESSMENT (TABLE 6-1)

A. Infant[1]

1. Physiologic response: Seen primarily in acute pain; subsides with continuing/chronic pain. Characterized by increase in blood pressure, heart rate, and respiratory rate; oxygen desaturation; crying; diaphoresis; flushing or pallor
2. Behavioral response:
   a. Observe characteristics and duration of cry, facial expressions, visual tracking, body movements, and response to stimuli
   b. Neonatal Infant Pain Scale (NIPS): Behavioral assessment tool for the preterm neonate (gestational age <37 weeks) and full-term neonate (gestational age >37 weeks up to 6 weeks after birth)
   c. FLACC scale (Table 6-2): Measures and evaluates pain interventions by quantifying pain behaviors, such as facial expression, leg movement, activity, cry, and consolability, with scores ranging from 0 to 10.[2] Revised FLACC scale reliable for children with cognitive impairment[3]

B. Preschooler

In addition to physiologic and behavioral responses, use the **FACES** pain rating scale to assess pain intensity in children as young as age 3 years.

C. School-Age and Adolescent

Evaluate physiologic and behavioral responses; ask about description, location, and character of pain. Children age 7–8 years can use the standard pain rating scale (0 is no pain and 10 is the worst pain ever experienced).

III. ANALGESICS[1,4]

A. Nonopioid Analgesics

Weak analgesics with antipyretic activity are commonly used to manage mild to moderate pain of nonvisceral origin. Administer alone or in

TABLE 6-1

DEVELOPMENTAL RESPONSES TO PAIN

Stage	Age	Response
Infant	<6 mo	No expression of anticipatory fear. Level of anxiety reflects that of the parent.
	6–18 mo	Anticipatory fear of painful experiences begins to develop.
Preschooler	18–24 mo	Verbalization. Children express pain with words such as "hurt" and "boo-boo."
	3 yr	Localization and identification of external causes. Children more reliably assess their pain but continue to depend on visual cues for localization and are unable to understand a reason for pain.
School-age child	5–7 yr	Cooperation. Children have improved understanding of pain and ability to localize it and cooperate.

Data from Hsu DC: Pain control and sedation in children. Uptodate Online version 18.2. www.utdol.com.

TABLE 6-2

FLACC: PAIN ASSESSMENT TOOL

FACE
0—No particular expression or smile
1—Occasional grimace or frown, withdrawn, disinterested
2—Frequent to constant frown, quivering chin, clenched jaw
LEGS
0—Normal position or relaxed
1—Uneasy, restless, tense
2—Kicking or legs drawn up
ACTIVITY
0—Lying quietly, normal position, moves easily
1—Squirming, shifting back and forth, tense
2—Arched, rigid or jerking
CRY
0—No cry (awake or asleep)
1—Moans or whimpers, occasional complaint
2—Crying steadily, screams or sobs, frequent complaints
CONSOLABILITY
0—Content, relaxed
1—Reassured by occasional touching, hugging or being talked to; distractible
2—Difficult to console or comfort

Adapted from Manworren R, Hynan L: Clinical validation of FLACC: preverbal patient pain scale. Pediatr Nurs 2003;29(2):140–146.

combination with opiates. Drugs, routes of administration, and specific comments are as follows:

1. **Acetaminophen** (by mouth [PO]/per rectum [PR]): Weak analgesic with no anti-inflammatory activity; no platelet inhibition or gastrointestinal (GI) irritation

2. **Aspirin (PO/PR):** Associated with platelet inhibition and GI irritation. Avoid due to risk of Reye syndrome
3. **Choline magnesium trisalicylate (PO):** No platelet inhibition. Also associated with Reye syndrome
4. **Nonsteroidal anti-inflammatory drugs (NSAIDs):** Ibuprofen (PO), ketorolac (intravenous [IV]/intramuscular [IM]/PO), naproxen (PO)
   a. Especially useful for sickle cell, bony, rheumatic, and inflammatory pain
   b. Associated with GI symptoms (epigastric pain, gastritis, GI bleeding): Recommend histamine-2-receptor blocker concurrently with prolonged use
   c. Other adverse effects: Interference with platelet aggregation, bronchoconstriction, hypersensitivity reactions, and azotemia. May interfere with bone healing. Should be avoided in patients with severe renal disease, dehydration, or heart failure

NOTE: Ketorolac is a potent analgesic (1 mg/kg IV is equivalent to 0.1 mg/kg morphine). Only parenteral NSAID available.

See the Quick Reference to Analgesics Drugs in Table EC 6-A on Expert Consult.

B. Opioids (Table 6-3)

1. Produce analgesia by binding mu receptors in the brain and spinal cord
2. Most flexible and widely used analgesics
3. Side effects: Pruritus, nausea, vomiting, constipation, urine retention, and (rarely) respiratory depression and hypotension
4. Morphine: Gold (unit) standard of this drug class

C. Local Anesthetics[4–7]

Used primarily to anesthetize areas for minor procedures. Administered topically, subcutaneously, into peripheral nerves (e.g., digital nerve, penile nerve block), or centrally (epidural/spinal). They act by blocking nerve conduction at the sodium channel.

1. For all local anesthetics, 1% solution = 10 mg/mL
2. Topical local anesthetics (Table 6-4)[8]
3. Injectable local anesthetics (Table 6-5):
   a. Infiltration of the skin at the site: Used for painful procedures such as wound closure, IV line placement, or lumbar puncture
   b. To reduce stinging from injection: Use a small needle (27- to 30-gauge). Alkalinize anesthetic: add 1 mL (1 mEq) sodium bicarbonate to 9 mL lidocaine (or 29 mL bupivacaine), use lowest concentration of anesthetic available, warm solution (between 37° and 42°C), inject anesthetic slowly, and rub skin at injection site first
   c. To enhance efficacy and duration: Add epinephrine to decrease vascular uptake. **Never use local anesthetics with epinephrine in areas supplied by end arteries** (e.g., pinna, digits, nasal tip, and penis)
   d. Toxicity: Central nervous system (CNS) and cardiac toxicity are of greatest concern. CNS symptoms are seen before cardiovascular

TABLE 6-3

COMMONLY USED OPIATES

Drug	Route; Equi-analgesic Doses (mg/kg/dose)	Onset (min)	Duration (hr)	Side Effects	Comments
Codeine	PO; 1.2	30–60	3–4	• Can cause severe nausea and vomiting • Histamine release	Converted in liver to morphine (10%). Newborns and 10% of U.S. population cannot make this conversion.
Meperidine (Demerol)	IV; 1.0 PO; 1.5–2.0	5–10 30–60	3–4 2–4	• Catastrophic interaction with MAO inhibitors • Tachycardia, histamine release • Metabolite can cause seizures; avoid in predisposed patients	Euphoric effects are greater than with morphine. Low doses (0.1–0.25 mg/kg) stop shivering. Not recommended for prolonged use or patient-controlled analgesia.
Oxycodone	PO; 0.1	30–60	3–4		Available in sustained-release form for chronic pain. Much less nauseating than codeine.
Methadone	IV; 0.1 PO; 0.1	5–10 30–60	4–24 4–24		Initial dose may produce analgesia for 3–4 hr; duration of action is increased with repeated dosing.
Morphine	IV; 0.1 IM/SC; 0.1–0.2 PO; 0.3–0.5	5–10 10–30 30–60	3–4 4–5 4–5	• Seizures in neonates • Can cause significant histamine release	The "gold standard" against which all other opioids are compared. Available in sustained-release form for chronic pain.
Hydromorphone	IV/SC; 0.015 PO; 0.02–0.1	5–10 30–60	3–4		Less sedation, nausea, pruritus than morphine
Fentanyl	IV; 0.001 Transdermal; 0.001 Transmucosal; 0.01	1–2 12 15	0.5–1 2–3	• Pruritus • Bradycardia • Chest wall rigidity with doses >5 mcg/kg (but can occur at all doses); treat with naloxone or neuromuscular blockade	Rarely causes cardiovascular instability (relatively safer in hypovolemia, congenital heart disease, or head trauma). Respiratory depressant effect much longer (4 hr) than analgesic effect. Levels of unbound drug are higher in newborns. Most commonly used opioid for short painful procedures.

IM, Intramuscular; IV, intravenous; PO, by mouth; SC, subcutaneous.

Adapted from Yaster M, Cote C, Krane E, et al: Pediatric pain management and sedation handbook. St. Louis, Mosby, 1997, pp. 29–50.

TABLE 6-4

COMMONLY USED TOPICAL LOCAL ANESTHETICS[8]

	Components	Indications	Peak Effect	Duration†	Cautions*
EMLA	Lidocaine 2.5% Prilocaine 2.5%	Intact skin only Venipuncture, circumcision, LP, abscess drainage, BMA	60 min	90 min	Methemoglobinemia: Not for use in patients who are predisposed to methemoglobinemia (e.g., G6PD deficiency, some medications) Infants <3 mo of age: Use sparingly (up to 1 g is safe)
LMX	Lidocaine 4%	Same as EMLA	30 min	60 min	Same as EMLA
LET	Lidocaine 4% Epinephrine 0.1% Tetracaine 0.5% Can be mixed with cellulose to create a gel	Safe for nonintact skin Lacerations Not for use in contaminated wounds	30 min	45 min	Vasoconstriction: Contraindicated in areas supplied by end-arteries (e.g., pinna, nose, penis, digits) Avoid contact with mucus membranes
Viscous Lidocaine	Lidocaine 2% May be mixed with Maalox and Benadryl elixir in a 1:1:1 ratio for palatability	Safe for nonintact skin Mucous membranes (e.g., urethral catheter placement, mucositis)	10 min	30 min	Overuse can lead to life threatening toxicity Not to be used for teething

*Maximum lidocaine dose is 5 mg/kg.

†Approximate.

BMA, Bone marrow aspiration; EMLA, eutectic mixture of local anesthetics; G6PD, glucose-6-phosphate dehydrogenase; LP, lumbar puncture.

TABLE 6-5

COMMONLY USED INJECTABLE LOCAL ANESTHETICS[1,5]

Agent	Concentration (%) (1% solution = 10 mg/mL)	Max dose (mg/kg)	Onset (min)	Duration (hr)
Lidocaine	0.5–2	5	3	0.5–2
Lidocaine with epinephrine	0.5–2	7	3	1–3
Bupivicaine	0.25–0.75	2.5	15	2–4
Bupivicaine with epinephrine	0.25–0.75	3	15	4–8

NOTE: Max volume = (max mg/kg × weight in kg)/(% solution × 10).

Data from St. Germaine Brent A: The management of pain in the emergency department. Pediatr Clin North Am 2000;47(3):651–679, and Yaster M et al: Pediatric pain management and sedation handbook. St. Louis, Mosby, 1997, pp. 51–72.

collapse. Progression of symptoms: Perioral numbness, dizziness, auditory disturbances, muscular twitching, unconsciousness, seizures, coma, respiratory arrest, cardiovascular collapse. It is important to calculate the volume limit of the local anesthetic and always draw up less than the maximum volume. (see Formulary for maximum doses)

NOTE: Bupivicaine is associated with more severe cardiac toxicity than lidocaine.

D. Nonpharmacologic Measures of Pain Relief[9,10]

1. Sucrose for neonates (Sweet Ease):
   a. Indications: Procedures such as heel sticks, immunizations, venipuncture, IV line insertion, arterial puncture, insertion of a Foley catheter, and lumbar puncture in neonates and infants. Strongest evidence exists for infants 0–1 month of age,[9] but more recent evidence suggests efficacy up to 12 months[10]
   b. Procedure: Administer up to 2 mL of 24% sucrose into the infant's mouth by syringe or from a nipple/pacifier ~2 min before the procedure. **NOTE:** Effective doses in very low birth weight infants may be as low as 0.05–0.1 mL 24% sucrose and in term neonates may be as high as 2 mL 24% sucrose
   c. May be given for more than one procedure within a relatively short period of time but should not be administered more than twice in 1 hour

   NOTE: Studies have suggested potential adverse neurocognitive effects with many repeated doses.[10]

   d. Effectiveness has been most often studied with adjunctive pacifier/nipple and parental holding which may contribute to stress/pain alleviation
   e. Avoid use if patient is under nothing by mouth (NPO) restrictions

2. Parental presence
3. Distraction with toys
4. Child life specialists strongly encouraged

IV. SEDATION[1,4–7,11]

A. Definitions

1. **Mild sedation (anxiolysis):** Intent is anxiolysis with maintenance of consciousness. Practically, obtained when a single drug is given once at a low dose (not chloral hydrate)
2. **Moderate sedation:** Formerly known as conscious sedation. A controlled state of depressed consciousness during which airway reflexes and airway patency are maintained. Patient responds appropriately to age-appropriate commands ("Open your eyes.") and light touch. Practically, obtained any time a combination of sedative-hypnotic and analgesic is used
3. **Deep sedation:** A controlled state of depressed consciousness during which airway reflexes and airway patency may not be maintained and the child is unable to respond to physical or verbal stimuli. Practically, required for most painful procedures in children. The following IV drugs always produce deep sedation: propofol, etomidate, thiopental, methohexital
4. **Dissociative sedation:** Unique state of sedation achieved with ketamine. Deep level of depressed consciousness but airway reflexes and patency are generally maintained

Mild and moderate sedation can easily progress to deep sedation.
See the Quick Reference to Sedative-Hypnotic Drugs in Table EC 6-A.

B. Preparation

1. Patient should be **NPO** for solids and clear liquids (Table 6-6 shows current American Society of Anesthesiologists recommendations)

NOTE: Some studies have suggested no increased incidence of adverse outcomes with shorter periods of fasting.[12]

See Figure EC 6-A on Expert Consult for more information on fasting recommendations.

TABLE 6-6

FASTING RECOMMENDATIONS FOR ANESTHESIA

Food Type	Minimum Fasting Period (hr)
Clear liquids	2
Breast milk	4
Nonhuman milk, formula	6
Solids	8

Data from Practice guidelines for preoperative fasting and the use of pharmacologic agents to reduce the risk of pulmonary aspiration: application to healthy patients undergoing elective procedures. A report by the American Society of Anesthesiologists Task Force on Preoperative Fasting and Use of Pharmacologic Agents to Reduce the Risk of Pulmonary Aspiration [Online]. http://www.asahq.org/publicationsAndServices/NPO.pdf

6

2. **Written informed consent**
3. **Focused patient history:**
   a. Allergies and medications
   b. Airway (asthma, acute respiratory disease, reactive airway disease), airway obstruction (mediastinal mass, history of noisy breathing, obstructive sleep apnea), craniofacial abnormalities (e.g., Pfeiffer, Crouzon, Apert, Pierre Robin syndromes), recent upper respiratory infection (suggests increased risk of laryngospasm)
   c. Aspiration risk (neuromuscular disease, gastroesophageal reflux disease, altered mental status, obesity, pregnancy)
   d. Prematurity, comorbidities, and adverse reactions to sedatives and anesthesia
4. **Physical examination:** With specific attention to head, ears, eyes, nose, and throat (HEENT); lungs; cardiac examination; and neuromuscular function. Assess ability to open mouth and extend neck. If risk for moderate sedation is too high, consider an anesthesia consultation and general anesthesia
5. **Determine American Society of Anesthesiologists Physical Status Classification:** See Table EC 6-B on Expert Consult. Class I and II patients are generally good candidates for mild, moderate or deep sedation outside of the operating room[13]
6. Have an **emergency plan** ready: Make sure qualified backup personnel and equipment are close by
7. **Personnel:** Two providers are required. One provider should perform the procedure and a separate provider should monitor the patient during sedation and recovery
8. Ensure **IV access**
9. Have **airway/intubation equipment available** (See Chapter 1)
10. **Medications** to have available: Those for rapid sequence intubation (see Chapter 1) or emergencies (e.g., epinephrine, atropine)
11. **Antagonist (*reversal*) agents** should be readily available (e.g. Naloxone, flumazenil)

C. Monitoring

1. **Vital signs:** Obtain baseline vital signs (including pulse oximetry). Continuously monitor heart rate and oxygen saturation; intermittently monitor blood pressure and respiratory rate. Record vital signs at least every 5 minutes until the patient returns to presedation level of consciousness

NOTE: Complications most often occur 5 to 10 min after administration of IV medication and immediately after a procedure is completed (when stimuli associated with the procedure are removed)[7]

2. **Airway:** Assess airway patency and adequacy of ventilation through capnography, auscultation, or direct visualization frequently

D. Pharmacologic Agents

1. Goal of sedation: To tailor drug combination to provide levels of analgesia, sedation-hypnosis, and anxiolysis deep enough to facilitate the procedure but shallow enough to avoid loss of airway reflexes
2. CNS, cardiovascular, and respiratory depression are potentiated by combining sedative drugs and/or opioids and by rapid drug infusion. Titrate to effect
3. Common sedative/hypnotic agents (Box 6-1):

BOX 6-1

PROPERTIES OF COMMON SEDATIVE/HYPNOTIC AGENTS

SEDATING ANTIHISTAMINES (DIPHENHYDRAMINE, HYDROXYZINE)

- Mild sedative-hypnotics with anti-emetic and antipruritic properties. Used for sedation and treatment of opiate side effects
- No anxiolytic or analgesic effects

BARBITURATES

- Contraindicated in patients with porphyria. Suitable only for nonpainful procedures
- No anxiolytic or analgesic effects

BENZODIAZEPINES

- Reversible with flumazenil
- + Anxiolytic effects. No analgesic effects

OPIATES

- Reversible with Naloxone
- + Analgesic effects. No anxiolytic effects

KETAMINE[1,5,9]

- Phencyclidine derivative that causes potent dissociative anesthesia, analgesia and amnesia
- Nystagmus indicates likely therapeutic effect
- Vocalizations/movement may occur even with adequate sedation
- Results in “dissociative sedation” by any route
- Onset: IV, 0.5–2 min; IM, 5–10 min; PO/PR, 20–45 min
- Duration: IV, 20–60 min; IM, 30–90 min; PO/PR, 60–120+ min
- ***CNS effects:*** increased ICP, emergence delirium with auditory, visual, and tactile hallucinations
- ***Cardiovascular effects:*** inhibits catecholamine reuptake, causing increased HR, BP, SVR, PVR, direct myocardial depression
- ***Respiratory effects:*** bronchodilation (useful in asthmatics), increased secretions (can result in laryngospasm), maintenance of ventilatory response to hypoxia, relative maintenance of airway reflexes
- ***Other effects:*** increased muscle tone, myoclonic jerks, increased IOP, nausea, emesis
- **Contraindications:** increased ICP, increased IOP, hypertension, pre-existing psychotic disorders

Continued

BOX 6-1

PROPERTIES OF COMMON SEDATIVE/HYPNOTIC AGENTS (Continued)

PROPOFOL

- Give 1 mg/kg followed by 0.5 mg/kg IV
- Extremely rapid onset and brief recovery (5–15 min) antiemetic and euphoric
- Caution: respiratory depression, apnea, hypotension
- + Anxiolytic and analgesic effects

CHLORAL HYDRATE[†]

- May be used to produce immobilization for painful procedures
- High risk of severe airway obstruction in children with OSA
- 30%–40% failure rate
- Long and unpredictable onset/duration of action
- No anxiolytic or analgesic effects

[†]High rate of failure of chloral hydrate combined with its adverse effects increase the risk/benefit profile of this agent. We recommend considering alternative sedatives whenever possible. See Formulary for dosing recommendations.

BP, Blood pressure; HR, heart rate; ICP, intracranial pressure; IM, intramuscular; IOP, intraocular pressure; IV, intravenous; OSA, obstructive sleep apnea; PO, by mouth; PR, per rectum; PVR, pulmonary vascular resistance; SVR, systemic vascular resistance.

Data from Yaster M, Cote C, Krane E, et al: Pediatric pain management and sedation handbook. St. Louis, Mosby, 1997, pp. 376–382; St Germaine Brent A: The management of pain in the emergency department. Pediatr Clin North Am 2000;47(3):651–679; and Cote CJ et al: A practice of anesthesia for infants and children. Philadelphia, WB Saunders, 2001.

See also Tables 6-3 and 6-7 for more information on opiates and barbiturates/benzodiazepines

4. Reversal agents:
   a. Naloxone: Opioid antagonist. See Box 6-2 for Narcan administration protocol
   b. Flumazenil: Benzodiazepine antagonist. See Formulary for dosing details

E. Discharge Criteria[13]

1. Airway is patent and cardiovascular function is stable
2. Easy arousability; intact protective reflexes (swallow and cough, gag reflex)
3. Ability to talk and sit up unaided (if age appropriate)
4. Alternatively for very young or intellectually disabled children, goal is to return as close as possible to presedation level of responsiveness
5. Adequate hydration
6. Recovery after sedation protocols varies but typically ranges from 60 to 120 minutes

TABLE 6-7

COMMONLY USED BENZODIAZEPINES* AND BARBITURATES[1,5,11]

Drug Class	Duration of Action	Drug	Route	Onset (min)	Duration (hr)	Comments
Benzodiazepines	Short	Midazolam (Versed)	IV	1–3	1–2	• Has rapid and predictable onset of action, a short recovery time
			IM/IN	5–10		• Causes amnesia
			PO/PR	10–30		• Results in mild depression of hypoxic ventilatory drive
	Intermediate	Diazepam (Valium)	IV (painful)	1–3	0.25–1	• Poor choice for procedural sedation
			PR	7–15	2–3	• Excellent for muscle relaxation or prolonged sedation
			PO	30–60	2–3	• Painful on IV injection
						• Faster onset than midazolam
	Long	Lorazepam (Ativan)	IV	1–5	3–4	• Poor choice for procedural sedation
			IM	10–20	3–6	• Ideal for prolonged anxiolysis, seizure treatment
			PO	30–60	3–6	
Barbiturates	Short	Methohexital	PR†	5–10	1–1.5	• PR form used as sedative for nonpainful procedures
		Thiopental	PR†	5–10	1–1.5	• IV form induces general anesthesia; do not use for sedation
	Intermediate	Pentobarbital	IV	1–10	1–4	• Predictable sedation and immobility for nonpainful procedures
			IM	5–15	2–4	• Minimal respiratory depression when used alone
			PO/PR	15–60	2–4	• Associated with slow wake up and agitation

*Use IV solution for PO, PR, and IN administration. Rectal diazepam gel (Diastat) is also available.

†IV administration produces general anesthesia; only PR should be used for sedation.

IM, Intramuscular; IN, intranasal; IV, intravenous; PO, by mouth; PR, per rectum.

Data from Yaster M, Cote C, Krane E, et al: Pediatric pain management and sedation handbook. St. Louis, Mosby, 1997, pp. 345–374; St Germaine Brent A: The management of pain in the emergency department. Pediatr Clin North Am 2000;47(3):651–679; and Cote CJ et al: A practice of anesthesia for infants and children. Philadelphia, WB Saunders, 2001.

BOX 6-2

NALOXONE (NARCAN) ADMINISTRATION

INDICATIONS: PATIENTS REQUIRING NALOXONE (NARCAN) USUALLY MEET ALL OF THE FOLLOWING CRITERIA*

- Unresponsive to physical stimulation
- Shallow respirations or respiratory rate <8 breaths/min[†]
- Pinpoint pupils

PROCEDURE

1. **Stop opioid administration** (as well as other sedative drugs), start the **ABCs** (**A**irway, **B**reathing, **C**irculation), and call for **HELP**
2. **Dilute naloxone:** Mix 0.4 mg (1 ampule) of naloxone with 9 mL of normal saline (final concentration 0.04 mg/mL = 40 mcg/mL)
   (If child <40 kg, dilute 0.1 mg (one-fourth ampule) in 9 mL of normal saline to make 0.01 mg/mL solution = 10 mcg/mL)
3. **Administer and observe response:** Administer dilute naloxone slowly (1–2 mcg/kg/dose IV over 2 min). Observe patient response
4. **Titrate to effect:** Within 1–2 min, patient should open eyes and respond. If not, continue until a total dose of 10 mcg/kg is given. If no response is obtained, evaluate for other cause of sedation/respiratory depression
5. **Discontinue naloxone administration:** Discontinue naloxone as soon as patient responds (e.g., takes deep breaths when directed)
6. **Caution:** Another dose of naloxone may be required within 30 min of first dose (duration of action of naloxone is shorter than that of most opioids)
7. **Monitor patient:** Assign a staff member to monitor sedation/respiratory status and to remind the patient to take deep breaths as necessary
8. **Alternative analgesia:** Provide nonopioids for pain relief. Resume opioid administration at half the original dose when the patient is easily aroused and respiratory rate is >9 breaths/min.

*Patients with significant opiate exposure (sickle cell, cancer) should be carefully evaluated for the need for naloxone. The reversal of analgesia could produce hypertension, tachycardia, ventricular arrhythmias, and pulmonary edema. If necessary, give at the lowest dose possible and titrate carefully.

[†]Respiratory rates that require naloxone vary according to infant's/child's usual rate.

Modified from McCaffery M, Pasero C: Pain: clinical manual. St. Louis, Mosby, 1999, pp. 269–270.

F. Examples of Sedation Protocols (Tables 6-8 and 6-9)

V. PATIENT-CONTROLLED ANALGESIA (PCA)

A. Definition

PCA is a device that enables a patient to receive continuous (basal) opioids and/or self-administer small supplemental doses (bolus) of analgesics on an as-needed basis. In children younger than age 6 years, a family member, caregiver, or nurse may administer doses.

B. Indications

Moderate to severe pain of acute or chronic nature. Commonly used in sickle cell disease, postsurgery, post-trauma, burns, and cancer. Also for preemptive pain management (e.g., to facilitate dressing changes).

TABLE 6-8
EXAMPLES OF SEDATION PROTOCOLS*

Protocol/Doses	Comments
Ketamine (1 mg/kg/dose IV × 1–2 doses)	Lowest rates of adverse events when ketamine used alone[‡]
Ketamine + midazolam + atropine ("ketodazzline") **IV route:** Ketamine 1 mg/kg/dose × 1–2 doses Midazolam 0.05 mg/kg × 1 dose Atropine 0.02 mg/kg × 1 dose **IM route:** combine (use smallest volume possible) Ketamine 1.5–2.0 mg/kg Midazolam 0.15–0.2 mg/kg Atropine 0.02 mg/kg	Atropine = antisialogogue Midazolam = counter emergence delirium
Midazolam + fentanyl Midazolam 0.1 mg/kg IV × 3 doses PRN Fentanyl 1 mcg/kg IV × 3 doses PRN	High likelihood of respiratory depression Infuse fentanyl no more frequently than q3min

*These examples reflect commonly used current protocols at the Johns Hopkins Children's Center; variations are found at other institutions.

‡Green, SM, Roback MG, Krauss B, et al: Predictors of emesis and recovery agitation with emergency department ketamine sedation: an individual-patient data meta-analysis of 8,282 children. Ann Emerg Med. 2009;54(2):171–180.

Adapted from Yaster M, Cote C, Krane E, et al: Pediatric pain management and sedation handbook. St. Louis, Mosby, 1997.

TABLE 6-9
SUGGESTED ANALGESIA AND SEDATION PROTOCOLS

Pain Threshold	Procedure	Suggested Choices
Non Painful	CT/MRI/EEG/ECHO	Midazolam*
Mild	Phlebotomy/IV	EMLA
	LP	EMLA (± midazolam)
	Pelvic exam	Midazolam
	Minor laceration, well vascularized	LET
	Minor laceration, not well vascularized	Lidocaine
Moderate	BM aspiration	EMLA (± midazolam)
	Arthrocentesis	Lidocaine (local) for cooperative child or Ketamine† for uncooperative child
	Fracture reduction	Ketamine
	Major laceration	Ketamine or fentanyl + midazolam
	Burn débridement	Ketamine or fentanyl + midazolam
	Long procedures (>30 min)	Consider general anesthesia
Severe	Fracture reduction	Ketamine
	Long procedures (>30 min)	Consider general anesthesia

*Caution for antiepileptics for EEG.

†Ketamine should not be chosen with head injury or open globe eye injury.

BM, Bone marrow; CT, computed tomography; ECHO, echocardiogram; EEG, electroencephalogram; EMLA, eutectic mixture of local anesthetics; LP, lumbar puncture; LET, lidocaine, epinephrine, tetracaine; MRI, magnetic resonance imaging.

Adapted from Yaster M, Cote C, Krane E, et al: Pediatric pain management and sedation handbook. St. Louis, Mosby, 1997, pp. 551–552.

TABLE 6-10

ORDERS FOR PATIENT-CONTROLLED ANALGESIA

Drug	Basal Rate (mcg/kg/hr)	Bolus Dose (mcg/kg)	Lockout Period (min)	Boluses (hr)	Max Dose (mcg/kg/hr)
Morphine	10–30	10–30	6–10	4–6	100–150
Hydromorphone	3–5	3–5	6–10	4–6	15–20
Fentanyl	0.5–1	0.5–10	6–10	2–3	2–4

Data from Yaster M, Cote C, Krane E, et al: Pediatric pain management and sedation handbook. St. Louis, Mosby, 1997, p. 100.

C. Routes of Administration

IV, subcutaneous, or epidural

D. Agents (Table 6-10)

E. Complications

1. Pruritus, nausea, constipation, urine retention, excessive drowsiness, respiratory depression
2. Consider a low-dose naloxone (Narcan) infusion (0.25 mcg/kg/hr) to reduce pruritus and nausea[14]

VI. OPIOID TAPERING[4]

A. Indication

Tapering schedule is required if the patient has received frequent opioid analgesics for >5–10 days due to development of dependence and potential for withdrawal

B. Withdrawal

1. See Box 18-1 for symptoms of opiate withdrawal
2. Onset of signs and symptoms: 6–12 hours after last dose of morphine, 36–48 hours after last dose of methadone
3. Duration: 7–14 days; peak intensity reached within 2–4 days

C. Guidelines

1. **Conversion:** Convert all drugs to a single equi-analgesic member of that group (Table 6-11)
2. **PCA wean:** Change drug dosing from continuous/intermittent IV infusion to oral (PO) bolus therapy around the clock. If on PCA, administer first PO dose, then stop basal infusion 30–60 minutes later. Keep bolus doses, but reduce by 25%–50%. Discontinue PCA if no boluses are required in next 6 hours, increase PO dose, or add adjuvant analgesic (e.g., NSAID)
3. Slow dose decrease: During an intermittent IV/PO wean, decrease total daily dose by 10%–20% of original dose every 1–2 days (e.g., to taper a morphine dose of 40 mg/day, decrease the daily dose by 4–8 mg every 1–2 days)

4. **Oral regimen:** If not done previously, convert IV dosing to equivalent PO administration 1–2 days before discharge, and continue titration as outlined previously
5. **Adjunctive therapy:** α_2 agonists (e.g., clonidine, dexmedetomidine)
   a. Clonidine in combination with opioid has been shown to decrease the length of time needed for opioid weaning in neonatal abstinence syndrome with few short term side effects. Long term safety has yet to be thoroughly investigated[15]
   b. Limited data exist evaluating use of oral clonidine in iatrogenic opioid abstinence syndrome in critically ill patients, but both transdermal clonidine and dexmedetomidine have shown promise[16]
   c. Several studies have examined the use of clonidine in treating opioid dependence but insufficient data exist to support its routine use outside of possibly the neonatal setting[17]

D. Examples (Box 6-3)

6

TABLE 6-11

RELATIVE POTENCIES AND EQUIVALENCE OF OPIOIDS

Drug	Morphine Equivalence Ratio	IV Dose (mg/kg)	Equivalent PO Dose (mg/kg)
Meperidine	0.1	1	1.5–2
Methadone	0.25–1	0.1	0.1
Morphine	1	0.1	0.3–0.5
Hydromorphone	5–7	0.015	0.02–0.1
Fentanyl	80–100	0.001	NA

NOTE: Removing a transdermal fentanyl patch does not stop opioid uptake from the skin, and fentanyl will continue to be absorbed for 12–24 hr after patch removal; fentanyl 25-mcg patch administers 25 mcg/hr of fentanyl.

NA, not applicable.

From Yaster M, Cote C, Krane E, et al: Pediatric pain management and sedation handbook. St. Louis, Mosby, 1997, p. 40.

BOX 6-3

EXAMPLES OF OPIOID TAPERING

EXAMPLE 1

Patient on morphine PCA to be converted to PO morphine with home weaning.

For example: Morphine PCA basal rate = 2 mg/hr, average bolus rate = 0.5 mg/hr

Step 1: Calculate daily dose: Basal + bolus = (2 mg/hr × 24 hr) + (0.5 mg/hr × 24 hr) = 60 mg IV morphine

Step 2: Convert according to drug potency: Morphine IV/morphine oral = approx 3:1 potency. 3 × 60 mg = 180 mg PO morphine

Step 3: Prescribe 90 mg bid or 60 mg tid; wean 10%–20% of original dose (30 mg) every 1–2 days

Continued

BOX 6-3

EXAMPLES OF OPIOID TAPERING (Continued)

Example 2

Patient on morphine PCA to be converted to transdermal fentanyl. Morphine PCA basal rate = 2 mg/hr. No boluses.

Step 1: Convert according to drug potency: Fentanyl/morphine = approx 100:1 potency; 2 mg/hr morphine = 2000 mcg/hr morphine = 20 mcg/hr fentanyl

Step 2: Prescribe 25 mcg fentanyl patch (delivers 25 mcg/hr fentanyl)

Step 3: Stop IV morphine 8 hr after patch is applied; prescribe second patch at 72 hr

Step 4: Prescribe PRN IV morphine with caution

IV, Intravenous; PCA, patient-controlled analgesia; PO, by mouth; PRN, as needed.
Data from Yaster M, Cote C, Krane E, et al: Pediatric pain management and sedation handbook. St. Louis, Mosby, 1997, pp. 29–50.

REFERENCES

1. Yaster M, Cote C, Krane E, et al. *Pediatric pain management and sedation handbook*. St. Louis: Mosby; 1997.
2. Manworren R, Hynan L. Clinical validation of FLACC: preverbal patient pain scale. *Pediatr Nurs* 2003;29(2):140–146.
3. Malviya S, Voepel-Lewis T. The revised FLACC observational pain tool: improved reliability and validity for pain assessment in children with cognitive impairment. *Paediatr Anaesth* 2006;16(3):258–265.
4. Yaster M, Maxwell LG. Pediatric regional anesthesia. *Anesthesiology* 1989;70:324–338.
5. St. Germain Brent A. The management of pain in the emergency department. *Pediatr Clin North Am* 2000;47(3):651–679.
6. Krauss B, Green S. Procedural sedation and analgesia in children. *Lancet* 2006;367:766–780.
7. Krauss B, Green SM. Sedation and analgesia for procedures in children. *N Engl J Med* 2000;342:938.
8. Zempsky W, Cravero J. Relief of pain and anxiety in pediatric patients in emergency medical systems. *Pediatrics* 2004;114(5):1348–1356.
9. Stevens B, Yamada J, Ohlsson A. Sucrose for analgesia in newborn infants undergoing painful procedures (review). *The Cochrane Library* 2010;Issue 1.
10. Harrison D, Stevens B, Bueno M, et al. Efficacy of sweet solutions for analgesia in infants between 1 and 12 months of age: a systematic review. *Arch Dis Child* 2010;95:406–413.
11. Cote CJ, Lerman J, Todres ID. *A practice of anesthesia for infants and children*. 4th ed. Philadelphia: WB Saunders; 2008.
12. Agrawal D, Manzi SF, Gupta R, Krauss B. Preprocedural fasting state and adverse events in children undergoing procedural sedation and analgesia in a pediatric emergency department. *Ann Emerg Med* 2003;42:636–646.
13. American Academy of Pediatrics Committee on Drugs. Guidelines for monitoring and management of pediatric patients during and after sedation for diagnostic and therapeutic procedures: an update. *Pediatrics* 2006;118(6):2587–2602.
14. Maxwell LG, Kaufmann SC, Bitzer S, et al. The effects of a small-dose naloxone infusion on opioid-induced side effects and analgesia in children and

adolescents treated with intravenous patient-controlled analgesia: a double-blind, prospective, randomized, controlled study. *Anesth Analg* 2005;100: 953–958.

15. Agthe AG, Kim GR, Mathias KB, et al. Clonidine as an adjunct therapy to opioids for neonatal abstinence syndrome: a randomized, controlled trial. *Pediatrics* 2009;123(5):e849–e856.
16. Honey BL, Benefield RJ, Miller JL, et al. α2-Receptor agonists for treatment and prevention of iatrogenic opioid abstinence syndrome in critically ill patients. *Ann Pharmacother* 2009;43(9):1506–1511.
17. Gowing L, Farrell M, Ali R, et al. Alpha-2 adrenergic agonists for the management of opioid withdrawal (review). *The Cochrane Library* 2009;3.

Chapter 7

Cardiology

Elaine Giannakos Lennox, MD

See additional content on Expert Consult

I. WEBSITES

Heart and stroke encyclopedia: http://www.americanheart.org
http://www.cincinnatichildrens.org/health/heart-encyclopedia/anomalies/
http://www.pted.org
http://www.murmurlab.org

II. THE CARDIAC CYCLE (FIG. 7-1)

III. PHYSICAL EXAMINATION

A. Blood Pressure

1. **Blood pressure:**
a. Four limb blood pressure measurements can be used to assess for coarctation of the aorta; pressure must be measured in both the right and left arms because of the possibility of an aberrant right subclavian artery
b. Pulsus paradoxus: An exaggeration of the normal drop in systolic blood pressure (SBP) seen with inspiration. Determine the SBP at the end of exhalation and then during inhalation; if the difference is >10 mmHg, consider pericardial effusion, tamponade, pericarditis, severe asthma, or restrictive cardiomyopathies
c. Blood pressure norms[1,2]: Tables 7-1 and 7-2; Figures 7-2 and 7-3
2. **Pulse pressure** = systolic pressure – diastolic pressure
a. Wide pulse pressure (>40 mmHg): Differential diagnosis includes aortic insufficiency, arteriovenous fistula, patent ductus arteriosus, thyrotoxicosis
b. Narrow pulse pressure (<25 mmHg): Differential diagnosis includes aortic stenosis, pericardial effusion, pericardial tamponade, pericarditis, significant tachycardia
3. **Mean arterial pressure (MAP)** = diastolic pressure + (pulse pressure/3). In preterm infants and newborns, generally a normal MAP = gestational age in weeks + 5

See Figure 7-4 for systolic blood pressure norms in preterm infants

B. Heart Sounds

1. S_1: Associated with closure of mitral and tricuspid valves; best heard at the apex or left lower sternal border (LLSB)

Text continued on page 164

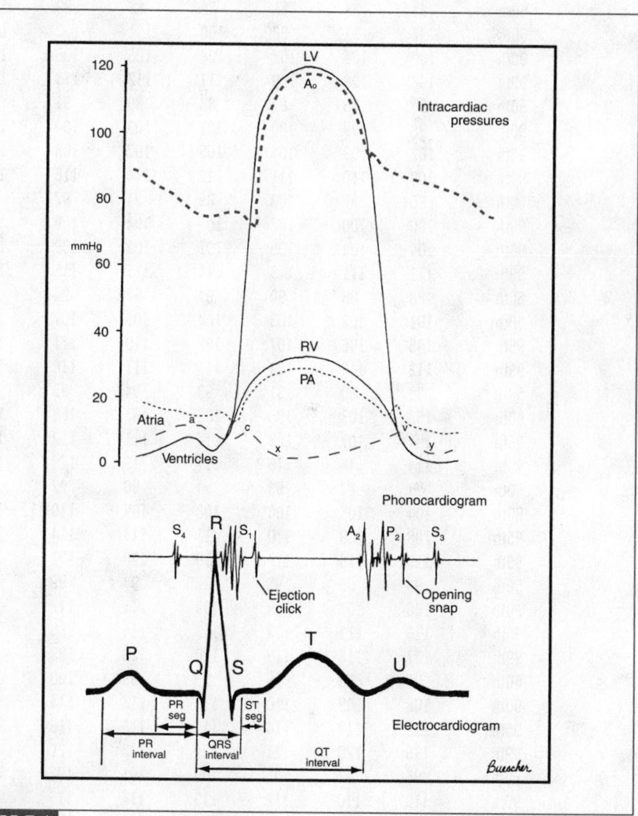

FIGURE 7-1
The cardiac cycle.

TABLE 7-1

BLOOD PRESSURE LEVELS FOR THE 50TH, 90TH, 95TH, AND 99TH PERCENTILES OF BLOOD PRESSURE FOR GIRLS AGE 1–17 YEARS BY PERCENTILES OF HEIGHT[2]

		SBP, mmHg						
		Percentile of Height*						
Age, y	**BP Percentile†**	**5th**	**10th**	**25th**	**50th**	**75th**	**90th**	**95th**
1	50th	83	84	85	86	88	89	90
	90th	97	97	98	100	101	102	103
	95th	100	101	102	104	105	106	107
	99th	108	108	109	111	112	113	114
2	50th	85	85	87	88	89	91	91
	90th	98	99	100	101	103	104	105
	95th	102	103	104	105	107	108	109
	99th	109	110	111	112	114	115	116
3	50th	86	87	88	89	91	92	93
	90th	100	100	102	103	104	106	106
	95th	104	104	105	107	108	109	110
	99th	111	111	113	114	115	116	117
4	50th	88	88	90	91	92	94	94
	90th	101	102	103	104	106	107	108
	95th	105	106	107	108	110	111	112
	99th	112	113	114	115	117	118	119
5	50th	89	90	91	93	94	95	96
	90th	103	103	105	106	107	109	109
	95th	107	107	108	110	111	112	113
	99th	114	114	116	117	118	120	120
6	50th	91	92	93	94	96	97	98
	90th	104	105	106	108	109	110	111
	95th	108	109	110	111	113	114	115
	99th	115	116	117	119	120	121	122
7	50th	93	93	95	96	97	99	99
	90th	106	107	108	109	111	112	113
	95th	110	111	112	113	115	116	116
	99th	117	118	119	120	122	123	124
8	50th	95	95	96	98	99	100	101
	90th	108	109	110	111	113	114	114
	95th	112	112	114	115	116	118	118
	99th	119	120	121	122	123	125	125
9	50th	96	97	98	100	101	102	103
	90th	110	110	112	113	114	116	116
	95th	114	114	115	117	118	119	120
	99th	121	121	123	124	125	127	127

DBP, mmHg						
Percentile of Height*						
5th	10th	25th	50th	75th	90th	95th
38	39	39	40	41	41	42
52	53	53	54	55	55	56
56	57	57	58	59	59	60
64	64	65	65	66	67	67
43	44	44	45	46	46	47
57	58	58	59	60	61	61
61	62	62	63	64	65	65
69	69	70	70	71	72	72
47	48	48	49	50	50	51
61	62	62	63	64	64	65
65	66	66	67	68	68	69
73	73	74	74	75	76	76
50	50	51	52	52	53	54
64	64	65	66	67	67	68
68	68	69	70	71	71	72
76	76	76	77	78	79	79
52	53	53	54	55	55	56
66	67	67	68	69	69	70
70	71	71	72	73	73	74
78	78	79	79	80	81	81
54	54	55	56	56	57	58
68	68	69	70	70	71	72
72	72	73	74	74	75	76
80	80	80	81	82	83	83
55	56	56	57	58	58	59
69	70	70	71	72	72	73
73	74	74	75	76	76	77
81	81	82	82	83	84	84
57	57	57	58	59	60	60
71	71	71	72	73	74	74
75	75	75	76	77	78	78
82	82	83	83	84	85	86
58	58	58	59	60	61	61
72	72	72	73	74	75	75
76	76	76	77	78	79	79
83	83	84	84	85	86	87

Continued

TABLE 7-1

BLOOD PRESSURE LEVELS FOR THE 50TH, 90TH, 95TH, AND 99TH PERCENTILES OF BLOOD PRESSURE FOR GIRLS AGE 1–17 YEARS BY PERCENTILES OF HEIGHT[2] (Continued)

		SBP, mmHg						
		Percentile of Height*						
Age, y	BP Percentile†	5th	10th	25th	50th	75th	90th	95th
10	50th	98	99	100	102	103	104	105
	90th	112	112	114	115	116	118	118
	95th	116	116	117	119	120	121	122
	99th	123	123	125	126	127	129	129
11	50th	100	101	102	103	105	106	107
	90th	114	114	116	117	118	119	120
	95th	118	118	119	121	122	123	124
	99th	125	125	126	128	129	130	131
12	50th	102	103	104	105	107	108	109
	90th	116	116	117	119	120	121	122
	95th	119	120	121	123	124	125	126
	99th	127	127	128	130	131	132	133
13	50th	104	105	106	107	109	110	110
	90th	117	118	119	121	122	123	124
	95th	121	122	123	124	126	127	128
	99th	128	129	130	132	133	134	135
14	50th	106	106	107	109	110	111	112
	90th	119	120	121	122	124	125	125
	95th	123	123	125	126	127	129	129
	99th	130	131	132	133	135	136	136
15	50th	107	108	109	110	111	113	113
	90th	120	121	122	123	125	126	127
	95th	124	125	126	127	129	130	131
	99th	131	132	133	134	136	137	138
16	50th	108	108	110	111	112	114	114
	90th	121	122	123	124	126	127	128
	95th	125	126	127	128	130	131	132
	99th	132	133	134	135	137	138	139
17	50th	108	109	110	111	113	114	115
	90th	122	122	123	125	126	127	128
	95th	125	126	127	129	130	131	132
	99th	133	133	134	136	137	138	139

*Height percentile determined by standard growth curves.

†Blood pressure percentile determined by a single measurement.

Adapted from National High Blood Pressure Education Program Working Group on High Blood Pressure in Children and Adolescents: The fourth report on the diagnosis, evaluation, and treatment of high blood pressure in children and adolescents. Pediatrics 2004;114(2 Suppl):555–576.

DBP, mmHg						
Percentile of Height*						
5th	10th	25th	50th	75th	90th	95th
59	59	59	60	61	62	62
73	73	73	74	75	76	76
77	77	77	78	79	80	80
84	84	85	86	86	87	88
60	60	60	61	62	63	63
74	74	74	75	76	77	77
78	78	78	79	80	81	81
85	85	86	87	87	88	89
61	61	61	62	b3	64	64
75	75	75	76	77	78	78
79	79	79	80	81	82	82
86	86	87	88	88	89	90
62	62	62	63	64	65	65
76	76	76	77	78	79	79
80	80	80	81	82	83	83
87	87	88	89	89	90	91
63	63	63	64	65	66	66
77	77	77	78	79	80	80
81	81	81	82	83	84	84
88	88	89	90	90	91	92
64	64	64	65	66	67	67
78	78	78	79	80	81	81
82	82	82	83	84	85	85
89	89	90	91	91	92	93
64	64	65	66	66	67	68
78	78	79	80	81	81	82
82	82	83	84	85	85	86
90	90	90	91	92	93	93
64	65	65	66	67	67	68
78	79	79	80	81	81	82
82	83	83	84	85	85	86
90	90	91	91	92	93	93

TABLE 7-2

BLOOD PRESSURE LEVELS FOR THE 50TH, 90TH, 95TH, AND 99TH PERCENTILES OF BLOOD PRESSURE FOR BOYS AGE 1–17 YEARS BY PERCENTILES OF HEIGHT[2]

		SBP, mmHg Percentile of Height*						
Age, y	**BP Percentile[†]**	**5th**	**10th**	**25th**	**50th**	**75th**	**90th**	**95th**
1	50th	80	81	83	85	87	88	89
	90th	94	95	97	99	100	102	103
	95th	98	99	101	103	104	106	106
	99th	105	106	108	110	112	113	114
2	50th	84	85	87	88	90	92	92
	90th	97	99	100	102	104	105	106
	95th	101	102	104	106	108	109	110
	99th	109	110	111	113	115	117	117
3	50th	86	87	89	91	93	94	95
	90th	100	101	103	105	107	108	109
	95th	104	105	107	109	110	112	113
	99th	111	112	114	116	118	119	120
4	50th	88	89	91	93	95	96	97
	90th	102	103	105	107	109	110	111
	95th	106	107	109	111	112	114	115
	99th	113	114	116	118	120	121	122
5	50th	90	91	93	95	96	98	98
	90th	104	105	106	108	110	111	112
	95th	108	109	110	112	114	115	116
	99th	115	116	118	120	121	123	123
6	50th	91	92	94	96	98	99	100
	90th	105	166	108	110	111	113	113
	95th	109	110	112	114	115	117	117
	99th	116	117	119	121	123	124	125
7	50th	92	94	95	97	99	100	101
	90th	106	107	109	111	113	114	115
	95th	110	111	113	115	117	118	119
	99th	117	118	120	122	124	125	126
8	50th	94	95	97	99	100	102	102
	90th	107	109	110	112	114	115	116
	95th	111	112	114	116	118	119	120
	99th	119	120	122	123	125	127	127
9	50th	95	96	98	100	102	103	104
	90th	109	110	112	114	115	117	118
	95th	113	114	116	118	119	121	121
	99th	120	121	123	125	127	128	129

DBP, mmHg						
Percentile of Height*						
5th	10th	25th	50th	75th	90th	95th
34	35	36	37	38	39	39
49	50	51	52	53	53	54
54	54	55	56	57	58	58
61	62	63	64	65	66	66
39	40	41	42	43	44	44
54	55	56	57	58	58	59
59	59	60	61	62	63	63
66	67	68	69	70	71	71
44	44	45	46	47	48	48
59	59	60	61	62	63	63
63	63	64	65	66	67	67
71	71	72	73	74	75	75
47	48	49	50	51	51	52
62	63	64	65	66	66	67
66	67	68	69	70	71	71
74	75	76	77	78	78	79
50	51	52	53	54	55	55
65	66	67	68	69	69	70
69	70	71	72	73	74	74
77	78	79	80	81	81	82
53	53	54	55	56	57	57
68	68	69	70	71	72	72
72	72	73	74	75	76	76
80	80	81	82	83	84	84
55	55	56	57	58	59	59
70	70	71	72	73	74	74
74	74	75	76	77	78	78
82	82	83	84	85	86	86
56	57	58	59	60	60	61
71	72	72	73	74	75	76
75	76	77	78	79	79	80
83	84	85	86	87	87	88
57	58	59	60	61	61	62
72	73	74	75	76	76	77
76	77	78	79	80	81	81
84	85	86	87	88	88	89

Continued

TABLE 7-2

BLOOD PRESSURE LEVELS FOR THE 50TH, 90TH, 95TH, AND 99TH PERCENTILES OF BLOOD PRESSURE FOR BOYS AGE 1–17 YEARS BY PERCENTILES OF HEIGHT[2] (Continued)

		SBP, mmHg						
		Percentile of Height*						
Age, y	BP Percentile[†]	5th	10th	25th	50th	75th	90th	95th
10	50th	97	98	100	102	103	105	106
	90th	111	112	114	115	117	119	119
	95th	115	116	117	119	121	122	123
	99th	122	123	125	127	128	130	130
11	50th	99	100	102	104	105	107	107
	90th	113	114	115	117	119	120	121
	95th	117	118	119	121	123	124	125
	99th	124	125	127	129	130	132	132
12	50th	101	102	104	106	108	109	110
	90th	115	116	118	120	121	123	123
	95th	119	120	122	123	125	127	127
	99th	126	127	129	131	133	134	135
13	50th	104	105	106	108	110	111	112
	90th	117	118	120	122	124	125	126
	95th	121	122	124	126	128	129	130
	99th	128	130	131	133	135	136	137
14	50th	106	107	109	111	113	114	115
	90th	120	121	123	125	126	128	128
	95th	124	125	127	128	130	132	132
	99th	131	132	134	136	138	139	140
15	50th	109	110	112	113	115	117	117
	90th	122	124	125	127	129	130	131
	95th	126	127	129	131	133	134	135
	99th	134	135	136	138	140	142	142
16	50th	111	112	114	116	118	119	120
	90th	125	126	128	130	131	133	134
	95th	129	130	132	134	135	137	137
	99th	136	137	139	141	143	144	145
17	50th	114	115	116	118	120	121	122
	90th	127	128	130	132	134	135	136
	95th	131	232	134	136	138	139	140
	99th	139	140	141	143	145	146	147

*Height percentile determined by standard growth curves.

[†]Blood pressure percentile determined by a single measurement.

Adapted from National High Blood Pressure Education Program Working Group on High Blood Pressure in Children and Adolescents: The fourth report on the diagnosis, evaluation, and treatment of high blood pressure in children and adolescents. Pediatrics 2004;114(2 Suppl):555–576.

DBP, mmHg						
Percentile of Height*						
5th	10th	25th	50th	75th	90th	95th
58	59	60	61	61	62	63
73	73	74	75	76	77	78
77	78	79	80	81	81	82
85	86	86	88	88	89	90
59	59	60	61	62	63	63
74	74	75	76	77	78	78
78	78	79	80	81	82	82
86	86	87	88	89	90	90
59	60	61	62	63	63	64
74	75	75	76	77	78	79
78	79	80	81	82	82	83
86	87	88	89	90	90	91
60	60	61	62	63	64	64
75	75	76	77	78	79	79
79	79	80	81	82	83	83
87	87	88	89	90	91	91
60	61	62	63	64	65	65
75	76	77	78	79	79	80
80	80	81	82	83	84	84
87	88	89	90	91	92	92
61	62	63	64	65	66	66
76	77	78	79	80	80	81
81	81	82	83	84	85	85
88	89	90	91	92	93	93
63	63	64	65	66	67	67
78	78	79	80	81	82	82
82	83	83	84	85	86	87
90	90	91	92	93	94	94
65	66	66	67	68	69	70
80	80	81	82	83	84	84
84	85	86	87	87	88	89
92	93	93	94	95	96	97

7

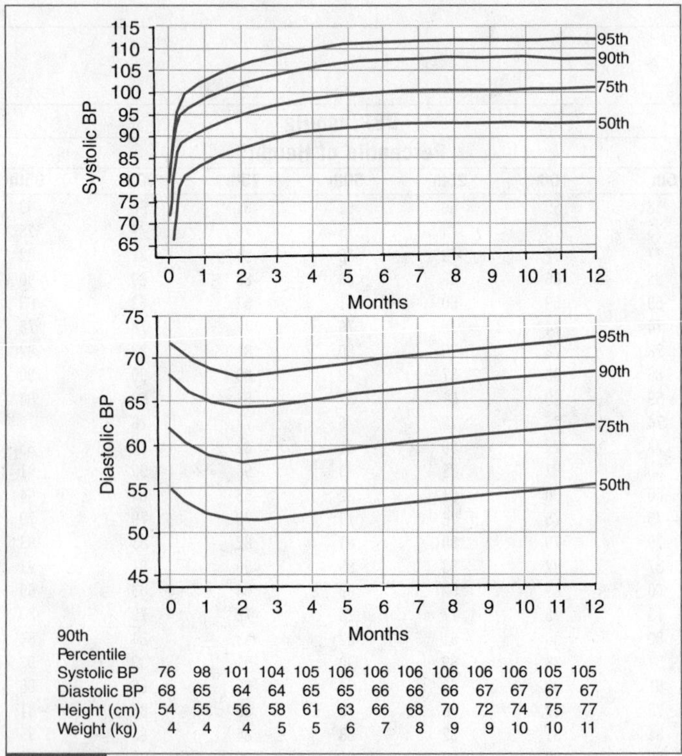

90th Percentile													
Systolic BP	76	98	101	104	105	106	106	106	106	106	106	105	105
Diastolic BP	68	65	64	64	65	65	66	66	66	67	67	67	67
Height (cm)	54	55	56	58	61	63	66	68	70	72	74	75	77
Weight (kg)	4	4	4	5	5	6	7	8	9	9	10	10	11

FIGURE 7-2

Age-specific percentiles of blood pressure (BP) measurements in boys from birth to 12 months of age; Korotkoff phase IV (K4) used for diastolic BP. *(From Task Force on Blood Pressure Control in Children: Report of the Second Task Force on Blood Pressure Control in Children. Pediatrics 1987;79[1]:1–25.)*

2. S_2: Associated with closure of pulmonary and aortic valves, heard best at the left upper sternal border (LUSB) and has normal physiologic splitting that increases with inspiration
3. S_3: Heard best at the apex or LLSB
4. S_4: Heard at the apex

See Box 7-1 for abnormal heart sounds.[3]

C. Systolic and Diastolic Sounds

1. **Ejection click:** Sounds like splitting of S_1 but is most audible at the apex, in contrast to the normal finding of a split S_1, which is best heard at the LLSB. May also be heard at the LUSB with valvular pulmonary stenosis (PS). Associated with stenosis of the semilunar

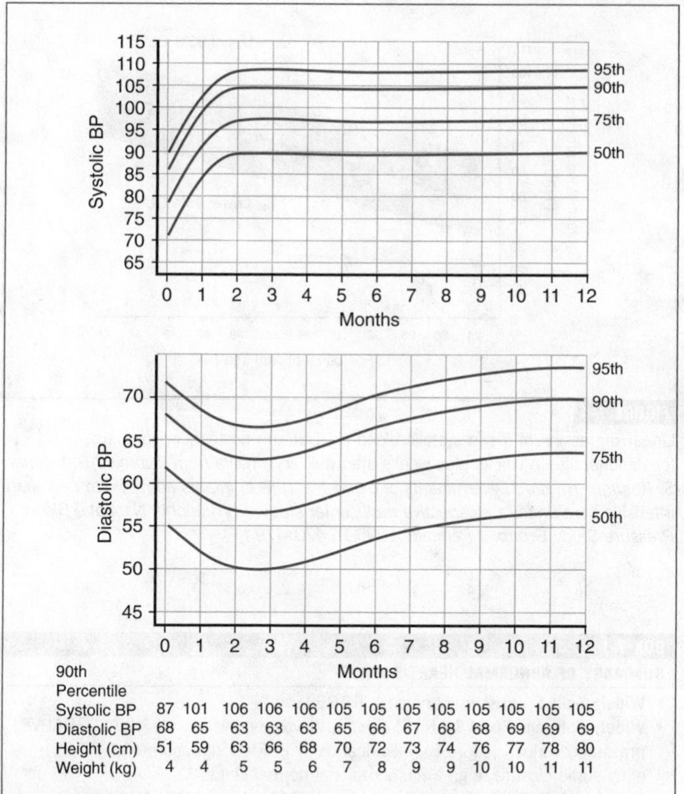

90th Percentile	0	1	2	3	4	5	6	7	8	9	10	11	12
Systolic BP	87	101	106	106	106	105	105	105	105	105	105	105	105
Diastolic BP	68	65	63	63	63	65	66	67	68	68	69	69	69
Height (cm)	51	59	63	66	68	70	72	73	74	76	77	78	80
Weight (kg)	4	4	5	5	6	7	8	9	9	10	10	11	11

FIGURE 7-3

Age-specific percentile of blood pressure (BP) measurements in girls from birth to 12 months of age; Korotkoff phase IV (K4) used for diastolic BP. *(From Task Force on Blood Pressure Control in Children: Report of the Second Task Force on Blood Pressure Control in Children. Pediatrics 1987;79[1]:1–25.)*

valves and large great arteries (e.g., systemic hypertension; pulmonary hypertension; idiopathic dilation of the pulmonary artery; tetralogy of Fallot [TOF], in which the aorta is dilated; and persistent truncus arteriosus)

2. **Midsystolic click with or without a late systolic murmur:** Heard near the apex in mitral valve prolapse
3. **Diastolic opening snap:** Audible at the apex or LLSB in mitral stenosis

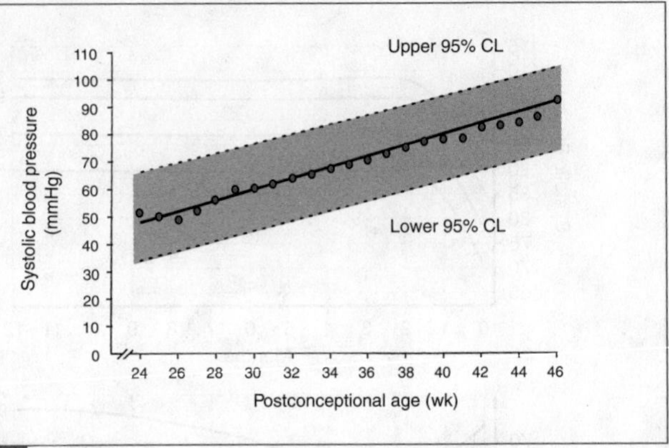

FIGURE 7-4

Linear regression of mean systolic blood pressure on postconceptional age (gestational age in weeks plus weeks after delivery). *(Data from Zubrow AB, Hulman S, Kushner H, et al: Determinants of blood pressure in infants admitted to neonatal intensive care units: a prospective multicenter study. Philadelphia Neonatal Blood Pressure Study Group. J Perinatol 1995;15:470–479.)*

BOX 7-1

SUMMARY OF ABNORMAL HEART SOUNDS

- **Widely Split S_1:** Ebstein's anomaly, RBBB
- **Widely Split and Fixed S_2:** Right ventricular volume overload (e.g., ASD, PAPVR), pressure overload (e.g., PS), electrical delay in RV contraction (e.g., RBBB), early aortic closure (e.g., MR), occasional normal child
- **Narrowly Split S_2:** Pulmonary hypertension, AS, delay in LV contraction (e.g., LBBB), occasional normal child
- **Single S_2:** Pulmonary hypertension, one semilunar valve (e.g., pulmonary atresia, aortic atresia, truncus arteriosus), P2 not audible (e.g., TGA, TOF, severe PS), severe AS, occasional normal child
- **Paradoxically Split S_2:** Severe AS, LBBB, Wolff-Parkinson-White syndrome (type B)
- **Abnormal Intensity of P2:** Increased P2 (e.g., pulmonary hypertension), decreased P2 (e.g., severe PS, TOF, TS)
- **S_3:** Occasionally heard in healthy children or adults, or may indicate dilated ventricles (e.g., large VSD, CHF)
- **S_4:** Always pathologic, decreased ventricular compliance

AS, Aortic stenosis; ASD, atrial septal defect; LBBB, left bundle-branch block; MR, mitral regurgitation; PAPVR, partial anomalous pulmonary venous return; PS, pulmonary stenosis; RBBB, right bundle-branch block; TGA, transposition of the great arteries; TOF, tetralogy of Fallot; TS, tricuspid stenosis.

Modified from Park MK: Pediatric cardiology for practitioners, 5th ed. St. Louis, Mosby, 2008, p. 25.

D. Murmurs[4] (http://www.murmurlab.org)

1. **Benign heart murmurs:** Caused by a disturbance of the laminar flow of blood, frequently produced as the diameter of the blood's pathway decreases and the velocity increases

a. Present in more than 80% of children sometime during childhood, most commonly beginning at age 3 to 4 years

b. Accentuated in high-output states, especially with fever and anemia

c. Normal electrocardiogram (ECG) and radiographic findings

NOTE: ECG and chest radiograph are not routinely useful or cost-effective screening tools for distinguishing benign from pathologic murmurs.

d. Clinical characteristics summarized in Table 7-3[3]

2. **Likely pathologic murmur** when one or more of the following are present: Symptoms; cyanosis; systolic murmur that is loud (grade ≥3/6), harsh, pansystolic, or long in duration; diastolic murmur; abnormal heart sounds; presence of a click; abnormally strong or weak pulses

3. **Systolic and diastolic heart murmurs** (Box 7-2)

7

TABLE 7-3

COMMON INNOCENT HEART MURMURS

Type (Timing)	Description of Murmur	Age Group
Classic vibratory murmur (Still's murmur; systolic)	Maximal at LMSB or between LLSB and apex Grade 2–3/6 in intensity Low-frequency vibratory, twanging string, groaning, squeaking, or musical	3–6 yr; occasionally in infancy
Pulmonary ejection murmur (systolic)	Maximal at LUSB Early to midsystolic Grade 1–3/6 in intensity Blowing in quality	8–14 yr
Pulmonary flow murmur of newborn (systolic)	Maximal at LUSB Transmits well to left and right chest, axilla, and back Grade 1–2/6 in intensity	Premature and full-term newborns Usually disappears by 3–6 mo
Venous hum (continuous)	Maximal at right (or left) supraclavicular and infraclavicular areas Grade 1–3/6 in intensity Inaudible in supine position Intensity changes with rotation of head and disappears with compression of jugular vein	3–6 yr
Carotid bruit (systolic)	Right supraclavicular area over carotids Grade 2–3/6 in intensity Occasional thrill over carotid	Any age

LLSB, Left lower sternal border; LMSB, left middle sternal border; LUSB, left upper sternal border.
From Park MK: Pediatric cardiology for practitioners, 5th ed. St. Louis, Mosby, 2008, p. 36.

BOX 7-2

SYSTOLIC AND DIASTOLIC HEART MURMURS

RUSB

Aortic valve stenosis (supravalvar, subvalvar)
Aortic regurgitation

LUSB

Pulmonary valve stenosis
Atrial septal defect
Pulmonary ejection murmur, innocent
Pulmonary flow murmur of newborn
Pulmonary artery stenosis
Aortic stenosis
Coarctation of the aorta
Patent ductus arteriosus
Partial anomalous pulmonary venous return (PAPVR)
Total anomalous pulmonary venous return (TAPVR)
Pulmonary regurgitation

LLSB

Ventricular septal defect, including atrioventricular septal defect
Vibratory innocent murmur (Still's murmur)
HOCM (IHSS)
Tricuspid regurgitation
Tetralogy of Fallot
Tricuspid stenosis

APEX

Mitral regurgitation
Vibratory innocent murmur (Still's murmur)
Mitral valve prolapse
Aortic stenosis
HOCM (IHSS)
Mitral stenosis

The location at which various murmurs may be heard. Diastolic murmurs are in italics. HOCM, Hypertrophic obstructive cardiomyopathy; IHSS, idiopathic hypertrophic subaortic stenosis; LLSB, left lower sternal border; LUSB, left upper sternal border; RUSB, right upper sternal border. From Park MK: Pediatric cardiology for practitioners, 5th ed. St. Louis, Mosby, 2008, p. 30.

IV. LIPID MONITORING RECOMMENDATIONS (AMERICAN ACADEMY OF PEDIATRICS RECOMMENDATIONS)

A. Screening of Children and Adolescents[5]

Perform targeted screening of fasting lipid profile in children >2 years of age who fulfill one of the following criteria:

1. Parents or grandparents with premature cardiovascular disease (≤55 years of age for men and ≤65 years of age for women)
2. Parent with elevated blood cholesterol level (≥240 mg/dL) or other pattern of dyslipidemia

3. Parental history is unobtainable; particularly for those with other risk factors such as smoking, obesity/overweight, or diabetes mellitus
4. Patients with diseases that increase risk of premature cardiovascular disease (CVD): Diabetes, kidney disease, congenital/acquired heart disease, history of Kawasaki's disease, childhood cancer survivors

B. Goals for Lipid Levels in Childhood

1. **Total cholesterol**
a. Acceptable (<170 mg/dL): Repeat measurement in 3–5 years
b. Borderline (170–199 mg/dL): Repeat cholesterol and average with previous measurement. If <170 repeat in 3–5 years. If ≥170, obtain lipoprotein analysis
c. High (≥200 mg/dL): Obtain lipoprotein analysis
2. **Low-density lipoprotein (LDL) cholesterol**
a. Acceptable (<110 mg/dL)
b. Borderline (110–129 mg/dL)
c. High (≥130 mg/dL)

C. Management of Hyperlipidemia[5]

1. **Normal and borderline elevated LDL levels:** Education, risk factor intervention including diet, smoking cessation, and an exercise program. For borderline levels, reevaluate in 1 year
2. **High LDL levels:** Examine for secondary causes (liver, thyroid, renal disorders) and familial disorders. Initiate low-fat, low-cholesterol diet; reevaluate in 3 months
3. **Drug therapy:** Should be considered in children >8 years of age after failure of 6–12 month trial of diet therapy as follows:
a. LDL >190 mg/dL without other cardiovascular disease risk factors
b. LDL >160 mg/dL with risk factors (diabetes, obesity, hypertension, positive family history of premature cardiovascular disease)
c. LDL >130 mg/dL in children with diabetes mellitus
d. Bile acid sequestrants and statins are the usual first-line drugs for treatment in children
4. **Persistently high triglycerides (>150 mg/dL) and reduced HDL (<35 mg/dL):** Evaluate for secondary causes (diabetes, alcohol abuse, renal or thyroid disease). Treatment is diet and exercise

V. ELECTROCARDIOGRAPHY

A. Basic Electrocardiography Principles

1. **Lead placement** (Fig. 7-5)
2. **ECG complexes** (see Fig. 7-1)
a. P wave: Represents atrial depolarization
b. QRS complex: Represents ventricular depolarization
c. T wave: Represents ventricular repolarization
d. U wave: May follow T wave, representing late phases of ventricular repolarization

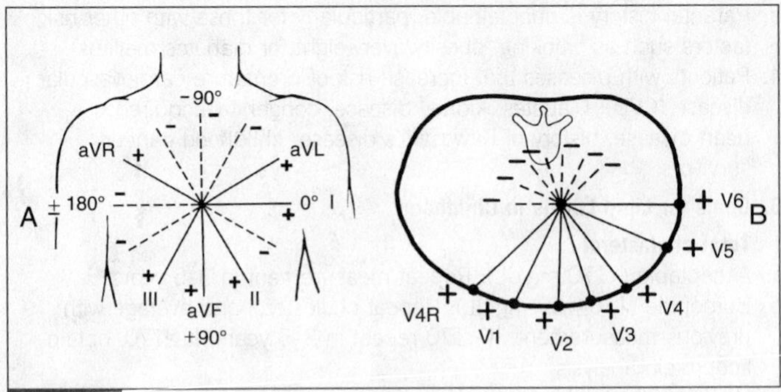

FIGURE 7-5

A, Hexaxial reference system. **B,** Horizontal reference system. *(Modified from Park MK, Guntheroth WG: How to read pediatric ECGs, 4th ed. Philadelphia, Mosby, 2006, p. 3.)*

TABLE 7-4

NORMAL PEDIATRIC ELECTROCARDIOGRAM (ECG) PARAMETERS

Age	Heart Rate (bpm)	QRS Axis*	PR Interval (sec)*	QRS Duration (sec)†
0–7 days	95–160 (125)	+30 to 180 (110)	0.08–0.12 (0.10)	0.05 (0.07)
1–3 wk	105–180 (145)	+30 to 180 (110)	0.08–0.12 (0.10)	0.05 (0.07)
1–6 mo	110–180 (145)	+10 to +125 (+70)	0.08–0.13 (0.11)	0.05 (0.07)
6–12 mo	110–170 (135)	+10 to +125 (+60)	0.10–0.14 (0.12)	0.05 (0.07)
1–3 yr	90–150 (120)	+10 to +125 (+60)	0.10–0.14 (0.12)	0.06 (0.07)
4–5 yr	65–135 (110)	0 to +110 (+60)	0.11–0.15 (0.13)	0.07 (0.08)
6–8 yr	60–130 (100)	−15 to +110 (+60)	0.12–0.16 (0.14)	0.07 (0.08)
9–11 yr	60–110 (85)	−15 to +110 (+60)	0.12–0.17 (0.14)	0.07 (0.09)
12–16 yr	60–110 (85)	−15 to +110 (+60)	0.12–0.17 (0.15)	0.07 (0.10)
>16 yr	60–100 (80)	−15 to +110 (+60)	0.12–0.20 (0.15)	0.08 (0.10)

*Normal range and (mean).

†Mean and (98th percentile).

Adapted from Park MK: Pediatric cardiology for practitioners, 5th ed. St. Louis, Mosby, 2008 and Davignon A et al: Normal ECG standards for infants and children. Pediatr Cardiol 1979;1:123–131.

3. **Systematic approach for evaluating ECGs** (Table 7-4 shows normal ECG parameters)[3,6]:
   a. Rate
      (1) Standardization: Paper speed is 25 mm/sec. One small square = 1 mm = 0.04 sec. One large square = 5 mm = 0.2 sec. Amplitude standard: 10 mm = 1 mV
      (2) Calculation: Heart rate (beats per minute) = 60 divided by the average R-R interval in seconds, or 1500 divided by the R-R interval in millimeters
   b. Rhythm
      (1) Sinus rhythm: Every QRS complex is preceded by a P wave, normal PR interval (although the PR interval may be prolonged, as in first-degree atrioventricular [AV] block), and normal P-wave axis (upright P in lead I and aVF)
      (2) There is normal respiratory variation of the R-R interval without morphologic changes of the P wave or QRS complex

Lead V_1			Lead V_6		
R Wave Amplitude (mm)†	**S Wave Amplitude (mm)†**	**R/S Ratio**	**R Wave Amplitude (mm)†**	**S Wave Amplitude (mm)†**	**R/S Ratio**
13.3 (25.5)	7.7 (18.8)	2.5	4.8 (11.8)	3.2 (9.6)	2.2
10.6 (20.8)	4.2 (10.8)	2.9	7.6 (16.4)	3.4 (9.8)	3.3
9.7 (19)	5.4 (15)	2.3	12.4 (22)	2.8 (8.3)	5.6
9.4 (20.3)	6.4 (18.1)	1.6	12.6 (22.7)	2.1 (7.2)	7.6
8.5 (18)	9 (21)	1.2	14 (23.3)	1.7 (6)	10
7.6 (16)	11 (22.5)	0.8	15.6 (25)	1.4 (4.7)	11.2
6 (13)	12 (24.5)	0.6	16.3 (26)	1.1 (3.9)	13
5.4 (12.1)	11.9 (25.4)	0.5	16.3 (25.4)	1.0 (3.9)	14.3
4.1 (9.9)	10.8 (21.2)	0.5	14.3 (23)	0.8 (3.7)	14.7
3 (9)	10 (20)	0.3	10 (20)	0.8 (3.7)	12

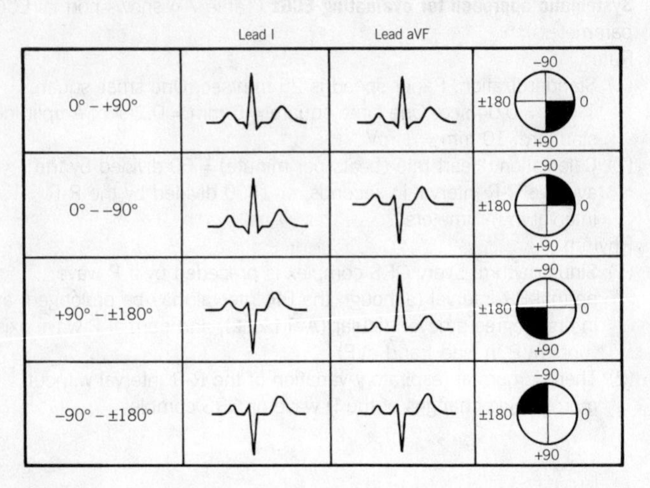

FIGURE 7-6

Locating quadrants of mean QRS axis from leads I and aVF. *(From Park MK, Guntheroth WG: How to read pediatric ECGs, 4th ed. Philadelphia, Mosby, 2006, p. 17.)*

c. Axis: Determine quadrant and compare with age-matched normal values (Fig. 7-6; see Table 7-4)
d. Intervals (PR, QRS, QTc): See Table 7-4 for normal PR and QRS intervals. The QTc is calculated using the Bazett formula

$$\text{QTc} = \text{QT (sec) measured}/\sqrt{\text{R-R}}$$

(average 3 measurements taken from same lead)

The R-R interval should extend from the R wave in the QRS complex in which you are measuring QT to the preceding R wave. Normal values for QTc are as follows:
(1) 0.44 sec is 97th percentile for infants 3 to 4 days old[7]
(2) ≤0.45 sec in all males >1 week of age and prepubescent females
(3) ≤0.46 sec for postpubescent females
e. P-wave size and shape: Normal P wave should be <0.10 sec in children, <0.08 sec in infants, with amplitude <0.3 mV (3 mm in height, with normal standardization)
f. R-wave progression: There is generally a normal increase in R-wave size and decrease in S-wave size from leads V_1 to V_6 (with dominant S waves in right precordial leads and dominant R waves in left precordial leads), representing dominance of left ventricular forces. However, newborns and infants have a normal dominance of the right ventricle

g. Q waves: Normal Q waves are usually <0.04 sec in duration and <25% of the total QRS amplitude. Q waves are <5 mm deep in left precordial leads and aVF and ≤8 mm deep in lead III for children <3 years of age
h. ST-segment and T-wave evaluation: ST-segment elevation or depression >1 mm in limb leads and >2 mm in precordial leads is consistent with myocardial ischemia or injury. Tall, peaked T waves may be seen in hyperkalemia. Flat or low T waves may be seen in hypokalemia, hypothyroidism, normal newborn, and myocardial and pericardial ischemia and inflammation (Table 7-5 and Fig. 7-7)
i. Hypertrophy/enlargement
   (1) Atrial enlargement (Fig. 7-8)
   (2) Ventricular hypertrophy: Diagnosed by QRS axis, voltage, and R/S ratio (Box 7-3; see also Table 7-4)

TABLE 7-5
NORMAL T-WAVE AXIS

Age	V_1, V_2	AVF	I, V_5, V_6
Birth–1 day	±	+	±
1–4 days	±	+	+
4 days to adolescent	–	+	+
Adolescent to adult	+	+	+

+, T wave positive; –, T wave negative; ±, T wave normally either positive or negative.

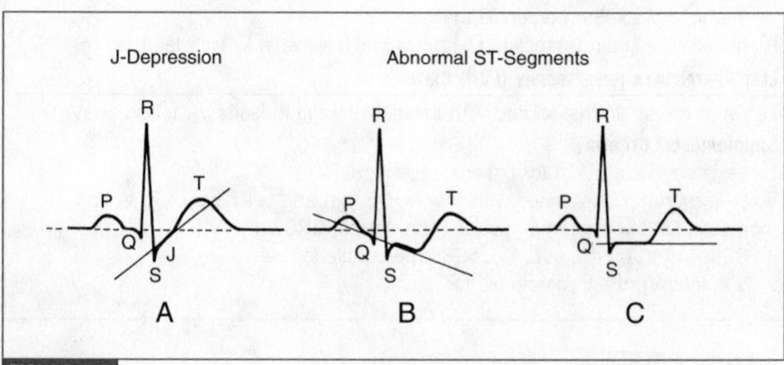

FIGURE 7-7
Nonpathologic (nonischemic) and pathologic (ischemic) ST and T changes. **A,** Characteristic nonischemic ST-segment alteration called J depression; note that the ST slope is upward. **B** and **C,** Ischemic or pathologic ST-segment alterations. **B,** Downward slope of the ST segment. **C,** Horizontal segment is sustained. *(From Park MK, Guntheroth WG: How to read pediatric ECGs, 4th ed. Philadelphia, Mosby; 2006, p. 107.)*

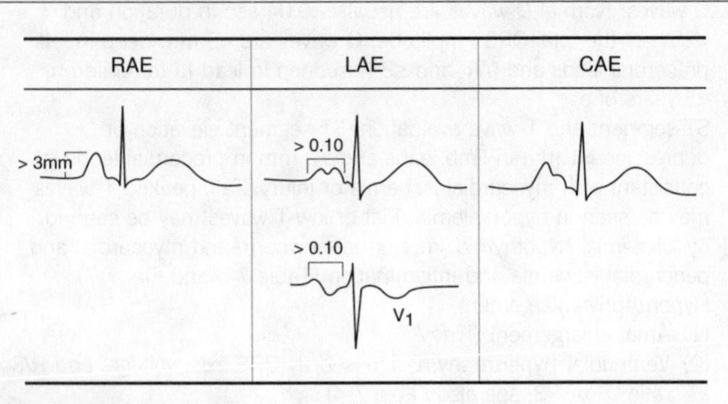

FIGURE 7-8
Criteria for atrial enlargement. CAE, combined atrial enlargement; LAE, left atrial enlargement; RAE, right atrial enlargement. *(From Park MK: Pediatric cardiology for practitioners, 5th ed. St. Louis, Mosby, 2008, p. 53.)*

BOX 7-3

VENTRICULAR HYPERTROPHY CRITERIA

RIGHT VENTRICULAR HYPERTROPHY (RVH) CRITERIA

Must Have at Least One of the Following:

Upright T wave in lead V_1 after 3 days of age to adolescence
Presence of Q wave in V_1 (QR or QRS pattern)
Increased right and anterior QRS voltage (with normal QRS duration):
- R in lead V_1, >98th percentile for age
- S in lead V_6, >98th percentile for age

Right ventricle strain (associated with inverted T wave in V_1 with tall R wave)

LEFT VENTRICULAR HYPERTROPHY (LVH) CRITERIA

Left ventricle strain (associated with inverted T wave in leads V_6, I, and/or aVF)

Supplemental Criteria

Left axis deviation (LAD) for patient's age
Volume overload (associated with Q wave >5 mm and tall T waves in V_5 or V_6)
Increased QRS voltage in left leads (with normal QRS duration):
- R in lead V_6 (and I, aVL, V_5), >98th percentile for age
- S in lead V_1, >98th percentile for age

B. ECG Abnormalities

1. Nonventricular arrhythmias (Table 7-6; Figs. 7-9 and 7-10)[8]
2. Ventricular arrhythmias (Table 7-7; Fig. 7-11)
3. Nonventricular conduction disturbances (Fig. 7-12 and Table 7-8)[9]
4. Ventricular conduction disturbances (Table 7-9)

Text continued on page 180

TABLE 7-6

NONVENTRICULAR ARRHYTHMIAS

Name/Description	Cause	Treatment
SINUS		
TACHYCARDIA		
Normal sinus rhythm with HR >95th percentile for age (usually <230 beats/min)	Hypovolemia, shock, anemia, sepsis, fever, anxiety, CHF, PE, myocardial disease, drugs (e.g., β-agonists, albuterol, caffeine, atropine)	Address underlying cause
BRADYCARDIA		
Normal sinus rhythm with HR <5th percentile for age	Normal (especially in athletic individuals), increased ICP, hypoxia, hyperkalemia, hypercalcemia, vagal stimulation, hypothyroidism, hypothermia, drugs (e.g., digoxin, β-blockers), long QT	Address underlying cause; if symptomatic, refer to inside back cover for bradycardia algorithm
SUPRAVENTRICULAR*		
PREMATURE ATRIAL CONTRACTION (PAC)		
Narrow QRS complex; ectopic focus in atria with abnormal P wave morphology	Digitalis toxicity, medications (e.g., caffeine, theophylline, sympathomimetics), normal variant	Treat digitalis toxicity; otherwise no treatment needed
ATRIAL FLUTTER		
Atrial rate 250–350 beats/min; characteristic sawtooth or flutter pattern with variable ventricular response rate and normal QRS complex	Dilated atria, previous intra-atrial surgery, valvular or ischemic heart disease, idiopathic in newborns	Synchronized cardioversion or overdrive pacing; treat underlying cause
ATRIAL FIBRILLATION		
Irregular; atrial rate 350–600 beats/min, yielding characteristic fibrillatory pattern (no discrete P waves) and irregular ventricular response rate of about 110–150 beats/min with normal QRS complex	Wolff-Parkinson-White syndrome and those listed previously for atrial flutter (except not idiopathic), alcohol exposure, familial	Synchronized cardioversion; then may need anticoagulation pretreatment
SVT		
Sudden run of three or more consecutive premature supraventricular beats at >230 beats/min, with narrow QRS complex and abnormal P wave; either sustained (>30 sec) or nonsustained	Most commonly idiopathic, but may be seen in congenital heart disease (e.g., Ebstein's anomaly, transposition)	Vagal maneuvers, adenosine; if unstable, need immediate synchronized cardioversion (0.5 j/kg up to 1 j/kg). Consult cardiologist. See "Tachycardia with Poor Perfusion" or "Tachycardia with Adequate Perfusion" algorithms in back of handbook

Continued

TABLE 7-6

NONVENTRICULAR ARRHYTHMIAS (Continued)

Name/Description	Cause	Treatment
I. AV Reentrant: Presence of accessory bypass pathway, in conjunction with AV node, establishes cyclic pattern of reentry independent of SA node; most common cause of nonsinus tachycardia in children (see Wolff-Parkinson-White syndrome, Table 7-9 and Fig. 7-10)		
II. Junctional: Automatic focus; simultaneous depolarization of atria and ventricles yields invisible P wave or retrograde P wave	Cardiac surgery, idiopathic	Adjust for clinical situation; consult cardiology
III. Ectopic atrial tachycardia: Rapid firing of ectopic focus in atrium	Idiopathic	AV nodal blockade, ablation
NODAL ESCAPE/JUNCTIONAL RHYTHM		
Abnormal rhythm driven by AV node impulse, giving normal QRS complex and invisible P wave (buried in preceding QRS or T wave) or retrograde P wave (negative in lead II, positive in aVR), seen in sinus bradycardia	Common after surgery of atria	Often requires no treatment. If rate is slow enough, may require pacemaker

*Abnormal rhythm resulting from ectopic focus in atria or AV node, or from accessory conduction pathways. Characterized by different P-wave shape and abnormal P-wave axis. QRS morphology usually normal. See Figure 7-9, 7-10.7

AV, Atrioventricular; CHF, congestive heart failure; HR, heart rate; ICP, intracranial pressure; PE, pulmonary embolism; SA, sinoatrial; SVT, supraventricular tachycardia.

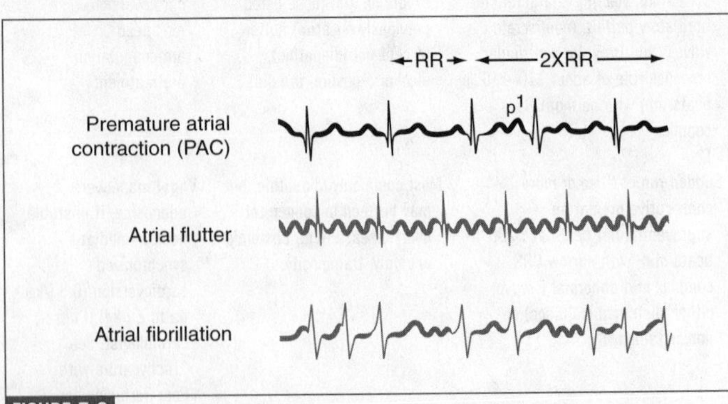

FIGURE 7-9

Supraventricular arrhythmias. p1, Premature atrial contraction. *(From Park MK, Guntheroth WG: How to read pediatric ECGs, 4th ed. Philadelphia, Mosby, 2006, p. 129.)*

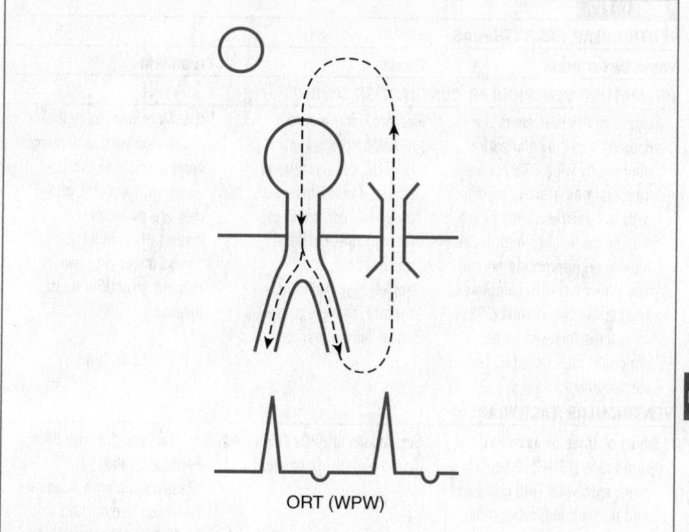

FIGURE 7-10

Supraventricular tachycardia pathway: Mechanism for orthodromic reentry (Wolff-Parkinson-White syndrome). Diagram shows the sinoatrial (SA) node (upper left circle), with the atrioventricular (AV) node (above the horizontal line) and bundle branches crossing to the ventricle (below the horizontal line). *(Adapted from Walsh EP: Cardiac arrhythmias. In Fyler DC [ed]: Nadas' pediatric cardiology. Philadelphia, Hanley & Belfus, 1992, p. 384.)*

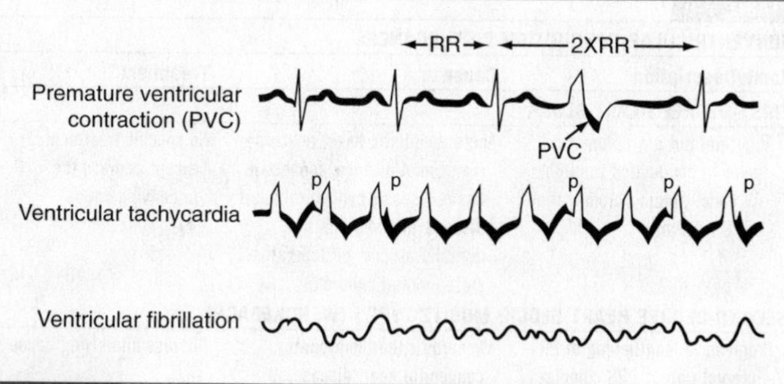

FIGURE 7-11

Ventricular arrhythmias. P, P wave. *(From Park MK, Guntheroth WG: How to read pediatric ECGs, 4th ed. Philadelphia, Mosby, 2006, p. 138.)*

TABLE 7-7

VENTRICULAR ARRHYTHMIAS

Name/Description	Cause	Treatment
PREMATURE VENTRICULAR CONTRACTION (PVC)		
Ectopic ventricular focus causing early depolarization. Abnormally wide QRS complex appears prematurely, usually with full compensatory pause. May be unifocal or multifocal. **Bigeminy:** Alternating normal and abnormal QRS complexes; **Trigeminy:** Two normal QRS complexes followed by an abnormal one. **Couplet:** Two consecutive PVCs	Myocarditis, myocardial injury, cardiomyopathy, long QT, congenital and acquired heart disease, drugs (catecholamines, theophylline, caffeine, anesthetics), MVP, anxiety, hypokalemia, hypoxia, hypomagnesemia Can be normal variant	None. More worrisome if associated with underlying heart disease or syncope, if worse with activity, or if they are multiform (especially couplets). Address underlying cause, rule out structural heart disease
VENTRICULAR TACHYCARDIA		
Series of three or more PVCs at rapid rate (120–250 beats/min), with wide QRS complex and dissociated, retrograde, or no P wave.	See causes of PVCs (70% have underlying cause)	See "Tachycardia with Poor Perfusion" and "Tachycardia with Adequate Perfusion" algorithms in back of handbook
VENTRICULAR FIBRILLATION		
Depolarization of ventricles in uncoordinated, asynchronous pattern, yielding abnormal QRS complexes of varying size and morphology with irregular, rapid rate. Rare in children.	Myocarditis, MI, postoperative state, digitalis or quinidine toxicity, catecholamines, severe hypoxia, electrolyte disturbances, long QT	Requires immediate defibrillation. See algorithm for "Asystole and Pulseless Arrest" at back of book

MI, Myocardial infarction; MVP, mitral valve prolapse.

TABLE 7-8

NONVENTRICULAR CONDUCTION DISTURBANCES

Name/Description*	Cause	Treatment
FIRST-DEGREE HEART BLOCK		
Abnormal but asymptomatic delay in conduction through AV node, yielding prolongation of PR interval	Acute rheumatic fever, tickborne (i.e., Lyme) disease, connective tissue disease, congenital heart disease, cardiomyopathy, digitalis toxicity, postoperative state, normal children	No specific treatment except address the underlying cause
SECOND-DEGREE HEART BLOCK: MOBITZ TYPE I (WENCKEBACH)		
Progressive lengthening of PR interval until a QRS complex is not conducted. Does not usually progress to complete heart block	Myocarditis, cardiomyopathy, congenital heart disease, postoperative state, MI, toxicity (digitalis, β-blocker), normal children, Lyme disease, lupus	Address underlying cause

TABLE 7-8

NONVENTRICULAR CONDUCTION DISTURBANCES (Continued)

Name/Description*	Cause	Treatment
SECOND-DEGREE HEART BLOCK: MOBITZ TYPE II		
Loss of conduction to ventricle without lengthening of the PR interval. May progress to complete heart block	Same as for Mobitz Type I	Address underlying cause; may need pacemaker
THIRD-DEGREE (COMPLETE) HEART BLOCK		
Complete dissociation of atrial and ventricular conduction. P wave and PP interval regular; RR interval regular and much slower. Width of QRS complex will be narrow and faster with underlying junctional pacemaker, wide and slower with ventricular pacemaker	Congenital due to maternal lupus or other connective tissue disease, structural heart disease; acquired (acute rheumatic fever, myocarditis, Lyme carditis, postoperative, cardiomyopathy, MI, drug overdose)	If bradycardic and symptomatic, consider pacing; see bradycardia algorithm on inside back cover

*High-degree AV block: Conduction of atrial impulse at regular intervals, yielding 2:1 block (two atrial impulses for each ventricular response), 3:1 block, etc.

AV, Atrioventricular; MI, myocardial infarction.

7

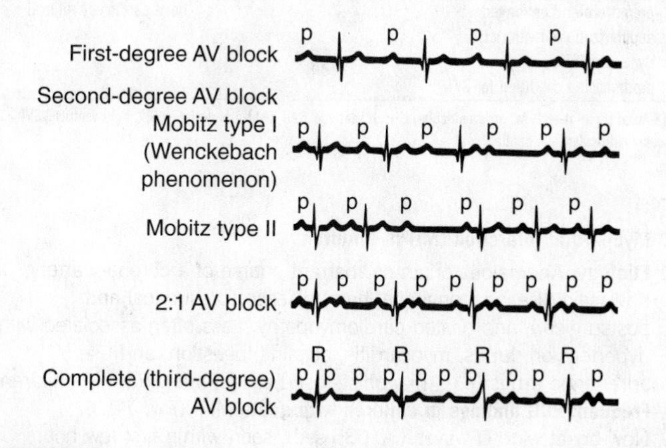

FIGURE 7-12

Conduction blocks. P, P wave; R, QRS complex. *(From Park MK, Guntheroth WG: How to read pediatric ECGs, 4th ed. Philadelphia, Mosby, 2006, p. 141.)*

TABLE 7-9

VENTRICULAR CONDUCTION DISTURBANCES

Name/Description	Criteria	Causes/Treatment
RIGHT BUNDLE-BRANCH BLOCK (RBBB)		
Delayed right bundle conduction prolongs RV depolarization time, leading to wide QRS	1. RAD 2. Prolonged or wide QRS with terminal slurred R′ (m-shaped RSR′ or RR′) in V_1, V_2, aVR 3. Wide and slurred S wave in leads I and V_6	ASD, surgery with right ventriculostomy, Ebstein's anomaly, coarctation in infants <6 mo, endocardial cushion defect, and partial anomalous pulmonary venous return; occasionally occurs in normal children
LEFT BUNDLE-BRANCH BLOCK (LBBB)		
Delayed left bundle conduction prolongs septal and LV depolarization time, leading to wide QRS with loss of usual septal signal; there is still a predominance of left ventricle forces. Rare in children	1. Wide negative QS complex in lead V_1 with loss of septal R wave 2. Entirely positive wide R or RR′ complex in lead V_6 with loss of septal Q wave	Hypertension, ischemic or valvular heart disease, cardiomyopathy
WOLFF-PARKINSON-WHITE (WPW)		
Atrial impulse transmitted via anomalous conduction pathway to ventricles, bypassing AV node and normal ventricular conduction system. Leads to premature and prolonged depolarization of ventricles. Bypass pathway is a predisposing condition for SVT.	1. Shortened PR interval 2. Delta wave 3. Wide QRS	Acute management of SVT if necessary as previously described; consider ablation of accessory pathway if recurrent SVT. All patients need cardiology referral

ASD, Atrial septal defect; AV, atrioventricular; LV, left ventricle; RAD, right axis deviation; RV, right ventricle; SVT, supraventricular tachycardia.

C. Myocardial Infarction (MI) in Children

1. **Etiology:** Anomalous origin or aberrant course of a coronary artery, Kawasaki disease, congenital heart disease (presurgical and postsurgical), and dilated cardiomyopathy. Less often associated with hypertension, lupus, myocarditis, cocaine ingestion, and use of adrenergic drugs (e.g., β-agonists used for asthma). Rare in children
2. **Frequent ECG findings in children with acute MI**[10] (Fig. 7-13):

a. New-onset wide Q waves (>0.035 sec), seen within first few hours (persist over several years)
b. ST-segment elevation (>2 mm), seen within first few hours
c. Diphasic T waves, seen within first few days (becoming sharply inverted, then normalizing over time)
d. Prolonged QTc interval (>0.44 sec) with abnormal Q waves

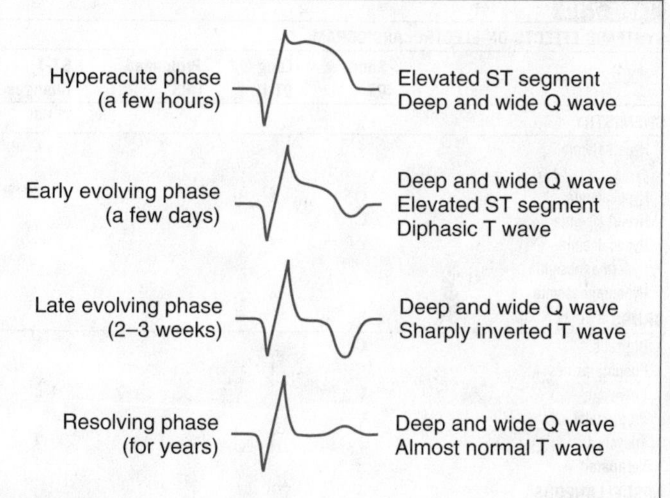

FIGURE 7-13

Sequential changes during myocardial infarction. *(From Park MK, Guntheroth WG: How to read pediatric ECGs, 4th ed. Philadelphia, Mosby, 2006, p. 115.)*

e. Deep, wide Q waves in leads I, aVL, or V_6, without Q waves in II, III, aVF, suggest anomalous origin of the left coronary artery

3. **Other criteria:**

a. Elevated creatinine kinase (CK)/MB fraction: Not specific for acute MI in children

b. Cardiac troponin I: More sensitive indicator of early myocardial damage in children.[11] Becomes elevated within hours of cardiac injury, persists for 4 to 7 days, is specific for cardiac injury

D. ECG Findings Secondary to Electrolyte Disturbances, Medications, and Systemic Illnesses

1. **Digitalis:**

a. Digitalis effect: Associated with shortened QTc interval, ST depression (*scooped* or *sagging*), mildly prolonged PR interval, and flattened T waves

b. Digitalis toxicity: Primarily arrhythmias (bradycardia, supraventricular tachycardia, ectopic atrial tachycardia, ventricular tachycardia, atrioventricular [AV] block)

2. **Other conditions** (Table 7-10)[7,12]

E. Long QT

1. **Diagnosis:** See Section V for normal QTc ranges. Elevated QTc in the absence of other underlying causes (electrolyte disturbances,

TABLE 7-10

SYSTEMIC EFFECTS ON ELECTROCARDIOGRAM

	Short QT	Long QT-U	Prolonged QRS	ST-T Changes
CHEMISTRY				
Hyperkalemia			X	X
Hypokalemia		X		X
Hypercalcemia	X			
Hypocalcemia		X		
Hypermagnesemia				
Hypomagnesemia		X		
DRUGS				
Digitalis	X			X
Phenothiazines		T		
Phenytoin	X			
Propranolol	X			
Tricyclics		T	T	T
Verapamil				
MISCELLANEOUS				
CNS injury		X		X
Friedreich's ataxia				X
Duchenne's muscular dystrophy				
Myotonic dystrophy			X	X
Collagen vascular disease				X
Hypothyroidism				
Hyperthyroidism			X	X
Lyme disease			X	
Holt-Oram, maternal lupus				

CNS, Central nervous system; T, present only with drug toxicity; X, present.

Adapted from Garson A Jr: The Electrocardiogram in Infants and Children: A Systematic Approach. Philadelphia, Lea & Febiger, 1983, p. 172, and Walsh EP: Cardiac arrhythmias. In Fyler DC, Nadas A (eds): Pediatric Cardiology. Philadelphia, Hanley & Belfus, 1992, pp 141–143.

prematurity). The diagnosis may be supported by associated bradycardia, second-degree AV block, multiform premature ventricular contractions (PVCs), ventricular tachycardia, or abnormal T-wave morphologies. In approximately 10% of cases, patients may have a normal QTc on ECG. Patients may also have a family history of long QT with unexplained syncope, seizure, or cardiac arrest without prolongation of QTc on ECG. Treadmill exercise test may prolong the QTc and will sometimes incite arrhythmias

2. **Complications:** Associated with the ventricular arrhythmias (torsades de pointes), syncope, and sudden death
3. **Management:**

a. Congenital long QT: β-blockers and/or defibrillators; rarely require cardiac sympathetic denervation or cardiac pacemakers

Sinus Tachycardia	Sinus Bradycardia	AV Block	Ventricular Tachycardia	Miscellaneous
		X	X	Low-voltage Ps; peaked Ts
	X	X	X	
X		X		
		X		
	T	X	T	
			T	
	X	X		
T		T	T	
	X	X		
X	X	X		
X				Atrial flutter
X	X			Atrial flutter
X		X		
		X	X	
	X			Low voltage
X		X		
		X		
		X		

b. Acquired long QT: Treatment of arrhythmias, discontinue precipitating drug, correction of metabolic abnormalities

VI. CONGENITAL HEART DISEASE

Table 7-11 shows common syndromes associated with cardiac lesions.

A. Acyanotic Lesions (Table 7-12)

B. Cyanotic Lesions (Table 7-13)

An oxygen challenge test is used to evaluate the etiology of cyanosis in neonates. Obtain baseline arterial blood gas (ABG) with saturation at $FiO_2 = 0.21$, then place infant in an oxygen hood at $FiO_2 = 1$ for a minimum of 10 min, and repeat ABG. Pulse oximetry will not be useful for following the change in oxygenation once the saturations reach 100% (approximately PaO_2 >90 mmHg).[13–16]

1. See Table EC 7-A on Expert Consult for **interpretation of oxygen challenge test**
2. Table EC 7-B on Expert Consult shows acute **management of hypercyanotic spells in TOF**

TABLE 7-11

MAJOR SYNDROMES ASSOCIATED WITH CARDIAC DEFECTS

Syndrome	Dominant Cardiac Defect
CHARGE	TOF, truncus arteriosus, aortic arch abnormalities
DiGeorge	Aortic arch anomalies, TOF, truncus arteriosus, VSD, PDA
Trisomy 21	Atrioventricular septal defects, VSD
Marfan	Aortic root dissection, mitral valve prolapse
Loeys-Dietz	Aortic root dissection with higher risk of rupture at smaller dimensions
Noonan	Supravalvular pulmonic stenosis, LVH
Turner	COA, bicuspid aortic valve
Williams	Supravalvular aortic stenosis, Pulmonary artery stenosis
FAS	Occasional: VSD, PDA, ASD, TOF
IDM	TGA, VSD, COA, cardiomyopathy
VATER/VACTERL	VSD
VCFS	Truncus arteriosus, TOF, pulmonary atresia with VSD, TGA, interrupted aortic arch

ASD, Atrial septal defect; CHARGE, a syndrome of associated defects, including **c**oloboma of the eye, **h**eart anomaly, choanal **a**tresia, **r**etardation, and **g**enital and **e**ar anomalies; COA, coarctation of aorta; FAS, fetal alcohol syndrome; IDM, infant of diabetic mother; LVH, left ventricular hypertrophy; PDA, patent ductus arteriosis; TGA, transposition great arteries; TOF, tetralogy of Fallot; VATER/VACTERL, association of **V**ertebral anomalies, **A**nal atresia, **C**ardiac anomalies, **T**rache**oe**sophageal fistula, **R**enal/radial anomalies, **L**imb defects; VCFS, velocardiofacial syndrome; VSD, ventricular septal defect.

Adapted from Park MK: Pediatric Cardiology for Practitioners, 5th ed. St. Louis, Mosby, 2008, p. 10–12.

C. Surgeries and Other Interventions

1. **Atrial septostomy:** Creates an intra-atrial opening to allow for mixing or shunting between atria of systemic and pulmonary venous blood. (used for transposition of the great arteries [TGA], tricuspid, mitral, tricuspid and pulmonary atresia, and sometimes total anomalous pulmonary venous return). Most commonly performed percutaneously with a balloon-tipped catheter (Rashkind procedure)
2. **Palliative systemic-to-pulmonary artery shunts,** such as the Blalock-Taussig shunt (subclavian artery to pulmonary artery [PA]): Use systemic arterial flow to increase pulmonary blood flow in cardiac lesions with impaired pulmonary perfusion (e.g., TOF, hypoplastic right heart, tricuspid atresia, pulmonary atresia) (Fig. 7-14)
3. **Palliative superior vena cava-to-pulmonary artery shunts** such as the Glenn shunt (superior vena cava [SVC] to the right pulmonary artery [RPA]) or Hemi-Fontan: Directs a portion of the systemic venous return directly into the pulmonary blood flow (usually performed outside of the neonatal period in infants with lower pulmonary vascular resistance) as an intermediate step to a Fontan procedure (see Fig. 7-14)
4. **Fontan procedure:** Glenn shunt, together with anastomosis of the right atria and/or inferior vena cava (IVC) to pulmonary arteries via conduits; separates systemic and pulmonary circulations in patients with functionally single ventricles (tricuspid atresia, hypoplastic left heart syndrome)

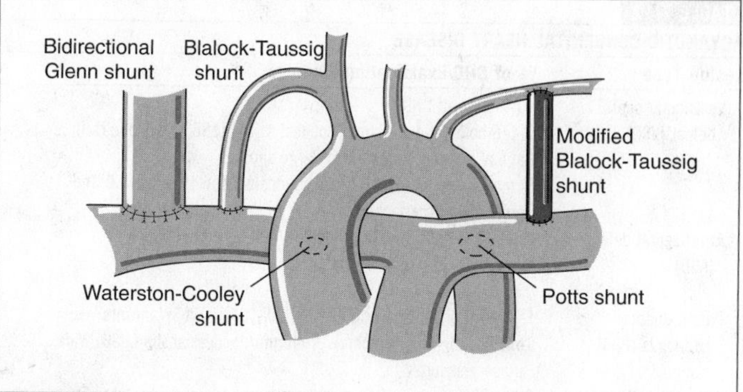

FIGURE 7-14
Schematic diagram of cardiac shunts.

5. **Norwood procedure:** Used for hypoplastic left heart syndrome
   a. Stage 1 (neonatal period): Anastomosis of the proximal main pulmonary artery (MPA) to the aorta, with aortic arch reconstruction and transection and patch closure of the distal MPA; a modified right Blalock-Taussig shunt (subclavian artery to RPA) to provide pulmonary blood flow; alternatively, a right ventricle to pulmonary artery conduit can be used for pulmonary blood flow (Sano modification). An atrial septal defect is created to allow for adequate left to right flow
   b. Stage 2 (3–6 months of age): Bidirectional Glenn shunt or Hemi-Fontan to reduce volume overload of single right ventricle
   c. Modified Fontan (12–18 months of age)
6. **Repair of TGA:**
   a. Atrial inversion (Mustard or Senning operation) (rarely performed today)
   b. Arterial switch
7. **Ross procedure:** Pulmonary root autograft for aortic stenosis; autologous pulmonary valve replaces aortic valve, and aortic or pulmonary allograft replaces pulmonary valve

VII. IMAGING

A. Chest radiograph

1. **Evaluate the heart:**
   a. Size: Cardiac shadow should be less than 50% of thoracic width (the maximal width between the inner margins of the ribs, as measured on a posteroanterior radiograph during inspiration)
   b. Shape: Can aid in the diagnosis of chamber/vessel enlargement and some congenital heart disease (Fig. 7-15)
   c. Situs (levocardia, mesocardia, dextrocardia)

Text continued on page 190

TABLE 7-12

ACYANOTIC CONGENITAL HEART DISEASE

Lesion Type	% of CHD/Examination Findings
Ventricular septal defect (VSD)	20%–25% of CHD 2–5/6 holosystolic murmur, loudest at the LLSB, ± systolic thrill ± apical diastolic rumble with large shunt S_2 may be narrow and P2 may be increased, with large VSD and pulmonary hypertension
Atrial septal defect (ASD)	Wide, fixed split S_2 with grade 2–3/6 SEM at the LUSB May have mid-diastolic rumble at LLSB
Patent ductus arteriosus (PDA)	5%–10% of CHD in term infants; 40–60% in VLBW infants 1–4/6 continuous "machinery" murmur loudest at the LUSB. Wide pulse pressure
Atrioventricular septal defects	30%–60% occur in Down syndrome Hyperactive precordium with systolic thrill at the LLSB and loud S_2 ± grade 3–4/6 holosystolic regurgitant murmur along the LLSB ± systolic murmur of MR at apex ± mid-diastolic rumble at LLSB or at apex ± Gallop rhythm
Pulmonary stenosis (PS)	Ejection click at LUSB with valvular PS—click intensity varies with respiration, decreasing with inspiration and increasing with expiration S_2 may split widely with P2 diminished in intensity SEM (2–5/6) ± thrill at LUSB with radiation to back and sides
Aortic stenosis (AS)	Systolic thrill at RUSB, suprasternal notch, or over carotids Ejection click, which does not vary with respiration, if valvular AS Harsh SEM (2–4/6) at second RICS or third LICS with radiation to the neck and apex ± early diastolic decrescendo murmur as a result of AR Narrow pulse pressure if severe stenosis
Coarctation of the aorta May present as (1) Infant in CHF (2) Child with HTN (3) Child with murmur	8%–10% of CHD with male/female ratio of 2 : 1. 2–3/6 SEM at the LUSB radiating to the left interscapular area Bicuspid valve is often associated and thus may have systolic ejection click at the apex and RUSB BP in lower extremities will be lower than in upper extremities Pulse oximetry discrepancy of >5% between upper and lower extremities is also suggestive of coarctation

ECG Findings	Chest Radiograph Findings
Small VSD: Normal *Medium VSD:* LVH ± LAE *Large VSD:* BVH ± LAE, pure RVH	May show cardiomegaly and increased PVMs dependent on the amount of left to right shunting
Small ASD: Normal *Large ASD:* RAD and mild RVH or RBBB with RSR′ in V_1	May show cardiomegaly with increased PVMs if hemodynamically significant ASD
Small–moderate PDA: Normal or LVH *Large PDA:* BVH	May have cardiomegaly and increased PVMs, depending on size of shunt (see Chapter 18 for treatment)
Superior QRS axis RVH and LVH may be present	Cardiomegaly with increased PVMs
Mild PS: Normal *Moderate PS:* RAD and RVH *Severe PS:* RAE and RVH with strain	Normal heart size with normal to decreased PVMs
Mild AS: Normal *Moderate–severe AS:* LVH ± strain	Usually normal
In infancy: RVH or RBBB *In older children:* LVH	Marked cardiomegaly and pulmonary venous congestion. Rib notching from collateral circulation usually not seen in children younger than 5 years because collaterals not yet established

AR, Aortic regurgitation; BP, blood pressure; BVH, biventricular hypertrophy; CHD, congenital heart disease; CHF, congestive heart failure; HTN, hypertension; LAE, left atrial enlargement; LICS, left intercostal space; LLSB, left lower sternal border; LUSB, left upper sternal border; LVH, left ventricular hypertrophy; MR, mitral regurgitation; PVM, pulmonary vascular markings; RAD, right axis deviation; RAE, right atrial enlargement; RICS, right intercostal space; RBBB, right bundle-branch block; RUSB, right upper sternal border; RVH, right ventricular hypertrophy; SEM, systolic ejection murmur. VLBW, very low birth weight i.e. <1500 g.

TABLE 7-13

CYANOTIC CONGENITAL HEART DISEASE

Lesion	**Examination Findings**	**ECG Findings**	**Chest Radiograph Findings**
Tetralogy of Fallot: 1. Large VSD 2. RVOT obstruction 3. RVH 4. Overriding aorta Degree of RVOT obstruction will determine whether there is clinical cyanosis. If there is only mild PS, there will be a left to right shunt, and the child will be acyanotic. Increased obstruction leads to increased right to left shunting across the VSD and cyanosis	Loud SEM at LMSB and LUSB and a loud, single S_2 ± thrill at the LMSB and LLSB. *Tet spells:* Occur in young infants. As RVOT obstruction increases or systemic resistance decreases, right to left shunting across the VSD occurs. May present with tachypnea, increasing cyanosis, and decreasing murmur. See Table EC 7-B for treatment	RAD and RVH	Boot-shaped heart with normal heart size ± decreased PVMs
Transposition of great arteries	Nonspecific. Extreme cyanosis. Loud, single S_2. No murmur unless there is associated VSD or PS	RAD and RVH (due to RV acting as systemic ventricle). Upright T wave in V_1 after age 3 days may be only abnormality.	Classic finding: "egg on a string" with cardiomegaly; possible increased PVMs
Tricuspid atresia: Absent tricuspid valve and hypoplastic RV and PA. Must have ASD, PDA, or VSD to survive	Single S_2 + grade 2–3/6 systolic regurgitation murmur at the LLSB if VSD is present. Occasional PDA murmur	Superior QRS axis; RAE or CAE, and LVH	Normal or slightly enlarged heart size; may have boot-shaped heart

TABLE 7-13

CYANOTIC CONGENITAL HEART DISEASE (Continued)

Lesion	Examination Findings	ECG Findings	Chest Radiograph Findings
Total anomalous pulmonary venous return Instead of draining into LA, pulmonary veins drain into the following locations. Must have ASD or PFO for survival 1. *Supracardiac (most common):* SVC 2. *Cardiac:* coronary sinus or RA 3. *Subdiaphragmatic:* IVC, portal vein, ductus venosus, or hepatic vein 4. *Mixed type*	Hyperactive RV impulse, quadruple rhythm, S_2 fixed and widely split, 2–3/6 SEM at LUSB, and mid-diastolic rumble at LLSB	RAD, RVH (RSR′ in V_1). May see RAE	Cardiomegaly and increased PVMs; classic finding is "snowman in a snowstorm," but this is rarely seen until after age 4 months
OTHER			
Cyanotic CHDs that occur at a frequency of <1% each include pulmonary atresia, Ebstein's anomaly, truncus arteriosus, single ventricle, and double outlet right ventricle.			

ASD, Atrial septal defect; CAE, common atrial enlargement; ECG, electrocardiogram; IVC, inferior vena cava; LA, left atrium; LLSB, left lower sternal border; LMSB, left mid-sternal border; LUSB, left upper sternal border; LVH, left ventricular hypertrophy; PA, pulmonary artery; PDA, patent ductus arteriosus; PFO, patent foramen ovale; PVM, pulmonary vascular markings; PS, pulmonary stenosis; RA, right atrium; RAD, right axis deviation; RAE, right atrial enlargement; RV, right ventricle; RVH, right ventricular hypertrophy; RVOT, right ventricular outflow tract; SEM, systolic ejection murmur; SVC, superior vena cava; VSD, ventricular septal defect.

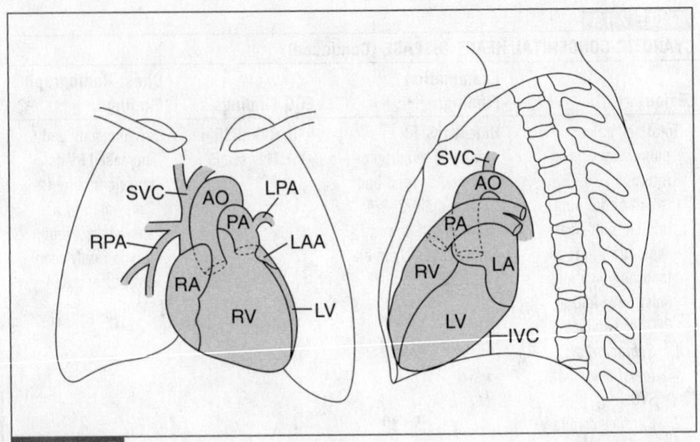

FIGURE 7-15

Radiologic contours of the heart. AO, Aorta; IVC, inferior vena cava; LA, left atrium; LAA, left atrial appendage; LPA, left pulmonary artery; LV, left ventricle; PA, pulmonary artery; RA, right atrium; RPA, right pulmonary artery; RV, right ventricle; SVC, superior vena cava.

2. **Evaluate the lung fields:**
   a. Decreased pulmonary blood flow: Seen in pulmonary or tricuspid stenosis/atresia, TOF, pulmonary hypertension (*peripheral pruning*)
   b. Increased pulmonary blood flow: Seen as increased pulmonary vascular markings (PVMs) with redistribution from bases to apices of lungs and extension to lateral lung fields (see Tables 7-12 and 7-13)
   c. Venous congestion, or congestive heart failure (CHF): Increased PVMs centrally, interstitial and alveolar pulmonary edema (air bronchograms), septal lines, and pleural effusions (see Tables 7-12 and 7-13)
3. **Evaluate the trachea:** Usually bends slightly to the right above the carina in normal patients with a left-sided aortic arch. A perfectly straight or left-bending trachea suggests a right aortic arch, which may be associated with other defects (TOF, truncus arteriosus, vascular rings, chromosome 22 microdeletion)
4. **Skeletal anomalies:**
   a. Rib notching (e.g., from collateral vessels in patients >5 years of age with coarctation of the aorta)
   b. Sternal abnormalities (e.g., Holt-Oram syndrome, pectus excavatum in Marfan, Ehlers-Danlos, and Noonan syndromes)
   c. Vertebral anomalies (e.g., VATER/VACTERL syndrome: **V**ertebral anomalies, **A**nal atresia, **T**racheo**e**sophageal fistula, **R**adial and **R**enal, **C**ardiac, and **L**imb anomalies)

Please see Chapter 25 for more information on the chest radiograph.

B. Echocardiography

1. **Approach:**

a. Transthoracic echocardiography (TTE): Does not require general anesthesia, is simpler to perform than transesophageal echocardiography (TEE), but does have limitations in some patients (e.g., uncooperative, obese, or those with suspected endocarditis)

b. TEE: Uses an ultrasound transducer on the end of a modified endoscope to view the heart from the esophagus and stomach, allowing for better imaging of intracardiac structures. It allows for better imaging in obese and intraoperative patients. TEE is also useful for visualizing very small lesions such as some vegetations

2. **Shortening fraction:** Very reliable index of left ventricular function. Normal values range from approximately 30% to 45%, depending on age[16]

See more information on echocardiography on Expert Consult, Chapter 7.

C. Cardiac Catheterization

See Figure EC 7-A on Expert Consult for Diagram of normal pressure values.

VIII. EXERCISE RECOMMENDATIONS FOR CONGENITAL HEART DISEASE (TABLE 7-14)[17]

IX. ACQUIRED HEART DISEASE

A. Endocarditis

1. **Common causative organisms:** About 70% of causes of endocarditis are streptococcal species (*Streptococcus viridans,* enterococci); 20% are staphylococcal species (*Staphylococcus aureus, Staphylococcus epidermidis*); 10% are other organisms (*Haemophilus influenzae,* gram-negative bacteria, fungi)
2. **Clinical findings:** New heart murmur, recurrent fever, splenomegaly, petechiae, fatigue, Osler nodes (tender nodules at fingertips), Janeway lesions (painless hemorrhagic areas on palms or soles), splinter hemorrhages, and Roth spots (retinal hemorrhages)

B. Bacterial Endocarditis Prophylaxis[18]

1. All dental procedures that involve treatment of gingival tissue or periapical region of the teeth or oral mucosal perforation
2. Invasive procedures that involve incision or biopsy of respiratory mucosa, such as tonsillectomy and adenoidectomy
3. Not recommended for genitourinary or gastrointestinal tract procedures; solely for bacterial endocarditis prevention

See Table 7-15 and Box 7-4.

C. Myocardial Disease

1. **Dilated cardiomyopathy:** End result of myocardial damage, leading to atrial and ventricular dilation with decreased systolic contractile function of the ventricles

7

TABLE 7-14

EXERCISE RECOMMENDATIONS FOR CONGENITAL HEART DISEASE AND SPORTS ALLOWED FOR SOME SPECIFIC CARDIAC LESIONS[18]

Diagnosis	Sports Allowed
Small ASD or VSD	All
Mild aortic stenosis	All
MVP (without other risk factors)	All
Moderate aortic stenosis	IA, IB, IIA
Mild LV dysfunction	IA, IB, IC
Moderate LV dysfunction	IA only
Long QT syndrome	IA only
Hypertrophic cardiomyopathy	None (or IA only)
Severe aortic stenosis	None

Sports Classification	Low Dynamic (A)	Moderate Dynamic (B)	High Dynamic (C)
I. Low static	Billiards Bowling Golf Riflery	Baseball/Softball Table tennis Volleyball Fencing	Racket sports Cross-country skiing Field hockey* Race walking Running (long distance) Soccer*
II. Moderate static	Archery Auto racing*,† Diving*,† Equestrian*,† Motorcycling*,†	Fencing Field events (jumping) Figure skating* Football (American)* Surfing Rugby* Running (sprint) Synchronized swim†	Basketball* Ice hockey* Cross-country skiing (skating technique) Swimming Lacrosse* Running (middle distance) Team handball
III. High static	Bobsledding Field events Gymnastics*,† Rock climbing Sailing Windsurfing*,† Waterskiing*,† Weight lifting*,†	Body building*,† Downhill skiing*,† Skateboarding*,†	Boxing/Wrestling* Martial Arts* Rowing Speed skating Cycling*,†

*Danger of bodily collision.

†Increased risk if syncope occurs.

ASD, Atrial septal defect; LV, left ventricular; MVP, mitral valve prolapse; VSD, ventricular septal defect.

Adapted from Maron BJ, Zipes DP: 36th Bethesda Conference: Eligibility recommendations for competitive athletes with cardiovascular abnormalities. J Am Coll Cardiol 2005;45(8):1313–1375; and Committee on Sports Medicine and Fitness, American Academy of Pediatrics: Medical conditions affecting sports participation. Pediatrics 2001;107(5):1205–1209.

TABLE 7-15

PROPHYLACTIC REGIMENS FOR DENTAL AND RESPIRATORY TRACT PROCEDURES

Drug	Dosing* (not to exceed adult dose)
Amoxicillin**	Adult: 2 g; Child: 50 mg/kg PO
Ampicillin	Adult: 2 g; Child: 50 mg/kg IM/IV
Cefazolin or ceftriaxone[†]	Adult: 1 g; Child: 50mg/kg IM/IV
Cephalexin[†]	Adult: 2 g; Child: 50 mg/kg PO
Clindamycin	Adult: 600 mg; Child: 20 mg/kg PO/IM/IV
Azithromycin/clarithromycin	Adult: 500 mg; Child 15 mg/kg PO

*PO medications should be given 1 hour before procedure; IM/IV medications should be given within 30 min prior to procedure.

**Standard general prophylaxis.

[†]Cephalosporins should not be used in persons with intermediate-type hypersensitivity reaction to penicillins or ampicillin.

Adapted from Wilson W, Taubert KA, Gewitz M, et al: Prevention of Infective Endocarditis: Guidelines from the American Heart Association: A Guideline from the American Heart Association Rheumatic Fever, Endocarditis, and Kawasaki Disease Committee, Council on Cardiovascular Disease in the Young, and the Council on Clinical Cardiology, Council on Cardiovascular Surgery and Anesthesia, and the Quality of Care and Outcomes Research Interdisciplinary Working Group. Circulation 2007;116:1736–1754.

BOX 7-4

CARDIAC CONDITIONS FOR WHICH ANTIBIOTIC PROPHYLAXIS IS RECOMMENDED FOR DENTAL, RESPIRATORY TRACT, INFECTED SKIN, SKIN STRUCTURES, OR MUSCULOSKELETAL TISSUE PROCEDURES

- Prosthetic cardiac valve
- Previous bacterial endocarditis
- Congenital heart disease (CHD)—Limited to the following conditions*
  - Unrepaired cyanotic defect, including palliative shunts and conduits
  - Completely repaired CHD with prosthetic material/device (placed by surgery or catheterization), during first 6 months after procedure[†]
  - Repaired CHD with residual defects at or adjacent to the site of prosthetic patch or device (which inhibit endothelialization)
  - Cardiac transplantation patients who develop cardiac valvulopathy

*Conditions associated with the highest risk of adverse outcome from endocarditis.

[†]Endothelialization process of prosthetic material occurs within 6 months after the procedure.

Adapted from Wilson W, Taubert KA, Gewitz M, et al: Prevention of infective endocarditis: guidelines from the American Heart Association: a guideline from the American Heart Association Rheumatic Fever, Endocarditis, and Kawasaki Disease Committee, Council on Cardiovascular Disease in the Young, and the Council on Clinical Cardiology, Council on Cardiovascular Surgery and Anesthesia, and the Quality of Care and Outcomes Research Interdisciplinary Working Group. Circulation 2007;116:1736–1754.

a. Etiology: Infectious, toxic (alcohol, anthracyclines), metabolic (hypothyroidism, muscular dystrophy), immunologic, collagen vascular disease, nutritional deficiency (kwashiorkor, beriberi)
b. Symptoms: Fatigue, weakness, shortness of breath
c. Examination: Look for signs of CHF, including tachycardia, tachypnea, rales, cold extremities, jugular venous distention, hepatomegaly,

peripheral edema, S_3 gallop, and displacement of point of maximal impulse to the left and inferiorly

d. Chest radiograph: Generalized cardiomegaly, pulmonary congestion
e. ECG: Sinus tachycardia, left ventricular hypertrophy (LVH), possible atrial enlargement, arrhythmias, conduction disturbances, ST-segment and T-wave changes
f. Echocardiography: Enlarged ventricles (increased end-diastolic and end-systolic dimensions) with little or no wall thickening; decreased shortening fraction
g. Treatment: Management of CHF (digoxin, diuretics, vasodilation, angiotensin-converting enzyme [ACE] inhibitors, rest). Consider anticoagulants to decrease risk for thrombus formation

2. **Hypertrophic cardiomyopathy:** Abnormality of myocardial cells leading to significant ventricular hypertrophy, particularly of the left ventricle, with small to normal ventricular dimensions. Increased contractile function, but impaired filling secondary to stiff ventricles. The most common type is asymmetrical septal hypertrophy, also called idiopathic hypertrophic subaortic stenosis (IHSS), with varying degrees of obstruction. A 4% to 6% incidence of sudden death in children and adolescents with hypertrophic obstructive cardiomyopathy (HOCM)
   a. Etiology: Genetic (autosomal dominant, 60% of cases) or sporadic (40% of cases)
   b. Symptoms: Easy fatigability, anginal pain, shortness of breath, occasional palpitations
   c. Examination: Usually in adolescents or young adults; signs include left ventricular heave, sharp upstroke of arterial pulse, murmur of mitral regurgitation, midsystolic ejection murmur along left midsternal border (LMSB) that increases in intensity in the standing position (in patients with midcavity left ventricular obstruction)
   d. Chest radiograph: Globular-shaped heart with left ventricular enlargement
   e. ECG: LVH, prominent Q waves (septal hypertrophy), ST-segment and T-wave changes, arrhythmias
   f. Echocardiography: Extent and location of hypertrophy, obstruction, increased contractility
   g. Treatment: Moderate restriction of physical activity, administration of negative inotropes (β-blocker, calcium channel blocker) to help improve filling and subacute bacterial endocarditis prophylaxis. If at increased risk for sudden death, may consider implantable defibrillator. If symptomatic with subaortic obstruction, may benefit from myectomy
3. **Restrictive cardiomyopathy:** Myocardial or endocardial disease (usually infiltrative or fibrotic) resulting in stiff ventricular walls, with restriction of diastolic filling but normal contractile function. Results in atrial enlargement. Associated with a high mortality rate. Very rare in children

a. Etiology: Scleroderma, amyloidosis, sarcoidosis, mucopolysaccharidosis
b. Treatment: Supportive, poor prognosis. Diuretics, anticoagulants, calcium channel blockers, pacemaker for heart block, cardiac transplantation if severe

4. **Myocarditis:** Inflammation of myocardial tissue
a. Etiology: Viral (coxsackievirus, echovirus, adenovirus, poliomyelitis, mumps, measles, rubella, cytomegalovirus, HIV, arbovirus, influenza); bacterial, rickettsial, fungal, or parasitic infection; immune-mediated disease (Kawasaki disease, acute rheumatic fever); collagen vascular disease; toxin-induced
b. Symptoms: Nonspecific and inconsistent, depending on severity of disease. Variably anorexia, lethargy, emesis, lightheadedness, cold extremities, shortness of breath
c. Examination: Look for signs of CHF (tachycardia, tachypnea, jugular venous distention, rales, gallop, hepatomegaly); occasionally, a soft, systolic murmur or arrhythmia may be noted
d. Chest radiograph: Variable cardiomegaly and pulmonary edema
e. ECG: Low QRS voltages throughout (<5 mm), ST-segment and T-wave changes (e.g., decreased T-wave amplitude), prolongation of QT interval, arrhythmias (especially premature contractions, first- or second-degree AV block)
f. Laboratory tests: CK, troponin
g. Echocardiography: Enlargement of heart chambers, impaired left ventricular function
h. Treatment: bed rest, diuretics, inotropes (dopamine, dobutamine, milrinone), digoxin, gamma globulin (2 g/kg over 24 hours), ACE inhibitors, possibly steroids. May require heart transplantation if no improvement (about 20% to 25% of cases)

D. Pericardial Disease

1. **Pericarditis:** Inflammation of visceral and parietal layers of pericardium
a. Etiology: Viral (especially echovirus, coxsackievirus B), tuberculosis, bacterial, uremic, neoplastic, collagen vascular, post-MI or postpericardiotomy, radiation induced, drug induced (e.g., procainamide, hydralazine), or idiopathic
b. Symptoms: Chest pain (retrosternal or precordial, radiating to back or shoulder, pleuritic in nature, alleviated by leaning forward, aggravated by supine position), dyspnea
c. Examination: Pericardial friction rub, distant heart sounds, fever, tachypnea
d. ECG: Diffuse ST-segment elevation in almost all leads (representing inflammation of adjacent myocardium); PR-segment depression
e. Treatment: Often self-limited. Treat underlying condition, and provide symptomatic treatment with rest, analgesia, and anti-inflammatory drugs

2. **Pericardial effusion:** Accumulation of excess fluid in pericardial sac
a. Etiology: Associated with acute pericarditis (exudative fluid) or serous effusion resulting from increased capillary hydrostatic pressure (e.g., CHF), decreased plasma oncotic pressure (e.g., hypoproteinemia), and increased capillary permeability (transudative fluid)
b. Symptoms: Can present with no symptoms, dull ache in left chest, abdominal pain, or symptoms of cardiac tamponade, discussed subsequently
c. Examination: Muffled distant heart sounds, dullness to percussion of posterior left chest (secondary to atelectasis from large pericardial sac), hemodynamic signs of cardiac compression
d. Chest radiograph: Globular, symmetrical cardiomegaly
e. ECG: Decreased voltage of QRS complexes, electrical alternans (variation of QRS axis with each beat secondary to swinging of heart within pericardial fluid)
f. Echocardiography shows extent and location of hypertrophy, obstruction, increased contractility
g. Treatment: Address underlying condition. Observe if asymptomatic; use pericardiocentesis if there is sudden increase in volume or hemodynamic compromise. Nonsteroidal anti-inflammatory drugs or steroids may be of benefit, depending on etiology

3. **Cardiac tamponade:** Accumulation of pericardial fluid under high pressure, causing compression of cardiac chambers, limiting filling, and decreasing stroke volume and cardiac output
a. Etiology: As for pericardial effusion. Most commonly associated with viral infection, neoplasm, uremia, and acute hemorrhage
b. Symptoms: Dyspnea, fatigue, cold extremities
c. Examination: Jugular venous distention, hepatomegaly, peripheral edema, tachypnea, rales (from increased systemic and pulmonary venous pressure), hypotension, tachycardia, pulsus paradoxus (decrease in systolic blood pressure by >10 mmHg with each inspiration), decreased capillary refill (from decreased stroke volume and cardiac output), quiet precordium, and muffled heart sounds
d. ECG: Sinus tachycardia, decreased voltage, electrical alternans
e. Echocardiography: Right ventricle collapse in early diastole, right atrial/left atrial collapse in end-diastole and early systole
f. Treatment: Pericardiocentesis with temporary catheter left in place if necessary (see Chapter 3), pericardial window or stripping if it is a recurrent condition

E. Kawasaki Disease

Leading cause of acquired heart disease in children in developed countries. Seen almost exclusively in children <8 years of age. Patients present with acute febrile vasculitis, which may lead to long-term cardiac complications from vasculitis of coronary arteries. The number of cases peaks in winter and spring.

1. Etiology: Unknown. Thought to be immune-regulated, in response to infectious agents or environmental toxins
2. Diagnosis: Based on clinical criteria. These include high fever lasting 5 days or more, plus at least four of the following five criteria:
   a. Bilateral bulbar conjunctival injection without exudate
   b. Erythematous mouth and pharynx, strawberry tongue, or red, cracked lips
   c. Polymorphous exanthem (may be morbilliform, maculopapular, or scarlatiniform)
   d. Swelling of the hands and feet, with erythema of the palms and soles.
   e. Cervical lymphadenopathy (>1.5 cm in diameter), usually single and unilateral

NOTE: Incomplete Kawasaki disease, more often seen in infants, consists of fever with fewer than four of the criteria just cited but findings of coronary artery abnormalities. Echocardiography should be considered in any infant <6 months with fever of >7 days' duration, laboratory evidence of systemic inflammation, and no other explanation for the febrile illness. See Figure EC 7-B on Expert Consult for evaluation of incomplete Kawasaki disease.

3. Other clinical findings: Often associated with extreme irritability, abdominal pain, diarrhea, vomiting. Also seen are anterior uveitis (80%), arthritis and arthralgias (35%), aseptic meningitis (25%), pericardial effusion or arrhythmias (20%), gallbladder hydrops (<10%), carditis (<5%), and perineal rash with desquamation
4. Laboratory findings: Leukocytosis with left shift, neutrophils with vacuoles or toxic granules, elevated C-reactive protein (CRP) or erythrocyte sedimentation rate (ESR) (seen acutely), thrombocytosis (after first week, peaking at 2 weeks), normocytic and normochromic anemia, sterile pyuria (70%), increased transaminases (40%)
5. Subacute phase (11 to 25 days after onset of illness): Resolution of fever, rash, and lymphadenopathy. Often, desquamation of the fingertips or toes and thrombocytosis occur
6. Cardiovascular complications: If untreated, 15% to 25% develop coronary artery aneurysms and dilation in subacute phase (peak prevalence occurs about 2 to 4 weeks after onset of disease; rarely appears after 6 weeks) and are at risk for coronary thrombosis acutely and coronary stenosis chronically. Carditis; aortic, mitral, and tricuspid regurgitation; pericardial effusion; CHF; MI; left ventricular dysfunction; and ECG changes may also occur
7. Convalescent phase: ESR, CRP, and platelet count return to normal. Those with coronary artery abnormalities are at increased risk for MI, arrhythmias, and sudden death
8. Management (See also Table EC 7-C on Expert Consult)[19]:
   a. Intravenous immune globulin (IVIG)
      (1) Shown to reduce incidence of coronary artery dilation to <3% and decrease duration of fever if given in the first 10 days of illness.

Current recommended regimen is a single dose of IVIG, 2 g/kg over 10 to 12 hours

(2) 10% of patients treated with IVIG fail to respond (persistent or recurrent fever ≥36 hr after IVIG completion). Retreat with second dose

b. Aspirin is recommended for both its anti-inflammatory and its antiplatelet effects. American Heart Association (AHA) recommends initial high-dose aspirin (80 to 100 mg/kg/day divided in four doses) until 48–72 hours after defervescence. Given with IVIG. Then continue with low-dose aspirin (3 to 5 mg/kg/day as a single daily dose) for 6 to 8 weeks or until platelet count and ESR are normal (if there are no coronary artery abnormalities) or indefinitely if coronary artery abnormalities persist

c. Dipyridamole, 4 mg/kg divided in three doses, is sometimes used as alternative to aspirin, particularly if symptoms of influenza or varicella arise while on aspirin (concern for Reye's syndrome)

d. Follow-up: Serial echocardiography is recommended to assess coronary arteries and left ventricular function (at time of diagnosis, at 2 weeks, at 6 to 8 weeks, and at 12 months [optional]). More frequent intervals and long-term follow-up are recommended if abnormalities are seen on echocardiography. Cardiac catheterization may be necessary

F. Rheumatic Heart Disease

1. Etiology: Believed to be immunologically mediated delayed sequela of group A streptococcal pharyngitis
2. Clinical findings: History of streptococcal pharyngitis 1 to 5 weeks before onset of symptoms. Often with pallor, malaise, easy fatigability
3. Diagnosis: Jones criteria (Box 7-5)

BOX 7-5

GUIDELINES FOR THE DIAGNOSIS OF INITIAL ATTACK OF RHEUMATIC FEVER (JONES CRITERIA)

Major Manifestations	**Minor Manifestations**
Carditis	Clinical findings
Polyarthritis	Arthralgia
Chorea	Fever
Erythema marginatum	Laboratory findings
Subcutaneous nodule	Elevated acute phase reactants (erythrocyte sedimentation rate, C-reactive protein)
	Prolonged PR interval

Plus

Supporting evidence of antecedent group A streptococcal infection

Positive throat culture or rapid streptococcal antigen test

Elevated or rising streptococcal antibody titer

NOTE: If supported by evidence of preceding group A streptococcal infection, the presence of two major manifestations or of one major and two minor manifestations indicates a high probability of acute rheumatic fever.

4. Management: Penicillin, bed rest, salicylates, supportive management of CHF (if present) with diuretics, digoxin, morphine

G. Lyme Disease

1. Etiology: Following infection with *Borrelia burgdorferi*
2. Clinical symptoms: Approximately 8% to 10% of patients will get AV block. Other possible cardiac symptoms include myocarditis and pericarditis

X. CARDIOVASCULAR SCREENING

See Expert Consult, Chapter 7, including Table EC 7-D for sports participation screening and screening recommendations for ADHD medications.

REFERENCES

1. Zubrow AB, Hulman S, Kushner H, et al. Determinants of blood pressure in infants admitted to neonatal intensive care units: a prospective multicenter study. Philadelphia Neonatal Blood Pressure Study Group. *J Perinatol.* 1995;15:470.
2. National High Blood Pressure Education Program Working Group on High Blood Pressure in Children and Adolescents. The fourth report on the diagnosis, evaluation, and treatment of high blood pressure in children and adolescents. *Pediatrics.* 2004;114(2 Suppl):555–576.
3. Park MK. *Pediatric cardiology for practitioners.* 5th ed. St. Louis: Mosby; 2008.
4. Sapin SO. Recognizing normal heart murmurs: a logic-based mnemonic. *Pediatrics.* 1997;99(4):616–619.
5. Daniels SR, Greer FR. Committee on nutrition: lipid screening and cardiovascular health in childhood. *Pediatrics.* 2008;122:198–206.
6. Davignon A, Rautaharju P, Boisselle E, et al. Normal ECG standards for infants and children. *Pediatr Cardiol.* 1979;1:123–131.
7. Schwartz PJ, Stramba-Badiale M, Segantini A, et al. Prolongation of the QT interval and the sudden infant death syndrome. *N Engl J Med.* 1998;338: 1709–1714.
8. Garson A Jr. *The electrocardiogram in infants and children: a systematic approach.* Philadelphia: Lea & Febiger; 1983.
9. Park MK, Guntheroth WG. *How to read pediatric ECGs.* 4th ed. Philadelphia: Mosby; 2006.
10. Towbin JA, Bricker JT, Garson A Jr. Electrocardiographic criteria for diagnosis of acute myocardial infarction in childhood. *Am J Cardiol.* 1992;69:1545–1548.
11. Hirsch R, Landt Y, Porter S, et al. Cardiac troponin I in pediatrics: normal values and potential use in assessment of cardiac injury. *J Pediatr.* 1997;130: 872–877.
12. Walsh EP. Cardiac arrhythmias. In: Fyler DC, Nadas A, eds. *Pediatric cardiology.* Philadelphia: Hanley & Belfus; 1992:384.
13. Lees MH. Cyanosis of the newborn infant: recognition and clinical evaluation. *J Pediatr.* 1970;77:484–498.
14. Kitterman JA. Cyanosis in the newborn infant. *Pediatr Rev.* 1982;4:13–24.
15. Jones RW, Baumer JH, Joseph MC, et al. Arterial oxygen tension and response to oxygen breathing in differential diagnosis of heart disease in infancy. *Arch Dis Child.* 1976;51:667–673.

16. Colan SD, Parness IA, Spevak PJ, et al. Developmental modulation of myocardial mechanics: age- and growth-related alterations in afterload and contractility. *J Am Coll Cardiol.* 1992;19:619–629.
17. Maron BJ, Zipes DP. Introduction: eligibility recommendations for competitive athletes with cardiovascular abnormalities. *J Am Coll Cardiol.* 2005;45(8): 1313–1375.
18. Wilson W, Taubert KA, Gewitz M, et al. Prevention of infective endocarditis: guidelines from the American Heart Association: a guideline from the American Heart Association Rheumatic Fever, Endocarditis, and Kawasaki Disease Committee, Council on Cardiovascular Disease in the Young, and the Council on Clinical Cardiology, Council on Cardiovascular Surgery and Anesthesia, and the Quality of Care and Outcomes Research Interdisciplinary Working Group. *Circulation.* 2007;116:1736–1754.
19. Newburger JW, Takahashi M, Gerber MA, et al. Diagnosis, treatment, and long term management of Kawasaki disease. *Circulation.* 2004;110:2747–2771.
20. Maron BJ, Thompson PD, Ackerman MJ, et al. Recommendations and considerations related to preparticipation screening for cardiovascular abnormalities in competitive athletes: 2007 update: a scientific statement from the American Heart Association Council on Nutrition, Physical Activity, and Metabolism: endorsed by the American College of Cardiology foundation. *Circulation.* 2007;115:1643–1655.

Chapter 8

Dermatology

Nisha Kapadia, MD

See additional content on Expert Consult

I. WEBSITE

Derm Atlas: http://dermatlas.med.jhmi.edu/derm/

NOTE: Please refer to the color plates in this chapter for photographic examples of dermatologic findings.

8

II. EVALUATION AND CLINICAL DESCRIPTIONS OF SKIN FINDINGS

A. Primary Skin Lesions (Fig. 8-1A)

1. Macule/patch: Small flat lesion with altered color (<1 cm); large macule (>1 cm)
2. Papule/plaque: Elevated, well-circumscribed lesion (<1 cm); large papule (>1 cm)
3. Nodule/tumor: Mass located in dermis or subcutaneous fat (may be solid or soft); large nodule
4. Vesicle/bulla: Blister with transparent fluid; large vesicle
5. Wheal: Erythematous, well-circumscribed, raised, edematous lesion that appears and disappears quickly

B. Secondary Skin Lesions (Fig. 8-1B)

1. Scale: Small, thin plate of horny epithelium
2. Pustule: Well-circumscribed elevated lesion filled with pus
3. Crust: Exudative mass consisting of blood, scale, and pus from skin erosions or ruptured vesicles/papules
4. Ulcer: Erosion of dermis and cutis with clearly defined edges
5. Scar: Formation of new connective tissue after damage to epidermis and cutis, leaving permanent change in skin
6. Excoriation: Surface marks often linear secondary to scratching
7. Fissure: Linear skin crack with inflammation and pain

III. SKIN LUMPS: DIAGNOSIS AND TREATMENT

A. Hemangiomas

1. Pathogenesis

A benign vascular tumor of infancy with a phase of rapid proliferation followed by spontaneous involution. During proliferative phase, densely packed endothelial cells form small capillaries; subsequent vessels develop from existing vasculature.

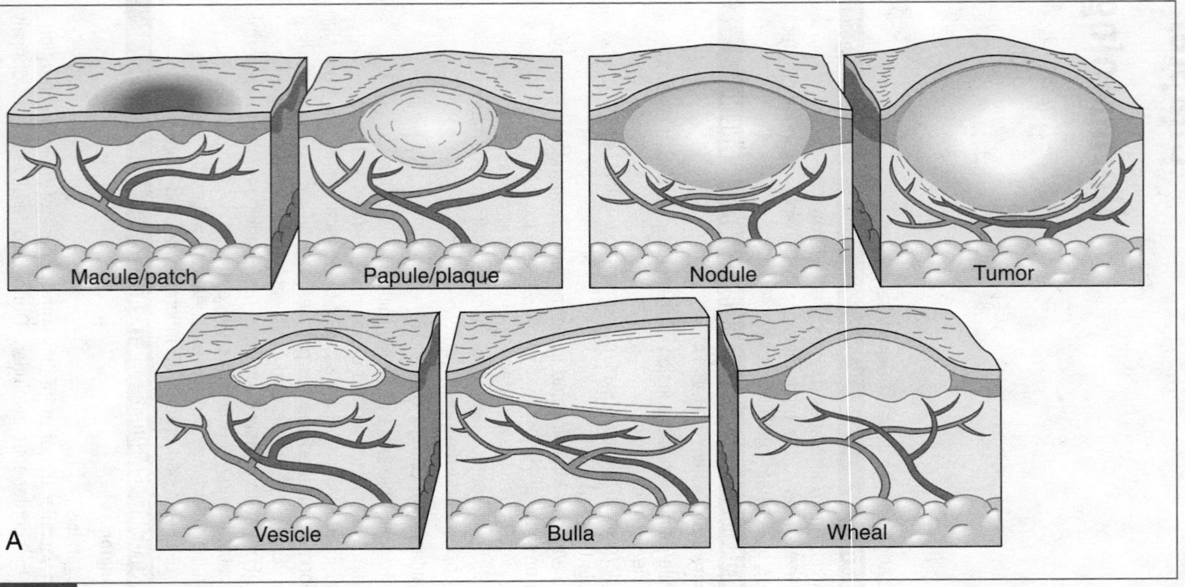

FIGURE 8-1 Pattern diagnosis. **A,** Primary skin lesions.

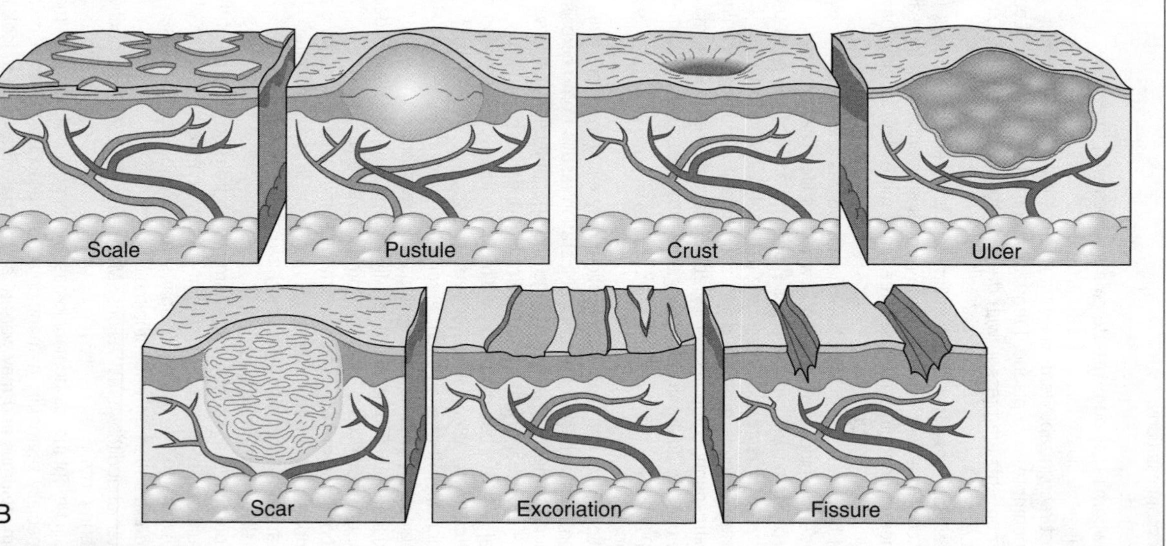

FIGURE 8-1 (Continued)

B, Secondary skin lesions. (***A and B,*** *From Cohen BA: Pediatric dermatology, 2nd ed. St. Louis, Mosby, 1999, p. 5.*)

2. Clinical manifestations:
a. Appearance:
    (1) Newborns may demonstrate pale macules with threadlike telangiectasias
    (2) Most recognizable form is a bright red, slightly elevated, noncompressible plaque. Frequently, both superficial and deep components are present, with deep components appearing bluish in color
    (3) Size: Can range from a few millimeters to several centimeters
b. Incidence: Most common soft tissue tumors in infancy, with increased incidence in premature infants; three times more likely in girls than boys
c. Natural history: About 5%–10% of hemangiomas are present at birth; remainder develop within the first 4 weeks of life. The most rapid growth phase occurs between ages 2 and 4 months, 85% peak by 3 months, with regression beginning at age 4–12 months
d. Diagnosis: Although most are diagnosed clinically, imaging techniques (e.g., ultrasound, computed tomography, magnetic resonance imaging) can be used to differentiate hemangiomas from vascular malformations or neoplastic processes
3. Complications:
a. Ulceration: Most common complication; may result in severe pain, infection, hemorrhage, or scarring; ulceration results from necrosis of superficial components. Hemorrhage and superinfection may also occur. Hemorrhage, although alarming in appearance, is usually minimal and can be controlled by direct pressure. Superinfection may lead to cellulitis, osteomyelitis, or septicemia
b. Kasabach-Merritt phenomenon: A complication of rare hemangiopericytoma, tufter angiomas, or Kaposiform hemangioendotheliomas which rapidly enlarge, and are usually deep lesions; characterized by anemia, thrombocytopenia, and coagulopathy, requiring aggressive medical management. Lesions are differentiated from benign hemangiomas by their deep red-blue appearance, marked firmness, and histologic appearance
c. Regionally important lesions:
    (1) Periorbital lesions: May cause amblyopia from obstruction of the visual axis or astigmatism from insidious compression of the globe or extension into the retrobulbar space. Require careful observation and evaluation by an ophthalmologist
    (2) External auditory canal lesions: May result in otitis or conductive hearing loss
    (3) Multiple cutaneous hemangiomas and large facial hemangiomas, especially segmental hemangiomas, are associated with visceral hemangiomas and may warrant abdominal ultrasound to look for organ involvement (i.e., liver hemangiomas). A high occurrence of hemangiomas in the cervical-tracheal region (PHACES syndrome:

posterior cranial fossa malformations, facial hemangiomas, arterial anomalies, aortic coarctation and other cardiac disorders, ocular abnormalities and stenotic arterial disease)[1] may be associated with abnormalities of the urogenital system[2]

(4) Visceral hemangiomas: Often characterized by high-flow patterns; may result in high-output cardiac failure and anemia. Large facial hemangiomas are also associated with posterior fossa vascular malformations, and thus patients should have neuroimaging with special attention to the posterior fossa

(5) Airway hemangiomas: Often located in the subglottic region; may cause hoarseness and stridor. Infants with cutaneous lesions in a beard distribution (chin, lips, mandibular region, and neck) are at greatest risk for airway involvement

(6) Lumbosacral hemangiomas that span the midline are associated with spinal malformations, dysraphism, and anomalies of the anorectal and urogenital regions. An ultrasound of the L5 spine in infants <6 months of age is an effective noninvasive screening study

4. Management:

a. Most require no intervention. Decision to treat should be based on location and depth of the lesion, age of patient, and likelihood of complication. Photodocumentation is used to follow the growth and regression process

b. Systemic corticosteroids previously was the mainstay of therapy to prevent subsequent complication (i.e., periorbital or subglottic lesions). Usually, 2 to 3 mg/kg/day of prednisone or prednisolone. One third of lesions demonstrate dramatic shrinkage, one third demonstrate stabilization of growth, and one third show no response

c. Propranolol for treating infantile hemangiomas is considered an *off-label* use. Below treatment is based on preliminary data. Protocol should be used under careful supervision of a pediatric dermatologist in an inpatient hospital setting[3–5]

(1) Propranolol is a new treatment for hemangiomas with growing clinical evidence but is still considered *off-label*

(2) Treatment is indicated for hemangiomas that are blocking visual fields or other concerning areas

(3) It is imperative to screen patients for history of asthma and/or cardiac disease

(a) Always obtain a baseline electrocardiogram (ECG)

(b) Discuss with cardiologist prior to initiating treatment if cardiac conditions are present

(4) Dose escalation schedule:

(a) Propranolol 0.33 mg/kg/dose q8 hours for 24 hours with a total daily dose 1 mg/kg/day then

(b) Propranolol 0.67 mg/kg/dose q8 hours for 24 hours with a total daily dose 2 mg/kg/day

This will be goal home dose

(5) Monitor the following during administration:
   (a) Blood pressure, heart rate, and blood glucose 1 hour after each dose
   (b) Ensure infants <6 months are fed q4 hours
   (c) Assess patients immediately if heart rate (HR) <120 bpm for infants <6 months or <100 for patients >6 months, if systolic blood pressure (SBP) <80 or diastolic blood pressure (DBP) <40

(6) The patient can be discharged once the goal dose has been reached and observed for 3 doses. Must follow up with pediatrician every 48 hours for blood pressure (BP) and HR checks for first week after discharge and then weekly for one month, followed by monthly evaluation until treatment is complete

(7) In older patients, (>12 months) for whom approval for admission cannot be obtained, may very cautiously start at initial dose as outpatient with very close monitoring and slower increase in dose over 2–4 weeks

(8) Average length of treatment is 6–9 months, but depends on the regression of the lesion and age. Younger infants tend to have a longer treatment course secondary to higher rates of recurrence

d. Laser ablation: Evidence-based research suggests this is not effective
e. Interferon: Not often used because of neurologic complications
f. Embolization: Can be used to treat cutaneous hemangiomas that have not responded to medical therapy
g. Surgical excision[6]: Used in rare circumstances

B. Warts

1. Pathogenesis: Caused by more than 100 types of human papillomavirus (HPV). The virus enters the skin through breaks in the epithelium, causing hyperplasia of the squamous epithelium
2. Morphology:

a. Common warts: Lesions are skin-colored, rough, minimally scaly papules and nodules found on the exposed surfaces of the hands, face, arms, and legs. Lesions can be solitary or multiple, a few millimeters to several centimeters in diameter, and may form large plaques or a confluent, linear pattern secondary to autoinoculation
b. Flat warts: Occur over the hands, arms, and face; are usually <2 mm wide. Often present in clusters
c. Plantar warts: Found on the soles of the feet as sometimes painful but often asymptomatic, inward-growing, hyperkeratotic plaques and papules. Trauma on weight-bearing surfaces results in small black dots (*seeds* from thrombosed vessels on the surface of the wart)
d. Anogenital warts: See Chapter 5

3. Treatment (Table 8-1)[7,8]:

a. Spontaneous resolution occurs in >75% of warts in otherwise healthy individuals within 3 years

TABLE 8-1
WART THERAPY

Treatment	Advantages	Disadvantages
Keratolytics (lactic acid, salicylic acid, tretinoin)	Available without prescription, home therapy, low cost, low risk, little pain	Slow response, irritation
DESTRUCTIVE AGENTS		
Cryotherapy	Quick office procedure, relatively low cost	Pain, scarring, recurrence
Caustics (topical acids)	Home or office therapy, relatively low cost	Irritation, recurrence, systemic toxicity (podophyllin)
Cantharidin (vesicant)	Occasionally effective	High risk for recurrence, prominent pigmentary changes
Electrocautery and laser	Usually effective	Pain, scarring, recurrence, requires anesthesia, moderate cost

From Cohen BA: Warts and children: can they be separated? Contemp Pediatr 1997;2:128–149.

b. Keratolytics (i.e., topical salicylates): Work by removing excess scale within and around warts and by triggering an inflammatory reaction. Particularly effective in combination with adhesive tape occlusion; response may take 4 to 6 months
c. Destructive techniques depend on destruction of wart and surrounding normal skin and should be used only with the consent of the patient
   (1) There is no good data that shows destructive methods are better than placebo and, therefore, they are not recommended for children

See more treatment options on Expert Consult, Chapter 8

NOTE: As with molluscum contagiosum (discussed subsequently), recalcitrant or widespread lesions should be screened for immunodeficiency (congenital and acquired)

C. Molluscum Contagiosum

1. Morphology (Color Plate 1): Caused by the pox virus; consists of dome-shaped, often umbilicated, translucent to white papules that range from 1 mm to 1 cm, with a tiny keratotic core at the center. Lesions are often surrounded by scaling and erythema that resemble eczema. They may appear inflamed and secondarily infected when undergoing spontaneous involution. Often occur in children on the trunk, axillary region, face, and diaper regions, often spreading by autoinoculation. In teens, lesions may occur in the genital area as a sexually transmitted infection
2. Treatment: Lesions are benign and self-limited. Treatment, with the consent of the child, is directed toward symptomatic lesions, because destruction of the individual lesions may lead to scarring and recurrences of new papules are common despite treatment. No treatment has been proven to be more effective than placebo

See more treatment options on Expert Consult, Chapter 8

8

D. Pyogenic Granuloma (Color Plate 2)

1. Morphology: A benign erythematous, sessile or pedunculated papule, also known as a *lobular capillary hemangioma.* Usually solitary, bright red, soft papules; surface may be weepy, crusty, or completely epithelialized. Papules range in size from 2 mm to 2 cm, and may initially grow rapidly and bleed easily when traumatized. Relatively common in children (especially toddlers, commonly affecting the face) and young adults (especially during pregnancy); most commonly found on the head and neck, followed by the trunk, upper extremities, and lower extremities, respectively. Biopsy shows proliferating capillaries in a loose edematous fibrous matrix
2. Treatment:
   a. Surgical excision: May lead to scarring and frequently recurs
   b. Cauterization with silver nitrate: Also may lead to scarring and frequently recurs
   c. Laser ablation
   d. Shave excision: Electrodesiccation of the base or pedunculated papule that often has a discernible epithelial collarette. This is a relatively simple, effective, and cheap treatment with good results

E. Scabies

1. Pathogenesis: Mites are eight-legged arachnids about the size of a grain of sand. The infecting organism is most commonly *Sarcoptes scabiei.* Spread by skin-to-skin contact and through fomites, as they are able to live for 2 days away from the human body. Activated by warmth, the mite burrows under the skin to the stratum corneum in 2.5 min. Female moves 2–3 mm/day and lays eggs as she tunnels
2. Clinical manifestations: Small papules over female mite bite and/or linear or wavy burrows. Most commonly located in interdigital webs, wrist folds, elbows, axilla, buttocks, and belt line. May cause severe itching, especially at night. May result in secondary phenomena such as urticaria, excoriation, impetigo, and eczematous plaques
3. Treatment[9]:
   a. Permethrin cream: 5% cream applied from neck down to feet, including under fingernails, and left on for 8–14 hours. In infants, treatment should include scalp, neck, and forehead. Treat all family members with symptoms simultaneously, and advise parents to use topical lubricants generously to treat dryness of the skin produced by scabicide

See more treatment options on Expert Consult, Chapter 8

F. Reactive Erythema (Fig. 8-2; Color Plates 3 to 9)

1. Morphology: Group of disorders characterized by erythematous patches, plaques, and nodules that vary in size, shape, and distribution
2. Etiology: Represent cutaneous reaction patterns triggered by endogenous and environmental factors

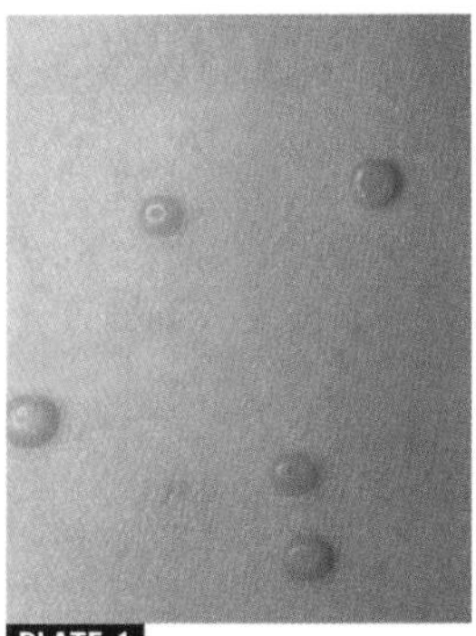

PLATE 1

Molluscum contagiosum. *(From Cohen BA: Pediatric dermatology, 3rd ed. St. Louis, Mosby, 2005, p. 126.)*

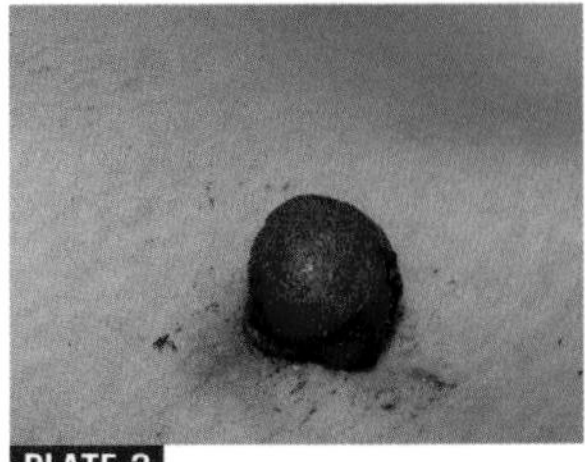

PLATE 2

Pyogenic granuloma. *(From Cohen BA: Dermatology image atlas. Available at www.med.jhu.edu/peds/dermatlas, 2001.)*

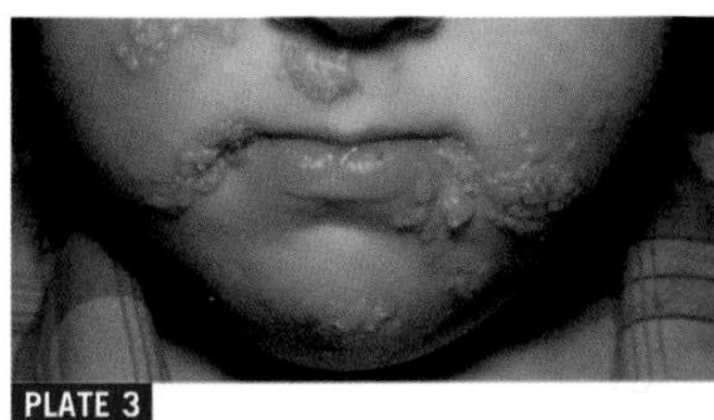

PLATE 3

Herpetic gingivostomatitis. *(From Cohen BA: Pediatric dermatology, 3rd ed. St. Louis, Mosby, 2005, p. 103.)*

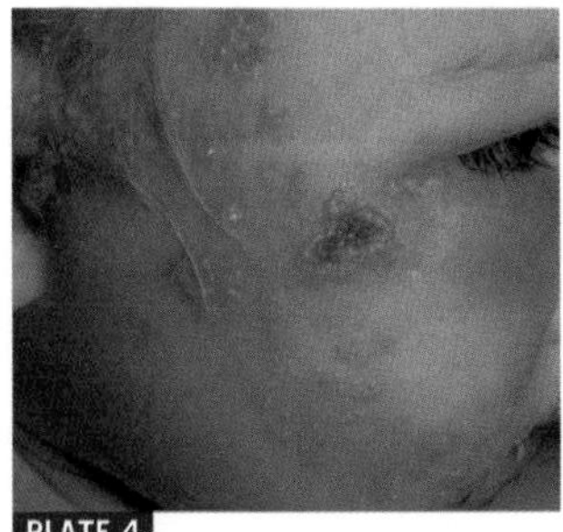

PLATE 4

Herpes zoster. *(From Cohen BA: Pediatric dermatology, 3rd ed. St. Louis, Mosby, 2005, p. 106.)*

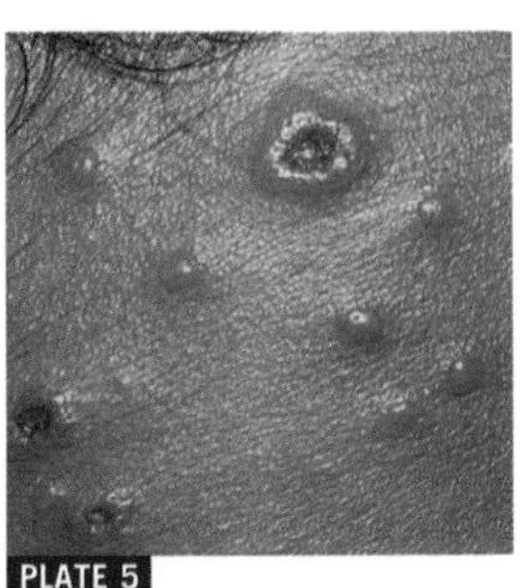

PLATE 5

Varicella. *(From Cohen BA: Pediatric dermatology, 3rd ed. St. Louis, Mosby, 2005, p. 104.)*

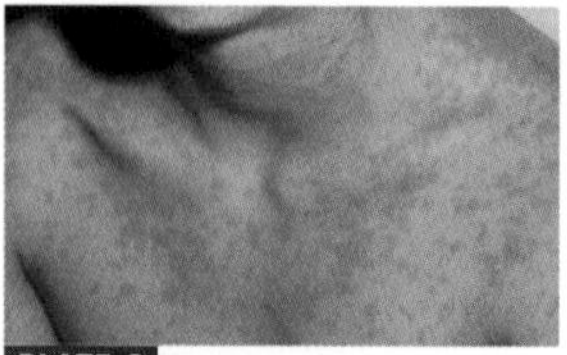

PLATE 6

Measles. *(From Cohen BA: Pediatric dermatology, 3rd ed. St. Louis, Mosby, 2005, p. 166.)*

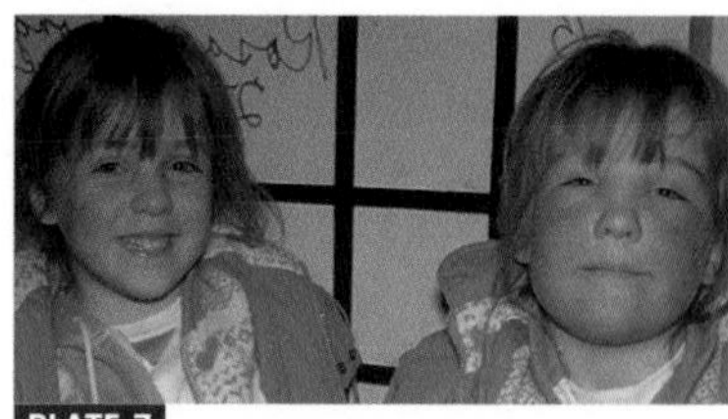

PLATE 7

Fifth disease. *(From Cohen BA: Pediatric dermatology, 3rd ed. St. Louis, Mosby, 2005, p. 167.)*

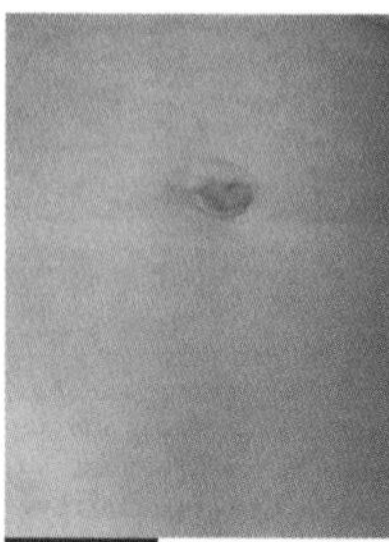

PLATE 8

Roseola. *(From Cohen BA: Pediatric dermatology, 3rd ed. St. Louis, Mosby, 2005, p. 168.)*

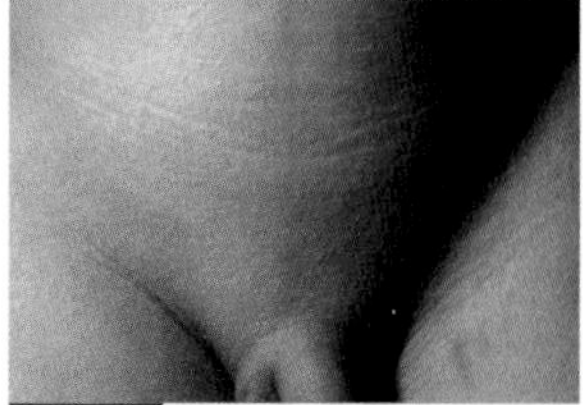

PLATE 9

Scarlet fever. *(From Cohen BA: Dermatology image atlas. Available at www.med.jhu.edu/peds/dermatlas, 2001.)*

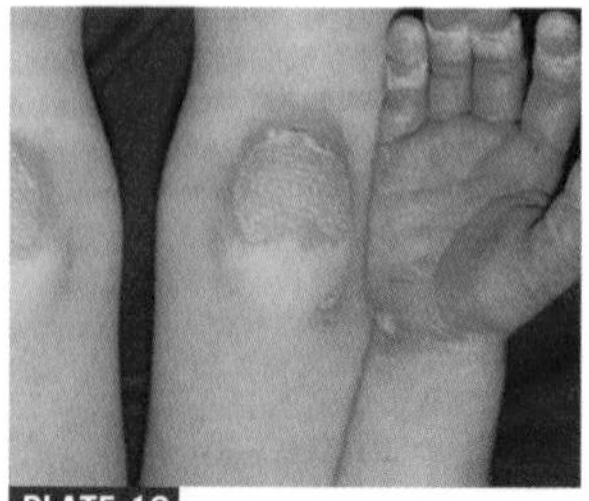

PLATE 10

Psoriasis. *(From Cohen BA: Pediatric dermatology, 3rd ed. St. Louis, Mosby, 2005, p. 67.)*

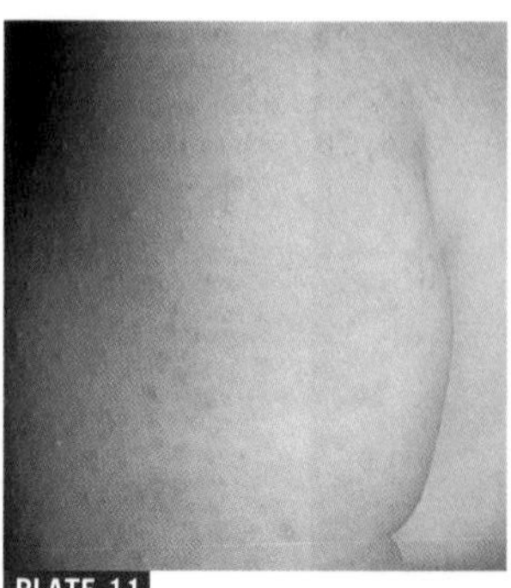

PLATE 11

Keratosis pilaris. *(From Cohen BA: Pediatric dermatology, 3rd ed. St. Louis, Mosby, 2005, p. 81.)*

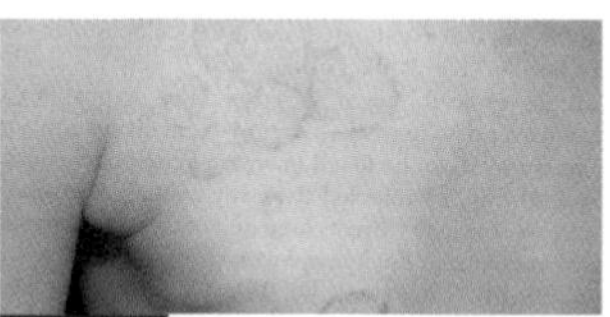

PLATE 12

Tinea corporis. *(From Cohen BA: Pediatric dermatology, 3rd ed. St. Louis, Mosby, 2005, p. 94.)*

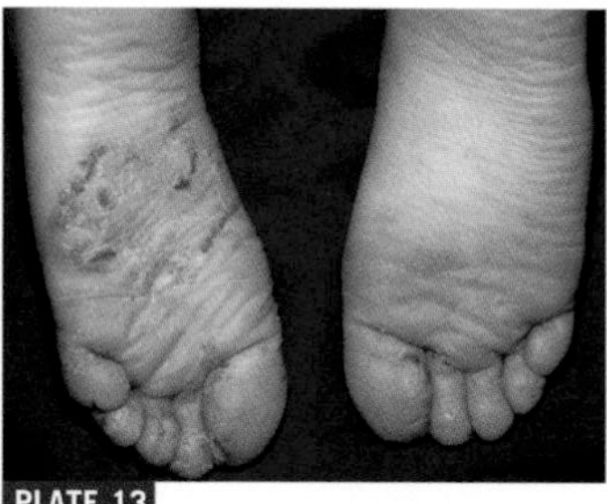

PLATE 13

Tinea pedis. *(From Cohen BA: Dermatology image atlas. Available at www.med.jhu.edu/peds/dermatlas, 2001.)*

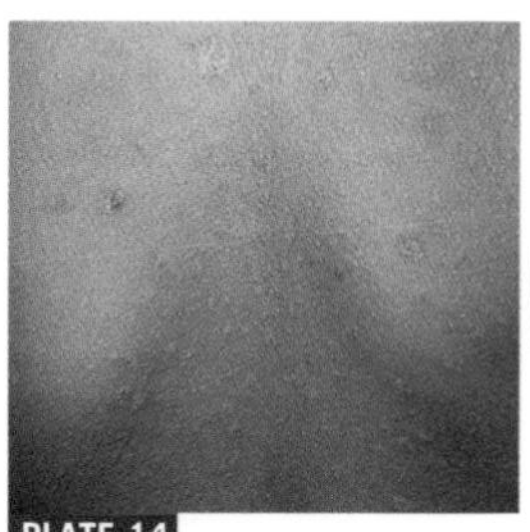

PLATE 14

Pityriasis rosea. *(From Cohen BA: Pediatric dermatology, 3rd ed. St. Louis, Mosby, 2005, p. 87.)*

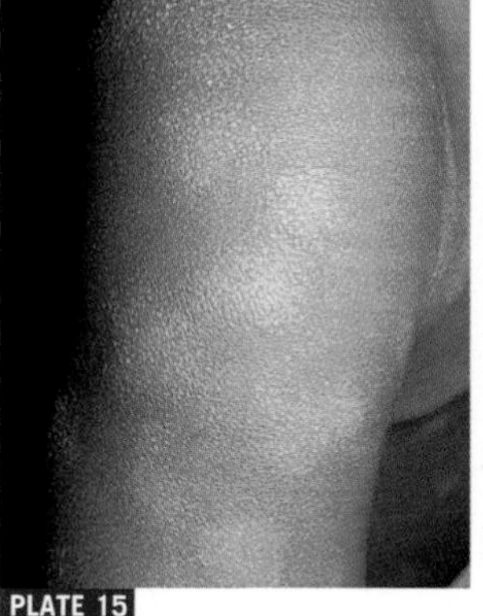

PLATE 15

Pityriasis alba. *(From Cohen BA: Pediatric dermatology, 3rd ed. St. Louis, Mosby, 2005, p. 82.)*

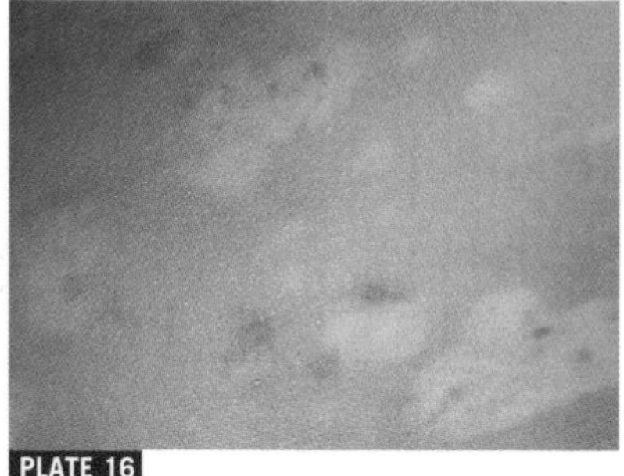

PLATE 16

Postinflammatory hyperpigmentation. *(From Cohen BA: Atlas of pediatric dermatology. St. Louis, Mosby, 1993.)*

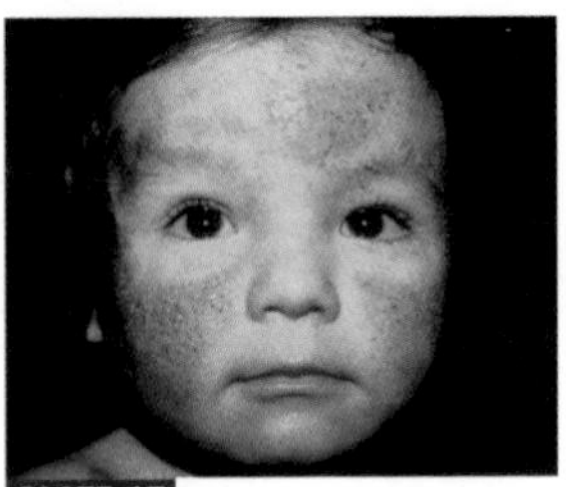

PLATE 17

Infantile eczema. *(From Cohen BA: Pediatric dermatology, 3rd ed. St. Louis, Mosby, 2005, p. 79.)*

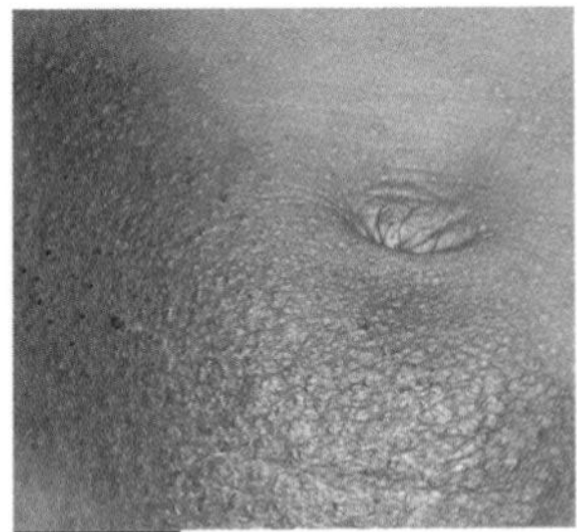

PLATE 18

Childhood eczema. *(From Cohen BA: Dermatology image atlas. Available at www.med.jhu.edu/peds/dermatlas, 2001.)*

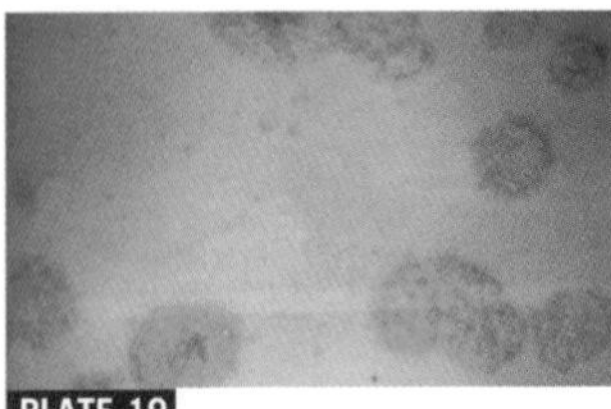

PLATE 19

Nummular eczema. *(From Cohen BA: Pediatric dermatology, 3rd ed. St. Louis, Mosby, 2005, p. 80.)*

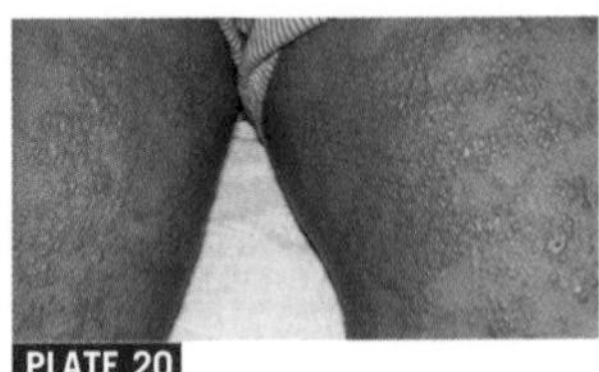

PLATE 20

Follicular eczema. *(From Cohen BA: Pediatric dermatology, 3rd ed. St. Louis, Mosby, 2005, p. 80.)*

PLATE 21

Childhood eczema with lesion in suprapubic area. *(From Cohen BA: Pediatric dermatology, 3rd ed. St. Louis, Mosby, 2005, Fig. 3.20c.)*

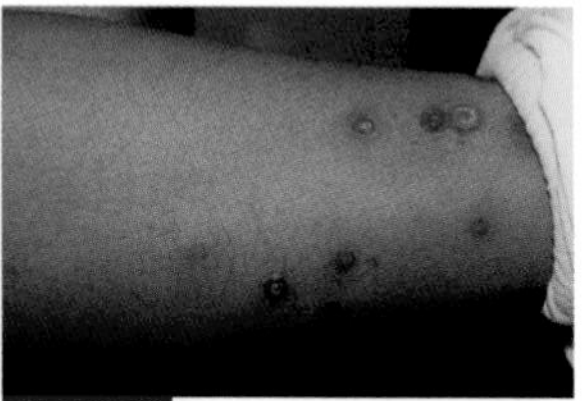

PLATE 22

Papular urticaria. *(From Cohen BA: Dermatology image atlas. Available at www.med.jhu.edu/peds/dermatlas, 2001.)*

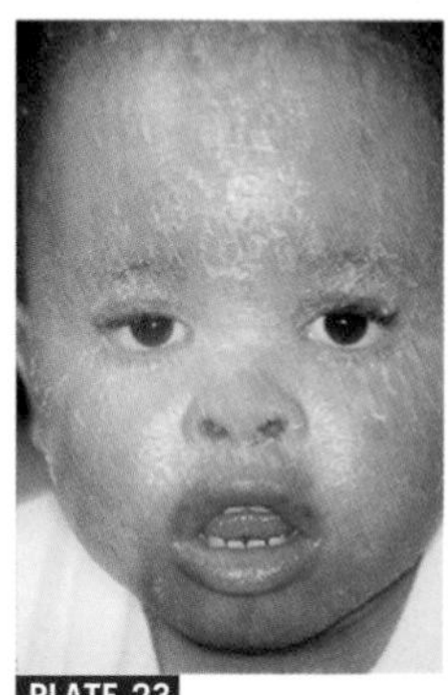

PLATE 23

Congenital ichthyosis erythroderma. *(From Cohen BA: Pediatric dermatology, 3rd ed, St. Louis, Mosby, 2005, p. 29.)*

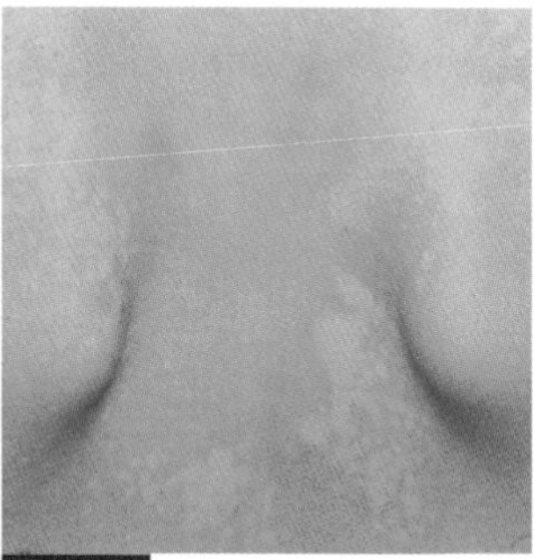

PLATE 24

Tinea versicolor. *(From Cohen BA: Atlas of pediatric dermatology. St. Louis, Mosby, 1993.)*

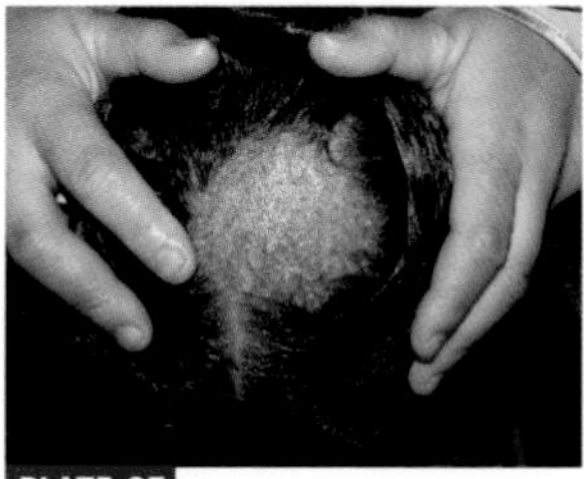

PLATE 25

Tinea capitis. *(From Cohen BA: Atlas of pediatric dermatology. St. Louis, Mosby, 1993.)*

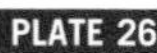

PLATE 26

Kerion. *(From Cohen BA: Pediatric dermatology, 3rd ed. St. Louis, Mosby, 2005, p. 207.)*

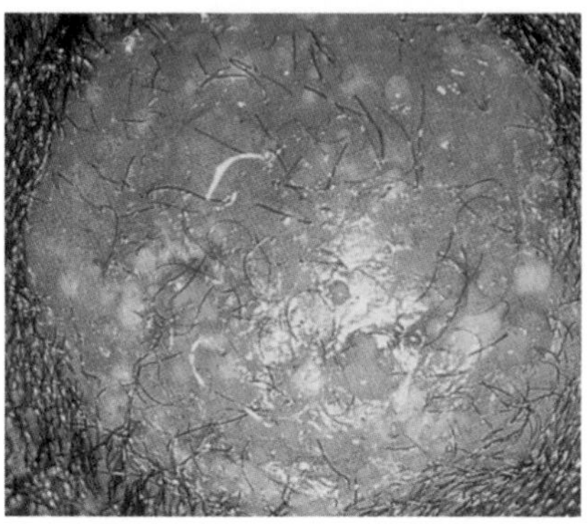

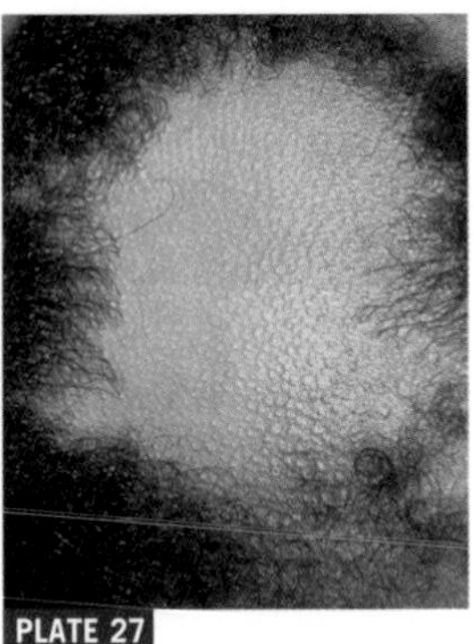

PLATE 27

Alopecia areata. *(From Cohen BA: Pediatric dermatology, 3rd ed. St. Louis, Mosby, 2005, p. 208.)*

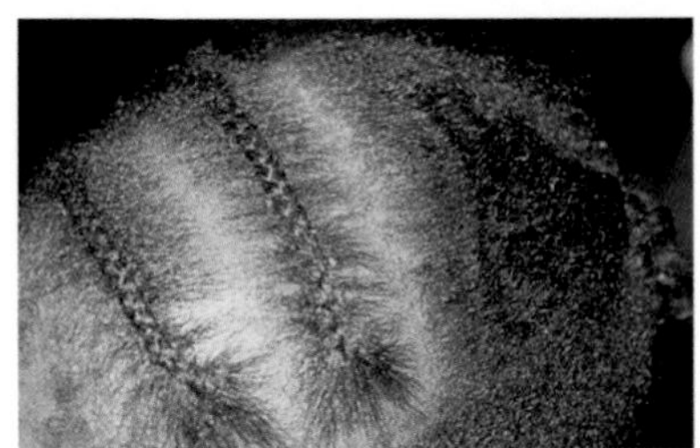

PLATE 28

Traction alopecia. *(From Cohen BA: Pediatric dermatology, 3rd ed. St. Louis, Mosby, 2005, p. 209.)*

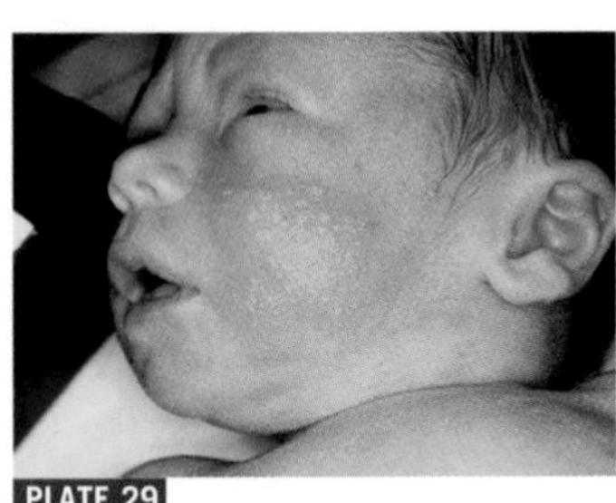

PLATE 29

Erythema toxicum neonatorum. *(From Cohen BA: Pediatric dermatology, 2nd ed. St. Louis, Mosby, 1999, p. 18.)*

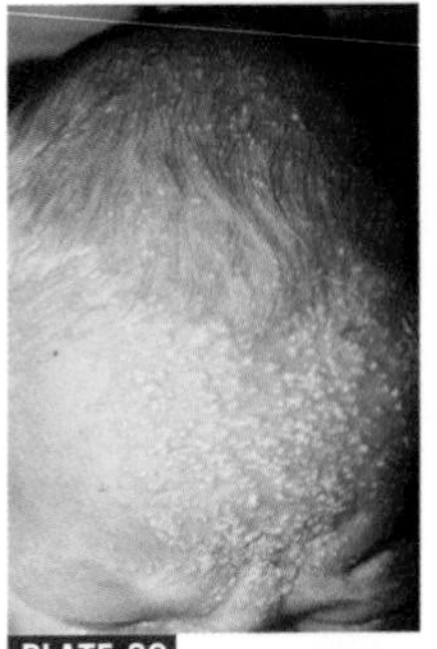

PLATE 30

Transient neonatal pustular melanosis. *(From Cohen BA: Pediatric dermatology, 3rd ed, St. Louis, Mosby, 2005, p. 20.)*

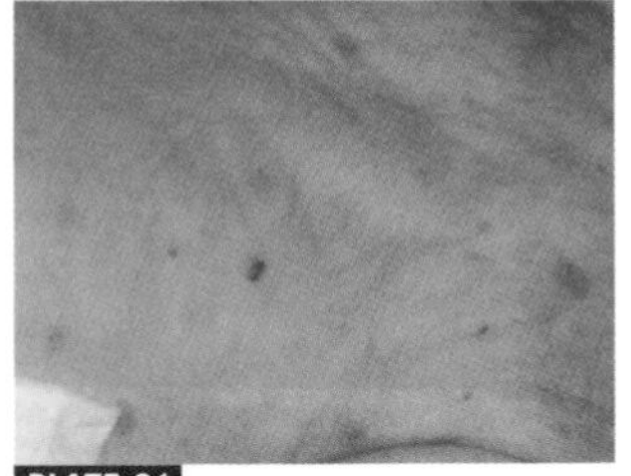

PLATE 31

Hyperpigmentation from resolving transient neonatal pustular melanosis. *(From Cohen BA: Pediatric dermatology, 3rd ed. St. Louis, Mosby, 2005, p. 20.)*

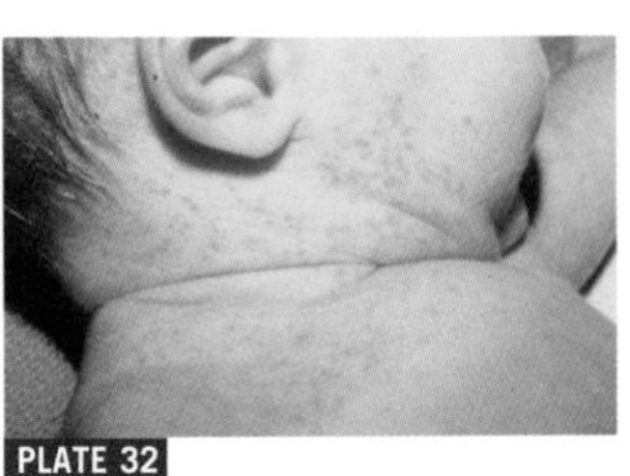

PLATE 32

Miliaria rubra. *(From Cohen BA: Pediatric dermatology, 3rd ed, St. Louis, Mosby, 2005, p. 22.)*

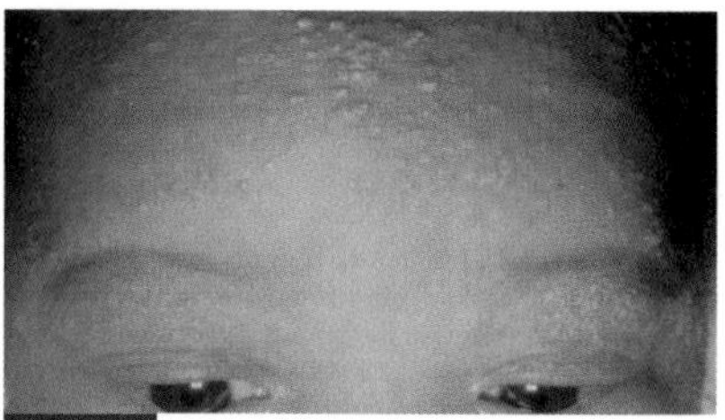

PLATE 33

Milia. *(From Cohen BA: Pediatric dermatology. St. Louis, 3rd ed, Mosby, 2005, p. 22.)*

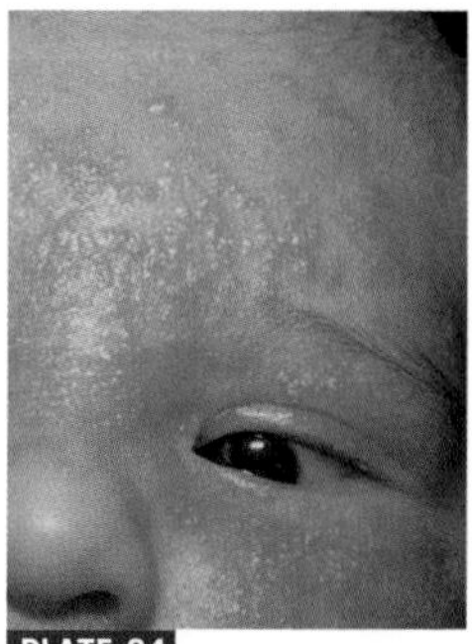

PLATE 34

Neonatal acne. *(From Cohen BA: Pediatric dermatology, 3rd ed. St. Louis, Mosby, 2005, p. 23.)*

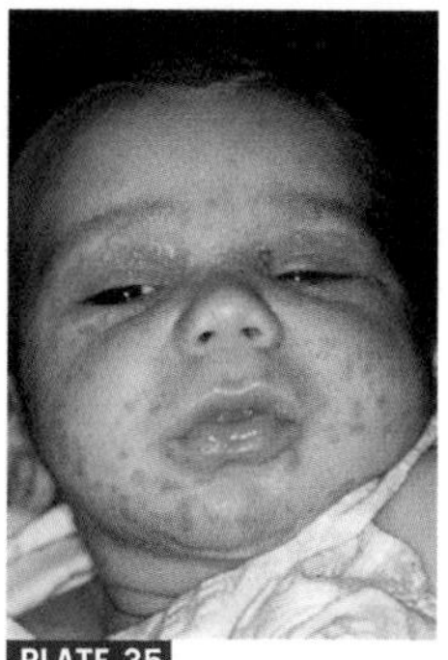

PLATE 35

Seborrheic dermatitis. *(From Cohen BA: Pediatric dermatology, 3rd ed, St. Louis, Mosby, 2005, p. 33.)*

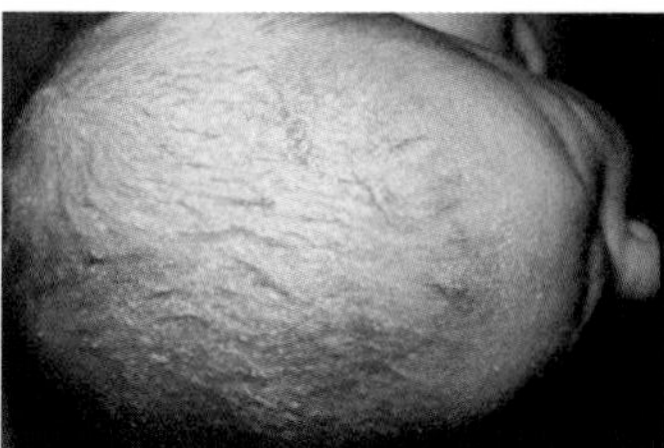

PLATE 36

Seborrheic dermatitis. *(From Cohen BA: Pediatric dermatology, 3rd ed, St. Louis, Mosby, 2005, p. 33.)*

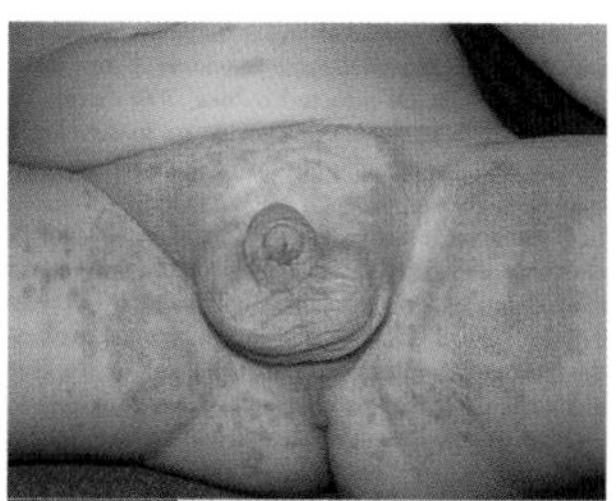

PLATE 37

Diaper candidiasis. *(From Cohen BA: Pediatric dermatology, 3rd ed. St. Louis, Mosby, 2005, p. 34.)*

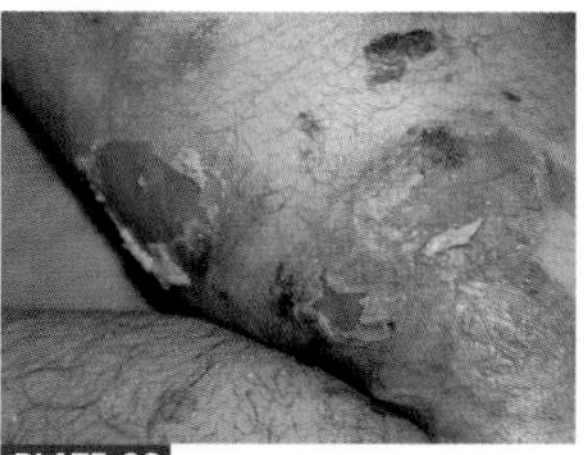

PLATE 38

Pemphigus vulgaris. *(From Cohen BA: Dermatology image atlas. Available at www.med.jhu.edu/peds/dermatlas, 2001.)*

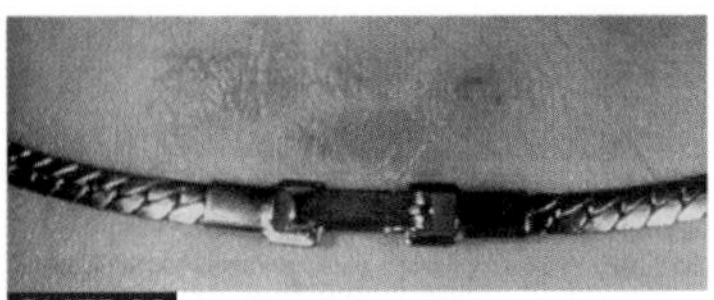

PLATE 39

Allergic contact dermatitis. *(From Cohen BA: Pediatric dermatology, 3rd ed. St. Louis, Mosby, 2005, p. 75.)*

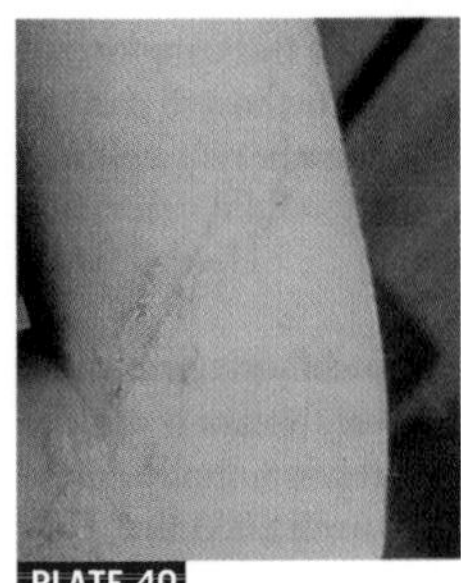

PLATE 40

Poison ivy. *(From Cohen BA: Dermatology image atlas. Available at www.med.jhu.edu/peds/dermatlas, 2001.)*

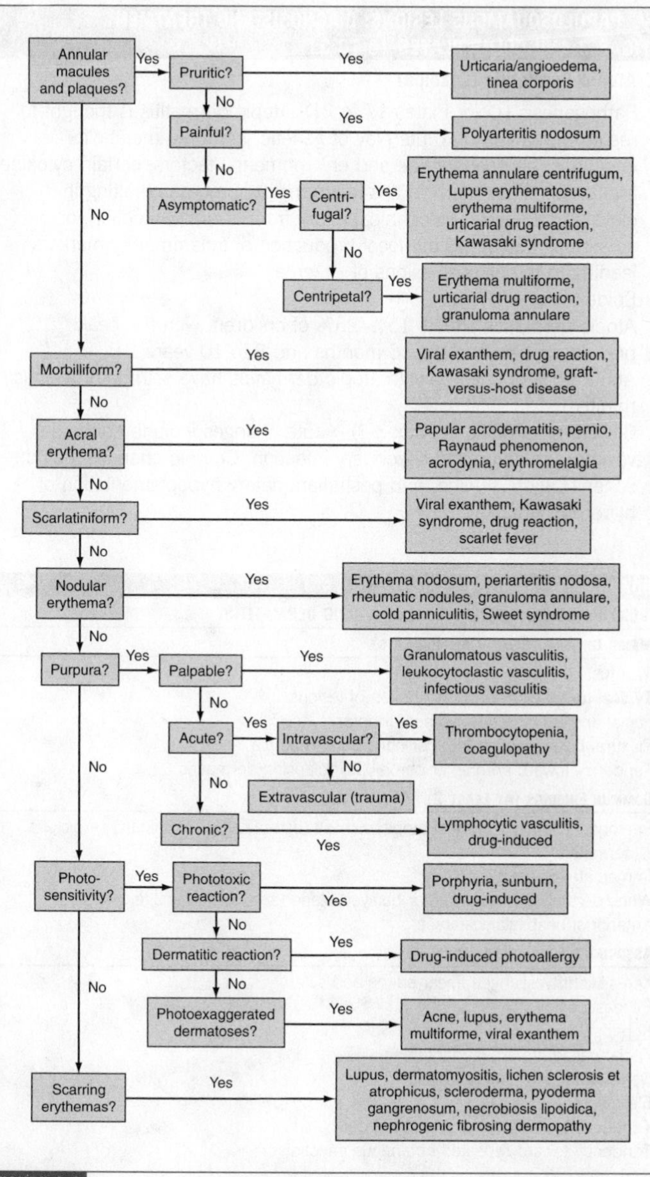

FIGURE 8-2

Reactive erythema. *(Modified from Cohen BA: Atlas of pediatric dermatology, 3rd ed. St. Louis, Mosby, 2005, p. 196.)*

8

IV. PAPULOSQUAMOUS LESIONS: DIAGNOSIS AND TREATMENT (FIG. 8-3 AND COLOR PLATES 10 TO 21)

A. Atopic Dermatitis (Eczema)

1. Pathogenesis (Color Plates 17 to 21): Atopic dermatitis is thought to result from a complex interplay of genetic, immune, metabolic, infectious, neuroendocrine and environmental factors; certain cytokines and chemokines mediate this inflammatory process resulting in elevated IgE levels. Mechanical injury from trauma, infection, or scratching stimulates the local production of inflammatory markers leading to the clinical lesions of eczema
2. Epidemiology:
   a. Atopic dermatitis affects 15%–25% of children, with the peak prevalence between ages 6 months and 8 to 10 years
   b. About 95% of children with atopic dermatitis have asthma or allergic rhinitis
3. Clinical presentations (Box 8-1): Acute changes include erythema, vesicles, crusting, and secondary infection. Chronic changes include lichenification, scaling, and postinflammatory hypopigmentation or hyperpigmentation

BOX 8-1

IDENTIFYING CHARACTERISTICS OF ATOPIC DERMATITIS

MAJOR CRITERIA (SEEN IN ALL PATIENTS)

Pruritus
Typical morphology and distribution of lesions
Facial and extensor involvement in infants
Flexural lichenification in older children and adults
Tendency toward chronic or chronically relapsing dermatitis

COMMON FINDINGS (AT LEAST 2)

Personal or family history of atopic disease (asthma, allergic rhinitis, atopic dermatitis)
Immediate skin test reactivity
White dermatographism and/or delayed blanch to cholinergic agents
Anterior subcapsular cataracts

ASSOCIATED FINDINGS (AT LEAST 4)

Xerosis/ichthyosis/hyperlinear palms and soles
Pityriasis alba
Keratosis pilaris
Facial pallor/infraorbital darkening
Dennie-Morgan infraorbital fold
Elevated serum IgE
Tendency toward nonspecific hand dermatitis
Tendency toward repeated cutaneous infections

From Cohen BA: Atopic dermatitis: Breaking the itch-scratch cycle. *Contemp Pediatr* 1992;7:64–81.

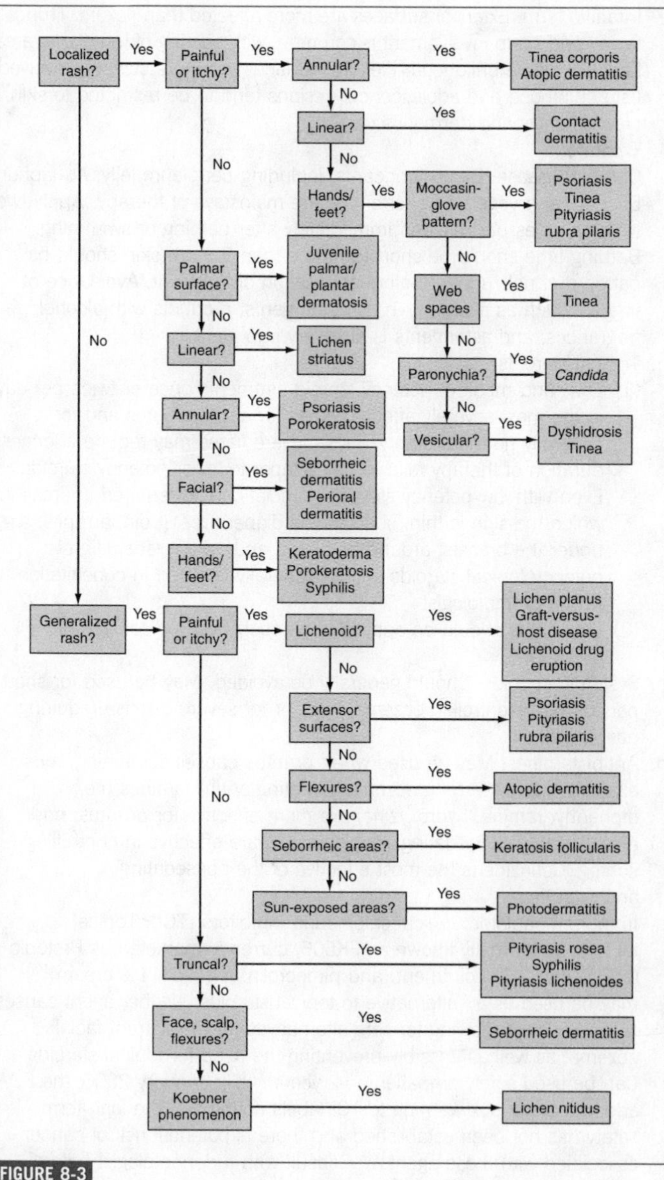

FIGURE 8-3

Papulosquamous disorders algorithm. *(Modified from Cohen BA: Atlas of pediatric dermatology, 3rd ed. St. Louis, Mosby, 2005, p. 97.)*

a. Infantile form: Extensor surfaces are more affected than flexors. Truncal, facial, and scalp involvement is common, with sparing of the diaper area
b. Early to middle childhood: Flexural surfaces are more severely involved
c. Late childhood and adolescence: Lesions tend to be restricted to skin creases and hand dermatitis

4. Treatment:

a. Chronic disease: Bland lubricants, including petroleum jelly, Aquaphor, Eucerin, and vegetable shortening, are mainstays of therapy. Apply two to three times per day and immediately after bathing or swimming. Bathing time should be short (no more than 5 min); skin should be patted dry, not rubbed, before application of lubricant. Avoidance of triggers such as allergens, harsh detergents, products with alcohol, fragrances, and astringents is also very important
b. Topical steroids:
   (1) Low- and medium-potency steroid ointments once or twice per day in the most severely affected areas for eczema flares and for generally no more than 7 days. Severe flares may require a longer duration of therapy followed by a taper to lower-potency steroids. Even with low-potency steroids, special care is required in areas in which the skin is thin, such as the diaper area, groin, armpits, under the breasts, around the neck, and on the face. High-potency topical steroids should generally be used in consultation with a dermatologist
   (2) Lubricants should be applied generously over topical steroid ointment
c. Systemic steroids: Should generally be avoided. May be used for short periods of uncontrolled eczema flares or for severe disease requiring hospitalization
d. Antihistamines: May be used when pruritus causes scratching, thus exacerbating underlying eczema. Sedating antihistamines (i.e., diphenhydramine, hydroxyzine) are more effective for pruritus; no evidence that nonsedating antihistamines are effective in controlling itching. Cetirizine is the most effective of the nonsedating antihistamines
e. Immunomodulators-topical calcineurin inhibitors (TCI): Topical tacrolimus (formally known as FK506, currently marketed as Protopic 0.03% and 0.1% ointment) and pimecrolimus (Elidel 1% cream)[10,11] may be used as an alternative to topical steroids. Neither agent causes skin atrophy,[12] allowing for safe alternatives for recalcitrant facial eczema, as well as possibly preventing the need for topical steroids. Can be used safely on patients >2 years[13–15] In January 2006, the FDA added a black box warning to TCI labels noting that the long-term safety has not been established and there is potential risk of cancer associated with these agents.[16] Consult with a dermatologist before considering this treatment
f. Protective clothing should be worn

5. Complications[17]: Most common complications include blistering of lesions, bacterial infections, and eczema herpeticum

See more information about eczema complications on Expert Consult, Chapter 8

B. Papular Urticaria (Color Plate 22)

Insect bite-induced hypersensitivity (IBIH)

1. Morphology: Characterized by chronic or recurrent eruptions of pruritic papules, vesicles, and wheals resulting from a hypersensitivity reaction to biting and stinging insects. Predominance of a T-cell mediated response characterizes its chronic nature. Most commonly grouped in linear clusters and present on exposed areas with sparing of the genital, perianal, and axillary regions. Intense pruritus, resulting in excoriation, secondary infection. Scarring and permanent hyperpigmentation and/or hypopigmentation in some patients, particularly in darkly pigmented individuals
2. SCRATCH principles[18]:

S: Symmetrical eruption: Usually in exposed areas; sparing of the diaper region

C: Clustering: Described as *meal cluster;* linear or triangular groupings of lesions that reflect the biting insect's path along the skin

R: Rover not required: A history of pets in the home is not a requirement for considering IBIH; exposure may be remote

A: Age: Rarely seen before age 2 years. Peak age range: 2–10 years, with most children developing tolerance by age 10 years. If patient is <2 years old, rethink diagnosis

T: Target lesions: Common appearance, especially in darker pigmented patients
Time: Emphasize chronic nature of eruption and need for watchful waiting

C: Confused pediatrician/parent: Often diagnosis is met with disbelief by parent and/or referring pediatrician

H: Household: Because it is a hypersensitivity reaction IBIH often affects only one family member, unlike atopic dermatitis and scabies, in which multiple family members may have a history of symptoms

3. Management (The 3 Ps):

a. **P**revention: Advise patients to wear protective clothing and use insect repellent when outside, launder bedding and mattress pads for bed mites, and maximize flea control for pets

b. **P**ruritus control: Antihistamines if symptoms are acute and suggest a type 1 nature; not very effective in chronic stages. Topical steroids may also be used for acute lesions; extension into the dermis and fat may make these ineffective. Second-generation antihistamines such as cetirizine may be helpful for pruritus

c. **P**atience: Advise patients of the frustrating, recurrent nature of IBIH reactions; ensure parents of the eventual development of tolerance and resolution of symptoms

C. Ichthyosis (Color Plate 23)

A group of scaling disorders consisting of five major variants: congenital ichthyosiform erythroderma, lamellar ichthyosis, epidermolytic hyperkeratosis, ichthyosis vulgaris, and X-linked ichthyosis. There are also six separate ichthyotic syndromes, of which these lesions are a feature.

D. Tinea Versicolor (Color Plate 24)

1. Epidemiology: Infecting organism is *Pityrosporum (Malassezia)*; commonly colonizes skin by age 4–6 months
2. Clinical presentation: Multiple small oval scaly patches that measure 1–3 cm in diameter in a raindrop pattern on upper chest, back, and proximal portions of the upper extremities of adolescents and young adults. Usually asymptomatic, but some patients may complain of pruritus. Lesions appear light tan, reddish, or white in color; appear hyperpigmented in light-skinned patients and hypopigmented in darker-skinned patients
3. Diagnosis: Based on physical appearance; "*spaghetti and meatball*" short pseudohyphae on potassium hydroxide (KOH) microscopy
4. Treatment: Selenium sulfide and propylene glycol; rapidly clear infection; pigmentary changes may take a prolonged time to clear, and recurrence is common

E. Tinea Corporis

1. Epidemiology: Most commonly caused by *Trichophyton* species
2. Clinical presentation: Patients typically present with annular patch or plaque with an advancing, raised, scaling border and a central clearing. Typically affects glabrous skin (smooth and bare) and is often pruritic
3. Diagnosis: Most patients are diagnosed clinically, but KOH microscopy of a skin scraping can determine if hyphae are present. Culture confirmation is usually not required
4. Treatment: Topical treatment is often sufficient for treatment, but oral antifungals can be added for severe infections. Traditional topical antifungals include clotrimazole and miconazole, but newer antifungals such as butenafine and terbinafine have been shown to be more effective because of their stronger fungicidal properties. Topical treatment is recommended until the lesion resolves plus 1–2 additional weeks[19]

V. HAIR LOSS: DIAGNOSIS AND TREATMENT

A. Tinea Capitis (Color Plate 25)

1. Epidemiology:

a. *Trichophyton tonsurans* accounts for >90% of tinea capitis in North America. An anthropophilic organism with no known natural reservoir; persists for long periods on fomites such as hairbrushes, combs, furniture, stuffed toys, and clothing

b. Most patients are age 1–10 years, but infection may occur at any age
c. Incidence is highest in African American children and second highest in Hispanic youths. This predisposition is not completely understood, but may be the result of the character of the hair follicle, tight braiding, or the use of pomades
2. Clinical presentations:
a. Classic tinea capitis: Presents as one or more round to oval patches of partial to complete alopecia, with varying degrees of erythema. Scale is present, and the border is slightly raised and more erythematous than the central area
b. Kerion (Color Plate 26): Inflammatory presentation of tinea capitis. A boggy, tender, edematous plaque or cluster of nodules with erythema; usually solitary and is frequently accompanied by cervical or occipital adenopathy and papular morbilliform eruption, classified as an *id reaction*
c. Seborrheic dermatitis-like pattern (most common): May produce minimal or no alopecia and show diffuse scaling over the scalp, with pruritus
d. Follicular pustules with crusting and scaling scattered over the scalp. Pattern seen predominantly in African American children with tight braiding and constant pomade use; often resembles bacterial folliculitis, but bacterial culture is negative
3. Diagnosis: The presumptive clinical diagnosis may be confirmed by either direct microscopic examination or culture of scale (may be collected with a toothbrush on a culture plate or on a moistened culturette swab)
4. Treatment:
a. Success requires oral therapy; griseofulvin is the agent of choice. It is best taken with fatty food to promote absorption (see Formulary for dosage information). Standard references suggest 4–6 weeks of therapy, although 8–12 weeks may be required for eradication. Patients should be reevaluated monthly; repeat culture may be obtained 2 weeks *before* therapy is discontinued to document cure. Patients will often develop an eczema-like rash associated with the fungal infection (id reaction); not a drug reaction, and griseofulvin therapy should be continued[19]
b. Terbinafine (Lamisil granules) can be used for a 4-week treatment course and has been shown to be just as effective as an 8-week course of griseofulvin against *Trichophyton* infections; however, it is not as effective against *Microsporum*[20]
c. Fluconazole is an alternative oral therapy that has been shown to be effective for treatment of tinea capitis either for continuous use for 3 to 6 weeks or once-weekly dosing for 8 weeks; however this has not been approved for treatment of tinea in children by the FDA. The other azoles (itraconazole and ketoconazole) have also been used to treat

8

superficial and systemic fungal infections, but have not been approved by the FDA for treatment of tinea

d. Kerions: Treat with prednisone or prednisolone (0.5 mg/kg/day for 10–14 days) if no contraindication exists in addition to standard griseofulvin therapy
e. The use of sporicidal shampoos in addition to oral therapy promotes rapid elimination of spores, thus decreasing the contagion risk to family members and schoolmates. Selenium sulfide 2.5% shampoo twice weekly is recommended. Ketoconazole 1% and 2% shampoo is also available for this purpose

B. Alopecia Areata (Color Plate 27)

1. Clinical presentation: Common condition characterized by the sudden onset of asymptomatic, noninflammatory, round, bald patches located on any hair-bearing part of the body, most commonly the scalp. Course is irregular and unpredictable; most patients develop good regrowth of hair within 1 or 2 years
2. Diagnosis: Differentiated by the absence of hair follicles in the bald spot. There is also a lack of scaly erythema, pustules, and crusts
3. Treatment: Topical corticosteroids, topical minoxidil, tar preparations, anthralin, topical sensitizers, and ultraviolet light therapy.[21] Although there is some thought that these treatments may be helpful, there is no research-based evidence that these interventions improve the disease course. Likewise, systemic steroids should generally not be used because they do not alter prognosis. In adolescents and adults, hair loss often resolves over months to years; in younger children, the prognosis is more guarded

C. Telogen Effluvium

1. Pathogenesis: Growing hair follicles respond to physiologic and pathologic stress (e.g., high fever, severe influenza, infection, surgery, drugs, pregnancy, hypothyroidism) by regressing to the resting, or telogen, state
2. Clinical presentation: A form of alopecia characterized by diffuse hair loss that is usually not clinically obvious to anyone but the patient and parent
3. Treatment: Usually occurs 3–5 months after the stressor and is self-limited

D. Traction Alopecia (Color Plate 28)

1. Pathogenesis: Often a result of hairstyles that apply tension for long periods of time
2. Clinical presentation: Noninflammatory linear areas of hair loss at the margins of the hairline, part line, or scattered regions, depending on hair styling procedures used
3. Treatment: Avoidance of styling products or styles resulting in traction

E. Hair Pulling

Hair pulling is a benign, self-limited activity common in young children.

F. Trichotillomania

1. Pathogenesis: Alopecia caused by the compulsion to pull out one's own hair, resulting in irregular areas of incomplete hair loss, mainly on the scalp; eyebrows and eyelashes may also be involved
2. Clinical presentation: Characterized by areas of hair loss within which are short, broken hair shafts of varying lengths
3. Treatment: Most cases spontaneously resolve, but in severe cases a psychiatric evaluation may be warranted

VI. ACNE VULGARIS

A. Pathogenesis

Four primary factors contribute to the development of acne lesions: abnormal desquamation of keratinocytes within the pilosebaceous unit, increased sebum production, proliferation of *Propionibacterium acnes,* and inflammation

1. Noninflammatory = closed comedo (whitehead) or open comedo (blackhead)
   a. Obstructive lesions: Open comedones are dilated follicles and closed comedones are white or skin-colored papules without surrounding erythema
2. Inflammatory = papules, pustules, nodules or cysts
   a. Typically appear later in the course of acne and vary from 1 to 2 mm micropapules to nodules larger than 5 mm; nodulocystic presentations are more likely to lead to permanent scarring/ hyperpigmentation

B. Treatment[22] (Table 8-2 and Table 8-3)

1. Gentle, nonabrasive cleaning is best. Vigorous scrubbing, abrasive cleaners, and mechanical devices can promote the development of inflammatory lesions
2. Dietary factors play no role in sebum production
3. Topical retinoids are the first-line of therapy for both comedonal and inflammatory acne. Retinoids prevent the formation of new lesions, enhance penetration of topical antibiotics and benzoyl peroxide and are thus considered an essential part of therapy
   a. Starting with topical retinoid therapy is standard for comedonal acne, but therapy with retinoids combined with either a topical or oral antibiotic and benzoyl peroxide (BPO) is considered standard of care for patients with both inflammatory and comedonal acne
4. Topical antibiotic therapy is indicated for mild inflammatory acne; antibiotic resistance is fairly common with prolonged use without concomitant use of BPO. Topical antibiotics are no longer recommended as monotherapy for acne

TABLE 8-2

TOPICAL AND SYSTEMIC ANTIBIOTICS USED TO TREAT ACNE

Antibiotic	Characteristics
TOPICAL	
Erythromycin	*P. acnes* very sensitive; least lipophilic
Clindamycin	*P. acnes* very sensitive; more lipophilic than erythromycin, but less than benzoyl peroxide
Benzoyl peroxide plus erythromycin	*P. acnes* very sensitive; most lipophilic topical agent; less irritating than benzoyl peroxide alone
Benzoyl peroxide plus clindamycin	Similar to characteristics for previous benzoyl peroxide plus erythromycin
Azelaic acid	*P. acnes* sensitive; minimal lipophilia; can reduce abnormal desquamation
Metronidazole	*P. acnes* not sensitive; has anti-inflammatory properties
Benzoyl peroxide plus glycolic acid	Glycolic acid may enhance penetration and reduce abnormal desquamation
SYSTEMIC	
Tetracycline	*P. acnes* sensitive; inexpensive; usually needs to be taken two to four times a day; compliance can be a problem because of need to take on an empty stomach
Erythromycin	*P. acnes* very sensitive; resistance emerging; gastrointestinal upset common; inexpensive
Doxycycline	Lipophilic; *P. acnes* very sensitive; resistance not yet seen; photosensitivity can occur; more expensive than tetracycline and erythromycin
Minocycline	Lipophilic; *P. acnes* very sensitive; resistance not yet seen; no photosensitivity; abnormal pigmentation in oral mucosa and skin; vertigo-like symptoms; most expensive
Trimethoprim-sulfamethoxazole	Lipophilic; *P. acnes* very sensitive; severe erythema multiforme and toxic epidermal necrolysis limit use
Clindamycin	*P. acnes* very sensitive; somewhat lipophilic; pseudomembranous colitis limits use

From Leyden JJ: Therapy for acne vulgaris. N Engl J Med 1997;16:1156–1162.

5. Moderate to severe acne: Oral antibiotic therapy should be instituted along with a topical retinoid and BPO
   a. Tetracycline, doxycycline, and minocycline are the standard first-line choice
6. Hormonal therapy, oral contraceptives, and spironolactone are appropriate for females who have sudden onset of severe acne who have not responded to conventional first-line therapy, or have persistent inflammatory papules and nodules involving primary the lower face and neck. Hormonal therapy is integral for treating women with hyperandrogenism
7. Systemic isotretinoin: Reserved for patients with nodular, cystic lesions who do not respond to systemic antibiotics and other combination acne treatments
   a. Should be used in consultation with a dermatologist in order for labs to be followed secondary to risk for leukocytosis, to screen for depression,

TABLE 8-3

ACNE TREATMENT ALGORITHM

	Acne Severity				
	Mild		Moderate		Severe
	Comedonal	**Papular/Pustular**	**Papular/Pustular**	**Nodular**	**Nodular/Conglobate**
1st-Line Treatment	Topical Retinoid	Topical Retinoid + Topical Antibiotic	Oral Antibiotic + Topical Retinoid +/– BPO	Oral Antibiotic + Topical Retinoid +/– BPO	Oral Isotretinoin
Alternative Treatments	Alternative Topical Retinoid OR Salicylic Acid	Alternative Topical Antimicrobial Agent + Alternative Topical Retinoid OR Azelaic Acid	Alternative Oral Antibiotic + Alternative Topical Retinoid +/– BPO	Oral Isotretinoin OR Alternative Oral Antibiotic + Alternative Topical Retinoid +/– BPO	High-Dose Oral Antibiotic + Topical Retinoid +BPO
Alternative Treatments for Females			Oral Antiandrogen + Topical Retinoid +/– Topical Antimicrobial	Oral Antiandrogen + Topical Retinoid +/– Oral Antibiotic +/– Topical Antimicrobial	High Dose Oral Antiandrogen + Topical Retinoid +/– Topical Antimicrobial
Maintenance Treatment	Topical Retinoid		Topical Retinoid +/– BPO		

BPO, Benzoyl Peroxide.

Adapted from Gollnick, H et al. AAD Management of Acnes: A Report from the Global Alliance to Improve Outcomes in Acne. p38.

8

and to ensure that two forms of effective and reliable contraception for women are in place secondary to the medication's teratogenic effects

b. Use in patients with acute promyelocytic leukemia (APL) is extremely dangerous. APL syndrome is characterized by respiratory distress, fever, weight gain, and effusions of the heart and lungs[23]
c. iPledge Program: Computer-based risk management program; designed to eliminate fetal exposure to isotretinoin through special restricted distribution program approved by the FDA

VII. COMMON NEONATAL DERMATOLOGIC CONDITIONS (FIG. 8-4 AND COLOR PLATES 29 TO 37; SEE ALSO COLOR PLATE 23)

A. Erythema Toxicum Neonatorum (ET) (Color Plate 29)

Most common rash (pustular) in infants. It is described as a papular rash (2–3 mm in diameter at first), often evolving into vesicles. Rash occurs most often on the second or third days of life (but can emerge as late as 2–3 weeks). Lesions may be clustered and usually resolve in 5–7 days from emergence; recurrences may occur. Vesicular fluid is significant for the presence of eosinophils; treatment is supportive only because rash is self-limited.

B. Transient Neonatal Pustular Melanosis (Color Plates 30 and 31)

Occurs in 4% of infants, especially infants with darker skin tones, and is usually present at birth. This vesicular rash is described as 2–5 mm pustules with a hyperpigmented, nonerythematous base, which over time develops a central crust and leaves a hyperpigmented macule with concurrent scale. Self-limiting, as the name implies.

C. Miliaria (Color Plate 32)

Noted commonly on the nose, these (often erythematous) lesions occur secondary to obstruction of eccrine sweat ducts. May also occur as small papules and pustules secondary to obstruction of these ducts in the mid-epidermis (also known as *prickly heat*). Often occur after the first week of life in areas of high heat production and occlusion by clothes or coverings; course is self-limiting and can be hastened by removal of tight wraps or clothing.

D. Milia (Color Plate 33)

Common lesions (up to 50% occurrence) are 1–3 mm papules (white to yellow in color), occurring mostly on the upper body and face of newborns, usually within the first month of life. Can persist for several months and are epidermal inclusion cysts requiring no treatment.

E. Neonatal Acne (Color Plate 34)

Often present at birth, these common (occurring in up to 20% of infants), open or closed comedones are thought to be triggered by maternal and endogenous androgens. No treatment is necessary because these lesions are self-limiting.

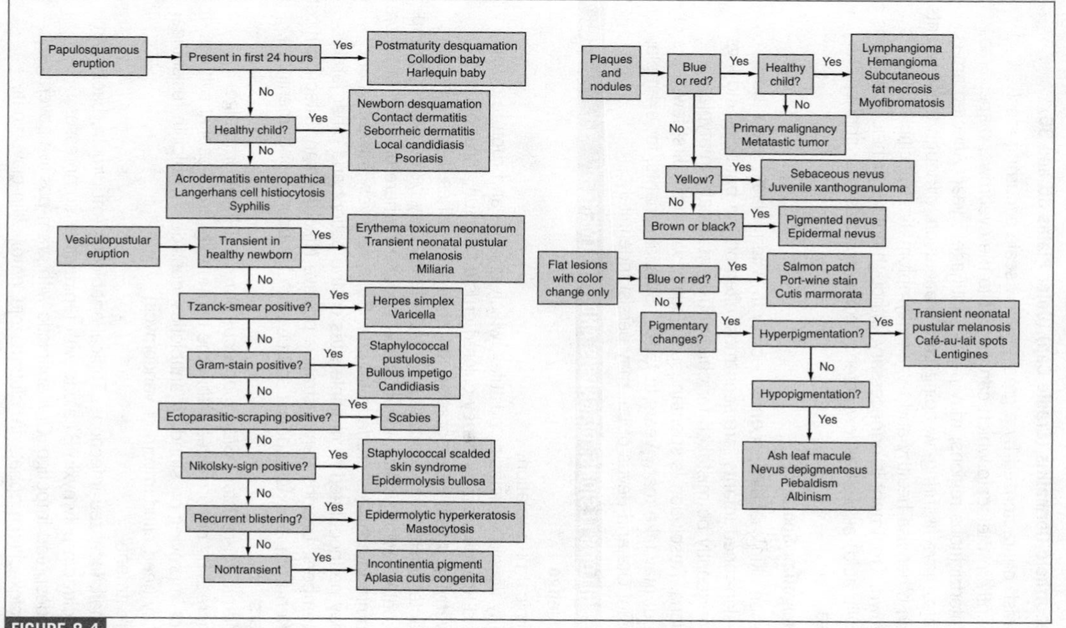

FIGURE 8-4 Evaluation of neonatal rashes. *(Modified from Cohen BA: Atlas of pediatric dermatology, 3rd ed. St. Louis, Mosby, 2005, p. 62.)*

F. Seborrheic Dermatitis (Cradle Cap) (Color Plates 35 and 36)

Skin rash characterized by a greasy yellow scale occurring most frequently in the scalp which can extend to the eyebrows, diaper area, and intertriginous regions; may persist until age 1 year. Affected areas may also have fissuring, weeping, and maceration, although these infants remain otherwise healthy and largely asymptomatic. Specific etiology is unknown. Treatment is unnecessary, although antiseborrheic shampoos (salicylic acid) as well as low-potency corticosteroids may shorten the course.

G. Mongolian Spots

Common skin macules, seen especially in Asian, black, and other dark-skin-toned infants; are seen most often on the buttocks and legs. Can frequently be mistaken for child abuse, especially in atypical locations. Resolution is spontaneous, usually within the first few years of life, but may take many years to fade.[24] Special variants, for example, nevus of Ota and nevus of Ita, may persist indefinitely.

VIII. BULLOUS LESIONS: DIAGNOSIS AND TREATMENT

A. Impetigo

1. Clinical presentation:
   a. Tiny flaccid vesicles or pustules, which enlarge and rupture quickly and are followed by honey-colored crusted plaque, most often overlying insect bite, abrasion, or other skin rashes. Most common bacteria is *Staphylococcus aureus;* at times may be caused by group A beta-hemolytic streptococci. May occur anywhere on skin, but more common are sites prone to trauma. Bullae are very infectious and may be inoculated to multiple sites on the patient and other family members. Lesions demonstrate a positive Nikolsky sign. Infection most often from a noncutaneous source such as lungs, bone, meninges, ears
   b. Methicillin-resistant *Staphylococcus aureus* (MRSA) impetigo: Increasing occurrences within the community and hospital settings. If not improving on standard antibiotics, consider methicillin resistance; may need clindamycin or vancomycin
2. Treatment:
   a. Small, localized infections: Topical antibiotics (mupirocin, bacitracin, bacitracin-polymyxin B) along with tepid water compresses
   b. Widespread impetigo: Oral antibiotic with gram-positive coverage (dicloxacillin, cephalexin, clotrimazole, amoxicillin-clavulanate potassium)
   c. Parenteral antibiotics, hospitalization and supportive care if any signs of progression to cellulitis or visceral dissemination

B. Autoimmune-Bullous Lesions

These lesions include pemphigus vulgaris (Color Plate 38), pemphigus foliaceus, bullous pemphigoid, dermatitis herpetiformis, and epidermolysis bullosa acquisita. Generally rare in children, but should be considered with bullous lesions that do not respond to standard therapy.

See more information about Autoimmune-Bullous Lesions on Expert Consult, Chapter 8.

C. Insect Bites (See Papular Urticaria, Section IV.B)

D. Burns (see also Chapter 4)

1. Chemical: Produce dry eschar, crust, and form necrotic blisters
2. Thermal: Flame, scald/contact, electrical, cold/frostbite. May produce erythema, moist blistering
3. Nonaccidental burns: Important to evaluate burns for their shape, distribution, inconsistent history, and delay in care, which may point toward a concern for abuse. Symmetrical burns, those from hot water immersion (top of feet and hands may be more involved because skin on palms and soles is thicker), cigarette lesions (punched-out ulcers with dry purple crusts). See Plates 1 and 5 in Chapter 4 which details non-accidental burns

NOTE: All burns are susceptible to becoming secondarily infected, which may make it difficult to distinguish the type of burn you are encountering.

E. Contact Dermatitis

1. Irritant dermatitis: Usually caused by caustic agents such as acid, alkalis, and hydrocarbons. Defined on the premise that anyone exposed to these agents for long enough in a high enough concentration would develop a reaction
2. Allergic dermatitis (Color Plate 39):

a. Pathogenesis: T-cell mediated immune reaction in response to an environmental trigger that comes into contact with the skin. After a sensitization reaction with the initial exposure, an allergic response occurs with subsequent exposures

b. Allergens: Most common antigen is poison ivy. Other common allergens include nickel, rubber, glues, dyes in shoes, ethylenediamine in topical lubricants

c. Clinical presentation: Most often presents as abrupt erythema, pruritus, and vesiculation; may progress to a chronic stage involving scaling, lichenification, and pigmentary changes. Initial reaction occurs after a sensitization period of 7–10 days in susceptible individuals. Re-exposure to the antigen will cause a more rapid reactivation reaction

3. Poison ivy (Color Plate 40):

a. Pathogenesis: Often causes a contact dermatitis, which erupts after exposure to a causative plant, most usually of the *Toxicodendron* or *Rhus* genus. Culprit plant is a three-leaved tall shrub or woody rope–like vine that grows within grasses, on trees, on fences, and in vacant areas. Exposure may also occur from contact with item of clothing or pet that has brushed up against the plant

b. Clinical presentation: Appears often as streaks of erythematous pustules and vesicles; in highly sensitized individuals may appear as large patches. Impressive swelling can ensue. Areas with highest concentration of antigen develop first, and lower doses react in succession. Once on the skin antigen becomes fixed to epithelial cells in 20 minutes and cannot be spread further. Immediate washing after exposure can reduce eruption; barrier creams may afford some protection

4. Diagnosis of contact dermatitis: *Careful history;* in some cases, patch testing is helpful
5. Treatment:

a. Remove causative agent
b. Topical steroids for local areas of inflammation
c. If widespread or severe local inflammation involving eyelids, parts of face, genitals, hands, or other areas where swelling can be incapacitating, treat with 2–3 week tapering course of systemic corticosteroids starting at 0.5–1 mg/kg/day

REFERENCES

1. Bhattacharya JJ, Luo CB, Alvarez H, et al. PHACES syndrome: a review of eight previously unreported cases with late arterial occlusions. *Neuroradiology.* 2004;46:227–233.
2. Faranoff AA. *Neonatal-perinatal medicine: diseases of the fetus and infant.* 7th ed. St. Louis: Mosby; 2002.
3. Léauté-Labrèze C, Dumas de la Roque E, Hubiche T, et al. Propranolol for severe hemangiomas of infancy. *N Engl J Med* 2008;358:2649–2651.
4. Sans V, Dumas de la Roque E, Berge J, et al. Propranolol for severe infantile hemangiomas: follow-up report. *Pediatrics* 2009;124:e423–e431.
5. Truong MT, Chang KW, Berk DR, et al. Propranolol for the treatment of a life-threatening subglottic and mediastinal infantile hemangioma. *J Pediatr* 2010;156:335–338.
6. Drolet BA, Esterly NB, Frieden IJ. Hemangiomas and children. *Primary Care* 1999;3:173–181.
7. Dasher DA, Burkhart CN, Morrell DS. Immunotherapy for childhood warts. *Pediatr Ann* 2009;38(7):373–379.
8. Gladsjo JA, Alió Sáenz AB, Bergman J, et al. 5% 5-Fluorouracil cream for treatment of verruca vulgaris in children. *Pediatr Dermatol* 2009;26: 279–285.
9. Diamantis SA, Morrell DS, Burkhart CN. Pediatric infestations. *Pediatric Ann* 2009;38:326–332.
10. Eichenfield LF, Lucky AW, Boguniewicz M, et al. Safety and efficacy of pimecrolimus (ASM 981) cream 1% in the treatment of mild and moderate atopic dermatitis in children and adolescents. *J Am Acad Dermatol* 2002;46:495–504.
11. Wahn U, Bos JD, Goodfield M, et al. Efficacy and safety of pimecrolimus cream in the long-term management of atopic dermatitis in children. *Pediatrics* 2002;110:e2, 1–8.
12. Rikkers SM, Holland GN, Drayton GE, et al. Topical tacrolimus treatment of atopic eyelid disease. *Am J Ophthalmol* 2003;135:297–302.

13. Boguniewicz M, Fiedler VC, Raimer S, et al for the Pediatric Tacrolimus Study Group: A randomized, vehicle-controlled trial of tacrolimus ointment for treatment of atopic dermatitis in children. *J Allergy Clin Immunol* 1998;102: 637–644.
14. Reitamo S, Van Leent EJ, Ho V, et al. Efficacy and safety of tacrolimus ointment compared with that of hydrocortisone acetate ointment in children with atopic dermatitis. *J Allergy Clin Immunol* 2002;109:547–555.
15. Wollenberg A, Sharma S, von Bubnoff D, et al. Topical tacrolimus (FK506) leads to profound phenotypic and functional alterations of epidermal antigen-presenting dendritic cells in atopic dermatitis. *J Allergy Clin Immunol* 2001;107: 519–525.
16. Krakowski AC. Management of atopic dermatitis in the pediatric population. *Pediatrics* 2008;122:812–824.
17. Cohen BA. Atopic dermatitis: breaking the itch-scratch cycle. *Contemp Pediatr* 1992;7:64–81.
18. Hernandez RG, Cohen BA. Insect bite-induced hypersensitivity and the SCRATCH principles: a new approach to papular urticaria. *Pediatrics* 2006;118(1):e189–196.
19. Shy R. Tinea corporis and tinea capitis. *Pediatr Rev* 2007;28:164–174.
20. Andrews MD, Burns M. Common tinea infections in children. *Am Fam Physician* 2008;77:1415–1420.
21. Cohen BA. *Pediatric Dermatology*. 3rd ed. London: Mosby; 2005.
22. Zaenglein AL, Thiboutot DM. Expert committee recommendations for acne management. *Pediatrics* 2006;118:1188–1199.
23. *Mosby's Drug Consult*. St. Louis: Mosby; 2004.
24. Behrman RE, Kliegman RM, Jenson HB. *Nelson Textbook of Pediatrics*. 17th ed. Philadelphia: Elsevier; 2003.

8

Chapter 9

Development, Behavior, and Mental Health

Jessica Perniciaro, MD

See additional content on Expert Consult

I. WEBSITES

ADHD: www.chadd.org
American Academy of Pediatrics—Developmental and Behavioral Pediatrics: www.dbpeds.org
www.disability.gov
Learning Disabilities Association of America: www.ldanatl.org
Intellectual Disability: www.thearclink.org
Bright Futures: www.brightfutures.org
National Early Childhood Technical Assistance Center: www.nectac.org
Reach Out and Read: www.reachoutandread.org
Child and Adolescent Psychiatry Practice Parameters: www.aacap.org
Mental health patient and provider handouts: www.nimh.nih.gov

II. INTRODUCTION

A. Chapter Focus

This chapter describes the assessment of normal and abnormal development and behavior through infancy, childhood, and adolescence. It focuses on recognition and management of developmental disabilities, which are a group of interrelated, nonprogressive, neurologic disorders occurring in childhood. There is also a focus on the most common mental health issues that occur in the pediatric population.

B. Development

1. Development can be divided into five major streams: Visual-motor, language (the cognitive streams), motor, social, and adaptive. Abnormal development in one stream increases the risk for deficit in another and should prompt a careful assessment of all streams. A developmental diagnosis is a functional description and classification that does not specify an etiology or medical diagnosis
2. Developmental assessment is based on the premise that milestone acquisition occurs at a specific rate and in an orderly and sequential manner. A good milestone is one that can be easily assessed by parents or a provider, and also one that occurs in a narrow time window. When development is not progressing normally, the pattern of abnormal development usually includes delay, deviancy, or dissociation

III. DEFINITIONS[1]

A. Developmental Quotient (DQ)

1. A calculation that reflects the rate of development in any given stream. DQ represents the percentage of normal development present at the time of testing. Can be calculated for any given stream as follows:

$$DQ = (\text{developmental age}/\text{chronologic age}) \times 100$$

2. Two separate developmental assessments over time are more predictive than a single assessment

B. Delay

Performance significantly below average (DQ <70) in a given area of skill. May occur in a single stream or several streams.

C. Deviancy

Atypical development within a single stream, such as developmental milestones occurring out of sequence. Deviancy does not necessarily imply abnormality, but should alert one to the possibility that problems may exist. Example: An infant who rolls at an early age may have abnormally increased tone. Deviancy may also denote the emergence of a presentation that is not typically part of the developmental sequence. Example: A toddler showing no interest in peers.

D. Dissociation

A substantial difference in the rate of development between two or more streams. Example: Motor delay relative to cognition is seen in some children with cerebral palsy.

IV. GUIDELINES FOR NORMAL DEVELOPMENT AND BEHAVIOR

A. Developmental Milestones (Table 9-1)

B. Reach Out and Read Milestones of Early Literacy (Table 9-2)

C. Age-Appropriate Behavioral Issues in Infancy and Early Childhood (Table 9-3)

V. DEVELOPMENTAL SCREENING AND EVALUATION

A. Developmental Screening Guidelines

1. In assessing for delay, an individual DQ can be calculated for any given developmental stream; if the quotient is <70%, a diagnosis of delay can be made and warrants further evaluation or referral. Example: A 13-month-old child who does not yet walk alone, but is able to walk when led with two hands held (i.e., a 10-month level of motor development) has a DQ of 10/13 = 77% and is not considered delayed
2. Developmental surveillance should occur at every well-child visit. Developmental screening using standardized tools should be administered at 9-month, 18-month, and 30-month well-child visits. If a 30-month visit is not possible, this screening can be done at the 24-month visit. Also, specific screening for autism should occur at the 18-month and 24-month visits[2]

TABLE 9-1

DEVELOPMENTAL MILESTONES

Age	Gross Motor	Visual-Motor/ Problem Solving	Language	Social/Adaptive
1 mo	Raises head from prone position	Visually fixes, follows to midline, has tight grasp	Alerts to sound	Regards face
2 mo	Holds head in midline, lifts chest off table	No longer clenches fists tightly, follows object past midline	Smiles socially (after being stroked or talked to)	Recognizes parent
3 mo	Supports on forearms in prone position, holds head up steadily	Holds hands open at rest, follows in circular fashion, responds to visual threat	Coos (produces long vowel sounds in musical fashion)	Reaches for familiar people or objects, anticipates feeding
4 mo	Rolls over, supports on wrists, shifts weight	Reaches with arms in unison, brings hands to midline	Laughs, orients to voice	Enjoys looking around
6 mo	Sits unsupported, puts feet in mouth in supine position	Unilateral reach, uses raking grasp, transfers objects	Babbles, ah-goo, razz, lateral orientation to bell	Recognizes that someone is a stranger
9 mo	Pivots when sitting, crawls well, pulls to stand, cruises	Uses immature pincer grasp, probes with forefinger, holds bottle, throws objects	Says "mama, dada" indiscriminately, gestures, waves bye-bye, understands "no"	Starts exploring environment, plays gesture games (e.g., pat-a-cake)
12 mo	Walks alone	Uses mature pincer grasp, can make a crayon mark, releases voluntarily	Uses two words other than "mama, dada" or proper nouns, jargoning (runs several unintelligible words together with tone or inflection), one-step command with gesture	Imitates actions, comes when called, cooperates with dressing
15 mo	Creeps up stairs, walks backward independently	Scribbles in imitation, builds tower of 2 blocks in imitation	Uses 4–6 words, follows one-step command without gesture	15–18 mo: Uses spoon and cup
18 mo	Runs, throws objects from standing without falling	Scribbles spontaneously, builds tower of 3 blocks, turns two or three pages at a time	Mature jargoning (includes intelligible words), 7–10 word vocabulary, knows 5 body parts	Copies parent in tasks (sweeping, dusting), plays in company of other children

TABLE 9-1

DEVELOPMENTAL MILESTONES (Continued)

Age	Gross Motor	Visual-Motor/ Problem Solving	Language	Social/Adaptive
24 mo	Walks up and down steps without help	Imitates stroke with pencil, builds tower of 7 blocks, turns pages one at a time, removes shoes, pants, etc.	Uses pronouns (I, you, me) inappropriately, follows two-step commands, 50-word vocabulary, uses 2-word sentences	Parallel play
3 yr	Can alternate feet going up steps, pedals tricycle	Copies a circle, undresses completely, dresses partially, dries hands if reminded, unbuttons	Uses minimum of 250 words, 3-word sentences, uses plurals, knows all pronouns, repeats two digits	Group play, shares toys, takes turns, plays well with others, knows full name, age, gender
4 yr	Hops, skips, alternates feet going down steps	Copies a square, buttons clothing, dresses self completely, catches ball	Knows colors, says song or poem from memory, asks questions	Tells "tall tales," plays cooperatively with a group of children
5 yr	Skips alternating feet, jumps over low obstacles	Copies triangle, ties shoes, spreads with knife	Prints first name, asks what a word means	Plays competitive games, abides by rules, likes to help in household tasks

From Capute AJ, Biehl RF: Functional developmental evaluation: prerequisite to habilitation. Pediatr Clin North Am 1973;20:3; Capute AJ, Accardo PJ: Linguistic and auditory milestones during the first two years of life: a language inventory for the practitioner. Clin Pediatr 1978;17:847; and Capute AJ et al: The Clinical Linguistic and Auditory Milestone Scale (CLAMS): identification of cognitive defects in motor delayed children. Am J Dis Child 1986;140:694. Rounded norms from Capute AJ et al: Clinical Linguistic and Auditory Milestone Scale: prediction of cognition in infancy. Dev Med Child Neurol 1986;28:762.

B. Commonly Used Developmental Screening and Assessment Tools

1. Appropriate screening tests vary with age and suspected diagnosis. Significant delays on screening merit referral for formal assessment. Several developmental screening and assessment tools are available (Table 9-4)
2. Capute Scales: An assessment tool that gives quantitative developmental quotients for visual-motor/problem-solving and language abilities. The CLAMS (Clinical Linguistic and Auditory Milestone Scale) was developed for the assessment of language milestones from birth to age 36 months. The CAT (Clinical Adaptive Test) consists of problem-solving items for ages from birth to 36 months, adapted from standardized infant psychological tests

TABLE 9-2

REACH OUT AND READ MILESTONES OF EARLY LITERACY

Age	Motor	Cognitive
6–12 mo	Reaches for books, turns pages with help	Looks at pictures, pats pictures
12–18 mo	Carries book, holds book with help, turns several board pages at a time	Points to pictures with a single finger, points to specific items on page, gives book to adult
18–24 mo	Turns one board page at a time	Repeats and retells parts of known stories
24–36 mo	Begins to turn paper pages	Looks at favorite books on own, repeats and retells whole phrases and stories, associates pictures with text of story
3 yr	Turns paper pages easily	Growing attention span, recites favorite stories, begins to identify single letters
4 yr and above	Writes name	Uses past tense and plurals, answers "what will happen next"

From Reach Out and Read National Center: www.reachoutandread.org.

TABLE 9-3

AGE-APPROPRIATE BEHAVIORAL ISSUES IN INFANCY AND EARLY CHILDHOOD

Age	Behavioral Issue	Symptoms	Guidance
1–3 mo	Colic	Paroxysms of fussiness/crying, 3+ hr per day, 3+ days per wk, may pull knees up to chest, pass flatus	Crying usually peaks at 6 wk and resolves by 3–4 mo. Prevent overstimulation; swaddle infant; use white noise, swing, or car rides to soothe. Avoid medication and formula changes. Encourage breaks for the primary caregiver.
3–4 mo	Trained night feeding	Night awakening	Comfort quietly, avoid reinforcing behavior (i.e., avoid night feeds). Do not play at night. Introducing cereal or solid food does not reduce awakening. Develop a consistent bedtime routine. Place baby in bed while drowsy and not fully asleep.
9 mo	Stranger anxiety/ separation anxiety	Distress when separated from parent or approached by a stranger	Use a transitional object, such as a special toy or blanket; use routine or ritual to separate from parent; may continue until 24 mo but can reduce intensity.
	Developmental night waking	Separation anxiety at night	Keep lights off. Avoid picking child up or feeding. May reassure verbally at regular intervals or place a transitional object in crib.
12 mo	Aggression	Biting, hitting, kicking in frustration	Say "no" with negative facial cues. Begin time out (1 minute per year of age). No eye contact or interaction, place in a nonstimulating location. May restrain child gently until cooperation is achieved.

TABLE 9-3

AGE-APPROPRIATE BEHAVIORAL ISSUES IN INFANCY AND EARLY CHILDHOOD (Continued)

Age	Behavioral Issue	Symptoms	Guidance
	Need for limit setting	Exploration of environment, danger of injury	Avoid punishing exploration or poor judgment. Emphasize child-proofing and distraction.
18 mo	Temper tantrums	Occur with frustration, attention seeking rage, negativity/refusal	Try to determine cause and react appropriately (i.e., help child who is frustrated, ignore attention-seeking behavior). Make sure child is in a safe location.
24 mo	Toilet training	Child needs to demonstrate readiness: shows interest, neurologic maturity (i.e., recognizes urge to urinate or defecate), ability to walk to bathroom and undress self, desire to please/imitate parents, increasing periods of daytime dryness	Age range for toilet training is usually 2–4 yr. Give guidance early; may introduce potty seat but avoid pressure or punishment for accidents. Wait until the child is ready. Expect some periods of regression, especially with stressors.
24–36 mo	New sibling	Regression, aggressive behavior	Allow for special time with parent, 10–20 min daily of one-on-one time exclusively devoted to the older sibling(s). Child chooses activity with parent. No interruptions. May not be taken away as punishment.
36 mo	Nightmares	Awakens crying, may or may not complain of bad dream	Reassure child, explain that he or she had a bad dream. Leave bedroom door open, use a nightlight, demonstrate there are no monsters under the bed. Discuss dream the following day. Avoid scary movies or television shows.
	Night terrors	Agitation, screaming 1–2 hr after going to bed. Child may have eyes open but not respond to parent. May occur at same time each night	May be familial, not volitional. *Prevention:* For several nights, awaken child 15 min before terrors occur. Avoid overtiredness. *Acute:* Be calm; speak in soft, soothing, repetitive tones; help child return to sleep. Protect child against injury.

From Dixon SD, Stein MT: Encounters with children: pediatric behavior and development. St. Louis, Mosby, 2000.

TABLE 9-4

DEVELOPMENTAL AND MENTAL HEALTH SCREENING TESTS BY DIAGNOSIS

Diagnosis	Screening Tests	Age	Administration Time	Completed by	Weblink
Cognitive/motor development	Ages and Stages Questionnaire (ASQ)	4–60 mo	10–15 min	Parent	http://www.agesandstages.com
	Parents Evaluation of Developmental Status (PEDS)	0–8 yr	2–10 min	Parent	http://www.pedstest.com
	Denver II Developmental Screening Test	0–6 yr	10–12 min	Clinician	
	Capute Scales (CAT/CLAMS)	3–36 mo	15–20 min	Clinician	
Autism spectrum disorders	Modified Checklist for Autism in Toddlers (M-CHAT)	16–48 mo	5–10 min	Parent	http://www.firstsigns.org/downloads/m-chat.PDF
	Childhood Autism Rating Scale (CARS)	>2 yr	20–30 min	Clinician	
Attention deficit/hyperactivity disorder (ADHD)	Vanderbilt Scales Connors Scales	6–12 yr	10–15 min	Parent and teachers	http://www.brightfutures.org/mentalhealth/pdf/professionals/bridges/adhd.pdf
Mental health	Pediatric Symptom Checklist (PSC)	4–18 yr	5–10 min	Parent or child/adolescent	http://psc.partners.org/psc_english.pdf
Depression	Center for Epidemiological Studies Depression Scale for Children (CES-DC)		5–10 min	Child/adolescent	http://www.brightfutures.org/mentalhealth/pdf/professionals/bridges/ces_dc.pdf

Partially adapted from American Academy of Pediatrics. Identifying infants and young children with developmental disorders in the medical home: an algorithm for developmental surveillance and screening. Pediatrics 2006;118:405–420.

3. Denver II Developmental Assessment: A tool for screening the apparently normal child between ages 0 and 6 years. The test screens the child in four areas: personal-social, fine motor, gross motor, and language. For children born before 38 weeks' gestation, age should be corrected for prematurity, up to age 2 years. A child fails a Denver screen if he or she has two or more delays noted. Indications for referral are a failed test or a classification of untestable on two consecutive screenings. See Figure EC 9-A on Expert Consult
4. Ages and Stages Questionnaire: Parent-based questionnaire for ages 4 months to 60 months. The benefits of parent-based questionnaires include increased time efficiency since parents can fill these out while waiting, as well as providing an opportunity to document milestones that are difficult to assess in the office or that children are less likely to perform in an unfamiliar setting
5. PEDS: Parent-based questionnaire for up to 8 years of age
6. Goodenough-Harris Draw-a-Person Test: Give the child a pencil and a sheet of blank paper. Instruct the child to "draw a person; draw the best person you can." Use scoring guidelines to assess drawing and compare with norms for age. See Box EC 9-A on Expert Consult
7. Gesell figures (Fig. 9-1): When using Gesell figures, the examiner is not supposed to demonstrate the drawing of the figures for the patient
8. Gesell block skills (Fig. 9-2): The block structures should be demonstrated for the child. Figure 9-2 includes the developmental age at which each structure can usually be accomplished

VI. MEDICAL EVALUATION OF DEVELOPMENTAL DISORDERS

A. History

A thorough past medical history should include assessment of risk.

1. Prenatal and birth: Toxins, trauma, prematurity, infection
2. Past medical problems or trauma: Infection, medication
3. Developmental history: Inquire about timing of milestone achievement, delayed skills, and loss of skills in all streams
4. Behavioral history: Social skills, eye contact, affection, hyperactivity, impulsivity, inattention, distractibility, self-regulation, perseveration, worries/avoidance, stereotypies, peculiar habits
5. Educational history: Need for special services, retention, established educational plans
6. Family history: Developmental disabilities, late talkers or walkers, trouble with education, ADHD, seizures, tics

B. Physical Examination

1. General: Height, weight, head circumference, cardiac murmurs, midline defects
2. Review for dysmorphic features

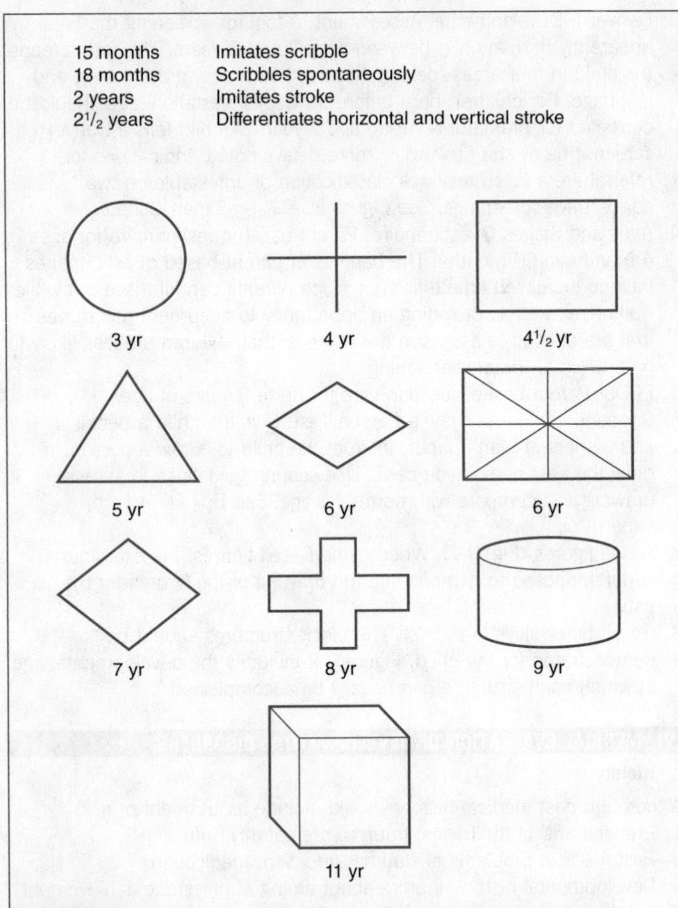

FIGURE 9-1

Gesell figures. *(From Illingsworth RS: The development of the infant and young child, normal and abnormal, 5th ed. Baltimore, Williams & Wilkins, 1972, pp. 229–232, and Cattel P: The measurement of intelligence of infants and young children. New York, Psychological Corporation, 1960, pp. 97–261.)*

3. Age-directed neurologic examination: Exam should be tailored to the age of the patient, including primitive reflexes for infants. See Tables EC 9-A and 9-B on Expert Consult

C. Laboratory Investigations, Imaging Studies, Other Tests

1. Audiologic testing: Indicated for all children with global developmental delay, or any delay in communication or language

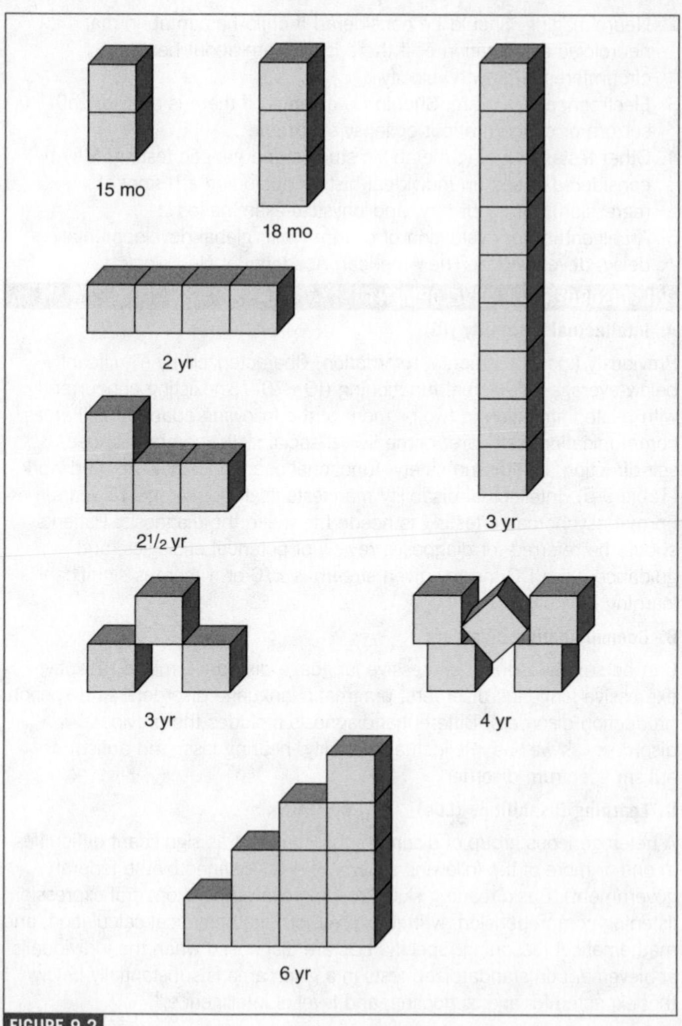

FIGURE 9-2

Block skills. *(From Capute AJ, Accardo PJ: The pediatrician and the developmentally disabled child: a clinical textbook on mental retardation. Baltimore, University Park Press, 1979, p. 122.)*

2. Neuroimaging: Should be considered if child has an abnormal neurologic examination or if there is concern about head circumference growth velocity
3. Electroencephalogram: Should be obtained if there is a history of seizure or concern about epilepsy syndrome
4. Other tests, including metabolic studies and genetic testing: May be considered based on individual history (including a history of regression), family history, and physical examination
5. An algorithm for evaluation of children with global developmental delay, developed by The American Academy of Neurology[3]

VII. DISORDERS OF DEVELOPMENT

A. Intellectual Disability (ID)

Previously known as mental retardation. Characterized by significantly below-average intellectual functioning (IQ <70–75) existing concurrently with related limitation in two or more of the following adaptive skill areas: communication, self-care, home living, social skills, community use, self-direction, health and safety, functional academics, leisure, and work (Table 9-5). Intellectual disability manifests itself before age 18 years. Formal psychometric testing is needed to make the diagnosis. Patients should be referred for diagnosis, review of potential etiologies, and guidance if the DQ for any given stream is <70 or if there is significant learning difficulty.

B. Communication Disorders

Can be subdivided into expressive language disorders, mixed receptive-expressive language disorders, pragmatic language disorders, and speech production disorders. Differential diagnosis includes the previous disorders, as well as intellectual disability, hearing loss, and autism or autism spectrum disorder.

C. Learning Disabilities (LDs)

A heterogeneous group of disorders that manifest as significant difficulties in one or more of the following seven areas (as defined by the federal government): Basic reading skills, reading comprehension, oral expression, listening comprehension, written expression, mathematical calculation, and mathematical reasoning. Specific LDs are diagnosed when the individual's achievement on standardized tests in a given area is substantially below that expected for age, schooling, and level of intelligence.[4]

D. Cerebral Palsy (CP)

A disorder of movement and posture resulting from a permanent, nonprogressive lesion of the immature brain. Manifestations may change with brain growth and development. The diagnosis of CP is made at a mean age of 13 months. CP is classified in terms of physiologic and topographic characteristics as well as severity (Table 9-6).[5] Classification is important because different classifications often have very different etiologies and associated deficits.

TABLE 9-5

INTELLECTUAL DISABILITY—DSM-IV-TR CLASSIFICATIONS*

Level	IQ	Academic Potential	Daily Living/Work	Expected Mental Age as an Adult (yr)	Intensity of Support
Mild	70–80	Educable to about the 6th grade level	Fully independent and employable	—	Intermittent
	50–69	Reading and writing to 4th–5th grade level or less	Relatively independent; employable, often need training	9–11	Intermittent
Moderate	35–49	Limited reading to 1st–2nd grade level	Dress without help, use toilet, prepare food; likely need sheltered employment	5–8	Limited
Severe	20–34	Very unlikely to read or write	Can be toilet trained, dress with help; sheltered employment	3–5	Extensive
Profound	<20	None	Occasionally can be toilet trained, dress with help, often nonverbal, very limited employment potential	<3	Pervasive

*The American Association on Intellectual and Developmental Disabilities has moved away from the use of strict categories. It instead advocates an individualized approach that addresses specific limitations in capabilities and functioning.

Adapted from American Association on Mental Retardation. Mental retardation: definition, classification and systems of supports, 9th ed. Washington, DC, AAMR, 1992, pp. 5–34, and American Psychiatric Association: Diagnostic and Statistical Manual of Mental Disorders (DSM-IV-TR), 4th ed., text revision. Washington, DC, American Psychiatric Press, 2000, pp. 41–45.

E. Autism Spectrum Disorders (ASD)

Includes autism, pervasive developmental disorder NOS, Asperger disorder, childhood disintegrative disorder, and Rett disorder. See the *DSM-IV-TR* for full diagnostic criteria.[6] For more detailed guidelines on the evaluation for ASD, see the American Academy of Pediatrics (AAP) practice guidelines.[7]

1. Autism: Essential features are impaired social interaction and communication and a restricted group of activities and interests, with stereotyped behaviors, rituals, or mannerisms. Onset of abnormal functioning occurs before age 3 years. A large proportion of autistic children function in the range of intellectual disability. Siblings of children with autism appear to be at greater risk and males are disproportionately affected. Assessment scales such as M-CHAT and CARS are available for screening (Table 9-4)
2. Pervasive developmental disorder NOS: Characterized by impaired social interaction and communication skills and/or repetitive,

TABLE 9-6

CLINICAL CLASSIFICATION OF CEREBRAL PALSY[5]

Type	Pattern of Involvement
I. Spastic (Increased Tone, Clasped Knife, Clonus, Further Classified by Distribution)	
Hemiplegia	Ipsilateral arm and leg; arm worse than leg
Diplegia	Legs primarily affected
Quadriplegia	All four extremities impaired; legs worse than arms
Double hemiplegia	All four extremities; arms notably worse than legs
Monoplegia	One extremity, usually upper; probably reflects a mild hemiplegia
Triplegia	One upper extremity and both lower; probably represents a hemiplegia plus a diplegia or incomplete quadriplegia
II. Extrapyramidal (Lead Pipe or Candle Wax Rigidity, Variable Tone, ± Clonus)	
Choreoathetosis, rigidity, dystonia	Complex movement/tone disorders reflecting basal ganglia pathology
Ataxia, tremor	Movement and tone disorders reflecting cerebellar origin
Hypotonia	Usually related to diffuse, often severe, cerebral and/or cerebellar cortical damage

From Capute AJ, Accardo PJ (eds): Cerebral palsy: developmental disabilities in infancy and childhood, 2nd ed., vol 2. Baltimore, Paul H. Brookes, 1996, pp. 83–86.

stereotyped behaviors, that does not meet diagnostic criteria for autism or other mental health disorder

3. Asperger disorder: Characterized by impairment in social interactions and restricted, repetitive patterns of behavior with no general delay in language, cognition, or attainment of self-help skills. More common in boys. Those affected have difficulty understanding and responding to social conventions and nonverbal cues and are therefore often unable to develop peer relationships

VIII. DISORDERS OF BEHAVIOR

A. Attention Deficit/Hyperactivity Disorder (ADHD)

1. A neurobehavioral disorder characterized by inattention, distractibility, impulsivity, and hyperactivity, that are more frequent and severe than typically observed in children of the same developmental age. ADHD is a mental health disorder that manifests in a predominantly behavioral presentation. Symptoms must persist for at least 6 months, occur before age 7 years, and be evident in two or more settings. ADHD is further organized into inattentive, hyperactive/impulsive, and combined subtypes. See the *DSM-IV-TR* for full diagnostic criteria[6]
2. Proper diagnosis, evaluation, and treatment are paramount to ensuring academic, behavioral, emotional, and social function. Diagnosis is made using history, observation, and behavioral checklists such as the Vanderbilt Assessment Scale. The Vanderbilt Assessment scale may be downloaded from: http://www.brightfutures.org/mentalhealth/pdf/professionals/bridges/adhd.pdf

TABLE 9-7

COMMONLY USED ATTENTION DEFICIT/HYPERACTIVITY DISORDER (ADHD) MEDICATIONS

Medication	Examples	Duration	Comments
Amphetamine	Adderall, Dexedrine, DextroStat	Short-acting	Short-acting stimulants often used for initial treatment for younger children. Generally need BID-TID dosing for control.
	Adderall XR, Dexedrine Spansule, Lisdexamfetamine	Long-acting	Long-acting stimulants with daily dosing offer increased convenience and compliance. May have increased side effects in regards to sleep and appetite.
Methylphenidate	Focalin, Methylin, Ritalin	Short-acting	Short-acting stimulants often used for initial treatment for younger children. Generally need BID-TID dosing for control.
	Metadate CD, Metadate ER, Methylin ER, Ritalin LA, Ritalin SR	Intermediate-acting	
	Concerta, Daytrana patch, Focalin XR	Long-acting	Long-acting stimulants with daily dosing offer increased convenience and compliance. May have increased side effects in regards to sleep and appetite.
Selective norepinephrine reuptake inhibitor	Atomoxetine (Strattera)	Intermediate-acting	Nonstimulant. Not a schedule II medication. Can be given once daily or BID. Often used when there are significant side effects with stimulants or in setting of substance abuse. Monitor closely for changes in mood or behavior.

Adapted from American Academy of Child and Adolescent Psychiatry. Practice parameter for the assessment and treatment of children and adolescents with attention-deficit/hyperactivity disorder. J Am Acad Child Adolesc Psychiatry 2007;46(7):894–921.

If there is an unremarkable medical history current recommendations say that no laboratory or neurological evaluations need to be done. It is important however to screen for comorbid psychiatric conditions[8]

3. Once diagnosis is made, psychopharmacological and/or behavioral therapy can be used to manage ADHD. See Table 9-7 for commonly used ADHD medications

IX. DISORDERS OF MENTAL HEALTH

A. Overview

Screening for mental health issues should occur at all routine well-child visits from early childhood through adolescence, including history of mood symptoms and any behavioral issues. The Pediatric Symptom Checklist

(PSC) is a general mental health checklist for ages 4–18 years that is filled out by a parent and can be found at http://psc.partners.org/psc_english.pdf (Table 9-4). It screens for a broad array of mental health disorders, including conduct disorders, attention disorders, depression, anxiety, and adjustment disorders. See the *DSM-IV-TR* for a more complete list of psychiatric diagnoses and full diagnostic criteria.[6]

B. Anxiety Disorders

1. Anxiety is one of the most common mental health issues that presents in the general pediatric setting. Pediatric patients with anxiety often present with nonspecific and/or chronic pain or other somatic complaints
2. The anxiety disorders in the *DSM-IV-TR* include generalized anxiety disorder, separation anxiety disorder, social phobia, specific phobia, panic disorder, agoraphobia, posttraumatic stress disorder, and obsessive compulsive disorder.[9] In general children with anxiety disorders have fear and anxiety outside the realm of normal for their age, and often have somatic complaints as well. See the *DSM-IV-TR* for specific criteria for each disorder[6]
3. Treatment of anxiety disorders generally warrants referral. Psychotherapy is often the initial treatment, in particular exposure-based cognitive-behavioral therapy has the most empirical support for treatment of anxiety disorders in pediatric patients. This may also be supplemented with the use of SSRIs.[9] Refer to the Psychiatric Drug Formulary (Table 30-8) in the Formulary Adjunct section for anxiolytics, starting doses, and side effects

C. Depression

1. Major depression is defined as 5 or more depressive symptoms for at least 2 weeks, with those symptoms causing significant impairment in functioning. Also symptoms are not due to effects of substance use or a medical condition, and there is no history of manic episodes. Depressive symptoms include depressed or irritable mood (adolescents more likely to manifest as irritable mood compared to adults), anhedonia, change in appetite or weight, change in sleep (hypersomnia or insomnia), psychomotor slowing or restlessness, fatigue, decreased concentration, feelings of guilt or worthlessness, and recurrent thoughts of death or suicide[10]
2. Screening for depression can be done through history, can also use standardized screening tools such as the PSC, or the Center for Epidemiological Studies Depression Scale for Children (CES-DC) can be given to an older adolescent. It is a 20-item self-report questionnaire that screens for depressive symptoms and can be found at http://www.brightfutures.org/mentalhealth/pdf/professionals/bridges/ces_dc.pdf
   a. This initial evaluation must include an assessment of thoughts/plans of self-harm or harm to others

3. Treatment of depression may be initiated in the primary care setting or may require referral depending on severity. The literature has shown that a combination of antidepressant medication and cognitive-behavioral therapy (CBT) is most effective, followed by medication alone and then CBT alone (although each of these alone as treatment have generally similar rates of reducing symptoms). There is a black box warning in place for concern that selective serotonin reuptake inhibitors (SSRIs) may increase suicidal thoughts or behaviors in children and adolescents following the initiation of these medications. Patients should therefore be followed closely during the 4–8 weeks after SSRIs are started (once weekly for the first 2–4 weeks, then every other week thereafter), but does not mean that SSRIs cannot be initiated in the primary care setting.[11] Refer to the Psychiatric Drug Formulary (Table 30-8) in the Formulary Adjunct section for common antidepressant medications, starting doses, and side effects, and the Physicians Med Guide prepared by the American Psychological Association (APA) and American Academy of Child and Adolescent Psychiatry (AACAP) for guidelines regarding medication use for depression in adolescent patients[11]

9

D. Bipolar Disorder

1. Bipolar disorder type I (relatively rare in the pediatric population) is defined by a manic episode of at least 7 days, with symptoms such as elevated mood, grandiosity, decreased need for sleep, rapid speech, racing thoughts, agitation, distractibility, increased spending, risky behaviors, and possibly hallucinations or delusions (although these are rare). The DSM definition does not require a depressive episode although most people do experience depressive episodes as well. Bipolar generally presents in young adulthood, and there is currently some controversy surrounding the diagnosis of childhood or juvenile bipolar disorder[12]
2. Treatment of mania that is well-defined by the DSM criteria is pharmacotherapy, and warrants referral to a mental health provider. Lithium is the only Food and Drug Administration (FDA)-approved medication for the pediatric population, ages 12 and older, for bipolar disorder, although many mood stabilizers and antipsychotic medications are used in the adult population. Psychotherapy is an important adjunct for long-term management

X. REFERRAL AND INTERVENTION

A. State Support

1. The Individuals with Disabilities Education Act (IDEA) requires states to provide early intervention services to children
2. Early intervention services eligibility criteria vary from state to state. The National Early Childhood Technical Assistance Center (www.nectac.org) provides information about criteria in each state

B. Recommendations

1. Facilitate communication between family and school
2. Advocate for appropriate services and monitor their effectiveness regularly
3. Medical workup when indicated
4. Provide pharmacologic intervention as needed
5. Refer to an appropriate specialist when indicated

REFERENCES

1. Capute AJ, Shapiro BK, Palmer FB. Spectrum of developmental disabilities: continuum of motor dysfunction. *Orthop Clin North Am.* 1981;12:15–21.
2. American Academy of Pediatrics. Identifying infants and young children with developmental disorders in the medical home: an algorithm for developmental surveillance and screening. *Pediatrics.* 2006;118:405–420.
3. American Academy of Neurology. Practice parameter: evaluation of the child with global developmental delay. *Neurology.* 2003;60:367–380.
4. Shapiro BK, Gallico RP. Learning disabilities. *Pediatr Clin North Am.* 1993;40:491–505.
5. Capute AJ, Accardo PJ, eds. *Cerebral palsy: developmental disabilities in infancy and childhood,* 2nd ed, vol 2. Baltimore: Paul H. Brookes; 1996.
6. American Psychiatric Association. *Diagnostic and statistical manual of mental disorders,* 4th ed, text revision. Arlington, VA: American Psychiatric Publishing; 2000.
7. Johnson CP, Myers SM. American Academy of Pediatrics: identification and evaluation of children with autism spectrum disorders. *Pediatrics.* 2007;120:1183–1215.
8. Practice parameter for the assessment and treatment of children and adolescents with attention-deficit/hyperactivity disorder. *J Am Acad Child Adolesc Psychiatry.* 2007;46(7):894–921.
9. Practice parameter for the assessment and treatment of children and adolescents with anxiety disorders. *J Am Acad Child Adolesc Psychiatry.* 2007;46(2):267–283.
10. Practice parameter for the assessment and treatment of children and adolescents with depressive disorders. *J Am Acad Child Adolesc Psychiatry.* 2007;46(11):1503–1526.
11. Physicians Med Guide. *The use of medication in treating childhood and adolescent depression: information for physicians.* Prepared by the American Psychiatric Association and the American Academy of Child and Adolescent Psychiatry. October 7, 2009. http://www.physicianmedguide.org/physiciansmedguide.htm
12. Practice parameter for the assessment and treatment of children and adolescents with bipolar disorder. *J Am Acad Child Adolesc Psychiatry.* 2007;46(1):107–125.

Chapter 10

Endocrinology

Lauren Cohee, MD

See additional content on Expert Consult

I. WEBSITES

www.childrenwithdiabetes.com

Pediatric Endocrine Society (formerly Lawson Wilkins Pediatric Endocrine Society): http://www.lwpes.org/

II. DIABETES

A. Diagnostic Criteria (American Diabetes Association)[1]

Must meet one of four criteria:

1. Symptoms of diabetes (polyuria, polydipsia, or weight loss) *and* random blood glucose ≥200 mg/dL
2. A fasting blood glucose (no caloric intake for at least 8 hours) ≥126 mg/dL*
3. An oral glucose tolerance test (OGTT) with a 2-hr postload blood glucose of ≥200 mg/dL* (See Section VI.A for more information on OGTT.)
4. Hemoglobin A_{1c} (HbA_{1c}) ≥6.5%

B. Diabetes Classification[2,3]

1. Type I or type II (most common types, polygenic)
a. Patient characteristics (Table 10-1)
b. Laboratory characteristics:
   (1) Islet cell autoantibodies: (GAD-65, insulin, islet cell antibodies) Suggestive of type 1; however, ~15% of children with type 1 diabetes will not have autoantibodies to a specific islet cell antigen and ~5% will not have any detectable islet cell autoantibodies.

NOTE: Some children with type 2 diabetes will have measurable islet cell autoantibodies

   (2) Ketoacidosis: Usually associated with type 1, but does not exclude type 2 (see Sections C and D). Recurrent ketosis, especially diabetic ketoacidosis (DKA), in a type 2 patient should prompt reevaluation of classification
   (3) C-peptide: In a type 1 patient, elevation >2 years after diagnosis should prompt reevaluation of classification

---

*In absence of unequivocal hyperglycemia, these values should be repeated on another day

TABLE 10-1

CHARACTERISTICS SUGGESTIVE OF TYPE 1 VERSUS TYPE 2 DIABETES AT PRESENTATION

Characteristic	Type 1	Type 2
Onset	Usually prepuberty	Usually postpuberty
Polydipsia and polyuria	Present for days to weeks	Absent; or present for weeks to months
Ethnicity	Caucasian	African American, Hispanic, Asian, Native American
Weight	Weight loss	Obese
Other physical findings		Acanthosis nigricans
Family history	Autoimmune diseases	Type 2 diabetes
Ketoacidosis	More common	Less common

(4) Insulin and C-peptide: Not helpful in initial classification. At presentation, levels usually low in type 1 but there is significant overlap with type 2

2. Other forms of diabetes: Monogenic diabetes of youth (MODY) and neonatal diabetes mellitus (NDM) (rare, monogenic)

a. MODY: (Specific subtypes and mutations not differentiated here)

(1) Suspect when there is a strong family history of young onset diabetes mellitus (DM), mild persistent hyperglycemia with a HbA_{1c} at the upper limit of normal, glucosuria at low blood glucose, type II-like disease in a nonobese host, or type I-like disease in a host who has never had DKA or is still producing insulin beyond the honeymoon phase (up to 3 years)

(2) Significance is better understanding of clinical course; some types are responsive to sulfonylureas

b. NDM: Suspect when presentation is at ≤12months of age. Diabetes may be persistent or transient ± relapse. Subset is responsive to sulfonylureas

C. Diabetic Ketoacidosis (DKA)[4]

1. **Definition:** Hyperglycemia, ketonemia, ketonuria, and metabolic acidosis (pH <7.30, bicarbonate <15 mEq/L)

2. **Assessment:**

a. History: In a *suspected* diabetic, determine whether there is a history of polydipsia, polyuria, polyphagia, weight loss, vomiting, or abdominal pain as well as history of infection or inciting event. In a *known* diabetic, also determine the usual insulin regimen, timing and amount of last dose

b. Examination: Assess for dehydration, Kussmaul respirations, fruity breath, change in mental status, and current weight

c. Laboratory tests: See Figure 10-1. Also consider HbA_{1c} to assess for chronic hyperglycemia (normal values are 4.5%–5.9%); in a new-onset diabetic, consider islet cell antibodies, insulin antibodies, thyroid

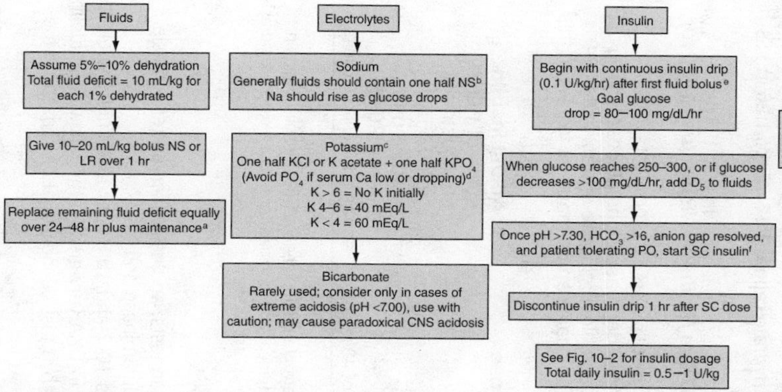

Fluids

Assume 5%–10% dehydration
Total fluid deficit = 10 mL/kg for each 1% dehydrated

↓

Give 10–20 mL/kg bolus NS or LR over 1 hr

↓

Replace remaining fluid deficit equally over 24–48 hr plus maintenance[a]

Electrolytes

Sodium
Generally fluids should contain one half NS[b]
Na should rise as glucose drops

↓

Potassium[c]
One half KCl or K acetate + one half KPO_4
(Avoid PO_4 if serum Ca low or dropping)[d]
K > 6 = No K initially
K 4–6 = 40 mEq/L
K < 4 = 60 mEq/L

↓

Bicarbonate
Rarely used; consider only in cases of extreme acidosis (pH <7.00), use with caution; may cause paradoxical CNS acidosis

Insulin

Begin with continuous insulin drip (0.1 U/kg/hr) after first fluid bolus[e]
Goal glucose drop = 80–100 mg/dL/hr

↓

When glucose reaches 250–300, or if glucose decreases >100 mg/dL/hr, add D_5 to fluids

↓

Once pH >7.30, HCO_3 >16, anion gap resolved, and patient tolerating PO, start SC insulin[f]

↓

Discontinue insulin drip 1 hr after SC dose

↓

See Fig. 10–2 for insulin dosage
Total daily insulin = 0.5–1 U/kg

Laboratory values

Check blood glucose q1h

↓

Check VBG and electrolytes, including calcium and phosphate, q2h until stable, then monitor q4h

↓

Monitor urine for ketones and glucose with each void

[a] If urine output is high, include in maintenance until osmotic diuresis slows; therefore maintenance = urine output + insensible losses (one third of standard maintenance calculations).
[b] Some DKA protocols recommend using NS rather than half NS during part of the replacement period in an effort to further decrease risk of cerebral edema.
[c] Patients with DKA are total body K^+ depleted and are at risk for severe hypokalemia during DKA therapy. However, serum K^+ levels may be normal or elevated as a result of the shift of K^+ to the extracellular compartment in the setting of acidosis.
[d] Phosphate is depleted in DKA and will drop further with insulin therapy. Consider replacing half of K as KPO_4 for first 8 hr, then all as KCl. Excessive phosphate may induce hypocalcemic tetany.
[e] Lower dose insulin infusions can be considered in very young patients.
[f] Some protocols recommend also waiting for urine ketones to decrease or clear before starting SC insulin.

FIGURE 10-1

Management of diabetic ketoacidosis. *(Modified from Cooke DW, Plotnick L. Management of diabetic ketoacidosis in children and adolescents. Pediatr Rev 2008; 29(12):431–436.)*

Example: A-32 kg patient

***Total daily SC insulin dose* = 0.5–1.0 units/kg/day**
0.75 x 32 = 24 units/day

***Basal insulin dose* = ½ of total daily SC dose:**
24 ÷ 2 = 12 units at bedtime as glargine insulin (Lantus) in this example

***Carbohydrate coverage:* 450 ÷ total daily SC insulin dose:**
450 ÷ 24 = 18.75;
Insulin (lispro): carbohydrate ratio = 1:18.75, or 1:20 in this example

Correction factor: 1800 rule for insulin lispro (use 1500 for regular insulin)
1800 ÷ total daily SC insulin dose = 1800 ÷ 24 = 75
1 unit of insulin lispro will decrease blood glucose 75 mg/dL, or 0.5 units will decrease blood glucose approximately 40 mg/dL, so that a sliding scale can be made as follows in this example

For blood glucose	Adjust insulin
<70 mg/dL	subtract 1 unit
71–120	no adjustment
121–160	add 0.5 units
161–200	add 1 unit
201–240	add 1.5 units
each additional increase of 40 mg/dL	add an additional 0.5 units

FIGURE 10-2
Calculations for a starting intermittent subcutaneous (SC) insulin regimen. Calculations are based on empirically determined formulas. Doses are adjusted once responses to starting doses are assessed.

antibodies, thyroid function tests, and celiac screen (endomesial antibody or tissue transglutaminase and total IgA)

3. **Management:** See Figures 10-1 and 10-2. Because fluid and electrolyte requirements of patients in DKA vary greatly, the following guidelines are a starting point; therapy must be individualized based on the dynamics of the patient
   a. Acidosis: pH is an indicator of insulin deficiency; if acidosis is not resolving, the patient may need more insulin. **NOTE:** Initial insulin administration will cause transient worsening of acidosis as potassium is driven into the cells in exchange for hydrogen ions
   b. Hyperglycemia: Blood glucose is an indicator of hydration status
4. **Cerebral edema:** Most severe complication of DKA. Overly aggressive hydration and rapid correction of hyperglycemia may play a role in its development

D. Type II Diabetes Mellitus[2,3,5]

1. Prevalence: Increasing among children, especially among African Americans, Hispanics, and Native Americans; increase is related to increased prevalence of childhood obesity
2. Etiology: Abnormality in glucose levels caused by insulin resistance and insulin secretory defect
3. Presentation: Although not typical, can present in ketoacidosis (chronic high glucose impairs β-cell function and increases peripheral insulin resistance)
4. Screening:
a. Consider screening by measuring fasting blood glucose levels among children who are overweight (body mass index >85th percentile for age and gender) *and* have two of the following risk factors:
   (1) Family history of type 2 DM in a first- or second-degree relative
   (2) Race/ethnicity: African American, Native American, Hispanic, or Asian or Pacific Islander
   (3) Signs associated with insulin resistance (acanthosis nigricans, hypertension, dyslipidemia, polycystic ovarian disease)
b. Begin at age 10 years or onset of puberty (whichever occurs first) and repeat every 2 years
c. Based on adult data, HbA_{1c} may be used as a screening tool: HbA_{1c} = 5.7%–6.4% indicates increased risk of future diabetes; 6.0%–6.5% is abnormal and indicates need for further testing (OGTT, fasting plasma glucose); >6.5% is diagnostic of diabetes
5. Treatment: Primarily diet and exercise; pharmacologic agents are often necessary for those who fail conservative management or are symptomatic at presentation
a. Metformin has been used for patients with serum glucose levels <350 mg/dL without ketones (see Formulary)
b. Minimal data exists on the use of medications other than insulin and metformin in children and adolescents. Until data on the efficacy and safety of these agents are demonstrated in studies in children, treatment with GLP-1 agonists, dipeptidyl-proteinase 4 inhibitors, pramlintide, and thiazolidinediones should not be used routinely in children

E. Monitoring of All Diabetics

1. Glucose control: Daily blood glucoses; HbA_{1c} level every 3 months
2. Other involved organ systems: Frequent eye examinations and screening for hypertension, proteinuria, and hyperlipidemia (Monitor q2 years with goals of low-density lipoprotein [LDL] <100 mg/dL, high-density [HDL] >35 mg/dL, triglycerides [TGs] <150 mg/dL)

III. THYROID AND PARATHYROID FUNCTION[6–8]

A. Thyroid Tests

1. Interpretation of thyroid function tests (Table 10-2). See reference values for age (Tables 10-3 and 10-4)

10

TABLE 10-2

THYROID FUNCTION TESTS: INTERPRETATION

Disorder	TSH	T_4	Free T_4
Primary hyperthyroidism	L	H	High N to H
Primary hypothyroidism	H	L	L
Hypothalamic/pituitary hypothyroidism	L, N, H*	L	L
TBG deficiency	N	L	N
Euthyroid sick syndrome	L, N, H*	L	L to low N
TSH adenoma or pituitary resistance	N to H	H	H
Compensated hypothyroidism[†]	H	N	N

*Can be normal, slightly low, or slightly high.

[†]Treatment may not be necessary.

H, High; L, low; N, normal; T_4, thyroxine; TBG, thyroxine-binding globulin; TSH, thyroid-stimulating hormone.

2. Thyroid scan: Used to assess thyroid clearance and to study structure and function of the thyroid. Localizes ectopic thyroid tissue and hyperfunctioning and nonfunctioning thyroid nodules
3. Technetium uptake: Measures uptake of technetium by thyroid gland; levels are increased in hyperthyroidism and decreased in thyroxine-binding globulin deficiency and in hypothyroidism (except dyshormonogenesis, when it may be increased)

B. Hypothyroidism (Table 10-5)

NOTE: Do not begin treatment of central hypothyroidism until documenting normal adrenocorticotropic hormone (ACTH)/cortisol function due to risk of inducing adrenal crisis if there is ACTH deficiency.

C. Hyperthyroidism

1. **General**

a. Symptoms: Hyperactivity, irritability, altered mood, insomnia, heat intolerance, increased sweating, pruritus, tachycardia, palpitations, fatigue, weakness, weight loss despite increased appetite (or weight gain), increased stool frequency, oligomenorrhea or amenorrhea, fine tremor, hyperreflexia, hair loss

b. Epidemiology: Prevalence increases with age beginning in adolescence. 4:1 female-to-male predominance

c. Etiology: Most common cause in childhood is Graves disease (see later). Other causes: subacute thyroiditis, factitious hyperthyroidism (intake of exogenous hormone), rarely a thyroid-stimulating hormone (TSH)-secreting pituitary tumor. Pituitary resistance to thyroid hormone (compensatory rise in T_4, but TSH remains within normal range)

d. Lab findings: ↑ T_4, ↑ T_3, usually ↓ TSH. Further tests include TSH receptor stimulating antibody, thyroid-stimulating immunoglobulin (TSI), antithyroglobulin and antimicrosomal antibodies, free T_4, and free T_3

TABLE 10-3

ROUTINE STUDIES (THYROID)

Test	Age	Normal	Comments
Total T_4 (mcg/dL)	Birth–3 d	11.0–21.5	Measures total T_4 by radioimmunoassay
	4d–4 wk	8.0–20.0	
	1–12 mo	7.2–15.6	
	1–5 yr	7.3–15.0	
	5y 1d–adult	4.5–12.5	
Free T_4 (ng/dL)	0–3 d	0.66–2.71	Metabolically active form; the normal range for free T_4 is very assay dependent
	4–30 d	0.83–3.09	
	31 d–12 mo	0.48–2.34	
	13 mo–5 yr	0.85–1.75	
	6–10 yr	0.90–1.67	
	11–19 yr	0.93–1.60	
	>19 yr	0.93–1.71	
Total T_3 (ng/dL)	0–3 d	96–292	Measures T_3 by RIA
	4–30 d	62–243	
	31 d–12 mo	81–281	
	13 mo–5 yr	83–252	
	6–10 yr	92–219	
	>10 yr	71–180	
TSH (mIU/mL)	0–3 d	5.17–14.6	TSH surge peaks from 80–90 mIU/mL in term newborn by 30 min after birth. Values after 1 wk are within adult normal range. Elevated values suggest primary hypothyroidism, whereas suppressed values are the best indicator of hyperthyroidism
	4–30 d	0.430–16.1	
	31 d–12 mo	0.62–8.05	
	13 mo–5 yr	0.54–4.53	
	6–10 yr	0.66–4.14	
	>10 yr	0.45–4.50	
TBG (mcg/mL)	1–11 mo	Male 16–33; female 18–32	
	1–3 yr	Male 16–32; female 19–34	
	4–6 yr	Male 17–30; female 18–31	
	7–12 yr	Male 17–29; female 15–29	
	13–18 yr	Male 13–26; female 14–29	
	>18 yr	Male 13–39; female 13–39	

RIA, Radioimmune assay; T_3, triiodothyronine; T_4, thyroxine; TBG, thyroxine-binding globulin; TSH, thyroid-stimulating hormone.

Free T_4, TBG, total T_3, and TSH ranges are from: Labcorp https://www.labcorp.com/wps/portal/provider. Total T_4 range is from: Quest Diagnostics http://www.questdiagnostics.com/. **NOTE:** If age specific reference ranges are provided by the lab that runs the test, please refer to those ranges.

TABLE 10-4

SERUM T_4 IN PRETERM AND TERM INFANTS

Age (days)	VLBW (mg/dL)	LBW (mg/dL)	Term (mg/dL)
1–3	7.9 ± 3.3	11.4 ± 2.5	12 ± 1.9
4–6	6.5 ± 2.9	9.9 ± 2.5	11 ± 2.5
7–10	6.3 ± 3.0	9.5 ± 2.3	
11–14	5.7 ± 2.8	9.2 ± 2.1	
15–28	7.0 ± 2.5	9.1 ± 2.3	
29–56	7.8 ± 2.5	9.3 ± 3.3	

Low birth weight (LBW): 1500–2499 g; term: 2500–5528 g; very low birth weight (VLBW): 400–1499 g.
From Frank JE, Faix JE, Hermos RJ, et al: Thyroid function in very low birth weight infants: effects on neonatal hypothyroid screening. J Pediatrics 1996;128(4):548–555.

2. **Graves disease**
   a. Physical exam: Diffuse goiter, a feeling of grittiness and discomfort in the eye, retrobulbar pressure or pain, eyelid lag or retraction, periorbital edema, chemosis, scleral injection, exophthalmos, extraocular muscle dysfunction, localized dermopathy, and lymphoid hyperplasia
   b. Epidemiology: Peak incidence: age 11–15 years. 5 : 1 female-to-male ratio. Family history of autoimmune thyroid disease
   c. Etiology: Autoimmune (positive TSI, may also have low titers of thyroglobulin ± microsomal antibodies)
   d. Lab findings: ↑ T_4, ↑ T_3, ↓ TSH (↑ I^{123} uptake distinguishes from Hashimoto's thyroiditis)
   e. Treatment and monitoring: Methimazole (inhibits formation of thyroid hormone). Propylthiouracil (PTU) should not be used as first-line treatment in children due to higher risk of liver dysfunction than with methimazole; PTU can be considered for those with mild reactions to methimazole. Radioactive iodine (^{131}I) or surgical thyroidectomy are options for initial treatment or refractory cases. Follow symptoms and level of T_4 and TSH
3. **Hashimoto's thyroiditis**
   a. Presentation: ± initial hyperthyroidism followed by eventual burn out of the thyroid and hypothyroidism
   b. Etiology: Autoimmune (significantly elevated thyroglobulin and/or microsomal antibody)
   c. Lab findings: Mild to moderate ↑ T_4 (↓ I^{123} uptake distinguishes from Graves)
   d. Treatment: Hyperthyroid phase is usually self-limited, may eventually need thyroid replacement. Propranolol if symptomatic
4. **Thyroid storm**
   a. Presentation: Acute onset of hyperthermia, tachycardia, and restlessness. May progress to delirium, coma, and death
   b. Treatment: Propranolol is used to relieve signs and symptoms of thyrotoxicosis. Potassium iodide may also be used for acute hyperthyroid management. Long-term management as for Graves disease

TABLE 10-5

HYPOTHYROIDISM

Disease and Clinical Symptoms	Onset	Etiology	Management	Follow-up
Primary/Congenital				
Large fontanelles, lethargy, constipation, hoarse cry, hypotonia, hypothermia, jaundice	Symptoms usually develop within first 2 weeks of life; almost always present by 6 weeks. Some infants may be relatively asymptomatic if the cause is other than absence of the thyroid gland. Treated patients are still at risk for developmental delay.	Primary hypothyroidism: Most common cause is defect of fetal thyroid development. Other causes include TSH receptor mutation or thyroid dyshormonogenesis. *or* Central hypothyroidism: deficiency of thyrotropin-releasing hormone or thyrotropin (TSH)	Goal is to achieve T_4 in the upper half of normal range. In primary hypothyroidism, TSH should be kept <5. A minority of infants maintain persistently high TSH despite correction of T_4. Replacement with L-thyroxine as soon as diagnosis is confirmed.	Monitor T_4 and TSH at the end of weeks 1 and 2 of therapy and 3–4 weeks after any dose change. If levels are adequate, follow every 1–3 months during the first 12 months.
Acquired				
Growth deceleration; other signs may include coarse, brittle hair; dry, scaly skin; delayed tooth eruption; cold intolerance	Can occur as early as the first 2 years of life.	Hashimoto thyroiditis (diagnosis supported by presence of antithyroglobulin or antimicrosomal antibodies) Head/neck radiation Central hypothyroidism (pituitary/ hypothalamic insult).	Replacement with L-thyroxine.	As for primary/congenital. After 2 years, monitor levels every 6 to 12 months as dose changes become less frequent.

NOTE: Thyroid hormone levels in premature infants are lower than those seen in full-term infants. Further, the TSH surge seen at approximately 24 hours of age in full-term babies does not appear in preterm infants. In this population, lower levels are associated with increased illness, but the effect of replacement therapy remains controversial.

TSH, Thyroid-stimulating hormone.

5. **Neonatal thyrotoxicosis**
a. Presentation: Microcephaly, frontal bossing, intrauterine growth retardation (IUGR), tachycardia, systolic hypertension leading to widened pulse pressure, irritability, failure to thrive, exophthalmos, goiter, flushing, vomiting, diarrhea, jaundice, thrombocytopenia, and cardiac failure or arrhythmias. Onset from immediately after birth to weeks
b. Etiology: Exclusively in infants born to mothers with Graves disease. Caused by transplacental passage of maternal TSI. Occasionally, mothers are unaware that they have Graves. Also, note that if a mother has received definitive treatment (thyroidectomy or radiation therapy), the passage of TSI remains possible
c. Treatment and monitoring: Propranolol for control of symptoms. Methimazole to lower thyroxine levels. Digoxin may be indicated for heart failure. Disease usually resolves by age 6 months

D. Hyperparathyroidism and Hypoparathyroidism

1. Parathyroid hormone (PTH) function: Increases serum calcium by increasing bone resorption, increasing calcium and magnesium reuptake in the kidney, increasing phosphorus excretion in the kidney, increasing 25-hydroxy vitamin D conversion to 1,25-dihydroxy vitamin D in order to increase calcium absorption in the intestine
2. **Hypoparathyroidism:**
a. Presentation: Asymptomatic or mild muscle cramps to hypocalcemic tetany, prolonged QTc, and convulsions
b. Etiology: Results from a decrease in PTH due to decreased function or absence of the parathyroid gland. This can be due to transient hypoparathyroidism in infants, autoimmune disease, DiGeorge syndrome, iatrogenic removal of the parathyroid gland during other surgical procedures. Pseudohypoparathyroidism results from PTH resistance; is distinguished by normal or elevated PTH
c. Laboratory findings: ↓ PTH; ↓ serum Ca^{2+}, ↑ serum phos, normal/↓ alkaline phosphatase, ↓ 1,25-OH– vitamin D_3
d. Treatment and monitoring: Calcium supplementation for documented hypocalcemia, Vitamin D supplementation with calcitriol. Carefully monitor serum calcium and phosphorus during therapy. Monitor urine calcium levels to avoid hypercalciuria
3. **Hyperparathyroidism:**
a. Presentation: Hypercalcemia leading to vomiting, constipation, abdominal pain, weakness, paresthesias, malaise, and bone pain. Uncommon in childhood
b. Etiology: Associated with multiple endocrine neoplasia syndromes (see Expert Consult, Box EC 10-A). Secondary hyperparathyroidism more common; develops in response to hypocalcemic states, such as renal failure or rickets

c. Laboratory Findings: ↑ PTH, ↑ serum Ca^{2+}; ↓ serum phos; normal/↑ alkaline phosphatase. In secondary hyperparathyroidism, Ca^{2+} normal/↓
d. Treatment: Hydration is mainstay of treatment; enhances calciuria. Furosemide may be used with caution if adequate hydration. Hydrocortisone (1 mg/kg q6h), reduces intestinal absorption of calcium. Calcitonin transiently opposes bone resorption. In severe hypercalcemia, bisphosphates may be considered. Surgical removal of parathyroid glands (may result in hypoparathyroidism)

E. Vitamin D Deficiency (Table 10-6) (Dosing per Formulary)

F. Multiple Endocrine Neoplasias

See Box EC 10-A.

IV. ADRENAL AND PITUITARY FUNCTION[9–11]

A. Adrenal Insufficiency

1. Etiology:
a. Common causes: Congenital adrenal hyperplasia (CAH) and chronic glucocorticoid treatment (suppression of ACTH secretion)
b. Other causes: Addison's disease and hypothalamic or pituitary disease secondary to tumors, surgery, radiation therapy, or congenital defects
2. Evaluation:
a. AM cortisol level (see Table 10-7 for interpretation)
b. ACTH stimulation test (see Section VI.B.)

TABLE 10-6

VITAMIN D DEFICIENCY

Disease, Clinical Symptoms, and Onset	Etiology	Evaluation	Management
Rickets (infancy/childhood): Failure of adequate bone mineralization leading to soft bones/skeletal deformities **Osteomalacia** (adults): Bone pain and muscle weakness	Decreased dietary intake Inadequate exposure to sunlight Increased melanin Impaired renal function Fat malabsorption (celiac disease, cystic fibrosis, Crohn's disease)	↓ 25–OH vitamin D	Supplementation for: • Breast-fed infants • Those with celiac disease, cystic fibrosis, Crohn's disease, pancreatic deficiency Repletion per Formulary

TABLE 10-7

CORTISOL, 8 AM

Interpretation	Cortisol (mcg/dL)
Suggestive of adrenal insufficiency	<5 mcg/dL
Indeterminate	5–14 mcg/dL
Adrenal insufficiency unlikely	>14 mcg/dL

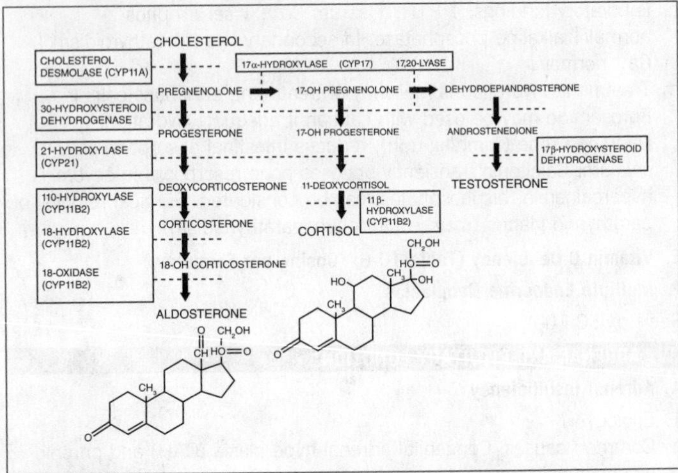

FIGURE 10-3

Biosynthetic pathway for steroid hormones. *(From Marshall I, Nimkarn S, New MI: Endocrine hypertension in childhood. Available at www.endotext.org/pediatrics/pediatrics9/index.html. Accessed December 21, 2007.)*

3. **Congenital adrenal hyperplasia**[10,11]**:**
   a. Group of autosomal recessive disorders characterized by a defect in one of the enzymes required in the synthesis of cortisol from cholesterol (Fig. 10-3). Cortisol deficiency results in oversecretion of ACTH and hyperplasia of the adrenal cortex
   b. The most common cause of ambiguous genitalia in females
   c. 21-Hydroxylase deficiency accounts for 90% of cases
   d. The enzymatic defect results in impaired synthesis of adrenal steroids beyond the enzymatic block and overproduction of the precursors before the block. Two major classifications:
      (1) Classic (complete enzyme deficiency):
         (a) Occurs with or without salt loss
         (b) Symptoms occur in the absence of stress
         (c) Adrenal crisis in untreated patients occurs at 1 to 2 weeks of life, with signs and symptoms of adrenal insufficiency rarely occurring before 3 to 4 days of life. (Non-salt-losing forms have a less severe risk for adrenal crisis owing to preservation of mineralocorticoid synthesis.)
         (d) Diagnosis: Elevated 17-hydroxyprogesterone (17-OHP) levels (often on newborn screen)
         (e) Elevated testosterone in girls and androstenedione in boys and girls

(f) For apparent male infants presenting with classic CAH, a karyotype should be evaluated to rule out the possibility of a severely masculinized female infant

(2) Nonclassic or simple virilizing form (partial enzyme deficiency):

(a) Adrenal insufficiency tends to occur only under stress; manifests as androgen excess after infancy (precocious pubarche, irregular menses, hirsutism, acne, advanced bone age)

(b) Morning 17-OHP levels may be elevated, but diagnosis may require an ACTH stimulation test (see Section VI.B). A significant rise in the 17-OHP level 60 min after ACTH injection is diagnostic. Cortisol response will be decreased

4. **Management of adrenal insufficiency:**

a. **Glucocorticoid maintenance:**

(1) Adrenal insufficiency—replacement of physiologic glucocorticoid production: Approximately 6–9 mg/m^2/day hydrocortisone (or equivalent glucocorticoid dose of another steroid). See Formulary Adjunct for forms of steroids used

(2) CAH—higher doses are required to achieve suppression of ACTH axis: 10–20 mg/m^2/day of hydrocortisone orally (PO) is recommended

(3) Doses often are titrated to preserve normal skeletal growth and rate of skeletal maturation and in CAH to suppress production of excess androgen

b. **Mineralocorticoid maintenance:**

(1) These patients should have ready access to salt

(2) For salt-losing forms of adrenal insufficiency (e.g., CAH, Addison's): 0.1–0.2 mg oral fludrocortisone acetate once daily is recommended. (**NOTE:** Intravenous [IV] hydrocortisone at 50 mg/m^2/day will supply a maintenance amount of mineralocorticoid activity. Synthetic steroids such as prednisone and dexamethasone do not supply appropriate mineralocorticoid effects.)

(3) Infants also require 1–2 g (17–34 mEq) of sodium supplementation per day

(4) Always monitor blood pressure and electrolytes when supplementing mineralocorticoids

c. **Stress dose glucocorticoids:**

(1) The dose of glucocorticoid should increase in patients with fever or other illness to mimic normal physiologic cortisol response to stress

(2) Stress dose: 25–50 mg/m^2/day of hydrocortisone IV/intramuscular [IM] (as a continuous drip or divided q3–6hr) or 50–75 mg/m^2/day PO divided q6–8hr

(3) For surgery or severe illness, hydrocortisone doses of 50–125 mg/m^2/day IV may be indicated

5. **Acute adrenal crisis:**
a. Often precipitated by acute illness, trauma, surgery, or exposure to excess heat
b. Presentation: Emesis, diarrhea, dehydration, hypotension, metabolic acidosis, and shock
c. Laboratory values: Often hypoglycemia, hyponatremia, and hyperkalemia. In addition, serum cortisol and aldosterone are decreased, and ACTH and renin are elevated. In infants with CAH, 17-OHP is increased

NOTE: These studies are useful to perform before steroid administration to confirm the diagnosis, but treatment should not be delayed.

d. Management includes rapid volume expansion to support blood pressure, sufficient dextrose to maintain blood glucose, close monitoring of electrolytes, and corticosteroid administration
   (1) Give 50 mg/m^2 of hydrocortisone by IV bolus (rapid estimate: infants = 25 mg; children = 50–100 mg), followed by 50 $mg/m^2/24$ hr by continuous drip (preferable) or divided q3–4hr
   (2) Hydrocortisone and cortisone are the only glucocorticoids that provide the necessary mineralocorticoid effects

B. Syndrome of Inappropriate Antidiuretic Hormone Secretion (SIADH)

1. Presentation: Hyponatremia (Na^+ <135 mEq/L) with inappropriately concentrated urine in the setting of euvolemia or mild hypervolemia
2. Etiology: Central nervous system (CNS) trauma, CNS infection, CNS or other types of surgery, particularly tonsillectomy and adenoidectomy, pneumonia
3. Laboratory findings: ↓ serum Na^+ and Cl^- with normal HCO_3^-, hypouricemia, inappropriately concentrated urine
4. Treatment: Correct hyponatremia slowly with fluid restriction (~10% rise in Na^+ per 24 hours). *In the setting of coma or seizures,* use hypertonic saline to rapidly correct Na^+ to ~120–125 mEq/L. Definitive therapy: identify and treat the underlying cause

C. Diabetes Insipidus (DI)[12]

1. **General:** Inability to concentrate urine
a. Presentation: Infants may present with failure to thrive, vomiting, constipation, unexplained fevers; severe dehydration, hypovolemic shock, and seizure may occur in more severe cases
b. Etiology: May be central or nephrogenic (see below)
c. Diagnosis: Water-deprivation test (Section VI.C). Vasopressin test (Section VI.D) differentiates between central and nephrogenic DI

2. **Central DI**
a. Etiology: Caused by vasopressin deficiency, associated with CNS injury, including trauma and tumors. Following trauma to axons of vasopressin containing neurons, a temporary or permanent DI may result. Due to the initial edema occurring in the area of the hypothalamus and

pituitary, a short-lived period (2–5 days) of DI is observed. This is succeeded by a stage of SIADH, as dying neurons release vasopressin. The final stage results in permanent DI, if a significant number of neurons are injured

b. Laboratory findings: Low urine specific gravity (<1.005), low urine osmolarity (50–200), low vasopressin (<0.5 pg/mL)
c. Treatment: IV, PO, subcutaneous (SC) or nasal desmopressin acetate (DDAVP). Titrate dosage to urine output, goal is ≥1-hour period of diuresis per day that stimulates thirst. Monitor electrolytes. Infants are often not treated with DDAVP due to difficulty monitoring input and output. Rather, they can be treated with increased free water and salt restriction

3. **Nephrogenic DI**
a. Etiology: Caused by renal tubular resistance to vasopressin; genetic or acquired
b. Laboratory findings: Low urine specific gravity (<1.005), low urine osmolarity (50–200 mOsm/L)
c. Treatment: Increase free water and a low-salt diet

V. GROWTH AND SEXUAL DEVELOPMENT[12–21]

A. Growth

1. **Target height range:** Calculated as midparental stature ± 2 SD (1 SD = 2 inches)
a. Midparental stature for boys: (paternal height + maternal height + 5 inches)/2
b. Midparental stature for girls: (paternal height + maternal height – 5 inches)/2

2. **Short stature (Fig. 10-4):**
a. Definition: Height less than the 3rd percentile; decreasing growth velocity; height percentile below the target height range
b. Differential diagnosis: Constitutional growth delay (CGD) and familial short stature (FSS) must be distinguished from pathologic causes of short stature
   (1) FSS: Characterized by slow growth rate during the first 2 to 3 years of life followed by a low-normal growth velocity. Bone age x-rays may be within normal limits for age
   (2) CGD: Typically characterized by similar growth charts as those with FSS; however, a delay in the onset of puberty and skeletal maturation allows for a period of catch-up growth. Family history of delayed puberty is often present. Bone age x-rays may be delayed for age
   (3) Pathologic short stature (see Fig. 10-4)
c. Initial evaluation: Detailed history/physical examination, evaluation of growth curves, and pubertal stage. Initial screening tests include complete blood count, liver function tests, electrolytes, erythrocyte

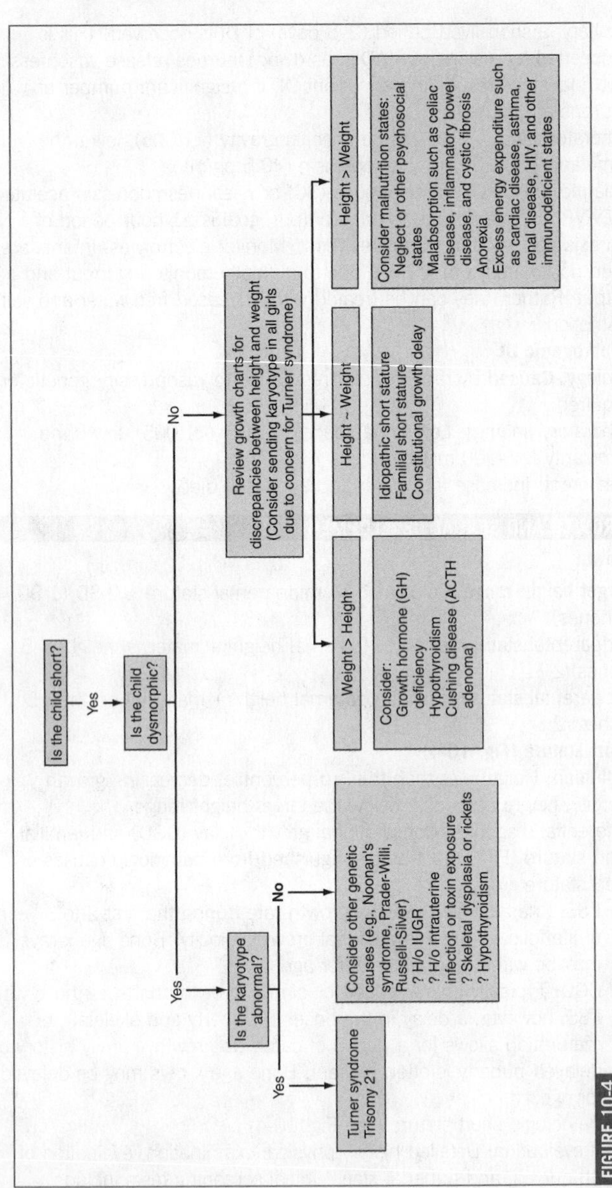

FIGURE 10-4 Differential diagnosis of short stature.

sedimentation rate, and urinalysis (including pH and specific gravity). Also consider thyroid function tests, serum insulin-like growth factor-1 (IGF-1) and IGF binding protein (IGFBP-3), tissue transglutaminase for celiac disease, bone age (radiograph of left wrist and hand), and karyotype (in girls). Consider a skeletal survey in a patient with disproportionate features

3. **Tall stature:** Most common cause is familial tall stature or precocious puberty. Bone age may be helpful
4. **Obesity:** A growing problem among the pediatric population. Although the majority do not have endocrine etiology, two disease categories may be addressed when approaching the obese patient
   a. Hypothyroidism: May be evaluated with serum thyroid function tests
   b. Cushing syndrome: Unlikely without linear growth failure in addition to obesity (see Section VI for laboratory testing details)
5. **Polycystic ovarian syndrome (PCOS)**
   a. Syndrome of hyperandrogenism and menstrual dysfunction
   b. Diagnostic criteria:
      (1) Hyperandrogenism: Clinical characteristics are hirsutism, acne, and female pattern alopecia. Biochemical characteristic is elevated free testosterone, calculated from total serum testosterone and sex hormone binding protein (SHBG)
      (2) Menstrual dysfunction: Amenorrhea or oligomenorrhea
      (3) Polycystic ovaries: Ultrasound (US) characteristics are increased ovarian volume (reliable in adolescents via transabdominal US) or follicular phase with ≥12 follicles measuring 2–9 mm (reliable via transvaginal US only)
   c. Management:
      (1) Weight reduction and other lifestyle changes increase SHBG (therefore decreasing free testosterone), can restore ovulation, and increase insulin sensitivity
      (2) Treatment of hirsutism/acne: Hormonal contraceptives
      (3) Insulin sensitizing agents, such as metformin, may help mitigate metabolic consequences
      (4) Prevention of endometrial hyperplasia (increased risk of endometrial cancer) by intermittent induction of menstruation or prevention of endometrial proliferation by hormonal contraception

B. Sexual Development

1. **Delayed puberty:** For girls, no pubertal development by age 14 years, or >5 year between thelarche and adrenarche. Primary amenorrhea: No menarche by age 16 years in the presence of secondary sexual characteristics or no menarche and no secondary sexual characteristics by age 14 years. For boys, no testicular enlargement by age 14 years, or >5 year for genital development

a. Delayed puberty may be divided according to luteinizing hormone (LH) and follicle-stimulating hormone (FSH) levels:
   (1) **Hypergonadotropic hypogonadism** (high LH and FSH): Primary gonadal failure, possibly due to Turner syndrome, Klinefelter syndrome, androgen insensitivity, tumor, chemotherapy
   (2) **Hypogonadotropic hypogonadism** (low or normal LH/FSH) may be secondary to constitutional delay, or central gonadotropin deficiency. Of the latter cause, etiologies include Kallman's (most common cause of isolated gonadotropin deficiency), central nervous system (CNS) tumors, hypopituitarism
b. Evaluation of delayed puberty may also be divided into the following categories (Fig. 10-5):
   (1) Constitutional delay
   (2) Hypopituitarism
   (3) Chromosomal abnormality
c. Initial evaluation: LH and FSH, bone age and thyroid studies. A gonadotropin-releasing hormone (GnRH) stimulation test can be obtained to rule out hypogonadotropic hypogonadism (See Chapter 10, G, on Expert Consult)

2. **Precocious puberty:** Traditionally defined as any sign of secondary sexual maturation before age 8 years in girls and age 9 years in boys. More recent data suggest early puberty may not warrant extensive evaluation or intervention if it occurs after age 6 years in African American girls or after age 7 years in Caucasian girls
a. Central, true, isosexual, *or* complete precocious puberty (CPP): Involves premature activation of the hypothalamic-pituitary-gonadal axis, leading to increased GnRH and therefore increased LH/FSH; five times more likely to occur in females, and often represents an idiopathic variant of normal puberty. In the majority of males with CPP, a CNS insult or structural anomaly is the cause
b. Peripheral *or* pseudoprecocious puberty: GnRH-independent puberty; involves adrenal, gonadal, ectopic, or exogenous sources of hormone production. Most common causes are CAH, adrenal tumors, McCune-Albright syndrome, gonadal tumors, human chorionic gonadotropin (hCG)-producing tumors, and exogenous sex hormones. Hypothyroidism can also cause GnRH-independent precocity. Penile length is disproportionately greater than testicular size in pseudo-precocious puberty, whereas testicular volume is disproportionately greater than penile size in normal puberty and in CPP
c. Initial evaluation: Begin with history (assessing for premature thelarche/adrenarche) physical examination, and growth curves
   (1) Bone age (generally >2 year in advance of chronologic age in long-standing precocious puberty due to the action of sex hormones)
   (2) Assess degree of estrogenization or virilization: Check plasma estradiol or plasma testosterone/DHEAS, respectively. Check basal and/or GnRH-stimulated LH levels (see Chapter 10 EC), estradiol

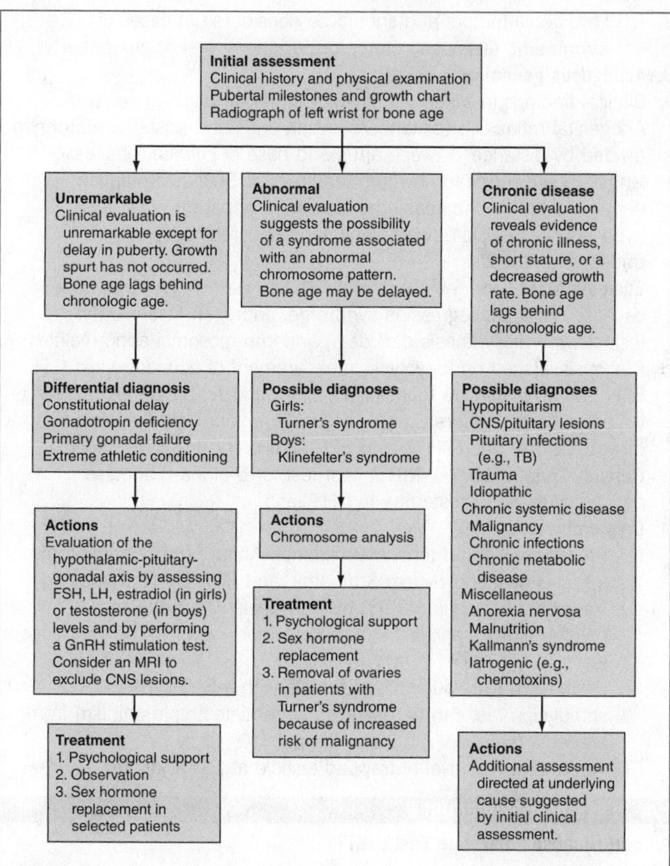

FIGURE 10-5

An approach to the child presenting with delayed puberty. CNS, central nervous system; FSH, follicle-stimulating hormone; GnRH, gonadotropin-releasing hormone; LH, luteinizing hormone; MRI, magnetic resonance imaging; TB, tuberculosis.[20] *(From Blondell R Foster MB, Dave KC: Disorders of puberty. Am Family Phys 1999;60(1):209–218.)*

measurement in girls, testosterone levels in boys, 17-OHP levels, dehydroepiandrosterone (DHEA) levels, and urinary 17-ketosteroids (see Section VII for normal values)

(3) Imaging: Magnetic resonance imaging of the brain may help identify a CNS lesion. In girls, pelvic ultrasonography may identify ovarian cysts, whereas in boys it may detect non-palpable

Leydig-cell tumors and should be considered in cases of asymmetric testicular volume or peripheral precocious puberty

3. **Ambiguous genitalia:**

a. Clinical findings in a neonate suspicious for ambiguous genitalia: Anogenital ratio >0.5 (distance between anus and posterior fourchette divided by distance between anus and base of clitoris), phallus length <1.9 cm (mean newborn length—2.5 SD), clitoromegaly (length >1 cm), nonpalpable gonads in an apparent male, and hypospadias associated with separation of scrotal sacs or undescended testis

b. Etiology: Most common cause is CAH (See Section IV.A.3). Other causes: Testicular regression syndrome, androgen insensitivity, testosterone biosynthesis disorders, and chromosomal abnormalities

c. Diagnosis: Based on karyotype, measurement of gonadotropins (LH, FSH), adrenal steroids (cortisol, 17-OHP, and ACTH stimulation test), testosterone precursors (DHEA, androstenedione), testosterone, dihydrotestosterone (DHT), and hCG stimulation test (see Expert Consult Chapter 10, H). **NOTE:** best test for 5-alpha-reductase deficiency is the testosterone to DHT ratio.

d. **Cryptorchidism:**

(1) Prevalence: 3% of term male infants. About 50% of cryptorchid testicles descend by age 3 months, and 80% by 12 months. Neoplasm occurs in 48.9% of individuals with untreated cryptorchidism, and 25% of those tumors occur in the contralateral testis

(2) Evaluation: Rule out virilized female with a karyotype. hCG stimulation test can be used to differentiate cryptorchidism from anorchia (see Expert Consult Chapter 10, H)

(3) Treatment: Removal of trapped testicle at 1 year of life

VI. TESTS AND PROCEDURES

A. Oral Glucose Tolerance Test (OGTT)

1. Pretest preparation:

a. Calorically adequate diet required for 3 days before the test, with 50% of total calories taken as carbohydrate

b. Delay test 2 weeks after illness

c. Discontinue all hyperglycemic and hypoglycemic agents (e.g., salicylates, diuretics, oral contraceptives, phenytoin)

2. Procedure: Give 1.75 g/kg (maximum of 75 g) of glucose PO after a 12-hour fast, allowing up to 5 min for ingestion. Mix glucose with water and lemon juice as a 20% dilution. Quiet activity is permissible during the OGTT. Draw blood samples at 0 and 120 minutes after ingestion

3. Interpretation: 2-hour blood glucose <140 mg/dL = normal; 140–199 mg/dL = impaired glucose tolerance; ≥200 mg/dL = diabetes mellitus

B. ACTH Stimulation Test

1. Purpose: Measures the ability of the adrenal gland to produce cortisol in response to ACTH. Most useful in diagnosis of adrenal insufficiency
2. Interpretation: Normally, there is a rise in serum cortisol after ACTH administration. With ACTH deficiency or prolonged adrenal suppression, there is no rise in cortisol after a single ACTH dose. A blunted cortisol response can be indicative of CAH. A lack of response after 3 consecutive days of ACTH stimulation is pathognomonic of Addison disease
3. Standard-dose ACTH stimulation test (250 mcg IV); cortisol measured at 30 minutes (Used to evaluate for primary adrenal insufficiency, although may be used to evaluate for central adrenal insufficiency):
   a. For evaluation of primary adrenal insufficiency:
      <18 mcg/dL highly suggestive of adrenal insufficiency
      >18 mcg/dL normal (rules out adrenal insufficiency)
   b. For evaluation of central adrenal insufficiency:
      <16 mcg/dL highly suggestive of adrenal insufficiency
      16–30 mcg/dL adrenal insufficiency less likely but not excluded
      >30 mcg/dL normal (rules out adrenal insufficiency)
4. Low-dose ACTH stimulation test (1 mcg per $1.73m^2$); cortisol measured at 30 minutes (Used to evaluate for central adrenal insufficiency, where it may have higher sensitivity compared to the standard-dose test):

Level <16 mcg/dL suggestive of adrenal insufficiency
Level 16–22 mcg/dL adrenal insufficiency less likely but not excluded
Level >22 mcg/dL adrenal insufficiency unlikely

NOTE: None of the tests of adrenal insufficiency has perfect sensitivity or specificity, so results must be interpreted in the individual clinical context.

C. Water Deprivation Test

1. Purpose: Determines ability to concentrate urine, useful in the diagnosis of DI. Risk of dehydration and hypernatremia, so careful supervision is required
2. Method:
   a. Begin the test after a 24-hour period of adequate hydration and stable weight
   b. Obtain a baseline weight after bladder emptying
   c. Restrict fluids. Measure body weight and urine specific gravity and volume hourly
   d. Check serum Na and urine and serum osmolality every 2 hours. (Hematocrit and blood urea nitrogen (BUN) levels may also be obtained but are not critical.) Monitor carefully to ensure that fluids are not ingested during the test
   e. Terminate the test if weight loss approaches 5%

3. Interpretation:

a. Normal individuals and those with psychogenic DI: Urine will be concentrated to 500–1400 mOsm/L; plasma osmolality will be 288–291 mOsm/L. Urine specific gravity rises to at least 1.010, urine-to-plasma osmolality ratio is >2, urine volume decreases significantly, and there should be no appreciable weight loss. Urine osmolarity >1000 mOsm/L (or >600 mOsm/L for >1 hour) generally excludes a diagnosis of DI

b. Central or nephrogenic DI: Specific gravity remains <1.005. Urine osmolality remains <150 mOsm/L, with no significant reduction of urine volume. A weight loss of up to 5% usually occurs. At the end of the test, a serum osmolality >290 mOsm/L, Na >150 mEq/L, and a rise of BUN and hematocrit provide evidence that the patient has DI

D. Vasopressin Test

1. Purpose: Used to differentiate between central (ADH-deficient) and nephrogenic DI
2. Method: Vasopressin is given subcutaneously, preferably at the end of the water deprivation test. Urine output, urine specific gravity, and water intake are monitored
3. Interpretation:

a. Central DI: Patients concentrate their urine (>1.010), demonstrate a reduction of urine volume and decreased fluid intake in response to exogenous vasopressin

b. Nephrogenic DI: No significant change in fluid intake, urine volume or specific gravity

c. Psychogenic DI: Continued fluid intake, decreased urine output and increased specific gravity

E. Cushing Evaluation

1. 24-hour urine collection for excess cortisol (normal value range by mass spectrometry is ≤27–30 ng/mL)
2. Salivary cortisol level: Measured at 11 PM (*spit in a tube*); levels are akin to free serum cortisol. Normal range is <0.2 mcg/dL
3. Dexamethasone suppression test:

a. Dexamethasone suppresses secretion of ACTH by the normal pituitary, decreasing endogenous production of cortisol. Useful in determining the etiology of glucocorticoid or androgen overproduction

b. Overnight dexamethasone suppression test: Measure serum cortisol at 8 AM; preceded by 1 mg of dexamethasone PO given at 11 PM the night before; level <1.8 mcg/dL (50 nanomol/L) is within normal range of suppression

NOTE: Random cortisol is not useful in evaluation for Cushing syndrome.

F. Neonatal Hypoglycemia and Glucagon Stimulation Test[23]

1. Definition of hypoglycemia: Serum glucose level that is insufficient to meet metabolic requirements; can vary with perinatal stress, birth

weight, and maternal factors. For practical purposes value is defined as <45 mg/dL

NOTE: Bedside glucometer is inaccurate at levels <40 mg/dL; stat serum glucose must be sent.

2. Symptoms: Abnormal cry, seizures, apnea, hypotonia, bradycardia, hypothermia.
3. Treatment: Do not delay treatment for serum glucose results
   a. Plasma glucose 25–45 mg/dL (1.4–2.5 mM), asymptomatic: Breast-feed or nipple/gavage with formula
   b. Plasma glucose level <25 mg/dL (<1.4 mM) with or without symptoms, asymptomatic infants who do not tolerate enteral feeding, or symptomatic infants:
      (1) Give IV bolus of glucose 0.25 g/kg (2.5 mL/kg of 10% glucose, or 1.0 mL/kg of 25% glucose) over 1 to 2 minutes
      (2) Continue IV glucose at a rate of 6–8 mg/kg/min (3.6–4.8 mL/kg/hr of 10% glucose)
      (3) Monitor blood glucose q30–60 minutes and increase glucose delivery by 1–2 mg/kg/min if blood glucose is consistently <50 mg/dL
4. If serum glucose is consistently <45 mg/dL: Further endocrine workup is warranted. At the time of hypoglycemia (serum glucose <45 mg/dL) obtain serum levels of glucose, insulin, growth hormone, free fatty acids, and β-hydroxybutyrate
5. Glucagon stimulation test: At the time of hypoglycemia, obtain above labs, administer glucagon and obtain serum glucose levels q10 minutes × 4. Repeat growth hormone and cortisol levels 30 minutes after documented hypoglycemia
   a. A rise in glucose secondary to glucagon ≥30mg/dL along with elevated insulin levels, low serum levels of free fatty acids and β-hydroxybutyrate and a glucose requirement >8 mg/kg/min suggests a diagnosis of hyperinsulinemia
   b. Hypoglycemia with midline defects and micropenis in a male suggest hypopituitarism, supported by low serum levels of growth hormone and cortisol at the time of hypoglycemia

See Expert Consult, Chapter 10, for additional information about serum-free fractionated metanephrines

See Expert Consult, Chapter 10, G and H, for additional information about GNRH and hCG stimulation tests.

VII. NORMAL VALUES (TABLES 10-7, 10-8, 10-9, 10-10, 10-11, 10-12, 10-13, 10-14, 10-15, 10-16, 10-17, AND 10-18)

Normal values may differ among laboratories because of variation in technique and in type of radioimmunoassay used. Unless otherwise noted, the values in these tables are reference ranges from the Johns Hopkins Hospital Laboratories or from SmithKline Beecham clinical laboratories in Baltimore, Maryland.

10

TABLE 10-8

VITAMIN D

Compound	Value
25-Hydroxy-vitamin D	(ng/mL)
Severe deficiency	<10
Mild/moderate deficiency	10–20
Optimal level	20–50*
1,25-Dihydroxy-vitamin D	(pg/mL)
Newborns	8–72
Children	15–90
Adults	24–64

NOTE: 1,25-dihydroxy-vitamin D is the physiologically active form; however, 25-hydroxy-vitamin D is the value to monitor for vitamin D deficiency, because this approximates body stores of vitamin D.

*Controversy exists with regard to the optimal 25-hydroxy-vitamin D level. Some experts recommend a level >30 ng/mL as optimal.

Ross AC, Manson JE, Abrams SA. The 2011 Report on Dietary Reference Intakes for Calcium and Vitamin D from the Institute of Medicine: What clinicians need to know. J Clin Endocrinol Metab. 2010 Nov 29. [Epub ahead of print]"

TABLE 10-9

TESTOSTERONE

Age	Testosterone, Serum Total (ng/dL)	Testosterone, Unbound (pg/mL)
Prepubertal children	10–20	0.15–0.6
Men	275–875	52–280
Women	23–75	1.1–6.3
Pregnancy	35–195	

NOTE: Normal Testosterone/Dihydrotestosterone (T/DHT) ratio is <18 in adults and older children, <10 in neonates. T/DHT ratio of >20 suggests 5-alpha-reductase deficiency or androgen insensitivity syndrome.

TABLE 10-10

ESTRADIOL

Age	Level (pg/mL)
Prepubertal children	<25
Men	6–44
Women	
Luteal phase	None detected–266
Follicular phase	118–355
Midcycle	None detected–102
Adult women on OCP	26–165

NOTE: Normal infants have an elevated estradiol at birth, which decreases to prepubertal values during the first week of life. Estradiol levels increase again between age 1 and 2 months and return to prepubertal values by age 6–12 months.

OCP, Oral contraceptive pill.

TABLE 10-11

DEHYDROEPIANDROSTERONE (DHEA)

Age	DHEA (ng/dL)	DHEA Sulfate (mg/dL)
Prepubertal children	25 ± 8	2.3–15
Men	643 ± 112	223 ± 93
Women	516 ± 106	138 ± 51

Adapted from Bertrand J et al: Pediatric endocrinology, 2nd ed. Baltimore, Williams & Wilkins, 1993.

TABLE 10-12

17-HYDROXYPROGESTERONE, SERUM

Age	Baseline (ng/dL)	60 Min Post ACTH Stimulation (ng/dL)
Term infants (3 d)	≤420	
1–12 mo	11–170	85–465
1–5 yr	4–115	50–350
6–12 yr	7–69	75–220
Males, Tanner II–III	12–130	69–310
Females, Tanner II–III	18–220	80–420
Male, Tanner IV–V	51–190	105–230
Females, Tanner IV–V	36–200	80–225
Male (18–30 yr)	32–307	
Adult female		
Follicular phase	≤185	
Midcycle phase	≤225	
Luteal phase	≤285	

NOTE: 8 AM level is most accurate given diurnal variation. Levels are normally increased in newborns for the first few days of life. Be aware that infant serum contains substances that may cross-react in the assay for 17-hydroxyprogesterone and artificially elevate the level, unless they are separated by chromatography. Before interpreting results on infants, be sure that the laboratory has prepared samples appropriately.

ACTH, Adrenocorticotropic hormone.

For preterm infants or infants born small for gestational age, see: Olgemöller et al. Screening for congenital adrenal hyperplasia: adjustment of 17-hydroxyprogesterone cut-off values to both age and birth weight markedly improves the predictive value. J Clin Endocrinol Metab 2003;88:5790–5794.

TABLE 10-13

INSULIN-LIKE GROWTH FACTOR 1 (IGF-1)

Age	Males (ng/mL)	Females (ng/mL)
2 mo–6 yr	17–248	17–248
6–9 yr	88–474	88–474
9–12 yr	110–565	117–771
12–16 yr	202–957	261–1096
16–26 yr	182–780	182–780
>26 yr	123–463	123–463

NOTE: A clearly normal IGF-1 level argues against growth hormone (GH) deficiency, except in young children, where there is considerable overlap between normals and those with GH deficiency.

TABLE 10-14

INSULIN-LIKE GROWTH FACTOR-BINDING PROTEIN (IGF-BP3)

Age (yr)	Males (mg/L)	Females (mg/L)
0–2	0.94–1.76	0.66–2.51
2–4	1.12–2.33	0.84–3.77
4–6	1.16–3.13	1.32–3.60
6–8	1.32–3.38	1.21–4.66
8–10	1.35–3.94	1.58–3.99
10–12	1.53–5.02	1.93–6.46
12–14	1.73–5.11	1.78–6.08
14–16	1.90–6.40	2.02–5.44
16–18	1.70–6.04	1.88–5.29
18–20	1.52–6.01	1.63–6.02
20–22	1.79–5.41	1.82–5.35
Adult (continues to vary with age)	1.15–5.18	1.19–5.69

NOTE: Levels below the 5th percentile suggest growth hormone deficiency. This test may have greater discrimination than the IGF-1 test in younger patients.

TABLE 10-15

MEAN STRETCHED PENILE LENGTH (cm)

Age	Mean ± SD	–2.5 SD
Birth		
30 wk gestation	2.5 ± 0.4	1.5
34 wk gestation	3.0 ± 0.4	2.0
Full term	3.5 ± 0.4	2.5
0–5 mo	3.9 ± 0.8	1.9
6–12 mo	4.3 ± 0.8	2.3
1–2 yr	4.7 ± 0.8	2.6
2–3 yr	5.1 ± 0.9	2.9
3–4 yr	5.5 ± 0.9	3.3
4–5 yr	5.7 ± 0.9	3.5
5–6 yr	6.0 ± 0.9	3.8
6–7 yr	6.1 ± 0.9	3.9
7–8 yr	6.2 ± 1.0	3.7
8–9 yr	6.3 ± 1.0	3.8
9–10 yr	6.3 ± 1.0	3.8
10–11 yr	6.4 ± 1.1	3.7
Adult	13.3 ± 1.6	9.3

NOTE: Measured from the pubic ramus to the tip of the glans while traction is applied along the length of the phallus to the point of increased resistance.

SD, Standard deviation.

From Feldman KW, Smith DW: Fetal phallic growth and penile standards for newborn male infants. J Pediatr 1975;86:395.

TABLE 10-16

TESTICULAR SIZE

Tanner Stage (Genital)	Length (cm) (Mean ± SD)	Volume (mL)
I	2.0 ± 0.5	2
II	2.7 ± 0.7	5
III	3.4 ± 0.8	10
IV	4.1 ± 1.0	20
V	5.0 ± 0.5	29

NOTE: Testicular volume of >4 mL or a long axis >2.5 cm is evidence that pubertal testicular growth has begun.
SD, Standard deviation.

TABLE 10-17

GONADOTROPINS

Age	FSH (mIU/mL)	LH (mIU/mL)
Prepubertal children	0.0–2.8	0.0–1.6
Men	1.4–14.4	1.0–10.2
Women, follicular phase	3.7–12.9	0.9–14

NOTE: Normal infants have a transient rise in follicle-stimulating hormone (FSH) and luteinizing hormone (LH) to pubertal levels or higher within the first 3 mo, which then declines to prepubertal values by the end of the first year.

TABLE 10-18

ANDROSTENEDIONE, SERUM

Age	Males (ng/dL)	Females (ng/dL)
Preterm infants		
26–28 wk to day 4 of life	92–892	92–892
31–35 wk to day 4 of life	80–446	80–446
Full-term infants		
1–7 day	20–290	20–290
1–12 mo	6–68	6–68
Prepubertal children	8–50	8–50
Tanner II	31–65	42–100
Tanner III	50–100	80–190
Tanner IV	48–140	77–225
Tanner V	65–210	80–240
Adults	78–205	85–275

See Expert Consult, Chapter 10, for normal values of:
Table EC 10-A, Dihydrotestosterone (DHT)
Table EC 10-B, Catecholamines, urine
Table EC 10-C, Catecholamines, serum

REFERENCES

1. American Diabetes Association. Diagnosis and classification of diabetes mellitus. *Diabetes Care*. 2010;33:S62–S69.
2. Alberti G, Zimmet P, Shaw J, et al. Type 2 diabetes in the young: the evolving epidemic: the international diabetes federation consensus workshop. *Diabetes Care*. 2004;27(7):1798–1811.

10

3. Hattersley A, Bruining J, Shield J, et al. ISPAD Clinical Practice Consensus Guidelines 2006–2007. The diagnosis and management of monogenic diabetes in children. *Pediatr Diabetes.* 2006;7(6):352–360.
4. Cooke DW, Plotnick L. Management of diabetic ketoacidosis in children and adolescents. *Pediatr Rev.* 2008;29(12):431–436.
5. International Expert Committee report on the role of the A1c assay in the diagnosis of diabetes. *Diabetes Care.* 2009;32:1327–1334.
6. Fisher DA. The thyroid. In *Rudolf's pediatrics.* New York: The McGraw-Hill Companies; 2003.
7. Fisher DA. Thyroid function and dysfunction in premature infants. *Pediatr Endocrinol Rev.* 2007;4(4):317–328.
8. Büyükgebiz A. Newborn screening for congenital hypothyroidism. *J Pediatr Endocrinol Metab.* 2006;19(11):1291–1298.
9. Stewart PM. The adrenal cortex. In: Kronenberg HM, et al. ed. *Williams textbook of endocrinology.* Philadelphia: Saunders; 2008.
10. American Academy of Pediatrics, Section on Endocrinology and Committee on Genetics. Technical report: congenital adrenal hyperplasia. *Pediatrics.* 2000;106(6):1511–1518.
11. Levine LS. Congenital adrenal hyperplasia. *Pediatr Rev.* 2000;21(5):159–170.
12. Robinson AG, Verbalis JG. Posterior pituitary. In: Kronenberg HM, Melmed S, Polonsky KS, et al. ed. *Williams textbook of endocrinology.* Philadelphia: Saunders; 2008.
13. Plotnick L, Miller R. Growth, growth hormone, and pituitary disorders. In: McMillan J, ed. *Oski's pediatrics principles and practice.* Philadelphia: Lippincott Williams & Wilkins; 2006:2084–2092.
14. MacGillivray MH. The basics for the diagnosis and management of short stature: a pediatric endocrinologist's approach. *Pediatr Ann.* 2000;29(9):570–575.
15. Norman RJ, Dewailly D, Legro RS, et al. MD Polycystic ovary syndrome. *Lancet.* 2007;370(9588):685–697.
16. Styne DM. New aspects in the diagnosis and treatment of pubertal disorders. *Pediatr Endocrinol.* 1997;44(2):505–529.
17. Rosen DS, Foster C. Delayed puberty. *Pediatr Rev.* 2001;22(9):309–314.
18. Carel JC, Leger J. Clinical practice. Precocious puberty. *N Engl J Med.* 2008;358(22):2366–2377.
19. American Academy of Pediatrics, Committee on Genetics, Sections on Endocrinology and Urology. Evaluation of newborn with developmental anomalies of the external genitalia. *Pediatrics.* 2000;106(1):138–142.
20. Blondell R, Foster MB, Dave KC. Disorders of puberty. *Am Family Phys.* 1999;60(1):209–218.
21. Master-Hunter T, Heiman DL. Amenorrhea: evaluation and treatment. *Am Family Phys.* 2006;73(8):1374–1382.
22. Carel JC, Eugster EA, Rogol A, et al. Consensus statement on the use of gonadotropin-releasing hormone analogs in children. *Pediatrics.* 2009;123(4): e752–762.
23. Cooke DW. Metabolism and endocrinology. In: Seidel HM, Rosenstein BJ, Pathak A, eds. *Primary care of the newborn,* 4th ed. Philadelphia: Mosby; 2006.
24. Lenders JWM, Pacak K, Walther MM, et al. Biomedical diagnosis of pheochromocytoma: which test is best? *JAMA.* 2002;287:1427–1434.
25. Weise M, Merke DP, Pacak K, et al. Utility of plasma free metanephrines for detecting childhood pheochromocytoma. *JCEM.* 2002;87:1955–1960.

Chapter 11

Fluids and Electrolytes

Elizabeth Quaal Hines, MD

See additional content on Expert Consult

I. OVERALL GOALS OF FLUID AND ELECTROLYTE MANAGEMENT

Fluid therapy is an essential component of the care of hospitalized children. Appropriate fluid management involves the calculation and administration of water volume and electrolyte concentration of:

A. Maintenance Requirements

B. Initial Deficit Repletion

C. Ongoing Losses

This basic principle should be followed whether providing oral or parenteral fluids.

II. MAINTENANCE REQUIREMENTS

The amount of water and electrolytes lost during normal basal metabolism. Metabolism creates two by-products, heat and solute, that need to be eliminated to maintain homeostasis. The amount of heat dissipated through insensible water losses and the amount of solute excreted in urine is directly related to caloric expenditure.

Metabolic demands do not increase in direct proportion to body mass (weight) across the continuum. The metabolic rate per kg body weight declines with age; an infant generates significantly more solute and heat per kg than a child or adolescent. However, the volume of water and concentration of solute required per kcal burned remains constant across all ages. To correctly calculate maintenance needs, it is necessary to determine calories burned. The relationship between caloric expenditure and normal volume losses (Fig. 11-1)[1]

A. Maintenance Volume: Caloric Calculations

There are three basic methods to calculate maintenance fluid volume needs.

1. **Basal calorie method:** Useful for all ages, types of body habitus, and clinical states
   a. Determine the child's estimated energy requirements based on age and activity level (see Table 21-2)
   b. Adjust caloric expenditure needs by various factors (e.g., fever) as described in Chapter 21
   c. For each 100 calories metabolized in 24 hr, the average patient will need 100–120 mL H_2O, 2–4 mEq Na^+, and 2–3 mEq K^+

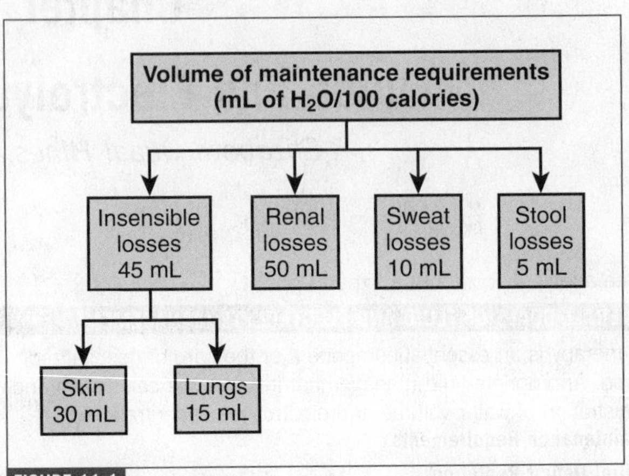

FIGURE 11-1

For each 100 calories metabolized in 24 hours, about 55–60 mL of fluid is required to provide for insensible losses as well as basal stool and sweat losses, and 50 mL of fluid is required for the kidneys to excrete an ultrafiltrate of plasma at 300 mOsm/L without having to concentrate the urine. *(Redrawn from Roberts KB: Fluids and electrolytes: parenteral fluid therapy. Pediatr Rev 2001;22:380–387.)*

TABLE 11-1

HOLLIDAY-SEGAR METHOD

	Water		
Body Weight	**mL/kg/day**	**mL/kg/hr**	**Electrolytes (mEq/100 mL H_2O)**
First 10 kg	100	~4	Na^+ 3
Second 10 kg	50	~2	Cl^- 2
Each additional kg	20	~1	K^+ 2

2. **Holliday-Segar method** (Table 11-1 and Box 11-1)[2]: Estimates caloric expenditure in fixed weight categories and makes the same assumption for water and electrolyte needs based on 100 kcal burned as above

NOTE: The Holliday-Segar method is not suitable for neonates <14 days old; generally, it overestimates fluid needs in neonates compared with the caloric expenditure method. (See Chapter 18 for further neonatal fluid management)

3. **Body surface area (BSA) method:** Based on the assumption that caloric expenditure is related to BSA (Table 11-2). It should not be used for children <10 kg. See BSA calculation in Formulary Adjunct

BOX 11-1

HOLLIDAY-SEGAR METHOD

Example: Determine the correct fluid rate for an 8-year-old child weighing 25 kg:

First 10 kg:	4 mL/kg/hr × 10 kg = 40 mL/hr	100 mL/kg/day × 10 kg = 1000 mL/day
Second 10 kg:	2 mL/kg/hr × 10 kg = 20 mL/hr	50 mL/kg/day × 10 kg = 500 mL/day
Each Additional 1 kg:	1 ml/kg/hr × 5 kg = 5 mL/hr	20 mL/kg/day × 5 kg = 100 mL/day
	Answer: 65 mL/hr	Answer: 1600 mL/day

TABLE 11-2

STANDARD VALUES FOR USE IN BODY SURFACE AREA METHOD

H_2O	1500 mL/m^2/24 hr
Na^+	30–50 mEq/m^2/24 hr
K^+	20–40 mEq/m^2/24 hr

Data from Finberg L, Kravath R, Fleischman A: Water and electrolytes in pediatrics. Philadelphia, WB Saunders, 1982; and Hellerstein S: Fluids and electrolytes: clinical aspects. Pediatr Rev 1993;14(3):103–115.

B. Maintenance Solute

1. For the purposes of fluid calculation, fluid lost via insensible losses through the skin and respiratory tract can be considered electrolyte-free. Urine represents the primary source of electrolyte loss with variability based on the kidney's ability to dilute and concentrate. Average electrolyte requirements per 100 mL H_2O are seen in Table 11-1 with the addition of 5%–10% dextrose depending on need to prevent ketosis

Solute needs can thus be met by administering D5 ¼ normal saline (NS) with 20 mEq/L KCl.

2. Cautions regarding hypotonic fluid administration:

a. Regarding hypotonic fluids, the Holliday-Segar Method is based on the maintenance caloric, fluid and electrolyte needs of healthy, milk-fed infants and children that can be met with hypotonic fluids. Many hospitalized patients have water and electrolyte deficits and may retain free water due to various disease processes. Therefore, hypotonic fluids (i.e., 0.225% NS) should be used for maintenance needs only. Prior or ongoing losses of water or electrolytes require further volume and electrolyte deficit calculations and appropriate adjustment of replacement fluids in their management

b. Due to >50 reported deaths or severe neurologic injury from iatrogenic hyponatremia since the mid-1990s, some experts have suggested using NS in all patients receiving maintenance intravenous (IV) fluids.[3] NS may be used to provide water and electrolytes for certain patients (i.e., postoperative neurosurgical and traumatic brain injury patients), but the safety of routinely using NS as maintenance fluid has not been adequately studied in randomized, controlled trials

III. DEFICIT REPLETION[4]

The following equations are numbered and can be used to calculate fluid management per Figure 11-2.

Based on the amount of fluid/electrolytes lost prior to a patient's hospital presentation.

A. Fluid Deficit Volume

1. **Calculated assessment:** The most precise method of assessing fluid deficit is weight loss. If this is not known, clinical observation may be used, as described subsequently

Fluid deficit (L) = pre-illness weight (kg) – illness weight (kg) (Equation A.1)

% Dehydration = (pre-illness weight – illness weight)/pre-illness weight × 100%

2. **Clinical assessment** (Table 11-3): Each 1% dehydration corresponds with 10 mL/kg fluid deficit

TABLE 11-3

CLINICAL OBSERVATIONS IN DEHYDRATION*

		Older Child	
	3% (30 mL/kg)	**6% (60 mL/kg)**	**9% (90 mL/kg)**
		Infant	
	5% (50 mL/kg)	**10% (100 mL/kg)**	**15% (150 mL/kg)**
EXAMINATION			
Dehydration	Mild	Moderate	Severe
Skin turgor	Normal	Tenting	None
Skin (touch)	Normal	Dry	Clammy
Buccal mucosa/lips	**Dry**	Dry	Parched/cracked
Eyes	Normal	Deep set	Sunken
Tears	Present	Reduced	None
Fontanelle	Flat	Soft	Sunken
CNS	Consolable	Irritable	Lethargic/obtunded
Pulse rate	Normal	**Slightly increased**	Increased
Pulse quality	Normal	Weak	**Feeble/impalpable**
Capillary refill	Normal	~2 sec	**>3 sec**
Urine output	Normal to **Decreased**	Decreased	Anuric

*Serum sodium concentration affects the clinical manifestations of dehydration, such as skin turgor and mucous membranes. For example, hyponatremia exaggerates instability and hypernatremia maintains intravascular volume at the expense of intracellular volume.

CNS, Central nervous system.

Data from Kliegman RM, Behrman RE, Jenson HB, et al: Nelson textbook of pediatrics, 18th ed. Philadelphia, WB Saunders, 2007; and Oski FA: Principles and practice of pediatrics, 4th ed. Philadelphia, JB Lippincott, 2006.

Isonatremic Dehydration

	F.#	First 8 hours	Next 16 hours
Fluid deficit volume	A.1	Replace ½ of calculated deficits divided evenly over 8 hours.	Replace remaining ½ of calculated deficits divided evenly over 16 hours.
Na^+ deficit	F.1		
K^+ deficit	F.2		
Maintenance		To be given in addition to above calculated deficits at hourly rate.	

Hyponatremic Dehydration

	F.#	First 8 hours	Next 16 hours
Fluid deficit volume	A.1	Replace ½ of calculated deficits divided evenly over 8 hours.	Replace remaining ½ of calculated deficits divided evenly over 16 hours.
Na^+ deficit	F.1		
Excess Na^+ deficit	F.3		
K^+ deficit	F.2		
Maintenance		To be given in addition to above calculated deficits at hourly rate.	

Hypernatremic Dehydration

	F.#	First 8 hours	Next 16 hours	Next 24 hours
Free water deficit	F.4	Replace ½ of deficit over first 24 hours.		Replace remaining ½ of calculated deficit over next 24 hours.
Solute fluid deficit	F.5	Replace ½ of calculated deficits divided evenly over 8 hours.	Replace remaining ½ of calculated deficits divided evenly over 16 hours.	
Solute Na^+ deficit	F.6			
Solute K deficit	F.7			
Maintenance		To be given in addition to above calculated deficits at hourly rate.		

FIGURE 11-2

Fluid and solute replacement in isonatremic, hyponatremic, and hypernatremic dehydration.

TABLE 11-4

INTRACELLULAR AND EXTRACELLULAR FLUID COMPOSITION

	Intracellular (mEq/L)	Extracellular (mEq/L)
Na^+	20	133–145
K^+	150	3–5
Cl^-	—	98–110
HCO_3^-	10	20–25
PO_4^{3-}	110–115	5
Protein	75	10
% Bodyweight	80	15 (interstitial), 5 (intravascular)

B. Solute Deficit Based on Solute Fluid Deficit (Isonatremic Dehydration)

Fluid losses from intracellular and extracellular compartments are used to determine electrolyte deficit and replacement.

NOTE: These calculations hold true for isonatremic dehydration. To calculate solute deficit in hypernatremic dehydration, see Section E.

1. Extracellular fluid compartment: ~20% of the body's weight (40% in the newborn), divided 3:1 between interstitial and intravascular compartments, respectively[5]
2. In dehydration, there are variable losses from the extracellular and intracellular compartments. The percentage deficit from these compartments is based on the total duration of illness
   a. Illness <3 days: 80% (0.8) extracellular fluid (ECF) deficit, 20% (0.2) intracellular fluid (ICF) deficit
   b. Illness ≥3 days: 60% (0.6) ECF deficit, 40% (0.4) ICF deficit
3. Composition of intracellular and extracellular fluid (Table 11-4)
4. **Na^+ deficit:** The amount of Na^+ lost from the Na^+-containing ECF compartment during the dehydration period. Intracellular Na^+ is negligible as a proportion of total and can be disregarded (Table 11-4)

$$\textbf{Na}^+\textbf{ deficit (mEq)} = \textbf{fluid deficit (L)} \times \textbf{proportion from ECF} \times \textbf{Na}^+\textbf{ concentration (mEq/L) in ECF} \quad \text{(Equation F.1)}$$

A 25-kg (pre-illness weight) child who has been ill >3 days, is 9% dehydrated, with serum [Na^+] 137 mEq/L.

$$Fluid\ deficit = (90\ mL/kg)(25\ kg) = 2250\ mL$$

$$Na^+\ deficit = (2.25\ L)(0.6)(137\ mEq/L) = 184\ mEq$$

5. **K^+ deficit:** The amount of K^+ lost from the K^+-containing ICF compartment during the dehydration period. Extracellular K^+ is negligible as a proportion of total and can be disregarded (Table 11-4).

$$\textbf{K}^+\textbf{ deficit (mEq)} = \textbf{fluid deficit (L)} \times \textbf{proportion from ICF} \times \textbf{K}^+\textbf{ concentration (mEq/L) in ICF} \quad \text{(Equation F.2)}$$

A 25-kg (pre-illness weight) child who has been ill >3 days and is 9% dehydrated.

$$K^+\ deficit = (2.25\ L)(0.4)(150\ mEq/L) = 135\ mEq$$

C. Excess Electrolyte Deficits—Hyponatremic Dehydration

The amount of additional Na^+ or K^+ deficit calculated based on serum laboratory findings. Typically calculated in hyponatremic dehydration.

mEq required = [concentration desired (mEq/L) − concentration present (mEq/L)] × fD × weight (kg, pre-illness) (Equation F.3)

fD = distribution factor as fraction of body weight (L/kg): HCO_3^- (0.4 − 0.5); Cl^- (0.2 − 0.3); Na^+ (0.6 − 0.7)

A 25-kg (pre-illness weight) child who has been ill >3 days and is 9% dehydrated with serum [Na+] 117 mEq/L

$$\text{Excess } Na^+ \text{ deficit} = (135\ mEq/L - 117\ mEq/L)(0.6)(25\ kg) = 270\ mEq$$

D. Free Water Deficit (FWD)

The amount of additional free water loss in a patient with **hypernatremic dehydration.** Based on estimates that it requires 4 mL/kg to decrease serum Na^+ by 1 mEq/L. **NOTE:** If serum Na^+ is >170, estimate decreases to 3 mL/kg.

FWD (mL) = 4 mL/kg × weight (kg) × [concentration present (mEq/L) − concentration desired (mEq/L)] (Equation F.4)

A 25-kg (pre-illness weight) child who has been ill >3 days and is 9% dehydrated with serum [Na⁺] 160 mEq/L.

$$FWD = (4\ mL/kg)(25\ kg)(160\ mEq/L - 145\ mEq/L) = 1500\ mL$$

E. Solute Fluid Deficit (SFD):

The amount of additional fluid volume loss beyond free water loss in a patient with **hypernatremic dehydration.** The SFD is subsequently used to calculate Na^+ and K^+ deficits in these patients.

SFD = total fluid deficit − FWD (Equation F.5)

A 25-kg (pre-illness weight) child who has been ill >3 days and is 9% dehydrated with serum [Na] 160 mEq/L.

$$\text{Total fluid deficit} = (90\ mL/kg)(25\ kg) = 2250\ mL$$

$$SFD = 2250\ mL - 1500\ mL = 750\ mL$$

Solute Na⁺ deficit (mEq/L) = SFD (L) × proportion from ECF × Na⁺ concentration (mEq/L) in ECF (Equation F.6)

$$\text{Solute } Na^+ \text{ deficit} = (0.75\ L)(0.6)(145\ mEq/L) = 65\ mEq$$

Solute K⁺ deficit (mEq/L) = SFD (L) × proportion from ICF × K⁺ concentration (mEq/L) in ICF (Equation F.7)

$$\text{Solute } K^+ \text{ deficit} = (0.75\ L)(0.4)(150\ mEq/L) = 45\ mEq$$

F. Deficit Replacement Strategy:

1. **Phase I.** Rapid fluid resuscitation with isotonic fluid (normal saline [NS] or Lactated Ringers [LR])

11

a. Should be reserved for hemodynamic compromise (See Chapter 1). Generally, administration of isotonic fluid expands intravascular volume without causing significant fluid shifts, however isotonic fluids can be dangerous in patients with hyperosmolarity (i.e., diabetic ketoacidosis [DKA] with hyperglycemia)
b. Recognize that a bolus of 20 mL/kg represents only a 2% body weight replacement; a child calculated to be above 2% dehydrated will not be sufficiently repleted following an initial single bolus
c. Consider subtracting fluid and electrolyte given during resuscitation from the total deficits when calculating replacement of fluid and electrolytes

2. **Phase II.** Deficit repletion, maintenance and ongoing losses

Following initial stabilization, the remaining deficit is replaced over the next 24–48 hours. Replace one-half of the remaining deficit over the first 8 hours and the second-half over the following 16 hours (with the exception of free water deficit which is replaced over 48 hours) in addition to the previously calculated maintenance fluid rate. See Figure 11-2 for calculation of fluid and solute replacement in isonatremic, hyponatremic, and hypernatremic dehydration

a. **Hyponatremic dehydration:** Excess Na^+ loss (Na^+ <130 mEq/L). Rapid correction of serum Na^+ could result in central pontine myelinolysis and should be reserved for symptomatic patients. In asymptomatic patients, the rate of rise should not exceed 2–4 mEq/L q4h, or 10–20 mEq/L in 24 hours
b. **Isonatremic dehydration:** Proportional losses of Na and free water (Na^+ 130–149 mEq/L)
c. **Hypernatremic dehydration:** Excess free water loss (Na^+ >150 mEq/L). Avoid dropping the serum Na^+ by >15 mEq/L per 24 hours, to minimize the risk of cerebral edema
d. See Tables EC 11-A, 11-B, and 11-C (on Expert Consult) for sample calculations of fluid and solute replacement in isonatremic, hyponatremic, and hypernatremic dehydration

G. Calculation of Appropriate Fluids

After completing the previous calculations for the patient, then divide the desired amount of each solute by the total volume of fluid required in order to calculate the concentration of fluid and additives. Choose the appropriate corresponding fluid from Table 11-5 and add any other necessary solute components.

1. Parenteral fluid composition (Table 11-5)
2. Oral fluid composition (Table 11-5)

Oral rehydration therapy should be utilized in patients with mild to moderate dehydration without signs of shock, coma, acute abdomen, gastric distension, intractable vomiting, or excess stool losses

TABLE 11-5

COMPOSITION OF FREQUENTLY USED PARENTERAL AND ORAL REHYDRATION FLUIDS

	D% CHO (g/100 mL)	Protein* (g/100 mL)	Cal/L	Na^+ (mEq/L)	K^+ (mEq/L)	Cl^- (mEq/L)	HCO_3^-[†] (mEq/L)	Ca^{2+} (mEq/L)	mOsm/L
PARENTERAL FLUID									
D_5W	5	—	170	—	—	—	—	—	252
$D_{10}W$	10	—	340	—	—	—	—	—	505
NS (0.9% NaCl)	—	—	—	154	—	154	—	—	308
½ NS (0.45% NaCl)	—	—	—	77	—	77	—	—	154
D_5 ¼ NS (0.225% NaCl)	5	—	170	34	—	34	—	—	329
3% NaCl	—	—	—	513	—	513	—	—	1027
8.4% sodium bicarbonate (1 mEq/mL)	—	—	—	1000	—	—	1000	—	2000
Ringer's solution	0–10	—	0–340	147	4	155.5	—	≈4	—
Lactated Ringer's	0–10	—	0–340	130	4	109	28	3	273
Amino acid 8.5% (Travasol)	—	8.5	340	3	—	34	52	—	880
Plasmanate	—	5	200	110	2	50	29	—	—
Albumin 25% (salt poor)	—	25	1000	100–160	—	<120	—	—	300
Intralipid[‡]	2.25	—	1100	2.5	0.5	4.0	—	—	258–284
ORAL FLUID									
Pedialyte	2.5	—	—	45	20	35	30	—	250
WHO Solution	2	—	—	90	20	80	30	—	310
Rehydralyte	2.5	—	—	75	20	65	30	—	310

Continued

TABLE 11-5

COMPOSITION OF FREQUENTLY USED PARENTERAL AND ORAL REHYDRATION FLUIDS (Continued)

	D% CHO (g/100 mL)	Protein* (g/100 mL)	Cal/L	Na^+ (mEq/L)	K^+ (mEq/L)	Cl^- (mEq/L)	HCO_3^-† (mEq/L)	Ca^{2+} (mEq/L)	mOsm/L
APPROXIMATE ELECTROLYTE COMPOSITION OF COMMONLY CONSUMED FLUIDS (NOT RECOMMENDED FOR ORAL REHYDRATION THERAPY)**									
Apple juice	11.9	—	—	0.4	26	—	—	—	700
Coca-Cola	10.9	—	—	4.3	0.1	—	13.4	—	656
Gatorade	5.9	—	—	21	2.5	17	—	—	377
G2	4.7	—	—	20	3.2	—	—	—	
Ginger ale	9	—	—	3.5	0.1	—	3.6	—	565
Milk	4.9	—	—	22	36	28	30	—	260
Orange juice	10.4	—	—	0.2	49	—	50	—	654

*Protein or amino acid equivalent.

†Bicarbonate or equivalent (citrate, acetate, lactate).

‡Values are approximate; may vary from lot to lot. Also contains <1.2% egg-phosphatides.

**Values vary slightly depending on source.

CHO, Carbohydrate; HCO_3^-, bicarbonate; NS, normal saline.

a. Method: Give 5–10 mL of oral rehydration solution (ORS) every 5–10 minutes, gradually increasing volume
b. Deficit replacement:
Mild dehydration = 50 mL/kg over 4 hours
Moderate dehydration = 100 mL/kg over 4 hours
c. Maintenance: Infants should resume formula/breastmilk by mouth (PO) ad lib. Children should continue with regular diet
d. Ongoing losses: Regardless of the degree of dehydration, give additional 10 mL/kg of ORS for each additional diarrheal stool

IV. ONGOING LOSSES

Represent continued losses of fluid and solute following initial presentation, as in persistent vomiting, high fever with diuresis, or nasogastric suction. These losses can be measured directly and appropriately replaced based on known electrolyte concentrations (Table 11-6)

V. SERUM ELECTROLYTE DISTURBANCES

A. Sodium

1. **Hyponatremia:**
a. Etiologies, diagnostic studies, and management (Table 11-7)
b. Factitious etiologies
(1) Hyperlipidemia: Na^+ decreased by 0.002 × lipid (mg/dL)
(2) Hyperproteinemia: Na^+ decreased by 0.25 × [protein (g/dL) – 8]
(3) Hyperglycemia: Na^+ decreased 1.6 mEq/L for each 100-mg/dL rise in glucose
c. Clinical manifestations: Nausea, headache, lethargy, seizure, coma
2. **Hypernatremia:** Etiologies, diagnostic studies, and management (Table 11-8)

11

TABLE 11-6
ELECTROLYTE COMPOSITION OF VARIOUS BODY FLUIDS

Fluid	Na^+ (mEq/L)	K^+ (mEq/L)	Cl^- (mEq/L)	Replacement Fluid
Gastric	20–80	5–20	100–150	½ NS
Pancreatic	120–140	5–15	90–120	NS
Small bowel	100–140	5–15	90–130	NS
Bile	120–140	5–15	80–120	NS
Ileostomy	45–135	3–15	20–115	
Diarrhea	10–90	10–80	10–110	½ NS
Burns*	140	5	110	NS or LR
Sweat				
Normal	10–30	3–10	10–35	
Cystic fibrosis	50–130	5–25	50–110	

*3–5 g/dL of protein may be lost in fluid from burn wounds.
LR, Lactated Ringer's; NS, normal saline.
Modified from Kliegman RM, Behrman RE, HB Jenson, et al: Nelson Textbook of Pediatrics, 18th ed. Philadelphia, WB Saunders, 2007.

TABLE 11-7

HYPONATREMIA*

Decreased Weight		
Renal Losses	**Extrarenal Losses**	**Increased or Normal Weight**
Na^+-losing nephropathy	GI losses	Nephrotic syndrome
Diuretics	Skin losses	Congestive heart failure
Adrenal insufficiency	Third spacing	SIADH (see Chapter 10)
Cerebral salt-wasting syndrome	Cystic fibrosis	Acute/chronic renal failure
		Water intoxications
		Cirrhosis
		Excess salt-free infusions
LABORATORY DATA		
↑ Urine Na^+	↓ Urine Na^+	↓ Urine Na^{+}[†]
↑ Urine volume	↓ Urine volume	↓ Urine volume
↓ Specific gravity	↑ Specific gravity	↑ Specific gravity
↓ Urine osmolality	↑ Urine osmolality	↑ Urine osmolality
MANAGEMENT (in addition to treating underlying cause)		
Replace losses	Replace losses	Restrict fluids

*Hyperglycemia and hyperlipidemia cause spurious hyponatremia.

†Urine Na^+ may be appropriate for level of Na^+ intake in patients with SIADH and water intoxication.

GI, Gastrointestinal; SIADH, syndrome of inappropriate antidiuretic hormone secretion.

TABLE 11-8

HYPERNATREMIA

Decreased Weight		
Renal Losses	**Extrarenal Losses**	**Increased Weight**
Nephropathy	GI losses	Exogenous Na^+
Diuretic use	Skin losses	Mineralocorticoid excess
Diabetes insipidus	Respiratory*	Hyperaldosteronism
Postobstructive diuresis		
Diuretic phase of ATN		
LABORATORY DATA		
↑ Urine Na^+	↓ Urine Na^+	Relative ↓ urine Na^{+}[†]
↑ Urine volume	↓ Urine volume	Relative ↓ urine volume
↓ Specific gravity	↑ Specific gravity	Relative ↑ specific gravity
CLINICAL MANIFESTATIONS		
Predominantly neurologic symptoms: Lethargy, weakness, altered mental status, irritability, and seizures.[6,7] Additional symptoms may include muscle cramps, depressed deep tendon reflexes, and respiratory failure.		
MANAGEMENT		
Replace free water losses based on calculations in text and treat cause. Consider a natriuretic agent if there is increased weight.		

*This cause of hypernatremia is usually secondary to free water loss, so that the fractional excretion of sodium may be decreased or normal.

†Exogenous Na^+ administration will cause an increase in the fractional excretion of sodium.

ATN, Acute tubular necrosis; GI, gastrointestinal.

TABLE 11-9

CAUSES OF HYPOKALEMIA

Decreased Stores			
	Normal Blood Pressure		
Hypertension	**Renal**	**Extrarenal**	**Normal Stores**
Renovascular disease	RTA	Skin losses	Metabolic alkalosis
Excess renin	Fanconi syndrome	GI losses	Hyperinsulinemia
Excess mineralocorticoid	Bartter syndrome	High CHO diet	Leukemia
Cushing Syndrome	DKA	Enema abuse	β_2 Catecholamines
	Antibiotics	Laxative abuse	Familial hypokalemic periodic paralysis
	Diuretics	Anorexia nervosa	
	Amphotericin B	Malnutrition	Familial
LABORATORY DATA			
↑ Urine K^+	↑ Urine K^+	↓ Urine K^+	↑ Urine K^+

CHO, Carbohydrate; DKA, diabetic ketoacidosis; GI, gastrointestinal; RTA, renal tubular acidosis.

B. Potassium

1. **Hypokalemia:**
   a. Etiologies and laboratory data (Table 11-9)
   b. Clinical manifestations: Skeletal muscle weakness or paralysis, ileus, cardiac arrhythmias.[6,7] Electrocardiogram (ECG) changes include delayed depolarization, with flat or absent T waves and, in extreme cases, U waves
   c. Diagnostic studies:
      (1) Blood: Electrolytes, blood urea nitrogen/creatinine (BUN/Cr), creatine kinase (CK), glucose, renin, arterial blood gas (ABG)
      (2) Urine: Urinalysis, K^+, Na^+, Cl^-, osmolality, 17-ketosteroids
      (3) Other: ECG, consider evaluation for Cushing syndrome (Chapter 10)
   d. Management: Rapidity of treatment should depend on symptom severity. See Formulary for dosage information
      (1) Acute: Calculate deficit and replace with potassium acetate or potassium chloride. Enteral replacement is safer when feasible, with less risk for iatrogenic hyperkalemia. Follow serum K^+ closely
      (2) Chronic: Determine daily requirement and replace with potassium chloride or potassium gluconate
2. **Hyperkalemia:**
   a. Etiologies (Table 11-10)
   b. Clinical manifestations: Skeletal muscle weakness, paresthesias, and ECG changes. Typical ECG changes of hyperkalemia progress with increasing serum K+ values:
      (1) peaked T waves
      (2) loss of P waves with widening of QRS
      (3) ST-segment depression with further widening of QRS

11

TABLE 11-10

CAUSES OF HYPERKALEMIA

Increased Stores		
Increased Urine K^+	**Decreased Urine K^+**	**Normal stores**
Transfusion with aged blood	Renal failure	Tumor lysis syndrome
Exogenous K^+ (e.g., salt substitutes)	Hypoaldosteronism	Leukocytosis (>100 K/μL)
Spitzer syndrome	Aldosterone insensitivity	Thrombocytosis (>750 K/μL)
	↓ Insulin	Metabolic acidosis*
	K^+-sparing diuretics	Blood drawing (hemolyzed sample)
	Congenital adrenal hyperplasia	Type IV RTA
		Rhabdomyolysis/crush injury
		Malignant hyperthermia
		Theophylline intoxication

*For every 0.1-unit reduction in arterial pH, there is an approximately 0.2–0.4 mEq/L increase in plasma K^+.
RTA, Renal tubular acidosis.

(4) bradycardia, atrioventricular (AV) block, ventricular arrhythmias, torsades de pointes, and cardiac arrest

c. Management: Stop all IV infusions containing potassium; see algorithm in Figure 11-3

C. Calcium

1. **Hypocalcemia:**

a. Etiologies (Box 11-2)

b. Clinical manifestations: Tetany, neuromuscular irritability with weakness, paresthesias, fatigue, cramping, altered mental status, seizures, laryngospasm, cardiac arrhythmias[6,7]
   (1) ECG changes (prolonged QT interval)
   (2) Trousseau's sign (carpopedal spasm after arterial occlusion of an extremity for 3 minutes)
   (3) Chvostek sign (muscle twitching with percussion of facial nerve)

c. Diagnostic studies:
   (1) Blood: Total and ionized Ca^{2+}, phosphate, alkaline phosphatase, Mg^{2+}, total protein, BUN, creatinine, 25-OH vitamin D, parathyroid hormone (PTH)
      (a) Albumin: Δ of 1 g/dL changes total serum Ca^{2+} in the same direction by 0.8 mg/dL
      (b) pH: Acidosis increases ionized calcium
   (2) Urine: Ca^{2+}, phosphate, creatinine
   (3) Other: Chest x-ray (visualize thymus), ankle and wrist films (assess for rickets), ECG (QT interval)

d. Management: See Formulary for dosing information
   (1) Acute: Consider IV replacement (calcium gluconate, calcium gluceptate, or calcium chloride [cardiac arrest dose])

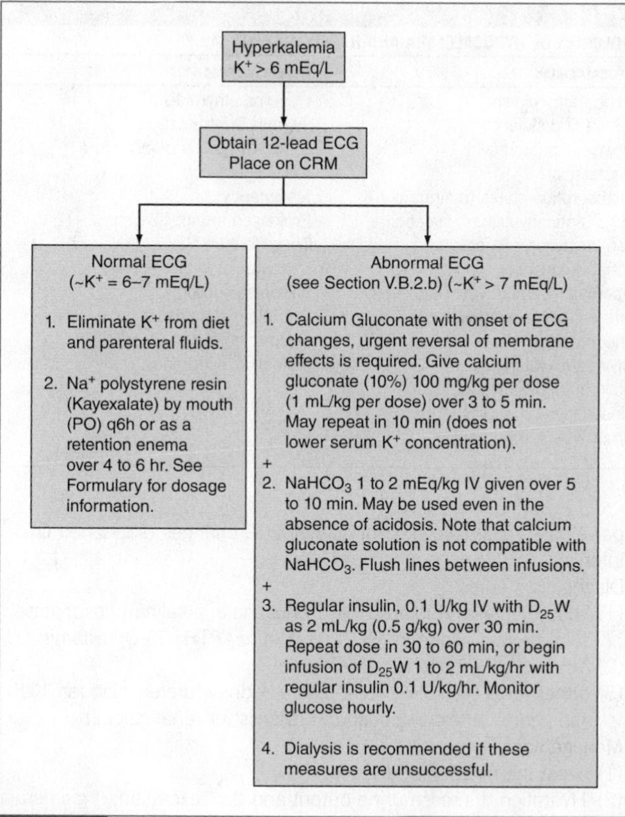

FIGURE 11-3
Algorithm for hyperkalemia.

(2) Chronic: Consider use of oral supplements of calcium carbonate, calcium gluconate, calcium glubionate, or calcium lactate

e. Special considerations:
   (1) Symptoms of hypocalcemia refractory to Ca^{2+} supplementation may be caused by hypomagnesemia
   (2) Significant hyperphosphatemia should be corrected before correction of hypocalcemia because renal calculi or soft tissue calcification may occur if total $[Ca^{2+}] \times [PO_4^{3-}] \geq 55$

2. **Hypercalcemia:**

a. Etiologies (see Box 11-2).

b. Clinical manifestations: Weakness, irritability, lethargy, seizures, coma, abdominal cramping, anorexia, nausea, vomiting, polyuria,

BOX 11-2

ETIOLOGIES OF HYPOCALCEMIA AND HYPERCALCEMIA

Hypocalcemia	**Hypercalcemia**
Hypoparathyroidism	Hyperparathyroidism
Vitamin D deficiency	Vitamin D intoxication
Hyperphosphatemia	Excessive exogenous calcium administration
Pancreatitis	Malignancy
Malabsorption states (malnutrition)	Prolonged immobilization
Drugs (anticonvulsants, cimetidine, aminoglycosides, calcium channel blockers)	Thiazide diuretics
Hypomagnesemia/hypermagnesemia	Subcutaneous fat necrosis
Maternal hyperparathyroidism (in neonates)	Williams syndrome
Ethylene glycol ingestion	Granulomatous disease (i.e., sarcoidosis)
Calcitriol (activated vitamin D) insufficiency	Hyperthyroidism
Tumor lysis syndrome	Milk-alkali syndrome

polydipsia, renal calculi, pancreatitis, ECG changes (shortened QT interval)

c. Diagnostic studies:
   (1) Blood: Total and ionized Ca^{2+}, phosphate, alkaline phosphatase, total protein, albumin, BUN, creatinine, PTH, 25-OH vitamin D
   (2) Urine: Ca^{2+}, phosphate, creatinine
   (3) Other: ECG (calculate QT interval), kidney, ureter, bladder (KUB) radiograph or renal ultrasound (assess for renal calculi)[8]

d. Management:
   (1) Treat the underlying disease
   (2) Hydration: Increase urine output and Ca^{2+} excretion. If glomerular filtration rate and blood pressure are stable, give NS with maintenance K^+ at two to three times maintenance rate until Ca^{2+} is normalized
   (3) Diuresis with furosemide
   (4) Consider hemodialysis for severe or refractory cases
   (5) Consider steroids in malignancy, granulomatous disease, and vitamin D toxicity to decrease vitamin D and Ca^{2+} absorption in consultation with appropriate specialists
   (6) Severe or persistently elevated Ca^{2+}. Consider calcitonin or bisphosphonate in consultation with endocrinologist

D. Magnesium

1. **Hypomagnesemia:**

a. Etiologies (Box 11-3)

b. Clinical manifestations: Anorexia, nausea, weakness, malaise, depression, nonspecific psychiatric symptoms, hyperreflexia,

BOX 11-3

ETIOLOGIES OF HYPOMAGNESEMIA AND HYPERMAGNESEMIA

HYPOMAGNESEMIA	HYPERMAGNESEMIA
Increased Urinary Losses Diuretic use, renal tubular acidosis, hypercalcemia, chronic adrenergic stimulants, chemotherapy **Increased Gastrointestinal Losses** Malabsorption syndromes, severe malnutrition, diarrhea, vomiting, short bowel syndromes, enteric fistulas **Endocrine Etiologies** Diabetes mellitus, parathyroid hormone disorders, hyperaldosterone states **Decreased Intake** Prolonged parenteral fluid therapy with Mg^{2+}-free solutions	**Renal Failure** **Excessive Administration** Status asthmaticus, eclampsia/pre-eclampsia, cathartics, enemas, phosphate binders

carpopedal spasm, clonus, tetany, ECG changes (atrial and ventricular ectopy; torsades de pointes)

c. Diagnostic studies:
 (1) Blood: Mg^{2+}, total and ionized Ca^{2+}
 (2) Other: Consider evaluation for renal/gastrointestinal losses or endocrine etiologies
d. Management: See Formulary for dosing and side effects
 (1) Acute: Magnesium sulfate
 (2) Chronic: Magnesium oxide or magnesium sulfate

2. **Hypermagnesemia:**
a. Etiologies (see Box 11-3)
b. Clinical manifestations: Depressed deep tendon reflexes, lethargy, confusion, respiratory failure (in extreme cases)

NOTE: Neonates born prematurely after tocolysis with magnesium sulfate are at high risk for respiratory sequelae, but serum magnesium levels tend to normalize within 72 hours

c. Diagnostic studies: Mg^{2+}, total and ionized Ca^{2+}, BUN, creatinine
d. Management:
 (1) Stop supplemental Mg^{2+}
 (2) Diuresis
 (3) Ca^{2+} supplements such as calcium chloride (cardiac arrest doses), or calcium gluconate (see Formulary for dosing)
 (4) Dialysis if life-threatening levels are present

11

BOX 11-4

ETIOLOGIES OF HYPOPHOSPHATEMIA AND HYPERPHOSPHATEMIA

Hypophosphatemia	Hyperphosphatemia
Starvation Protein-energy malnutrition Malabsorption syndromes Intracellular shifts associated with respiratory or metabolic alkalosis Treatment of diabetic ketoacidosis Corticosteroid administration Increased renal losses (i.e., renal tubular defects, diuretic use) Vitamin D-deficient and vitamin D-resistant rickets Very-low-birth weight infants when intake does not meet demand	Hypoparathyroidism (rarely in the absence of renal insufficiency) Excessive administration of phosphate (PO, IV, or enemas) Tumor lysis syndrome Reduction of glomerular filtration rate to <25% (may occur at smaller reductions in neonates)

E. Phosphate

1. **Hypophosphatemia:**
a. Etiologies (Box 11-4)
b. Clinical manifestations: Symptomatic only at very low levels (<1 mg/dL) with irritability, paresthesias, confusion, seizures, myocardial depression, apnea in very low birth weight infants, and coma
c. Diagnostic studies
(1) Blood: Phosphate, total and ionized Ca^{2+}, BUN, creatinine, Na, K, Mg^{2+}. Consider PTH and vitamin D
(2) Urine: Ca^{2+}, phosphate, creatinine, pH
d. Management:
(1) Insidious onset of symptoms: PO potassium phosphate or sodium phosphate (see Formulary for dosing)
(2) Acute onset of symptoms: IV potassium phosphate or sodium phosphate (see Formulary for dosing)

2. **Hyperphosphatemia**
a. Etiologies (see Box 11-4)
b. Clinical manifestations: Symptoms of resulting hypocalcemia (see previous)
c. Diagnostic studies:
(1) Blood: Phosphate, total and ionized Ca^{2+}, BUN, creatinine, Na, K, Mg^{2+}. Consider PTH, vitamin D, complete blood count, ABG
(2) Urine: Ca^{2+}, phosphate, creatinine, urinalysis

d. Management:
   (1) Restrict dietary phosphate
   (2) Phosphate binders (calcium carbonate, aluminum hydroxide; use with caution in renal failure). See Formulary for dosing
   (3) For cell lysis (with normal renal function), give an NS bolus and IV mannitol. See Chapter 22 for management of tumor lysis syndrome
   (4) If patient has poor renal function, consider dialysis

VI. ACID-BASE/OSMOLAR GAP DISTURBANCES

A. Definitions

1. **Serum osmolality:** Number of particles per liter. Can be calculated as follows:

$$2[Na^+] + \text{glucose (mg/dL)}/18 + \text{BUN (mg/dL)}/2.8$$

a. Normal range: 275 to 295 mOsm/L
b. Serum osmolar gap = calculated serum osmolality – laboratory measured osmolality.

NOTE: May be elevated in some anion gap acidosis, but a markedly elevated osmolar gap in the setting of an anion gap acidosis is highly suggestive of acute methanol or ethylene glycol intoxication.

2. **Anion gap (AG):** Represents anions other than bicarbonate and chloride required to balance the positive charge of Na^+. (K^+ is considered negligible in AG calculations.)

$$AG = Na^+ - (Cl^- + HCO_3^-) \text{ (Normal: 12 mEq/L} \pm \text{2 mEq/L)}$$

3. **Acidosis:** pH <7.35:
a. Respiratory acidosis: Pco_2 >45 mmHg
b. Metabolic acidosis: Arterial bicarbonate <22 mmol/L
4. **Alkalosis:** pH >7.45:
a. Respiratory alkalosis: Pco_2 <35 mmHg
b. Metabolic alkalosis: Arterial bicarbonate >26 mmol/L

B. Rules for Determining Primary Acid-Base Disorders[9]

1. **Determine the pH:** The body does not fully compensate for primary acid-base disorders; therefore, the primary disturbance will shift the pH away from 7.40. Examine the Pco_2 and HCO_3^- to determine whether the primary disturbance is a metabolic acidosis/alkalosis or respiratory acidosis/alkalosis
2. **Calculate the anion gap:** If the anion gap is >20 mmol/L, there is a primary metabolic acidosis regardless of pH or serum bicarbonate concentration. (The body does not generate a large anion gap to compensate for a primary disorder.)

C. Etiology of Acid-Base Disturbances (Fig. 11-4)

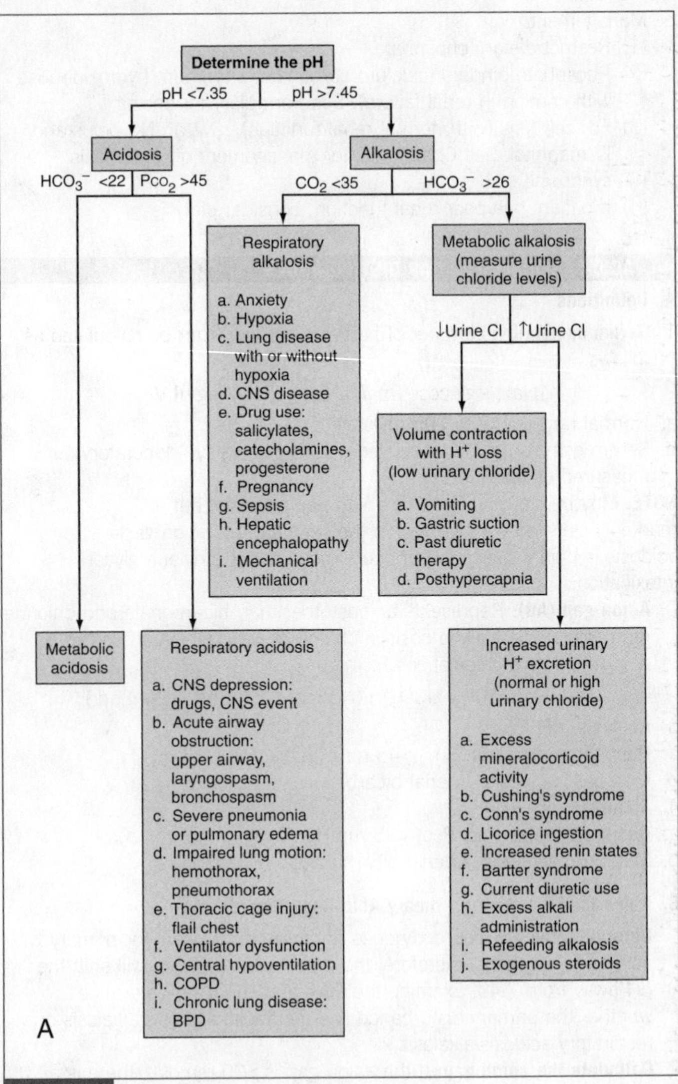

FIGURE 11-4

A and B, Etiology of acid-base disturbances.

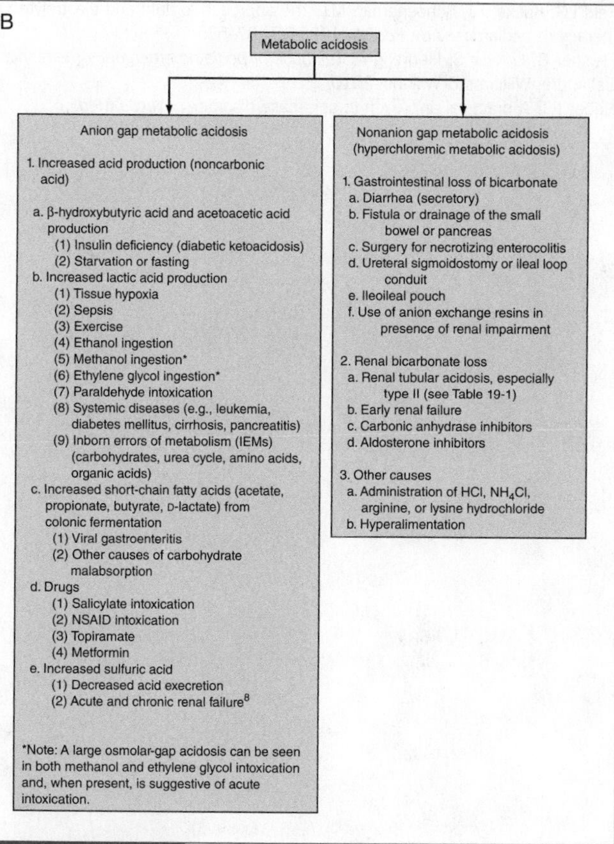

FIGURE 11-4 (Continued)

REFERENCES

1. Roberts KB. Fluids and electrolytes: parenteral fluid therapy. *Pediatr Rev.* 2001;22:380–387.
2. Segar WE. Parenteral fluid therapy. *Curr Probl Pediatr.* 1972;3:23–40.
3. Moritz ML, Ayus JC. Prevention of hospital-acquired hyponatremia: a case for using isotonic saline. *Pediatrics.* 2003;111:227–230.
4. Hellerstein S. Fluids and electrolytes: clinical aspects. *Pediatr Rev.* 1993;14(3):103–115.
5. Nichols DG, Yaster M, Lappe DG, et al. *Golden hour: the handbook of advanced pediatric life support.* St. Louis: Mosby; 1996.
6. Barkin R: *Pediatric emergency medicine*, 2nd ed. St. Louis: Mosby; 1997.

7. Feld LG, Kaskel FJ, Schoeneman MJ. The approach to fluid and electrolyte therapy in pediatrics. *Adv Pediatr.* 1988;35:497–535.
8. Fleisher G, Ludwig S, Henretig F. *Textbook of pediatric emergency medicine.* Baltimore: Williams & Wilkins; 2010.
9. Haber RJ. A practical approach to acid-base disorders. *West J Med.* 1991;155:146–151.

Chapter 12

Gastroenterology

Rebecca F. Rabin, MD, MHS

See additional content on Expert Consult

I. WEBSITES

American Academy of Pediatrics: www.aap.org

North American Society for Pediatric Gastroenterology, Hepatology, and Nutrition: www.naspghan.org

American College of Gastroenterology: www.acg.gi.org

II. GASTROINTESTINAL EMERGENCIES

A. Gastrointestinal Bleeding

1. **Presentation**—Blood loss from the gastrointestinal (GI) tract occurs in four ways: Hematemesis, hematochezia, melena, and occult bleeding
2. **Differential diagnosis of GI bleeding:** Table 12-1.
3. **Initial evaluation and management**

a. Assess airway, breathing, circulation, and hemodynamic stability

b. Perform physical examination, looking for evidence of bleeding

c. Verify bleeding with rectal examination, testing of stool or emesis for occult blood, and/or gastric lavage. If possible, differentiate between upper vs. lower GI bleeding and assess for ongoing bleeding

d. Obtain baseline laboratory tests. Complete blood count (CBC), prothrombin time/partial thromboplastin time (PT/PTT), blood type and cross-match, reticulocyte count, blood smear, blood urea nitrogen/ creatinine, electrolytes, and a panel to assess for disseminated intravascular coagulation (D-dimer, fibrinogen)

e. Begin initial fluid resuscitation with normal saline or lactated Ringer's solution. Consider transfusion if there is continued bleeding, symptomatic anemia, and/or a hematocrit level <20%. Initiate intravenous acid suppression therapy, preferably with a proton pump inhibitor (PPI)

f. Further evaluation and therapy based on assessment and site of bleeding:

(1) + Gastric lavage: Consider esophagogastroduodenoscopy (EGD). Treatment may include H2 blocker, PPI (use nasogastric tube with caution if esophageal varices are suspected)

(2) + Stool hemoccult: Abdominal film, upper GI study (± small bowel follow-through), air-contrast barium enema, colonoscopy, Meckel scan, tagged red cell scan. If signs/symptoms of infection exist,

TABLE 12-1

DIFFERENTIAL DIAGNOSIS OF GI BLEEDING

Age	Upper GI Tract	Lower GI Tract
Newborns (0–30 days)	Swallowed maternal blood Gastritis	Necrotizing enterocolitis Malrotation with midgut volvulus Anal fissure Hirschsprung disease
Infant (30 days–1 year)	Gastritis Esophagitis Peptic ulcer disease	Anal fissure Allergic proctocolitis Intussusception Meckel's diverticulum Lymphonodular hyperplasia Intestinal duplication Infectious colitis
Preschool (1–5 years)	Gastritis Esophagitis Peptic ulcer disease Esophageal varices Epistaxis	Juvenile polyps Lymphonodular hyperplasia Meckel's diverticulum Hemolytic-uremic syndrome Henoch-Schönlein purpura Infectious colitis Anal fissure
School age and adolescent	Esophageal varices Peptic ulcer disease Epistaxis Gastritis	Inflammatory bowel disease Infectious colitis Juvenile polyps Anal fissure Hemorrhoids

Modified from Pearl R: The approach to common abdominal diagnoses in infants and children. Part II. Pediatr Clin North Am 1998;45:1287–1326.

consider stool culture, stool ova & parasites, *Clostridium difficile* toxin

B. Acute Abdomen[1]

1. **Definition:** Severe abdominal pain (localized or generalized).[2] May require emergency surgical evaluation/intervention
2. **Differential diagnosis:**

a. GI source: Appendicitis, pancreatitis, intussusception, malrotation with volvulus, inflammatory bowel disease, gastritis, bowel obstruction, mesenteric lymphadenitis, irritable bowel syndrome, abscess, hepatitis, perforated ulcer, Meckel diverticulitis, cholecystitis, choledocholithiasis, constipation, gastroenteritis
b. Renal source: Urinary tract infection, pyelonephritis, nephrolithiasis
c. Gynecologic source: Ectopic pregnancy, ovarian cyst/torsion, pelvic inflammatory disease
d. Oncologic source: Wilms tumor, neuroblastoma, rhabdomyosarcoma, lymphoma
e. Other sources: Henoch-Schönlein purpura, pneumonia, sickle cell anemia, diabetic ketoacidosis, juvenile rheumatoid arthritis

3. **Evaluation:**
a. History: Course and characterization of pain, diarrhea, melena, hematochezia, fever, last oral intake, menstrual history, vaginal discharge/bleeding, urinary symptoms, and respiratory symptoms. Assess past GI history, travel history, and diet
b. Physical examination: Vital signs, toxicity, rashes, arthritis, jaundice. Abdominal tenderness on palpation, rebound/guarding, rigidity, masses, change in bowel sounds. Rectal exam with stool hemoccult test. Pelvic exam (discharge, masses, adnexal/cervical motion tenderness)
c. Radiologic studies: First obtain plain abdominal radiographs to assess for obstruction, constipation, free air, gallstones, and kidney stones. Consider chest radiograph to evaluate for pneumonia, abdominal/pelvic ultrasonography, abdominal spiral computed tomography with contrast (include rectal contrast for appendicitis evaluation), other contrast studies, and endoscopy
d. Laboratory studies: Electrolytes, chemistry panel, CBC, liver and kidney function tests, coagulation studies, blood type and screen/cross-match, urinalysis, amylase, lipase, gonorrhea/chlamydia cultures (or polymerase chain reaction probes), beta-human chorionic gonadotropin (β-hCG), erythrocyte sedimentation rate (ESR), C-reactive protein

4. **Management:**
a. Immediate: Patient should be placed on nothing by mouth (NPO) status. Begin rehydration. Consider nasogastric decompression, serial abdominal examinations, surgical/gynecologic/GI evaluation as indicated, pain control, and antibiotics as indicated
b. Definitive: Surgical or endoscopic exploration as warranted

III. CONDITIONS OF THE GI TRACT (ESOPHAGUS/STOMACH/BOWEL)

A. Vomiting

See Table 12-2 for evaluation of vomiting.

B. Diarrhea[3]

1. **Definition:** Usual stool output is 10 g/kg/day in children and 100 g/day in adults. Stool loss of >10 g/kg/day in infants and young children or >200 g/day in older children or adults is considered diarrhea.[4] Diarrhea is characterized by passage of loose or watery stools. The volume of fluid lost through stools can vary from 10 mL/kg/day (approximately normal) to >200 mL/kg/day. Acute diarrhea is >3 loose or watery stools per day. Chronic diarrhea is diarrhea lasting more than 14 days
2. **Diagnosis/evaluation:** History to assess acute vs. chronic, travel, recent antibiotic use, immune status. Consider laboratory evaluation: electrolytes, CBC, stool hemoccult, urine culture (young, febrile children), stool culture (febrile, ± bloody stools), stool tests for leukocytes, *C. difficile* toxin, ova and parasites, viral antigens (e.g., rotavirus)

TABLE 12-2

EVALUATION OF VOMITING

Type	
Typically bilious	**Etiology:** Obstruction, intussusception, malrotation ± volvulus, pancreatitis, intestinal dysmotility, peritoneal adhesions, incarcerated inguinal hernia, intestinal atresia/stenosis, superior mesenteric artery syndrome **Evaluation:** Review feeding and medication history; NG/OG tube for decompression if GI obstruction is suspected; if bilious and/or hematemesis, consider surgical consultation, BMP, CBC, ± UA, β-hCG, pancreatic enzymes, plain abdominal film with upright or cross-table lateral views to rule out obstruction, free air; abdominal ultrasound if pyloric stenosis is suspected; upper GI series to rule out pyloric stenosis, obstruction, anomalies and evaluate GI motility, neurologic evaluation and imaging
Typically nonbilious	**Etiology:** Overfeeding, GERD, milk-protein sensitivity, infection (GU, respiratory, GI), peptic disease, drugs, electrolyte imbalance, eating disorders, necrotizing enterocolitis, metabolic abnormality, pyloric stenosis, CNS lesion, esophageal/gastric atresia/stenosis, Hirschsprung disease, annular pancreas, web, pregnancy **Evaluation:** Consider feeding modifications ± medications if GERD is suspected; avoid antiemetics unless a specific benign etiology is identified
Either bilious or nonbilious	**Etiology:** Ileus, appendicitis

BMP, Basic metabolic panel; CBC, complete blood count; CNS, central nervous system; GERD, gastroesophageal reflux disease; GI, gastrointestinal; GU, genitourinary; hCG, human chorionic gonadotropin; NG/OG, nasogastric/orogastric; UA, urinalysis.

Modified from Saavedra J: Gastroenterology. In Seidel H et al (eds): Primary care of the newborn, 4th ed. St. Louis, Mosby, 2006; and Sondheimer JM: Vomiting. In Walker WA et al (eds): Pediatric gastrointestinal disease, 3rd ed. New York, BC Decker, 2000.

3. **Etiology:** Infectious or malabsorptive with osmotic or secretory mechanism
   a. Osmotic diarrhea: Water is drawn into intestinal lumen by maldigested nutrients (e.g., celiac or pancreatic disease, lactose) or other osmotic compounds. Stool volume depends on diet and decreases with fasting (stool osmolar gap ≥100 mOsm/kg)
   b. Secretory diarrhea: Water accompanies secreted or unabsorbed electrolytes into the intestinal lumen (e.g., excessive secretion of chloride ions caused by cholera toxin). Stool volume is increased and does not vary with diet (stool osmolar gap <100 mOsm/kg)
   c. Stool osmolar gap = Stool Osm − (2 × (stool [Na]mEq/L + stool [K] mEq/L)). Stool Osm is infrequently measured: standard value is 290 mOsm/kg[5]
4. **Management**
   a. Oral rehydration therapy (ORT): Mainstay of initial management regardless of etiology. Parenteral hydration is indicated in severe dehydration, hemodynamic instability, or failure of ORT. See Chapter

11 for oral rehydration solutions and for calculation of deficit and maintenance fluid requirements

b. Diet: Continue breastfeeding. Restart regular diet once patient is rehydrated, unless found to be the source of the diarrhea (e.g., gluten in Celiac Disease (CD), lactose in lactose intolerance)

c. Other: Nonspecific antidiarrheal agents (e.g., adsorbents such as kaolin-pectin), antimotility agents (e.g., loperamide), antisecretory drugs, and toxin binders (e.g., cholestyramine) have limited data regarding efficacy. If infectious, antimicrobial therapy may be indicated. If malabsorptive (e.g., celiac disease, inflammatory bowel disease), therapy should be tailored to disease process (e.g., gluten-free diet, steroids)

d. Probiotics: Evidence supporting the use of probiotics (live microorganisms in fermented foods that promote optimal health by establishing an improved balance in intestinal microflora) is limited but efficacy has been demonstrated in the following circumstances: antibiotic-associated diarrhea, mild to moderate acute diarrhea, *C. difficile* diarrhea (severe recurrent disease only), and prevention of atopic dermatitis. Probiotics are not regulated by the Food and Drug Administration; thus, there is no oversight of quality control (including potency)[6]

C. Constipation and Encopresis[7]

Normal stooling patterns by age: Infants 0–3 months: 2–3 bowel movements (BMs)/day, 6–12 months: 1.8/day, 1–3 years: 1.4/day, >3 years: 1/day

1. Definitions:

a. **Constipation:** Delay or difficulty in defecation for 2 or more weeks. Functional causes of constipation are most common. (See Table EC 12-A on Expert Consult for differential diagnosis)

b. **Encopresis:** Leakage of stool around impaction occurring in chronic constipation with loss of sensation in a distended rectal vault

2. **Diagnosis/evaluation:**

a. History: Timing of first meconium stool, family's definition of constipation, duration of condition and age of onset, toilet training experience, frequency/consistency/size of stools, pain or bleeding with defecation, presence of abdominal pain, soiling of underwear, stool withholding behavior, change in appetite, abdominal distension, anorexia, nausea, vomiting, weight loss, or poor weight gain, allergies, dietary history, medications, developmental history, psychosocial history, peer interactions, possibility of abuse, toilet habits at school, family history (constipation, thyroid disorders, cystic fibrosis)

b. Physical Exam: External perineum and perianal exam, digital anorectal exam (perianal sensation, anal tone, rectal size, presence of anal wink, amount/consistency/location of stool within the rectum). Stool occult blood test for all infants with constipation, any child with abdominal pain, failure to thrive, intermittent diarrhea, or family history of colon cancer or colonic polyps. Fecal impaction may be diagnosed with physical exam (hard mass within abdomen), digital exam (dilated rectal vault filled with stool), and/or abdominal radiography

3. **Treatment of functional constipation:**
a. Disimpaction (2–5 days)
   (1) Oral/nasogastric approach: Polyethylene glycol electrolyte solutions are effective for initial disimpaction. May also use magnesium hydroxide, magnesium citrate, lactulose, sorbitol, senna, or bisacodyl laxatives (avoid magnesium-containing products in infants due to potential toxicity, beware of overdose in children)
   (2) Rectal approach: Saline or mineral oil enemas. Avoid soap suds, tap water, and magnesium enemas due to potential toxicity. Avoid enemas in infants, may use glycerin suppositories. Avoid phosphate-containing products due to risk of acute phosphate nephropathy (reported with use of oral sodium phosphate products)
b. Maintenance therapy (usually 3–12 months): Goal is to prevent recurrence
   (1) Dietary changes: Increase intake of fluids and absorbable and nonabsorbable carbohydrates to soften stools. A balanced diet that includes whole grains, fruits, and vegetables is recommended. Data are too weak to support a definitive recommendation for fiber supplementation in the treatment of constipation in children
   (2) Behavioral modifications: Regular toilet habits, positive reinforcement, and proper toilet positioning (stable seating, feet firmly planted, knees and hips at 90-degree angle). Referral to mental health for help with motivational or behavioral concerns
   (3) Medications: Polyethylene glycol (osmotic laxatives), lactulose, magnesium hydroxide, or sorbitol is recommended. Avoid prolonged use of stimulant laxatives. Discontinue therapy gradually only after return of regular bowel movements with good evacuation

4. **Special considerations in infants <1 year of age:** Increased intake of fluids, particularly of juices containing sorbitol, such as prune, pear, and apple juices, is recommended within the context of a healthy diet. Barley malt extract, corn syrup, lactulose, or sorbitol can be used as stool softeners. Glycerin suppositories may be useful. Avoid mineral oil, stimulant laxatives, and phosphate enemas

D. Inflammatory Bowel Disease (IBD)[8,9]

1. Classification/types:
a. **Crohn's disease:** Transmural inflammatory process affecting any segment of the GI tract from mouth to anus in discontinuous fashion. Clinical presentation is variable and frequently non-specific. Abdominal pain in majority of cases, minority of children with "classical triad" of abdominal pain, weight loss, and diarrhea. Other symptoms include

lethargy, anorexia, fever, nausea, vomiting, growth retardation, malnutrition, delayed puberty, psychiatric symptoms, arthropathy, and erythema nodosum[9]

b. **Ulcerative colitis (UC):** Chronic relapsing inflammatory disease of the colon and rectum. Symptoms (present for at least 2 weeks) include gross or occult rectal bleeding, diarrhea, abdominal pain with or around time of defecation. Exclusion of enteric pathogens (e.g., *Salmonella, Shigella, Yersinia, Campylobacter, Escherichia coli* 0157:H7, *C. difficile*) is necessary.[10] Weight loss, anorexia, lethargy are less common than in Crohn's disease

2. **Evaluation:**
   a. Complete history and physical exam including family history, exposure to infectious agents or antibiotic treatment, assessment of hydration and nutritional status, signs of peritoneal inflammation, signs of systemic chronic disease. Stomatitis, perianal skin tags, fissures, fistulas are suggestive of Crohn's Disease. Presence of fever, orthostasis, tachycardia, abdominal tenderness, distension, or masses suggests moderate to severe disease and need for hospitalization
   b. Laboratory assessment: CBC, ESR, CRP, serum urea and creatinine, serum albumin, liver function tests. IBD is associated with decreased hemoglobin and albumin, rise in platelet count, ESR, CRP (although children with UC may have normal hemoglobin, platelets, and ESR). Anti-neutrophil cytoplasmic antibodies (ANCA) may be elevated in UC. Diagnostic endoscopy is typically used to make diagnosis
3. **Management:**
   a. First-line therapy: Corticosteroids, 5-aminosalicylates, antibiotics
   b. Second-line: Immunosuppression includes azathioprine, methotrexate Crohn's, cyclosporine, tacrolimus and anti-tumor necrosis factor (TNF) monoclonal antibodies
   c. Surgical intervention is indicated only after medical management has failed in both Crohn's and UC. In Crohn's, surgery is indicated for localized disease (strictures), abscess, or disease refractory to medical management

E. Gastrointestinal Reflux Disease[11]

1. **Definitions:** Gastroesophageal reflux (GER) is passage of gastric contents into the esophagus, and gastroesophageal reflux disease (GERD) is defined as symptoms or complications of GER
2. **Evaluation/diagnosis:**
   a. History and physical examination: Usually sufficient to reliably diagnose GER, identify complications, and initiate management
   b. Esophageal pH monitoring: Valid and reliable method of measuring acid reflux
   c. Esophageal impedance monitoring: Combine with esophageal pH monitoring to detect both acid as well as nonacid reflux with greater sensitivity than pH monitoring alone[12]

d. Upper GI series: Neither sensitive nor specific for GER but may be useful for the evaluation of anatomic abnormalities

3. **Management:**

a. Diet: Milk protein sensitivity is one cause of unexplained crying and vomiting in formula-fed infants; evidence supports 2–4 week trial of extensively hydrolyzed protein formula. Milk-thickening agents decrease visible regurgitation but do not decrease GER. No evidence to support routine elimination of specific foods to treat GERD in older children

b. Lifestyle: Prone or left-side sleeping position, elevation of head of bed may improve GER symptoms in adolescents. Infants up to 12 months should continue to sleep supine—sudden infant death syndrome (SIDS) risk far outweighs benefit of prone or lateral sleeping in GERD. (May consider prone positioning for infants while awake and monitored). Obesity and large meal volume are associated with increased GER in adults

c. Acid-suppressant therapy: Both PPIs and histamine-2 receptor antagonists (H_2RAs) are effective in relieving symptoms and promoting mucosal healing. PPIs are superior to H_2RAs. The smallest effective dose should be utilized for acid suppression

d. Prokinetic therapy: Potential side effects of each currently available prokinetic agent outweigh the potential benefits. There is insufficient evidence to support the routine use of metoclopramide, erythromycin, bethanechol, or domperidone for GERD

F. Eosinophilic Esophagitis (EE)[13]

1. **Definition:** Symptoms of esophageal dysfunction with ≥15 eosinophils/high-power field (hpf) on peripheral blood smear, and absence of pathologic GERD as evidenced by lack of responsiveness to high-dose PPI or normal pH monitoring of distal esophagus
2. **Presentation:** Dysphagia, food impaction, chest pain, food refusal or intolerance, GER symptoms, emesis, abdominal pain, failure to thrive. High rate of atopy in children with EE
3. **Diagnosis:** Endoscopy and esophageal biopsy, allergic evaluation for other atopic conditions
4. **Management:** Dietary therapy (elemental formula or removal of specific foods identified by skin prick or atopy patch testing), PPI therapy (as co-treatment), may consider systemic steroids for emergencies (e.g., dysphagia leading to dehydration, weight loss), topical steroids for less severe symptoms (6–8 week course of Fluticasone or Budesonide metered dose inhaler (MDI) administered orally *without* spacer). There are limited data on the use of steroids in EE—recommendation based on expert opinion and current literature
5. **Differential diagnosis** of esophageal eosinophilia: GERD, EE, eosinophilic gastroenteritis, Crohn's disease, connective tissue disease, hypereosinophilic syndrome, infection, drug hypersensitivity

G. Celiac Disease[14]

1. **Definition:** An immune-mediated enteropathy caused by a permanent sensitivity to gluten of the GI tract in genetically susceptible individuals. Increased occurrence in children with type 1 diabetes mellitus, autoimmune thyroiditis, Down syndrome, Turner syndrome, Williams syndrome, selective IgA deficiency, and in first-degree relatives of those with celiac disease
2. **Presentation:** Diarrhea, vomiting, abdominal pain, constipation, abdominal distension, failure to thrive. Non-GI symptoms include dermatitis herpetiformis, dental enamel hypoplasia of permanent teeth, osteoporosis, short stature, delayed puberty, and iron-deficient anemia resistant to oral iron
3. **Diagnosis:** Measure IgA antibody to human recombinant tissue transglutaminase (TTG) and serum IgA (high prevalence of IgA deficiency in celiac disease). Endomysial antibody is subject to interpretation error and adds cost. If there is known selective IgA deficiency and symptoms are suggestive of celiac disease, testing with TTG IgG is recommended. Confirmation requires an intestinal biopsy in all cases with findings of villous atrophy as a characteristic histopathologic feature
4. **Management:** Lifetime gluten-free diet

IV. CONDITIONS OF THE LIVER

A. Liver Function Studies: (See Table 12-3)

1. **Synthetic function:** Albumin, prealbumin, PT, activated PTT, cholesterol. Elevated NH_3 is evidence of decreased ability to detoxify ammonia
2. **Liver cell injury:** Elevation of aspartate aminotransferase, alanine aminotransferase, lactate dehydrogenase
3. **Cholestasis:** Increased bilirubin, urobilinogen, γ-glutamyltransferase, alkaline phosphatase, 5′-nucleotidase, serum bile acids

B. Acute Liver Failure (ALF)[15]

1. **Definition:** Biochemical evidence of liver injury with no history of known chronic liver disease, presence of coagulopathy not corrected by vitamin K administration, and international normalized ratio (INR) >1.5 if the patient has encephalopathy or >2.0 if the patient does not have encephalopathy. Causes of ALF vary in reversibility (with treatment or withdrawal of offending agent) and in age of presentation
2. **Etiologies:** (incidence varies by age):
   a. Infection: Herpes virus, hepatitis A, hepatitis B, adenovirus, cytomegalovirus, Epstein-Barr virus, enterovirus, indeterminate
   b. Vascular: Budd-Chiari syndrome, portal vein thrombosis, veno-occlusive disease, ischemic hepatitis
   c. Immune dysregulation: Natural killer (NK) cell dysfunction (hemophagocytic lymphohistiocytosis), autoimmune

TABLE 12-3

EVALUATION OF LIVER FUNCTION TESTS

Enzyme	Source	Increased	Decreased	Comments
AST/ALT	Liver Heart Skeletal muscle Pancreas RBCs Kidney	Hepatocellular injury Rhabdomyolysis Muscular dystrophy Hemolysis Liver cancer	Vitamin B_6 deficiency Uremia	ALT more specific than AST for liver AST >ALT in hemolysis AST/ALT >2 in 90% of alcohol disorders in adults
Alkaline phosphatase	Liver Osteoblasts Small intestine Kidney Placenta	Hepatocellular injury Bone growth, disease, trauma Pregnancy Familial	Low phosphate Wilson disease Zinc deficiency Hypothyroidism Pernicious anemia	Highest in cholestatic conditions Must be differentiated from bone source
GGT	Bile ducts Renal tubules Pancreas Small intestine Brain	Cholestasis Newborn period Induced by drugs	Estrogen therapy Artificially low in hyperbilirubinemia	Not found in bone Increased in 90% primary liver disease Biliary obstruction Intrahepatic cholestasis Induced by alcohol Specific for hepatobiliary disease in nonpregnant patient

5′-NT	Liver cell membrane Intestine Brain Heart Pancreas	Cholestasis		Specific for hepatobiliary disease in nonpregnant patient
NH_3	Bowel Bacteria Protein metabolism	Hepatic disease secondary to urea cycle dysfunction Hemodialysis Valproic acid therapy Urea cycle enzyme deficiency Organic acidemia and carnitine deficiency		Converted to urea in liver

AST/ALT, Aspartate aminotransferase/alanine aminotransterase; 5′-NT, 5′-nucleotidase; GGT, γ-glutamyl transpeptidase; RBCs, red blood cells.

d. Inherited/metabolic: Wilson's disease, mitochondrial, tyrosinemia, galactosemia, fatty acid oxidation defect, iron storage disease
e. Drugs/toxins: Acetaminophen, anticonvulsants
f. Other: Unknown, cancer/leukemia

3. **Presentation:** Prodrome of malaise, nausea, emesis, and anorexia; jaundice and encephalopathy (hyperammonemia, cerebral edema) may be delayed by hours to weeks; glucose instability with hypoglycemia, coagulopathy
4. **Evaluation:**

a. Clinical: Neurologic status, signs of chronic liver disease, other chronic disease
b. Laboratory: Electrolytes, BUN, creatinine, blood glucose, calcium, magnesium, phosphorous, blood gas, CBC with peripheral smear, reticulocyte count, liver function/production (albumin, aspartate aminotransferase [AST], alanine aminotransferase [ALT], alkaline phosphatase), INR, PT, PTT, ammonia, factors V, VII (depleted first in ALF), VIII, fibrinogen. Urine toxicology screen, serum acetaminophen level. Consider viral studies

NOTE: See Table 12-4 for interpretation of serologic markers of Hepatitis B.

c. Imaging: Abdominal ultrasound with Doppler flows, head computed tomography (CT) scan to exclude hemorrhage/edema, chest radiograph
d. Studies to explore causation: Viral studies, immune function, metabolic studies, tissue biopsies

C. Hyperbilirubinemia[16,17]

Bilirubin is the product of hemoglobin metabolism. There are two forms: direct (conjugated) and indirect (unconjugated). Hyperbilirubinemia is usually the result of increased hemoglobin load, reduced hepatic uptake, reduced hepatic conjugation, or decreased excretion. Direct hyperbilirubinemia is defined as direct bilirubin >20% of total or direct

TABLE 12-4

INTERPRETATION OF THE SEROLOGIC MARKERS OF HEPATITIS B IN COMMON SITUATIONS

Serologic Marker				
HB*s*Ag	**Total HB*c*Ab**	**IgM HB*c*Ab**	**HB*s*Ab**	**Interpretation**
–	–	–	–	No prior infection, not immune
–	–	–	+	Immune after hepatitis B vaccination (if concentration ≥10 mIU/mL or passive immunization from HBIG administration)
–	+	–	+	Immune after recovery from HBV infection
+	+	+	–	Acute HBV infection
+	+	–	–	Chronic HBV infection

HB*s*Ag, Hepatitis B surface antigen; HB*c*Ab, antibody to hepatitis B core antigen; HB*s*Ab, antibody to hepatitis B surface antigen; HBIG, hepatitis B immune globulin.

From Davis AR, Rosenthal P: Hepatitis B in children. Pediatr Rev 2008;29;111–120.

TABLE 12-5

DIFFERENTIAL DIAGNOSIS OF HYPERBILIRUBINEMIA

INDIRECT HYPERBILIRUBINEMIA	
Transient neonatal jaundice	Breast milk jaundice, physiologic jaundice Polycythemia, reabsorption of extravascular blood
Hemolytic disorders	Autoimmune disease, blood group incompatibility, hemoglobinopathies, microangiopathies, red cell enzyme deficiencies, red cell membrane disorders
Enterohepatic recirculation	Cystic fibrosis, Hirschsprung disease, ileal atresia, pyloric stenosis
Disorders of bilirubin metabolism	Acidosis, Crigler-Najjar syndrome, Gilbert syndrome, hypothyroidism, hypoxia
Miscellaneous	Dehydration, drugs, hypoalbuminemia, sepsis
DIRECT HYPERBILIRUBINEMIA	
Biliary obstruction	Biliary atresia, choledochal cyst, fibrosing pancreatitis, gallstones or biliary sludge, inspissated bile syndrome, neoplasm, primary sclerosing cholangitis
Infection	Cholangitis, cytomegalovirus, Epstein-Barr virus, herpes simplex virus, histoplasmosis, HIV, leptospirosis, liver abscess, sepsis, syphilis, toxocariasis, toxoplasmosis, tuberculosis, urinary tract infection, varicella-zoster virus, viral hepatitis
Genetic/metabolic disorders	α1-Antitrypsin deficiency, Alagille syndrome, Caroli disease, cystic fibrosis, Dubin-Johnson syndrome, galactokinase deficiency, galactosemia, glycogen storage disease, hereditary fructose intolerance, hypothyroidism, Niemann-Pick disease, rotor syndrome, tyrosinemia, Wilson disease
Chromosomal abnormalities	Trisomy 18, trisomy 21, Turner syndrome
Drugs	Acetaminophen, aspirin, erythromycin, ethanol, iron, isoniazid, methotrexate, oxacillin, rifampin, steroids, sulfonamides, tetracycline, vitamin A
Miscellaneous	Neonatal hepatitis syndrome, parenteral alimentation, Reye syndrome

bilirubin >2 mg/dL. See Table 12-5 for differential diagnosis of hyperbilirubinemia. Refer to Chapter 18 for evaluation and treatment of neonatal hyperbilirubinemia

V. PANCREATITIS[18,19]

Inflammatory disease of the pancreas; falls into two major categories, acute and chronic.

A. Acute Pancreatitis

1. **Presentation:** Sudden onset of abdominal pain associated with rise of pancreatic digestive enzymes in serum or urine with or without radiographic changes in the pancreas. It is a reversible process. Most common etiologies: trauma, multisystem disease, drugs, infections, idiopathic, and congenital anomalies. See Table 12-6 for conditions associated with acute pancreatitis

TABLE 12-6

CONDITIONS ASSOCIATED WITH ACUTE PANCREATITIS

SYSTEMIC DISEASES	
Infections	Coxsackie, CMV, cryptosporidium, EBV, hepatitis, influenza A or B, leptospirosis, mycoplasma, mumps, rubella, typhoid fever, varicella
Inflammatory and vasculitic disorders	Collagen vascular diseases, hemolytic uremic syndrome, Henoch-Schönlein purpura, inflammatory bowel disease, Kawasaki disease
Sepsis/peritonitis/shock	
Transplantation	
IDIOPATHIC (UP TO 25% OF CASES)	
MECHANICAL STRUCTURAL	
Trauma	Blunt trauma, child abuse, ERCP
Perforation	
Anomalies	Annular pancreas, choledochal cyst, pancreatic divisum, stenosis, other
Obstruction	Parasites, stones, tumors
METABOLIC AND TOXIC FACTORS	
Cystic fibrosis	
Diabetes mellitus	
Drugs/toxins	Salicylates, cytotoxic drugs (L-asparaginase), corticosteroids, chlorothiazides, furosemide, oral contraceptives (estrogen), tetracyclines, sulfonamides, valproic acid, azathioprine, 6-mercaptopurine
Hypercalcemia	
Hyperlipidemia	
Hypothermia	
Malnutrition	
Organic acidemia	
Renal disease	

CMV, Cytomegalovirus; EBV, Epstein-Barr virus; ERCP, endoscopic retrograde cholangiopancreatography.
Modified from Robertson MA: Pancreatitis. In Walker WA et al (eds): Pediatric gastrointestinal disease, 3rd ed. New York, BC Decker, 2000, pp. 1321–1344; and Werlin SL: Pancreatitis. In McMillan, JA et al (eds.), Oski's pediatrics. Philadelphia, PA, Lippincott Williams & Wilkins, 2006, pp. 2010–2012.

2. **Diagnosis/evaluation:**
   a. Clinical signs/symptoms: Abdominal pain (sudden or gradual, most commonly epigastric), anorexia, nausea, vomiting, tachycardia, fever, hypotension, guarding/rebound tenderness/decreased bowel sounds, sonographic or radiologic evidence of pancreatic inflammation. Gray-Turner and Cullen's sign are rare in children
   b. Laboratory findings:
      (1) Elevated lipase and amylase: ≥3 times above normal limit (but no correlation with disease severity); lipase is more sensitive and specific for acute pancreatitis but normalizes more slowly so it may be preferable to follow amylase after establishment of diagnosis[8]
      (2) Additional findings: Leukocytosis, hyperglycemia, glucosuria, hypocalcemia, hyperbilirubinemia

TABLE 12-7

PROPOSED ETIOLOGIES OF CHRONIC PANCREATITIS IN CHILDHOOD

Calcific	Cystic fibrosis, hereditary pancreatitis (e.g. PRSS1 and SPINK1 mutations), hypercalcemia, hyperlipidemia, idiopathic, juvenile tropical pancreatitis
Obstructive (noncalcific)	Congenital anomalies, idiopathic fibrosing pancreatitis, renal disease, sclerosing cholangitis, sphincter of Oddi dysfunction, trauma

3. **Management:**
a. Pancreatic rest: Nasogastric decompression, analgesia, IV fluid hydration, and oral intake restriction. Enteral feeding via naso-jejunal tube may be used for nutrition. (In adults, enteral nutrition is associated with lower incidence of infection, surgical intervention and shorter hospital stay. There is minimal pediatric evidence available)
b. Antibiotics are reserved for only the most severe cases

B. Chronic Pancreatitis

1. **Definition:** A progressive, inflammatory process causing irreversible changes in the architecture and function of the pancreas. Common complications include chronic abdominal pain, loss of exocrine function (malabsorption, malnutrition) and/or endocrine function (diabetes mellitus). Two major morphologic forms: Calcific and obstructive. See Table 12-7
2. **Management:** (for acute exacerbations) Same as management of acute pancreatitis; See Section V.A.3

C. Miscellaneous Tests (for Descriptions, See Expert Consult, Chapter 12)

12

REFERENCES

1. Moir CR. Abdominal pain in infants and children. *Mayo Clin Proc.* 1996;71(10):984–989.
2. World Health Organization. ICD-10, 2007, World Health Organization, Available online. http://www.who.int/classifications/icd/en/.
3. King CK, Glass R, Bresee JS, et al. Managing acute gastroenteritis among children: oral rehydration, maintenance, and nutritional therapy. *MMWR Recomm Rep.* 2003;52:1–16.
4. Vanderhoof JA. Chronic diarrhea. *Pediatr Rev.* 1998;19(12):418.
5. Thomas PD, Forbes A, Green J, et al. Guidelines for the investigation of chronic diarrhoea, 2nd ed. *Gut.* 2003;52(suppl 5):v1–15.
6. Clinical Practice Guideline. Clinical efficacy of probiotics: review of the evidence with focus on children. NASPGHAN Nutrition Committee Report. *J Pediatr Gastroenterol Nutr.* 2006:43:550–557.
7. Constipation Guideline Committee of the North American Society for Pediatric Gastroenterology, Hepatology and Nutrition. Evaluation and treatment of constipation in infants and children: recommendations of the North American Society for Pediatric Gastroenterology, Hepatology and Nutrition. *J Pediatr Gastroenterol Nutr.* 2006;43:e1–e13.

8. McMillan JA, Feigin RD, DeAngelis CD. *Oski's pediatrics*, 4th ed. 2006, pp. 1926, 1954, Philadelphia, PA: Lippincott Williams & Wilkins; 2011.
9. Beattie RM, Croft NM, Fell JM, et al. Inflammatory bowel disease. *Arch Dis Child.* 2006;91:426–432.
10. Clinical Report: Differentiating ulcerative colitis from Crohn disease in children and young adults: report of a working group of the North American Society for Pediatric Gastroenterology, Hepatology, and Nutrition and the Crohn's and Colitis Foundation of America. *J Pediatr Gastroenterol Nutr.* 2007;44:653–674.
11. Vandenplas Y, Rudolph CD, Di Lorenzo C, et al. Pediatric gastroesophageal reflux clinical practice guidelines: joint recommendations of the North American Society of Pediatric Gastroenterology, Hepatology, and Nutrition and the European Society of Pediatric Gastroenterology, Hepatology, and Nutrition. *J Pediatr Gastroenterol Nutr.* 2009;49:498–547.
12. Hirano I, Richter JE; Practice Parameters Committee of the American College of Gastroenterology. ACG practice guidelines: esophageal reflux testing. *Am J Gastroenterol.* 2007;102:668–685.
13. Furuta GT, Liacouras CA, Collins MH, et al. Eosinophilic esophagitis in children and adults: a systematic review and consensus recommendations for diagnosis and treatment. *Gastroenterology.* 2007;133:1342–1363.
14. Hill ID, Dirks MH, Liptak GS, et al. Guideline for the diagnosis and treatment of celiac disease in children: recommendations of the North American Society for Pediatric Gastroenterology, Hepatology and Nutrition. *J Pediatr Gastroenterol Nutr.* 2005;40:1–19.
15. Bucuvalas J, Yazigi N, Squires RH Jr. Acute liver failure in children. *Clin Liver Dis.* 2006;10:149–168.
16. Harb R, Thomas DW. Conjugated hyperbilirubinemia: screening and treatment in older infants and children. *Pediatr Rev.* 2007;28:83–91.
17. Moyer V, Freese DK, Whitington PF, et al. Guideline for the evaluation of cholestatic jaundice in infants: Recommendations of the North American Society for Pediatric Gastroenterology, Hepatology and Nutrition. *J Pediatr Gastroenterol Nutr.* 2004;39:115–128.
18. Lowe ME. Pancreatitis in childhood. *Curr Gastroenterol Rep.* 2004;6:240–246.
19. Nydegger A, Couper RTL. Childhood pancreatitis. *J Gastroenterol Hepatol.* 2006;21(3):499–509.

Chapter 13

Genetics

Emily Spengler, MD

When evaluating a child for a genetic disorder, the three-generation pedigree is a valuable tool. Specifically ask about family history of neonatal or childhood deaths, mental retardation, developmental delay, birth defects, seizure disorders, known genetic disorders, ethnicity, consanguinity, infertility, miscarriages, and stillbirths.

I. WEBSITES

National Newborn Screening and Genetics Resource Center: genes-r-us.uthscsa.edu/resources.htm

Online Mendelian Inheritance in Man (OMIM): www.ncbi.nlm.nih.gov/omim (includes a search engine for identifying genetic diseases based on clinical phenotype, gene, and OMIM number)

Gene Tests: www.genetests.org (includes information on genetic diagnostic tests, genetic clinics in the United States and laboratories that perform genetic testing)

American College of Medical Genetics: www.acmg.net/resources/policies/ACT/condition-analyte-links.htm (includes ACT sheets and algorithm to help guide physicians after a positive newborn metabolic screen)

National Organization for Rare Disorders: www.rarediseases.org

II. NEWBORN METABOLIC SCREEN[1–3]

All states screen for phenylketonuria (PKU), hypothyroidism, congenital adrenal hyperplasia (CAH), galactosemia, and hemoglobinopathies among others. (For a list of screening tests and number of states that use each test, see website: http://genes-r-us.uthscsa.edu/resources.htm)

A. Timing

Screen all infants before hospital discharge.

1. Normal-term infants: Screen as close as possible to hospital discharge, and preferably after at least 24 hours of normal protein and lactose feeding. Formula-fed infants may not have a diagnostic abnormality before 36 hours of age. Breast-fed infants may not have a diagnostic abnormality before 48 to 72 hours of age
2. Premature or ill infants: Perform initial screen at or near 7 days of age regardless of feeding status and repeat screen at 28 days of age or at hospital discharge, whichever comes first
3. All infants should be screened by 7 days of age. If first screen is before 24 hours of age, send repeat by 14 days of age. Most

13

geneticists recommend rescreening all infants at 2–4 weeks of age. Some tests are affected by blood transfusions and require a repeat test at least 90 days after transfusion

B. Results

1. Positive results: Immediate follow-up and confirmatory testing, including more specific testing for the particular disease. If a genetic disease is suspected, a consult with a geneticist is recommended. See ACT sheets for more information (www.acmg.net/resources/policies/ACT/condition-analyte-links.htm)
2. Negative results: A normal newborn screen does not imply that there are no genetic abnormalities

III. MANAGEMENT OF GENETIC DISEASES WITH ACUTE PRESENTATION: INBORN ERRORS OF METABOLISM[1,2,4,5]

Inborn errors of metabolism (IEMs) may present any time from the neonatal period to adulthood. Although often thought of as rare, when considered collectively, these disorders represent significant treatable causes of morbidity and mortality.

A. Presentations

1. Neonatal onset: Often presents with anorexia, lethargy, vomiting, seizures, and/or shock. Symptoms often develop at 24–72 hours of age. One in five sick full-term neonates with no risk factors for infection will have metabolic disease
2. Late onset (>28 days old): Some IEMs characteristically present late, whereas other IEMs may present late if the defect is partial
   a. Typical findings: Failure to thrive, developmental delay, vomiting, respiratory distress, psychomotor abnormalities, and changes in mental status, including confusion, lethargy, irritability, aggressive behavior, hallucinations, seizures, and coma
   b. Symptoms are usually brought on by intercurrent illness, prolonged fast, dietary indiscretion, or any process causing increased catabolism

B. Evaluation of Suspected Metabolic Disease

1. For laboratory tests recommended to detect IEMs, see Box 13-1. For sample collection requirements, see Table 13-1
2. If the initial evaluation is suspicious for metabolic disease, obtain further testing as listed in Box 13-1 and consult a geneticist. Early diagnosis and appropriate therapy are essential for preventing irreversible brain damage and death

C. Differential Diagnosis

1. Differential diagnosis of hyperammonemia (Fig. 13-1)
2. Differential diagnosis of hypoglycemia (see Section III.E and Fig. 13-2)
3. Positive urine reducing substances (Box 13-2)

BOX 13-1

LABORATORY TESTS FOR INBORN ERRORS OF METABOLISM

Initial Tests

Complete blood count with differential
Serum electrolytes (calculate anion gap)
Blood glucose
Aspartate aminotransferase (AST)
Alanine aminotransferase (ALT)
Total and direct bilirubin
Blood gas
Plasma ammonium
Plasma lactate
Urine dipstick: pH, ketones, glucose, protein, bilirubin
Urine-reducing substances (Clinitest tablet [Ames Co.], identifies all reducing substances in urine; see Box 13-2)
Acylcarnitine profile

Further Testing If Workup Is Suspicious

Plasma amino acids
Quantitative plasma carnitine
Urine organic acids
Carbohydrate deficient glycoprotein testing
If lactate level is elevated, serum pyruvate and repeat lactate level.

BOX 13-2

DISORDERS ASSOCIATED WITH A POSITIVE URINE-REDUCING SUBSTANCES TEST

Galactose: Galactosemia, galactokinase deficiency, severe liver disease
Fructose: Hereditary fructose intolerance, essential fructosuria
Glucose: Diabetes mellitus, renal tubular defects
p-Hydroxyphenylpyruvic acid: Tyrosinemia
Xylose: Pentosuria

13

D. General Acute Management of IEM

1. Stop dietary sources of protein
2. Start intravenous (IV) fluids: 10% dextrose (D_{10}) at 1.5 to 2 times maintenance dose delivers 10 to 15 mg/kg/min of glucose to stop catabolism. Add Na^+/K^+ based on the degree of dehydration and electrolyte levels. In severe dehydration, give a normal saline bolus in addition to D_{10} at 1.5 to 2 times the maintenance dose
3. Provide HCO^-_3 replacement for severe acidosis (pH <7.1) only
4. In cases of hyperammonemia, the following drugs may be used only in consultation with a geneticist (**overdoses may be lethal**): Sodium benzoate 250 mg/kg (5.5 g/m^2) IV; sodium phenylacetate 250 mg/kg (5.5 g/m^2) IV; and arginine HCl (10% solution) 6 mL/kg (12 g/m^2) IV. Give these doses as a bolus over 90 minutes. Repeat the same doses

TABLE 13-1

SAMPLE COLLECTION

Specimen	Volume (mL)	Tube*	Handling
Plasma ammonia	1–3	Green or purple top (check with your lab)	On ice; immediate transport to laboratory; levels rise rapidly on standing
Plasma amino acids†	1–3	Green top	On ice; if must store, spin down, separate plasma, and freeze
Plasma carnitine	1–3	Green top	On ice
Acylcarnitine profile	Saturate newborn screen filter paper with blood		Dry and mail to reference laboratory
Lactate	3	Gray top	On ice
Karyotype	3	Green top	Room temperature
Very-long-chain fatty acids	3	Purple top	Room temperature
White blood cells for enzymes/DNA	3	Purple top (For enzymes check with your lab)	Room temperature
Urine organic acids	5–10	—	Deliver immediately or freeze
Urine amino acids	5–10	—	Deliver immediately or freeze
Carbohydrate deficient glycoprotein testing	1–3	Red top	Frozen and sent on dry ice
Skin biopsy		Tissue culture medium or patient's plasma	Refrigerate; do not freeze

*Additives in tubes: purple, K3EDTA; green, lithium heparin; gray, potassium oxalate and sodium fluoride.

†Obtain after a 3-hour fast.

over 24 hours as a maintenance dose. Ondansetron may be used to decrease nausea and vomiting associated with these drugs. (Benzoate and phenylacetate are substrates for alternate pathways of nitrogen excretion; arginine supplementation allows continued operation of the urea cycle in defects in which the block is proximal to arginine.)

5. If the patient's condition is unresponsive to this management, hemodialysis should be initiated. Hemodialysis is often required in neonates because of their inherently catabolic state. Exchange transfusion should not be used

E. Hypoglycemia

1. Definitions: Glucose concentration <40 mg/dL typically is considered hypoglycemia. Potential causes include endocrine disorders or IEMs, including defects in gluconeogenesis, glycogen breakdown (glycogen storage diseases), and fatty acid oxidation, or toxic impairment of gluconeogenesis (organic acidemias). See Fig. 13-2 for evaluation.[5–7]

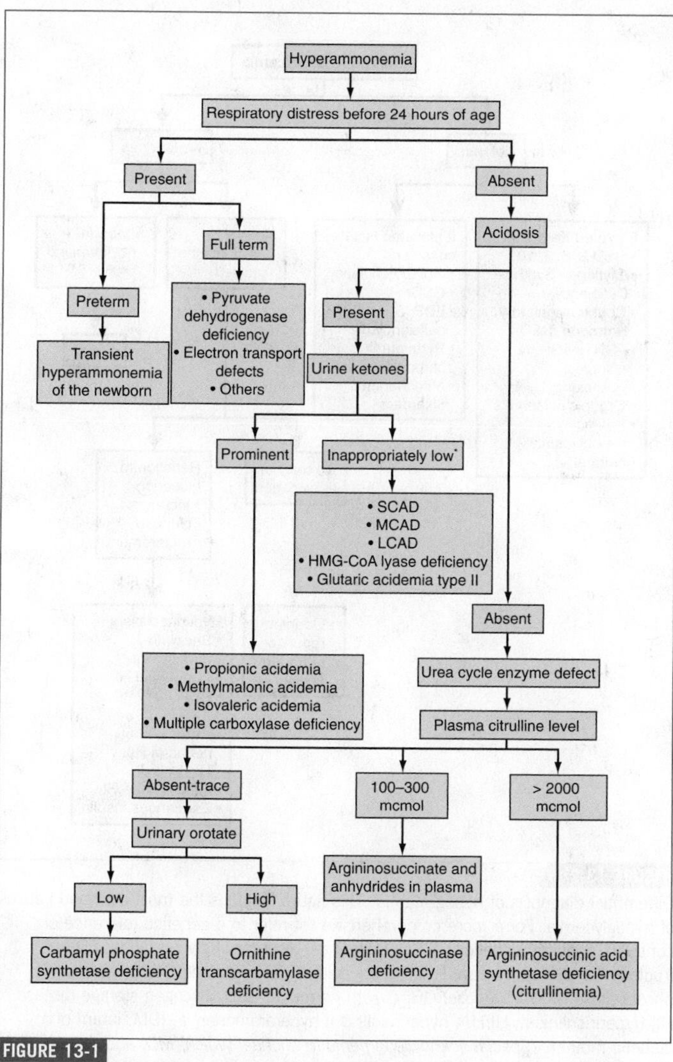

FIGURE 13-1

Differential diagnosis of hyperammonemia. *Indicates inappropriately low urinary ketones in setting of symptomatic hypoglycemia. HMG-CoA, Hydroxymethylglutaryl-CoA; LCAD, long-chain acyl-CoA dehydrogenase; MCAD, medium-chain acyl-CoA dehydrogenase; SCAD, short-chain acyl-CoA dehydrogenase.

13

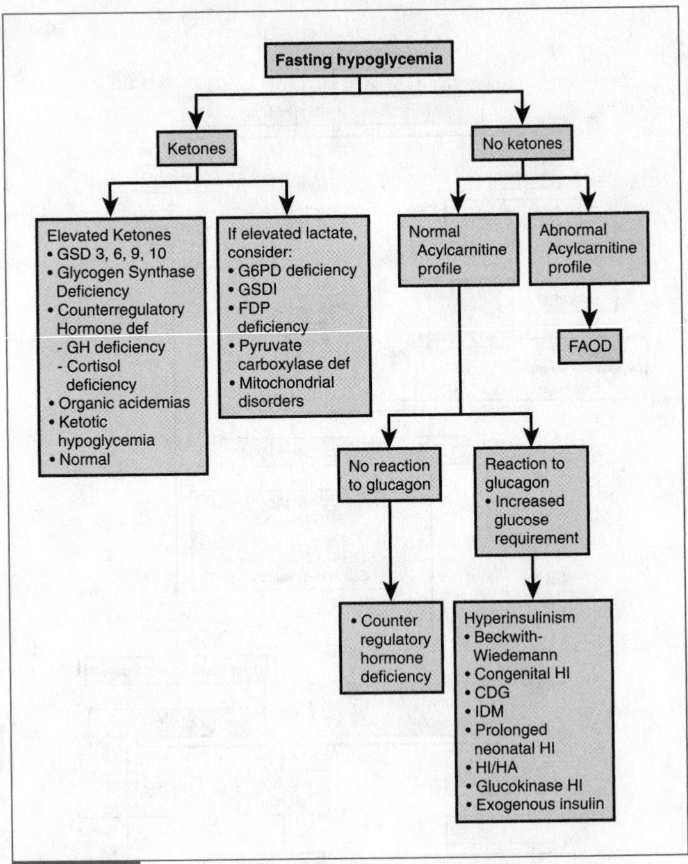

FIGURE 13-2[5–7]

Differential diagnosis of hypoglycemia. This figure includes the most common causes of hypoglycemia. For a more comprehensive list refer to a genetics reference or consult a pediatric geneticist. CDG, Congenital disorder of glycosylation; FDP, fructose 1,6-diphosphatase; FAOD, fatty acid oxidation defect; G6PD, glucose-6-phosphatase dehydrogenase; GH, growth hormone; GSD, glycogen storage disease; HI, hyperinsulinism; HI/HA, hyperinsulinism hyperammonemia; IDM, infant of a diabetic mother. *(Special acknowledgments to Michael Walsh, MD, and Ada Hamosh, MD, MPH, for lending their expertise to the design of this figure.)*

2. History questions: What is the patient's age? What is the relationship between the hypoglycemia and caloric intake? (Does it occur postprandially or after prolonged fasting, or is it constant?) Is the patient septic? Does the patient have hepatomegaly?
3. Laboratory evaluation (ideally obtained in setting of fasting hypoglycemia): Glucose, complete metabolic panel, including liver function tests (LFTs), insulin, c-peptide, cortisol, growth hormone, β-Hydroxybutyrate, free fatty acids, lactate, ammonia, acylcarnitine profile, total and free carnitine, urinary ketones and organic acids, glucose response to glucagon. Consult a geneticist to help interpret laboratory results and guide the workup

IV. DYSMORPHOLOGY

The suspicion for many syndromes and chromosomal anomalies is often raised by major or minor anomalies noted on physical examination. The most common anomalies and commonly used diagnostic tests are listed here. More complete information can be found in reference works by Hall and colleagues[8] and Jones.[9] In addition to well-known syndromes, many rare genetic disorders are listed in reference works.[9,10]

A. Physical Examination

1. Major anomalies: Defined as those that have medical, surgical, or cosmetic consequences; include structural brain abnormalities, mental retardation, failure to thrive, cleft lip and palate, congenital heart defects, abnormal secondary sexual development, urogenital defects, skeletal dysplasias, and severe limb anomalies
2. Minor anomalies: Defined as not having any serious medical, surgical, or severe cosmetic consequence; include abnormally shaped ears or eyes, inverted nipples, birth marks, abnormal structures of the hands and feet, and abnormal skin folds or creases. For complete list, see Jones text[9]

B. Genetic Diagnostic Tests

1. Karyotype: Detects abnormal numbers of chromosomes and deletions, duplications, translocations, and inversions that are large enough to be seen by light microscopy. Indicated in every patient with two major malformations or one major and two minor malformations
2. Fluorescence in situ hybridization (FISH): Hybridization of a fluorescently tagged DNA probe to chromosomes allows detection of submicroscopic deletions and duplications. FISH assays are commonly available for the following syndromes: Williams (7q11), Prader-Willi and Angelman (15q11), Miller-Dieker (17p13.3), Smith-Magenis (17p11.2), velocardiofacial and DiGeorge (22q11). For a complete, updated online list of genetic diagnostic tests, see www.genetests.org
3. Deoxyribonucleic acid (DNA) analysis: Many monogenic disorders now have DNA tests available. Contact your laboratory or www.genetests.org for a list of those available

4. BAC-CGH arrays: In addition to conventional chromosomal analysis, the suggestion has been made to send the patient's DNA for BAC-CGH arrays. This novel technology has been developed to detect chromosomal copy number changes on a genome wide and/or high-resolution scale, allowing the detection of very small chromosomal abnormalities. Unable to detect balanced translocations

C. Structural Diagnostic Tests

1. Brain magnetic resonance imaging (MRI)
2. Ophthalmologic examination: Optic atrophy, coloboma, cataracts, retinal abnormalities, lens subluxation, corneal abnormalities
3. Echocardiogram
4. Abdominal ultrasound: Polysplenia or asplenia, absent or horseshoe kidney, ureteral or bladder defects, abdominal situs inversus
5. Skeletal survey: Abnormalities of bone length or structure

V. COMMON SYNDROMES

For more information on common syndromes and other chromosomal abnormalities and syndromes, see Jones text.[9]

A. Trisomy 21[9,11]

1. Prevalence: 1 in 660 newborns
2. Features: Presence of 6 of the following 10 cardinal features in the neonate is highly suggestive of the diagnosis: hypotonia, poor Moro reflex, hyperflexibility, excess skin on back of the neck, flat facies, slanted palpebral fissures, anomalous auricles, pelvic dysplasia, dysplasia of the mid-phalanx of the fifth finger, and a single transverse palmar (simian) crease
3. Associated findings: Mental retardation (100%), hearing loss (66%), eye disease (60%), serous otitis media (60%–80%), cardiac defects (40%), thyroid disease (15%), gastrointestinal atresias (12%), atlantoaxial instability (12%–20%), and leukemia (1%)
4. Testing: Karyotype for diagnosis, echocardiogram, thyroid function tests (newborn, 6 months, then annually), yearly complete blood count, ophthalmologic and audiologic evaluation; radiographs of the atlanto-occipital junction by age 3 to 5 years
5. Health care: Information about ongoing health care can be found at www.ndss.org

B. Turner Syndrome—45,X[9,12]

1. Prevalence: 1 in 2,500 live born females
2. Features: Short female with broad chest, wide-spaced nipples, webbed neck, congenital lymphedema, pubertal delay, and left-sided heart defects
3. Associated findings: Gonadal dysgenesis (90%), renal anomalies (60%), cardiac defects (10%–30%), hearing loss (50%)

4. Testing: Karyotype for diagnosis. Baseline echocardiogram, electrocardiogram (ECG), renal ultrasound, pediatric ophthalmologic evaluation; blood pressure, hearing, growth parameters, and scoliosis screen with each examination; lipids, glucose, thyroid and liver function tests annually and echocardiogram every 5 to 10 years or as clinically indicated. Celiac screening every 2–5 years

C. Fragile X Syndrome[9,13]

1. Prevalence: 1 in 1,250 to 2,500 males and 1 in 1,600 to 5,000 females
2. Features: Boys: Mild to profound mental retardation, cluttered speech, autism (60%), macrocephaly, large ears, prognathism, postpubertal macro-orchidism, and tall stature. Phenotype most prominent in boys; girls may have only learning disabilities
3. Testing: X-linked inheritance; caused by an expansion of a CGG nucleotide repeat in the *FMR1* gene. The size of the repeat correlates with disease severity. Diagnosis is established by DNA analysis

D. Marfan Syndrome[1,9,14,15]

1. Prevalence: 1 in 10,000 individuals
2. Features: Major and minor diagnostic criteria involving the skeletal, ocular, cardiovascular, and pulmonary systems, and skin or integument. Features include, but are not limited to tall stature, low upper-to-lower segment ratio, arachnodactyly, joint laxity, scoliosis, pectus excavatum or carinatum, lens subluxation, glaucoma, retinal detachment, dilation with or without dissecting aneurysm of ascending aorta, mitral valve prolapse, lumbosacral dural ectasia by computed tomography or magnetic resonance imaging (MRI) scans, and inguinal and/or femoral hernias. For a complete list of criteria for diagnosis in both an index case and a family member, see Scriver and associates[5] and De Paepe and colleagues[14]
3. Testing: Genetic evaluation; routine ophthalmologic evaluation, including slit-lamp examination; and echocardiogram

E. 22q11 Syndrome[1,9]

1. Prevalence: 1 in 4,000 to 5,000 live births
2. Synonyms: DiGeorge syndrome, velocardiofacial syndrome (VCFS), Shprintzen syndrome, conotruncal anomaly face syndrome (CTAF)
3. Features: Congenital heart defects (85%), palatal abnormalities, immune deficiency (defective T-cell function), hypocalcemia (parathyroid involvement), and characteristic facial features
4. Testing: FISH analysis for 22q11.2 deletion and routine cytogenetics to evaluate for chromosomal rearrangement (<1% cases). Measure serum calcium, absolute lymphocyte count, B- and T-cell subsets if lymphopenic, renal ultrasound for structural abnormalities, chest x-ray

for thoracic vertebral anomalies, baseline cardiac evaluation, including echocardiogram. Parents should also be tested to determine whether they are carriers of the deletion

F. Prader-Willi Syndrome[9,16]

1. Prevalence: 1 in 15,000 newborns
2. Features: Hypotonia, poor feeding, and failure to thrive during infancy; short stature, mental retardation, obesity (onset 6 months to 6 years), bizarre and binge-type eating habits, small hands and feet, small genital structures, and characteristic facial features
3. Testing: High-resolution karyotype followed by methylation studies specific for Prader-Willi syndrome
4. Management: Follow growth parameters, routine ophthalmologic evaluation, dietary supervision, and physical activity plans

G. Trisomy 18[1]

1. Prevalence: 1 in 3,000 to 7,000 live births
2. Features: Clenched hand (index finger overlapping third and fifth fingers overlapping fourth), intrauterine growth retardation, decreased fetal activity, low-arch dermal ridge pattern, inguinal or umbilical hernia, cardiac defects, prominent occiput, low-set ears, micrognathia, and rocker-bottom feet
3. Testing: Karyotype with FISH analysis
4. Natural history: Apnea, severe failure to thrive; 50% die by 1 week, 90% by 1 year

H. Trisomy 13[1]

1. Prevalence: 1 in 5,000 to 12,000 live births
2. Features: Holoprosencephaly, polydactyly, scalp skin defects, seizures, deafness, microcephaly, sloping forehead, cleft lip, cleft palate, retinal anomalies, microphthalmia, abnormal ears, single umbilical artery, inguinal hernia, omphalocele, cardiac defects, and urinary tract malformations
3. Testing: Karyotype with FISH analysis
4. Natural history: 44% die within 1 month; 70% die by 1 year

I. Klinefelter Syndrome—47,XXY[9]

1. Prevalence: 1 in 500 males
2. Features: Mean full scale IQ 85–90, behavior problems, low upper to lower body ratio, small testes, inadequate testosterone production, infertility, gynecomastia, and increased risk of extragonadal germ cell tumors
3. Testing: Karyotype
4. Management: Testosterone replacement therapy

VI. DEGENERATIVE DISORDERS

NOTE: Many are progressive neurodegenerative disorders; an exhaustive list is beyond the scope of this chapter.

A. Lysosomal Disorders (e.g., the Mucopolysaccharidoses)

Include: Neurodegeneration with systemic storage resulting from lysosomal enzyme defects (e.g., Hurler, Hunter, Scheie, Sanfilippo, and Sly syndromes).

1. Presentation: Hepatosplenomegaly, corneal clouding (except Hunter syndrome), dysostosis multiplex, coarse features, neurologic deterioration
2. Laboratory findings: Inclusion bodies on peripheral blood smear, positive urine mucopolysaccharide spot; characteristic findings on eye examination and skeletal survey
3. Definitive diagnosis: Assay of skin fibroblasts for specific lysosomal hydrolases
4. Therapy: Enzyme replacement therapy; bone marrow transplantation may provide some enzyme activity, but cannot reverse brain damage

B. Peroxisomal Disorders

Include: Refsum syndrome, X-linked adrenoleukodystrophy, Zellweger syndrome, and others.

1. Presentation: Seizures, loss of milestones, loss of white matter on MRI scans. Progressive neurodegeneration and eventually death
2. Laboratory findings: Elevated very-long-chain fatty acids, pipecolic acid, phytanic acid, and plasmalogens
3. Definitive diagnosis: Enzyme assays in cultured skin fibroblasts and microscopy of peroxisomes
4. Therapy: Treat adrenal insufficiency if present; provide vitamin K. Research protocols include dietary lipid therapy, bone marrow transplantation, and immunosuppression

C. Mitochondrial Disorders[17,18]

Include: Leigh syndrome, MELAS (Mitochondrial encephalopathy, lactic acidosis, and stroke), Leber hereditary optic neuropathy, and several less specific syndromes associated with increased fatigue and decreased endurance.

Respiratory chain genes are encoded in both nuclear and mitochondrial DNA. Defects in mitochondrial DNA are more likely to result in disease because they are only maternally inherited. Nuclear defects present more often in childhood.

1. Presentation: Can affect any system, most commonly the nervous system. Increased suspicion if: short stature, sensorineural hearing loss, axonal neuropathy, progressive external ophthalmoplegia, diabetes mellitus, hypertrophic cardiomyopathy, or renal tubular acidosis
2. Findings: Elevated lactate and pyruvate levels in blood, urine or cerebrospinal fluid (CSF), abnormal pattern of plasma amino acids, brain imaging with stroke like lesions, lesions in basal ganglia and cerebellum, muscle biopsies with red ragged fibers or cytochrome oxidase negative fibers, decreased respiratory chain function as

determined by polarographic and spectrophotometric assays of muscle tissue
3. Definitive diagnosis: Mitochondrial DNA gene testing low yield in children (only 10% are due to mitochondrial DNA defects whereas 90% are nuclear defects). Clinical diagnosis is based on presentation and laboratory findings. However, often a specific molecular diagnosis cannot be determined
4. Therapy: Symptomatic, directed at treating energy deficiencies and prevention of complications. Supplementary therapy may include Coenzyme Q10, carnitine, creatine, and arginine (for MELAS)

VII. GENETIC CONSULTATION

A. Indications for Referral

1. Known or suspected hereditary disorder
2. Major physical anomalies, unusual body proportions, short stature, dysmorphic features
3. Major organ malformation
4. Developmental delay or mental retardation; learning disabilities in females who have brothers with mental retardation
5. Complete or partial blindness or hearing loss
6. Deterioration of motor or speech abilities in a previously thriving child
7. Maternal exposure to drugs, alcohol, or radiation during pregnancy
8. Strong family history of cancer
9. Failure to thrive if routine evaluation is unrevealing

B. Indications for Prenatal Counseling[1]

1. Genetic disorder or birth defect in one partner
2. Known carrier of a genetic disorder
3. Parent with balanced translocation
4. Previous child with known or suspected genetic disorder
5. Maternal age >35 years
6. Abnormal results on triple screening
7. Family history of known or suspected chromosomal anomaly
8. Multiple early miscarriages, stillbirths, or neonatal deaths
9. Member of an ethnic group known to have a high incidence of a specific genetic disorder
10. Exposures to teratogen or infections

C. Indications for Karyotype

1. Two major *or* one major and two minor malformations (include small for gestational age and mental retardation as major)
2. Features of a specific chromosomal syndrome
3. At risk for familial chromosomal aberration
4. Ambiguous genitalia
5. More than two spontaneous abortions or infertility (karyotype both partners)
6. Girls with short stature

REFERENCES

1. McMillan JA, Feigin RD, DeAngelis C, et al. *Oski's pediatrics: principles and practice.* 4th ed. Philadelphia: Lippincott Williams & Wilkins; 2006.
2. Seidel HM, Rosenstein B, Pathak A, et al. *Primary care of the newborn.* 4th ed. St. Louis: Mosby; 2006.
3. Kaye CI and Committee on Genetics. Introduction to the newborn screening fact sheets. *Pediatrics.* 2006;118:1304–1312.
4. Fernandes J, Saudubray J, van den Berghe G, et al. *Inborn metabolic diseases.* 4th ed. Berlin: Springer-Verlag; 2006.
5. Scriver CR, Sly WS, Childs B, et al. *The metabolic and molecular bases of inherited disease.* 8th ed. New York: McGraw-Hill; 2001.
6. Hoe FM. Hypoglycemia in infants and children. *Adv Pediatr.* 2008;55:367–384.
7. Sperling MA. *Pediatric endocrinology.* 3rd ed. Saunders, 2008.
8. Hall JG, Allanson J, Gripp K, et al. *Handbook of physical measurements.* 2nd ed. Oxford, UK: Oxford University Press; 2007.
9. Jones KL. *Smith's recognizable patterns of human malformation.* 6th ed. Philadelphia: Elsevier; 2006.
10. Hennekam R, Allanson J, Krantz I. *Gorlin's syndromes of the head and neck.* 5th ed. New York: Oxford University Press; 2010.
11. American Academy of Pediatrics, Committee on Genetics. Health supervision for children with Down syndrome. *Pediatrics.* 2001;107(2):442–449. Statement of reaffirmation September 2007.
12. Bondy, CA for the Turner Syndrome Consensus Group. Care of girls and women with Turner syndrome: a guideline of the Turner Syndrome Study Group. *J Clin Endocrinol Metab.* 2007;92(1):10–25.
13. American Academy of Pediatrics, Committee on Genetics. Health supervision for children with Fragile X syndrome. *Pediatrics.* 1996;98(2):297–300. Statement of reaffirmation May 2007.
14. De Paepe A, Devereux RB, Dietz HC, et al. Revised diagnostic criteria for the Marfan syndrome. *Am J Med Genet.* 1996;62(4):417–426.
15. American Academy of Pediatrics, Committee on Genetics. Health supervision for children with Marfan syndrome. *Pediatrics.* 1996;98(5):978–982. Statement of reaffirmation May 2007.
16. Wattendorf DJ, Muenke M. Prader-Willi syndrome. *Am Fam Phys.* 2005;72(5): 827–830.
17. Koenig MK. Presentation and diagnosis of mitochondrial disorders in children. *Pediatr Neurol.* 2008;38(5):305–313.
18. Rahman S, Hanna MG. Diagnosis and therapy in neuromuscular disorders: diagnosis and new treatments in mitochondrial diseases. *J Neurol Neurosurg Psychiatry.* 2009;80:943–953.

Chapter 14

Hematology

Sama Ahsan, MD, and Julia Noether, MD

I. ANEMIA

A. General Evaluation

Anemia is defined by age-specific norms (Table 14-1 and Fig. 14-1). Evaluation includes the following:

1. Complete history: Includes blood loss, fatigue, pica, medication exposure, growth and development, nutritional history, menstrual history, ethnic background, history of hyperbilirubinemia and family history of anemia, splenectomy, or cholecystectomy
2. Physical examination: Includes pallor, jaundice, glossitis, tachypnea, tachycardia, cardiac murmur, hepatosplenomegaly, and signs of systemic illness
3. Initial laboratory tests: May include a complete blood count with red blood cell (RBC) indices, reticulocyte count, blood smear, stool for occult blood, urinalysis, and serum bilirubin

B. Diagnosis

Anemias may be categorized as macrocytic, microcytic, or normocytic. Table 14-2 gives an approach to diagnosis based on RBC production and cell size. Note that normal ranges for hemoglobin (Hb) and mean corpuscular volume (MCV) are age dependent.

C. Evaluation of Specific Causes of Anemia

1. Iron-deficiency anemia: Hypochromic/microcytic anemia with a low reticulocyte count and an elevated red cell distribution width (RDW)

a. Serum ferritin reflects total body iron stores after age 6 months and is the first value to fall in iron deficiency; may be falsely elevated with inflammation or infection

b. Other indicators: Low serum iron, an elevated total iron-binding capacity (TIBC), low mean cell hemoglobin concentration (MCHC), elevated transferrin receptor level, and low reticulocyte Hb content

c. Iron therapy should result in an increased reticulocyte count in 2–3 days and an increase in hematocrit (HCT) after 1–4 weeks of therapy. Iron stores are generally repleted with 3 months of therapy

d. Mentzer index (MCV/RBC): Index >13.5 suggests iron deficiency; Mentzer index <11.5 suggests thalassemia minor. Increased RDW also helps distinguish iron-deficiency anemia from thalassemia

TABLE 14-1

AGE-SPECIFIC BLOOD CELL INDICES

Age	Hb (g/dL)*	HCT (%)*	MCV (fL)*	MCHC (g/dL RBC)*	Reticulocytes	WBCs (×10³/mL)†	Platelets (10³/mL)†
26–30 wk gestation‡	13.4 (11)	41.5 (34.9)	118.2 (106.7)	37.9 (30.6)	—	4.4 (2.7)	254 (180–327)
28 wk	14.5	45	120	31.0	(5–10)	—	275
32 wk	15.0	47	118	32.0	(3–10)	—	290
Term§ (cord)	16.5 (13.5)	51 (42)	108 (98)	33.0 (30.0)	(3–7)	18.1 (9–30)‖	290
1–3 day	18.5 (14.5)	56 (45)	108 (95)	33.0 (29.0)	(1.8–4.6)	18.9 (9.4–34)	192
2 wk	16.6 (13.4)	53 (41)	105 (88)	31.4 (28.1)	—	11.4 (5–20)	252
1 mo	13.9 (10.7)	44 (33)	101 (91)	31.8 (28.1)	(0.1–1.7)	10.8 (4–19.5)	—
2 mo	11.2 (9.4)	35 (28)	95 (84)	31.8 (28.3)	—	—	—
6 mo	12.6 (11.1)	36 (31)	76 (68)	35.0 (32.7)	(0.7–2.3)	11.9 (6–17.5)	—
6 mo–2 yr	12.0 (10.5)	36 (33)	78 (70)	33.0 (30.0)	—	10.6 (6–17)	(150–350)
2–6 yr	12.5 (11.5)	37 (34)	81 (75)	34.0 (31.0)	(0.5–1.0)	8.5 (5–15.5)	(150–350)
6–12 yr	13.5 (11.5)	40 (35)	86 (77)	34.0 (31.0)	(0.5–1.0)	8.1 (4.5–13.5)	(150–350)

Continued

14

TABLE 14-1

AGE-SPECIFIC BLOOD CELL INDICES (Continued)

Age	Hb (g/dL)*	HCT (%)*	MCV (fL)*	MCHC (g/dL RBC)*	Reticulocytes	WBCs ($\times 10^3$/mL)[†]	Platelets (10^3/mL)[†]
12–18 yr							
Male	14.5 (13)	43 (36)	88 (78)	34.0 (31.0)	(0.5–1.0)	7.8 (4.5–13.5)	(150–350)
Female	14.0 (12)	41 (37)	90 (78)	34.0 (31.0)	(0.5–1.0)	7.8 (4.5–13.5)	(150–350)
ADULT							
Male	15.5 (13.5)	47 (41)	90 (80)	34.0 (31.0)	(0.8–2.5)	7.4 (4.5–11)	(150–350)
Female	14.0 (12)	41 (36)	90 (80)	34.0 (31.0)	(0.8–4.1)	7.4 (4.5–11)	(150–350)

*Data are mean (−2 SD).

†Data are mean (± 2 SD).

‡Values are from fetal samplings.

§1 mo, capillary hemoglobin exceeds venous: 1 hr: 3.6 g difference; 5 day: 2.2 g difference; 3 wk: 1.1 g difference.

‖Mean (95% confidence limits).

Hb, Hemoglobin; HCT, hematocrit; MCHC, mean cell hemoglobin concentration; MCV, mean corpuscular volume; RBC, red blood cell; WBC, white blood cell.

Data from Forestier F, Dattos F, Galacteros F, et al: Hematologic values of 163 normal fetuses between 18 and 30 weeks of gestation. Pediatr Res 1986;20:342; Oski FA, Naiman JL: Hematological problems in the newborn infant. Philadelphia, WB Saunders, 1982; Nathan D, Oski FA: Hematology of infancy and childhood. Philadelphia; WB Saunders, 1998; Matoth Y, Zaizor K, Varsano I, et al: Postnatal changes in some red cell parameters. Acta Paediatr Scand 1971;60:317; and Wintrobe MM: Clinical hematology. Baltimore, Williams & Wilkins, 1999.

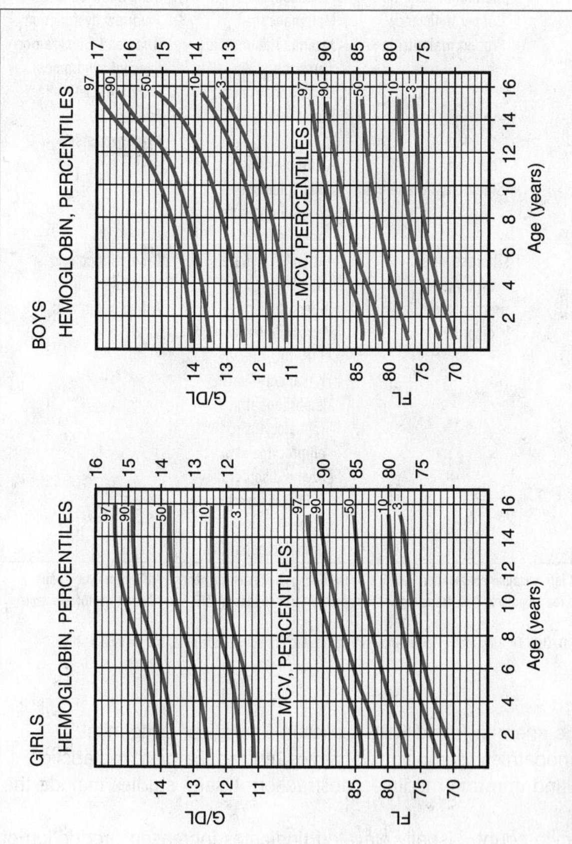

FIGURE 14-1 Hemoglobin and mean corpuscular volume (MCV) by age and gender. *(Data from Dallman PR, Siimes MA: Percentile curves for hemoglobin and red cell volume in infancy and childhood. J Pediatr 1979;94:26.)*

TABLE 14-2

CLASSIFICATION OF ANEMIA

Reticulocyte Count	Microcytic Anemia	Normocytic Anemia	Macrocytic Anemia
Low	Iron deficiency Lead poisoning Chronic disease Aluminum toxicity Copper deficiency Protein malnutrition	Chronic disease RBC aplasia (TEC, infection, drug induced) Malignancy Juvenile rheumatoid arthritis Endocrinopathies Renal failure	Folate deficiency Vitamin B_{12} deficiency Aplastic anemia Congenital bone marrow dysfunction (Diamond-Blackfan or Fanconi syndromes) Drug induced Trisomy 21 Hypothyroidism
Normal	Thalassemia trait Sideroblastic anemia	Acute bleeding Hypersplenism Dyserythropoietic anemia II	—
High	Thalassemia syndromes Hemoglobin C disorders	Antibody-mediated hemolysis Hypersplenism Microangiopathy (HUS, TTP, DIC, Kasabach-Merritt) Membranopathies (spherocytosis, elliptocytosis) Enzyme disorders (G6PD, pyruvate kinase) Hemoglobinopathies	Dyserythropoietic anemia I, III Active hemolysis

DIC, Disseminated intravascular coagulation; G6PD, glucose-6–phosphate dehydrogenase; HUS, hemolytic-uremic syndrome; RBC, red blood cell; TEC, transient erythroblastopenia of childhood; TTP, thrombotic thrombocytopenic purpura.

Data from Nathan D, Oski FA: Hematology of infancy and childhood, 6th ed. Philadelphia, WB Saunders, 2003.

2. Hemolytic anemia: Rapid RBC turnover. Etiologies: Congenital membranopathies, hemoglobinopathies, enzymopathies, metabolic defects, and immune-mediated destruction. Useful studies include the following:

a. Reticulocyte count: Usually elevated; indicates increased production of RBCs to compensate for increased destruction. Corrected reticulocyte count (CRC) accounts for differences in HCT and is an indicator of erythropoietic activity. A CRC >1.5 suggests increased RBC production as a result of hemolysis or blood loss

$$CRC = \% \text{ reticulocytes} \times \text{patient HCT/normal HCT}$$

b. Plasma aspartate aminotransferase and lactate dehydrogenase: Increased from release of intracellular enzymes

c. Haptoglobin: Binds free Hb; decreased with intravascular and extravascular hemolysis. Also, can be decreased in patients with liver dysfunction secondary to decreased synthesis, as well as in neonates
d. Direct Coombs test: Tests for the presence of antibody or complement on patient RBCs. Can be falsely negative if affected cells have already been destroyed or antibody titer is low
e. Indirect Coombs test: Tests for free autoantibody in the patient's serum after RBC antibody binding sites are saturated
f. Osmotic fragility test: Useful in diagnosis of hereditary spherocytosis. Can also be positive in ABO incompatibility, autoimmune hemolytic anemia, or anytime spherocytes are present
g. Glucose-6-phosphate dehydrogenase (G6PD) assay: Quantitative test used to diagnose G6PD deficiency, an X-linked disorder affecting 10%–14% of African American males. May be normal immediately after a hemolytic episode because older, more enzyme-deficient cells have been lysed. See Chapter 30 for a list of oxidizing drugs
h. Heinz body preparation: Detects precipitated Hb within RBCs; present in unstable hemoglobinopathies and enzymopathies during oxidative stress (e.g., G6PD deficiency)
i. Lactate dehydrogenase (LDH): An enzyme found in RBCs; serum levels significantly elevated in intravascular hemolysis and mildly elevated in extravascular hemolysis

3. Red cell aplasia: Variable cell size, low reticulocyte count, variable platelet and white blood cell (WBC) counts. Bone marrow aspiration evaluates RBC precursors in the marrow to look for marrow dysfunction, neoplasm, or specific signs of infection

a. Acquired aplasias:
   (1) Infectious causes: Include parvovirus in children with rapid RBC turnover (infects RBC precursors), Epstein-Barr virus (EBV), cytomegalovirus (CMV), human herpesvirus type 6, or human immunodeficiency virus (HIV)
   (2) Transient erythroblastopenia of childhood (TEC): Occurs from age 6 months to 4 years, with >80% of cases presenting after age 1 year with a normal or slightly low MCV and low reticulocyte count. Spontaneous recovery usually within 4–8 weeks
   (3) Exposures: Include radiation and various drugs and chemicals
b. Congenital aplasias: Typically macrocytic anemias
   (1) Fanconi anemia: Autosomal recessive disorder, usually presents before 10 years of age; may present with pancytopenia. Patients may have thumb abnormalities, renal anomalies, microcephaly, or short stature. Chromosomal fragility studies may be diagnostic
   (2) Diamond-Blackfan anemia: Autosomal recessive pure RBC aplasia; presents in the first year of life. Associated with congenital anomalies in one third of cases, including triphalangeal thumb, short stature, and cleft lip
c. Aplastic anemia: Idiopathic bone marrow failure, usually macrocytic

4. Physiologic anemia of infancy (physiologic nadir): Decrease in Hb until oxygen needs are greater than oxygen delivery, usually at Hb of 9–11 mg/dL. Normally occurs between age 8–12 weeks for full-term infants and age 3–6 weeks for preterm infants
5. Anemia of chronic inflammation: Usually normocytic with normal to low reticulocyte count. Iron studies reveal low iron, TIBC, and transferrin, and elevated ferritin

II. HEMOGLOBINOPATHIES

A. Hemoglobin Electrophoresis

Involves separation of Hb variants based on molecular charge and size. All positive sickle preparations and solubility tests for sickle Hb (e.g., Sickledex) should be confirmed with electrophoresis or isoelectric focusing (a component of the mandatory newborn screen in many states). See Table 14-3 for interpretation of neonatal Hb electrophoresis patterns.

B. Sickle Cell Anemia

Caused by a genetic defect in β-globin. 8% of African Americans are carriers; 1 in 500 African Americans have sickle cell anemia.

1. Diagnosis: Often made on newborn screen with Hb electrophoresis. The sickle preparation and Sickledex: Rapid tests that are positive in

TABLE 14-3

NEONATAL HEMOGLOBIN (Hb) ELECTROPHORESIS PATTERNS*

FA	Fetal Hb and adult normal Hb; the normal newborn pattern.
FAV	Indicates the presence of both HbF and HbA. However, an anomalous band (V) is present, which does not appear to be any of the common Hb variants.
FAS	Indicates fetal Hb, adult normal HbA, and HbS, consistent with benign sickle cell trait.
FS	Fetal and sickle HbS without detectable adult normal HbA. Consistent with clinically significant homozygous sickle Hb genotype (S/S) or sickle β-thalassemia, with manifestations of sickle cell anemia during childhood.
FC[†]	Designates the presence of HbC without adult normal HbA. Consistent with clinically significant homozygous HbC genotype (C/C), resulting in a mild hematologic disorder presenting during childhood.
FSC	HbS and HbC present. This heterozygous condition could lead to the manifestations of sickle cell disease during childhood.
FAC	HbC and adult normal HbA present, consistent with benign HbC trait.
FSA	Heterozygous HbS/β-thalassemia, a clinically significant sickling disorder.
F[†]	Fetal HbF is present without adult normal HbA. Although this may indicate a delayed appearance of HbA, it is also consistent with homozygous β-thalassemia major, or homozygous hereditary persistence of fetal HbF.
FV[†]	Fetal HbF and an anomalous Hb variant (V) are present.
AF	May indicate prior blood transfusion. Submit another filter paper blood specimen when the infant is 4 mo of age, at which time the transfused blood cells should have been cleared.

NOTE: HbA: $\alpha_2\beta_2$; HbF: $\alpha_2\gamma_2$; HbA$_2$: $\alpha_2\delta_2$.

*Hemoglobin variants are reported in order of decreasing abundance; for example, FA indicates more fetal than adult hemoglobin.

[†]Repeat blood specimen should be submitted to confirm the original interpretation.

all sickle hemoglobinopathies. False-negative test results may be seen in neonates and other patients with a high percentage of fetal Hb

2. Complications (Table 14-4): A hematologist should generally be consulted
3. Health maintenance[1,2]: Ongoing consultation and clinical involvement with a pediatric hematologist and/or with a sickle cell program are essential. See Table 14-5
4. Hemoglobin electrophoresis (outside neonatal period): Hemoglobin SF, SCF, SAF—other Hb combinations may sickle

C. Thalassemias

Defects in α- or β-globin production. Imbalance in production of globin chains leads to precipitation of excess chains, causing ineffective erythropoiesis and shortened survival of mature RBCs.

1. α-Thalassemias:

a. Hb Bart's hydrops fetalis (—/—): Hb Barts (γ_4) cannot deliver oxygen; usually fatal

b. HbH disease (β_4) (α–/—): Causes moderately severe anemia

c. α-Thalassemia trait (α–/α–) or (αα/–): Causes mild microcytic anemia, childhood and adult hemoglobin electrophoresis usually normal. Hb Barts can be seen in infancy (e.g., on state newborn screens) in patients with α-thalassemia trait

TABLE 14-4

SICKLE CELL DISEASE COMPLICATIONS

Complication	Evaluation	Treatment
Fever (T ≥38.5°C)	History and physical CBC with differential Reticulocyte count Blood cultures Chest x-ray Other cultures as indicated	IV antibiotics (third-generation cephalosporin, other antibiotics as indicated, especially if penicillin-resistant pneumococcus suspected) Admit if ill appearing, <3 yr of age, concerning lab results, or complications Some centers use antibiotics with a long half-life and re-evaluate in 24 hr as an outpatient
Vaso-occlusive Crisis Children <2 yr, dactylitis Children >2 yr, unifocal or multifocal pain	History and physical CBC with differential Reticulocyte count Type and screen	Oral analgesics as an outpatient, as tolerated IV analgesics and IV fluids if outpatient therapy fails (parenteral narcotics in form of PCA and parenteral NSAIDs usually used in combination) Aggressive early treatment of pain is essential

Continued

14

TABLE 14-4

SICKLE CELL DISEASE COMPLICATIONS (Continued)

Complication	Evaluation	Treatment
Acute chest syndrome New pulmonary infiltrate with fever, cough, chest pain, tachypnea, dyspnea, or hypoxia	History and physical CBC with differential Reticulocyte count Blood cultures Chest x-ray Type and screen	Admit O_2, incentive spirometry, bronchodilators IV antibiotics (third-generation cephalosporin and macrolide) Analgesia, IV fluids Simple transfusion or partial exchange for moderately severe illness, double the packed cell volume exchange transfusion (see above) for severe or rapidly progressing illness High-dose dexamethasone controversial (risk of readmission for pain or other SCD-related issues)[7]
Splenic sequestration Acutely enlarged spleen and Hb level ≥2 g/dL below patient's baseline	History and physical CBC Reticulocyte count Type and hold	Serial abdominal exams IV fluids and fluid resuscitation as necessary RBC transfusion or, in severe cases, exchange transfusion for cardiovascular compromise and Hb <4.5 g/dL. (Autotransfusion may occur with recovery, leading to increased Hb and CHF. Transfuse cautiously.)
Aplastic crisis Acute illness with Hb below patient's baseline and low reticulocyte count May follow viral illnesses, especially parvovirus B19	History and physical CBC with differential Reticulocyte count Type and screen Parvovirus serology and polymerase chain reaction	Admit IV fluids PRBCs for symptomatic anemia Isolation to protect susceptible individuals and women of childbearing age until parvovirus excluded
Other complications Priapism, CVA, TIA, gallbladder disease, avascular necrosis, hyphema*		

NOTE: CVA requires emergency transfusion guided by a hematologist and a neurologist experienced with sickle cell disease. Exchange transfusion preferable to simple transfusion, if possible.[8]

*Hyphema in a patient with sickle cell trait is an ophthalmologic emergency

CBC, Complete blood count; CHF, congestive heart failure; CVA, cerebrovascular accident; Hb, hemoglobin; IV, intravenous; NSAIDs, nonsteroidal anti-inflammatory drugs; PCA, patient-controlled analgesia; PRBCs, packed red blood cells; RBC, red blood cells; SCD, sickle cell disease; T, temperature; TIA, transient ischemic attack.

TABLE 14-5

SICKLE CELL DISEASE HEALTH MAINTENANCE

IMMUNIZATIONS	Maintenance
Pneumococcal vaccine	Vaccinate with 13-valent conjugate vaccine as per routine childhood schedule 23-valent polysaccharide vaccine at 2 years of age, booster at 5 years of age and every 5–7 years thereafter
Meningococcal vaccine	Give at 2 years of age and then every 10 years thereafter
Influenza vaccine	Vaccinate yearly once 6 months of age and older
MEDICATIONS	
PCN	Begin as soon as SCD diagnosis made (125 mg BID and increase dose to 250 mg at 3 yr of age*)
Folic acid	Recommend supplementation, start by 1 year of age
Hydroxyurea	Consider with frequent crises or in severe disease†
IMAGING	
Transcranial Doppler (TCD)	Perform annually from 2 to 16 years of age to evaluate for increased risk of cerebrovascular accident (CVA)
OTHER	
Ophthalmology	Perform annually from 10 years of age to evaluate for sickle retinopathy
Growth and development, school/social issues, counseling regarding fevers	Review closely at all visits

*Prophylaxis may be discontinued by age 5 years if patient has had no prior severe pneumococcal infections or splenectomy and has documented pneumococcal vaccinations, including second 23-valent vaccination. Practice patterns vary. Some continue penicillin indefinitely.

†Increases levels of fetal Hb and decreases HbS content in cells. Has been shown to significantly decrease episodes of vaso-occlusive crises, hemolytic crises, acute chest syndrome, number of transfusions, and days spent in the hospital.[9] May decrease mortality in adults.

PCN, Penicillin; SCD, sickle cell disease.

d. Silent carriers (α–/αα): Not anemic, childhood and adult hemoglobin electrophoresis usually normal

2. β-Thalassemia: Found throughout the Mediterranean, Middle East, India, and Southeast Asia. Ineffective erythropoiesis is more severe in β-thalassemia than α-thalassemia because excess α chains are more unstable than β chains. Adult hemoglobin electrophoresis with increased hemoglobin A_2, decreased hemoglobin A, and increased hemoglobin F

a. Thalassemia major/Cooley's anemia (β0/β0, β+/β0, or β+/β+): Presence of anemia within the first 6 months of life with hepatosplenomegaly and progressive bone marrow expansion, which may lead to frontal bossing and other skeletal deformities. Regular transfusions required to avoid anemia

b. Thalassemia intermedia (β+/β+): Presents at about age 2 years with moderate, compensated anemia, which may become symptomatic, leading to heart failure, pulmonary hypertension, splenomegaly, and bony expansion, usually in the second or third decade of life

c. Thalassemia trait/thalassemia minor (β/β+)or (β/β0): Usually asymptomatic with microcytosis out of proportion to anemia, sometimes with erythrocytosis

III. NEUTROPENIA

An absolute neutrophil count (ANC) <1500/μL, although neutrophil counts vary with age (Table 14-6). Severe neutropenia is defined as an ANC <500/μL. Children with significant neutropenia are at risk for bacterial and fungal infections. Granulocyte colony-stimulating factor may be indicated. Transient neutropenia secondary to viral illness rarely causes significant morbidity. For management of fever and neutropenia in oncology patients, see Chapter 22. See Box 14-1 for causes.

IV. THROMBOCYTOPENIA

A. Definition

A platelet count <150,000/μL. Clinically significant bleeding is unlikely with platelet counts >20,000/μL in the absence of other complicating factors.

B. Causes of Thrombocytopenia

1. Idiopathic thrombocytopenic purpura (ITP): A diagnosis of exclusion; can be acute or chronic. WBC count, Hb levels and peripheral blood smear are normal. Many require no therapy and even indications for treatment of patients without significant bleeding are not well established

a. Treatment options:
   (1) Rh (D) immune globulin (WinRho; useful only in Rh-positive, nonsplenectomized patients)
   (2) Intravenous immune globulin (see Formulary for IVIG dosing)
   (3) Corticosteroids (i.e., prednisone 2 mg/kg/day or up to 30 mg/kg methylprednisolone for up to 3 days)

BOX 14-1

DIFFERENTIAL DIAGNOSIS OF CHILDHOOD NEUTROPENIA

Acquired	Congenital
Infection	Cyclic neutropenia
Immune-mediated	Severe congenital neutropenia (Kostmann syndrome)
Hypersplenism	Chronic benign neutropenia of childhood
Vitamin B_{12}, folate, copper deficiency	Shwachman-Diamond syndrome
Drugs or toxic substances	Fanconi anemia
Aplastic anemia	Metabolic disorders (amino acidopathies, Barth syndrome, glycogen storage disorders)
Malignancies or preleukemic disorders	Osteopetrosis
Ionizing radiation	Neutropenia with pigmentation abnormalities, e.g., Chediak-Higashi

TABLE 14-6

AGE-SPECIFIC LEUKOCYTE DIFFERENTIAL

	Total Leukocytes*	Neutrophils†		Lymphocytes		Monocytes		Eosinophils	
Age	Mean (range)	Mean (range)	%	Mean (range)	%	Mean	%	Mean	%
Birth	18.1 (9–30)	11 (6–26)	61	5.5 (2–11)	31	1.1	6	0.4	2
12 hr	22.8 (13–38)	15.5 (6–28)	68	5.5 (2–11)	24	1.2	5	0.5	2
24 hr	18.9 (9.4–34)	11.5 (5–21)	61	5.8 (2–11.5)	31	1.1	6	0.5	2
1 wk	12.2 (5–21)	5.5 (1.5–10)	45	5.0 (2–17)	41	1.1	9	0.5	4
2 wk	11.4 (5–20)	4.5 (1–9.5)	40	5.5 (2–17)	48	1.0	9	0.4	3
1 mo	10.8 (5–19.5)	3.8 (1–8.5)	35	6.0 (2.5–16.5)	56	0.7	7	0.3	3
6 mo	11.9 (6–17.5)	3.8 (1–8.5)	32	7.3 (4–13.5)	61	0.6	5	0.3	3
1 yr	11.4 (6–17.5)	3.5 (1.5–8.5)	31	7.0 (4–10.5)	61	0.6	5	0.3	3
2 yr	10.6 (6–17)	3.5 (1.5–8.5)	33	6.3 (3–9.5)	59	0.5	5	0.3	3
4 yr	9.1 (5.5–15.5)	3.8 (1.5–8.5)	42	4.5 (2–8)	50	0.5	5	0.3	3
6 yr	8.5 (5–14.5)	4.3 (1.5–8)	51	3.5 (1.5–7)	42	0.4	5	0.2	3
8 yr	8.3 (4.5–13.5)	4.4 (1.5–8)	53	3.3 (1.5–6.8)	39	0.4	4	0.2	2
10 yr	8.1 (4.5–13.5)	4.4 (1.5–8.5)	54	3.1 (1.5–6.5)	38	0.4	4	0.2	2
16 yr	7.8 (4.5–13.0)	4.4 (1.8–8)	57	2.8 (1.2–5.2)	35	0.4	5	0.2	3
21 yr	7.4 (4.5–11.0)	4.4 (1.8–7.7)	59	2.5 (1–4.8)	34	0.3	4	0.2	3

*Numbers of leukocytes are $\times 10^3/\mu L$; ranges are estimates of 95% confidence limits; percents refer to differential counts.

†Neutrophils include band cells at all ages and a small number of metamyelocytes and myelocytes in the first few days of life.

Adapted from Cairo MS, Brauho F: Blood and blood-forming tissues. In Randolph AM (ed): Pediatrics, 21st ed. New York, McGraw-Hill, 2003.

(4) Consider Rituximab in chronic cases[3]
(5) Splenectomy or chemotherapy may be considered in chronic cases. Platelet transfusions are not generally helpful but are necessary in life-threatening bleeding

2. Neonatal thrombocytopenia: May be caused by the following:
a. Decreased production: Results from aplastic disorders, congenital malignancy such as leukemia, and viral infections
b. Increased consumption: Usually result of disseminated intravascular coagulation (DIC) from infection or asphyxia
c. Immune mediated: IgG or complement attach to platelets and cause destruction. Specific causes include pre-eclampsia, sepsis, maternal ITP, and platelet alloimmunization

3. Neonatal alloimmune thrombocytopenia (NAIT): Transplacental maternal antibodies (usually against PLA-1 antigen/HPA-1a) cause fetal platelet destruction. If severe, a transfusion of maternal platelets will be more effective in raising the platelet count than random donor platelets
a. Evaluation/diagnosis:
(1) Check maternal platelet count and platelet-associated IgG. Mother's platelet count should be normal and platelet-associated IgG usually negative
(2) Absence of maternal PLA-1 antigen/HPA-1a or other specific antigens
(3) Study of mother's or infant's plasma with a panel of known minor platelet antigens
(4) Mixing study of maternal or neonatal plasma and paternal platelets

4. Other causes of thrombocytopenia include microangiopathic hemolytic anemias, such as DIC and hemolytic-uremic syndrome (HUS), infection causing marrow suppression, malignancy, HIV, drug-induced thrombocytopenia, marrow infiltration, cavernous hemangiomas (Kasabach-Merritt syndrome), thrombocytopenia with absent radii syndrome (TAR), thrombosis, hypersplenism, and other rare inherited disorders (e.g., Wiskott-Aldrich, Paris-Trousseau, Noonan, and DiGeorge syndromes, myosin-9 associated megaplatelet disorders, chromosomal abnormalities)

V. COAGULATION (FIG. 14-2)

A. Tests of Coagulation

An incorrect anticoagulant-to-blood ratio will give inaccurate results. See Table 14-7 for normal hematologic values.

1. Activated partial thromboplastin time (aPTT): Measures intrinsic system; requires factors V, VIII, IX, X, XI, XII, fibrinogen, and prothrombin. May be prolonged in heparin administration, in hemophilia, in von Willebrand disease (vWD), in DIC, and in the presence of circulating inhibitors (e.g., lupus anticoagulants)
2. Prothrombin time (PT): Measures extrinsic pathway; requires factors V, VII, X, fibrinogen, and prothrombin. May be prolonged in warfarin

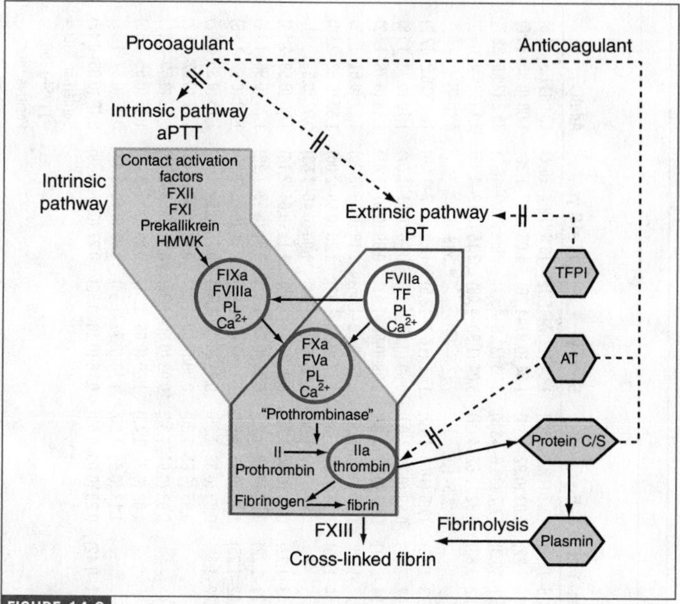

FIGURE 14-2

Coagulation cascade. AT, antithrombin; F, factor; HMWK, high molecular weight kininogen; PL, phospholipid; TF, tissue factor; TFPI, tissue factor pathway inhibitor. *(Adaptation courtesy of James Casella and Clifford Takemoto.)*

administration, deficiencies of vitamin K–associated factors, malabsorption, liver disease, DIC, and the presence of circulating inhibitors

3. Bleeding time (BT): Evaluates clot formation, including platelet number and function, and von Willebrand factor (vWF). Performed at patient's bedside. Always assess the platelet number and history of ingestion of platelet inhibitors, such as nonsteroidal anti-inflammatory drugs, before a BT test. Platelet aggregations and the Platelet Function Analyzer-100 (PFA-100) system are other in vitro methods for measuring platelet function

B. Hypercoagulable States

Present clinically as venous or arterial thrombosis (Box 14-2).

1. Laboratory evaluation[4,5]:

a. Initial laboratory screening includes PT, high-sensitivity aPTT, circulating anticoagulants, and, if the PT or aPTT are prolonged, a mixing study to look for circulating anticoagulants

b. Extended workup for hypercoagulable states (Box 14-3): A hematologist should be consulted

TABLE 14-7

AGE-SPECIFIC COAGULATION VALUES

Coagulation Test	Preterm Infant (30–36 wk), Day of Life 1*	Term Infant, Day of Life 1	Day of Life 3	1 Month–1 yr	1–5 yr	6–10 yr	11–16 yr	Adult
PT (sec)	13.0 (10.6–16.2)	15.6 (14.4–16.4)	14.9 (13.5–16.4)	13.1 (11.5–15.3)	13.3 (12.1–14.5)	13.4 (11.7–15.1)	13.8 (12.7–16.1)	13.0 (11.5–14.5)
INR		1.26 (1.15–1.35)	1.20 (1.05–1.35)	1.00 (0.86–1.22)	1.03 (0.92–1.14)	1.04 (0.87–1.20)	1.08 (0.97–1.30)	1.00 (0.80–1.20)
aPTT (sec)[†]	53.6 (27.5–79.4)	38.7 (34.3–44.8)	36.3 (29.5–42.2)	39.3 (35.1–46.3)	37.7 (33.6–43.8)	37.3 (31.8–43.7)	39.5 (33.9–46.1)	33.2 (28.6–38.2)
Fibrinogen (g/L)	2.43 (1.50–3.73)	2.80 (1.92–3.74)	3.30 (2.83–4.01)	2.42 (0.82–3.83)	2.82 (1.62–4.01)	3.04 (1.99–4.09)	3.15 (2.12–4.33)	3.1 (1.9–4.3)
Bleeding time (min)*					6 (2.5–10)	7 (2.5–13)	5 (3–8)	4 (1–7)
Thrombin time (sec)	14 (11–17)	12 (10–16)*		17.1 (16.3–17.6)	17.5 (16.5–18.2)	17.1 (16.1–18.5)	16.9 (16.2–17.6)	16.6 (16.2–17.2)
Factor II (U/mL)	0.45 (0.20–0.77)	0.54 (0.41–0.69)	0.62 (0.50–0.73)	0.90 (0.62–1.03)	0.89 (0.70–1.09)	0.89 (0.67–1.10)	0.90 (0.61–1.07)	1.10 (0.78–1.38)
Factor V (U/mL)	0.88 (0.41–1.44)	0.81 (0.64–1.03)	1.22 (0.92–1.54)	1.13 (0.94–1.41)	0.97 (0.67–1.27)	0.99 (0.56–1.41)	0.89 (0.67–1.41)	1.18 (0.78–1.52)
Factor VII (U/mL)	0.67 (0.21–1.13)	0.70 (0.52–0.88)	0.86 (0.67–1.07)	1.28 (0.83–1.60)	1.11 (0.72–1.50)	1.13 (0.70–1.56)	1.18 (0.69–2.00)	1.29 (0.61–1.99)
Factor VIII (U/mL)	1.11 (0.50–2.13)	1.82 (1.05–3.29)	1.59 (0.83–2.74)	0.94 (0.54–1.45)	1.10 (0.36–1.85)	1.17 (0.52–1.82)	1.20 (0.59–2.00)	1.60 (0.52–2.90)
vWF (U/mL)*	1.36 (0.78–2.10)	1.53 (0.50–2.87)			0.82 (0.47–1.04)	0.95 (0.44–1.44)	1.00 (0.46–1.53)	0.92 (0.5–1.58)
Factor IX (U/mL)	0.35 (0.19–0.65)	0.48 (0.35–0.56)	0.72 (0.44–0.97)	0.71 (0.43–1.21)	0.85 (0.44–1.27)	0.96 (0.48–1.45)	1.11 (0.64–2.16)	1.30 (0.59–2.54)
Factor X (U/mL)	0.41 (0.11–0.71)	0.55 (0.46–0.67)	0.60 (0.46–0.75)	0.95 (0.77–1.22)	0.98 (0.72–1.25)	0.97 (0.68–1.25)	0.91 (0.53–1.22)	1.24 (0.96–1.71)
Factor XI (U/mL)	0.30 (0.08–0.52)	0.30 (0.07–0.41)	0.57 (0.24–0.79)	0.89 (0.62–1.25)	1.13 (0.65–1.62)	1.13 (0.65–1.62)	1.11 (0.65–1.39)	1.12 (0.67–1.96)
Factor XII (U/mL)	0.38 (0.10–0.66)	0.58 (0.43–0.80)	0.53 (0.14–0.80)	0.79 (0.20–1.35)	0.85 (0.36–1.35)	0.81 (0.26–1.37)	0.75 (0.14–1.17)	1.15 (0.35–2.07)
PK (U/mL)*	0.33 (0.09–0.57)	0.37 (0.18–0.69)			0.95 (0.65–1.30)	0.99 (0.66–1.31)	0.99 (0.53–1.45)	1.12 (0.62–1.62)
HMWK (U/mL)*	0.49 (0.09–0.89)	0.54 (0.06–1.02)			0.98 (0.64–1.32)	0.93 (0.60–1.30)	0.91 (0.63–1.19)	0.92 (0.50–1.36)
Factor XIIIa (U/mL)*	0.70 (0.32–1.08)	0.79 (0.27–1.31)			1.08 (0.72–1.43)	1.09 (0.65–1.51)	0.99 (0.57–1.40)	1.05 (0.55–1.55)
Factor XIIIs (U/mL)*	0.81 (0.35–1.27)	0.76 (0.30–1.22)			1.13 (0.69–1.56)	1.16 (0.77–1.54)	1.02 (0.60–1.43)	0.97 (0.57–1.37)
D-Dimer		1.47 (0.41–2.47)	1.34 (0.58–2.74)	0.22 (0.11–0.42)	0.25 (0.09–0.53)	0.26 (0.10–0.56)	0.27 (0.16–0.39)	0.18 (0.05–0.42)
FDPs*								Borderline titer = 1:25–1:50. Positive titer <1:50

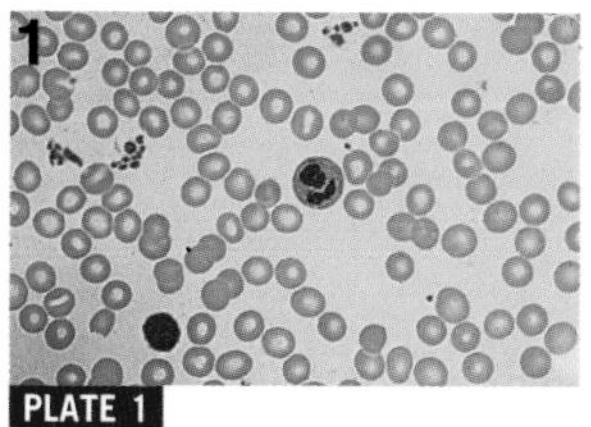

PLATE 1

Normal smear. Round RBCs with central pallor about one third of the cell's diameter, scattered platelets, occasional white blood cells.

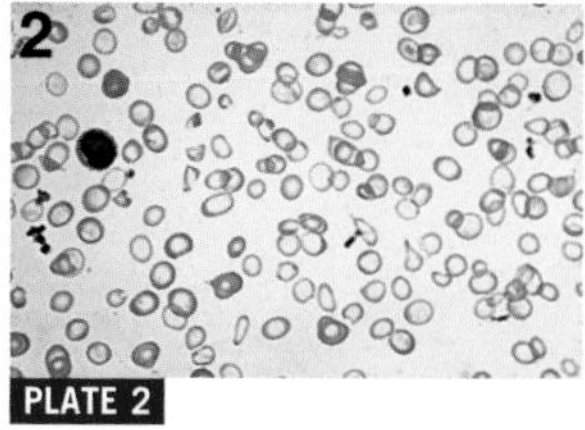

PLATE 2

Iron deficiency. Hypochromic/microcytic RBCs, poikilocytosis, plentiful platelets, occasional ovalocytes and target cells.

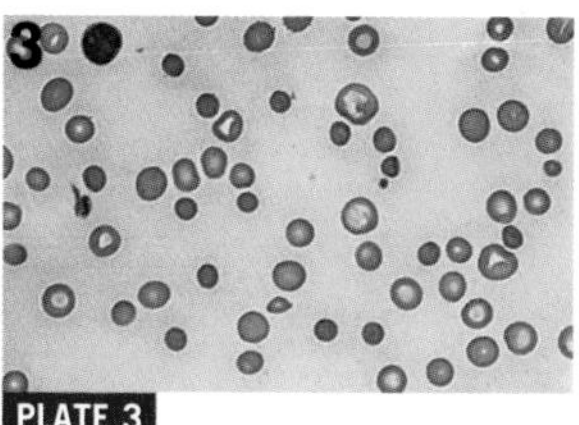

PLATE 3

Spherocytosis. Microspherocytes a hallmark (densely stained RBCs with no central pallor).

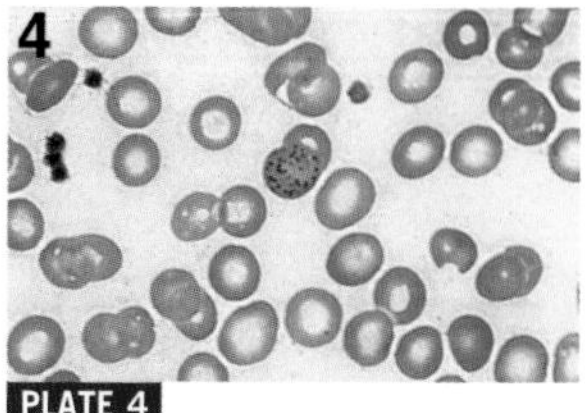

PLATE 4

Basophilic stippling as a result of precipitated RNA throughout the cell; seen with heavy metal intoxication, thalassemia, iron deficiency, and other states of ineffective erythropoesis.

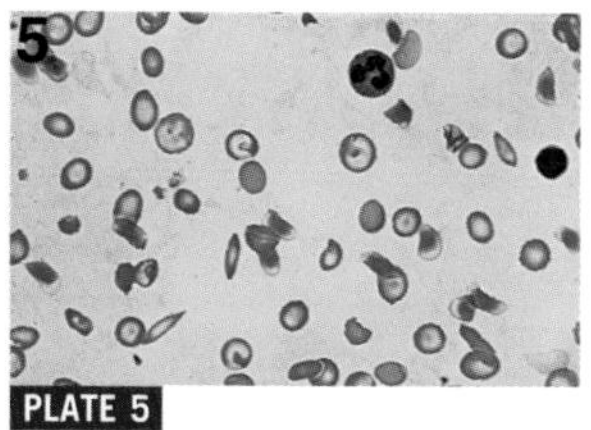

PLATE 5

Hemoglobin SS disease. Sickled cells, target cells, hypochromia, poikilocytosis, Howell-Jolly bodies; nucleated RBCs common (not shown).

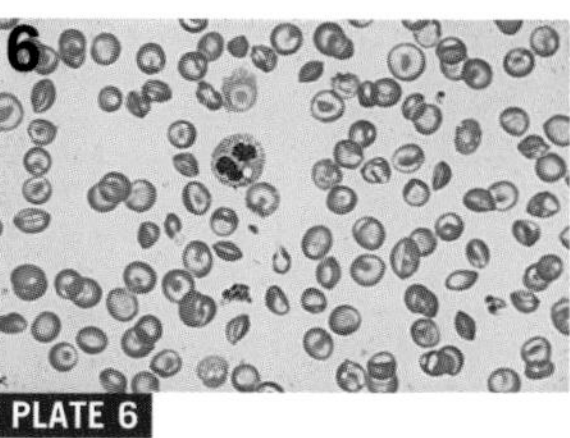

PLATE 6

Hemoglobin SC disease. Target cells, *oat cells*, poikilocytosis; sickle forms rarely seen.

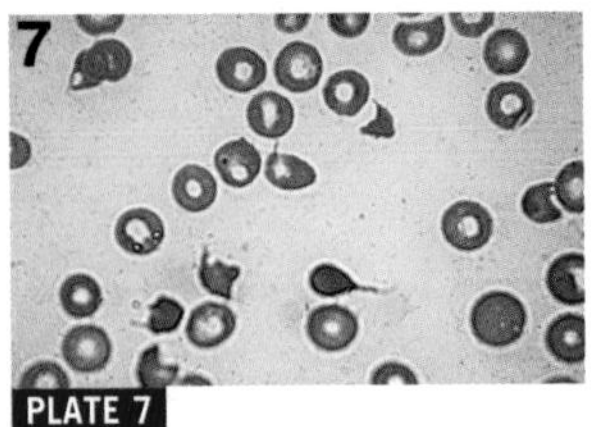

PLATE 7

Microangiopathic hemolytic anemia. RBC fragments, anisocytosis, polychromasia, decreased platelets.

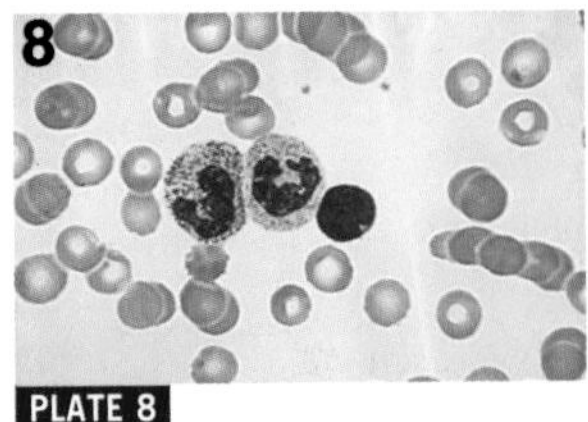

PLATE 8

Toxic granulations. Prominent dark blue primary granules; commonly seen with infection and other toxic states, such as Kawasaki disease.

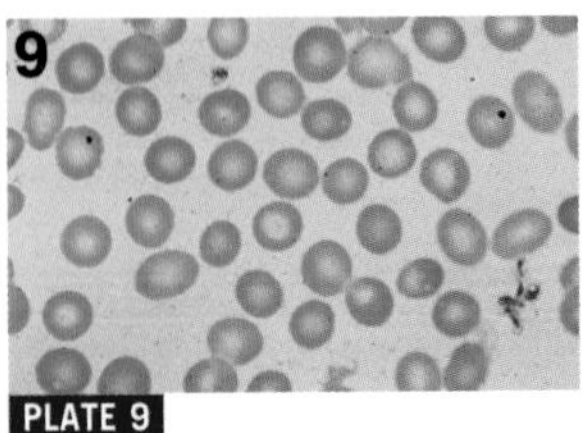

PLATE 9

Howell-Jolly body. Small, dense nuclear remnant in an RBC; suggests splenic dysfunction or asplenia.

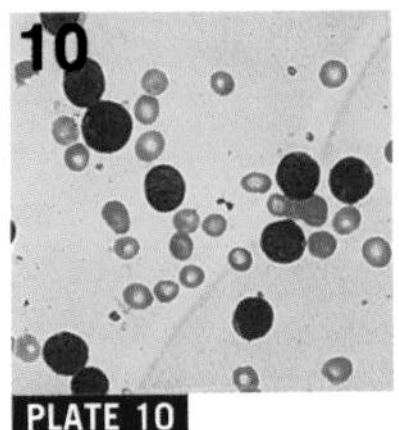

PLATE 10

Leukemic blasts showing large nucleus-to-cytoplasm ratio.

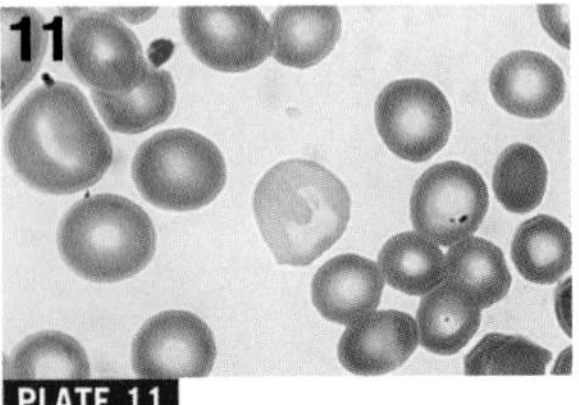

PLATE 11

Polychromatophilia. Diffusely basophilic because of RNA staining; seen with early release of reticulocytes from the marrow.

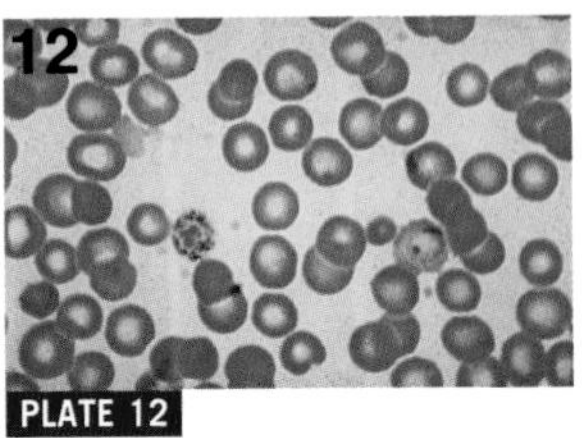

PLATE 12

Malaria. Intraerythrocytic parasites.

Coagulation Test	Preterm Infant (30–36 wk), Day of Life 1*	Term Infant, Day of Life 1	Day of Life 3	1 Month–1 yr	1–5 yr	6–10 yr	11–16 yr	Adult
COAGULATION INHIBITORS								
ATIII (U/mL)*	0.38 (0.14–0.62)	0.63 (0.39–0.97)			1.11 (0.82–1.39)	1.11 (0.90–1.31)	1.05 (0.77–1.32)	1.0 (0.74–1.26)
α_2 –M (U/mL)*	1.10 (0.56–1.82)	1.39 (0.95–1.83)			1.69 (1.14–2.23)	1.69 (1.28–2.09)	1.56 (0.98–2.12)	0.86 (0.52–1.20)
C1-Inh (U/mL)*	0.65 (0.31–0.99)	0.72 (0.36–1.08)			1.35 (0.85–1.83)	1.14 (0.88–1.54)	1.03 (0.68–1.50)	1.0 (0.71–1.31)
α_2 –AT (U/mL)*	0.90 (0.36–1.44)	0.93 (0.49–1.37)			0.93 (0.39–1.47)	1.00 (0.69–1.30)	1.01 (0.65–1.37)	0.93 (0.55–1.30)
Protein C (U/mL)	0.28 (0.12–0.44)	0.32 (0.24–0.40)	0.33 (0.24–0.51)	0.77 (0.28–1.24)	0.94 (0.50–1.34)	0.94 (0.64–1.25)	0.88 (0.59–1.12)	1.03 (0.54–1.66)
Protein S (U/mL)	0.26 (0.14–0.38)	0.36 (0.28–0.47)	0.49 (0.33–0.67)	1.02 (0.29–1.62)	1.01 (0.67–1.36)	1.09 (0.64–1.54)	1.03 (0.65–1.40)	0.75 (0.54–1.03)
FIBRINOLYTIC SYSTEM*								
Plasminogen (U/mL)	1.70 (1.12–2.48)	1.95 (1.60–2.30)			0.98 (0.78–1.18)	0.92 (0.75–1.08)	0.86 (0.68–1.03)	0.99 (0.7–1.22)
TPA (ng/mL)					2.15 (1.0–4.5)	2.42 (1.0–5.0)	2.16 (1.0–4.0)	4.90 (1.40–8.40)
α_2–AP (U/mL)	0.78 (0.4–1.16)	0.85 (0.70–1.0)			1.05 (0.93–1.17)	0.99 (0.89–1.10)	0.98 (0.78–1.18)	1.02 (0.68–1.36)
PAI (U/mL)					5.42 (1.0–10.0)	6.79 (2.0–12.0)	6.07 (2.0–10.0)	3.60 (0–11.0)

*Data from Andrew M et al: Development of the human anticoagulant system in the healthy premature infant. Blood 1987;70:165–172; Andrew M et al: Development of the human anticoagulant system in the healthy premature infant. Blood 1988;72:1651–1657; and Andrew M et al: Maturation of the hemostatic system during childhood. Blood 1992;8:1998–2005.

†aPTT values may vary depending on reagent.

α_2–AP, α_2–Antiplasmin; α_2–AT, α_2–antitrypsin; α_2–M, α_2–macroglobulin; aPTT, activated partial thromboplastin time; ATIII, antithrombin III; FDPs, fibrin degradation products; HMWK, high-molecular-weight kininogen; INR, international normalized ratio; PAI, plasminogen activator inhibitor; PK, prekallikrein; PT, prothrombin time; TPA, tissue plasminogen activator; VIII, factor VIII procoagulant; vWF, von Willebrand factor.

Adapted from Monagle et al: Developmental haemostasis. Impact for clinical haemostasis laboratories. Thromb Haemost 2006;95;362–372.

BOX 14-2

HYPERCOAGULABLE CONDITIONS

Congenital

Protein C and S deficiency: Hereditary, autosomal dominant disorder. Heterozygotes have threefold to sixfold increased risk for venous thrombosis.

Antithrombin III deficiency: Hereditary, autosomal dominant disorder. Homozygotes die in infancy.

Factor V Leiden (activated protein C resistance): 2%–5% of whites are heterozygotes with fivefold to tenfold increased risk for venous thrombosis; 1 in 1,000 are homozygotes, with 80-fold to 100-fold increased risk for venous thrombosis.

Homocystinemia: Increased levels of homocystine associated with arterial and venous thromboses, often due to MTHFR abnormalities.

Others: Prothrombin mutation (*G20210A*), plasminogen abnormalities, fibrinogen abnormalities.

Acquired

Endothelial damage: Causes include vascular catheters, smoking, diabetes, hypertension, surgery, hyperlipidemia.

Hyperviscosity: Macroglobulinemia, polycythemia, sickle cell disease.

Antiphospholipid syndromes: Common in patients with systemic lupus erythematosus; can occur with infections or idiopathically. Associated with venous and arterial thromboses and spontaneous abortions.

Platelet activation: Caused by essential thrombocytosis, oral contraceptives, heparin-induced thrombocytopenia.

Others: Drugs, malignancy, liver disease, inflammatory disease such as inflammatory bowel disease, paroxysmal nocturnal hemoglobinuria, lipoprotein A.

MTHFR, Methyltetrahydrofolate reductase.

BOX 14-3

EXTENDED WORKUP FOR HYPERCOAGULABLE STATES*

Factors VIII, IX, XI
Activated protein C resistance assay (screening test for factor V Leiden)
Factor V Leiden (DNA-based assay for factor V Leiden)
Factor II 20210A (prothrombin mutation)
Homocysteine
Methyltetrahydrofolate reductase (MTHFR) genetic testing if homocysteine elevated
Dilute Russell viper venom test (antiphospholipid antibody syndrome)
Platelet neutralization procedure (lupus anticoagulant)
Anticardiolipin screening ELISA assay (anticardiolipin antibodies)
Protein C activity and antigen (protein C deficiency and dysfunction)
Protein S activity and antigen (protein S deficiency and dysfunction)
Antithrombin III activity and antigen (antithrombin III deficiency and dysfunction)
Plasminogen activity
Tissue plasminogen activator (TPA) antigen
Plasminogen activator inhibitor activity (PAI-1) measures activity of this TPA inhibitor
α_2–Antiplasmin activity (measures activity of this plasmin inhibitor)
Lipoprotein (a) (Lp(a)) promotes decreased fibrinolysis

*Where necessary, abnormality tested for is listed in parenthesis.
ELISA, Enzyme-linked immunosorbent assay.

c. The identification of one risk factor, such as an indwelling vascular catheter, does not preclude the search for others, especially when accompanied by a family or personal history of thrombosis
2. Treatment of thromboses:
a. Unfractionated heparin (UFH): Used for treatment for arterial or venous thromboembolism
   (1) See Table 14-8 for heparin bolus and drip adjustment guidelines for goal Heparin anti-Xa level range of 0.3–0.7 or aPTTr range of 1.5–2.5 (obtain CBC daily while on UFH infusion)

TABLE 14-8A

UNFRACTIONATED HEPARIN (UFH) INITIATION DOSING GUIDELINES FOR PEDIATRIC PATIENTS FOR GOAL ANTI-Xa LEVEL 0.3–0.7 U/mL OR aPTTr RANGE 1.5–2.5[10]

Age	Loading Dose	Initial Infusion Rate	Monitoring
Neonates and infants <1 year	75 units/kg IV (no bolus for stroke patients)	28 units/kg/hour	Obtain aPTTr or anti-Xa UFH activity 4 hours after loading dose and/or start of infusion. *Consider obtaining anti-Xa activity in neonates to confirm aPTTr is therapeutic*
Children ≥1 year old to 16 years old	75 units/kg IV (max dose = 7700 units) (no bolus for stroke patients)	20 units/kg/hour (max initial rate = 1650 units/hour)	Obtain aPTTr or anti-Xa UFH activity 4 hours after loading dose and/or start of infusion
Patients >16 years old	70 units/kg IV (max dose = 7700 units) (no bolus for stroke patients)	15 units/kg/hour (max initial rate = 1650 units/hour)	Obtain aPTTr or anti-Xa activity UFH 4 hours after loading dose and/or start of infusion

TABLE 14-8B

UNFRACTIONATED HEPARIN LABORATORY DOSE ADJUSTMENT ALGORITHM FOR GOAL aPTTr RANGE 1.5–2.5*,[10]

aPTTr	Bolus (units/kg)	Hold (minutes)	Rate Change (%)	Repeat aPTTr (hours)
<1.2	50	0	Increase 10%–20%	4 hours
1.2–1.4	0	0	Increase 10%	4 hours
1.5–2.5	0	0	0	4 hours until two consecutive values in range‡
2.6–3.2	0	0	Decrease 10%	6 hours
3.3–4	0	30–60	Decrease 10%–20%	6 hours
≥4.1†	0	60–120 until aPTTr <3.5	Decrease 15%–30%; restart when aPTTr <3.5	6 hours after infusion is restarted

14

TABLE 14-8C

ALTERNATIVE UNFRACTIONATED HEPARIN LABORATORY DOSE ADJUSTMENT ALGORITHM FOR GOAL ANTI-Xa UFH LEVEL OF 0.3–0.7 UNITS/mL[10]

Heparin Anti-Xa Activity	Bolus (units/kg)	Hold (minutes)	Rate Change (%)	Repeat Heparin Anti-Xa Activity (hours)
≤0.1	50	0	Increase 10%–20%	4 hours
0.2	0	0	Increase 10%	4 hours
0.3–0.7	0	0	0	4 hours until two consecutive values in range‡
0.8	0	0	Decrease 10%	6 hours
0.9–1.0	0	30–60	Decrease 10%–20%	6 hours
>1.0†	0	60–120 until anti-Xa UFH activity ≤1 unit/mL	Decrease 15%–30%; restart when anti-Xa UFH activity <1 unit/mL	6 hours after infusion restarted

NOTE: Obtain complete blood count (CBC) daily while on UFH infusion. If platelet count is >50% reduction from baseline consider hematology consult for heparin-induced thrombocytopenia (HIT).

*Assuming this reflects anti-Xa level of 0.3–0.7.

†Confirm that specimen was not drawn from heparinized line or same extremity as site of heparin.

‡Anti-Xa UFH activity every 4 hours until two consecutive anti-Xa UFH activities are in range, then check levels daily.

aPTTr, Activated partial thromboplastin time ratio.

From The Johns Hopkins Hospital Children's Center pediatric policies, procedures, and protocols general care (Policy Number GEN109), Baltimore, 2010.

NOTE: Table 14-8B is based on Johns Hopkins Hospital Children's Center policy prior to institution of monitoring anti-Xa levels instead of aPTTr.

(2) Heparin may be reversed with protamine
(3) Heparin therapy should continue for at least 5–7 days while initiating warfarin for treatment of venous thrombosis

b. Low-molecular-weight heparin (LMWH)[4,5]: LMWH is routinely used in children, although less studied and more costly than UFH. LMWH is administered subcutaneously, has a longer half-life, more predictable pharmacokinetics, and requires less monitoring. Also associated with lower risk for heparin-induced thrombocytopenia
   (1) Dose depends on preparation. See Formulary for enoxaparin dosage information
   (2) Monitor LMWH therapy by following anti-Xa activity. Therapeutic range is 0.5–1.0 U/mL for thrombosis treatment and 0.1–0.3 U/mL for prophylactic dosing. Anti-Xa activity should be drawn 4 hours after dose
   (3) LMWH-induced bleeding can be partially reversed with protamine. Consult hematologist for protamine reversal protocol

c. Warfarin: Used for long-term anticoagulation, although it carries significant risk for morbidity and mortality. Patient must receive heparin while initiating warfarin therapy secondary to hypercoagulability from decreased protein C and S levels

(1) Usually administered orally at an initiation dose for 1–2 days, followed by a daily dose sufficient to maintain the PT/INR in the desired range. Infants often require higher daily doses. In all patients, levels should be measured every 1–2 weeks. See Table 14-9 for dose adjustment guidelines and Table 14-10 for management of excessive anticoagulation

TABLE 14-9

ADJUSTMENT AND MONITORING OF WARFARIN TO MAINTAIN AN INTERNATIONAL NORMALIZED RATIO (INR) BETWEEN 2 AND 3*,[10]

I. Day 1 Initial Dosing

a. Newborn: For ages <3 months, there are limited data for the safety and efficacy of warfarin. Higher dose may be needed in neonates and infants.

b. Infants and children:
- If the baseline INR is 1–1.3, dose = 0.2 mg/kg/dose orally q24hr (max 7.5 mg/dose)‡
- If the baseline INR >1.3, liver dysfunction, postoperative cardiac Fontan procedure patients, NPO/poor nutrition, receiving broad spectrum antibiotics, receiving medications causing significant drug/drug interactions, receiving medications with CYP2C9 enzyme inhibition (e.g., amiodarone, metronidazole, fluconazole, Bactrim), or slow metabolizer of warfarin, dose = 0.1 mg/kg/dose q24 hours (max 5 mg/dose)

II. Days 2–4

Dose Adjustment for Goal INR of 2–3			
Day 2		**Day 3 and 4**	
INR Level	**Action**	**INR Level**	**Action**
1.1–1.3	Repeat initial dose	1.1–1.3	Repeat initial dose*
1.4–1.9	50% of initial dose	1.4–1.9	50% of initial dose*
≥2	Hold dose for 24 hours, then restart at 50% of initial dose	2–3	50% of initial dose†
		3.1–3.5	25% of initial dose†
		>3.5	Hold dose until INR <3.5 then restart at 50% of previous dose†

III. Day 5 and Maintenance

Maintenance Dosing	
	≥5 Days
INR Level	**Action**
1.1–1.4	Increase weekly dose by 20%
1.5–1.9	Increase weekly dose by 10%
2–3	Continue current dose
3.1–3.5	Decrease weekly dose by 10%
>3.5	Hold dose, recheck INR daily until INR <3.5 then restart at 20% less than previous dose

*If INR is not >1.5 on day 4, the patient should be reassessed and dose/kg should be adjusted on an individual basis.

†Consult pediatric hematology for patient-specific recommendations on reduced dosing.

‡The reported average daily dose to maintain INR of 2–3 for infants is 0.33 mg/kg, for adolescents 0.09 mg/kg, and for adults from 0.04–0.08 mg/kg.

Adapted from The Johns Hopkins Hospital Children's Center pediatric policies, procedures, and protocols general care (Policy Number GEN069), Baltimore, 2010.

14

TABLE 14-10

MANAGEMENT OF EXCESSIVE WARFARIN ANTICOAGULATION

INR <5 without serious bleeding	Hold warfarin Recheck INR daily When INR approaches therapeutic range, resume warfarin at lower dose and follow INR daily*
INR ≥5 but <8 without serious bleeding	Hold warfarin Recheck INR every 12–24 hours If high risk for bleeding, consider low dose of vitamin K oral or IV (30 mcg/kg for patients <40 kg in weight; 1–2.5 mg for patients >40 kg) When INR approaches therapeutic range, resume warfarin at a lower dose*
INR ≥8 without serious bleeding	Hold warfarin Recheck INR every 6–12 hours. Give vitamin K oral or IV (30 mcg/kg for patients <40 kg in weight; 1–2.5 mg for patients >40 kg). INR reduction expected to occur within 12–24 hours with IV or 24–48 hours with oral vitamin K. Repeat vitamin K as necessary When INR approaches therapeutic range, resume warfarin at a lower dose*
Serious bleeding at any INR elevation	Hold warfarin Monitor INR every 6 hours Give vitamin K IV (2.5–5 mg). Vitamin K may be repeated as needed Consider use of FFP (10–15 mL/kg IV), Recombinant factor VIIa (16 mcg/kg IV), or prothrombinase complex concentrate, or rhFVIIa (Novoseven) IV Restart warfarin when INR approaches therapeutic range and when clinically appropriate at a lower dose*
Life-threatening bleeding at any INR	Hold warfarin Monitor INR every 2–4 hours Administer vitamin K IV at 5 to 10 mg. Repeat vitamin K as needed Transfuse FFP (10–15 mL/kg IV), consider rhFVIIa (Novoseven), or prothrombinase complex concentrate Restart warfarin when INR approaches therapeutic range and when clinically appropriate at a lower dose*

*Refer to Table 14-9.

NOTE: Always evaluate for bleeding risks and potential drug interactions.

FFP, fresh frozen plasma; INR, international normalized ratio; IV, intravenous, rhVIIa, Activated recombinant human factor VII.

Adapted from The Johns Hopkins Hospital Children's Center pediatric policies, procedures, and protocols general care (Policy Number GEN069), Baltimore, 2010.

(2) Efficacy is greatly affected by dietary intake of vitamin K. Patients should receive appropriate dietary education

(3) See Box 14-4 for a list of medicines that influence warfarin therapy

d. Anticoagulant therapy alters many coagulation tests

(1) Heparin alters aPTT, thrombin time, heparin level (anti-Xa), dilute Russell Viper Venom test (dRVVT), and mixing studies

BOX 14-4

MEDICATIONS THAT INFLUENCE WARFARIN THERAPY*

Significant Increase in the INR	**Significant Decrease in the INR**
Amiodarone	Amobarbital
Anabolic steroids	Aprepitant
Bactrim (TMP/SMZ)	Butabarbital
Chloramphenicol	Carbamazepine
Disulfiram	Dicloxacillin
Fluconazole	Griseofulvin
Isoniazid	Methimazole
Metronidazole	Phenobarbital
Miconazole	Phenytoin
Phenylbutazone	Primidone
Quinidine	Propylthiouracil
Sulfinpyrazone	Rifabutin
Sulfisoxazole	Rifampin
Tamoxifen	Secobarbital
Moderate Increase in the INR	**Moderate Decrease in the INR**
Cimetidine	Atazanavir
Ciprofloxacin	Efavirenz
Clarithromycin	Nafcillin
Delavirdine	Ritonavir
Efavirenz	
Itraconazole	
Lovastatin	
Omeprazole	
Propafenone	
Ritonavir	

*Numerous medications not listed in this table can affect warfarin administration.
INR, International normalized ratio; TMP/SMZ, trimethoprim/sulfamethoxazole.

14

(2) Warfarin alters PT, aPTT, dRVVT, and vitamin K–dependent factors (II, VII, IX, X, protein C and S)

e. Consult a hematologist for thrombolytic therapy

NOTE: Children receiving anticoagulation therapy should be protected from trauma. Intramuscular injections are contraindicated. The use of antiplatelet agents and arterial punctures should be avoided.

C. Bleeding Disorders (Fig. 14-3 and Box 14-5)

1. Differential diagnosis of bleeding disorders (Tables 14-11 and Box 14-5)
2. Desired factor replacement goals in hemophilia (Table 14-12)

VI. BLOOD COMPONENT REPLACEMENT

A. Blood Volume

Requirements are age specific (Table 14-13).

Text continued on page 348

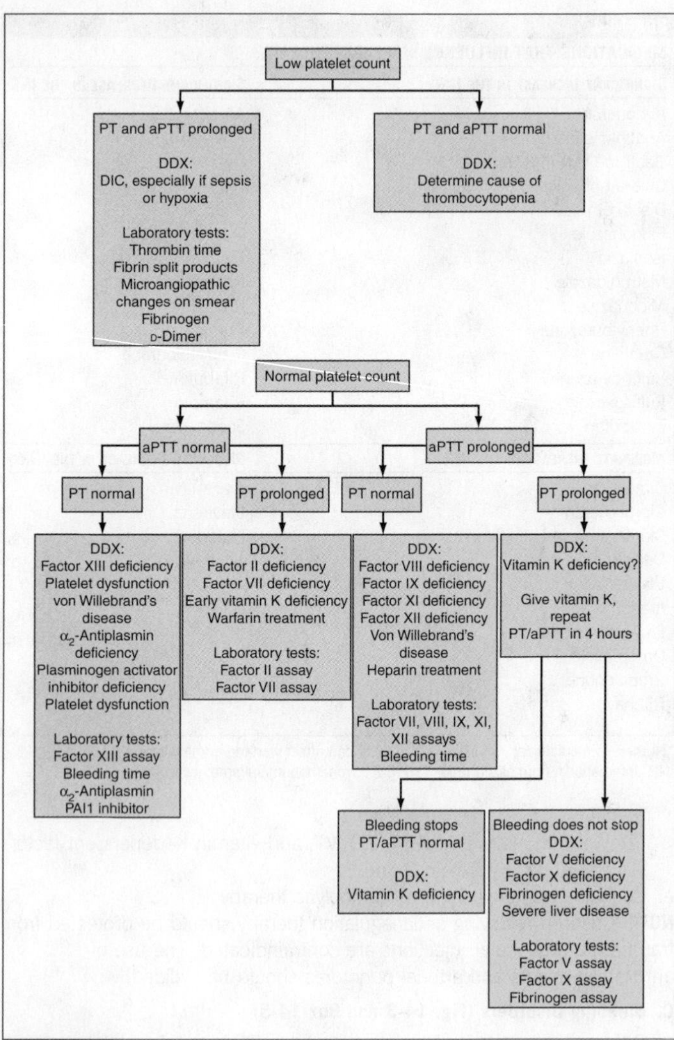

FIGURE 14-3

Differential diagnosis of bleeding disorders.

BOX 14-5

BLEEDING DISORDERS

Congenital	Acquired
Disorder of platelet number or function **Thrombocytopenia:** Secondary to bone marrow disease or defective megakaryocyte maturation. **Disorders of platelet function:** Bernard-Soulier syndrome, Glanzmann thrombasthenia, storage pool diseases **Factor VIII deficiency:** See Table 14-11 **Factor IX deficiency:** See Table 14-11 **von Willebrand disease:** See Table 14-11	**Disseminated intravascular coagulation:** Characterized by prolonged PT and aPTT, decreased fibrinogen and platelets, increased fibrin degradation products, and elevated D-dimer. Treatment includes identifying and treating underlying disorder. Replacement of depleted coagulation factors with FFP may be necessary in severe cases, especially when bleeding is present; 10–15 mL/kg will raise clotting factors 20%. Fibrinogen, if depleted, can be given as cryoprecipitate. Platelet transfusions may also be necessary. **Liver disease:** The liver is the major site of synthesis of factors V, VII, IX, X, XI, XII, XIII, prothrombin, plasminogen, fibrinogen, protein C and S, and ATIII. Treatment with FFP and platelets may be needed, but this will increase hepatic protein load. Vitamin K should be given to patients with liver disease and clotting abnormalities. **Vitamin K deficiency:** Factors II, VII, IX, X, protein C, and protein S are vitamin K dependent. Early vitamin K deficiency may present with isolated prolonged PT because factor VII has the shortest half-life. Fibrinogen should be normal. **Hemolytic-uremic syndrome/thrombotic thrombocytopenic purpura (HUS/TTP):** Characterized by the triad of microangiopathic hemolytic anemia, uremia, and thrombocytopenia. HUS is often triggered by bacterial enteritis, especially caused by *Escherichia coli* O157:H7, although there are a variety of causes. HUS does not typically include coagulation abnormalities, such as those seen in DIC. Avoid blood products in patients with HUS thought to be secondary to pneumococcal infection. TTP includes the triad of HUS in addition to fever and CNS changes and is more common in older adolescents and adults.

aPTT, Activated partial thromboplastin time; CNS, central nervous system; DIC, disseminated intravascular coagulation; FFP, fresh frozen plasma; PT, prothrombin time.

TABLE 14-11

COMMON BLEEDING DISORDERS

Factor VIII deficiency (hemophilia A)*	Characteristics: X-linked recessive, prolonged aPTT, reduced factor VIII activity, normal PT and BT Treatment: a. Treat with factor VIII concentrate, preferably recombinant Factor VIII to reduce risk of infection b. Factor level recovers by 2% per 1 unit of factor VIII per kg of body weight (Refer to Table 14-12) c. First dose has shorter half-life, so if redosing needed, second dose should be given after 4–8 hr. Subsequent doses can be given every 12 hr d. Continuous infusion often desirable, e.g., for surgical patients or prolonged therapy, usually require 50 U/kg loading dose, followed by 3–5 U/kg/hr e. For suspected intracranial bleeding, replace to 100% **before** diagnostic procedure (e.g., CT scan) f. Units of factor VIII = weight (kg) × desired % replacement × 0.5
Factor IX deficiency (hemophilia B or Christmas disease)*	Characteristics: X-linked recessive, prolonged aPTT, reduced factor IX activity Treatment: a. Treat with Factor IX concentrate, preferably recombinant to reduce risk of infection b. Factor level usually recovers by 1% for each unit of factor IX concentrate per kg of body weight c. Half-life of factor IX 18–24 hr. Similar to factor VIII, if second dose is needed, it should be given at a shorter interval d. Recombinant factor IX has a shorter half-life; consider evaluation of in vivo factor survival in patient e. Replace to 100% **before** diagnostic procedure if intracranial bleeding is suspected f. Units of factor IX = weight (kg) × desired % replacement (may be advisable to multiply by 1.2 for recombinant factor IX)

von Willebrand disease	Characteristics: vWF binds platelets to subendothelial surfaces and carries and stabilizes factor VIII Type 1: Decreased quantity vWF, may have an identifiable gene mutation, decreased ristocetin cofactor activity, but proportional to vWF, and mild to moderate bleeding. Prolonged BT, normal platelet count, mild to moderate prolongation of aPTT. Type 2: Characterized by four subtypes, all with various functional abnormalities of vWF, marked decrease in ristocetin cofactor activity compared to decrease in vWF, and moderate to severe bleeding. Type 3: More severe decrease in vWF and factor VIII secondary to genetic mutations and severe bleeding. Treatment: a. In patients with proven response to DDAVP (desmopressin acetate), bleeding or minor surgical procedures can be treated with DDAVP IV over 20–30 min, or intranasally b. DDAVP may be contraindicated in vWf type 2b, because it may exacerbate thrombocytopenia c. For more severe disease or patients with dysfunctional vWF (type 2), treatment of choice is Humate P (heat inactivated vWF-enriched concentrate: 40 IU/kg), a similar product containing active vWF, or cryoprecipitate. Concentrates are preferred because they are virally inactivated d. Aminocaproic acid 100 mg/kg IV or PO every 4–6 hr (up to 24 g/day) may be useful for treatment of oral bleeding and as prophylaxis for dental extraction

*All patients with hemophilia should be vaccinated with Hepatitis A and B vaccines.

aPTT, Activated partial thromboplastin time; BT, bleeding time; IV, intravenous; PO, per os; PT, prothrombin time; vWF, von Willebrand factor.

14

TABLE 14-12

DESIRED FACTOR REPLACEMENT IN HEMOPHILIA

Bleeding Site	Desired Level (%)
Joint or simple hematoma	20–70
Simple dental extraction	50
Major soft tissue bleed	80–100
Serious oral bleeding	80–100
Head injury	100+
Major surgery (dental, orthopedic, other)	100+

NOTE: A hematologist should be consulted for all major bleeding and before surgery.

TABLE 14-13

ESTIMATED BLOOD VOLUME (EBV)

Age	Total Blood Volume (mL/kg)
Preterm infants	90–105
Term newborns	78–86
1–12 mo	73–78
1–3 yr	74–82
4–6 yr	80–86
7–18 yr	83–90
Adults	68–88

Data from Nathan D, Oski FA: Hematology of infancy and childhood. Philadelphia, WB Saunders, 1998.

B. Blood Product Components

1. RBCs: The decision to transfuse RBCs should be made with consideration of clinical symptoms and signs, the degree of cardiorespiratory or central nervous system (CNS) disease, the cause and course of anemia, and options for alternative therapy, noting the risks for transfusion-associated infections and reactions.

a. Packed RBC (PRBC) transfusion: Concentrated RBCs, with HCT of 55%–70%. A typed and cross-matched blood product is preferred when possible; O-negative (or O-positive) blood may be used if transfusion cannot be delayed. O-negative is preferred for females of child-bearing age to reduce risk for Rh sensitization

(1) Unless rapid replacement is required for acute blood loss or shock, infuse no faster than 2–3 mL/kg/hr (generally 10–15 mL/kg aliquots over 4 hr) to avoid congestive heart failure

(2) A rule of thumb in severe compensated anemia is to give an X mL/kg aliquot, where X = patient Hb (g/dL); for example, if Hb = 5 g/dL, transfuse 5 mL/kg over 4 hours

(3) To calculate the volume of PRBC to achieve a desired HCT, use the following equation:

$$\text{Volume of PRBCs (mL)} = \frac{\text{EBV (mL)} \times (\text{desired HCT} - \text{actual HCT})}{\text{HCT of PRBCs}}$$

where EBV is the estimated blood volume (see Table 14-13 for age-specific EBV) and HCT of PRBCs is usually 55%–70%

(4) A unit of blood is 500 mL, but approximately 300 mL after processing without significant loss of red cells. This may vary with type of diluents used and time of storage, due to red cell compaction

b. Leukocyte-poor PRBCs:
   (1) Filtered RBCs: 99.9% of WBCs removed from product; used for cytomegalovirus (CMV)-negative patients to reduce risk for CMV transmission. Also reduces likelihood of a nonhemolytic febrile transfusion reaction
   (2) Washed RBCs: 92%–95% of WBCs removed from product. Similar advantages to leukocyte-poor filtered RBCs. Although filtered leukocyte-poor blood is now more commonly used, washing may be helpful if a patient has pre-existing antibodies to blood products (e.g., patients who have complete IgA deficiency or a history of urticarial transfusion reactions)
c. Irradiated blood products:
   (1) Many blood products (PRBCs, platelet preparations, leukocytes, fresh frozen plasma [FFP], and others) contain viable lymphocytes capable of proliferation and engraftment in the recipient, causing graft-versus-host disease (GVHD). Irradiation with 1500 cGy before transfusion may prevent GVHD but does not prevent antibody formation against donor white cells. Engraftment most likely in young infants, immunocompromised patients, and patients receiving blood from first-degree relatives
   (2) Indications: Intensive chemotherapy, leukemia, lymphoma, bone marrow transplantation, solid organ transplantation, known or suspected immune deficiencies, intrauterine transfusions, and transfusions in neonates
d. CMV-negative blood: Obtained from donors who test negative for CMV. May be given to neonates or other immunocompromised patients, including those awaiting organ or marrow transplant who are CMV negative

2. Platelets: Indicated to treat severe or symptomatic thrombocytopenia. Should not be refrigerated because this promotes premature platelet activation and clumping. Bacteremia secondary to contamination more common than with refrigerated blood product

a. Single-donor product: Preferred over pooled concentrate for patients with antiplatelet antibodies
b. Leukocyte-poor: Use if there is a history of significant acute, febrile platelet transfusion reactions
c. Usually give 4 U/m^2, or approximately 10 mL/kg of normally concentrated platelet product. The platelet count is raised by 10,000 to 15,000/μL by giving 1 U/m^2. For infants and children, 10 mL/kg will increase the platelet count by approximately 50,000/μL
d. Hemorrhagic complications are rare with platelet counts >20,000/μL. A transfusion *trigger* of 10,000/μL is recommended by many in the

absence of serious bleeding complications. A platelet count >50,000/μL is advisable for minor procedures; >100,000/μL is advisable for major surgery or intracranial operation

e. Usually unit = 50 mL after processing, ≥5.5 × 10^{11} plt/unit

3. FFP: Contains all clotting factors except platelets. Used in severe clotting factor deficiencies with active bleeding or in combination with vitamin K to achieve rapid reversal of effects of warfarin. Also replaces anticoagulant factors (antithrombin III, protein C, protein S). Used in treatment of DIC, vitamin K deficiency with active bleeding, or thrombotic thrombocytopenic purpura (TTP). One milliliter of FFP expected to provide 1 unit of activity of all factors except labile factor V and VIII, but individual units may vary. The usual amount is 10 to 15 mL/kg; repeat doses as needed. In acquired TTP, plasma exchange is the treatment of choice. Usually unit = 250–300 mL after processing
4. Cryoprecipitate: Enriched for factor VIII (5–10 U/mL), vWF, and fibrinogen. Historically useful for children with factor VIII or vWF deficiency in the context of active bleeding, but concentrates or recombinant products now preferred because of lower risk for viral transmission. Useful for raising fibrinogen when small volumes are required. Usually unit = 10–15 mL after processing (80 units factor VIII and 250 mg fibrinogen)
5. Monoclonal factor VIII: Highly purified factor, derived from pooled human blood
6. Recombinant factor VIII or IX: Highly purified, with less theoretical infectious risk than pooled human products. There is risk for inhibitor formation, as with other products

C. PRBC Exchange Transfusion

1. Partial PRBC exchange transfusion may be indicated for sickle cell patients with acute chest syndrome, stroke, intractable pain crisis, or refractory priapism. Replace with Sickledex-negative cells. Follow HCT carefully during transfusion to avoid hyperviscosity, maintaining HCT <35%
2. Indications for double packed volume PRBC exchange transfusion include severe acute chest and cerebrovascular accident (CVA). This is based on twice the patient's calculated packed cell volume. Goal is to reduce percentage of HbS to <30%. Expected reduction in percentage of circulating sickle cells is 60%–80%
3. To calculate the volume of PRBC needed for a double-volume exchange, use the following equation:

$$\frac{\text{EBV (mL)} \times \text{Patient HCT} \times 2}{\text{HCT of PRBC}}$$

where EBV is the age-dependent estimated blood volume (see Table 14-13) and HCT of PRBC is 55%–70%

D. Complications of Transfusions

1. Acute transfusion reactions:
 a. Acute hemolytic reaction: Most often the result of blood group incompatibility. Signs and symptoms include fever, chills, tachycardia, hypotension, and shock. Treatment includes immediate cessation of blood transfusion and institution of supportive measures. Laboratory findings include DIC, hemoglobinuria, and positive Coombs test
 b. Febrile nonhemolytic reaction: Usually the result of host antibody response to donor leukocyte antigens, common in previously transfused patients. Symptoms include fever, chills, and diaphoresis. Stop transfusion and evaluate. Prevention includes premedication with antipyretics, antihistamines, corticosteroids, and, if necessary, use of leukocyte-poor PRBCs
 c. Urticarial reaction: Reaction to donor plasma proteins. Stop transfusion immediately; treat with antihistamines, and epinephrine and steroids if there is respiratory compromise (see also treatment of anaphylaxis, Chapter 1). Use washed or filtered RBCs with the next transfusion
 d. Evaluation of acute transfusion reaction:
  (1) Patient's urine: Test for hemoglobin
  (2) Patient's blood: Confirm blood type, screen for antibodies, and repeat direct Coombs test (DCT) on pretransfusion and posttransfusion sera
  (3) Donor blood: Culture for bacteria
2. Delayed transfusion reaction: Usually due to minor blood group antigen incompatibility with low or absent titer of antibodies at time of transfusion. Occurs 3–10 days after transfusion. Symptoms include fatigue, jaundice, and dark urine. Laboratory findings include anemia, a positive Coombs test, new RBC antibodies, and hemoglobinuria. The need for acute intervention is much less likely than with acute reactions
3. Transmission of infectious diseases[6,11]: Blood supply is tested for HIV types 1 and 2, HTLV types I and II, hepatitis B, hepatitis C, syphilis, and West Nile virus. Data from *2009 Red Book*, estimates the risk for transmitting infection (estimated per unit) as follows: HIV (1 in 2,000,000); HTLV (1 in 641,000); hepatitis B (1 in 63,000–500,000); hepatitis C (1 in 100,000); parvovirus (1 in 10,000). CMV, hepatitis A, parasitic, tick-borne, and prion diseases may also be transmitted by blood products
4. Sepsis: Sepsis occurs with products that are contaminated with bacteria, particularly platelets, because they are stored at room temperature. Risk for transmitting bacteria in PRBCs is 1 in 5 million units and in platelets is 1 in 100,000

E. Reasons Not to Consider a Directed Donor

1. Donors less likely to be truthful about risk
2. Increase risk of transfusion related GVHD if from a relative
3. Can alloimmunize if potential bone marrow donor

F. Reasons to Consider a Directed Donor

1. Chronic transfusion programs (e.g., thalassemia or sickle cell disease), where donors provide antigen-matched red cells repetitively for the same patient
2. NAIT, where maternal platelets lack causative antigens and represent optimal therapy

VII. INTERPRETING BLOOD SMEARS

See Color Plates 1 to 12 in this chapter for examples of blood smears. Examine the blood smear in an area where the RBCs are nearly touching but do not overlap.

A. RBC

Examine size, shape, and color.

B. WBC

A rough estimate of the WBC count can be made by looking at the smear under high power (100× magnification). Each one cell per high-power field correlates with approximately 500 WBC/mm^3 (20× magnification).

C. Platelets

A rough estimate of platelet count is one platelet per high power field corresponds to 10,000–15,000/μL. Platelet clumps usually indicate >100,000 platelets/μL.

REFERENCES

1. American Academy of Pediatrics, Section on Hematology/Oncology Committee on Genetics. Health supervision in children with sickle cell disease. *Pediatrics.* 2002;109:526–535.
2. Driscoll MC. Sickle cell disease. *Pediatr Rev.* 2007;28:259–268.
3. Bennett CM, Rogers ZR, Kinnamon DD, et al. Prospective phase 1/2 study of rituximab in childhood and adolescent chronic immune thrombocytopenic purpura. *Blood.* 2006;107:2639–2642.
4. Streiff MB, Kickler TS. *The Johns Hopkins Hospital hemostatic testing and antithrombotic therapy manual*, 3rd ed. Baltimore, 2007.
5. The Johns Hopkins Hospital Children's Center pediatric policies, procedures, and protocols general care, Baltimore, 2010.
6. Red Book. *2009 Report of the Committee on Infectious Diseases*, 28th ed. Elk Grove Village, IL: American Academy of Pediatrics; 2009.
7. Strouse JJ, Takemoto CM, Keefer JR, et al. Corticosteroids and increased risk of readmission after acute chest syndrome in children with sickle cell disease. *Pediatr Blood Cancer.* 2008;50:1006–1012.
8. Hulbert ML, Scothorn DJ, Panepinto JA, et al. Exchange blood transfusion for first overt stroke is associated with a lower risk of subsequent stroke than simple transfusion: a retrospective cohort of 137 children with sickle cell anemia. *J Pediatr.* 2006;149:710–712.
9. Brawley OW, Cornelius LJ, Edwards LR, et al. National Institutes of Health Consensus Development Conference statement: hydroxyurea treatment for sickle cell disease. *Ann Intern Med.* 2008;148:932–938.

10. Monagle P, Chalmers E, Chan A, et al. Antithrombotic therapy in neonates and children. American College of Chest Physicians evidence-based clinical practice guidelines, 8th ed. *Chest.* 2008;133:887–968.
11. Red Cross Blood Testing. www.redcrossblood.org. Accessed December 10, 2010.

Chapter 15

Immunology and Allergy

Wonha Kim, MD

I. ALLERGIC RHINITIS[1–8]

A. Epidemiology

1. Most common chronic condition
2. Significant impact on quality of life including school performance and sleep patterns as demonstrated in multiple studies
3. Increases risk for recurrent otitis media and acute and chronic sinusitis
4. Risk factors: Atopic family history, serum IgE >100 IU/mL before age 6 years, higher socioeconomic status

B. Diagnosis

1. **History:**
   a. Symptoms: Nasal (congestion, rhinorrhea, pruritus), ocular (pruritus, tearing), postnasal drip (sore throat, cough, pruritus)
   b. Patterns: Seasonal (depending on local allergens) vs. perennial
   c. Coexisting atopic diseases common (eczema, asthma, food allergy)
2. **Physical examination:**
   a. *Allergic facies* with shiners, mouth breathing, transverse nasal crease
   b. Nasal mucosa may be normal to pink to pale gray
   c. Injected sclera with or without clear discharge, conjunctival cobblestoning
3. **Diagnostic studies:**
   a. Skin testing: Gold standard
   b. Total immunoglobulin E (IgE): Nonspecific. Limited value
   c. Peripheral blood eosinophil count
   d. Nasal smear for eosinophils: Quick, easy screen with good positive predictive value
   e. Radioallergosorbent testing (RAST): Identifies presence of serum IgE to selected antigens
   f. Imaging studies: Not useful
   g. Consider sleep study to evaluate for obstructive sleep apnea and pulmonary function tests (PFT) to evaluate for asthma

C. Differential Diagnosis

1. Vasomotor rhinitis: Symptoms made worse by scents, alcohol or changes in temperature or humidity
2. Episodic rhinitis: Allergic nasal symptoms elicited by sporadic exposures to inhalant aeroallergens
3. Adenoid hypertrophy

4. Rhinitis medicamentosa: Rebound rhinitis from prolonged use of nasal vasoconstrictors
5. Sinusitis: Acute or chronic
6. Nonallergic rhinitis with eosinophilia syndrome (NARES)
7. Nasal polyps

D. Treatment

1. **Allergen avoidance:**
   a. Relies on identification of triggers
   b. Difficult to avoid ubiquitous airborne allergens
   c. Thorough housecleaning and allergy-proof bed coverings can be useful
2. **Oral antihistamines** (diphenhydramine, cetirizine):
   a. First-line treatment
   b. Second-generation preparations preferable (loratadine, desloratadine, fexofenadine, cetirizine, levocetirizine)
   c. Adverse effects: Sedation, anticholinergic side effects with first-generation products
3. **Intranasal corticosteroids** (fluticasone, mometasone, budesonide, flunisolide, ciclesonide, triamcinolone):
   a. Second-line treatment
   b. Most effective maintenance therapy for nasal congestion
   c. Minimal benefit for ocular symptoms
   d. No proven adverse effect on long-term growth
   e. Adverse effects: Nasal irritation, sneezing, bleeding
   f. Recognize the potential risk of adrenal suppression at high doses of inhaled or intranasal steroids
4. **Leukotriene inhibitors** (montelukast): Alone or in combination with antihistamines
5. **Mast cell stabilizers** (cromolyn):
   a. Inexpensive and easily available
   b. Most effective as prophylaxis
   c. Few adverse effects
6. **Intranasal antihistamines** (azelastine, olopatadine):
   a. Effective for acute symptoms
   b. Not studied in children younger than 5 years
   c. Adverse effects: Bitter taste, systemic absorption with sedation
7. **Anticholinergics** (ipratropium):
   a. Useful for rhinorrhea only
   b. Adverse effects: Drying of nasal mucosa
8. **Immunotherapy:**
   a. Success rate is high when patients are chosen carefully and when performed by an allergy specialist
   b. Consider when drug side effects are limiting or triggering allergens are difficult to avoid
   c. Not recommended in poorly compliant patients or those with asthma

d. Not well studied in children younger than 5 years
e. May reduce risk for future development of asthma
9. **Nasal rinsing with hypertonic saline:** Tolerable and inexpensive

II. FOOD ALLERGY[9–14]

A. Epidemiology

1. Prevalence is 6%–8% in pediatric population
2. Most common allergens in children: Milk, eggs, peanuts, tree nuts such as cashew and walnut, soy, wheat

B. Manifestations of Food Allergy: Often a Combination of Several Syndromes

1. **Anaphylaxis:** (See Chapter 1, Section IV)
2. **Skin syndromes:**
   a. Urticaria/angioedema:
      (1) Chronic urticaria is rarely related to food allergy
      (2) Acute urticaria predicts risk for future anaphylaxis
   b. Atopic dermatitis/eczema:
      (1) Food allergy more common in patients with atopic dermatitis
      (2) Acute and chronic skin changes often coexist
3. **Gastrointestinal syndromes:**
   a. Oral allergy syndrome:
      (1) Edema of oral mucosa after ingestion of certain fresh fruits and vegetables in patients with pollen allergies
      (2) Inciting antigens destroyed by cooking
      (3) Caused by cross-reactivity of antibodies to pollens
      (4) Rarely progresses beyond the mouth
   b. Allergic eosinophilic gastroenteritis, esophagitis:
      (1) May cause gastroesophageal reflux, abdominal pain, diarrhea, early satiety
      (2) Characterized by eosinophilic infiltration of digestive tract
   c. Food-induced enterocolitis:
      (1) Presents in infancy
      (2) Vomiting and diarrhea (may contain blood); when severe, may lead to lethargy, dehydration, hypotension, acidosis
      (3) Most commonly associated with milk, soy
   d. Infantile proctocolitis:
      (1) Confined to distal colon and presents with only diarrhea
      (2) Symptoms usually resolve within 72 hours of stopping offending agent; rarely leads to anemia
4. **Respiratory syndromes:**
   a. Rhinitis (See Section I)
   b. Asthma (See Chapter 24)
   c. Heiner syndrome:
      (1) Precipitating IgG antibody to cow's milk
      (2) Results in pulmonary infiltrates, hemosiderosis, anemia, recurrent pneumonia, and failure to thrive

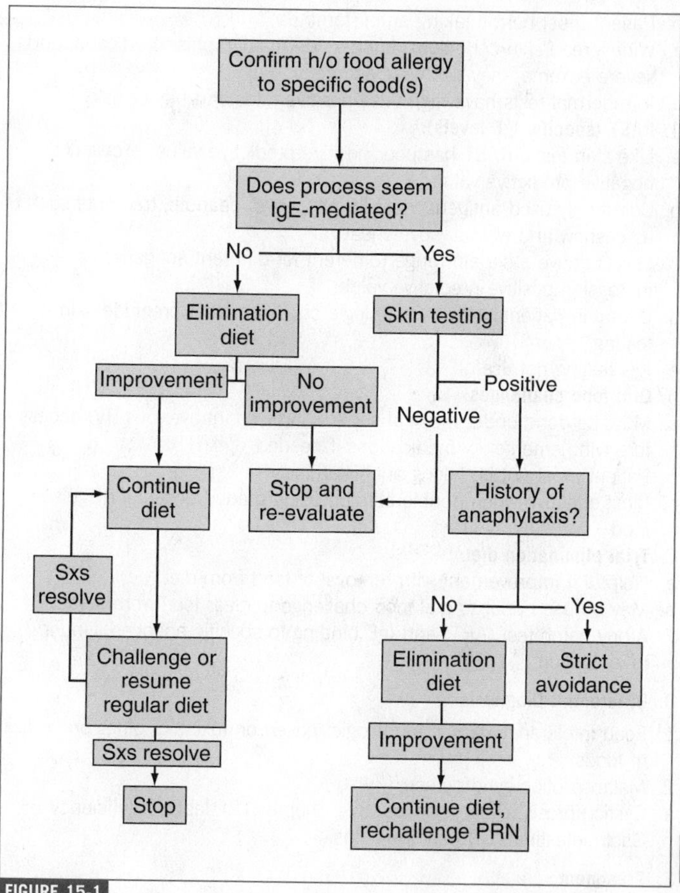

FIGURE 15-1

Evaluation and management of food allergy. *(Data from Wood RA: The natural history of food allergy. Pediatrics 2003;111[6]:1631–1637, and Wood RA: Up to Date 2009. http://www.uptodate.com.)*

15

C. Diagnosis of Food Allergy (Fig. 15-1)

1. **History:**
a. Identify specific foods and whether fresh vs. cooked
b. Establish timing and nature of reactions; patient should keep a food diary
2. **Physical examination**
3. **Skin testing:**
a. Skin prick test has poor positive predictive value, but very good negative predictive value

b. Patient must not be taking antihistamines
c. Widespread skin conditions, such as dermatographism, urticaria, and severe eczema, may decrease accuracy
d. Intradermal tests have high false-positive rates and higher risk

4. **RAST (specific IgE levels):**
a. Like skin tests, RAST has poor positive predictive value, excellent negative predictive value
b. Commonly used antigens include milk, eggs, peanuts, tree nuts such as cashew and walnut, soy, wheat
c. Levels above a certain range (different for different antigens) have increasing positive predictive value
d. Useful in patients with dermatologic conditions that preclude skin testing
e. IgG testing not useful

5. **Oral food challenges:**
a. Must be done under medical supervision with intravenous (IV) access for giving emergency medications if needed
b. Patient must not be taking antihistamines
c. Most effective when double-blinded using graded doses of disguised food

6. **Trial elimination diet:**
a. Helpful if improvement with removal of food from diet
b. May be used prior to oral food challenge to clear food from system

7. Atopy patch test (APT) and IgE binding to specific epitopes: Under investigation

D. Differential Diagnosis

1. Food intolerance: Nonimmunologic, based on toxins or other properties of foods
2. Malabsorption syndromes:
a. Cystic fibrosis, celiac disease (See Chapter 12), lactase deficiency
b. Gastrointestinal (GI) malformations

E. Treatment

1. **Allergen avoidance** is the most important intervention for all types of food allergy
a. Patients must pay close attention to food ingredients
b. Infants with milk, soy allergies may be placed on elemental formula
2. **For angioedema, urticaria:**
a. Antihistamines, corticosteroids
b. Broad differential
3. **Atopic dermatitis:** Symptomatic control (See Chapter 8)

F. Natural History

1. About one third of allergies are lost in a 1- to 2-year period (peanut, tree nut, and shellfish allergies are rarely outgrown)
2. Most likely to be outgrown with complete avoidance

3. Skin tests and RAST may remain positive even though symptoms resolve

III. PENICILLIN ALLERGY (FIG. 15-2)[15]

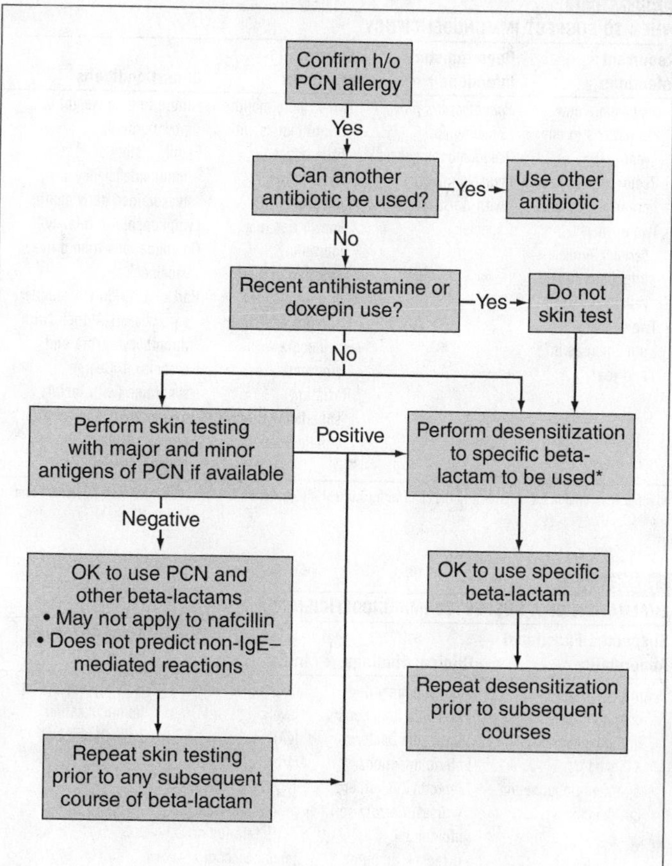

* May be performed orally (preferred) or parenterally, and multiple protocols are available. Should be done in an ICU setting where adverse reactions can be managed.

FIGURE 15-2

Evaluation and management of penicillin allergy. *(Adapted from Solensky R: Allergy to penicillins. Up to Date 2009. http://www.uptodate.com.)*

15

IV. EVALUATION OF A SUSPECTED IMMUNODEFICIENCY (TABLES 15-1 AND 15-2)[16–23]

TABLE 15-1

WHEN TO SUSPECT IMMUNODEFICIENCY

Recurrent Infections	Opportunistic Infections	Severe Infections	Other Conditions
Six or more new infections in one year Recurrent tissue or organ abscesses Two or more serious sinus infections in one year Two or more pneumonias in one year	*Pneumocystis jiroveci* pneumonia Pseudomonas sepsis Invasive infection with *Neisseria* species	Two or more months of antibiotics with little effect Sepsis in the absence of a known risk (e.g., indwelling vascular catheter or neutropenia) Bacterial meningitis Pneumonia with empyema Resistant superficial or oral candidiasis	Failure to gain weight or grow normally Family history of immunodeficiency or unexplained early deaths Lymphopenia in infancy Complications from a live vaccine Part of a syndrome complex: e.g., Wiskott-Aldrich (with thrombocytopenia and eczema), DiGeorge syndrome (with facial dysmorphism, congenital cardiac disease and hypoparathyroidism)

Adapted from Stiehm ER: Approach to the child with recurrent infections. Up to Date 2009. http://www.uptodate.com.

TABLE 15-2

EVALUATION OF A SUSPECTED IMMUNODEFICIENCY

Suspected Functional Abnormality	Clinical Findings	Initial Tests	More Advanced Tests
Antibody (e.g., common variable immunodeficiency, X-linked agammaglobulinemia, IgA deficiency)	Sinopulmonary and systemic infections (pyogenic bacteria) Enteric infections (enterovirus, other viruses, *Giardia* sp.) Autoimmune diseases (immune thrombocytopenia, hemolytic anemia, inflammatory bowel disease)	Immunoglobulin levels (IgG, IgM, IgA) Antibody levels to T-cell dependent protein antigens (e.g., tetanus or pneumococcal conjugate vaccines) Antibody levels to T-cell independent polysaccharide antigens in a child ≥2 yr (e.g., pneumococcal polysaccharide vaccine such as Pneumovax®)	B-cell enumeration Immunofixation electrophoresis

TABLE 15-2

EVALUATION OF A SUSPECTED IMMUNODEFICIENCY (Continued)

Suspected Functional Abnormality	Clinical Findings	Initial Tests	More Advanced Tests
Cell-mediated immunity (e.g., severe combined immunodeficiency, DiGeorge syndrome)	Pneumonia (pyogenic bacteria, fungi, *Pneumocystis jiroveci,* viruses)	Total lymphocyte counts HIV ELISA/Western blot/PCR	T-cell enumeration (CD3, CD4, CD8) In vitro T-cell proliferation to mitogens, antigens or allogeneic cells FISH 22q11 for DiGeorge deletion
Phagocytosis (chronic granulomatous disease, leukocyte adhesion deficiency, Chediak-Higashi syndrome)	Cutaneous infections, abscesses, lymphadenitis (staphylococci, enteric bacteria, fungi, mycobacteria), poor wound healing	WBC/neutrophil count and morphology	Nitroblue tetrazolium (NBT) test or dihydro-rhodamine (DHR) reduction test Chemotactic assay Phagocytic assay
Spleen	Bacteremia/hematogenous infection (pneumococcus, other streptococci, *Neisseria* sp.)	Peripheral blood smear for Howell-Jolly bodies Hemoglobin electrophoresis (HbSS)	Technetium-99 spleen scan or sonogram
Complement	Bacterial sepsis and other blood-borne infections (encapsulated bacteria, especially *Neisseria* sp.) Lupus, glomerulonephritis Angioedema	CH50 (total hemolytic complement)	Alternative pathway assay (AH50) Mannose-binding lectin level Individual complement component assays

ELISA, Enzyme-linked immunosorbent assay; FISH, fluorescent in situ hybridization; HIV, human immunodeficiency virus; PCR, polymerase chain reaction; WBC, white blood cell.

From Lederman HM: Clinical presentation of primary immunodeficiency diseases. In McMillan J: Oski's pediatrics. Philadelphia, Lippincott Williams & Wilkins, 2006, pp. 2441–2444.

15

V. IMMUNOGLOBULIN THERAPY[24,25]

A. Intravenous Immune Globulin (IVIG)

1. **Indications:**

a. *Replacement therapy for antibody-deficient disorders:*

(1) 400–500 mg/kg IV every 4 weeks to start

(2) Children with severe hypogammaglobulinemia (<100 mg/dL) may benefit from a total *loading* dose of 800 mg/kg given in two

separate doses a few days apart, followed by 400 to 500 mg/kg every month
   (3) Adjust dosing based on clinical response and to maintain trough IgG level of at least 500 mg/dL

b. *Immune thrombocytopenic purpura:*
   (1) Initially 400–2000 mg/kg (up to 1000 mg/kg given on a single day or in divided doses over 2–5 consecutive days)
   (2) Maintenance dose: 400–1000 mg/kg/dose every 3–6 weeks based on clinical response and platelet count
   (3) May also use Rh (D) immunoglobulin (WinRho) in Rh-positive patients

c. *Kawasaki disease:*
   (1) 2 g/kg × 1 dose over 8–12 hr
   (2) If signs and symptoms persist, consider second dose of 2 g/kg
   (3) Doses should be started within first 10 days of symptoms

d. *Pediatric human immunodeficiency virus (HIV) infection with antibody deficiency* (IgG concentration <400 mg/dL, failure to form antibodies to common antigens, recurrent serious bacterial infections, or measles prophylaxis): dosing same as for antibody-deficient disorders mentioned previously

e. *Bone marrow transplantation:*
   (1) 400–500 mg/kg/dose to start, adjust dosing to maintain trough IgG level of at least 400 mg/dL
   (2) May decrease incidence of infection and death but not acute graft-versus-host disease

f. *Other potential uses:*
   (1) Guillain-Barré syndrome
   (2) Refractory dermatomyositis and polymyositis
   (3) Chronic inflammatory demyelinating polyneuropathy

2. **Precautions and adverse reactions:**

a. Severe systemic symptoms (hemodynamic changes, respiratory difficulty, anaphylaxis)
b. Less severe systemic reactions (headache, myalgia, fever, chills, nausea, vomiting) may be alleviated by decreasing infusion rate or premedication with IV corticosteroids, antihistamines, and/or antipyretics
c. Aseptic meningitis syndrome
d. Acute renal failure (increased risk with preexisting renal insufficiency and with sucrose-containing IVIG)
e. Acute venous thrombosis (increased risk with sucrose-containing IVIG)
f. Use with caution in patients with undetectable IgA level due to trace amounts of IgA in IVIG, although routine screening for IgA deficiency is not recommended in potential recipients

B. Intramuscular Immune Globulin (IMIG)

1. **Indications:**
a. Hepatitis A prophylaxis
b. Measles prophylaxis
c. Rubella prophylaxis
d. Rabies prophylaxis
2. **Precautions and adverse reactions:**
a. Severe systemic symptoms (hemodynamic changes, anaphylaxis)
b. Local symptoms at the site of injection increase with repeated use
c. High risk for anaphylactoid reactions if given intravenously
d. Use with caution in patients with undetectable IgA levels due to trace amounts of IgA in IMIG
3. **Dose:**
a. Hepatitis A postexposure prophylaxis: 0.02 mL/kg given within 14 days of exposure. IG is not needed if at least one dose of hepatitis A vaccine was given at ≥1 month before exposure
b. Measles prophylaxis: 0.25 mL/kg/dose (maximum dose: 15 mL) given within 6 days of exposure in immunocompetent patient and 0.5 mL/kg (maximum dose: 15 mL) immediately following exposure in immunocompromised patients
c. Rubella prophylaxis during pregnancy: 0.55 mL/kg/dose within 72 hours of exposure
d. Rabies: 20 international units/kg single dose administered as soon as possible after exposure with the first dose of rabies vaccine
4. **Administration:**
a. No more than 5 mL should be given at one site in an adult or large child
b. Smaller amounts per site (1–3 mL) for smaller children and infants
c. Administration of >15 mL at one time is essentially never warranted
d. Peak serum levels achieved by 48 hours, and immune effect lasts 3 to 4 weeks
e. Intravenous or intradermal use of IMIG is absolutely contraindicated

C. Subcutaneous Immune Globulin

1. **Indication:** Replacement therapy for antibody deficiency
2. **Dose:**
a. 100–125 mg/kg weekly (maximum rate: 20 mL/hour; doses >15 mL usually should be divided between sites, but it depends on the amount of subcutaneous tissue)
b. Larger doses can be given simultaneously in multiple sites or more frequently than once per week
c. Using the same areas for injections improves tolerability
3. **Precautions and adverse reactions:** Similar to IMIG and IVIG
4. **Considerations:** Does not require venous access or special nursing (parents can administer) but may require multiple needlesticks in larger children due to volume restriction per site

D. Specific Immune Globulins

1. Hyperimmune globulins:
   a. Prepared from donors with high titers of specific antibodies
   b. Includes Hepatitis B immunoglobulin (HBIG), Varicella Zoster immunoglobulin (VZIG), Cytomegalovirus immunoglobulin (CMV-IG), Rho(D)IG, and others
2. Monoclonal antibody preparations (rituximab, palivizumab, and others)

VI. IMMUNOLOGIC REFERENCE VALUES

A. Serum IgG, IgM, IgA, and IgE Levels (Table 15-3)

B. Serum IgG, IgM, IgA, and IgE Levels for LBW Preterm Infants (Table 15-4)

C. Serum IgG Subclass Levels (Table 15-5)

D. Lymphocyte Enumeration (Table 15-6)

E. Serum Complement Levels (Table 15-7)

VII. COMPLEMENT PATHWAY (FIG. 15-3)

TABLE 15-3

SERUM IMMUNOGLOBULIN LEVELS*

Age	IgG (mg/dL)	IgM (mg/dL)	IgA (mg/dL)	IgE (IU/ml)
Cord blood (term)	1121 (636–1606)	13 (6.3–25)	2.3 (1.4–3.6)	0.22 (0.04–1.28)
1 mo	503 (251–906)	45 (20–87)	13 (1.3–53)	
6 wk				0.69 (0.08–6.12)
2 mo	365 (206–601)	46 (17–105)	15 (2.8–47)	
3 mo	334 (176–581)	49 (24–89)	17 (4.6–46)	0.82 (0.18–3.76)
4 mo	343 (196–558)	55 (27–101)	23 (4.4–73)	
5 mo	403 (172–814)	62 (33–108)	31 (8.1–84)	
6 mo	407 (215–704)	62 (35–102)	25 (8.1–68)	2.68 (0.44–16.3)
7–9 mo	475 (217–904)	80 (34–126)	36 (11–90)	2.36 (0.76–7.31)
10–12 mo	594 (294–1069)	82 (41–149)	40 (16–84)	
1 yr	679 (345–1213)	93 (43–173)	44 (14–106)	3.49 (0.80–15.2)
2 yr	685 (424–1051)	95 (48–168)	47 (14–123)	3.03 (0.31–29.5)
3 yr	728 (441–1135)	104 (47–200)	66 (22–159)	1.80 (0.19–16.9)
4–5 yr	780 (463–1236)	99 (43–196)	68 (25–154)	8.58 (1.07–68.9)†
6–8 yr	915 (633–1280)	107 (48–207)	90 (33–202)	12.89 (1.03–161.3)‡
9–10 yr	1007 (608–1572)	121 (52–242)	113 (45–236)	23.6 (0.98–570.6)§
14 yr				20.07 (2.06–195.2)
Adult	994 (639–1349)	156 (56–352)	171 (70–312)	13.2 (1.53–114)

*Numbers in parentheses are the 95% confidence intervals (CIs).

†IgE data for 4 yr.

‡IgE data for 7 yr.

§IgE data for 10 yr.

From Kjellman NM, Johansson SG, Roth A: Serum IgE levels in healthy children quantified by a sandwich technique (PRIST). Clin Allergy 1976;6:51–59; Jolliff CR, Cost KM, Stivrins PC, et al: Reference intervals for serum IgG, IgA, IgM, C3, and C4 as determined by rate nephelometry. Clin Chem 1982;28:126–128; and Zetterström O, Johansson SG: IgE concentrations measured by PRIST in serum of healthy adults and in patients with respiratory allergy: A diagnostic approach. Allergy 1981;36(8)537–547.

TABLE 15-4

SERUM IMMUNOGLOBULIN LEVELS FOR LOW BIRTH WEIGHT (LBW) PRETERM INFANTS

Age (mo)	Plasma IG Concentrations in 25–28 Wk Gestation Infants			Plasma IG Concentrations in 29–32 Wk Gestation Infants		
	IgG (mg/dL)*	IgM (mg/dL)*	IgA (mg/dL)*	IgG (mg/dL)*	IgM (mg/dL)*	IgA (mg/dL)*
0.25	251 (114–552)†	7.6 (1.3–43.3)	1.2 (0.07–20.8)	368 (186–728)†	9.1 (2.1–39.4)	0.6 (0.04–1.0)
0.5	202 (91–446)	14.1 (3.5–56.1)	3.1 (0.09–10.7)	275 (119–637)	13.9 (4.7–41)	0.9 (0.01–7.5)
1.0	158 (57–437)	12.7 (3.0–53.3)	4.5 (0.65–30.9)	209 (97–452)	14.4 (6.3–33)	1.9 (0.3–12.0)
1.5	134 (59–307)	16.2 (4.4–59.2)	4.3 (0.9–20.9)	156 (69–352)	15.4 (5.5–43.2)	2.2 (0.7–6.5)
2.0	89 (58–136)	16.0 (5.3–48.9)	4.1 (1.5–11.1)	123 (64–237)	15.2 (4.9–46.7)	3.0 (1.1–8.3)
3	60 (23–156)	13.8 (5.3–36.1)	3.0 (0.6–15.6)	104 (41–268)	16.3 (7.1–37.2)	3.6 (0.8–15.4)
4	82 (32–210)	22.2 (11.2–43.9)	6.8 (1.0–47.8)	128 (39–425)	26.5 (7.7–91.2)	9.8 (2.5–39.3)
6	159 (56–455)	41.3 (8.3–205)	9.7 (3.0–31.2)	179 (51–634)	29.3 (10.5–81.5)	12.3 (2.7–57.1)
8–10	273 (94–794)	41.8 (31.1–56.1)	9.5 (0.9–98.6)	280 (140–561)	34.7 (17–70.8)	20.9 (8.3–53)

*Geometric mean.

†Numbers in parentheses are ±2 SD.

From Ballow M, Cates KL, Rowe JC, et al: Development of the immune system in very low birth weight (less than 1500 g) premature infants: concentrations of plasma immunoglobulins and patterns of infections. Pediatr Res 1986;9:899–904.

15

TABLE 15-5

SERUM IgG SUBCLASS LEVELS*

Age (yr)	IgG1 (mg/dL)	IgG2 (mg/dL)	IgG3 (mg/dL)	IgG4 (mg/dL)
0.5–1	290 (140–620)	58 (41–130)	41 (11–85)	0.2 (0–0.8)
1–1.5	350 (170–650)	62 (40–140)	42 (12–87)	3 (0–26)
1.5–2	400 (220–720)	80 (50–180)	44 (14–91)	7 (0–41)
2–3	450 (240–780)	95 (55–200)	46 (15–93)	14 (0–69)
3–4	480 (270–810)	115 (65–220)	48 (16–96)	20 (1–94)
4–6	500 (300–840)	130 (70–250)	50 (17–97)	26 (2–116)
6–9	570 (350–910)	170 (85–330)	54 (20–100)	37 (3–158)
9–12	600 (370–930)	210 (10–400)	58 (22–109)	47 (4–190)
12–18	580 (370–910)	260 (110–480)	63 (24–116)	49 (5–196)
Adult	500 (280–800)	300 (115–570)	64 (24–120)	35 (5–125)

*Numbers in parentheses are the 95% confidence intervals (CIs).

From Schauer U, Stemberg F, Rieger CH, et al: IgG subclass concentrations in certified reference material 470 and reference values for children and adults determined with the binding site reagents. Clin Chem 2003;49(11):1924–1929.

TABLE 15-6

T AND B LYMPHOCYTES IN PERIPHERAL BLOOD

Age	CD3 (Total T cell) Count*,† (%)†	CD4 count*,† (%)†	CD8 Count*,† (%)†	CD19 (B cell) Count*,† (%)†
0–3 mo	2.50–5.50 (53–84)	1.60–4.00 (35–64)	0.56–1.70 (12–28)	0.30–2.00 (6–32)
3–6 mo	2.50–5.60 (51–77)	1.80–4.00 (35–56)	0.59–1.60 (12–23)	0.43–3.00 (11–41)
6–12 mo	1.90–5.90 (49–76)	1.40–4.30 (31–56)	0.50–1.70 (12–24)	0.61–2.60 (14–37)
1–2 yr	2.10–6.20 (53–75)	1.30–3.40 (32–51)	0.62–2.00 (14–30)	0.72–2.60 (16–35)
2–6 yr	1.40–3.70 (56–75)	0.70–2.20 (28–47)	0.49–1.30 (16–30)	0.39–1.40 (14–33)
6–12 yr	1.20–2.60 (60–76)	0.65–1.50 (31–47)	0.37–1.10 (18–35)	0.27–0.86 (13–27)
12–18 yr	1.00–2.20 (56–84)	0.53–1.30 (31–52)	0.33–0.92 (18–35)	0.11–0.57 (6–23)
Adult‡	0.70–2.10 (55–83)	0.30–1.40 (28–57)	0.20–0.90 (10–39)	

*Absolute counts (number of cells per microliter $\times 10^{-3}$).

†Normal values (10th to 90th percentile).

‡From Comans-Bitter WM, de Groot R, van den Beemd R, et al: Immunotyping of blood lymphocytes in childhood. Reference values for lymphocyte subpopulations. J Pediatr 1997; 130(3):388–393

From Shearer WT, Rosenblatt HM, Gelman RS, et al: Lymphocyte subsets in healthy children from birth through 18 years of age: the Pediatric AIDS Clinical Trials Group P1009 study. J Allergy Clin Immunol 2003;112: 973–980.

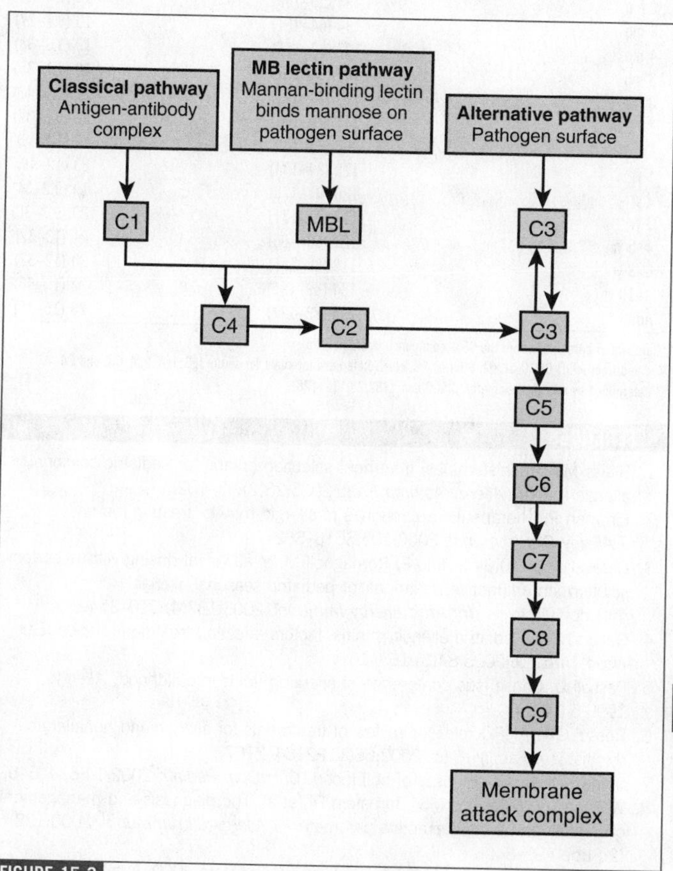

FIGURE 15-3
Complement pathway.

TABLE 15-7

SERUM COMPLEMENT LEVELS*

Age	C3 (mg/dL)	C4 (mg/dL)
Cord blood (term)	83 (57–116)	13 (6.6–23)
1 mo	83 (53–124)	14 (7.0–25)
2 mo	96 (59–149)	15 (7.4–28)
3 mo	94 (64–131)	16 (8.7–27)
4 mo	107 (62–175)	19 (8.3–38)
5 mo	107 (64–167)	18 (7.1–36)
6 mo	115 (74–171)	21 (8.6–42)
7–9 mo	113 (75–166)	20 (9.5–37)
10–12 mo	126 (73–180)	22 (12–39)
1 yr	129 (84–174)	23 (12–40)
2 yr	120 (81–170)	19 (9.2–34)
3 yr	117 (77–171)	20 (9.7–36)
4–5 yr	121 (86–166)	21 (13–32)
6–8 yr	118 (88–155)	20 (12–32)
9–10 yr	134 (89–195)	22 (10–40)
Adult	125 (83–177)	28 (15–45)

*Numbers in parentheses are the 95% confidence intervals (CIs).

Modified from Jolliff CR, Cost KM, Stivrins PC, et al: Reference intervals for serum IgG, IgA, IgM, C3, and C4 as determined by rate nephelometry. Clin Chem 1982;28:126–128.

REFERENCES

1. Blaiss MS. Antihistamines: treatment selection criteria for pediatric seasonal allergic rhinitis. *Allergy Asthma Proc*. 2005;26(2):95–102.
2. Fireman P. Therapeutic approaches to allergic rhinitis: treating the child. *J Allergy Clin Immunol*. 2000;105:S616–S621.
3. Garavello DW, DiBerardino F, Romagnoli M, et al. Nasal rinsing with hypertonic solution: an adjunctive treatment for pediatric seasonal allergic rhinoconjunctivitis. *Int Arch Allergy Immunol*. 2005;137(4):310–314.
4. Gelfand EW. Pediatric allergic rhinitis: factors affecting treatment choice. *Ear Nose Throat J*. 2005;84(3):163–168.
5. Passali D. Consensus conference of allergic rhinitis in childhood. *Allergy*. 1999;54:4–34.
6. Ressel GW. AHRQ releases review of treatments for allergic and nonallergic rhinitis. *Am Family Phys*. 2002;66(11):2164–2167.
7. Stone KD. Atopic diseases of childhood. *Curr Opin Pediatr*. 2002;14:634–646.
8. Wallace DV, Dykewicz MS, Bernstein DI, et al. The diagnosis and management of rhinitis: an updated practice parameter. *J Allergy Clin Immunol*. 2008;122 (2 Suppl):S1–84.
9. Burks W. Diagnostic tools for food allergy. Up to Date 2009. Available at www.uptodate.com.
10. Chapman JA. Food allergy: a practice parameter. *Ann Allergy Asthma Immunol*. 2006;96(3 Suppl 2):S1–68.
11. Lifschitz CH. Dietary protein-induced proctitis/colitis, enteropathy, and enterocolitis of infancy. Up to Date 2009. Available at www.uptodate.com.
12. Sampson HA, Sicherer SH, Birnbaum AH, et al. American Gastroenterology Association technical review on the evaluation of food allergy in gastrointestinal disorders. *Gastroenterology*. 2001;120(4):1023–1025.

13. Sicherer SH. Manifestations of food allergy: Evaluation and management. *Am Family Phys.* 1999;59(2):415–424.
14. Wood RA. The natural history of food allergy. *Pediatrics.* 2003;111(6): 1631–1637.
15. Solensky R. Allergy to penicillins. Up to Date 2009. Available at www.uptodate.com.
16. Bonilla FA, Bernstein IL, Khan DA, et al. Practice parameter for the diagnosis and management of primary immunodeficiency. *Ann Allergy Asthma Immunol.* 2005;94:S1.
17. Bonilla FA, Geha RS. Primary immunodeficiency diseases. *J Allergy Clin Immunol.* 2003;111(2 Suppl):S571–S581.
18. Bonilla FA, Geha RS. Update on primary immunodeficiency diseases. *J Allergy Clin Immunol.* 2006;117(2 Suppl Mini-Primer):S435–S441.
19. Fleisher TA. Back to basics: primary immune deficiencies: windows into the immune system. *Pediatr Rev.* 2006;27:363–372.
20. Geha RS, Notarangelo LD, Casanova JL, et al. International Union of Immunological Societies Primary Immunodeficiency Diseases Classification Committee. Primary immunodeficiency diseases: an update from the International Union of Immunological Societies Primary Immunodeficiency Diseases Classification Committee. *J Allergy Clin Immunol.* 2007;120:776–794.
21. Lederman HM. Clinical presentation of primary immunodeficiency diseases. In: McMillan J, ed. *Oski's pediatrics.* Philadelphia: Lippincott Williams & Wilkins; 2006:2441–2444.
22. Stiehm ER. Approach to the child with recurrent infections. Up to Date 2009. Available at www.uptodate.com.
23. Stiehm ER, Ochs HD, Winkelstein JA. Immunodeficiency disorders: general considerations. In: Stiehm ER, Ochs HD, Winkelstein JA, eds. *Immunologic disorders in infants and children.* 5th ed. Philadelphia: Elsevier/Saunders; 2004.
24. Garcia-Lloret M, McGhee S, Chatila TA, et al. Immunoglobulin replacement therapy in children. *Immunol Allergy Clin North Am.* 2008:28(4):833–849.
25. Orange J, Hossny EM, Weiler CR, et al. Use of intravenous immunoglobulin in human disease: a review of evidence by members of the Primary Immunodeficiency Committee of the American Academy of Allergy, Asthma, and Immunology. *J Allergy Clin Immunol.* 2006;117(4):S525–S553.

Chapter 16

Immunoprophylaxis

Kristin Santini Casasanta, MD

I. WEBSITES

American Academy of Pediatrics: Red Book: 2009 report of the Committee on Infectious Diseases, 28th ed. 2009: aapredbook.aappublications.org/

American Academy of Pediatrics: www.aap.org

Vaccine Adverse Event Reporting System: http://vaers.hhs.gov/index

Centers for Disease Control and Prevention, includes Morbidity and Mortality Weekly Reports pertaining to vaccines: http://www.cdc.gov/vaccines/

Influenza vaccines A and B: www.cdc.gov/flu/professionals/antivirals/index.htm

II. VACCINE ABBREVIATIONS (BOX 16-1)

BOX 16-1

VACCINE ABBREVIATIONS

BCG, bacilli Calmette–Guerin
DTaP, diphtheria and tetanus toxoids and acellular pertussis
DTP, diphtheria and tetanus toxoids and pertussis
Hep A or HAV, hepatitis A
Hep B or HBV, hepatitis B
Hep C or HCV, hepatitis C
Hib, *Haemophilus influenzae* type b
HPV or HPV4, human papillomavirus
IPV, inactivated poliovirus
LAIV, live attenuated influenza virus
MCV4, meningococcal conjugate
MMR, measles, mumps and rubella
MPSV4, meningococcal polysaccharide
OPV, oral (live attenuated) poliovirus
PCV7 or PCV13, pneumococcal conjugate
PPV23 or 23PS, 23 valent pneumococcal polysaccharide
Rota or RV1 or RV5, rotavirus
Td, tetanus and diphtheria toxoids
Tdap, tetanus and diphtheria toxoids and acellular pertussis
TIV, trivalent inactivated influenza vaccine

III. IMMUNIZATION SCHEDULES

A. Recommended Childhood Immunization Schedule (Fig. 16-1, A and B)[1]

B. Catch-up Immunization Schedules (Fig. 16-2)

1. Lapsed immunizations: Resume immunization schedule as if the usual interval had elapsed. Repeating doses is not indicated

C. Minimum Age for Initial Vaccination and Minimum Intervals between Doses of Various Vaccines (Table 16-1)

IV. IMMUNIZATION GUIDELINES

A. Vaccine Informed Consent

Vaccine information statements (VISes) can be obtained from local health departments, the Centers for Disease Control and Prevention (CDC), the American Academy of Pediatrics (AAP), and vaccine manufacturers. For vaccines that do not currently have VISes, the CDC produces *important information* statements. The most recent VIS must be provided to the patient (nonminor) or parent/guardian with documentation of version date and date vaccine administered.

B. Vaccine Administration

1. **Preferred sites of administration of intramuscular (IM) and subcutaneous (SC) vaccines:**
a. <18 months old: Anterolateral thigh
b. Toddlers: Anterolateral thigh or deltoid (deltoid preferred if large enough)
c. Adolescents and young adults: Deltoid
2. **Route:**
a. IM: Deep into muscle to avoid tissue damage from adjuvants, usually with a 22- to 25-gauge (22G to 25G) needle, ⅞-inch to 1-inch long in infants and toddlers and 1-inch to 2-inches long in adolescents and young adults
b. SC: Into pinched skin fold with a 23G to 25G needle ⅝-inch to ¾-inch long
3. **Simultaneous administration:**
a. Routine childhood vaccines are safe and effective when administered simultaneously at different sites, generally 1 inch to 2 inches apart. This includes inactivated and live vaccines
b. If two or more live vaccines are required but not administered at the same visit, an interval of 28 days should be allotted between them. This is not necessary for two or more inactivated vaccines or combination inactivated and live vaccines
4. **Misconceptions regarding vaccine administration: See Table 16-2**
a. Egg allergies
   (1) Skin testing is *not* needed in children with egg allergies before the administration of the measles/mumps/rubella (MMR) vaccine (refer to Section VI.H for details)

A

Recommended Immunization Schedule for Persons Aged 0–6 Years—UNITED STATES•2011

Vaccine ▼ Age ►	Birth	1 month	2 months	4 months	6 months	12 months	15 months	18 months	19–23 months	2–3 years	4–6 years
Hepatitis B[1]	HepB	HepB			HepB						
Rotavirus[2]			RV	RV	RV[2]						
Diphtheria, Tetanus, Pertussis[3]			DTaP	DTaP	DTaP	*see footnote*[3]	DTaP				DTaP
Haemophilus influenzae type b[4]			Hib	Hib	Hib[4]	Hib					
Pneumococcal[5]			PCV	PCV	PCV	PCV				PPSV	
Inactivated Poliovirus[6]			IPV	IPV	IPV						IPV
Influenza[7]					Influenza (Yearly)						
Measles, Mumps, Rubella[8]						MMR			*see footnote*[8]		MMR
Varicella[9]						Varicella			*see footnote*[9]		Varicella
Hepatitis A[10]						HepA (2 doses)				HepA Series	
Meningococcal[11]										MCV4	

Range of recommended ages for all children

Range of recommended ages for certain high-risk groups

This schedule includes recommendations in effect as of December 21, 2010. Any dose not administered at the recommended age should be administered at a subsequent visit, when indicated and feasible. The use of a combination vaccine generally is preferred over separate injections of its equivalent component vaccines. Considerations should include provider assessment, patient preference, and the potential for adverse events. Providers should consult the relevant Advisory Committee on Immunization Practices statement for detailed recommendations: **http://www.cdc.gov/vaccines/pubs/acip-list.htm**. Clinically significant adverse events that follow immunization should be reported to the Vaccine Adverse Event Reporting System (VAERS) at **http://www.vaers.hhs.gov** or by telephone, **800-822-7967**.

1. **Hepatitis B vaccine (HepB).** (Minimum age: birth)
   At birth:
   - Administer monovalent HepB to all newborns before hospital discharge.
   - If mother is hepatitis B surface antigen (HBsAg)-positive, administer HepB and 0.5 mL of hepatitis B immune globulin (HBIG) within 12 hours of birth.
   - If mother's HBsAg status is unknown, administer HepB within 12 hours of birth. Determine mother's HBsAg status as soon as possible and, if HBsAg-positive, administer HBIG (no later than age 1 week).

   Doses following the birth dose:
   - The second dose should be administered at age 1 or 2 months. Monovalent HepB should be used for doses administered before age 6 weeks.
   - Infants born to HBsAg-positive mothers should be tested for HBsAg and antibody to HBsAg 1 to 2 months after completion of at least 3 doses of the HepB series, at age 9 through 18 months (generally at the next well-child visit).
   - Administration of 4 doses of HepB to infants is permissible when a combination vaccine containing HepB is administered after the birth dose.
   - Infants who did not receive a birth dose should receive 3 doses of HepB on a schedule of 0, 1 and 6 months.
   - The final (3rd or 4th) dose in the HepB series should be administered no earlier than age 24 weeks.
2. **Rotavirus vaccine (RV).** (Minimum age: 6 weeks)
   - Administer the first dose at age 6 through 14 weeks (maximum age: 14 weeks, 6 days). Vaccination should not be initiated for infants aged 15 weeks, 0 days or older.
   - The maximum age for the final dose in the series is 8 months, 0 days.
   - If Rotarix is administered at ages 2 and 4 months, a dose at 6 months is not indicated.
3. **Diphtheria and tetanus toxoids and acellular pertussis vaccine (DTaP).** (Minimum age: 6 weeks)
   - The fourth dose may be administered as early as age 12 months, provided at least 6 months have elapsed since the third dose.
4. ***Haemophilus influenzae*type b conjugate vaccine (Hib).** (Minimum age: 6 weeks)
   - If PRP-OMP (PedvaxHIB or Comvax [HepB-Hib]) is administered at ages 2 and 4 months, a dose at age 6 months is not indicated.
   - Hiberix should not be used for doses at ages 2, 4 or 6 months for the primary series but can be used as the final dose in children aged 12 months through 4 years.
5. **Pneumococcal vaccine.** (Minimum age: 6 weeks for pneumococcal conjugate vaccine [PCV]; 2 years for pneumococcal polysaccharide vaccine [PPSV])
   - PCV is recommended for all children aged younger than 5 years. Administer 1 dose of PCV to all healthy children aged 24 through 59 months who are not completely vaccinated for their age.
   - A PCV series begun with 7-valent PCV (PCV7) should be completed with 13-valent PCV (PCV13).
   - A single supplemental dose of PCV13 is recommended for all children aged 14 through 59 months who have received an age-appropriate series of PCV7.
   - A single supplemental dose of PCV13 is recommended for all children aged 60 through 71 months with underlying medical conditions who have received an age-appropriate series of PCV7.
   - The supplemental dose of PCV13 should be administered at least 8 weeks after the previous dose of PCV7. See *MMWR.* 2010:59(No. RR-11).
   - Administer PPSV at least 8 weeks after last dose of PCV to children aged 2 years or older with certain underlying medical conditions, including a cochlear implant.
6. **Inactivated poliovirus vaccine (IPV).** (Minimum age: 6 weeks)
   - If 4 or more doses are administered prior to age 4 years, an additional dose should be administered at age 4 through 6 years.
   - The final dose in the series should be administered on or after the fourth birthday and at least 6 months following the previous dose.
7. **Influenza vaccine (seasonal).** (Minimum age: 6 months for trivalent inactivated influenza vaccine [TIV]; 2 years for live, attenuated influenza vaccine [LAIV])
   - For healthy children aged 2 years and older (i.e., those who do not have underlying medical conditions that predispose them to influenza complications), either LAIV or TIV may be used, except LAIV should not be given to children aged 2 through 4 years who have had wheezing in the past 12 months.
   - Administer 2 doses (separated by at least 4 weeks) to children aged 6 months through 8 years who are receiving seasonal influenza vaccine for the first time or who were vaccinated for the first time during the previous influenza season but only received 1 dose.
   - Children aged 6 months through 8 years who received no doses of monovalent 2009 H1N1 vaccine should receive 2 doses of 2010–2011 seasonal influenza vaccine. See *MMWR.* 2010;59(No. RR-8):33–34.
8. **Measles, mumps, and rubella vaccine (MMR).** (Minimum age: 12 months)
   - The second dose may be administered before age 4 years, provided at least 4 weeks have elapsed since the first dose.
9. **Varicella vaccine.** (Minimum age: 12 months)
   - The second dose may be administered before age 4 years, provided at least 3 months have elapsed since the first dose.
   - For children aged 12 months through 12 years, the recommended minimum interval between doses is 3 months. However, if the second dose was administered at least 4 weeks after the first dose, it can be accepted as valid.
10. **Hepatitis A vaccine (HepA).** (Minimum age: 12 months)
    - Administer 2 doses at least 6 months apart.
    - HepA is recommended for children aged older than 23 months who live in areas where vaccination programs target older children, who are at increased risk for infection, or for whom immunity against hepatitis A is desired.
11. **Meningococcal conjugate vaccine, quadrivalent (MCV4).** (Minimum age: 2 years)
    - Administer 2 doses of MCV4 at least 8 weeks apart to children aged 2 through 10 years with persistent complement component deficiency and anatomic or functional asplenia, and 1 dose every 5 years thereafter.
    - Persons with human immunodeficiency virus (HIV) infection who are vaccinated with MCV4 should receive 2 doses at least 8 weeks apart.
    - Administer 1 dose of MCV4 to children aged 2 through 10 years who travel to countries with highly endemic or epidemic disease and during outbreaks caused by a vaccine serogroup.
    - Administer MCV4 to children at continued risk for meningococcal disease who were previously vaccinated with MCV4 or meningococcal polysaccharide vaccine after 3 years if the first dose was administered at age 2 through 6 years.

The Recommended Immunization Schedules for Persons Aged 0 Through 18 Years are approved by the Advisory Committee on Immunization Practices (**http://www.cdc.gov/vaccines/recs/acip**), the American Academy of Pediatrics (**http://www.aap.org**), and the American Academy of Family Physicians (**http://www.aafp.org**).

Department of Health and Human Services • Centers for Disease Control and Prevention

FIGURE 16-1A

Recommended immunization schedule for persons aged 0–6 years–United States–2011. (These figures are available at www.cdc.gov. Centers for Disease Control and Prevention. Recommended immunization schedules for persons aged 0–6 years—United States, 2011. MMWR 2011;60(5).)

B

Recommended Immunization Schedule for Persons Aged 7–18 Yrs—UNITED STATES•2011

Vaccine ▼ Age ►	7–10 years	11–12 years	13–18 years
Tetanus, Diphtheria, Pertussis[1]		Tdap	Tdap
Human Papillomavirus[2]	*see footnote*[2]	HPV (3 doses)(females)	HPV series
Meningococcal[3]	MCV4	MCV4	MCV4
Influenza[4]	Influenza (Yearly)		
Pneumococcal[5]	Pneumococcal		
Hepatitis A[6]	HepA Series		
Hepatitis B[7]	Hep B Series		
Inactivated Poliovirus[8]	IPV Series		
Measles, Mumps, Rubella[9]	MMR Series		
Varicella[10]	Varicella Series		

Range of recommended ages for all children

Range of recommended ages for catch-up immunization

Range of recommended ages for certain high-risk groups

This schedule includes recommendations in effect as of December 21, 2010. Any dose not administered at the recommended age should be administered at a subsequent visit, when indicated and feasible. The use of a combination vaccine generally is preferred over separate injections of its equivalent component vaccines. Considerations should include provider assessment, patient preference, and the potential for adverse events. Providers should c onsult the relevant Advisory Committee on Immunization Practices statement for detailed recommendations: **http://www.cdc.gov/vaccines/pubs/acip-list.htm**. Clinically significant adverse events that follow immunization should be reported to the Vaccine Adverse Event Reporting System (VAERS) at **http://www.vaers.hhs.gov** or by telephone, **800-822-7967.**

1. **Tetanus and diphtheria toxoids and acellular pertussis vaccine (Tdap).** (Minimum age: 10 years for Boostrix and 11 years for Adacel)
   - Persons aged 11 through 18 years who have not received Tdap should receive a dose followed by Td booster doses every 10 years thereafter.
   - Persons aged 7 through 10 years who are not fully immunized against pertussis (including those never vaccinated or with unknown pertussis vaccination status) should receive a single dose of Tdap. Refer to the catch-up schedule if additional doses of tetanus and diphtheria toxoid–containing vaccine are needed.
   - Tdap can be administered regardless of the interval since the last tetanus and diphtheria toxoid–containing vaccine.
2. **Human papillomavirus vaccine (HPV).** (Minimum age: 9 years)
   - Quadrivalent HPV vaccine (HPV4) or bivalent HPV vaccine (HPV2) is recommended for the prevention of cervical precancers and cancers in females.
   - HPV4 is recommended for prevention of cervical precancers, cancers, and genital warts in females.
   - HPV4 may be administered in a 3-dose series to males aged 9 through 18 years to reduce their likelihood of genital warts.
   - Administer the second dose 1 to 2 months after the first dose and the third dose 6 months after the first dose (at least 24 weeks after the first dose).
3. **Meningococcal conjugate vaccine, quadrivalent (MCV4).** (Minimum age: 2 years)
   - Administer MCV4 at age 11 through 12 years with a booster dose at age 16 years.
   - Administer 1 dose at age 13 through 18 years if not previously vaccinated.
   - Persons who received their first dose at age 13 through 15 years should receive a booster dose at age 16 through 18 years.
   - Administer 1 dose to previously unvaccinated college freshmen living in a dormitory.
   - Administer 2 doses at least 8 weeks apart to children aged 2 through 10 years with persistent complement component deficiency and anatomic or functional asplenia, and 1 dose every 5 years thereafter.
   - Persons with HIV infection who are vaccinated with MCV4 should receive 2 doses at least 8 weeks apart.
   - Administer 1 dose of MCV4 to children aged 2 through 10 years who travel to countries with highly endemic or epidemic disease and during outbreaks caused by a vaccine serogroup.
   - Administer MCV4 to children at continued risk for meningococcal disease who were previously vaccinated with MCV4 or meningococcal polysaccharide vaccine after 3 years (if first dose administered at age 2 through 6 years) or after 5 years (if first dose administered at age 7 years or older).
4. **Influenza vaccine (seasonal).**
   - For healthy nonpregnant persons aged 7 through 18 years (i.e., those who do not have underlying medical conditions that predispose them to influenza complications), either LAIV or TIV may be used.
   - Administer 2 doses (separated by at least 4 weeks) to children aged 6 months through 8 years who are receiving seasonal influenza vaccine for the first time or who were vaccinated for the first time during the previous influenza season but only received 1 dose.
   - Children 6 months through 8 years of age who received no doses of monovalent 2009 H1N1 vaccine should receive 2 doses of 2010-2011 seasonal influenza vaccine. See *MMWR*. 2010;59(No. RR-8):33–34.
5. **Pneumococcal vaccines.**
   - A single dose of 13-valent pneumococcal conjugate vaccine (PCV13) may be administered to children aged 6 through 18 years who have functional or anatomic asplenia, HIV infection or other immunocompromising condition, cochlear implant or CSF leak. See *MMWR*. 2010;59(No. RR-11).
   - The dose of PCV13 should be administered at least 8 weeks after the previous dose of PCV7.
   - Administer pneumococcal polysaccharide vaccine at least 8 weeks after the last dose of PCV to children aged 2 years or older with certain underlying medical conditions, including a cochlear implant. A single revaccination should be administered after 5 years to children with functional or anatomic asplenia or an immunocompromising condition.
6. **Hepatitis A vaccine (HepA).**
   - Administer 2 doses at least 6 months apart.
   - HepA is recommended for children aged older than 23 months who live in areas where vaccination programs target older children, or who are at increased risk for infection, or for whom immunity against hepatitis A is desired.
7. **Hepatitis B vaccine (HepB).**
   - Administer the 3-dose series to those not previously vaccinated. For those with incomplete vaccination, follow the catch-up schedule.
   - A 2-dose series (separated by at least 4 months) of adult formulation Recombivax HB is licensed for children aged 11 through 15 years.
8. **Inactivated poliovirus vaccine (IPV).**
   - The final dose in the series should be administered on or after the fourth birthday and at least 6 months following the previous dose.
   - If both OPV and IPV were administered as part of a series, a total of 4 doses should be administered, regardless of the child's current age.
9. **Measles, mumps, and rubella vaccine (MMR).**
   - The minimum interval between the 2 doses of MMR is 4 weeks.
10. **Varicella vaccine.**
    - For persons aged 7 through 18 years without evidence of immunity (see *MMWR*. 2007;56[No. RR-4]), administer 2 doses if not previously vaccinated or the second dose if only 1 dose has been administered.
    - For persons aged 7 through 12 years, the recommended minimum interval between doses is 3 months. However, if the second dose was administered at least 4 weeks after the first dose, it can be accepted as valid.
    - For persons aged 13 years and older, the minimum interval between doses is 4 weeks.

The Recommended Immunization Schedules for Persons Aged 0 Through 18 Years are approved by the Advisory Committee on Immunization Practices (**http://www.cdc.gov/vaccines/recs/acip**), the American Academy of Pediatrics (**http://www.aap.org**), and the American Academy of Family Physicians (**http://www.aafp.org**).
Department of Health and Human Services • Centers for Disease Control and Prevention

FIGURE 16-1B

Recommended immunization schedule for persons aged 7 through 18 years–United States–2011. (Figures are available at www.cdc.gov. Centers for Disease Control and Prevention. Recommended immunization schedules for persons aged 7–18 years—United States, 2011. MMWR 2011;60(5).)

Catch-up Immunization Schedule for Persons Aged 4 Months Through 18 Years Who Start Late or Who Are More Than 1 Month Behind — United States • 2011

The table below provides catch-up schedules and minimum intervals between doses for children whose vaccinations have been delayed. A vaccine series does not need to be restarted, regardless of the time that has elapsed between doses. Use the section appropriate for the child's age.

Vaccine	Minimum Age for Dose 1	Minimum Interval Between Doses: Dose 1 to Dose 2	Dose 2 to Dose 3	Dose 3 to Dose 4	Dose 4 to Dose 5
PERSONS AGED 4 MONTHS THROUGH 6 YEARS					
Hepatitis B[1]	Birth	4 weeks	8 weeks (and at least 16 weeks after first dose)		
Rotavirus[2]	6 wks	4 weeks	4 weeks[2]		
Diphtheria, Tetanus, Pertussis[3]	6 wks	4 weeks	4 weeks	6 months	6 months[3]
Haemophilus influenzae type b[4]	6 wks	4 weeks if first dose administered at younger than age 12 months 8 weeks (as final dose) if first dose administered at age 12–14 months No further doses needed if first dose administered at age 15 months or older	4 weeks[4] if current age is younger than 12 months 8 weeks (as final dose)[4] if current age is 12 months or older and first dose administered at younger than age 12 months and second dose administered at younger than 15 months No further doses needed if previous dose administered at age 15 months or older	8 weeks (as final dose) This dose only necessary for children aged 12 months through 59 months who received 3 doses before age 12 months	
Pneumococcal[5]	6 wks	4 weeks if first dose administered at younger than age 12 months 8 weeks (as final dose for healthy children) if first dose administered at age 12 months or older or current age 24 through 59 months No further doses needed for healthy children if first dose administered at age 24 months or older	4 weeks if current age is younger than 12 months 8 weeks (as final dose for healthy children) if current age is 12 months or older No further doses needed for healthy children if previous dose administered at age 24 months or older	8 weeks (as final dose) This dose only necessary for children aged 12 months through 59 months who received 3 doses before age 12 months or for children at high risk who received 3 doses at any age	
Inactivated Poliovirus[6]	6 wks	4 weeks	4 weeks	6 months[6]	
Measles, Mumps, Rubella[7]	12 mos	4 weeks			
Varicella[8]	12 mos	3 months			
Hepatitis A[9]	12 mos	6 months			
PERSONS AGED 7 THROUGH 18 YEARS					
Tetanus, Diphtheria/ Tetanus, Diphtheria, Pertussis[10]	7 yrs[10]	4 weeks	4 weeks if first dose administered at younger than age 12 months 6 months if first dose administered at 12 months or older	6 months if first dose administered at younger than age 12 months	
Human Papillomavirus[11]	9 yrs	Routine dosing intervals are recommended (females)[11]			
Hepatitis A[9]	12 mos	6 months			
Hepatitis B[1]	Birth	4 weeks	8 weeks (and at least 16 weeks after first dose)		
Inactivated Poliovirus[6]	6 wks	4 weeks	4 weeks[6]	6 months[6]	
Measles, Mumps, Rubella[7]	12 mos	4 weeks			
Varicella[8]	12 mos	3 months if person is younger than age 13 years 4 weeks if person is aged 13 years or older			

1. **Hepatitis B vaccine (HepB).**
   - Administer the 3-dose series to those not previously vaccinated.
   - The minimum age for the third dose of HepB is 24 weeks.
   - A 2-dose series (separated by at least 4 months) of adult formulation Recombivax HB is licensed for children aged 11 through 15 years.
2. **Rotavirus vaccine (RV).**
   - The maximum age for the first dose is 14 weeks, 6 days. Vaccination should not be initiated for infants aged 15 weeks, 0 days or older.
   - The maximum age for the final dose in the series is 8 months, 0 days.
   - If Rotarix was administered for the first and second doses, a third dose is not indicated.
3. **Diphtheria and tetanus toxoids and acellular pertussis vaccine (DTaP).**
   - The fifth dose is not necessary if the fourth dose was administered at age 4 years or older.
4. ***Haemophilus influenzae* type b conjugate vaccine (Hib).**
   - 1 dose of Hib vaccine should be considered for unvaccinated persons aged 5 years or older who have sickle cell disease, leukemia or HIV infection, or who have had a splenectomy.
   - If the first 2 doses were PRP-OMP (PedvaxHIB or Comvax), and administered at age 11 months or younger, the third (and final) dose should be administered at age 12 through 15 months and at least 8 weeks after the second dose.
   - If the first dose was administered at age 7 through 11 months, administer the second dose at least 4 weeks later and a final dose at age 12 through 15 months.
5. **Pneumococcal vaccine.**
   - Administer 1 dose of 13-valent pneumococcal conjugate vaccine (PCV13) to all healthy children aged 24 through 59 months with any incomplete PCV schedule (PCV7 or PCV13).
   - For children aged 24 through 71 months with underlying medical conditions, administer 1 dose of PCV13 if 3 doses of PCV were received previously or administer 2 doses of PCV13 at least 8 weeks apart if fewer than 3 doses of PCV were received previously.
   - A single dose of PCV13 is recommended for certain children with underlying medical conditions through 18 years of age. See age-specific schedules for details.
   - Administer pneumococcal polysaccharide vaccine (PPSV) to children aged 2 years or older with certain underlying medical conditions, including a cochlear implant, at least 8 weeks after the last dose of PCV. A single revaccination should be administered after 5 years to children with functional or anatomic asplenia or an immunocompromising condition. See *MMWR*. 2010;59(No. RR-11).
6. **Inactivated poliovirus vaccine (IPV).**
   - The final dose in the series should be administered on or after the fourth birthday and at least 6 months following the previous dose.
   - A fourth dose is not necessary if the third dose was administered at age 4 years or older and at least 6 months following the previous dose.
   - In the first 6 months of life, minimum age and minimum intervals are only recommended if the person is at risk for imminent exposure to circulating poliovirus (i.e., travel to a polio-endemic region or during an outbreak).
7. **Measles, mumps, and rubella vaccine (MMR).**
   - Administer the second dose routinely at age 4 through 6 years. The minimum interval between the 2 doses of MMR is 4 weeks.
8. **Varicella vaccine.**
   - Administer the second dose routinely at age 4 through 6 years.
   - If the second dose was administered at least 4 weeks after the first dose, it can be accepted as valid.
9. **Hepatitis A vaccine (HepA).**
   - HepA is recommended for children aged older than age 23 months who live in areas where vaccination programs target older children, or who are at increased risk for infection, or for whom immunity against hepatitis A is desired.
10. **Tetanus and diphtheria toxoids (Td) and tetanus and diphtheria toxoids and acellular pertussis vaccine (Tdap).**
    - Doses of DTaP are counted as part of the Td/Tdap series.
    - Tdap should be substituted for a single dose of Td in the catch-up series for children aged 7 through 10 years or as a booster for children aged 11 through 18 years; use Td for other doses.
11. **Human papillomavirus vaccine (HPV).**
    - Administer the series to females at age 13 through 18 years if not previously vaccinated or have not completed the vaccine series.
    - Quadrivalent HPV vaccine (HPV4) may be administered in a 3-dose series to males aged 9 through 18 years to reduce their likelihood of genital warts.
    - Use recommended routine dosing intervals for series catch-up (i.e., the second and third doses should be administered at 1 to 2 and 6 months after the first dose). The minimum interval between the first and second doses is 4 weeks. The minimum interval between the second and third doses is 12 weeks, and the third dose should be administered at least 24 weeks after the first dose.

Information about reporting reactions after immunization is available online at http://www.vaers.hhs.gov or by telephone, 800-822-7967. Suspected cases of vaccine-preventable diseases should be reported to the state or local health department. Additional information, including precautions and contraindications for immunization, is available from the National Center for Immunization and Respiratory Diseases at http://www.cdc.gov/vaccines or telephone, **800-CDC-INFO** (800-232-4636).

Department of Health and Human Services • Centers for Disease Control and Prevention

FIGURE 16-2

Catch-up immunization schedule for persons aged 4 months through 18 years who start late or who are more than one month behind–United States 2011. (Figure is available at www.cdc.gov. Centers for Disease Control and Prevention. Catch-up immunization schedules for persons aged 4 months through 18 years who start late or who are more than 1 month behind—United States, 2011. MMWR 2011;60(5).)

(2) Skin testing with yellow fever vaccine is recommended before administration in children with a history of immediate hypersensitivity reaction (e.g., anaphylaxis or generalized urticaria) to eggs

(3) Immediate hypersensitivity reaction to eggs is a contraindication to both the parenteral and intranasal influenza vaccines. Less severe or local manifestations of allergy to egg are not contraindications to influenza vaccine

TABLE 16-1

MINIMUM AGE FOR INITIAL VACCINATION AND MINIMUM INTERVAL BETWEEN VACCINE DOSES, BY TYPE OF VACCINE

Vaccine	Minimum Age for First Dose*	Minimum Interval from Dose to Dose		
		1 to 2*	2 to 3*	3 to 4
DTaP[a,b]	6 wk	1 mo	1 mo	6 mo
Hib (PRP-OMP)[b]	6 wk	1 mo	1 mo[c]	2 mo
PCV13	6 wk	1 mo[d]	1 mo[d]	2 mo[d]
IPV	6 wk	1 mo	1 mo	6 mo[e]
MMR	12 mo[f]	1 mo	—	—
HBV[b]	Birth	1 mo	2 mo[g]	—
Varicella	12 mo	3 mo[h]	—	—
HAV	12 mo	6 mo	—	—
Influenza[i]	6 mo	1 mo	—	—
LAIV	2 y	1 mo		
Rotavirus	6 wk	1 mo	1 mo	—
MCV	2 y			
Tdap	11 y			
HPV	9 y	1 mo	3 mo[j]	

*These minimum acceptable ages and intervals may not correspond with the optimal recommended ages and intervals for vaccination. See Figure 16-1.

[a]The total number of doses of diphtheria and tetanus toxoids should not exceed six each before the seventh birthday. If the fourth dose is given after the fourth birthday, the fifth (booster) dose is not needed. If the fifth dose is needed, it should be given 6 months after the fourth dose.

[b]The combination vaccines Pediarix (DTaP/IPV/HepB) and Comvax (HepB-Hib) should not be given to infants <6 weeks.

[c]The booster dose, or fourth dose, of Hib vaccine recommended after the primary vaccination series should be administered no earlier than age 12 mo.

[d]See Figure 16-2 for recommendations of number of doses at different ages.

[e]If the third dose is given after the fourth birthday, the fourth (booster) dose is not needed. The final dose should be given after the age of 4 years regardless of number of previous doses.

[f]Although the age for measles vaccination may be as young as 6 mo in outbreak areas where cases are occurring in children 1 yr of age, children initially vaccinated before the first birthday should be revaccinated at 12–15 mo of age, and an additional dose of vaccine should be administered at the time of school entry or according to local policy. Doses of MMR or other measles-containing vaccine should be separated by at least 1 mo.

[g]This final dose is recommended at least 4 mo after the first dose, at least 2 mo after the second dose, and no earlier than 6 mo of age.

[h]A second dose of varicella is indicated for all children who received only one dose of the vaccine.

[i]Two doses of influenza are recommended for children 6 mo–9 yr of age who have never received the vaccine. Only one dose is required for children 9 yr or older, as well as children 6 mo–9 yr who have received the vaccine in the past.

[j]The third HPV dose must be given at least 24 weeks after the first dose.

Adapted from American Academy of Pediatrics: Red Book: 2009 Report of the Committee on Infectious Diseases, 28th ed. Elk Grove Village, IL, AAP,2009, Table 1.6 p. 29.

16

V. IMMUNOPROPHYLAXIS GUIDELINES FOR SPECIAL HOSTS

A. Immunocompromised Hosts

1. **Congenital immunodeficiency disorders:**

a. Live bacterial and live virus vaccines are generally contraindicated. See the *AAP Red Book*[2] for details regarding individual immunodeficiencies

Text continued on page 380

TABLE 16-2

GUIDE TO CONTRAINDICATIONS AND PRECAUTIONS TO IMMUNIZATIONS, 2009

Vaccine	Contraindications	Precautions*	Not Contraindications (Vaccines May Be Given)
General for all vaccines (DTaP, IPV, MMR, Hib, pneumococcal, hepatitis B, varicella, hepatitis A, influenza)	Anaphylactic reaction to a vaccine contraindicates further doses of that vaccine Anaphylactic reaction to a vaccine constituent contraindicates the use of vaccines containing that substance, including streptomycin and neomycin	Moderate or severe illnesses with or without a fever Latex allergy[†]	Mild to moderate local reaction (soreness, redness, swelling) after a dose of an injectable antigen Low-grade or moderate fever after a previous vaccine dose Mild acute illness with or without low-grade fever Current antimicrobial therapy Convalescent phase of illnesses Prematurity (same dosage and indications as for healthy, full-term infants) Recent exposure to an infectious disease Malnutrition Family history of adverse event to immunization History of penicillin or other nonspecific allergies or fact that relatives have such allergies Pregnancy of mother or household contact Unimmunized household contact Immunodeficient household contact Breast-feeding (nursing infant OR lactating mother)

DTaP	Encephalopathy within 7 days of administration of previous dose of DTaP/DTP Immediate anaphylactic reaction to DTaP Progressive neurologic disorder	Temperature of 40.5°C (104.8°F) within 48 hr after immunization with a previous dose of DTaP/DTP Collapse or shock-like state (hypotonic-hyporesponsive episode) within 48 hr of receiving a previous dose of DTaP/DTP Seizures within 3 days of receiving a previous dose of DTaP/DTP[‡] Persistent inconsolable crying lasting 3 hr, within 48 hr of receiving a previous dose of DTaP/DTP GBS within 6 wk after a dose[§]	Family history of seizures[‡] Family history of sudden infant death syndrome Family history of an adverse event after DTaP/DTP administration
IPV	Anaphylactic reactions to neomycin, streptomycin, or polymyxin B or previous dose of IPV	Pregnancy	

NOTE: This information is based on the recommendations of the Advisory Committee on Immunization Practices (ACIP) and the Committee on Infectious Diseases of the AAP. Sometimes, these recommendations vary from those in the manufacturers' package inserts. For more detailed information, health care professionals should consult the published recommendations of the ACIP, AAP, and the manufacturers' package inserts. These guidelines, originally issued in 1993, have been updated to give current recommendations as of 2009.

*The events or conditions listed as precautions, although not contraindications, should be reviewed carefully. The benefits and risks of administering a specific vaccine to a person under the circumstances should be considered. If the risks are believed to outweigh the benefits, the immunization should be withheld; if the benefits are believed to outweigh the risks (e.g., during an outbreak or foreign travel), the immunization should be given. Whether and when to administer DTaP to children with proven or suspected underlying neurologic disorders should be decided on an individual basis.

[†]If a person reports a severe (anaphylactic) allergy to latex, vaccines supplied in vials or syringes that contain natural rubber should not be administered unless the benefits of immunization outweigh the risks of an allergic reaction to the vaccine. For latex allergies other than anaphylactic allergies (e.g., a history of contact allergy to latex gloves), vaccines supplied in vials or syringes that contain dry natural rubber or latex can be administered.

[‡]Acetaminophen given before administering DTaP and thereafter q4hr for 24 hr should be considered for children with a personal or family (i.e., siblings or parents) history of seizures.

[§]The decision to give additional doses of DTaP should be made on the basis of consideration of benefit of further immunization versus risk of recurrence of GBS. For example, completion of the primary series in children is justified.

From American Academy of Pediatrics: Red Book: 2009 Report of the Committee on Infectious Diseases, 28th ed. Elk Grove Village, IL AAP, 2009, appendix VI, p. 848.

Continued

TABLE 16-2

GUIDE TO CONTRAINDICATIONS AND PRECAUTIONS TO IMMUNIZATIONS, 2009 (Continued)

Vaccine	Contraindications	Precautions*	Not Contraindications (Vaccines May Be Given)
MMR[‖,¶]	Pregnancy Anaphylactic reaction to neomycin or gelatin Known altered immune function (hematologic and solid tumors, congenital immunodeficiency, severe HIV infection, long-term immunosuppressive therapy)	Recent (within 3–11 mo, depending on product and dose) immune globulin administration[Δ] Thrombocytopenia or history of thrombocytopenic purpura[#] Tuberculosis or positive PPD[**] High dose steroid therapy	Simultaneous tuberculin skin testing[††] Breast-feeding Pregnancy of mother of recipient Immunodeficiency in a family member or household contact HIV infection Nonanaphylactic reactions to gelatin or neomycin
Hib	None	—	—
Hepatitis B	Anaphylactic reaction to baker's yeast	Prematurity[‡‡]	Pregnancy
Pneumococcal	Severe allergic reaction to previous dose/ component	Pregnancy Mod-severe acute illness	—
Varicella	Pregnancy Anaphylactic reaction to neomycin or gelatin Infection with HIV[§§] Known altered immune function (hematologic and solid tumors, congenital immunodeficiency, long-term immunosuppressive therapy)[‖‖]	Recent immune globulin administration[Δ] Family history of immunodeficiency[¶¶]	Pregnancy of mother of recipient Immunodeficiency in a household contact Household contact with HIV infection
Hepatitis A	Anaphylactic reaction to aluminum hydroxyphosphate sulfate, aluminum hydroxide or neomycin	Pregnancy	—
Influenza (TIV)	Anaphylactic reaction to eggs	GBS within 6 wk after a previous influenza immunization	Pregnancy
Tdap	Allergy to any vaccine component. Encephalopathy within 7 days of receiving previous vaccine	GBS Progressive neurologic disorder	Same as DTaP in addition to: pregnancy, breastfeeding, immunosuppression

Influenza (LAIV)	Pregnancy Underlying medical condition Wheezing in past 12 mo in a 2–4 yr old Aspirin treatment History of GBS		
Meningococcal	Severe allergic reaction to any component including diphtheria toxoid or any natural rubber latex	History of GBS	Pregnancy
HPV	Immediate hypersensitivity to yeast or vaccine component	Mod-severe acute illness Pregnancy	
Rotavirus	Severe allergic reaction to latex (RVI)	Mod-severe illness Pre existing chronic GI disease History of intussusception Spina bifida Bladder exstrophy	Breastfeeding Immunodeficient family member/contact

[‖]A theoretical risk exists that the administration of multiple live-virus vaccines within 30 days (4 weeks) of one another if not given on the same day will result in suboptimal immune response. No data substantiate this risk, however.

[¶]An anaphylactic reaction to egg ingestion previously was considered a contraindication unless skin testing and, if indicated, desensitization had been performed. However, skin testing is no longer recommended as of 1997.

[Δ]See *Red Book 2009* Table 3.34 for specific guidelines.[2]

[#]The decision to immunize should be made on the basis of consideration of the benefits of immunity to measles, mumps, and rubella versus the risk of recurrence or exacerbation of thrombocytopenia after immunization or from natural infections of measles or rubella. In most instances, the benefits of immunization will be much greater than the potential risks and justify giving MMR, particularly in view of the even greater risk of thrombocytopenia after measles or rubella disease. However, if previous episode of thrombocytopenia occurred in temporal proximity to immunization, not giving a subsequent dose may be prudent.

[**]A theoretical basis exists for concern that measles vaccine might exacerbate tuberculosis. Consequently, before administering MMR to people with untreated active tuberculosis, initiating antituberculosis therapy is advisable.

[††]Measles immunization may suppress tuberculin reactivity temporarily. MMR vaccine may be given after, or on the same day as, tuberculin testing. If MMR has been given recently, postpone the tuberculin skin test until 4–6 weeks after administration of MMR.

[‡‡]For preterm infants, see Figure 16-3.

[§§]Varicella vaccine should be considered for asymptomatic or mildly symptomatic HIV-infected children, see Section V.A2.

[‖‖]Varicella vaccine should not be administered to people who have cellular immunodeficiencies, but people with impaired humoral immunity may be immunized.

[¶¶]Varicella vaccine should not be administered to a person who has a family history of congenital or hereditary immunodeficiency in parents or siblings unless that person's immune competence has been substantiated clinically or verified by a laboratory.

GBS, Guillain-Barré syndrome; HIV, human immunodeficiency virus; PPD, purified protein derivative (tuberculin).

b. Inactivated vaccines should be given according to the routine schedule. Immune response may vary and may be inadequate
c. Immunoglobulin (Ig) therapy may be indicated
d. Household contacts: Immunize according to the routine childhood immunization schedule; yearly influenza vaccine is recommended

2. **Known or suspected human immunodeficiency virus (HIV) disease:**
a. Inactivated vaccines should be given according to the routine immunization schedule (see Fig. 16-1)
b. Immunize as soon as is age appropriate with inactivated vaccines. Do not administer oral polio vaccine (OPV) or bacilli Calmette-guerin (BCG)
c. Influenza vaccine should be given yearly. Do not administer the live attenuated influenza vaccine (LAIV)
d. MMR and varicella vaccines should be given to asymptomatic or mildly symptomatic patients with CD4 of 15% or greater.[3] Do not administer the MMRV combination vaccine. MMR vaccine can be given to a household member of a person with HIV. Varicella vaccine is encouraged in siblings and susceptible adult caregivers
e. Pneumococcal vaccine (PCV13): See Table 16-3

TABLE 16-3

RECOMMENDATIONS FOR PNEUMOCOCCAL IMMUNIZATION WITH PCV13 OR 23PS VACCINE FOR CHILDREN AT HIGH RISK FOR PNEUMOCOCCAL DISEASE*

Age	Previous Doses†	Recommendations
≤ 23 mo	Any	PCV13 according to Figure 16-1 (routine schedule) or Figure 16-2 (catch-up schedule)
24–71 mo	≤2 doses	2 doses of PCV13, 1 dose ≥8 weeks after most recent dose, and the second >8 weeks later 1 dose of 23PS ≥8 weeks after last dose of PCV13‡
	3 doses	1 dose of PCV13 ≥8 weeks after most recent dose 1 dose of 23PS ≥8 weeks after last dose of PCV13‡
	4 doses	1 supplemental dose of PCV13 ≥8 weeks after most recent dose 1 dose of 23PS ≥8 weeks after last dose of PCV13‡
6–18 y	Any	1 dose of PCV13

*Children at high risk include those who are immunocompetent including children with chronic heart disease, chronic lung disease, diabetes mellitus, cerebrospinal fluid (CSF) leaks, cochlear implants; those who have functional asplenia or anatomic asplenia including children with sickle cell disease (or other hemoglobinopathies), congenital or acquired asplenia; and those who have immunocompromising conditions including children with HIV, chronic renal failure or nephrotic syndrome, malignancy or diseases associated with immunosuppressive therapy, and congenital immunodeficiency.

†PCV7 or PCV13 or a combination.

‡A second dose of 23PS is indicated 5 years after the first in children who are immunocompromised (HIV, chronic renal failure or nephrotic syndrome, immunosupressed due to drugs or radiation therapy or with congenital immunodeficiency) but not with immunocompetent children with chronic illness.

Adapted from American Academy of Pediatrics: Red Book: 2009 Report of the Committee on Infectious Diseases, 28th ed., Elk Grove Village, IL, AAP, 2009.

TABLE 16-4

IMMUNIZATION FOR ONCOLOGY PATIENTS

Vaccine	Indications and Comments
DtaP	Indicated for incompletely immunized children <7 yr, even during active chemotherapy
Td	Indicated 1 yr after completion of therapy in children 7 yr
Hib	Indicated for incompletely immunized children if <7 yr
HBV	Indicated for incompletely immunized children
23PS	Indicated for asplenic patients
PCV13	Indicated for incompletely immunized children <5 yr (See Table 16-3)
Meningococcus	Consider in asplenic patients
IPV	Indicated for incompletely immunized children; also recommended for all household contacts requiring immunization to reduce the risk for vaccine-associated polio
MMR	Contraindicated until child is in remission and finished with all chemotherapy for 3–6 mo; may need to reimmunize after chemotherapy if titers have fallen below protective levels
Influenza	Defer in active chemotherapy; may give as early as 3–4 wk after remission and off chemotherapy if during influenza season; peripheral granulocyte and lymphocyte counts should be >1000/μL; should also be given to household contacts of children with cancer
Varicella	Consider immunizing children who have remained in remission and have finished chemotherapy for >1 yr; with absolute lymphocyte count of >700/μL and platelet count of >100,000/μL within 24 hr of immunization; check titers of previously immunized children to verify protective levels of antibodies

NOTE: Immune reconstitution is slower for oncology patients who have received bone marrow transplants. See Centers for Disease Control and Prevention: MMWR 2000;49(No. RR-10):1–147 for vaccine schedule.

f. Meningococcal vaccine (MCV4): Administer 2 doses at least 8 weeks apart
g. Passive immunoprophylaxis or chemoprophylaxis should be considered in all HIV-infected children after exposure to any vaccine-preventable disease

3. **Oncology patients** (See Table 16-4)

a. All live vaccines should be delayed at least 3 months after immunosuppressive therapy has been discontinued

4. **Functional or anatomic asplenia (including sickle cell disease):**

a. Penicillin prophylaxis: See Chapter 14
b. Pneumococcal vaccine: See Table 16-3
c. Meningococcal vaccine: At age 2 years or at diagnosis if ≥2 years old then a booster dose every 5 years
d. Ensure that *Haemophilus influenzae* type B (Hib) series is completed; children ≥5 years who never received Hib immunization should receive one dose
e. Children ≥2 years undergoing elective splenectomy should receive one or both of the pneumococcal vaccines and the meningococcal vaccine at least 2 weeks before surgery to ensure optimal immune response. Children <2 years should receive PCV13 before surgery

TABLE 16-5

LIVE-VIRUS IMMUNIZATION FOR PATIENTS RECEIVING CORTICOSTEROID THERAPY

Steroid Dose	Recommended Guidelines
Topical or inhaled therapy or local injection of steroids	Live-virus vaccines may be given unless there is clinical evidence of immunosuppression; if suppressed, wait 1 mo after cessation of therapy to give live-virus vaccines
Physiologic maintenance doses of steroids	Live-virus vaccines may be given
Low-dose steroids (<2 mg/kg/day prednisone or equivalent, or <20 mg/day if >10 kg, daily or on alternate days)	Live-virus vaccines may be given
High-dose steroids (≥2 mg/kg/day prednisone or equivalent, or 20 mg/day if >10 kg, daily or on alternate days)	
Duration of therapy <14 days	May give live-virus vaccines immediately after cessation of therapy (Consider 2-wk delay in administration.)
Duration of therapy ≥14 days	Do not give live-virus vaccines until therapy has been discontinued for 1 mo
Children with immunosuppressive disorders receiving steroid therapy	Live-virus vaccines are contraindicated, except in special circumstances

Adapted from American Academy of Pediatrics: Red Book: 2009. Report of the Committee on Infectious Diseases, 28th ed. Elk Grove Village, IL, AAP, 2009.

B. Corticosteroid Administration

Only live viral and live bacterial vaccines are potentially contraindicated (see Table 16-5 for details).

C. Patients Treated with Immunoglobulin or Other Blood Products

See the *AAP Red Book*[2] for suggested intervals between immunoglobulin or blood product administration and MMR or varicella immunization.

D. Preterm and Low Birth Weight Infants (<2500 g)

Immunize according to chronologic age using regular vaccine dosage.

1. **Hepatitis B virus (HBV):** Initiation of HBV vaccine may be delayed for infants of hepatitis B surface antigen (HBsAg)-negative mothers until the child is >2 kg or age 2 months, whichever is earlier. See Figure 16-3 for management of preterm infant born to mother with hepatitis B

FIGURE 16-3

Management of neonates born to mothers with unknown or positive HbsAg status. BW, birth weight. a, Only single antigen vaccine should be used. b, A fourth vaccine dose is required if using combination vaccines. (2 mo, 4 mo, 6 mo [Pediarix] or 12–15 mo [Comvax].) c, Reimmunization may be required based on anti-HBs. Test at 9–18 mo of age. *(Data from American Academy of Pediatrics: Red Book: 2009 Report of the Committee on Infectious Diseases, 28th ed. Elk Grove Village, IL, AAP, 2009, Table 3.19 p. 349 and Table 3.20 p. 351.)*

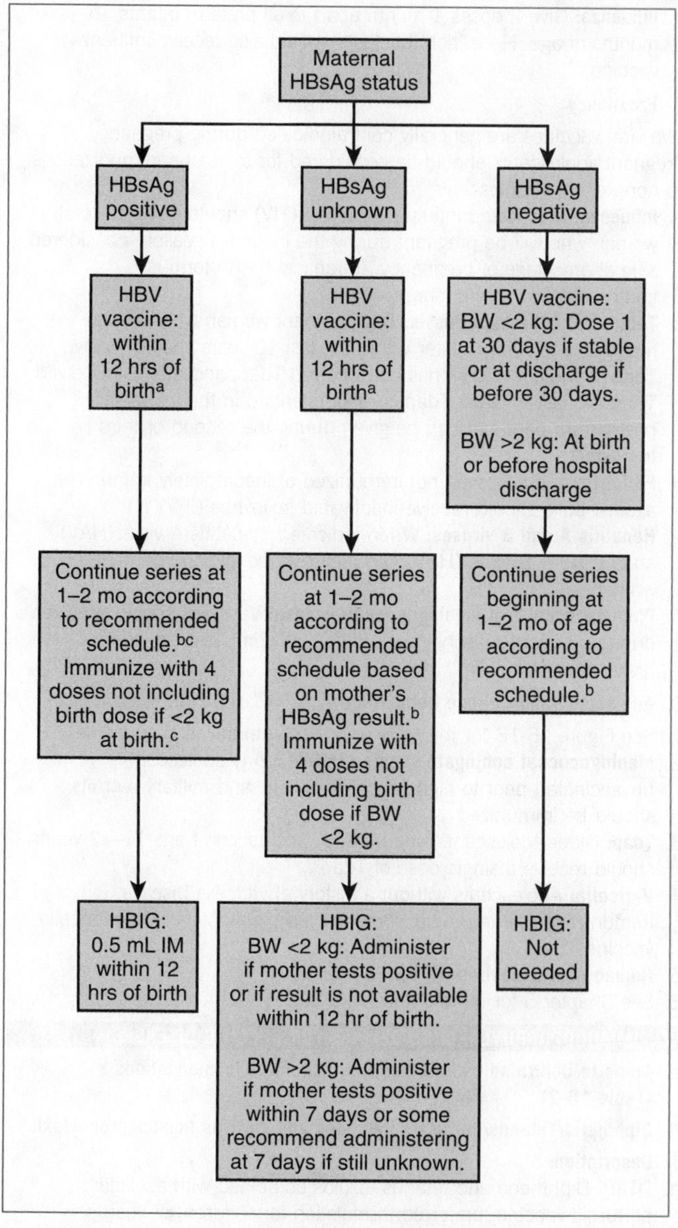

Maternal HBsAg status

HBsAg positive
- HBV vaccine: within 12 hrs of birth[a]
- Continue series at 1–2 mo according to recommended schedule.[b,c] Immunize with 4 doses not including birth dose if <2 kg at birth.[c]
- HBIG: 0.5 mL IM within 12 hrs of birth

HBsAg unknown
- HBV vaccine: within 12 hrs of birth[a]
- Continue series at 1–2 mo according to recommended schedule based on mother's HBsAg result.[b] Immunize with 4 doses not including birth dose if BW <2 kg.
- HBIG: BW <2 kg: Administer if mother tests positive or if result is not available within 12 hr of birth. BW >2 kg: Administer if mother tests positive within 7 days or some recommend administering at 7 days if still unknown.

HBsAg negative
- HBV vaccine: BW <2 kg: Dose 1 at 30 days if stable or at discharge if before 30 days. BW >2 kg: At birth or before hospital discharge
- Continue series beginning at 1–2 mo of age according to recommended schedule.[b]
- HBIG: Not needed

2. **Influenza:** Give 2 doses 1 month apart to all preterm infants >6 months of age. Household contacts should also receive influenza vaccine

E. Pregnancy

Live viral vaccines are generally contraindicated during pregnancy. Pregnant adolescents should be considered for the same immunizations as nonpregnant adolescents.

1. **Influenza:** Inactivated influenza vaccine (TIV) should be given to all women who will be pregnant during the influenza season; considered safe at any stage of pregnancy. Intranasal (LAIV) form is contraindicated during pregnancy
2. **Tetanus/diphtheria/pertussis:** Any pregnant woman who has not received a tetanus booster within the last 10 years should receive Tdap. If the adolescent has not received Tdap, and has not received Td in the last 2 years, Tdap is recommended in the immediate postpartum period or can be given during the second or third trimester[4]
3. **Polio:** Pregnant women not immunized or incompletely immunized against polio should receive inactivated poliovirus (IPV)
4. **Hepatitis A and B viruses:** When indicated, hepatitis A virus (HAV) and hepatitis B virus (HBV) vaccines may be given to pregnant women
5. **Pneumococcal and meningococcal disease:** Vaccines should be given during pregnancy if a high risk of serious complications due to these diseases exist

F. Adolescent and College Population

1. See Figure 16-1B for the recommended immunization schedule
2. **Meningococcal conjugate vaccine (MCV4):** Any adolescent unvaccinated prior to high school or college and military recruits should be immunized
3. **Tdap:** Older adolescents who missed vaccination at age 11–12 years should receive a single dose of Tdap[5]
4. **Varicella:** Adolescents without a history of varicella disease, immunization, or immunity should receive two doses of the varicella vaccine
5. **Human papillomavirus (HPV):** See section VI.F
6. See Chapter 5 for more details

VI. IMMUNOPROPHYLAXIS GUIDELINES FOR SPECIFIC DISEASES

A. Guide to Contraindications and Precautions to Immunizations (Table 16-2)

B. Diphtheria/Tetanus/Pertussis Vaccines and Tetanus Immunoprophylaxis

1. **Description:**

a. DTaP: Diphtheria and tetanus toxoids combined with acellular pertussis vaccine; preferred formulation for children <7 years

b. DT: Diphtheria and tetanus toxoids without pertussis vaccine; use in children <7 years in whom pertussis vaccine is contraindicated
c. Td: Tetanus toxoid with one third to one sixth the dose of diphtheria toxoid of other preparations; use in individuals ≥7 years
d. Tdap (Boostrix and Adacel): Tetanus and diphtheria toxoids combined with acellular pertussis vaccine. Boostrix can be given at age 10 years, Adacel at age 11 years

2. **Indications:**
a. Routine (Figure 16-1)
b. Children ages 7–10 yr who are not fully immunized against pertussis (including never being immunized or unknown status) should get a single dose of TdaP, regardless of interval since last tetanus immunization
c. Adolescents 11–18 years should receive a single dose of Tdap instead of Td for booster immunization. If they have received Td, it is recommended to administer a single dose of Tdap regardless of the interval since last tetanus immunization
d. Tetanus prophylaxis in wound management (Table 16-6)

3. **Precautions/contraindications** (Table 16-2)
4. **Children with neurologic disorders:**
a. Seizures:
(1) Poorly controlled or new-onset seizures: Defer pertussis immunization until seizure disorder is well controlled and progressive neurologic disorder is excluded; then give DTaP and antipyretics for 24 hours after immunization
(2) Personal or family history of febrile seizures: Give DTaP and antipyretics for 24 hours after immunization
b. Known or suspected progressive neurologic disorder: Defer pertussis immunization until diagnosis and treatment are established and neurologic condition is stable. Progressive disorders may merit

TABLE 16-6
INDICATIONS FOR TETANUS PROPHYLAXIS

	Clean, Minor Wounds		All Other Wounds	
Prior Tetanus Toxoid Doses	**Tetanus Vaccine***	**TIG**	**Tetanus Vaccine***	**TIG**
Unknown or <3	Yes	No	Yes	Yes
≥3, last <5 yr ago	No	No	No	No†
≥3, last 5–10 yr ago	No	No	Yes	No†
≥3, last >10 yr ago	Yes	No	Yes	No†

*Vaccine choice for child <7 yr is DTaP (DT if pertussis is contraindicated). For a child >7 years Tdap is the vaccine of choice if pertussis is not contraindicated.
†Any child with HIV infection or who is within the first year after bone marrow transplantation should receive TIG for any tetanus-prone wound regardless of vaccination status.
TIG, Tetanus immune globulin: 250 U IM.
Adapted from American Academy of Pediatrics: Red Book: 2009 Report of the Committee on Infectious Diseases, 28th ed. Elk Grove Village, IL, AAP, 2009, Table 3.77 p. 657.

16

permanent deferral of pertussis immunization. Reconsider pertussis immunization at each visit. Use DT if pertussis vaccine is permanently deferred

c. Children <1 year with neurologic disorders necessitating temporary deferment of pertussis vaccine should not receive DT because the risk for diphtheria and tetanus is low in the first year of life. After the first birthday, initiate either DT or DTaP immunization as clinically indicated

5. **Side effects:**

a. Minor side effects within 3 days: Erythema (26%–39%), drowsiness (40%–47%), swelling (15%–30%), anorexia (19%–25%), fussiness (14%–19%), vomiting (7%–13%), pain (4%–11%), body temperature >38.3°C (3%–5%)

b. Moderate to severe side effects of DTP: Allergic reactions 1/100,000, persistent crying >3 hours (1/100), seizures (1/1,750), hypotonic-hyporesponsive episode (1/1,750), anaphylaxis (1/50,000), body temperature >40.5°C (rare). These side effects are similar with DTaP, but significantly less frequent

6. **Administration:** DTaP, DT, Td, and TdaP are all given in a dose of 0.5 mL IM

7. **Special considerations:**

a. Pertussis exposure: Immunize all unimmunized or partially immunized close contacts <7 years and >10 years according to the recommended schedule
   (1) Give fourth dose of DTaP if third dose was given >6 months prior
   (2) Give booster dose of DTaP if last dose was given >3 years prior and child is <7 years

b. The total number of DT and DTaP immunizations should not exceed six by the seventh birthday

c. Treatment doses and duration vary by age. Recommended treatment includes azithromycin, erythromycin and clarithromycin. Alternatives include trimethoprim-sulfamethoxazole (See Table 3.44 of the *2009 Red Book* for more details[2])

C. Haemophilus Influenza Type B Immunoprophylaxis

1. **Description:** The three licensed vaccines consist of a capsular polysaccharide antigen (PRP) conjugated to a carrier protein. It is not necessary to use the same formulation for the entire series. Vaccines do not confer protection against the disease associated with the carrier (e.g., PRP-T does not protect against tetanus)

a. PRP-OMP (PedvaxHIB): Conjugated to outer membrane protein of *Neisseria meningitidis;* requires only two doses in primary series (2 and 4 months) plus booster at 12–15 months. If PRP-OMP is used only for part of the immunization series, the recommended number of doses to complete the series is based on the other Hib conjugate vaccine used. Children without prior DTaP vaccine may respond better to PRP-OMP than to other formulations

b. PRP-T (Hiberix): Conjugated to tetanus toxoid. Approved as a booster dose in ages 15 months to 4 years
c. PRP-T (ActHIB): Conjugated to tetanus toxoid. Approved for 2–18 months
d. See section VI.P for combination vaccines available
2. **Indications:**
a. Routine (Figure 16-1)
b. For catch-up schedule (Figure 16-2)
c. Children aged 12–59 months who are unimmunized or have received only one dose and have an underlying disease that predisposes them to Hib disease (HIV, IgG_2 deficiency, chemotherapy patients) should receive two doses separated by 2 months. If they have received two doses before 12 months they should receive a third dose. If they are unimmunized and >59 months they should receive two doses separated by 1–2 months
d. Children undergoing splenectomy: May benefit from an additional dose 7–10 days before procedure, even if series was previously completed
e. Children with invasive Hib disease at age <24 months: Begin Hib immunization 1 month after acute illness and continue as if previously unimmunized. Vaccination is not required if invasive disease develops after age 24 months. Consider immunologic workup for any child with invasive Hib disease after completing the immunization series
3. **Precautions/contraindications** (Table 16-2)
4. **Side effects:** Local pain, redness, and swelling in 25% of recipients (mild, lasting <24 hours)
5. **Administration:** Dose is 0.5 mL IM
6. **Exposure:** See the *AAP Red Book*[2] for details because this issue is controversial

D. Hepatitis A Virus Immunoprophylaxis

1. **Description:** HAV vaccine is an inactivated adsorbed vaccine. Two brands are available, Havrix and Vaqta (both are preservative-free). Licensed only for children ≥12 months
2. **Indications**[6]**:**
a. All children ≥12 months (see Figure 16-1 for schedule). Programs established to vaccinate children age 2–18 years should continue giving catch-up vaccinations during routine visits
b. Travelers to or residents of endemic areas
c. After exposure to HAV if future exposure is likely
d. Military personnel
e. Homosexual or bisexual men
f. Users of illicit injection and noninjection drugs
g. Patients with clotting factor disorders
h. Patients with chronic liver disease, including HBV and hepatitis C virus (HCV)
i. Persons at risk for occupational exposure

TABLE 16-7

RECOMMENDED DOSAGES AND SCHEDULES FOR HEPATITIS A VIRUS (HAV) VACCINES

Age (yr)	Vaccine	Antigen	Volume (mL)	No. of Doses	Schedule
1–18	Havrix (SB)	720 ELU	0.5	2	Initial and 6–12 mo later
	Vaqta (Merck)	25 U	0.5	2	Initial and 6–18 mo later
≥19	Havrix (SB)	1440 ELU	1.0	2	Initial and 6–12 mo later
	Vaqta (Merck)	50 U	1.0	2	Initial and 6–18 mo later
>18	Twinrix* (SB)	720 ELU	1.0	3–4	Initial and 1 and 6 mo later OR Initial, 7 and 21–30 days later, and 12 mo later

*Twinrix is a combination of hepatitis B (Energix-B, 20 mcg) and hepatitis A (Havrix, 720 ELU) vaccines.
ELU, Enzyme-linked immunoassay units; SB, SmithKline Beecham; U, antigen units.
Adapted from American Academy of Pediatrics: Red Book: 2009 Report of the Committee on Infectious Diseases, 28th ed. Elk Grove Village, IL, AAP, 2009, Table 3.14 p. 332.

j. Immunocompromised individuals; may be immunized, although efficacy is not established in immunocompromised children
k. Consider use in staff of institutions with ongoing or recurrent outbreaks
3. **Precautions/contraindications** (Table 16-2)
4. **Side effects:** Local reactions are typically mild; include injection site tenderness (21%), redness, swelling and warmth (4%), rash (1%), fever (11%), headache (<9%). No serious adverse events have been reported[7,8]
5. **Administration:** See Table 16-7 for dose and schedule; give IM
6. **Special considerations:**
a. Pre-exposure immunoprophylaxis for travelers
   (1) HAV vaccine is preferred for travelers ≥12 months old; a single dose usually provides adequate immunity if time does not allow further doses before travel
   (2) Ig, given IM, is protective for up to 5 months; see the *AAP Red Book*[2] for dosing. Ig can be given without vaccine to children <12 months before travel
b. Postexposure immunoprophylaxis: If exposed in the last 2 weeks and <12 months old should receive Ig. If 12 months or older, should receive HAV. If it has been >2 weeks since exposure, no prophylaxis is indicated if <12 months old, but HAV might be considered for 12 months and older if the exposure is ongoing. See the *AAP Red Book*[2] for Ig dosing and more information

E. Hepatitis B Virus Immunoprophylaxis

1. **Description:**
a. Hepatitis B immune globulin (HBIG): Prepared from plasma containing high-titer anti-HBsAg antibodies and negative for antibodies to HIV and HCV. Dose: Infants, 0.5 mL IM; older children, 0.06 mL/kg IM

TABLE 16-8

RECOMMENDED DOSE FOR HEPATITIS B VIRUS (HBV) VACCINES*

Patient Group	Recombivax Dose (mcg)†	Engerix-B Dose (mcg)‡
Up to 19 yr	5	10
11–15 yr§	10‡	—
≥20 yr	10	20
Patients undergoing dialysis and other immunosuppressed adults	40	40

*Vaccines are administered on a three- or four-dose schedule. Four doses are given if HBV is administered at birth, and a combination vaccine is used to complete the series.

†Recombivax HB is available from Merck & Co. in pediatric, adult, and dialysis patient formulations.

‡Engerix-B is available from GlaxoSmithKline Biologicals; it is also available as combination vaccines. See Section VI.P for details.

§May use alternative two-dose regimen 6 months apart.

Adapted from American Academy of Pediatrics: Red Book: 2009 Report of the Committee on Infectious Diseases, 28th ed. Elk Grove Village, IL, AAP, 2009, Table 3.17 p. 344.

b. HBV vaccine: Adsorbed HBsAg produced recombinantly. Different recombinant vaccines may be used interchangeably
c. See section VI.P for information on combination vaccines containing hepatitis B

2. **Indications:**
a. Routine (Figure 16-1)
b. Infants of mothers who are HBsAg positive or indeterminate (Figure 16-3)
3. **Precautions/contraindications** (Table 16-2)
4. **Side effects:** Pain at injection site (3%–29%) or fever >37.7°C (1%–6%); immediate hypersensitivity reaction is very rare
5. **Administration:**
a. See Table 16-8 for dose; give IM in the anterolateral thigh or deltoid; administration in the buttocks or intradermally is not recommended due to decreased immunogenicity
b. HBV vaccines are interchangeable between different manufacturers, but interchangeability of Pediarix may be limited by the DTaP component. See section VI.P
6. **Special considerations:** See Table 16-9 for HBV prophylaxis after percutaneous exposure to blood

F. Human Papillomavirus Immunoprophylaxis

1. **Description:** There are two approved vaccines. HPV4 (Gardasil by Merck) vaccine is an inactivated vaccine for HPV types 6, 11, 16, and 18 administered to females and males. It has proven efficacy against cervical, vulvar, and vaginal cancers caused by types 16 and 18, against genital warts in females and males caused by types 6 and 11, and against precancerous dysplastic lesions caused by all four types.[9] HPV2 (Cervarix by GlaxoSmithKline) has been approved for females and is an inactivated vaccine for HPV types 16 and 18

16

TABLE 16-9

HEPATITIS B VIRUS (HBV) PROPHYLAXIS AFTER PERCUTANEOUS EXPOSURE TO BLOOD

	HBsAg Status of Source of Blood		
Exposed Person	**Positive**	**Negative**	**Unknown**
Unimmunized	HBIG* and HBV series	HBV series	HBV series
Previously immunized			
Known responder	No treatment	No treatment	No treatment
Known nonresponder	HBIG and HBV series	No treatment	Treat as if positive if known high risk source Or HBIG × 2 (1 mo apart)†
Response unknown	Test exposed person for Anti-HBsAg and HBV booster dose	No treatment	Test exposed person for anti-HBs: If inadequate HBV booster dose If adequate (>10 mIU/mL)—no treatment

*HBIG dose is 0.06 mL/kg.

†Preferred if already received two vaccine series with failure to respond.

Adapted from American Academy of Pediatrics: Red Book: 2009 Report of the Committee on Infectious Diseases, 27th ed. Elk Grove Village, IL, AAP, 2009, Table 3.22, p 355.

2. **Indications:**
a. Routine (Figure 16-1)
b. Females age 11 to 26 years (can be given to girls as young as age 9 years and catch up can be given to girls aged 13–26) can receive Gardasil or Cervarix
c. Males age 9–26. Only Gardasil is approved for males
3. **Precautions/contraindications** (Table 16-2)
4. **Side effects:** Pain, swelling, and erythema at injection site (83%, 25%, and 25%, respectively), fever (10%), nausea (6%), dizziness (4%), syncope
5. **Administration:** Dose is 0.5 mL IM
a. First dose can be given at age 9 years but recommended to give the first dose at age 11–12 years. Second dose should be given 2 months after the first dose. Third dose should be given 6 months after the initial dose and 12 weeks after the second dose
b. Syncope has been reported after vaccination with Gardasil. Recommendations include observation for 15 minutes after administration
6. **Special considerations:**
a. Females or males with evidence of current HPV infection such as cervical dysplasia or warts of a positive HPV DNA test should still be immunized
b. Can be given to immunocompromised patients

G. Influenza Immunoprophylaxis

Influenza strains can change year to year, particularly in time of pandemic flu; please refer to the CDC for up to date guidelines.[1]

1. **Description:**
   a. Activated and inactivated influenza vaccines are produced in embryonated eggs
   b. Vaccines contain three viral strains (usually two type A strains and one type B strain), based on expected prevalent influenza strains for the upcoming winter
   c. Preparations:
      (1) Inactivated (TIV): Split-virus vaccines: Subvirion or purified surface antigen vaccines available; licensed for children ≥6 months
      (2) Live, attenuated intranasal vaccine (LAIV): Licensed for healthy children >2 years, nonpregnant adolescents and children free from asthma or wheezing who are 2 years of age and older. Not recommended for children with asthma or those <5 years with history of wheezing or possible reactive airway disease, pregnant adolescents, people with chronic illness, children on aspirin therapy, or immunocompromised children
2. **Indications:**
   a. All children 6 months and older and close contacts annually
   b. High-risk children:
      (1) Asthma and other chronic pulmonary diseases
      (2) Hemodynamically significant cardiac disease
      (3) Immunosuppressive disorders and therapy
      (4) HIV infection
      (5) Sickle cell anemia and other hemoglobinopathies
      (6) Diseases requiring long-term aspirin therapy
      (7) Chronic renal disease
      (8) Chronic metabolic disease, including diabetes mellitus
      (9) Conditions that compromise respiratory function or handling of secretions (e.g., spinal cord injury, neuromuscular disorders, cognitive dysfunction, or seizure disorder)
   c. Close contacts of high-risk children, children younger than 24 months, and adults, including household contacts, health care workers, and daycare providers. Consider chemoprophylaxis of these individuals
   d. Consider immunization for other high-risk persons
      (1) Women who are pregnant during influenza season (TIV only, not LAIV)
      (2) International travel to areas with influenza outbreaks
      (3) Institutional settings, including colleges and other residential facilities
3. **Precautions/contraindications** (Table 16-2)
4. **Side effects:**
   a. Fever 6–24 hours after immunization in children <2 years (10%–35%); rare in children >2 years
   b. Local reactions uncommon in children <13 years; 10% in children ≥13 years

16

TABLE 16-10

INFLUENZA VACCINE DOSAGE AND SCHEDULE

Vaccine	Age	Volume (mL)	Number of Doses
TIV	6–35 mo	0.25	1 or 2*
TIV	3–8 yr	0.5	1 or 2*
TIV	≥9 yr	0.5	1
LAIV	2–8 yr	0.2	1 or 2*
LAIV	≥9 yr	0.2	1

*Two doses, at least 1 mo apart, recommended for children <9 yr receiving influenza vaccine for the first time. Try to give the second dose before December.

Adapted from American Academy of Pediatrics: Red Book: 2009 Report of the Committee on Infectious Diseases, 28th ed. Elk Grove Village, IL, AAP, 2009, Table 3.30 and 3.31, p. 406–407.

c. Guillain-Barré syndrome (GBS): If there is an association between the influenza vaccine and GBS, the risk is rare and no more than 1–2 cases per million doses
d. LAIV: There are no statistically significant differences observed between placebo and LAIV recipients for fever, rhinitis, or nasal congestion

5. **Administration:**
a. Administer annually during the fall in preparation for winter influenza season
b. Dosage and schedule (Table 16-10); give TIV vaccine IM and LAIV intranasally

6. **Special considerations:**
a. Children receiving chemotherapy have poor seroconversion rates until chemotherapy is discontinued for 3–4 weeks and absolute neutrophil and lymphocyte counts are >1000/μL
b. Immunization may be delayed in patients on prolonged high-dose steroids (equivalent to 2 mg/kg/day or >20 mg/day of prednisone) until dose is decreased, only if time allows before the influenza season
c. Infants <6 months with high-risk conditions should not be immunized and should not receive chemoprophylaxis. However, close contacts of these infants should receive the vaccine
d. LAIV should not be administered until >48 hours after completing antiviral therapy for influenza[10]

7. **Chemoprophylaxis for influenza A and B:** High rates of resistance of influenza A and B to amantadine and rimantadine and of influenza A to oseltamivir cause recommendations to vary by season and location. Please refer to www.cdc.gov/flu/professionals/antivirals/index.htm
a. Oseltamivir and zanamivir: Approved for use in the United States for chemoprophylaxis against influenza A and B in children
(1) Oseltamivir: Approved for children ≥1 year
(2) Zanamivir: Approved for children ≥5 years

b. Amantadine and rimantadine: Approved for use in the United States for chemoprophylaxis against influenza A in children 1 year or older
c. Indications:
   (1) Unimmunized high-risk children including those for whom the vaccine is contraindicated or children immunized less than 2 weeks before influenza outbreak
   (2) Unimmunized individuals in close contact with or providing care to high-risk individuals
   (3) Immunodeficient individuals unlikely to have protective response to vaccine
   (4) Control of outbreaks in a closed setting
   (5) Immunized high-risk individuals if vaccine strain different from circulating strain
   (6) Healthy children with severe illness from influenza
d. Chemoprophylaxis is not a substitute for immunization and does not interfere with the immune response to the inactivated virus vaccine
e. Do not administer chemoprophylaxis until at least 2 weeks after administration of LAIV

H. Measles/Mumps/Rubella Immunoprophylaxis

1. **Description:**
a. MMR: Combination vaccine composed of live, attenuated viruses. Measles and mumps vaccines are grown in chick embryo cell culture; rubella vaccine is prepared in human diploid cell culture
b. Monovalent formulations are no longer available
c. Measles Ig: Intramuscular and intravenous immunoglobulin (IVIG) preparations contain similar concentration of measles antibody
d. Rubella Ig: There are limited data showing decreased clinical infection, viral shedding, and rate of viremia[2]
2. **Indications:**
a. Routine (Figure 16-1)
b. Postpubertal females without documentation or presumptive evidence of rubella immunity should be immunized unless they are pregnant. Serologic screening for susceptibility only delays vaccination
c. Screen all adolescents and young adults for susceptibility to measles. People are considered susceptible to measles unless they have had two measles-containing vaccines given 1 month apart after age 12 months, physician-diagnosed disease, or laboratory evidence of immunity
d. Immunize people traveling to foreign countries with MMR. Young children may need to be immunized at a younger age than recommended for routine immunization. See the *AAP Red Book*[2] for details
3. **Precautions/contraindications** (Table 16-2)

16

4. **Misconceptions:** The following are *not* contraindications to MMR administration:
a. Anaphylactic reaction to eggs: Consider observing patient for 90 minutes after vaccine administration. Skin testing is not predictive of hypersensitivity reaction and therefore is not recommended
b. Allergy to penicillin
c. History of seizures: There is a slightly increased risk for seizure after immunization. Temperature should be followed and treated with antipyretics
5. **Side effects[2]:**
a. Minor side effects 7–12 days after immunization: Fever to 39.4°C or higher develops in 5%–15% of immunized people, usually between 6 and 12 days after immunization and can last up to 5 days; transient rash (5%)
b. Moderate to severe side effects: Febrile seizures are rare and occur 8–14 days after the first dose; transient thrombocytopenia (1 in 25,000 to 1 in 2 million) 2–3 weeks after immunization; encephalitis and encephalopathy (<1 in 1 million)
6. **Administration:**
a. Dose is 0.5 mL SC
b. See *AAP Red Book*[2] for suggested intervals between Ig administration and MMR vaccination
c. Purified protein derivative (PPD) testing may be done on the day of immunization; otherwise, postpone PPD 4–6 weeks because of suppression of response
7. **Special considerations:**
a. Measles postexposure immunoprophylaxis:
   (1) Vaccine prevents or modifies disease if given within 72 hours of exposure; hence it is the intervention of choice for measles outbreak
   (2) Ig prevents or modifies disease if given within 6 days of exposure. It is indicated in susceptible household contacts, pregnant women, children <1 year, and immunocompromised individuals including HIV infected children regardless of immunization status. It is not indicated for contacts who have received one dose of the vaccine at 12 months or older unless the person is immunocompromised. Dosage is as follows:
      (a) Standard-dose Ig for children and pregnant women: 0.25 mL/kg (maximum dose, 15 mL) IM
      (b) High-dose Ig for immunocompromised children (including those with HIV infection): 0.5 mL/kg (maximum dose, 15 mL) IM. Not required if IVIG received within 3 weeks before exposure
b. Rubella postexposure immunoprophylaxis: Ig can be considered in rubella-susceptible women exposed to confirmed rubella early in pregnancy only if termination of the pregnancy is refused

I. Meningococcus Immunoprophylaxis

1. **Description:** Two meningococcal vaccines are available
a. A quadrivalent serogroup-specific vaccine made from purified capsular polysaccharide antigen from groups A, C, Y, and W-135 (MPSV4); intended for use in patients age 2 years and older
b. A tetravalent conjugate vaccine with antigen from groups A, C, Y, and W-135 (MCV4); intended for use in patients 2–55 years. This is the preferred vaccine
c. Immunogenicity of serogroup antigens varies with age of child. No vaccine is available for group B because of poor immunogenicity
2. **Indications:**
a. Routine immunization (Fig. 16-1)
   (1) Should receive first dose at 11–12 yrs with booster at 16 yrs. If first dose given at 13–15 yr give booster at age 16 to 18 years.
b. High-risk groups ≥2 years should receive 2 doses of MCV4 at least 8 weeks apart between 2–10 yr. Then 1 dose every 5 years. These groups include:
   (1) Functional or anatomic asplenia
   (2) Terminal complement or properdin deficiencies
c. Possible adjunct to postexposure chemoprophylaxis in an outbreak setting
d. College freshmen, particularly those living in dormitories or residence halls, should receive MCV4
e. Travelers to endemic or hyperendemic areas
f. U.S. military recruits
g. HIV infected children at least 2 years old should get 2 doses separated by 8 weeks
h. Outbreak control
3. **Precautions/contraindications** (Table 16-2)
4. **Side effects:** Mild; localized erythema and pain lasting 1–2 days occurs infrequently, fever (2%–5%), headache, irritability, fatigue
5. **Administration:** Dose is 0.5 mL SC for MPSV4 and 0.5 mL IM for MCV4
6. **Postexposure chemoprophylaxis:** Antibiotics should be given to those with contact with the index case within 7 days before the onset of illness including household, child care, and nursery school contacts, direct exposure to the index case's secretions including mouth-to-mouth and unprotected endotracheal intubation, those who frequently slept in the home of the index case, and passengers next to the index case during airline flights longer than 8 hours. Treatment should be given within 24 hours of primary case diagnosis
a. Rifampin is the drug of choice (see Formulary for dosage information)
b. Ciprofloxacin (20 mg/kg with a maximum of 500 mg single dose) may be given to persons ≥18 years. This may be justified in those <18 years old in certain circumstances
c. Ceftriaxone (125 mg single dose in children <15 years, 250 mg single dose in children ≥15 years)

J. Pneumococcal Immunoprophylaxis

1. **Description:**
a. PCV13: Pneumococcal conjugate vaccine includes 13 purified capsular polysaccharides of *Streptococcus pneumoniae,* each coupled to a variant of diphtheria toxin. Serotypes are 1, 3, 4, 5, 6A, 6B, 7F, 9V, 14, 18C, 19A, 19F, and 23F. This has taken the place of PCV7[11]
b. 23PS: Purified capsular polysaccharide includes antigen from 23 serotypes of *S. pneumoniae;* Approved for children 2 years and older with certain underlying medical conditions
2. **Indications:**
a. Routine (Figure 16-1)
b. See Figure 16-2 for catch-up schedule
c. See Table 16-3 for an immunization schedule of high-risk children and a list of underlying medical conditions causing children to be high risk[11]
3. **Precautions/contraindications** (Table 16-2)
4. **Side effects:** Pain and erythema at injection site (common); fever within 1–2 days after administration (less common); severe systemic reactions such as anaphylaxis (rare)
5. **Administration:**
a. Dose for both PCV13 and 23PS is 0.5 mL given IM
b. Concurrent administration of PCV13 and 23PS vaccines is not recommended. Either vaccine may be given concurrently with other vaccines in a separate syringe at a separate injection site
c. Give vaccine 2 weeks or more before elective splenectomy, chemotherapy, radiotherapy, or immunosuppressive therapy; or give 3 months after chemotherapy or radiotherapy
6. **Special considerations:**
a. Passive immunoprophylaxis with IVIG is recommended for some children with congenital or acquired immune deficiencies
b. See discussion of functional or anatomic asplenia in Section V.A
c. Catch up for PCV13: See Table 16-11

K. Poliomyelitis Immunoprophylaxis

1. **Description:**
a. IPV: Contains three types of poliovirus grown in Vero cells and inactivated in formaldehyde[12]
b. OPV: No longer available in the United States. Children who have received the appropriate number of doses of OPV in other countries should be considered adequately immunized
c. Combination vaccine: See Section VI.P
2. **Indications:**
a. Routine (Figure 16-1)
b. Unimmunized or partially immunized individuals who are at imminent risk for exposure to poliovirus (dose interval may be 4 weeks)
3. **Precautions/contraindications** (Table 16-2)

TABLE 16-11

TRANSITION FROM PNEUMOCOCCAL IMMUNIZATION PCV7 TO PCV13[11]

Age (months)	Previous Doses of PCV7 and/or PCV13	Recommended PCV13 Regimen
2–6	0	3 doses, 4 weeks apart, 4th dose at 12–15 mo*
	1	2 doses, 4 weeks apart, 4th dose at 12–15 mo
	2	1 dose, 4 weeks after most recent, 4th dose at 12–15 mo
7–11	0	2 doses, 4 weeks apart, 3rd dose at 12–15 mo (8 weeks apart)
	1–2 (before 7 mo)	1 dose, 2nd dose at 12–15 mo (8 weeks apart)
12–23	0 or 1 <12 mo	2 doses 8 weeks apart
	1 ≥12 mo or 2–3 <12 mo or 4	1 dose at least 8 weeks after most recent dose†
24–59	Any	1 dose at least 8 weeks after most recent dose

*Minimum interval between doses when given <12 mo is 4 weeks, but after 12 mo is 8 weeks.

†For ages 12–23 mo no additional PCV13 doses are required if the child received 2–3 doses of PCV7 <12 mo and one dose of PCV13 ≥12 mo.

4. **Side effects:** No serious side effects have been associated with use of IPV
5. **Administration:** Dose is 0.5 mL IM or SC

L. Rabies Immunoprophylaxis

1. **Description:**

a. Three rabies vaccines are available for prophylaxis:
   (1) Human diploid cell vaccine (HDCV)
   (2) Rabies vaccine adsorbed (RVA)
   (3) Purified chicken embryo cell vaccine (PCECV)

b. Human rabies immune globulin (RIG): Anti-rabies Ig prepared from plasma of donors hyperimmunized with rabies vaccine

2. **Indications:**

a. Pre-exposure prophylaxis: Indicated for high-risk groups, including veterinarians, animal handlers, laboratory workers, children living in high-risk environments, those traveling to high-risk areas, and spelunkers
   (1) Three injections of HDCV or PCEC vaccine on days 0, 7, and 21 or 28
   (2) Rabies serum antibody titers should be followed at 6-month intervals for those at continuous risk and at 2-year intervals for those with risk for frequent exposure; give booster doses only if titers are nonprotective

b. Postexposure prophylaxis (Table 16-12)

3. **Precautions/contraindications:** PCECV can be used if there is a serious allergic reaction to HDCV
4. **Side effects:** Uncommon in children. In adults, local reactions in 15%–25%; mild systemic reactions, such as headache, abdominal

TABLE 16-12

RABIES POSTEXPOSURE PROPHYLAXIS

Animal Type	Evaluation and Disposition of Animal	Postexposure Prophylaxis Recommendations
Dogs, cats, ferrets	Healthy and available for 10 days' observation	Do not begin prophylaxis unless animal develops signs of rabies.
	Rabid or suspected rabid; euthanize animal and test brain	Provide immediate immunization and RIG.
	Unknown (escaped)	Consult public health officials.
Skunk, raccoon, bat,* fox, woodchucks, most other carnivores	Regard as rabid unless geographic area is known to be free of rabies or until animal is euthanized and proven negative by testing.	Provide immediate immunization and RIG.†
Livestock, rodents, rabbit, other mammals	Consider individually	Consult public health officials; these bites rarely require treatment.

*In the case of direct contact between a human and a bat, consider prophylaxis even if a bite, scratch, or mucous membrane exposure is not apparent.

†Treatment may be discontinued if animal fluorescent antibody is negative.

RIG, Rabies immune globulin.

Adapted from American Academy of Pediatrics: Red Book: 2009 Report of the Committee on Infectious Diseases, 28th ed. Elk Grove Village, IL, AAP, 2009, Table 3.57 p. 554.

pain, nausea, muscle aches and dizziness in 10%–20%; neurologic illness similar to GBS or focal central nervous system (CNS) disorder (reported with HDCV, but not believed to be causally related); immune complex–like reaction (urticaria, arthralgia, angioedema, vomiting, fever, and malaise) 2–21 days after immunization with HDCV, rare in primary series, 6% after booster dose

5. **Administration:** Dose is 1 mL IM for HDCV, RVA, and PCECV
6. **Postexposure prophylaxis:**

a. General wound management:
   (1) Clean immediately with soap and water and flush thoroughly
   (2) Avoid suturing wound unless indicated for functional reasons
   (3) Consider tetanus prophylaxis and antibiotics if indicated

b. Indications: Infectious exposures include bites, scratches, or contamination of open wound or mucous membrane with infectious material of a rabid animal or human

NOTE: Report all patients suspected of rabies infection to public health authorities

c. Administration:
   (1) Vaccine and rabies immune globulin (RIG) should be given jointly except in previously immunized patients (no RIG required). If vaccine is not immediately available, give RIG alone and vaccinate later. If RIG is not available, give the vaccine alone. RIG may be given later, if it can be administered within 7 days after initiating immunization

(2) Vaccine for postexposure prophylaxis:
  (a) Do not administer in same part of body or in same syringe as RIG
  (b) Deltoid muscle, except in infants, in whom anterolateral thigh is appropriate
  (c) Routine serologic testing not indicated
  (d) Unimmunized: 1 mL IM on days 0, 3, 7, and 14. As of July 2009 according to the Advisory Committee on Immunization Practices (ACIP) provisional recommendations there is no longer a fifth dose required. The fifth dose is required for children who are immunosuppressed and should be given on day 28
  (e) Previously immunized including pre- and postexposure: 1 mL IM on days 0 and 3. Do not give RIG

(3) RIG: Recommended dose of 20 IU/kg should not be exceeded. Infiltrate around the wound and give remainder IM

M. Respiratory Syncytial Virus (RSV) Immunoprophylaxis

1. **Description:**

a. No vaccine available

b. Palivizumab (monoclonal RSV-Ig): Humanized mouse monoclonal IgG to RSV, recombinantly produced for IM administration

2. **Indications**[13]**:**

a. Infants and children <2 years with chronic lung disease (CLD) who have required medical therapy (oxygen, bronchodilators, diuretics, or corticosteroids) within the 6 months before the RSV season. These children should receive a maximum of five doses. Data are limited, but these patients may also benefit from prophylaxis during a second RSV season

b. Infants ≤32 weeks' estimated gestational age (EGA) at birth who do not have CLD: May benefit from prophylaxis with palivizumab. These children should receive a maximum of five doses
  (1) EGA ≤28 weeks: Consider during RSV season until age 12 months
  (2) EGA 29–32 weeks: Consider if younger than 6 months at the start of RSV season

c. Infants 32 weeks to <35 weeks EGA: Palivizumab should be limited in this group to those at the greatest risk of hospitalization due to RSV. This includes those infants <3 months at the start of the RSV season or born during the RSV season and who are likely to have increased RSV exposure including at least one risk factor (child care attendance or siblings younger than 5 years). These children should receive a maximum of three doses, none being after 3 months of age[13]

d. Infants with congenital abnormalities of the airway or neuromuscular disease born before 35 weeks EGA should be considered for prophylaxis and should receive a maximum of five doses during the first year of life

e. Infants with hemodynamically significant cyanotic or acyanotic congenital heart disease who are 24 months of age or less should be considered for prophylaxis. These children include those who:
   (1) Are receiving medication for the treatment of congestive heart failure
   (2) Have moderate to severe pulmonary hypertension
   (3) Have a cyanotic heart lesion. Children who have undergone a surgical procedure where bypass was used should receive a postoperative dose of palivizumab as soon as the patient is clinically stable
f. There are no specific recommendations for severely immunocompromised children, but they may benefit from prophylaxis

3. **Precautions/contraindications** (see Formulary)
4. **Side effects:**
   a. Palivizumab: Side effects are comparable to placebo
5. **Administration:** Give palivizumab at onset of RSV season (November 1 for most of the United States, July 1 for southeast Florida, and September 15 for north central and southwest Florida) and then monthly according to the indications reviewed previously
   a. Palivizumab: Dose is 15 mg/kg IM monthly

N. Rotavirus Immunoprophylaxis

1. **Description:** There are two vaccines licensed by the Food and Drug Administration (FDA)[14]
   a. RotaTeq (RV5, Merck): Pentavalent, live viral vaccine containing five reassortant human and bovine rotavirus strains in the form of an oral solution given in three doses
   b. Rotarix (RV1, GlaxoSmithKline): Live, human attenuated rotavirus in the form of an oral solution given in two doses. Contains latex rubber
2. **Indications** (Figure 16-1)
3. **Precautions/contraindications:** (Table 16-2)
4. **Side effects:** Diarrhea (24%), vomiting (15%), otitis media (14.5%), nasopharyngitis (7%), and bronchospasm (1%). Adverse events among Rotarix and placebo occurred at similar rates[15,16]
5. **Administration:**
   a. Rotateq: 2 mL PO. Vaccine is packaged in single-dose tubes to be administered directly to the patient without dilution. Should not be given with other liquids. Do not readminister if infant spits out or vomits dose. Given in three doses, typically at 2, 4, and 6 months of age. The final dose must be given by 32 weeks of age. Minimum interval between doses is 4 weeks
   b. Rotarix: 1 mL PO. Vaccine is packaged to be reconstituted only with the accompanying diluent. If the infant spits out or vomits a dose a single replacement dose at the same visit may be considered. Given in two doses, typically at 2 and 4 months of age. The final dose should be given by 24 weeks of age. Minimum interval between the doses is 4 weeks

6. **Special considerations:** Premature infants can begin the series at 6 weeks of chronologic age if clinically stable. Infants who received antibody-containing products can receive the first dose at least 42 days after the product was given

O. Varicella Immunoprophylaxis

1. **Description:**
a. Vaccine: Cell-free live attenuated varicella virus vaccine
b. Varicella-zoster immune globulin (VariZIG): Prepared from plasma containing high-titer anti-varicella antibodies
2. **Indications:**
a. Routine (Figure 16-1)
b. See Figure 16-2 for catch-up schedule
3. **Precautions/contraindications** (Table 16-2)
4. **Side effects:**
a. Injection site reactions (20%). Mild varicelliform rash within 5 to 26 days of vaccine administration (3% to 5%)
b. Vaccine rash often very mild, but patient may be infectious; reversion to wild-type virus has not been reported. Most varicelliform rashes that occur within 2 weeks of vaccination are due to wild-type varicella-zoster virus (VZV) infection
5. **Administration:**
a. Dose is 0.5 mL SC
b. May give simultaneously with MMR; otherwise, allow at least 1 month between MMR and varicella vaccines
c. Do not give for 5 months after VariZIG; do not give concurrently with VariZIG
d. Avoid salicylates for 6 weeks after vaccine administration if possible
e. Avoid antiviral treatment for 21 days after vaccination
6. **Special considerations:**
a. Live-virus vaccines are usually withheld for at least 3 months after discontinuing immunosuppressive therapy
b. Consider vaccine in household contacts of immunocompromised hosts: If a rash develops in the immunized child, avoid direct contact if possible
7. **Postexposure prophylaxis:**
a. Potential interventions for people without evidence of immunity include either varicella vaccine administered ideally within 3 days but up to 5 days after exposure or when indicated (see later). VariZIG is given as one dose up to 96 hours after exposure. IVIG can also be given if VariZIG is not available. IVIG is given as one dose up to 96 hours after exposure. Oral acyclovir can also be given beginning 7 days after exposure
b. Indications:
   (1) Significant exposures include the following:
      (a) Household contact

16

(b) Face-to-face indoor play
(c) Onset of varicella in the mother of a newborn from 5 days before to 2 days after delivery
(d) Hospital exposures: Roommate, face-to-face contact with infectious individual, visit by contagious individual or intimate contact with person with active zoster lesions

(2) Candidates for VariZIG or acyclovir who have had significant exposure include:
(a) Immunocompromised individuals without a history of varicella or varicella immunization
(b) Susceptible pregnant women
(c) Newborn infant with onset of varicella in mother from 5 days before to 2 days after delivery (even if mother received VariZIG during pregnancy)
(d) Hospitalized preterm infant who was born before 28 weeks' gestation or who weighs <1000 g, regardless of maternal history
(e) Hospitalized preterm infant who was born at ≥28 weeks' gestation to a susceptible mother

c. VariZIG dose is 125 units/10 kg body weight IM (maximum dose, 625 U; minimum dose, 125 U). Do not give intravenously. Local discomfort is common
d. IVIG dose is 400 mg/kg IV
e. Varicella vaccine should be administered to susceptible immunocompetent children within 72 hours after varicella exposure. If the child was exposed at the same time as the index case, the vaccine may not protect against the disease. Susceptible immunocompromised children should receive VariZIG as soon as possible

P. Combination Vaccines

1. **Comvax = PRP-OMP/HepB:**
a. Description: PRP-OMP and Recombivax (5 mcg)
b. Indications (Figure 16-1)
c. Approved for use between 6 weeks of age and 71 months of age
d. Licensed for use at 2, 4, and 12–15 months of age

2. **Kinrix = DTaP-IPV**
a. Description: DTaP and IPV
b. Indications: Available for children aged 4–6 years as the booster for the fifth dose of DTaP and the fourth dose of IPV

3. **Pediarix = DTaP/HepB/IPV:**
a. Description: DTaP, IPV, and Hepatitis B (Energix-B, 10 mcg)
b. Indications:
(1) Routine: Use when vaccine components are indicated, so long as other components are not contraindicated. Administered in a three-dose schedule, preferably at age 2, 4, and 6 months. See Figure 16-1

(2) Should not be administered to infants <6 weeks or to children >7 years

(3) Minimal time interval between doses is 6 weeks

c. If used as the third dose to complete the hepatitis B series, should be administered at age 6 months or older

d. Pediarix should not be used as a booster dose following the three-dose primary DTaP series; insufficient data on safety and efficacy of use as a booster dose

e. Side effects: Higher rates of fever are reported with combination vaccine than with three vaccines administered separately

f. Precautions/contraindications (Table 16-2)

4. **Pentacel = DTaP-IPV/Hib**

a. Description: DtaP, IPV and PRP-T

b. Indications: Available for ages 6 weeks through 4 years as a four dose series at 2, 4, 6, and 15–18 months

5. **Proquad = Measles/mumps/rubella/varicella[17]:**

a. Description: Measles, mumps, rubella, and varicella live viral vaccine

b. Indications: Use when vaccine components are indicated, so long as other component is not contraindicated. See Figure 16-1

c. Licensed for patients age 12 months to 12 years

d. Unless caregiver prefers MMRV vaccine, CDC recommends that MMR and varicella vaccines be administered separately for the first dose in 12–47 months due to studies showing increased risk for febrile seizure with combination vaccine in this younger age group. Then combination MMRV vaccine can be used for second dose for 15 mo–12 yrs or as first dose for >48 months

6. **TriHIBit = DTaP/Hib:**

a. Description: PRP-T and DTaP

b. Indications: Available for the fourth dose of Hib and DTaP series between 15 and 18 months

7. **Twinrix = HepA/HepB:**

a. Description: Energix-B (20 μg) and Havrix (720 ELU)

b. Licensed for use in patients ≥18 years

c. Administered in a three-dose schedule given at 0, 1 month, and at least 6 months later

REFERENCES

1. Centers for Disease Control and Prevention. Available at www.cdc.org
2. American Academy of Pediatrics: Red Book: *2009 Report of the Committee on Infectious Diseases*, 28th ed. Elk Grove Village, IL, AAP, 2009.
3. Pickering LK, Baker CJ, Freed GL, et al: Immunization programs for infants, children, adolescents, and adults: clinical practice guidelines by the Infectious Diseases Society of America. *Clin Infect Dis* 2009;49:817–840.
4. Centers for Disease Control and Prevention: Preventing tetanus, diphtheria, and pertussis among adolescents: use of tetanus toxoid, reduced diphtheria toxoid and acellular pertussis vaccines: recommendations of the Advisory Committee on Immunization Practices (ACIP). *MMWR* 2006;55(RR-3):1–30.

5. Policy Statement: Prevention of pertussis among adolescents: recommendation for use of tetanus toxoid, reduced diphtheria toxoid, and acellular pertussis (Tdap) vaccine. *Pediatrics* 2006;117:965–978.
6. Centers for Disease Control and Prevention: Prevention of hepatitis A through active or passive immunization: recommendations of the Advisory Committee on Immunization Practices (ACIP). *MMWR* 2006;55(RR-7):1–23.
7. GlaxoSmithKline package insert for Havrix (hepatitis A vaccine).
8. Merck package insert for Vaqta (hepatitis A vaccine).
9. Merck package insert for Gardasil (HPV vaccine).
10. Centers for Disease Control and Prevention: Prevention and control of seasonal influenza with vaccines: recommendations of the Advisory Committee on Immunization Practices (ACIP). *MMWR* 2009;58:1–52.
11. Centers for Disease Control and Prevention: Provisional recommendations for use of 13-valent pneumococcal conjugate vaccine (PCV13) among infants and children: recommendations of the Advisory Committee on Immunization Practices (ACIP). *MMWR* 2010;59(09):248–261.
12. Centers for Disease Control and Prevention: Updated recommendations of the Advisory Committee on Immunization Practices (ACIP) regarding routine poliovirus vaccination. *MMWR* 2009;58(30):829–830.
13. Meissner HC, Bocchini JA: Reducing RSV hospitalizations: AAP modifies recommendations for use of palivizumab in high-risk infants, young children. *American Academy of Pediatrics News* 2009;30:1.
14. Centers for Disease Control and Prevention: Prevention of rotavirus gastroenteritis among infants and children: recommendations of the Advisory Committee on Immunization Practices (ACIP). *MMWR* 2009;58(RR-2):1–28.
15. GlaxoSmithKline package insert for Rotarix (rotavirus vaccine).
16. Merck package insert for RotaTeq (rotavirus vaccine).
17. Merck package insert for ProQuad (measles, mumps, rubella, and varicella live virus vaccine).

Chapter 17

Microbiology and Infectious Disease

Benjamin Lee, MD, and Tracy McCallin, MD

See additional content on Expert Consult

I. MICROBIOLOGY

A. Collection of Specimens for Blood Culture

1. Preparation: Proper specimen collection is essential to minimize contamination. Clean venipuncture site with 70% isopropyl ethyl alcohol. Apply tincture of iodine or 10% povidone-iodine and allow to dry for at least 1 min, or scrub site with 2% chlorhexidine for 30 seconds and allow to dry for 30 seconds for dry sites, scrub for 2 minutes and allow to dry for 1 minute for moist sites. Clean blood culture bottle injection site with alcohol only
2. Collection: Ideally, two sets of cultures of equal blood volume should be obtained for each febrile episode, based on patient weight: <8 kg, 1–3 mL each; 8–13 kg, 4–5 mL; 14–25 kg, 10–15 mL each; >25 kg, 20–30 mL each (adapted from Kaditis et al., 1996[1]). Total blood volume drawn should not exceed more than 1% of the patient's total blood volume

B. Rapid Microbiologic Identification of Common Aerobic Bacteria (Fig. 17-1)

C. Choosing Appropriate Antibiotic Based on Sensitivities

1. Definitions[2,3]:
a. Minimum inhibitory concentration (MIC): Lowest concentration of an antimicrobial agent that prevents visible growth after an 18- to 24-hour incubation period
b. Minimum bactericidal concentration (MBC): Lowest concentration of an antimicrobial agent that kills the organism, as measured by subculturing to antibiotic-free media after 18- to 24-hour incubation
2. Mistakes to avoid when selecting antibiotics based on sensitivity profiles (Table 17-1): Clinically significant, common discrepancies between in vitro (laboratory reported) and in vivo antibiotic sensitivity profiles that may result in inappropriate antibiotic treatment

Text continued on page 410

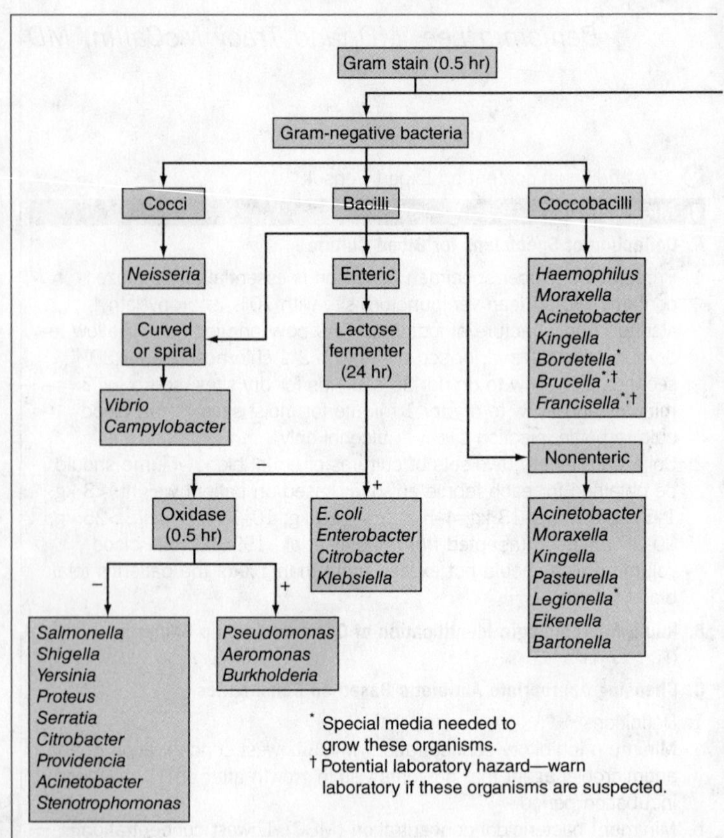

FIGURE 17-1

Algorithm demonstrating identification of aerobic bacteria. Numbers in parentheses indicate the time required for the tests.

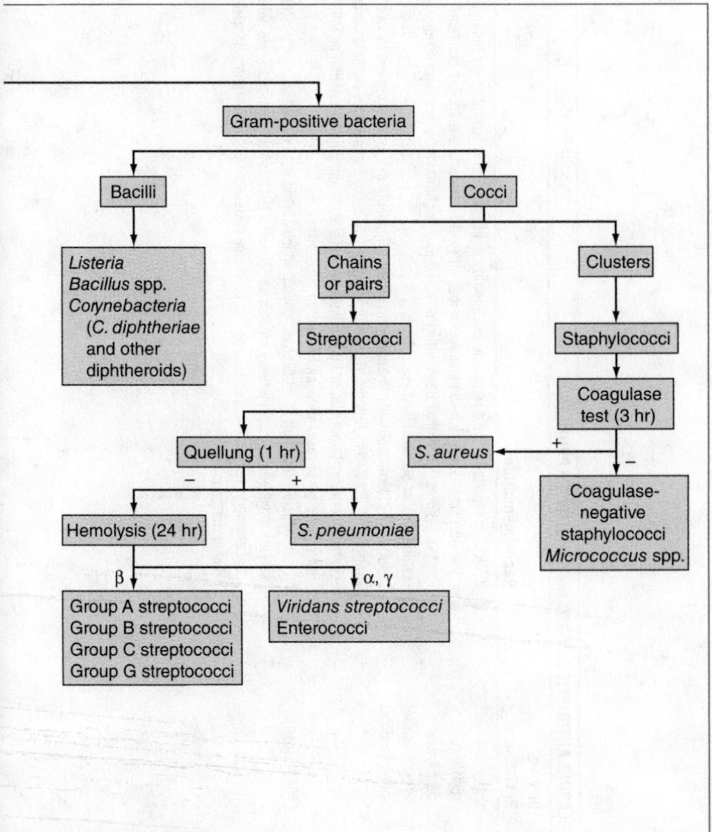

- Gram-positive bacteria
  - Bacilli
    - *Listeria*
    - *Bacillus* spp.
    - *Corynebacteria* (*C. diphtheriae* and other diphtheroids)
  - Cocci
    - Chains or pairs
      - Streptococci
        - Quellung (1 hr)
          - −: Hemolysis (24 hr)
            - β: Group A streptococci, Group B streptococci, Group C streptococci, Group G streptococci
            - α, γ: *Viridans streptococci*, Enterococci
          - +: *S. pneumoniae*
    - Clusters
      - Staphylococci
        - Coagulase test (3 hr)
          - +: *S. aureus*
          - −: Coagulase-negative staphylococci, *Micrococcus* spp.

FIGURE 17-1 (Continued)

TABLE 17-1

MISTAKES TO AVOID WHEN SELECTING ANTIBIOTICS BASED ON SENSITIVITY PROFILES

Bacteria	In Vivo Resistance	Recommendations
Staphylococci	Methicillin-resistant *Staphylococcus aureus* (MRSA)	If MRSA is reported to be susceptible to clindamycin in vitro, but resistant to erythromycin, a D test (double disk diffusion assay) is recommended to look for in vitro macrolide-inducible clindamycin resistance. If D test is positive, MRSA may have inducible resistance to clindamycin; consider using vancomycin, TMP-SMX, or linezolid for serious infections.
Salmonella	Aminoglycosides	Despite in vitro susceptibility to aminoglycosides, salmonella are not susceptible in vivo to this class of antibiotics. Treatment failures also occur with first- to second-generation cephalosporins. Third-generation cephalosporin, azithromycin, or fluoroquinolone preferred. Ampicillin/amoxicillin or TMP-SMX can be used if low prevalence of resistance, and based on susceptibilities.
Enterobacter spp. *Citrobacter* spp. *Pseudomonas aeruginosa* *Serratia* spp. *Providencia* spp. *Morganella* spp.	Cephalosporins	All are inducibly resistant to all cephalosporins, which should not be used as sole treatment for invasive or serious infections caused by these organisms. Because β-lactamase inhibitors are potent inducers of cephalosporin resistance, and they do not overcome resistance in these organisms, β-lactamase inhibitors should not be used.[4]

Burkholderia cepacia *Stenotrophomonas maltophilia*	Aminoglycosides	*Stenotrophomonas* species are often only susceptible to TMP-SMX, the drug of choice in most cases for these organisms. *Burkholderia* often requires a carbapenem plus additional agents.
P. aeruginosa *Acinetobacter* spp.	TMP-SMX	*P. aeruginosa* and *Acinetobacter* species are usually susceptible to aminoglycosides, but are resistant to TMP-SMX (despite reported in vitro susceptibility).
Enterococci	Most single-agent antibiotic classes	Usually requires double-agent therapy for synergy and bacterial killing for invasive infections. Recommended therapy is ampicillin (vancomycin if ampicillin resistant). Add an aminoglycoside (preferably gentamicin or streptomycin) for serious invasive infections. Nitrofurantoin can be used only for uncomplicated UTI. Other antibiotics with activity against enterococci include amoxicillin, penicillin, piperacillin, and imipenem.
	Vancomycin-resistant enterococcus (VRE)	VRE is usually *Enterococcus faecium,* although rarely *E. faecalis.* Linezolid is active against most enterococcal isolates, including VRE. Quinupristin/dalfopristin (Synercid) is active against most *E. faecium,* including VRE, but not against *E. faecalis.* The following antibiotics are *not* clinically active against enterococci: all cephalosporins, antistaphylococcal penicillins (e.g., oxacillin), macrolides, clindamycin, and quinolones.

TMP-SMX, Trimethoprim-sulfamethoxazole; UTI, urinary tract infection.

II. INFECTIOUS DISEASE

A. Fever without Localizing Source: Evaluation and Management Guidelines

1. Age ≤90 days: See Figure 17-2. Due to the greater risk of serious bacterial infections in young infants with fever, a conservative approach is warranted
   a. ≤28 days with fever should be hospitalized for full evaluation
   b. Infants >28 days who are well-appearing and meet low-risk criteria may potentially be managed as outpatients if reliable follow-up and monitoring is assured
2. Age >90 days: Traditionally, similar risk stratification strategies had been advocated and utilized to aid in evaluation and management of febrile children >90 days. However, the marked decline in invasive infections due to *Haemophilus influenzae* type B and *Streptococcus pneumoniae* since the introduction of conjugate vaccines has significantly reduced the likelihood of serious bacterial infection in a well-appearing child within this age group
   a. If ill-appearing without source of infection identified, consider admission and empiric antimicrobial therapy
   b. If source of infection identified, treat accordingly
   c. If well-appearing and without foci of infection, many experts now advocate urinalysis + urine culture as the only routine diagnostic test, if reliable follow-up and monitoring is assured, including all females and uncircumcised males <2 years, all circumcised males <6 months, and all children with known genitourinary tract abnormalities[5,6]

B. Intrauterine and Perinatal Infections (See Table 17-2 for Specific Clinical Features and Therapy)

1. **Intrauterine (congenital) infections:** TORCH infections (toxoplasmosis; other: syphilis, varicella-zoster virus [VZV]; rubella; cytomegalovirus [CMV]; and herpes simplex virus [HSV]) often present in the neonate with overlapping findings: intrauterine growth restriction (IUGR), hematologic involvement (anemia, neutropenia, thrombocytopenia, petechiae, purpura), ocular signs (chorioretinitis, keratoconjunctivitis, glaucoma, microphthalmos), central nervous system (CNS) signs (microcephaly, hydrocephalus, intracranial calcifications), other organ system involvement (pneumonitis, myocarditis, nephritis, hepatitis), and nonimmune hydrops.[7] Initial evaluation of a neonate depends on level of suspicion and severity of clinical findings[8] and may include head computed tomography or ultrasound (intracerebral calcifications), long-bone films (metaphyseal abnormalities), ophthalmologic examination (keratoconjunctivitis and chorioretinitis), brainstem evoked responses (hearing evaluation), and specific blood, urine, and cerebrospinal fluid (CSF) evaluation
2. **Perinatal viral infections:** Perinatal VZV, HSV, enterovirus, and CMV infections can be severe with profound morbidity and mortality.

Text continued on page 415

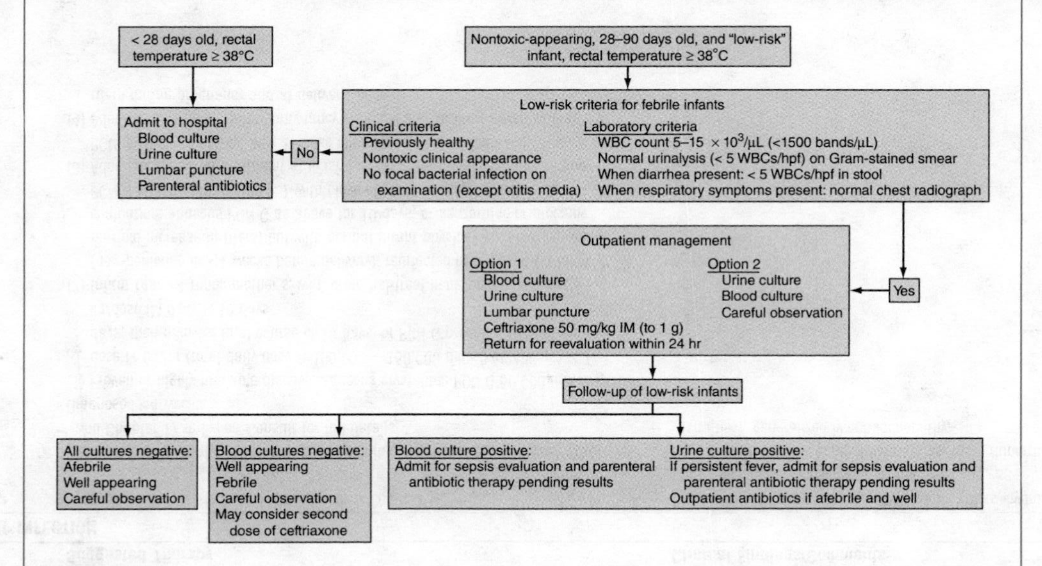

FIGURE 17-2

Algorithm for the management of a previously healthy infant ≤90 days of age with a fever without localizing signs. This algorithm is a suggested, but not exhaustive, approach to management. hpf, High-power field. *(Modified from Baraff LJ: Management of fever without source in infants and children. Ann Emerg Med 2000;36[6]:602–614; and Baraff LJ: Management of infants and young children with fever without source. Pediatr Ann 2008;37(10):673–679.)*

TABLE 17-2

CONGENITAL (INTRAUTERINE) AND PERINATAL VIRAL AND BACTERIAL INFECTIONS: NEONATAL MANAGEMENT

Etiology	Suggested Therapy	Clinical Findings/Comments
CONGENITAL INFECTION		
Toxoplasma	Pyrimethamine + sulfadiazine with leucovorin, up to 1 yr	Chorioretinitis, meningitis, cerebral calcifications, hydrocephalus, or significant organ damage may be seen
Syphilis	Depending on level of suspicion, various penicillin regimens. See *Red Book 2009*[9] and Chapter 17 in Expert Consult for full details. Diagnosed <4 weeks: (1) Proven or highly probable disease: aqueous crystalline PCN G 50,000 units/kg/dose IV q12hr (total daily dose = 100,000 – 150,000 units/kg/24hours) × 7 days, then q8hr for total course of 10 days; or PCN G procaine 50,000 units/kg/dose IM daily × 10 days (2) Infant titer <4 times mother's, with maternal treatment: none, inadequate (non-penicillin or <4 weeks before delivery), reinfected or relapsed (at least fourfold increase in titers) but with normal infant physical examination and/or evaluation: aqueous PCN G as above for 10 days, or benzathine or procaine PCN G 50,000 units/kg IM × 1 with close clinical, serological follow-up (3) Adequate maternal treatment at least 4 weeks prior to delivery: benzathine PCN G 50,000 units/kg IM × 1, close clinical, serological follow-up (4) Adequate treatment before pregnancy with low and stable nontreponemal titers during pregnancy and at delivery: none	Hepatosplenomegaly, bone abnormalities, rash, rhinorrhea (snuffles), generalized lymphadenopathy.

	Diagnosed >4 weeks of age: Aqueous crystalline PCN G 50,000 units/kg/dose IV Q4-6H (200,000–300,000 units/kg/day) × 10 days.	**NOTE:** Benzathine or procaine PCN G can be used only if FULL evaluation is completely normal without any equivocal results (e.g., uninterpretable CSF); otherwise, full course of crystalline PCN G is required.
Rubella	Supportive.	IUGR, cataracts, cardiac anomalies, deafness, blueberry muffin rash. Vaccinate all nonimmune mothers immediately postpartum.
CMV	Initiating ganciclovir IV within 1st mo of life for symptomatic CNS disease may protect against hearing loss, developmental impairment; limited data. No data for treatment of end-organ damage in preterm infants with perinatal infection; consider 2 weeks ganciclovir, assess response and continue therapy for additional 1–2 weeks if clinical improvement seen.[9]	IUGR, jaundice, hepatosplenomegaly, microcephaly, thrombocytopenia, intracranial calcifications, deafness.
Parvovirus	Infant treatment supportive. Consider intrauterine blood transfusions for hydrops fetalis.	Hydrops fetalis, IUGR, pleural or pericardial effusion, death.
PERINATAL VIRAL INFECTION		
HSV	Acyclovir 20 mg/kg/dose IV q8hr. Skin, eye, and mouth (SEM) disease: 14 days; CNS or disseminated disease: 21 days. Topical treatment (trifluridine, iododeoxyuridine, or vidarabine) for ocular involvement.	HSV can present any time within the first 4–5 weeks of life as: (1) Disease localized to SEM (2) Localized CNS infection (meningoencephalitis) or (3) Disseminated disease with severe pneumonitis and hepatitis. Disseminated disease often presents in 1st to 2nd week of life; CNS disease presents later, often 2nd to 3rd week of life.[9]

Continued

TABLE 17-2

CONGENITAL (INTRAUTERINE) AND PERINATAL VIRAL AND BACTERIAL INFECTIONS: NEONATAL MANAGEMENT (Continued)

Etiology	Suggested Therapy	Clinical Findings/Comments
Varicella	Maternal[10]: Acyclovir may be beneficial during pregnancy, especially 2nd to 3rd trimesters. VariZIG or IVIG after exposure for susceptible pregnant women is recommended. VariZIG is available under an investigational new drug protocol by calling 1-800-843-7477. Infant[10]: VariZIG and/or acyclovir if mother developed primary varicella (not zoster) between 5 days before and 2 days after delivery, and hospitalized preterm infants <28 weeks or >28 weeks if mother lacks historical or serologic evidence of protection.	If a mother develops varicella from 5 days before to 2 days after delivery, neonatal infection can be severe. Neonates initially look well, then develop rash within the first 2 weeks of life, generally in the second week. Disseminated disease may develop: pneumonitis, encephalitis, purpura fulminans, bleeding, hypotension, death. If mother develops varicella >5 days before delivery and gestational age >28 weeks, disease is milder secondary to transplacental transfer of antibody.
Enterovirus	IVIG	Neonates <2 weeks can develop severe infection: Hepatitis, myocarditis, meningitis, encephalitis, pneumonitis, NEC, DIC, death (usually from hepatic failure or myocarditis).
Hepatitis B	Appropriate immunoprophylaxis (see Chapter 16). Interferon alpha (2b and pegylated 2a) and lamivudine for children with chronic HBV with necroinflammatory disease.	Over 90% of perinatally infected children will develop chronic HBV, underscoring the need for appropriate prophylaxis. If mother is positive for both HBsAg and HBeAg, the risk for development of chronic HBV infection in the child is 70%–90% by age 6 mo in the absence of postexposure immunoprophylaxis.[11] However, appropriate prophylaxis is highly effective.
Hepatitis C	No therapy until HCV status ascertained. Non-pegylated interferon-alpha-2b plus ribavirin approved in children 3–17 years but no data for neonates	Transmission chiefly through blood. No evidence that breastfeeding increases risk of transmission, but consider abstaining if nipples cracked or bleeding.
HIV	See Section E.	See Section E.

CMV, Cytomegalovirus; CNS, central nervous system; CSF, cerebrospinal fluid; DIC, disseminated intravascular coagulation; HBV, hepatitis B virus; HCV, hepatitis C virus; HSV, herpes simplex virus; IM, intramuscular; IUGR, intrauterine growth retardation; IV, intravenous; IVIG, intravenous immunoglobulin; NEC, necrotizing enterocolitis; PCN, penicillin; VariZIG, varicella zoster immune globulin.

Although VZV, HSV, hepatitis B, and hepatitis C can all cause intrauterine (congenital) infection, perinatal infection around the time of birth are more common. It can be difficult to distinguish neonatal VZV and HSV lesions clinically

3. **Diagnosis of specific intrauterine and perinatal infections**[9]

a. **Toxoplasmosis:**
   (1) *Prenatal diagnosis:* Detection of parasite DNA (fetal blood, amniotic fluid) or isolation of parasite by mouse or tissue culture inoculation
   (2) *Postnatal diagnosis:* Toxoplasma IgG, IgM, IgA, and IgE (newborn and maternal serum) along with polymerase chain reaction (PCR) (white blood cells, CSF, amniotic fluid). Alternate: Detection of parasite (placenta, umbilical cord, blood) by mouse inoculation. Positive IgM, IgA, persistently elevated or rising IgG in infant compared to mother within first 12 months indicates congenital infection. Persistently positive IgG titer beyond first year confirms diagnosis
   (3) Increased suspicion in mothers co-infected with HIV due to increased likelihood of maternal reactivation

b. **Syphilis:**
   (1) Evaluation of congenital syphilis can be complicated and best achieved in conjunction with a specialist. For further details regarding maternal testing, infant testing, evaluation, and treatment, please refer to *Red Book 2009*[9] and in Expert Consult Chapter 17 and Table EC 17-A
   (2) Testing during pregnancy: All pregnant women should be screened with a nontreponemal antibody test (Venereal Disease Research Laboratory [VDRL] test or rapid plasma reagin [RPR] test) early in pregnancy and preferably again at delivery. In high prevalence areas and high-risk patients, a test early in the third trimester is also indicated. Positive RPR or VDRL should be confirmed with a treponemal antibody test (fluorescent treponemal antibody absorption [FTA-ABS] or T. pallidum particle agglutination [TP-PA]). If infected, treatment and serial RPR or VDRL titers to assess efficacy indicated
   (3) Evaluation of infants: No newborn should be discharged from the hospital without determining mother's serologic status. Testing of cord blood or infant serum not adequate for screening. Obtain venous VDRL or RPR for all infants of infected women. See Chapter 17 in Expert Consult and Table EC 17-A for evaluation of congenital syphilis

c. **Rubella:** IgM (infant serum) and culture (nasal, throat specimen). In congenital infection, infant should be virus positive at birth. Alternate: Culture (blood, urine, cataract specimens), RNA PCR (throat swab, urine). Infection confirmed by persistent or rising IgG over several months. Low-avidity IgG (vs. high-avidity) on avidity assay consistent with recent infection (where available). Maternal immune status at onset of pregnancy is most helpful information, but if checked late in pregnancy, infection early in pregnancy cannot be excluded. If suspected, laboratory personnel should be notified due to specialized testing required

d. **CMV:** Culture (urine, stool, respiratory tract, or CSF) within 2–4 weeks of birth. Alternate: IgM, PCR (CSF or blood) within 3 weeks of birth. Beyond this period, serology may indicate postnatal infection
e. **Parvovirus:** Serum IgM (preferred) or PCR
f. **HSV:** Surface culture (conjunctiva, nasopharynx, mouth, rectum, blood, CSF, skin vesicles); PCR (blood, CSF). CSF PCR is indicated for diagnosis of suspected CNS disease. Positive surface cultures from any site >12–24 hours after birth indicate viral replication suggestive of infection rather than contamination after intrapartum exposure. Radiography and liver function tests indicated in suspected disseminated disease to assess for pneumonitis, hepatitis
g. **VZV:** Direct fluorescent antigen (DFA, vesicle scraping, swab of lesion base), PCR (vesicle swabs, scrapings, scabs, tissue biopsy, or CSF). Alternate: Tissue culture (vesicular fluid, CSF, biopsy tissue) during first 3–4 days of eruption
h. **Enterovirus:** RNA PCR (throat, stool, rectal swab, urine, blood, and CSF). Alternate: Culture (same sites)
i. **Hepatitis B:** All mothers should be screened for HBsAg status and appropriate postexposure prophylaxis initiated in at-risk children (see Chapter 16). Children born to HBsAg-positive mothers should have the first HepB vaccine within 12 hours of life, concurrently with HBIG. Postimmunization testing for HBsAg and anti-HBs should be performed at 9 to 18 months of age, after completion of the primary HepB series. If HepBsAg is negative on follow-up, indicating lack of chronic infection, but anti-HBs concentration is <10 mIU/mL, then the infant did not have a vaccine response and should repeat an additional three doses of Hepatitis B vaccine (as if unimmunized) with testing of anti-HBs 1 month after third dose to assess for response to reimmunization
j. **Hepatitis C:** Check hepatitis C virus (HCV) IgG at 18 months, after maternal antibodies have waned. If symptomatic or earlier diagnosis needed, HCV RNA via nucleic acid amplification after 1–2 months of age preferred, but single negative test inconclusive due to intermittent viremia
k. **HIV:** See Section E

4. **Group B streptococcal (GBS) infection:**

a. Maternal intrapartum antibiotic prophylaxis: Figure 17-3
b. Evaluation and empiric management of the neonate born to a mother who received intrapartum prophylaxis for GBS: Figure 17-4
c. Presentation of and regimens for prophylaxis and/or treatment of early and late onset GBS: Table 17-3

Text continued on page 437

Recommended	Penicillin G, 5 million units IV initial dose, then 2.5 million units IV every 4 hours until delivery
Alternative	Ampicillin, 2 g IV initial dose, then 1 g IV every 4 hours until delivery
If penicillin allergic[†]	
Patients not at high risk for anaphylaxis	Cefazolin, 2 g IV initial dose, then 1 g IV every 8 hours until delivery
Patients at high risk for anaphylaxis[††]	
GBS susceptible to clindamycin and erythromycin[¶]	Clindamycin, 900 mg IV every 8 hours until delivery OR Erythromycin, 500 mg IV every 6 hours until delivery
GBS resistant to clindamycin or erythromycin or susceptibility unknown	Vancomycin,** 1 g IV every 12 hours until delivery

- Broader-spectrum agents, including an agent active against GBS, may be necessary for treatment of chorioamnionitis.

† History of penicillin allergy should be assessed to determine whether a high risk for anaphylaxis is present. Penicillin-allergic patients at high risk for anaphylaxis are those who have experienced immediate hypersensitivity to penicillin including a history of penicillin-related anaphylaxis; other high-risk patients are those with asthma or other diseases that would make anaphylaxis more dangerous or difficult to treat, such as persons being treated with beta-adrenergic–blocking agents.

†† If laboratory facilities are adequate,clindamycin and erythromycin susceptibility testing should be performed on prenatal GBS isolates from penicillin-allergic women at high risk for anaphylaxis.

¶ Resistance to erythromycin is often but not always associated with clindamycin resistance. If a strain is resistant to erythromycin but appears susceptible to clindamycin, it may still have inducible resistance to clindamycin.

** Cefazolin is preferred over vancomycin for women with a history of penicillin allergy other than immediate hypersensitivity reactions, and pharmacologic data suggest it achieves effective intraamniotic concentrations. Vancomycin should be reserved for penicillin-allergic women at high risk for anaphylaxis.

A

FIGURE 17-3 *Continued*

Indications and antibiotic selection for intrapartum antimicrobial prophylaxis (IAP) to prevent early-onset Group B streptococcal disease. *(From Morbidity and Mortality Weekly Report: MMWR Recommendations and Reports, Atlanta, GA, CDC 2002; 51[RR-11]:1–22.)*

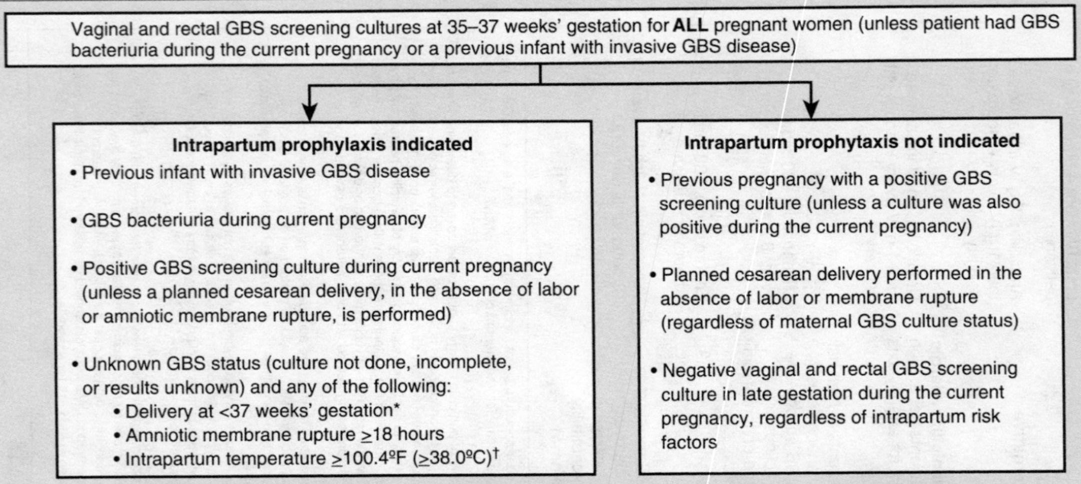

Vaginal and rectal GBS screening cultures at 35–37 weeks' gestation for **ALL** pregnant women (unless patient had GBS bacteriuria during the current pregnancy or a previous infant with invasive GBS disease)

Intrapartum prophylaxis indicated

- Previous infant with invasive GBS disease
- GBS bacteriuria during current pregnancy
- Positive GBS screening culture during current pregnancy (unless a planned cesarean delivery, in the absence of labor or amniotic membrane rupture, is performed)
- Unknown GBS status (culture not done, incomplete, or results unknown) and any of the following:
  - Delivery at <37 weeks' gestation*
  - Amniotic membrane rupture ≥18 hours
  - Intrapartum temperature ≥100.4ºF (≥38.0ºC)†

Intrapartum prophytaxis not indicated

- Previous pregnancy with a positive GBS screening culture (unless a culture was also positive during the current pregnancy)
- Planned cesarean delivery performed in the absence of labor or membrane rupture (regardless of maternal GBS culture status)
- Negative vaginal and rectal GBS screening culture in late gestation during the current pregnancy, regardless of intrapartum risk factors

* If onset labor or rupture of amniotic membrane occurs <37 weeks gestation and there is a significant risk for preterm delivery (as assessed by the clinician), a suggested algorithm for GBS prophylaxis management is provided.

B † If amnionitis is suspected, broad-spectrum antibiotic therapy that includes an agent known to be active against GBS should replace GBS prophylaxis.

FIGURE 17-3 (Continued)

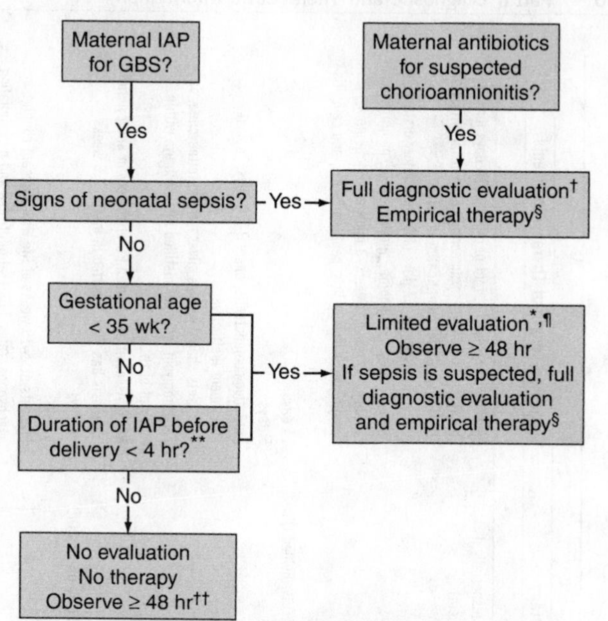

* If no maternal intrapartum prophylaxis for GBS was administered despite an indication being present, data are insufficient on which to recommend as a single management strategy.

† Includes complete blood cell count and differential, blood culture, and chest radiograph if respiratory abnormalities are present. When signs of sepsis are present, a lumbar puncture, if feasible, should be performed.

§ Duration of therapy varies depending on results of blood culture, cerebrospinal fluid findings, if obtained, and the clinical course of the infant. If laboratory results and clinical course do not indicate bacterial infection, duration may be as short as 48 hours.

¶ CBC with differential and blood culture.

** Applies only to penicillin, ampicillin, or cefazolin and assumes recommended dosing regimen.

†† A healthy-appearing infant who was ≥38 weeks' gestation at delivery and whose mother received ≥4 hours of intrapartum prophylaxis before delivery may be discharged home after 24 hours if other discharge criteria have been met and a person able to comply fully with instructions for home observation will be present. If any one of these conditions is not met, the infant should be observed in the hospital for at least 48 hours and until criteria for discharge are achieved.

FIGURE 17-4

Empirical management of neonate born to a mother who received intrapartum antimicrobial prophylaxis (IAP) to prevent early-onset group B streptococcal disease. This algorithm is a suggested, but not exclusive, approach to management. *(From Morbidity and Mortality Weekly Report: MMWR Recommendations and Reports, Atlanta, GA, CDC 2002;51[RR-11]:1–22.)*

TABLE 17-3

COMMON PEDIATRIC INFECTIONS: GUIDELINES FOR INITIAL MANAGEMENT

Infectious Syndrome	Usual Etiology	Suggested Empirical Therapy	Suggested Length of Therapy/Comments
Neonatal bacterial infections			
GBS infections	GBS	Ampicillin + aminoglycoside (especially if meningitis; usually gentamicin) Alternative: Cefotaxime	Duration depends on extent of disease: 10 days for bacteremia, 14 days for uncomplicated meningitis, up to 3–4 weeks for complicated infection Early onset disease (<7 days old): Respiratory distress, apnea, shock, pneumonia, and less often, meningitis. Late-onset disease (1 week–3 months): Bacteremia, meningitis, osteomyelitis, septic arthritis, and cellulitis
Chlamydial infections	*Chlamydia trachomatis*		
Conjunctivitis (ophthalmia neonatorum)		Erythromycin 50 mg/kg/day PO/IV divided QID Alternative: Azithromycin Regular saline irrigation	14 days 5 days Exudative conjunctivitis, onset 3–10 days. Topical treatment ineffective All infants should receive silver nitrate, tetracycline, or erythromycin ointment instilled into each eye within 1 hr of birth **NOTE:** Association between PO erythromycin and pyloric stenosis has been reported in infants <6 weeks
Pneumonia		Erythromycin 50 mg/kg/day PO/IV divided QID Alternative: Azithromycin	14 days 5 days Presents at 2–19 weeks of life with staccato cough, tachypnea, rales, bilateral infiltrates and hyperinflation on CXR, usually afebrile

Gonococcal infections	*Neisseria gonorrhoeae*		Infants born to mothers with active gonococcal infection should be empirically treated with a single dose of ceftriaxone
Conjunctivitis (ophthalmia neonatorum)		Ceftriaxone 25–50 mg/kg (max 125 mg) IV/IM Alternative: Cefotaxime Regular saline irrigation	Single dose 7 days Exudate conjunctivitis, onset 2–4 days. Admit for evaluation and treatment of possible disseminated disease All infants should receive silver nitrate, tetracycline, or erythromycin ointment instilled into each eye within 1 hr of birth
Sepsis, arthritis, scalp abscess		Ceftriaxone 25–50 mg/kg IV/IM q24hr or cefotaxime	7 days
Meningitis		Ceftriaxone or cefotaxime	14 days
Septic arthritis	*S. aureus*, GBS, gram-negative bacilli, *N. gonorrhoeae* (see above)	(Cefotaxime or gentamicin) + (nafcillin or oxacillin) Consider vancomycin instead of PCNs if MRSA prevalent	Drainage essential
Meningitis			
Neonate <1 mo	GBS, *E. coli, L. monocytogenes*	Ampicillin + (cefotaxime and/or gentamicin) Add gentamicin if gram-negative organisms	14–21 days for GBS and Listeria 21 days for gram negative organisms (Cefotaxime plus aminoglycoside)
Pneumonia			
Neonatal	*E. coli*, GBS, *Streptococcus* spp., *S. aureus, L. monocytogenes, C. trachomatis*	Ampicillin and gentamicin, ± cefotaxime Vancomycin if MRSA prevalent	10–21 days, depending on disease severity Blood cultures indicated. Effusions should be drained and gram stain of fluid obtained

Continued

17

TABLE 17-3

COMMON PEDIATRIC INFECTIONS: GUIDELINES FOR INITIAL MANAGEMENT (Continued)

Infectious Syndrome	Usual Etiology	Suggested Empirical Therapy	Suggested Length of Therapy/Comments
Bacteremia (outpatient)	*S. pneumoniae*, GAS, *Neisseria meningitidis, E. coli, Salmonella* spp.	Ceftriaxone or cefotaxime	7–10 days (longer for some pathogens) Occult bacteremia with susceptible *S. pneumoniae* may be treated with amoxicillin if afebrile, well, and without focal complications
Bacterial vaginosis	Polymicrobial, often *Gardnerella vaginalis*	Metronidazole 500 mg PO BID Alternatives: Metronidazole gel 0.75% 5 g intravaginally daily or clindamycin cream 2% 5 g intravaginally daily	7 days 5 days 7 days
Bites			
Human	*Streptococcus* spp., *S. aureus, S. epidermidis,* oral anaerobes, *Eikenella corrodens,* Haemophilus spp.	PO: Amoxicillin/clavulanic acid Alternative: Clindamycin + (3rd-generation cephalosporin or TMP/SMX) IV: Ampicillin/sulbactam Alternative: TMP/SMX + (clindamycin or cefoxitin or meropenem)	5–7 days Cleaning, irrigation, and débridement most important Assess tetanus immunization status, risk of hepatitis B and HIV Antibiotic prophylaxis routinely used for human bites
Dog/cat	Add *Pasteurella multocida, Capnocytophaga, Corynebacterium* spp., Neisseria spp.	Same	7–10 days Assess tetanus immunization status, risk of rabies Antibiotic prophylaxis for all cat bites and selected dog bites

Catheter-related bloodstream infections	*S. aureus,* CONS, enteric gram negative bacilli, Candida spp; Immuno-compromised patients: Add *Pseudomonas, Corynebacterium* spp.	Immunocompetent: Vancomycin + 3rd-generation cephalosporin or aminoglycoside Immunocompromised: Vancomycin + (ceftazidime or cefepime or piperacillin/tazobactam or aminoglycoside)	Consider catheter removal and fungal coverage as clinically indicated
Cellulitis	GAS, *S. aureus* (MSSA or MRSA)	PO: Cephalexin Alternative: Clindamycin if PCN-allergic or MRSA common IV: Oxacillin Alternative: Clindamycin or vancomycin if MRSA common	3 days after acute inflammation resolves (usually 7–10 days) TMP/SMX not active against GAS See Figure 17-5 for management of skin and soft tissue infections caused by community-acquired *S. Aureus*
Conjunctivitis (Suppurative, non-neonatal)	*S. pneumoniae, H. influenzae* (nontypeable) *Moraxella*	Ophthalmic: Erythromycin, bacitracin/polymyxin B, or polymyxin B/TMP	5 days Ointments preferred for infants or young children and eyedrops for older children and adolescents
Dacrocystitis	*S. pneumoniae, H. influenzae,* *S. aureus,* *S. pyogenes,* *P. aeruginosa,* CONS	Initial conservative management: warm compresses. PO: Nafcillin/oxacillin or cephalexin or clindamycin	Consider ophthalmologic evaluation to relieve obstruction
Dental abscesses	Oral flora, including anaerobes	Clindamycin or amoxicillin/clavulanic acid	Consider dental evaluation for surgical drainage

Continued

TABLE 17-3

COMMON PEDIATRIC INFECTIONS: GUIDELINES FOR INITIAL MANAGEMENT (Continued)

Infectious Syndrome	Usual Etiology	Suggested Empirical Therapy	Suggested Length of Therapy/Comments
Gastroenteritis			
Community	Viruses		Primary treatment: Fluid and electrolyte replacement
Acquired	*E. coli*	Antibiotic therapy strongly discouraged because of possible increased risk for hemolytic-uremic syndrome occurring in patients with E. coli 0157:H7 treated with antibiotics[12] Azithromycin or ciprofloxacin for traveler's diarrhea	
	Salmonella spp.	Cefotaxime or ceftriaxone Alternative: Azithromycin Ampicillin, amoxicillin, or TMP/SMX for susceptible strains	10–14 days for infants <3 mo, bacteremia, toxicity, hemoglobinopathy, or immunosuppressed. Antibiotics generally not indicated otherwise
	Shigella spp.	Ceftriaxone (IV), azithromycin, or fluoroquinolone	5 days for dysentery, immunosuppressed, or to prevent spread in mild disease. Oral cephalosporins not useful. Amoxicillin or TMP/SMX can be used if susceptible, but not recommended for empiric treatment due to high rates of resistance
	Yersinia spp.	TMP/SMX, aminoglycosides, cefotaxime, flouroquinolone, or tetracycline (≥8 yr)	Usually no antibiotic therapy is recommended except with bacteremia, extraintestinal infections, or immunocompromised hosts
	Campylobacter spp.	Azithromycin or erythromycin	5–7 days. Shortens duration of fecal excretion
Nosocomial	*Clostridium difficile*	Metronidazole Oral vancomycin for severe infection	7 days Stop the precipitating antibiotic therapy as soon as possible Community organisms unlikely after 72 hr of hospitalization

Condition	Organisms	Treatment	Comments
Influenza	Influenza A Influenza B	Neuraminidase inhibitors: Oseltamivir (≥1 yr) or Zanamivir (≥7 yr for treatment, ≥5 yr for chemoprophylaxis); Adamantine class: Rimantadine (>13 yr for treatment, >1 yr for prophylaxis) or Amantadine (>1 yr) for influenza A (no activity against influenza B) if circulating strain susceptible (novel H1N1 resistant)	Treatment: 5 days, greatest benefit when initiated within 48 hours of symptom onset Chemoprophylaxis: 5–10 days. Recommendations vary yearly based on characteristics and resistance patterns of circulating strains. See http://www.cdc.gov/flu/ for most up-to-date recommendations The FDA granted an Emergency Use Authorization for the use of oseltamivir in children <1 yr in 2009. However, none of the antivirals have been licensed for general use in children <1 yr
Lymphadenitis	Viruses, GAS, *M. tuberculosis, S. aureus*, anaerobes, atypical mycobacteria, *Actinomyces, Bartonella henselae* (cat scratch disease)	PO: Amoxicillin/clavulanic acid or clindamycin if MRSA prevalent Alternative: Cephalexin or dicloxacillin IV: Oxacillin or nafcillin or clindamycin if MRSA present Alternative: Cefazolin If PCN-allergic: Cefdinir, cefuroxime, or vancomycin	Surgical excision with *M. tuberculosis* Needle aspiration with *B. henselae*
Mastoiditis (acute)	*S. pneumoniae, S. pyogenes, S. aureus, H. influenzae* (nontypeable)	Ampicillin/sulbactam or clindamycin Alternative: Cefuroxime for PCN allergy	10 days Surgical management required, definitive therapy should be guided by culture obtained at surgery

Continued

17

TABLE 17-3

COMMON PEDIATRIC INFECTIONS: GUIDELINES FOR INITIAL MANAGEMENT (Continued)

Infectious Syndrome	Usual Etiology	Suggested Empirical Therapy	Suggested Length of Therapy/Comments
Meningitis (non-neonatal) Infants >1 mo and children	*S. pneumoniae*, N. meningitidis, *H. influenzae*, neonatal pathogens	Cefotaxime or ceftriaxone, + vancomycin (resistant *S. Pneumoniae*) For severe PCN allergy, consider chloramphenicol + vancomycin	Duration depends on organism See *Red Book 2009*[9] for chemoprophylaxis recommendations for contacts of meningococcal and Hib disease Dexamethasone use, except for *H. influenzae* uncertain
Orbital cellulitis	*S. pneumoniae*, *H. influenzae* (nontypeable), *Moraxella catarrhalis*, *S. aureus*, GAS	Ampicillin/sulbactam; or (cefotaxime or ceftriaxone) AND (clindamycin or oxacillin) Alternative: Cefuroxime PCN allergy: (vancomycin or clindamycin) + rifampin, OR aztreonam Consider vancomycin if concern for MRSA	10 days Recommend ophthalmologic consultation, CT to evaluate intracranial extension, cavernous thrombosis
Osteomyelitis			
Uncomplicated	*S. aureus*, GAS, *Streptococcus* spp., *Kingella*	Oxacillin or nafcillin or clindamycin Alternative: Vancomycin	4–6 wk Clindamycin ineffective as monotherapy for *Kingella* infections
Foot puncture	Add *Pseudomonas aeruginosa*	Add ceftazidime or anti-pseudomonal PCN and aminoglycoside	
Sickle cell disease	Add Salmonella spp.	Add cefotaxime or ceftriaxone	
Otitis media (acute)	*S. pneumoniae*, *H. influenzae* (nontypeable), *M. catarrhalis*, viruses	Not severe: "High dose" amoxicillin (80–90 mg/kg/day) Severe (moderate-severe otalgia or fever >39°C): Amoxicillin/clavulanic acid Alternative for PCN allergy: cefuroxime, cefdinir, or azithromycin Ceftriaxone IM if cannot take PO	10 days (5–7 days for healthy children >6 yr) Analgesia for otalgia 10 days If >6 mo, not severe, and uncertain diagnosis, or >2 yr and not severe, observation ("watchful waiting") may be employed with reassessment at 48–72 hours Single dose

		Persistent otitis media (after 3 days): Amoxicillin/clavulanic acid, cefuroxime, or ceftriaxone IM daily	Consider tympanocentesis 3 days (for IM Ceftriaxone)
Otitis externa (uncomplicated)	*Pseudomonas*, Enterobacteriaceae, Proteus spp, fungi	Eardrops: Polymyxin B/neomycin/hydrocortisone or ciprofloxacin or TMP/SMX	7–10 days Analgesics for pain Consider wick for moderate to severe cases
Parotitis	*S. aureus* most common. Also: oral flora, gram-negative rods, viruses (including mumps, HIV, EBV), or noninfectious causes	PO: Clindamycin or nafcillin/oxacillin/dicloxacillin or amoxicillin/clavulanic acid	Sialogogues, local heat, gentle massage of the gland from posterior to anterior, and hydration provide symptomatic relief. Surgical drainage may be required. Consider HIV test if chronic parotitis
Periorbital cellulitis (preseptal)	GAS and Streptococcus spp., *S. aureus, H. influenzae* (nontypeable), *M. catarrhalis*	Ampicillin/sulbactam or amoxicillin/clavulanic acid or clindamycin + 3rd-generation cephalosporin Alternative: Cefuroxime or fluoroquinolone Consider vancomycin, TMP/SMX, or clindamycin if concern for MRSA	10–14 days If secondary to local trauma and not associated sinusitis, treat as staph/strep cellulitis
Pharyngitis	GAS, *Group C and G streptococci, Arcanobacterium haemolyticum, Mycoplasma*, viruses (including coxsackievirus, other enteroviruses, Ebstein-Barr virus in infectious mononucleosis)	PCN V or amoxicillin Benzathine PCN G × 1 for GAS Alternative: Clindamycin, macrolide or cephalexin	10 days, regardless of promptness of recovery (to prevent acute rheumatic fever in GAS infection). TMP/SMX not effective Supportive treatment only for viral pharyngitis

Continued

TABLE 17-3

COMMON PEDIATRIC INFECTIONS: GUIDELINES FOR INITIAL MANAGEMENT (Continued)

Infectious Syndrome	Usual Etiology	Suggested Empirical Therapy	Suggested Length of Therapy/Comments
Pneumonia (non-neonatal)			
4 wk–3 mo	*C. trachomatis, S. pneumoniae, B. pertussis, S. aureus,* viruses	Erythromycin Alternative: Azithromycin Add cefotaxime if febrile, ill-appearing Consider adding clindamycin or vancomycin in severe infections	10 days For pertussis, azithromycin if <1 mo of age. Treatment during catarrhal stage may provide clinical benefit; during paroxysmal stage, treatment is to limit spread of disease. Chemoprophylaxis for close contacts
Infant/child (3 mo–5 yr):	*S. pneumoniae, Mycoplasma, C. pneumoniae,* GAS, *S. aureus,* viruses, influenza	Outpatient: Amoxicillin (high-dose), ± azithromycin Alternative: Clindamycin Inpatient: (ceftriaxone or cefotaxime) + azithromycin Alternative: (clindamycin or vancomycin) + azithromycin Vancomycin or clindamycin if severe Illness or features suggestive of *S. aureus* (pleural effusion, cavitation)	7–10 days See influenza section for treatment guidelines Atypical organisms are more likely with older age of the child
>5 yr	*S. pneumoniae, Mycoplasma, C. pneumoniae,* GAS, *S. aureus, M. tuberculosis,* viruses, influenza	Outpatient: Azithromycin ± amoxicillin Alternative: Azithromycin ± clindamycin Inpatient: (cetriaxone or cefotaxime) + azithromycin Vancomycin or clindamycin if severe Illness or features suggestive of *S. aureus* (pleural effusion, cavitation)	7–10 days See influenza section for treatment guidelines

Postspinal fusion	*Staphylococcus, Streptococcus* spp.; enteric or genitourinary gram-negative organisms	Vancomycin + piperacillin/tazobactam Consider adding gentamicin ± rifampin	Consider suction irrigation to wound initially. Deep tissue culture of wound may direct treatment. Removal of instrumentation may be necessary
Septic arthritis (non-neonatal)			
<5 yr	*S. aureus*, GAS, *S. pneumoniae, Kingella*, Haemophilus spp.	Cefotaxime + (nafcillin, oxacillin, or clindamycin) Add clindamycin or vancomycin if MRSA prevalent Alternative: Vancomycin + cefotaxime	3–4 wk IV Aspiration of affected joint recommended. Therapy should be guided by gram stain and culture, if available May switch to PO after response
>5 yr	*S. aureus*, GAS, *Streptococcus* spp.	Nafcillin, oxacillin, or clindamycin Alternative: Vancomycin	
Adolescent	Add *N. gonorrhoeae*	Add ceftriaxone	See sexually transmitted infections
Sexually transmitted infections			
Chlamydia infections	*C. trachomatis*		
Uncomplicated urethritis, endocervicitis, or proctitis		Azithromycin 1 g PO or doxycycline 100 mg PO BID (>8 yr) Alternative: Erythromycin PO QID (preferred for <6 mo) or ofloxacin or levofloxacin PO	Single dose 7 days 7 days
Epididymitis		Doxycycline 10 mg PO BID	10 days
Infection in pregnancy (may require second course due to low efficacy)		Azithromycin 1 g PO or Amoxicillin PO TID Alternative: Erythromycin base PO QID	Single dose 7 days 7 days

Continued

TABLE 17-3

COMMON PEDIATRIC INFECTIONS: GUIDELINES FOR INITIAL MANAGEMENT (Continued)

Infectious Syndrome	Usual Etiology	Suggested Empirical Therapy	Suggested Length of Therapy/Comments
Gonorrheal infections	*N. gonorrhoeae*		Fluoroquinolones are no longer recommended for presumptive treatment of gonorrhea. *All gonorrheal infections should be treated presumptively for Chlamydia as detailed.
Prepubertal children <100 lb (45 kg)			
Uncomplicated urethritis, vulvovaginitis, proctitis, or pharyngitis		Ceftriaxone 125 mg IM Alternative: Cefixime 8 mg/kg (max 400 mg) PO or spectinomycin 40 mg/kg (max 2 g) IM AND* azithromycin 20 mg/kg (max 1 g) PO or erythromycin PO QID	Single dose Single dose Single dose Single dose 14 days
Disseminated gonococcal infections (e.g. arthritis-dermatitis syndrome)		Ceftriaxone 50 mg/kg/day (max 1 gm) IV/IM Q24H AND* erythromycin PO QID	7 days 14 days
Meningitis or endocarditis		Ceftriaxone 50 mg/kg/day (max 2 g/day) IV/IM Q12H AND* erythromycin PO QID	Meningitis: 10–14 days Endocarditis: ≥28 days
Conjunctivitis		Ceftriaxone 50 mg/kg (max 125 mg) IM	Single dose

Patients >100 lb (45 kg) and >8 years		
Uncomplicated urethritis, endocervicitis, proctitis, or pharyngitis	Ceftriaxone 125 mg IM Alternative: (Cefixime or cefpodoxime 400 mg PO or spectinomycin 2 g IM) AND* (azithromycin 1 g PO or doxycycline 100 mg PO BID)	Single dose Single dose 7 days
Disseminated gonococcal infections (e.g. arthritis-dermatitis syndrome)	Ceftriaxone 1 gm IV/IM q24hr AND* (azithromycin 1 g PO or doxycycline 100 mg PO BID)	Single dose Single dose 7 days
Meningitis or endocarditis	Ceftriaxone 1–2 g IV/IM q12hr AND* (azithromycin 1 g PO or doxycycline 100 mg PO BID)	Meningitis: 10–14 days Single dose 7 days Endocarditis: ≥28 days
Conjunctivitis	Ceftriaxone 1 gm IM AND* (azithromycin 1 g PO or doxycycline 100 mg PO BID)	Single dose Single dose 7 days
Epididymitis	Ceftriaxone 250 mg IM AND* doxycycline 100 mg PO BID	Single dose 10 days

Continued

17

TABLE 17-3

COMMON PEDIATRIC INFECTIONS: GUIDELINES FOR INITIAL MANAGEMENT (Continued)

Infectious Syndrome	Usual Etiology	Suggested Empirical Therapy	Suggested Length of Therapy/Comments
Trichomoniasis	*Trichomonas vaginalis*	Metronidazole 2 g PO	Single dose (adult dosing)
Pelvic inflammatory disease (PID)	*C. trachomatis, N. gonorrhoeae,* lower genital tract flora: *H. influenzae,* gram-negative rods, anaerobes, *Streptococcus agalactiae,* Mycoplasma spp.	Parenteral regimens: Regimen A (Cefotetan 2 g IV q12hr or cefoxitin 2 g IV q6hr) AND doxycycline 100 mg IV/PO q12hr Regimen B Clindamycin 900 mg IV q8hr AND gentamicin 2 mg/kg loading dose, then 1.5 mg/kg IV q8hr maintenance, or single daily dosing	Switch to oral therapy 24 hours after clinical improvement, to complete 14 days of treatment with clindamycin QID or doxycycline BID Fluoroquinolones may be considered only if parenteral cephalosporin therapy is not feasible AND community prevalence and individual risk of gonorrhea are low
		Oral Regimen:	
		(Ceftriaxone 250 mg IM or other 3rd-generation cephalosporin) or	Single dose
		(cefoxitin 2 g IM + probenecid 1 g PO) AND	Single dose each
		doxycycline 100 mg PO BID	14 days
		± metronidazole 500 mg PO BID	14 days

Syphilis (not congenital, age >1 mo)	*Treponema pallidum*		**NOTE:** Must exclude asymptomatic neurosyphilis in children
Primary, secondary, or early latent syphilis (<1 yr duration)		Benzathine PCN G 50,000 units/kg (max 2.4×10^6 units) IM	Single dose
		Alternatives if >8 yr:	
		Tetracycline 500 mg PO QID or	14 days
		Doxycycline 100 mg PO BID	14 days
Late syphilis (>1 yr duration), tertiary syphilis		Benzathine PCN G 50,000 units/kg (max 2.4×10^6 units) IM Q1week	3 weeks
		Alternatives if >8 yr:	
		Tetracycline 500 mg PO QID or	28 days
		Doxycycline 100 mg PO BID	28 days
Neurosyphilis		Aqueous crystalline PCN G 50,000 units/kg/dose (max 4×10^6 units/dose) IV q4–6 hr (200,000–300,000 units/kg/day, max 24×10^6 units/day)	10–14 days If PCN-allergic, PCN desensitization required
		Alternatives:	
		Procaine PCN G 2.4×10^6 units IM daily AND	10–14 days
		probenecid 500 mg PO q6hr	10–14 days
		May be followed by benzathine PCN G 50,000 units/kg/dose (maximum 2.4×10^6 units) IM q week	3 weeks

Continued

17

TABLE 17-3

COMMON PEDIATRIC INFECTIONS: GUIDELINES FOR INITIAL MANAGEMENT (Continued)

Infectious Syndrome	Usual Etiology	Suggested Empirical Therapy	Suggested Length of Therapy/Comments
Sinusitis			
Acute	*S. pneumoniae, H. influenzae, M. catarrhalis*	Amoxicillin ("high dose") 80–90 mg/kg/day divided BID Alternative: Cefpodoxime, cefuroxime, cefdinir, azithromycin, or rifampin	10–14 days Add clavulanic acid if severe, risk factors for resistance (day care, recent antibiotics), or fails to respond in 48–72 hr. If severe and fails to respond, consider imaging and/or drainage. Parenteral therapy generally reserved for complicated sinusitis
Chronic	Add *S. aureus,* anaerobes (to acute pathogens)	Amoxicillin/clavulanic acid, cefpodoxime, cefuroxime, or cefdinir Alternatives: (ceftriaxone or cefotaxime) AND (clindamycin or vancomycin) or fluoroquinolone	21 days, or 7 days after resolution of symptoms
Seriously ill child or immunocompromised	Add *Pseudomonas,* gram negatives, *Mucor, Rhizopus, Aspergillus*	Cefepime or piperacillin/tazobactam ± amphotericin B	Consider surgical intervention

UTI			
Cystitis	*E. coli,* Enterobacteriaceae, Proteus spp., *S. saprophyticus,* Enterococcus spp.	PO: TMP/SMX, cefixime IV: (cefotaxime or ceftriaxone) OR (ampicillin and gentamicin) Alternatives: Nitrofurantoin OR ciprofloxacin	7–14 days Consider phenazopyridine for comfort (urine and other secretions may turn red) For severe PCN allergy or resistant organisms
Pyelonephritis	*E. coli,* Enterobacteriaceae, Proteus spp., Enterococcus spp.	Ceftriaxone OR (ampicillin + gentamicin) Alternative: Cefixime or ciprofloxacin	7–14 days Parenteral until afebrile for 24 hr. Consider outpatient treatment in selected patients
Abnormal host/urinary tract	Add *Pseudomonas,* resistant gram negatives	Piperacillin/tazobactam or ceftazidime	14–21 days
Ventriculoperitoneal shunt, infected	*S. epidermidis, S. aureus,* Enterobacteriaceae, *Propionibacterium acnes*	Vancomycin + (cefotaxime or ceftriaxone) Add aminoglycoside if culture suggests Enterobacteriaceae Consider adding rifampin	10–21 days, depending on organism and response Shunt removal or revision is often required for successful treatment

*All gonorrheal infections should be treated presumptively for Chlamydia as detailed.

CONS, Coagulase-negative staphylococcus; CXR, chest x-ray; FDA, Food and Drug Administration; GAS, group A streptococcus; GBS, group B streptococcus; IM, intramuscular; IV, intravenous; MSSA, methicillin-sensitive Staphylococcus aureus; MRSA, methicillin-resistant Staphylococcus aureus; PCN, penicillin; PO, by mouth; TMP/SMX, trimethoprim/sulfamethoxazole; UTI, urinary tract infection.

Recommendations adapted from American Academy of Pediatrics. Pickering LK, Baker CJ, Kimberlin DW, Long SS (eds): Red book: 2009 Report of the Committee on Infectious Diseases, 28th ed. Elk Grove Village, IL, American Academy of Pediatrics, 2009; and McMillan JA, Siberry GK, Dick JD, et al: The Harriet Lane handbook of pediatric antimicrobial therapy. Philadelphia, PA, Mosby Elsevier, 2009.

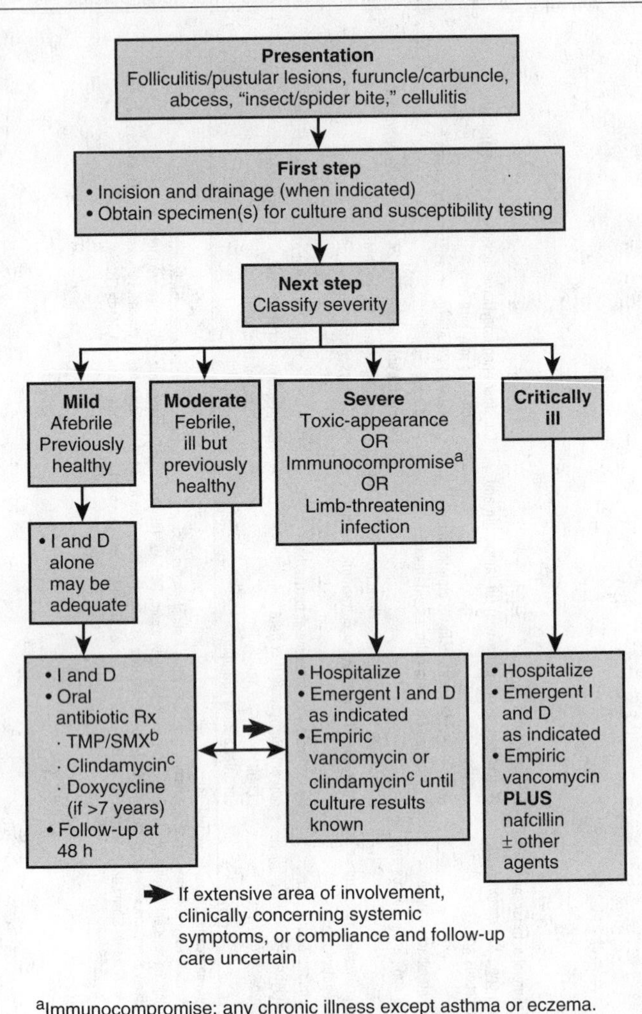

FIGURE 17-5

Algorithm for Initial Management of Skin and Soft Tissue Infections Caused by Community-Acquired *Staphylococcus Aureus* (MSSA and MRSA). *(From Pickering LK, Baker CJ, Kimberlin DW, et al. Red Book: 2009 Report of the Committee on Infectious Diseases. 28th ed. Elk Grove Village, IL. American Academy of Pediatrics, 2009, p. 609.)*

C. Common Pediatric Infections: Guidelines for Initial Management (Table 17-3)

D. Pelvic Inflammatory Disease (PID) (See Table 17-3 for Selected Sexually Transmitted Diseases)

1. Treatment: Empiric treatment indicated for all sexually active females if minimum diagnostic criteria are met
2. Minimum diagnostic criteria: Uterine or adnexal tenderness without other identifiable cause
3. Additional criteria that may improve specificity: Fever (>38.3°C); mucopurulent vaginal or cervical discharge, leukocytes on saline microscopy of vaginal secretions, increased erythrocyte sedimentation rate (ESR) or C-reactive protein (CRP), laboratory documentation of *Chlamydia* or gonorrhea infection
4. Diagnostic techniques for gonorrhea and *Chlamydia*
   a. In many locations, culture is the only method accepted for evaluation of child abuse (for legal purposes); please consider local requirements and clinical scenario when selecting diagnostic techniques. Gonorrhea culture requires selective media with carbon dioxide incubation for transport
   b. Presumptive diagnosis: Intracellular gram-negative diplococci on gram-stain (gonorrhea), nucleic acid amplification test from urine, male urethral, vaginal (transcription-mediated amplification test only for post-menarche females), or endocervical swab. DNA probe, enzyme immunoassay, and direct fluorescent antibody tests available, but not as sensitive
5. Organisms other than gonorrhea and chlamydia can cause PID; treatment should not be stopped for failure to isolate these organisms if clinical suspicion high and other causes excluded
6. Differential diagnosis is broad, but consider endometriosis, tubo-ovarian abscess, acute surgical abdomen
7. Admission criteria: Cannot exclude acute surgical abdomen (e.g., appendicitis, ovarian torsion, ectopic pregnancy), presence of tubo-ovarian abscess, pregnancy, immunodeficiency, severe illness (e.g., nausea, vomiting, anorexia), inability to tolerate or follow outpatient regimen, failure to respond to appropriate outpatient therapy, follow-up cannot be otherwise ensured

E. Human Immunodeficiency Virus (HIV) and Acquired Immunodeficiency Syndrome (AIDS)

For the most recent information on the diagnosis and management of children with HIV infection, check the recommendations at www.aidsinfo.nih.gov/

1. **Counseling and testing:** Legal requirements vary by state. Counseling includes informed consent for testing, implications of positive test results, and prevention of transmission

a. Prenatal testing:

(1) New guidelines from the Centers for Disease Control and Prevention (CDC), American College of Obstetrics and Gynecology (ACOG), and American Academy of Pediatrics (AAP) strengthen the recommendations for routine HIV testing during pregnancy to provide universal HIV screening of pregnant women with opt-out consent. The CDC also recommends that HIV screening be included in the routine panel of prenatal tests for all pregnant women. If a state requires written consent, the recommendation is that separate written consent for HIV testing should not be required[13]

(2) The CDC also recommends that repeat HIV antibody testing occur in the third trimester, preferably before 36 weeks of gestation for women with high risk of acquiring HIV, including the following: living in states with high HIV prevalence in women 15 to 45 years of age, delivering in hospitals with HIV prevalence greater than or equal to 1 in 1,000 pregnant women screened, or increasing risk of acquiring HIV (women with another sexually transmitted infection diagnosed during pregnancy, intravenous drug users and their partners, women who exchange sex or money for drugs, women whose sex partner is HIV infected, women who have had a new or more than one sex partner during pregnancy, or women with signs/symptoms of acute HIV infection)[13]

b. Perinatal and newborn testing:

(1) The current recommendation for women in labor with undocumented HIV-infection status during the pregnancy, is to perform maternal testing with opt-out consent, using a rapid HIV antibody test

(2) For newborn infants whose mother's HIV status is unknown, the mother and/or newborn should undergo rapid HIV antibody testing, with appropriate consent as required by state or local law

(3) See Table 17-4 for recommendations on HIV DNA PCR testing for newborns exposed to HIV in utero

c. Adolescent testing: The CDC recommends that universal HIV-1 screening with opt-out consent be part of routine clinical care in all health-care settings for patients beginning at age 13 years. Repeat HIV-1 antibody testing should be performed on a regular basis for adolescents who remain at risk of HIV-1 infection

2. **Management of perinatal HIV exposure**[13,14]: Recommendations provided are current at the time of publication; check the recent recommendations for most current therapy at www.aidsinfo.nih.gov/

a. Prevention of mother to child transmission: Three interventions are recommended to reduce transmission, including use of antiretroviral therapy during pregnancy, during delivery, and in the newborn, elective cesarean section for women with high viral load (greater than 1,000 copies per mL), and use of breastfeeding alternatives where

TABLE 17-4

DIAGNOSIS AND MANAGEMENT FOR INFANTS WITH IN UTERO HIV EXPOSURE

Age	Labs to Obtain*	Management	Comments
Newborn	(1) Optional HIV DNA PCR (or RNA assay)—consent signed by guardian and provider and placed in patient's chart (2) If testing is done, umbilical cord blood should not be used due to possible contamination with maternal blood	(1) Start Zidovudine (ZDV) (2 mg/kg/dose every 6 hours) × 6 weeks. Alternative dosing 4 mg/kg/dose every 12 hr may be considered for concern of adherence (2) Combination therapy may be considered in consultation with a specialist experienced in pediatric HIV treatment	Different dose of ZDV for premature (<35 wk GA) infants. Concern for bone marrow suppression
2–3 weeks	(1) HIV DNA PCR (or RNA assay)—consent signed if no prior consent for testing on chart (2) CBC with diff	Check ZDV dosing and administration. Assess psychosocial needs, consider case management referral	HIV antibody testing is not routine—only if lacking evidence of maternal HIV status (otherwise antibody is expected to be positive in HIV-exposed infants)
4–6 weeks	(1) HIV DNA PCR (or RNA assay)—consent signed if no prior consent for testing on chart (2) CBC with diff (use discretion, based on results of previous CBC)	(1) Discontinue ZDV regardless of PCR result (ZDV monotherapy is used during first 6 weeks for prophylaxis only) (2) Presumptively exclude HIV infection: If results of ≥2 weeks PCR and ≥4 weeks PCR both negative. No TMP-SMX is needed (3) If PCR results not yet known, begin TMP-SMX at 75 mg/m^2/dose BID for 3 consecutive days of week	(1) If TMP-SMX is not tolerated, alternatives are aerosolized pentamidine, dapsone, or atovaquone (see Table EC 17-B Chapter 17 Expert Consult for dosing guidelines) (2) TMP-SMX can be discontinued as soon as results of both ≥2 week PCR and ≥4 week PCR are negative (3) **NOTE:** One single HIV-1 DNA PCR test has a sensitivity of 95% and a specificity of 97% for samples collected from infected infants 1 to 36 months of age

Continued

TABLE 17-4

DIAGNOSIS AND MANAGEMENT FOR INFANTS WITH IN UTERO HIV EXPOSURE (Continued)

Age	Labs to Obtain*	Management	Comments
2 months		(1) Check TMP-SMX dosing and administration, if still needed (2) Discontinue TMP-SMX if meets criteria above for negative testing	Routine well-child check and immunizations
4 months	HIV DNA PCR (or RNA assay) to be performed at 4 months or older	Definitively exclude HIV infection: Two negative PCRs (one ≥1 month, one ≥4 months) as long as no signs/symptoms of HIV infection	(1) HIV is diagnosed (infected child) if any two separate DNA PCR assays result as positive (2) If HIV infection is definitively excluded, infant needs only routine, comprehensive well-child care including all routine immunizations
12, 15, 18 months	HIV antibody optional (to document clearance of maternal antibody—usually by 12 months, but may persist to 18 months)		(1) Routine TB risk assessment—especially if HIV-infected household contacts—to determine need for PPD (2) Routine well-child care and immunizations including MMR and varicella

CBC, Complete blood count; GA, gestational age; MMR, measles/mumps/rubella; PCR, polymerase chain reaction; PPD, purified protein derivative; TB, tuberculosis; TMP-SMX, trimethoprim-sulfamethoxazole.

*Any abnormal result requires prompt pediatric HIV specialist consultation

Adapted from DHHS guidelines for pediatric and perinatal HIV infection (see www.aidsinfo.nih.gov for more detailed information). Accessed December 7, 2010.

they are found to be affordable, feasible, acceptable, sustainable, and safe. Infants born to an HIV-infected mother who did not receive interventions to prevent transmission have a risk of infection estimated to range from 12% to 40%. Health care professionals who are treating HIV-infected pregnant women and their newborn infants should report all instances of prenatal exposure to antiretroviral drugs to the Antiretroviral Pregnancy Registry (1-800-258-4263 or www.apregistry.com)

(1) Pregnancy: All HIV-infected women should be offered antiretroviral therapy for their own health, consistent with the standards of nonpregnant adults. Current U.S. Public Health Service (USPHS) guidelines recommend use of combination regimens including at least three antiretroviral drugs during pregnancy and labor for all pregnant women with HIV infection. Zidovudine (ZDV) should be included in the pregnant woman's regimen. Use of ZDV alone is controversial but may be considered for HIV infected women with a low viral load of less than 1,000 copies per mL. ZDV given during pregnancy (initiated at 14–34 weeks' gestation) and then given to the infant at delivery and for 6 weeks postnatally significantly reduces vertical transmission of HIV (Table 17-5). ACOG and USPHS recommend elective cesarean section at 38 weeks for all HIV infected pregnant women with viral load greater than 1,000 copies per mL at time of delivery, or who have unknown viral load, regardless of the antiretroviral therapy being received. It is recommended for HIV-infected women in the United

TABLE 17-5

RECOMMENDED ZIDOVUDINE (ZDV) REGIMEN FOR PREVENTION OF MATERNAL TO CHILD TRANSMISSION OF HIV

Stage of Labor	Recommended Regimen
Antepartum*	Oral administration of ZDV 200 mg TID or 300 mg BID, initiated after 14 weeks gestation and continued throughout the pregnancy
Intrapartum	During labor, intravenous (IV) administration of ZDV in a 1-hr initial dose of 2 mg/kg, followed by continuous infusion of 1 mg/kg/hr until delivery. Administration should occur for 3 hr prior to cesarean section
Postpartum	Oral administration of ZDV to the newborn (ZDV at 2 mg/kg/dose q6hr) for the first 6 weeks of life, beginning as soon as possible after birth. Administration after the first 48 hours of life is not likely to be efficacious in preventing transmission of HIV†

*Most women will be treated with a three-drug regimen of highly active antiretroviral therapy (HAART) after the first trimester unless treatment is required sooner for maternal health reasons. Oral ZDV may be used as part of that regimen.

†Intravenous dosage for full-term infants who cannot tolerate oral intake is 1.5 mg/kg IV q6hr. ZDV dosing for infants <35 weeks' gestation at birth is 1.5 mg/kg/dose IV or 2.0 mg/kg/dose per os (PO) q12hr, advancing to q8hr at 2 weeks of age if >30 weeks' gestation at birth or at 4 weeks of age if <30 weeks' gestation at birth.

Adapted from Pickering LK (ed): 2009 Red book: Report of the Committee on Infectious Diseases, 28th ed. Elk Grove Village, IL, American Academy of Pediatrics, 2009, Table 3.28.

States not to breastfeed. However, in resource-poor countries, the morbidity associated with artificial feeding may be unacceptably high. If the criteria for breastfeeding alternatives listed in Section E. 2a are not met, HIV-infected women are recommended to breastfeed exclusively for the first 6 months of life, with weaning after that time when replacement feeding meets the affordable, feasible, acceptable, sustainable, and safe criteria. Testing for HIV infection in the newborn should continue throughout the period of breastfeeding and for 6 months after cessation when an infant is breastfed

(2) Labor: See Table 17-5 for ZDV regimen during labor. Invasive procedures such as fetal scalp electrode monitoring are generally avoided. For women with undetermined HIV status who are found to be positive on HIV rapid antibody test, antiretroviral prophylaxis should be administered to the mother (and newborn) without waiting for results of confirmatory HIV testing. Breastfeeding should not occur. However, if confirmatory test results are negative, then prophylaxis may be discontinued and breastfeeding can be initiated. In the United States, the addition of single-dose intrapartum/newborn nevirapine (NVP) to the standard regimen is not recommended because it does not appear to provide additional efficacy in reducing transmission, and may be associated with development of NVP resistance

(3) Newborn: See Table 17-5 for ZDV regimen in newborns. If infant prophylaxis with antiretrovirals in addition to ZDV is being considered, choice of drugs should be determined in consultation with an expert in pediatric HIV infection. Monitor ZDV toxicity with periodic complete blood count (CBC) with differential count. Main toxicities are anemia and neutropenia. If hematologic abnormalities are identified, decisions on whether to continue infant antiretroviral prophylaxis need to be individualized based on extent of the abnormality, risk of HIV infection, and availability of alternative treatments. Consultation with an expert in pediatric HIV infection is advised if discontinuation of antiretrovirals is considered

(4) Infant: In addition to breastfeeding, premastication of food for teething infants has been linked to late HIV-1 transmission in three infants in the United States. There was documentation of bleeding gums or oral sores in two of the three caregivers; therefore, transmission most likely occurred via blood and not via saliva. It is important to educate HIV-infected caregivers regarding the risks of premastication and recommend other methods of preparing food for infants

3. **Diagnosis and management of HIV-exposed infants (Table 17-4)**[15]
4. **Opportunistic Infections:**

a. *Pneumocystis jiroveci* pneumonia (PCP) is the most common of the opportunistic infections. Trimethoprim-sulfamethoxazole (TMP-SMX) is recommended for all HIV-exposed infants until HIV infection is reasonably excluded, for all HIV-infected infants until age 12 months, and for HIV-infected children and adolescents older than 1 year whose CD4 values fall into the severe immune suppression category (CD4 percentage <15% or CD4 count <200 cells/mm^3)[15]

b. For more detailed information, see Table EC 17-B on Expert Consult. Drug regimens for prevention and treatment of opportunistic infection in HIV infected children

5. **Management of HIV-infected infants and children[15,16]:**

NOTE: Primary care physicians are encouraged to participate in the care and management of HIV-infected children in consultation with specialists who have expertise in the care of such children. Knowledge about antiretroviral therapy is changing, and in areas where enrollment into clinical trials is possible, it should be encouraged. Since treatment guidelines change frequently, it is important to reference the most up-to-date guidelines at http://www.aidsinfo.nih.gov/

a. Criteria for initiation of antiretroviral therapy[9]:
   (1) Initiation of antiretroviral therapy depends on virologic, immunologic, and clinical status
   (2) All HIV-infected infants (<12 months) regardless of immunologic, virologic, or clinical status, should receive antiretroviral therapy
   (3) HIV-infected children 1 year of age or older should start antiretroviral therapy if they have AIDS or significant HIV-related symptoms
   (4) Asymptomatic or mildly symptomatic HIV-infected children between the ages of 1 and 4 years should start antiretroviral therapy for CD4 percentage of less than 25%
   (5) Asymptomatic or mildly symptomatic HIV-infected children 5 years of age or older should start antiretroviral therapy for CD4 count of less than 350 cell/mm^3
   (6) Recommendations to defer therapy for asymptomatic or mildly symptomatic HIV-infected children 1 year of age or older are based on degree of immunosuppression and height of viral load

b. Revised pediatric HIV classification system (Table 17-6)

TABLE 17-6

1994 REVISED PEDIATRIC HIV CLASSIFICATION SYSTEM: IMMUNOLOGIC CATEGORIES BASED ON AGE-SPECIFIC CD4+ LYMPHOCYTE COUNT AND PERCENT

	Age of Child		
	<12 mo	**1–5 yr**	**6–12 yr**
Immunologic Category	**Cells/mL (%)**	**Cells/mL (%)**	**Cells/mL (%)**
1. No suppression	≥1,500 (≥25)	≥1,000 (≥25)	≥500 (≥25)
2. Moderate suppression	750–1,499 (15–24)	500–999 (15–24)	200–499 (15–24)
3. Severe suppression	<750 (<15)	<500 (<15)	<200 (<15)

From Centers for Disease Control and Prevention: MMWR Recomm Rep 1994;43(RR-12):4.

c. Antiretroviral regimen: For most recent recommendations, refer to http://www.aidsinfo.nih.gov/. Data support the use of combination therapy with a three-drug regimen for initial and ongoing therapy. If an infant is identified as HIV infected while receiving ZDV prophylaxis, therapy should be changed to combination therapy
d. Clinical and laboratory monitoring in HIV-infected children: Immune status (CD4 count or percentage), viral load, and evidence of HIV progression (plasma HIV RNA) should be monitored at diagnosis and on a regular basis (every 3 to 4 months). In children younger than 5 years, CD4 percentage is preferred for monitoring immune status because of age-related changes in absolute CD4 count in this age group. Other testing to perform at diagnosis includes HIV genotype, CBC with differential, serum chemistry with liver and renal function, lipid profile, and urinalysis. Drug toxicity should also be monitored on a regular basis. More frequent monitoring of laboratory data may be considered in special cases including infants less than age 6 to 12 months, children with suspected clinical, immunologic, or virologic deterioration, or initiating or changing therapy. Careful attention to routine aspects of pediatric care, such as growth, development, and vaccines, is essential. Screening for hepatitis B and C infection, as well as, for tuberculosis is also recommended for all HIV-infected patients[15]

6. Immunizations in HIV-infected or HIV-exposed infants and children: Perinatally exposed infants should receive all scheduled US infant immunizations. Live vaccines, measles/mumps/rubella (MMR) and varicella vaccine, should be given to asymptomatic HIV-infected children and adolescents (see Chapter 16). HIV-infected children should receive PCV23 at age 2 and 5 years. Influenza vaccine should be given annually in the fall to all infected children ≥6 months as well as children ≥6 months who have HIV-infected household contacts

F. Tuberculosis

1. Recommended tuberculosis testing[9]:
a. Immunologic based testing with interferon gamma release assay (IGRA) is a new type of tuberculosis (TB) test that measures interferon-gamma production from T lymphocytes in response to stimulation with antigens that are fairly specific to *Mycobacterium tuberculosis* complex. The sensitivity of IGRA is similar to tuberculin skin test (TST) and specificity of IGRA is higher because the antigens used are not found in Bacille Calmette-Guérin (BCG) or most pathogenic nontuberculous mycobacteria
   (1) Current recommendations for use in children (from *2009 Red Book*):
      (a) Testing of immune competent children 5 years of age or older in place of a TST
      (b) May be useful to determine whether a BCG-immunized child with a reactive TST more likely has latent TB infection or has a false-positive TST reaction caused by the BCG

b. TST is the most common method for diagnosing latent TB infection in asymptomatic people. BCG immunization is not a contraindication to tuberculin skin testing. Recommendations on testing (from *2009 Red Book*)[9]:
   (1) Immediate testing:
      (a) Contacts of people with confirmed or suspected infectious TB (contact investigation)
      (b) Children with clinical or radiographic findings of TB
      (c) Children immigrating from or with history of travel to TB-endemic areas (e.g., Asia, the Middle East, Africa, Latin America, and countries of the former Soviet Union) including international adoptees; children with close contacts from TB-endemic areas. (If the child is well, TST should be delayed for up to 10 weeks after return.)
   (2) Annual testing (initial TST is at the time of diagnosis or circumstance, beginning as early as age 3 months):
      (a) HIV-infected children (TST only, not recommended to perform IGRA)
      (b) Incarcerated adolescents
   (3) Children at increased risk for progression of infection to disease: Medical conditions such as diabetes mellitus, chronic renal failure, malnutrition, and congenital or acquired immunodeficiencies. Immunodeficiency itself may increase risk for progression to severe disease; if exposure is likely, immediate and periodic TST should be considered; TST should always be performed before initiation of immunosuppressive therapy. For HIV infected children, annual TB testing with TST is recommended starting between 3 to 12 months of age
   (4) The incubation period from TB infection to a positive TST or IGRA is approximately 2 to 10 weeks

c. Standard TST is the Mantoux test. Tine test (multipuncture test) is not recommended.
   (1) Inject 5 tuberculin units (5 TU) of purified protein derivative (0.1 mL) intradermally with a 27-gauge needle and 1-mL syringe on the volar aspect of the forearm to form a 6- to 10-mm wheal. Results of skin testing (in millimeters of induration) should be read 48–72 hours later by qualified medical personnel
   (2) Definition of positive Mantoux test (regardless of whether BCG has been previously administered): Box 17-1

2. Drug therapy:

a. Treatment of latent TB infection
   (1) Indications:
      (a) Children with positive tuberculin tests but no evidence of clinical disease

BOX 17-1

DEFINITIONS OF POSITIVE TUBERCULIN SKIN TESTING[9]

INDURATION ≥5 mm

Children in close contact with known or suspected contagious cases of tuberculosis

Children suspected to have tuberculosis based on clinical or radiographic findings

Children on immunosuppressive therapy or with immunosuppressive conditions (including HIV infection)

INDURATION ≥10 mm

Children at increased risk for dissemination based on young age (<4 yr) or with other medical conditions (cancer, diabetes mellitus, chronic renal failure, or malnutrition)

Children with increased exposure: those born in or whose parents were born in endemic countries; those with travel to endemic countries; those exposed to HIV-infected adults, homeless persons, illicit drug users, nursing home residents, incarcerated or institutionalized persons, migrant farm workers

INDURATION ≥15 mm

Children ≥4 yr without any risk factors

(b) Recent contacts, especially HIV-infected children, of people with infectious tuberculosis, even if tuberculin test and clinical evidence are not indicative of disease

(2) Recommendations (see Formulary for specific doses and Table 17-7)

b. Treatment for active tuberculosis disease.[9] (For details, see *2009 Red Book*. See also Table 17-7.)

G. Selected Tick-borne Illnesses[9]

For all of the following illnesses, infection typically occurs between spring and fall seasons.

1. **Lyme disease**

a. Presentation:

(1) *Early localized disease:* 3–32 days after tick bite. Erythema migrans (annular rash at site of bite, target lesion with clear or necrotic center), fever, headache, myalgia, malaise

(2) *Early disseminated disease:* 3–10 wk after the tick bite. Secondary erythema migrans with multiple, smaller target lesions, cranioneuropathy (especially facial nerve palsy), systemic symptoms as previously listed, and lymphadenopathy; 1% may develop carditis with heart block or aseptic meningitis

(3) *Late disease:* Intermittent, recurrent symptoms occur 2–12 months from initial tick bite. Pauciarticular arthritis affecting large joints (7% of those untreated), peripheral neuropathy, encephalopathy

TABLE 17-7

RECOMMENDED TREATMENT REGIMENS FOR DRUG-SUSCEPTIBLE TUBERCULOSIS IN INFANTS, CHILDREN, AND ADOLESCENTS

Infection or Disease Category	Regimen	Remarks
Latent tuberculosis infection (positive skin test or IGRA, no disease)		
Isoniazid-susceptible	9 mo of isoniazid q24hr	If daily therapy is not possible, DOT twice a wk may be used for 9 mo
Isoniazid-resistant	6 mo of rifampin q24hr	If daily therapy is not possible, DOT twice a wk may be used for 6 mo
Isoniazid/ rifampin-resistant[a]	Consultation with a tuberculosis specialist	For management of neonates born to mothers with evidence of tuberculosis infection, see 2009 *Red Book*
Pulmonary and extrapulmonary (except meningitis)	2 mo of isoniazid, rifampin, ethambutol and pyrazinamide q24hr, followed by 4 mo of isoniazid and rifampin[b] by directly observed therapy (DOT)[c]	If possible drug resistance is a concern, another drug (ethambutol or an aminoglycoside) is added to the initial 3-drug therapy until drug susceptibilities are determined DOT is highly desirable
	9–12 mo of isoniazid and rifampin for drug-susceptible *Mycobacterium bovis*	If hilar adenopathy only, a 6-mo course of isoniazid and rifampin is sufficient Drugs can be given 2 or 3 times/wk under DOT in the initial phase if nonadherence is likely
Meningitis	2 mo of isoniazid, rifampin, pyrazinamide, and an aminoglycoside, ethambutol, or ethionamide q24hr, followed by 7–10 mo of isoniazid and rifampin q24hr or twice per wk (9–12 mo total) At least 12 mo of therapy without pyrazinamide for drug-susceptible *M. bovis*	A fourth drug, such as an aminoglycoside, is given with initial therapy until drug susceptibility is known. For patients who may have acquired tuberculosis in geographic areas where resistance to streptomycin is common, capreomycin (15–30 mg/kg/day), kanamycin (15–30 mg/kg/day) or amikacin may be used instead of streptomycin

[a]Duration of therapy is longer in HIV-infected persons, and additional drugs may be indicated.

[b]Medications should be administered daily for first 2 weeks to 2 months then can be administered 2 to 3 times per week by DOT.

[c]If initial chest x-ray shows cavitary lesions and sputum after 2 months of therapy remains positive, duration of therapy is extended to 9 months.

Modified from Pickering LK (ed): 2009 Red Book: Report of the Committee on Infectious Diseases, 28th ed. Elk Grove Village, IL, American Academy of Pediatrics, 2009, p. 688.

b. Transmission: Spirochete *Borrelia burgdorferi.* Inoculation occurs by the bite of a deer tick, *Ixodes scapularis* or *Ixodes pacificus;* disseminates systemically through blood and lymphatics. Transmission of *B. burgdorferi* requires 24–48 hours of tick attachment. Occurs commonly in New England and Middle Atlantic, Upper Midwest, and Pacific Northwest
c. Diagnosis:
   (1) Clinical exam: Most early Lyme disease can be diagnosed clinically by the characteristic erythema migrans rash or illness compatible with early or late disease (e.g., meningitis, facial palsy, arthritis)
   (2) Laboratory markers: Immunoassays for *B. burgdorferi*–specific IgM, which begins at 3–4 weeks and peaks at 6–8 weeks after disease onset. Only use IgG to confirm late diagnosis. False-positive results of these assays occur as result of cross-reactivity with viral infections, other spirochetal infections, and autoimmune diseases. Western blot assays should be used to confirm positive enzyme immunoassays (EIA). Lyme disease–specific antibodies can be isolated from CSF in patients with CNS involvement
d. Treatment: Antibiotic prophylaxis not routinely recommended for ticks attached <24–48 hours. For early localized disease, doxycycline 100 mg PO BID for 14–21 days is treatment of choice for patients ≥8 years. Amoxicillin or cefuroxime recommended for younger children. Early disseminated and late-onset disease manifestations are treated by the same oral regimen as early disease with time frames as indicated: multiple erythema migrans (21 days), isolated facial palsy (21–28 days), and arthritis (28 days). Persistent or recurrent arthritis (>2 months), carditis, meningitis, or encephalitis may be treated with ceftriaxone or parenteral penicillin (14–28 days)

2. **Rocky Mountain Spotted Fever**[9]

a. Presentation: Incubation period: 1–55 days. Fever, headache, and a characteristic rash that usually occurs by day 6 of illness; initially erythematous and macular and progresses to maculopapular and petechial due to vasculitis. The rash usually appears on wrists and ankles and spreads proximally. Palms and soles are often involved. Other symptoms: myalgia, nausea, anorexia, abdominal pain, diarrhea
   (1) Laboratory manifestations: Thrombocytopenia, hyponatremia, and anemia. White blood cell count usually normal. Severe disease may manifest in CNS, cardiac, pulmonary, gastrointestinal tract, renal involvement, disseminated intravascular involvement, and shock leading to death
b. Transmission: *Rickettsia rickettsii,* an obligate intracellular pathogen transmitted to humans by a tick bite. Most cases are reported in the south Atlantic, southeastern, and south central United States, although the disease is widespread
c. Diagnosis: Diagnosis is by rickettsial group-specific serologic tests, which may be negative early in the illness. A fourfold or greater change

between acute- and convalescent-phase serum specimens is diagnostic. Probable diagnosis can be established by a single serum titer of 1:64 or greater by IFA assay. Culture of *R. rickettsii* is generally not attempted because of danger of transmission to laboratory personnel. *R. rickettsii* can be obtained by immunohistochemical staining of tissue specimens obtained before initiation of antimicrobial therapy. This method is highly specific but not sensitive

d. Treatment: Doxycycline is recommended drug for children of any age. Treatment initiated on the basis of clinical features and epidemiologic considerations, most effective during first week of illness. Usually lasts 7–10 days and is continued until the patient is afebrile for ≥3 days and has demonstrated clinical improvement

e. For discussion of other rickettsial spotted fever infections that are clinically similar but epidemiologically distinct, see *2009 Red Book* (Section 3, Chapter 35)

3. **Ehrlichiosis**[9]

a. Presentation: Systemic febrile illness with headache, chills, rigors, malaise, myalgia, arthralgia, nausea, vomiting, anorexia, or acute weight loss. Rash is variable in location and appearance
   (1) Laboratory manifestations: Leukopenia, anemia, and hepatitis are common
   (2) More severe disease: Pulmonary infiltrates, bone marrow hypoplasia, respiratory failure, encephalopathy, meningitis, disseminated intravascular coagulation (DIC), spontaneous hemorrhage, and renal failure

b. Transmission: *Ehrlichia chaffeensis* (human monocytic ehrlichiosis [HME]) and *Ehrlichia ewingii* associated with the bite of a lone star tick *(Amblyomma americanum),* although other tick species may be vectors. Mammalian reservoirs include white-tailed deer and white-footed mice. Most HME infections occur in the southeastern, south central, and midwestern United States

c. Diagnosis: Confirmed by isolation of *Ehrlichia* organisms from blood or CSF, a fourfold or greater change in antibody titer by IFA assay between acute and convalescent serum specimens, PCR assay amplification of ehrlichial DNA from a clinical specimen, or detection of an intraleukocytoplasmic cluster of bacteria in conjunction with a single IFA titer ≥64. PCR from acute-phase peripheral blood of patients with ehrlichiosis seems sensitive, specific, and promising for early diagnosis

d. Treatment: Doxycycline 4 mg/kg/day q12hr intravenous (IV) or per os (PO) (maximum, 100 mg/dose). Ehrlichiosis may be severe or fatal in untreated patients; initiate treatment early. Failure to respond within first 3 days should suggest infection with an agent other than *Ehrlichia.* Treatment should be continued for at least 3 days after defervescence for a minimum total course of 7 days

4. **Anaplasmosis:** Per the *2009 Red Book,* ehrlichiosis and anaplasmosis are now described separately. The previous information on clinical presentation and treatment is the same for anaplasmosis. Differences from ehrlichiosis are as follows: caused by *Anaplasma phagocytophilum* (human granulocytotrophic anaplasmosis [HGA]), transmitted by the deer tick *(Ixodes scapularis)* or western black legged tick *(Ixodes pacificus),* diagnosis via *Anaplasma* organisms using techniques as described previously. Most cases are reported from the north central and northeastern United States, and from northern California

H. Fungal and Yeast Infections

1. Diagnosis:
a. Place specimen (nail or skin scrapings, biopsy specimens, fluids from tissues or lesions) in 10% potassium hydroxide (KOH) on glass slide to look for hyphae, pseudohyphae
b. Germ tube screen of yeast (3 hours) for *Candida albicans:* All germ tube-positive yeast are *C. albicans,* but not all *C. albicans* are germ tube positive
2. Common community-acquired fungal infections, etiology, and treatment (Table 17-8)

I. Exposures to Blood-borne Pathogens and Postexposure Prophylaxis (PEP)

1. **HIV**[9,17,18]**:**
a. Occupational exposure: Risk for occupational transmission of HIV:
   (1) Needlesticks: Three infections for every 1,000 exposures (0.3%). Risk is greater when the exposure involves a larger volume of blood and/or higher titer of HIV, as in a deep injury, visible blood on the device causing the injury, a device previously used in the source patient's vein or artery, or a source patient in the late stages of HIV infection
   (2) Mucous membrane exposure: One infection for every 1,000 exposures (0.1%). The risk may be higher when the exposure involves a larger volume of blood and a higher titer of HIV, prolonged skin contact, extensive surface area of exposure, or skin integrity that is visibly compromised
b. Nonoccupational HIV exposure in children and adolescents[18]:
   (1) Injury from needles of discarded syringes: No confirmed reports of HIV acquisition from percutaneous injury by a needle found in the community. Risk for transmission from a *found needle* (i.e., a needle discarded in a public place) is low. However, if the needle or syringe is found to have visible blood and the source is known to be HIV infected, PEP should be considered. Testing the syringe for HIV is not practical or reliable
   (2) Repeated sexual encounters or a single episode of sexual abuse: Risk is highest with unprotected receptive anal intercourse (50 per 10,000 exposures), intermediate with receptive vaginal intercourse

TABLE 17-8

COMMON COMMUNITY-ACQUIRED FUNGAL INFECTIONS

Disease	Usual Etiology	Suggested Therapy	Suggested Length of Therapy
Tinea capitis (ringworm of scalp)	*Trichophyton tonsurans, Microsporum canis*	Oral griseofulvin (ultramicro): Give with fatty foods Fungal shedding decreased with 1%–2.5% selenium sulfide shampoo Alt: Terbinafine, itraconazole (total 2–4 weeks), or fluconazole (once weekly)	4–8 wk or 2 wk after clinical resolution
Tinea corporis/pedis/cruris (ringworm of body/feet/genital region)	*Epidermophyton floccosum, Trichophyton rubrum, Trichophyton mentagrophytes, Microsporum canis*	Topical antifungal (miconazole, clotrimazole) (once daily or BID) Terbinafine (BID)	1–4 wks for either therapy
Oral candidiasis (thrush) in immunocompetent patients	*Candida albicans, Candida tropicalis*	Nystatin suspension or clotrimazole troche (only nystatin for infants)	7–10 days, then continue 3 days after clinical resolution
Candidal skin infections (intertriginous)	*Candida albicans*	Topical nystatin, miconazole, clotrimazole	3 days after clinical resolution
Tinea unguium (ringworm of nails)	*Trichophyton mentagrophytes, Trichophyton rubrum, Epidermophyton floccosum*	Oral griseofulvin Alt: Oral terbinafine Itraconazole Fluconazole	6–12 mo 4–6 mo for alternatives (once weekly for fluconazole)

Adapted from 2009 Harriet Lane handbook of pediatric antimicrobial therapy, See Table 1-5, p. 69 for more details regarding treatment of fungal infections.

(10 per 10,000 exposures), and even lower with insertive vaginal intercourse. If the exposure source has genital ulcer disease or another sexually transmitted infection or if there was tissue damage, the risk for HIV transmission is higher, increasing the benefit of PEP relative to the burden and risk for drug toxicity

(3) Human milk[13]: In the United States, women who are HIV infected should be counseled not to breastfeed. An infant who has a single exposure to human milk from a woman with HIV infection is estimated to have 100 times lower risk than that of other mucous membrane exposures, and PEP is likely not warranted

17

(4) Human bites: Transmission is extremely rare even when saliva is contaminated with blood; saliva inhibits HIV infectivity, HIV is rarely isolated from saliva, and concentrations of HIV in saliva of HIV-infected persons is low even in the presence of periodontal disease

c. Prophylaxis:
   (1) Optimally, PEP should be initiated as soon as possible, preferably within 1–3 hours of exposure but no later than 72 hours. The usual duration of PEP, if tolerated, is 28 days. The benefits of postexposure prophylaxis are greatest when risk of infection is high, intervention is prompt, and adherence is likely[9]
   (2) A clinician with experience in treatment of individuals with HIV infection should be consulted whenever possible (without causing PEP initiation delay) before initiating therapy. Decision about need for PEP is based on HIV status of source, type, and severity of potential exposure and individual risk tolerance. PEP is generally composed of two-drug or three-drug regimens, frequently available in fixed-dose combination pills for older children and adults. No clear evidence of superior efficacy of a three-drug regimen over a two-drug regimen in preventing HIV infection after exposure, but many experts prefer to use three drugs; this practice must be balanced against the increased toxicity potential when additional drugs are used. Typical regimens include two nucleoside reverse transcriptase inhibitors (NRTIs) (e.g., zidovudine+ lamivudine or, in adolescent/adults, tenofovir+ emtricitabine), two NRTIs plus a protease inhibitor (PI) (e.g., lopinavir/ritonavir) or two NRTIs plus a non-nucleoside reverse transcriptase inhibitor (NNRTI) (e.g., efavirenz). Full descriptions of potential regimens can be found in CDC and AAP guidelines
   (3) Use of zidovudine alone as PEP is no longer recommended. For most recent recommendations, refer to CDC and AAP guidelines. The CDC's postexposure prophylaxis hotline (open 24 hr/day) is 888-448-4911

2. **Hepatitis B:** Most readily transmitted of the blood-borne pathogens. Recommendations for hepatitis B prophylaxis in nonimmune person after percutaneous exposure to blood that contains (or might contain) HBsAg include hepatitis B immune globulin and initiation of hepatitis B vaccine series. For details, see Chapter 16
3. **Hepatitis C:** No preventive therapy available. Serologic testing and follow-up are important to document if infection occurs. Infections become chronic in the majority of patients

J. Infectious Diseases in Internationally Adopted Children

For more information, see American Academy of Pediatrics. Medical evaluation of internationally adopted children for infectious diseases. In *2009 Red Book*,[9] pp. 177–179.

REFERENCES

1. Kaditis A, O'Marcaigh A, Rhodes K, et al: Yield of positive blood cultures in pediatric oncology patients by a new method of blood culture collection. *Pediatr Infect Dis J* 1996;15(7):615–620.
2. Gilbert DN, Moellering RC, Eliopoulos GM, et al: *The Sanford guide to antimicrobial therapy*, 39th ed. Sperryville, VA, Antimicrobial Therapy, Incorporated, 2009.
3. Mandell GL, Bennett GL, Dolin R: *Principles of practice of infectious disease*, 6th ed. New York, Churchill Livingston, 2005.
4. Livermore DM: β-Lactamases in laboratory and clinical resistance. *Clin Microbiol Rev* 1995;8:557–584.
5. Shapiro ED: Fever without localizing signs. In Long SS, Pickering LK, Prober CG (eds): *Principles and practice of pediatric infectious disease*, 3rd ed. Philadelphia, PA, Churchill Livingstone Elsevier, 2008.
6. Barraff L: Management of infants and young children with fever without a source. *Pediatr Ann* 2008;27(1):673–679.
7. Kliegman RE, Stanton B, St Geme J, et al. *Nelson textbook of pediatrics*, 19th ed. Philadelphia, WB Saunders, 2010.
8. McMillan JA, Feigin RD, DeAngelis CD, et al (eds): *Oski's pediatrics: principles and practice*, 4th ed. Philadelphia, Lippincott Williams and Wilkins, 2006.
9. American Academy of Pediatrics, Pickering LK, Baker CJ, Kimberlin DW, et al: *Red Book: 2009 Report of the Committee on Infectious Diseases*. 28th ed. Elk Grove Village, IL. American Academy of Pediatrics, 2009.
10. Centers for Disease Control and Prevention: A new product (VariZIG) for postexposure prophylaxis of varicella available under an investigational drug application expanded access protocol. *MMWR* 2006; 55:209–210.
11. Wong VC, Reesink HW, Lelie PN, et al. Prevention of the HBsAg carrier state in newborn infants of mothers who are chronic carriers of HBsAG and HBeAg by administration of hepatitis-B vaccine and hepatitis-B immunoglobulin: double-blind randomized placebo-controlled study. *Lancet* 1984;1(8383): 921–926.
12. Wong CS, Jelacic S, Habeeb RL, et al: The risk of hemolytic-uremic syndrome after antibiotic treatment of Escherichia coli O157:H7 infections. *N Engl J Med* 2000;342:1930–1936.
13. AAP Committee on Pediatric AIDS: HIV testing and prophylaxis to prevent mother-to-child transmission in the United States. *Pediatrics* 2008;122(5): 1127–1134.
14. Perinatal HIV Guidelines Working Group: *Public Health Service Task Force recommendations for use of antiretroviral drugs in pregnant HIV-1-infected women for maternal health and interventions to reduce perinatal HIV-1 transmission in the United States.* Rockville (MD): Public Health Service Task Force, April 29, 2009, p. 111.
15. Simpkins EP, Siberry GK, Hutton N: Thinking about HIV Infection. *Pediatr Rev* 2009;30;337–349.
16. Working Group on Antiretroviral Therapy and Medical Management of HIV-Infected Children: *Guidelines for the use of antiretroviral agents in pediatric HIV infection.* Bethesda. MD. U.S. Department of Health and Human Services. February 23, 2008, p. 139.

17. Centers for Disease Control and Prevention: Updated U.S. Public Health Service guidelines for the management of occupational exposures to HIV and recommendations for postexposure prophylaxis. *MMWR* 2005;54(RR-09):1–17.
18. Havens P, American Academy of Pediatrics Committee on Pediatric AIDS: Postexposure prophylaxis in children and adolescents for nonoccupational exposure to human immunodeficiency virus. *Pediatrics* 2003;111(6): 1475–1489.

Chapter 18

Neonatology

Matthew H. Merves, MD

See additional content on Expert Consult

I. WEBSITES

www.nicuniversity.org

Outcomes calculator: http://www.nichd.nih.gov/about/org/cdbpm/pp/prog_epbo/epbo_case.cfm

Neonatal dermatology: http://www.adhb.govt.nz/newborn/TeachingResources/Dermatology/Dermatology.htm

II. FETAL ASSESSMENT

(See Box EC 18-A, Box EC 18-B, and Table EC 18-A on Expert Consult)

III. NEWBORN RESUSCITATION

A. NALS Algorithm for Neonatal Resuscitation (Fig. 18-1)

For infants with meconium in the amniotic fluid, routine intrapartum oropharyngeal and nasopharyngeal **suctioning is not recommended.** If the infant is not vigorous, endotracheal intubation should be performed immediately after birth and suction should be applied to the endotracheal tube as it is withdrawn.[1]

B. Endotracheal Tube Size and Depth of Insertion (See Table 18-1)

C. Ventilatory Support (See Chapter 4)

D. Vascular Access (See Chapter 3 for Umbilical Venous Catheter and Umbilical Artery Catheter Placement)

NOTE: During initial resuscitation, Umbilical Venous Catheter (UVC) should be inserted just far enough to obtain blood return; no measurement or verified placement necessary initially.

IV. NEWBORN ASSESSMENT

A. Vital Signs

1. Heart rate 120–160 bpm
2. Respiratory rate 40–60 breaths/min
3. Arterial blood pressure: related to birth weight, gestational age (see Chapter 7)
4. Core temperature: 36.5°–37.5°C rectally
5. See Chapter 21 for growth charts in the premature infant

B. Apgar Scores (Table 18-2)

Assessed at 1 and 5 minutes. May be repeated at 5-minute intervals for infants with 5-minute scores <7.[2]

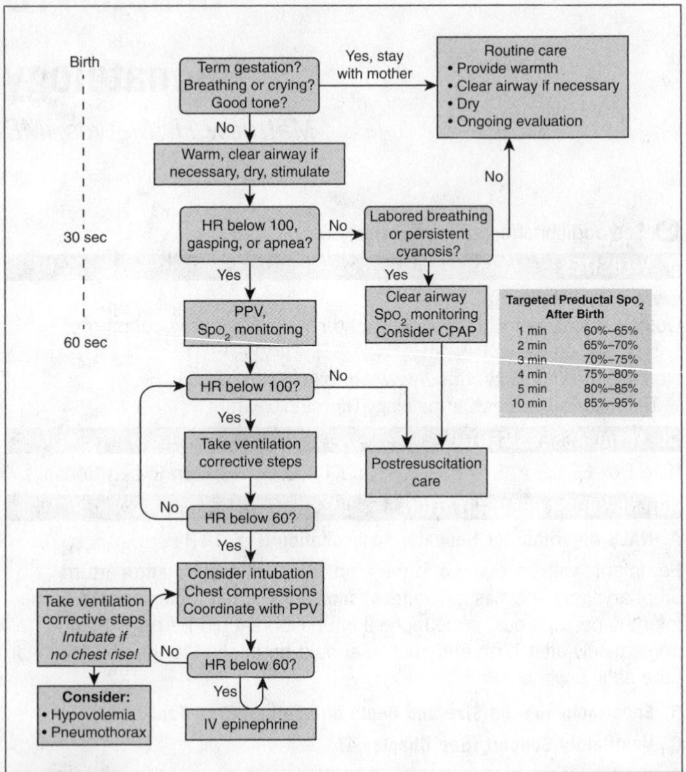

FIGURE 18-1

Overview of resuscitation in the delivery room. *(Kattwinkel J, Perlman JM, Aziz K, et al: Part 15: Neonatal Resuscitation: 2010 American Heart Association Guidelines for Cardiopulmonary Resuscitation and Emergency Cardiovascular Care Circulation. 2010;122:S909–S919.)*

C. New Ballard Gestational Age Estimation

The Ballard score is most accurate when performed between age 12 and 20 hours.[3] Approximate gestational age is calculated based on the sum of the neuromuscular and physical maturity ratings (Fig. 18-2).

1. **Neuromuscular maturity:**
   a. Posture: Observe infant quiet and supine. Score 0 for arms, legs extended; 1 for starting to flex hips and knees, arms extended; 2 for stronger flexion of legs, arms extended; 3 for arms slightly flexed, legs flexed and abducted; and 4 for full flexion of arms and legs

TABLE 18-1

PREDICTED ENDOTRACHEAL TUBE SIZE AND EXPECTED BIRTH WEIGHT BY GESTATIONAL AGE*

Gestational Age (wk)	Weight (g)*	ETT Size (mm)	ETT Depth of Insertion (cm from upper lip)
24	700	2.5	7
26	900	2.5	7
28	1100	2.5–3.0	7
30	1350	3.0	7
32	1650	3.0	7
34	2100	3.5	8
36	2600	3.5	8
38	3000	3.5–4.0	9

*Weight is the 50th percentile for age.

ETT, Endotracheal tube.

Data from Usher R, McLean F: Intrauterine growth of liveborn Caucasian infants at sea level: Standards obtained from measurements in seven dimensions of infants born between 25 and 44 week gestation. J Pediatr 1969;74:901–910; Welty SE: Intrauterine guidelines for neonatal resuscitation and emergency cardiovascular care—International Consensus on Science. Pediatrics 2000;106(3):e29.

TABLE 18-2

APGAR SCORES

Score	0	1	2
Heart rate	Absent	<100 bpm	>100 bpm
Respiratory effort	Absent, irregular	Slow, crying	Good
Muscle tone	Limp	Some flexion of extremities	Active motion
Reflex irritability (nose suction)	No response	Grimace	Cough or sneeze
Color	Blue, pale	Acrocyanosis	Completely pink

Data from Apgar V: Proposal for a new method of evaluation of the newborn infant. Anesth Analg 1953;32:260.

b. Square window: Flex hand on forearm enough to obtain fullest possible flexion without wrist rotation. Measure angle between the hypothenar eminence and the ventral aspect of the forearm
c. Arm recoil: With infant supine, flex forearms for 5 seconds, fully extend by pulling on hands, then release. Measure the angle of elbow flexion to which the arms recoil
d. Popliteal angle: Hold infant supine with pelvis flat, thigh held in the knee-chest position. Extend leg by gentle pressure and measure the popliteal angle
e. Scarf sign: With baby supine, pull infant's hand across the neck toward the opposite shoulder. Determine how far the elbow will go across. Score 0 if elbow reaches opposite axillary line; 1 if past midaxillary line; 2 if past midline; and 3 if elbow unable to reach midline
f. Heel-to-ear maneuver: With baby supine, draw foot as near to the head as possible without forcing it. Observe distance between foot and head and degree of extension at the knee

Neuromuscular maturity

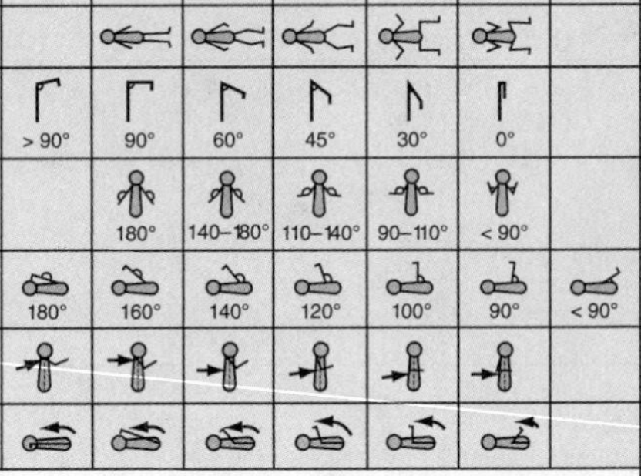

Neuromuscular maturity sign	Score −1	0	1	2	3	4	5	Record score here
Posture								
Square window (wrist)	> 90°	90°	60°	45°	30°	0°		
Arm recoil		180°	140–180°	110–140°	90–110°	< 90°		
Popliteal angle	180°	160°	140°	120°	100°	90°	< 90°	
Scarf sign								
Heel to ear								
							TOTAL NEUROMUSCULAR MATURITY SCORE	

Physical maturity

Physical maturity sign	Score −1	0	1	2	3	4	5	Record score here
Skin	Sticky, friable, transparent	Gelatinous, red, translucent	Smooth, pink, visible veins	Superficial peeling and/or rash, few veins	Cracking, pale areas, rare veins	Parchment, deep cracking, no vessels	Leathery, cracked, wrinkled	
Lanugo	None	Sparse	Abundant	Thinning	Bald areas	Mostly bald		
Plantar surface	Heel-toe: 40–50 mm: −1 <40 mm: −2	>50 mm, no crease	Faint red marks	Anterior transverse crease only	Creases anterior two thirds	Creases over entire sole		
Breast	Imperceptible	Barely perceptible	Flat areola, no bud	Stippled areola, 1–2 mm bud	Raised areola, 3–4 mm bud	Full areola, 5–10 mm bud		
Eye/ear	Lids fused: loosely: −1 tightly: −2	Lids open, pinna flat, stays folded	Sl. curved pinna, soft, slow recoil	Well-curved pinna, soft but ready recoil	Formed and firm, instant recoil	Thick cartilage, ear stiff		
Genitals (male)	Scrotum flat, smooth	Scrotum empty, faint rugae	Testes in upper canal, rare rugae	Testes descending, few rugae	Testes down, good rugae	Testes pendulous, deep rugae		
Genitals (female)	Clitoris prominent and labia flat	Prominent clitoris and small labia minora	Prominent clitoris and enlarging minora	Majora and minora equally prominent	Majora large, minora small	Majora cover clitoris and minora		
							TOTAL PHYSICAL MATURITY SCORE	

Score
Neuromuscular______
Physical______
Total______

Maturity rating

Score	−10	−5	0	5	10	15	20	25	30	35	40	45	50
Weeks	20	22	24	26	28	30	32	34	36	38	40	42	44

Gestational age (weeks)
By dates______
By ultrasound______
By exam______

FIGURE 18-2

Neuromuscular and physical maturity (New Ballard Score). *(Modified from Ballard JL et al: New Ballard Score, expanded to include extremely premature infants. J Pediatr 1991;119:417–423.)*

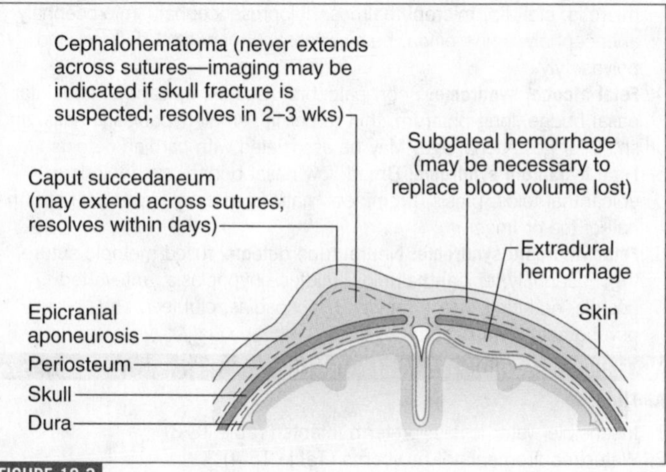

FIGURE 18-3

Types of extradural fluid collections seen in newborn infants.

2. **Physical maturity:** Based on the developmental stage of eyes, ears, breasts, genitalia, skin, lanugo, and plantar creases (see Fig. 18-2)

D. Birth Trauma

1. **Extradural fluid collections (Fig. 18-3):** Caput succedaneum, cephalohematoma, and subgaleal hemorrhage
2. **Fractured clavicle:** Perhaps crepitus on day 1 ± swelling/discomfort on day 2
3. **Brachial Plexus injuries:** Erb's palsy (C5-6) most common, but also possible to have Klumpke's (C8-T1; least common) and Total (C5-T1). See Section XII.E

E. Selected Anomalies, Syndromes, and Malformations (See Chapter 13 for Common Syndromes/Genetic Disorders)

1. **VATER association: V**ertebral anomalies, **A**nal anomalies and anal atresia, **T**racheoesophageal fistula, **E**sophageal atresia, and **R**adial and/or **R**enal defects. May also include vascular (cardiac) defects
2. **CHARGE syndrome** (associated with mutations in gene *CHD7* on chromosome 8q12): **C**oloboma, **H**eart disease, choanal **A**tresia, **R**etarded growth and development (may include central nervous system [CNS] anomalies), **G**enital anomalies (may include hypogonadism), **E**ar abnormalities or deafness
3. **Infant of a diabetic mother:** Sacral agenesis, femoral hypoplasia, heart defects, and cleft palate. May also include preaxial radial defects,

microtia, cleft lip, microphthalmos, holoprosencephaly, microcephaly, anencephaly, spina bifida, hemivertebra, urinary tract defects, and polydactyly

4. **Fetal alcohol syndrome:** Short palpebral fissures, epicanthal folds, flat nasal bridge, long philtrum, thin upper lip, small hypoplastic nails, and small for gestational age. May be associated with cardiac defects
5. **Fetal hydantoin syndrome:** Broad, low nasal bridge; hypertelorism, epicanthal folds, ptosis, prominent malformed ears, hypoplasia of fifth nail of toe or finger
6. **Fetal valproate syndrome:** Neural tube defects, fused metopic suture, trigonocephaly, epicanthal folds, midface hypoplasia, anteverted nostrils, oral cleft, heart defects, hypospadias, clubfeet, and psychomotor retardation

V. FLUIDS, ELECTROLYTES, AND NUTRITION

A. Fluids

1. Insensible water loss in preterm infants (Table 18-3)
2. Water requirements of newborns (Table 18-4)

B. Glucose

1. Requirements: Preterm neonates require about 5–6 mg/kg/min of glucose (40–100 mg/dL).[4] Term neonates require about 3–5 mg/kg/min of glucose. The formula to calculate glucose infusion rate (GIR) is as follows:

$$\begin{aligned} \text{GIR (mg/kg/min)} &= [(\%\text{ glucose in solution} \times 10) \times \\ &\quad (\text{rate of infusion per hour})]/[60 \times \text{weight (kg)}] \\ &= 0.167 \times (\%\text{ glucose}) \times (\text{infusion rate})/\text{weight (kg)} \end{aligned}$$

2. Management of hyperglycemia and hypoglycemia (Table 18-5).[5] See also Chapter 10

C. Electrolytes, Minerals, and Vitamins

1. **Electrolyte requirements (Table 18-6).**
2. **Mineral and vitamin requirements:**

a. Infants born at <34 weeks' gestation have higher calcium, phosphorus, sodium, iron, and vitamin D requirements and

TABLE 18-3

INSENSIBLE WATER LOSS IN PRETERM INFANTS*

Body Weight (g)	Insensible Water Loss (mL/kg/day)
<1000	60–70
1000–1250	60–65
1251–1500	30–45
1501–1750	15–30
1751–2000	15–20

*Estimates of insensible water loss at different body weights during the first few days of life.
Data from Veille JC: Clin Perinatol 1988;15:863.

TABLE 18-4

WATER REQUIREMENTS OF NEWBORNS

	Water Requirements (mL/kg/24 hr) by Age		
Birth Weight (g)	**1–2 days**	**3–7 days**	**7–30 days**
<750	100–250	150–300	120–180
750–1000	80–150	100–150	120–180
1000–1500	60–100	80–150	120–180
<1500	60–80	100–150	120–180

Data from Taeusch HW, Ballard RA (eds): Schaeffer and Avery's diseases of the newborn, 7th ed. Philadelphia, WB Saunders, 1998

TABLE 18-5

MANAGEMENT OF HYPERGLYCEMIA AND HYPOGLYCEMIA[5]

	Hypoglycemia	Hyperglycemia
Definition	Serum glucose <45 mg/dL in term and preterm infants	Serum glucose >125 mg/dL in term infants, >150 mg/dL in preterm infants
Differential diagnosis	Insufficient glucose delivery Decreased glycogen stores Increased circulating insulin (infant of a diabetic mother, maternal drugs, Beckwith-Wiedemann syndrome, tumors) Endocrine and metabolic disorders Sepsis Hypothermia Polycythemia Asphyxia Shock	Excess glucose administration Sepsis Hypoxia Hyperosmolar formula Neonatal diabetes mellitus Medications
Evaluation	Assess for symptoms Calculate glucose delivery to infant Serum glucose (to confirm bedside testing) Complete blood count with differential Blood, urine, ± CSF cultures Urinalysis Electrolytes Insulin and C-peptide levels if warranted	
Management	Change dextrose infusion rates gradually. Generally, it should not exceed 2 mg/kg/min in a 2-hr interval. (See Chapter 10 for further guidelines) Monitor glucose levels every 30–60 min until normal	Gradually decrease glucose infusion rate if receiving >5 mg/kg/min Monitor glucosuria. Consider insulin infusion for persistent hyperglycemia

require breast-milk fortifier or special preterm formulas with iron. Fortifier should be added to breast milk only after the second week of life

b. Iron: Enterally fed preterm infants require elemental iron supplementation of 2 mg/kg/day after age 4–8 weeks

TABLE 18-6

ELECTROLYTE REQUIREMENTS

	Before 48 Hours of Life	After 48–72 Hours of Life
Sodium	None, unless serum sodium <135 mEq/L without evidence of volume overload	Term infants: 2–3 mEq/kg/day Preterm infants: 3–5 mEq/kg/day
Potassium	None	1–2.5 mEq/kg/day if adequate urine output is established and serum level <4.5 mEq/L

D. Nutrition

1. **Growth and caloric requirements:**

a. Preterm infants (healthy and thermoneutral environments):
   (1) Caloric requirements: 115–130 kcal/kg/day (up to 150 kcal/kg/day for very low birth weight infants)
   (2) Growth (after 10 days of life): 15–20 g/kg/day

b. Term infants:
   (1) Caloric requirements: 100–120 kcal/kg/day
   (2) Growth (after 10 days of life): 10 g/kg/day

2. **Total parenteral nutrition (see Chapter 21)**

VI. CYANOSIS IN THE NEWBORN

A. Differential Diagnosis

1. General: Hypothermia, hypoglycemia, sepsis, shock
2. Neurologic: Central apnea, central hypoventilation, intraventricular hemorrhage (IVH), meningitis
3. Respiratory: Persistent pulmonary hypertension of the newborn (PPHN), diaphragmatic hernia, pulmonary hypoplasia, choanal atresia, pneumothorax, respiratory distress syndrome (RDS), transient tachypnea of the newborn (TTN), pneumonia, meconium aspiration
4. Cardiac: Congestive heart failure, congenital cyanotic heart disease
5. Hematologic: Polycythemia, methemoglobinemia
6. Medications: Respiratory depression from maternal medications (e.g., magnesium sulfate, narcotics)

B. Evaluation

1. **Physical examination:** Note central versus peripheral, persistent versus intermittent cyanosis; respiratory effort; single versus split S_2, presence of heart murmur. Acrocyanosis is often a normal finding in newborns
2. **Clinical tests:** Oxygen challenge test (see Chapter 7), pre/postductal arterial blood gases or pulse oximetry to assess for right-to-left shunt, and transillumination of chest for possible pneumothorax
3. **Other data:** Complete blood count with differential, serum glucose, chest radiograph, electrocardiogram (ECG), echocardiography. Consider blood, urine, and cerebrospinal fluid cultures if sepsis is suspected, and methemoglobin level if cyanosis is out of proportion to hypoxemia

VII. RESPIRATORY DISEASES

A. General Respiratory Considerations

1. **Exogenous surfactant therapy:**
a. Indications: Respiratory distress syndrome in preterm infants, meconium aspiration, pneumonia, persistent pulmonary hypertension
b. Administration: If the infant is ≤26 weeks' gestation, the first dose is typically given in the delivery room or as soon as stabilized; repeat dosing may follow at 6-hr intervals
c. Complications: Pneumothorax, pulmonary hemorrhage
2. **Supplemental O_2:** Adjust inspired oxygen to maintain O_2 saturation between 85% and 94% until the retina is fully vascularized, between 94% and 98% if the retinas are mature (see Section XIII), and >97% in cases of pulmonary hypertension

B. Respiratory Distress Syndrome (RDS)

1. **Definition:** Deficiency of pulmonary surfactant (a phospholipid protein mixture that decreases surface tension and prevents alveolar collapse). Produced by type II alveolar cells in increasing quantities from 32 weeks' gestation
a. Maternal administration of steroids antenatally has been shown to decrease neonatal morbidity and mortality. Risk for RDS is decreased in babies born >24 hours and <7 days after maternal steroid administration
b. Other factors that accelerate lung maturity: maternal hypertension, sickle cell disease, narcotic addiction, intrauterine growth retardation, prolonged rupture of membranes and fetal stress
2. **Incidence:**
a. <30 weeks' gestation: 60% without antenatal steroids, 35% in those who received antenatal steroids
b. 30 to 34 weeks' gestation: 25% in untreated infants, 10% in those who have received antenatal steroids
c. >34 weeks' gestation: 5%
3. **Risk factors:** Prematurity, maternal diabetes, cesarean section without antecedent labor, perinatal asphyxia, second twin, previous infant with RDS
4. **Clinical presentation:** Respiratory distress worsens during the first few hours of life, progresses over 48–72 hours, and subsequently improves
a. Recovery is accompanied by brisk diuresis
b. Chest x-ray findings: *reticulogranular* pattern to lung fields; may obscure heart borders
5. **Management:**
a. Support ventilation and oxygenation
b. Surfactant therapy

C. Persistent Pulmonary Hypertension of the Newborn (PPHN)

1. **Etiology:** Idiopathic or secondary to conditions leading to increased pulmonary vascular resistance. Most commonly seen in term or

post-term infants, infants born by cesarean section, and infants with a history of fetal distress and low Apgar scores. Usually presents within 12–24 hours of birth

a. Vasoconstriction secondary to hypoxemia and acidosis (e.g., neonatal sepsis)
b. Interstitial pulmonary disease (meconium aspiration syndrome, pneumonia)
c. Hyperviscosity syndrome (polycythemia)
d. Pulmonary hypoplasia, either primary or secondary to congenital diaphragmatic hernia or renal agenesis

2. **Diagnostic features:**

a. Severe hypoxemia (Pao_2 <35–45 mmHg in 100% O_2) disproportionate to radiologic changes
b. Structurally normal heart with right-to-left shunt at foramen ovale and/or ductus arteriosus; decreased postductal oxygenation compared with preductal. (Difference of at least 7–15 mmHg between preductal and postductal Pao_2 is significant.)
c. Must be distinguished from cyanotic heart disease. Infants with heart disease will have an abnormal cardiac examination and show little to no improvement in oxygenation with increased fraction of inspired O_2 (Fio_2) and hyperventilation. See Chapter 7 for interpretation of oxygen challenge test

3. **Principles of therapy:**

a. **Improve oxygenation:** Supplemental oxygen (Fio_2) to improve alveolar oxygenation; Optimize oxygen-carrying capacity with blood transfusions as needed
b. **Minimize pulmonary vasoconstriction**
   (1) Minimal handling and limited invasive procedures. Sedation and occasionally paralysis of intubated neonates may be necessary
   (2) Alkalosis (pH 7.45–7.55): Metabolic or respiratory (Pco_2 in low 30s); may improve oxygenation, although not noted to affect outcome. Avoid severe hypocarbia (Pco_2 <30), which can be associated with myocardial ischemia and decreased cerebral blood flow. Hyperventilation may result in barotrauma, predisposing to chronic lung disease, so should be minimized if possible. Consider high-frequency ventilation
c. **Maintenance of systemic blood pressure and perfusion:** reversal of right-to-left shunt through volume expanders and/or inotropes
d. **Consider pulmonary vasodilator therapy**
   (1) Inhaled nitric oxide (NO): Reduces pulmonary vascular resistance (PVR). Blended with ventilatory gases and titrated to effect. Typical starting dose is 20 parts per million (ppm). Unlikely to be efficacious >40 ppm. Complications include methemoglobinemia (reduce NO dose for methemoglobin >4%), NO_2 poisoning (reduce NO dose for NO_2 concentration >1–2 ppm)

(2) Prostaglandin I_2 (prostacyclin): A complex molecule made from arachidonic acid; major endogenous pulmonary vasodilator. Normally produced by lung when lung vessels are constricted

e. **Broad-spectrum antibiotics:** Sepsis is a common underlying cause of PPHN

f. **Consider extracorporeal membrane oxygenation (ECMO):** Reserved for cases of severe cardiovascular instability, oxygenation index (OI) >40 for >3 hour, or alveolar-arterial gradient (A-aO_2) ≥610 for 8 hours (see Chapter 4 for the calculation of OI and A-aO_2. PaO_2 should be postductal). Patients typically need to be >2000 g and >34 weeks' gestation; should have head ultrasound and echocardiogram before initiating ECMO

4. **Mortality depends on underlying diagnosis:** Mortality rates generally lower for RDS and meconium aspiration but higher in sepsis and diaphragmatic hernia

D. Spontaneous Pneumothorax

1. Seen in 1%–2% of normal newborns
2. Associated with use of high inspiratory pressures and underlying diseases such as RDS, meconium aspiration, and pneumonia
3. Patient should be monitored in an intensive care unit (ICU) setting

VIII. APNEA AND BRADYCARDIA

A. Apnea[6]

1. **Definition:** Respiratory pause >20 seconds, or a shorter pause associated with cyanosis, pallor, hypotonia, or bradycardia <100 bpm. In preterm infants, apnea may be central (no diaphragmatic activity), obstructive (upper airway obstruction), or mixed central and obstructive. Common causes of apnea in the newborn are listed in Figure 18-4
2. **Incidence:** Apnea of prematurity occurs in most infants born at <28 weeks' gestation, about 50% of infants born at 30–32 weeks' gestation, and <7% of infants born at 34–35 weeks' gestation. It usually resolves by 34–36 weeks' postconceptual age, but may persist after term in infants born at <25 weeks' gestation
3. **Management:**

a. Consider pathologic causes for apnea
b. Pharmacotherapy with caffeine or other stimulants
c. Continuous positive-airway pressure or mechanical ventilation (see Chapter 4 for details)

B. Bradycardia Without Central Apnea

Etiologies include obstructive apnea, mechanical airway obstruction, gastroesophageal reflux, increased intracranial pressure (ICP), increased vagal tone (defecation, yawning, rectal stimulation, placement of nasogastric [NG] tube), electrolyte abnormalities, heart block

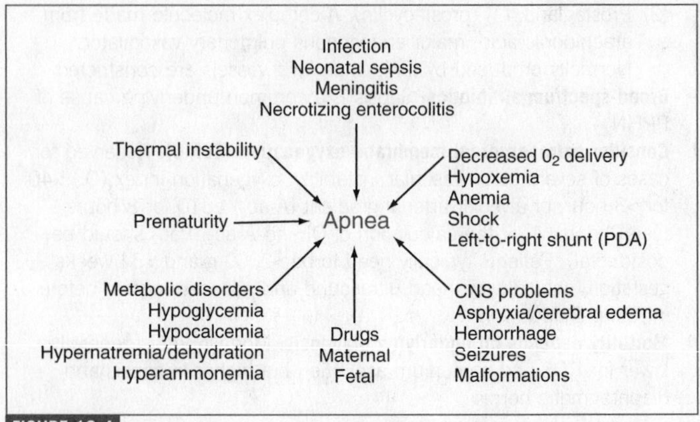

FIGURE 18-4

Causes of apnea in the newborn. *(From Klaus MH, Fanaroff AA: Care of the high-risk neonate, 5th ed. Philadelphia, WB Saunders, 2001, p. 268.)*

IX. CARDIAC DISEASES

A. Patent Ductus Arteriosus (PDA)

1. **Definition:** Failure of the ductus arteriosus to close in the first few days of life or reopening after functional closure. Typically results in left-to-right shunting of blood once PVR has decreased. If PVR remains high, blood may be shunted right to left, resulting in hypoxemia (see Section VII.C)
2. **Incidence:** Up to 60% in preterm infants weighing <1500 g, higher in those <1000 g. Female-to-male ratio is 2:1. Obligatory PDA is found in 10% of infants with congenital heart disease
3. **Risk factors:** Most often related to hypoxia and immaturity. Term infants with PDA usually have structural defects in the walls of the ductal vessel
4. **Diagnosis:**

a. Examination: A systolic murmur that may be continuous, best heard at the left upper sternal border or left infraclavicular area. May have apical diastolic rumble because of increased blood flow across the mitral valve in diastole. Bounding peripheral pulses with widened pulse pressure if large shunt. Hyperactive precordium and palmar pulses may be present

b. ECG: Normal or left ventricular hypertrophy in small to moderate PDA. Biventricular hypertrophy in large PDA

c. Chest radiograph: May have cardiomegaly and increased pulmonary vascular markings depending on size of the shunt

d. Echocardiogram

5. **Management:**
a. Indomethacin: A prostaglandin synthetase inhibitor; 80% closure rate in preterm infants
   (1) For dosage information and contraindications, see Formulary
   (2) Complications: Transient decrease in glomerular filtration rate and decreased urine output; transient gastrointestinal bleeding (not associated with an increased incidence of necrotizing enterocolitis [NEC]); prolonged bleeding time and disturbed platelet function for 7–9 days independent of platelet number (not associated with increased incidence of intracranial hemorrhage). Spontaneous isolated intestinal perforations are seen with indomethacin use. Rates are higher with concomitant hydrocortisone use
b. Ibuprofen[6,7]—As effective as indomethacin with fewer renal adverse effects
c. Surgical ligation of the duct

B. Cyanotic Heart Disease

See Chapter 7.

X. HEMATOLOGIC DISEASES

A. Unconjugated Hyperbilirubinemia in the Newborn[8]

1. **Overview:** During the first 3–4 days of life, serum bilirubin increases from 1.5 mg/dL in cord blood to 6.5 ± 2.5 mg/dL
a. Maximum rate of increase in bilirubin for normal infants with nonhemolytic hyperbilirubinemia: 5 mg/dL/24 hr, or 0.2 mg/dL/hr
b. Consider pathologic cause: Visible jaundice or a total bilirubin concentration >5 mg/dL on the first day of life
c. Risk factors: Birth weight <2500 g, breastfeeding, prematurity
2. **Evaluation:**
a. Maternal prenatal testing: ABO and Rh (D) typing and serum screen for isoimmune antibodies
b. Infant or cord blood: Blood smear, direct Coombs test, blood and Rh typing (if maternal blood type is O, Rh negative, or prenatal blood typing was not performed)
3. **Management:**
a. Phototherapy: Ideally, intensive phototherapy should produce a decline of the total serum bilirubin (TSB) level of 1–2 mg/dL within 4–6 hours with further decline subsequently
   (1) Preterm newborn (see Table 18-7)
   (2) Term newborn (see Fig. 18-5)
b. Intravenous immune globulin (IVIG) (>35 weeks gestational age [GA]): In isoimmune hemolytic disease, administration of IVIG (0.5–1 g/kg over 2 hours) is recommended if the TSB is rising despite intensive phototherapy or the TSB level is within 2–3 mg/dL of the exchange level. Repeat in 12 hours if needed

TABLE 18-7

GUIDELINES FOR USE OF PHOTOTHERAPY IN PRETERM INFANTS <1 WEEK OF AGE

Weight (g)	Phototherapy (mg/dL)	Consider Exchange Transfusion (mg/dL)
500–1000	5–7	12–15
1000–1500	7–10	15–18
1500–2500	10–15	18–20
>2500	>15	>20

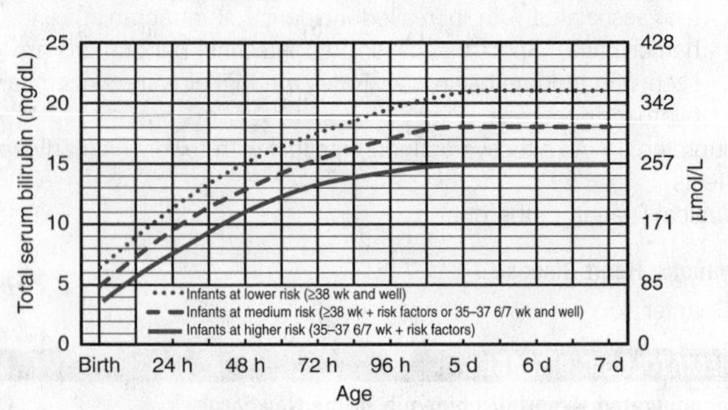

- Use total bilirubin. Do not subtract direct reacting or conjugated bilirubin.
- Risk factors: Isoimmune hemolytic disease, G6PD deficiency, asphyxia, significant lethargy, temperature instability, sepsis, acidosis, or albumin <3.0 g/dL (if measured).
- For well infants 35–37 6/7 wk can adjust TSB levels for intervention around the medium risk line. It is an option to intervene at lower TSB levels for infants closer to 35 wks and at higher TSB levels for those closer to 37 6/7 wk.
- It is an option to provide conventional phototherapy in hospital or at home at TSB levels 2–3 mg/dL (35–50 mmol/L) below those shown, but home phototherapy should not be used in any infant with risk factors.

FIGURE 18-5

Guidelines for phototherapy in infants born at 35 weeks' gestation or more.

c. Neonatal double-volume exchange transfusion (see Table 18-7 and Fig. 18-6):
   (1) Volume: 160 mL/kg for full-term infant; 160–200 mL/kg for preterm infant
   (2) Route: During the exchange, blood is removed through the umbilical arterial catheter (UAC) and an equal volume is infused through the umbilical venous catheter (UVC). If UAC is unavailable, use a single venous catheter
   (3) Rate: Exchange in 15 mL increments for vigorous, full-term infants. Exchange at 2–3 mL/kg/min in premature/less stable infants to avoid trauma to red blood cells
   (4) Complications: Emboli, thromboses, hemodynamic instability, electrolyte disturbances, coagulopathy, infection, and death

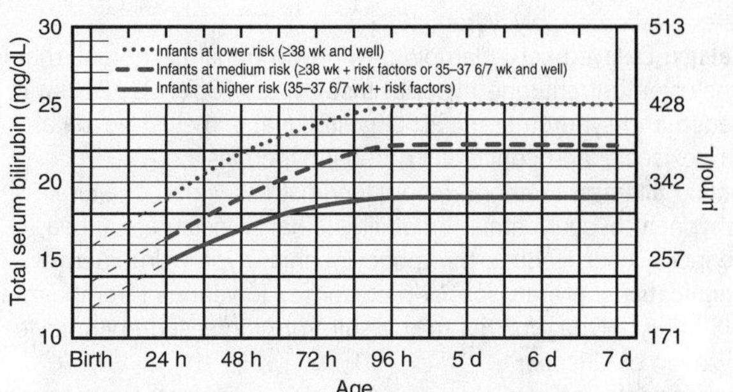

- The dashed lines for the first 24 hours indicate uncertainty due to a wide range of clinical circumstances and a range of responses to phototherapy.
- Immediate exchange transfusion is recommended if infant shows signs of acute bilirubin encephalopathy (hypertonia, arching, retrocollis, opisthotonos, fever, high-pitched cry) or if TBS is ≥5 mg/dL (85 μmol/L) above these lines.
- Risk factors: Isoimmune hemolytic disease, G6PD deficiency, asphyxia, significant lethargy, temperature instability, sepsis, acidosis.
- Measure serum albumin and calculate B/A ratio (see legend).
- Use total bilirubin. Do not subtract direct reacting or conjugated bilirubin.
- If infant is well and 35–37 6/7 wk (median risk) can individualize TSB levels for exchange based on actual gestational age.

FIGURE 18-6

Guidelines for exchange transfusion in infants born at 35 weeks' gestation or more.

NOTE: Complete blood count (CBC), reticulocyte count, peripheral smear, bilirubin, Ca^{2+}, glucose, total protein, infant blood type, Coombs test, and newborn screen should be performed on a pre-exchange sample of blood because they are of no diagnostic value on post-exchange blood. If indicated, save pre-exchange blood for serologic or chromosome studies.

B. Conjugated Hyperbilirubinemia

1. **Definition:** Direct bilirubin >2.0 mg/dL and >10% of the total serum bilirubin
2. **Etiology:** Biliary obstruction/atresia, choledochal cyst, hyperalimentation, α_1-antitrypsin deficiency, hepatitis, sepsis, infections (especially urinary tract infections), hypothyroidism, inborn errors of metabolism, cystic fibrosis, red blood cell abnormalities
3. **Management:** Phenobarbital for infants not on full feeds, ursodiol for infants on full feeds. Consider supplementation with fat-soluble vitamins—ADEK

C. Polycythemia

1. **Definition:** Venous hematocrit >65% confirmed on two consecutive samples. May be falsely elevated when sample obtained by heel stick.

Arterial hematocrit samples may be lower and should not be used for the evaluation of polycythemia

2. **Etiology:** Delayed cord clamping; twin-twin transfusion; maternal-fetal transfusion; intrauterine hypoxia; trisomy 13, 18, or 21; Beckwith-Wiedemann syndrome; maternal gestational diabetes; neonatal thyrotoxicosis; and congenital adrenal hyperplasia
3. **Clinical findings:** Plethora, respiratory distress, cardiac failure, tachypnea, hypoglycemia, irritability, lethargy, seizures, apnea, jitteriness, poor feeding, thrombocytopenia, hyperbilirubinemia
4. **Complications:** Hyperviscosity predisposes to venous thrombosis and CNS injury. Hypoglycemia may result from increased erythrocyte utilization of glucose
5. **Management:** Partial exchange transfusion for symptomatic infants with isovolemic replacement of blood with isotonic fluid. Blood is exchanged in 10- to 20-mL increments to reduce hematocrit to <55. (See Chapter 14 to calculate the amount of blood to be exchanged. Use birth weight (kg) × 90 mL/kg for estimated blood volume in mL.)

XI. GASTROINTESTINAL DISEASES

A. Necrotizing Enterocolitis

1. **Definition:** Serious intestinal inflammation and injury thought to be secondary to bowel ischemia, immaturity, and infection
2. **Incidence:** More common in preterm (3%–4% of infants <2000 g) and African-American infants. Occurs principally in infants who have been fed
3. **Risk factors:** Prematurity, asphyxia, hypotension, polycythemia-hyperviscosity syndrome, umbilical vessel catheterization, exchange transfusion, bacterial and viral pathogens, enteral feeds, PDA, congestive heart failure, cyanotic heart disease, RDS, intrauterine cocaine exposure
4. **Clinical findings:** See Table EC 18-B on Expert Consult for staging
   a. Systemic: Temperature instability, apnea, bradycardia, metabolic acidosis, hypotension, disseminated intravascular coagulation
   b. Intestinal: Elevated pregavage residuals with abdominal distention, blood in stool, absent bowel sounds, and/or abdominal tenderness or mass. Elevated pregavage residuals in the absence of other clinical symptoms rarely raise suspicion of NEC
   c. Radiologic: Ileus, intestinal pneumatosis, portal vein gas, ascites, pneumoperitoneum
5. **Management:** Nothing by mouth, NG tube decompression, maintain adequate hydration and perfusion, antibiotics for 7–14 days, surgical consultation. Surgery is performed for signs of perforation or necrotic bowel

B. Bilious Emesis Differential

(See Table EC 18-C on Expert Consult and Chapter 12)

1. Mechanical: Annular pancreas, intestinal atresia/duplication/malrotation/obstruction (including adjacent organomegaly), meconium plug or ileus, Hirschsprung, imperforate anus
2. Functional (i.e., poor motility): NEC, electrolyte abnormalities, sepsis

NOTE: Must eliminate malrotation as an etiology because its complication (volvulus) is a surgical emergency.

C. Abdominal Wall Defects

Omphalocele and gastroschisis (See Table EC 18-D on Expert Consult)

XII. NEUROLOGIC DISEASES

A. Intraventricular Hemorrhage (IVH)

1. **Definition:** Intracranial hemorrhage usually arising in the germinal matrix and periventricular regions of the brain
2. **Incidence:**
   a. 30–40% of infants <1500 g; 50–60% of infants <1000 g
   b. Highest incidence in first 72 hours of life: 60% within 24 hours, 85% within 72 hours, <5% after 1 week of age
3. **Diagnosis and classification:** Ultrasonography. Grade is based on the maximum amount of hemorrhage seen by age 2 weeks
   a. Grade I: Hemorrhage in germinal matrix only
   b. Grade II: IVH without ventricular dilatation
   c. Grade III: IVH with ventricular dilatation (30%–45% incidence of motor and cognitive impairment)
   d. Grade IV: IVH with periventricular hemorrhagic infarct (60%–80% incidence of motor and cognitive impairment)
4. **Screening:** Indicated in infants <32 weeks' gestational age within the first week of life; repeat in the second week
5. **Prophylaxis:** Maintain acid-base balance and avoid fluctuations in blood pressure. Indomethacin is considered for IVH prophylaxis in some newborns (<28 weeks' gestation, birth weight <1250 g) and is most efficacious if given in the first 6 hours of life, but has not been shown to impact long-term outcome[9]
6. **Outcome:** Infants with grade III and IV hemorrhages have a higher incidence of neurodevelopmental disabilities and an increased risk for posthemorrhagic hydrocephalus

B. Periventricular Leukomalacia

1. **Definition and ultrasound findings:** Ischemic necrosis of periventricular white matter characterized by CNS depression within first week and ultrasound findings of cysts with or without ventricular enlargement caused by cerebral atrophy
2. **Incidence:** More common in preterm infants but also occurs in term infants; 3.2% in infants <1500 g
3. **Etiology:** Primarily ischemia-reperfusion injury, hypoxia, acidosis, hypoglycemia, acute hypotension, low cerebral blood flow

4. **Outcome:** Commonly associated with cerebral palsy with or without sensory and cognitive deficit

C. Neonatal Seizures (See Chapter 20)

D. Neonatal Abstinence Syndrome

Onset of symptoms usually occurs within the first 24–72 hours of life (methadone may delay symptoms until 96 hours or later). Symptoms may last weeks to months. Box 18-1 shows signs and symptoms of opiate withdrawal

E. Peripheral Nerve Injuries

1. **Etiology:** Result from lateral traction on the shoulder (vertex deliveries) or the head (breech deliveries)
2. **Clinical features (see Table 18-8)**
3. **Management:** Evaluate for associated trauma (clavicular and humeral fractures, shoulder dislocation, facial nerve injury, and cord injuries). Treatment includes immobilization for 7–10 days. Full recovery is seen in 85%–95% of cases in the first year of life

BOX 18-1

OPIATE WITHDRAWAL

Signs and Symptoms of Opiate Withdrawal	
W	Wakefulness
I	Irritability, insomnia
T	Tremors, temperature variation, tachypnea, twitching (jitteriness)
H	Hyperactivity, high-pitched cry, hiccoughs, hyperreflexia, hypertonia
D	Diarrhea (explosive), diaphoresis, disorganized suck
R	Rubmarks, respiratory distress, rhinorrhea, regurgitation
A	Apnea, autonomic dysfunction
W	Weight loss
A	Alkalosis (respiratory)
L	Lacrimation (photophobia), lethargy
S	Seizures, sneezing, stuffy nose, sweating, sucking (nonproductive)

TABLE 18-8

PLEXUS INJURIES

Plexus Injury	Spinal Level Involved	Clinical Features
Erb-Duchenne palsy (90% of cases)	C5 to C6 Occasionally involves C4	Adduction and internal rotation of the arm. Forearm is pronated. Wrist is flexed. Diaphragm paralysis may occur if C4 is involved
Total palsy (8%–9% of cases)	C5 to T1 Occasionally involves C4	Upper arm, lower arm, and hand are involved. Horner syndrome (ptosis, anhydrosis, and miosis) exists if T1 is involved
Klumpke paralysis (<2% of cases)	C7 to T1	Hand flaccid with little control. Horner syndrome if T1 is involved

XIII. RETINOPATHY OF PREMATURITY (ROP)[10]

A. Definition

Interruption of the normal progression of retinal vascularization.

B. Etiology

Exposure of the immature retina to high oxygen concentrations can result in vasoconstriction and obliteration of the retinal capillary network, followed by vasoproliferation. Risk is greatest in the most immature infant.

C. Diagnosis—Dilated Funduscopic Exam

Dilated funduscopic exam should be performed in the following patients: (See Table 18-9 for timing)

1. All infants born ≤32 weeks gestational age
2. Infants born >32 weeks gestational age with unstable clinical course, including those requiring cardiorespiratory support
3. Any infant born weighing 1500–2000 grams

D. Classification

1. **Stage:**
   - a. Stage 1: Demarcation line separates avascular from vascularized retina
   - b. Stage 2: Ridge forms along demarcation line
   - c. Stage 3: Extraretinal fibrovascular proliferation tissue forms on ridge
   - d. Stage 4: Partial retinal detachment
   - e. Stage 5: Total retinal detachment
2. **Zone** (Fig. 18-7)
3. **Plus disease:** Increased venous dilatation and arteriolar tortuosity of the posterior retinal vessels; may be present at any stage
4. Number of clock hours or 30-degree sectors involved

TABLE 18-9

TIMING OF FIRST RETINAL EXAMINATION BASED ON GESTATIONAL AGE AT BIRTH

Gestational Age at Birth (wk)	Recommended Age for Initial Exam—Postmenstrual Age (wk)
≤27	31
28	32
29	33
30	34
31	35
32	36

Modified from American Academy of Pediatrics: Screening examination of premature infants for retinopathy of prematurity, AAP Policy statement. Pediatrics 2006;117(2):572–576.

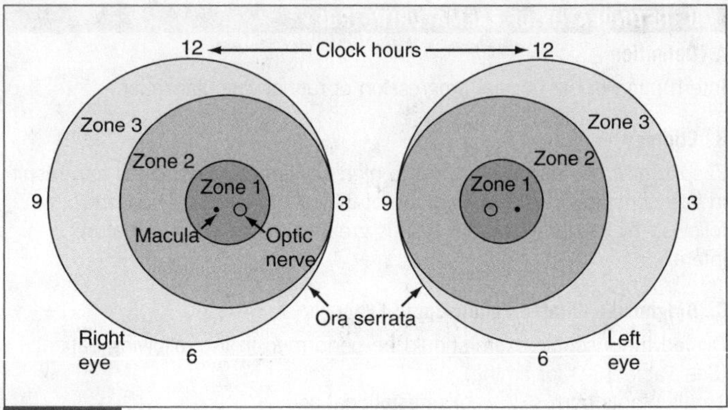

FIGURE 18-7

Zones of the retina. *(From American Academy of Pediatrics: Screening examination of premature infants for retinopathy of prematurity, AAP Policy Statement. Pediatrics 2006;117(2):572–576.)*

TABLE 18-10

SUGGESTED SCHEDULE FOR FOLLOW-UP OPHTHALMOLOGIC EXAM IN RETINOPATHY OF PREMATURITY

≤1 Week	1–2 Weeks	2 Weeks	2–3 Weeks
Stage 1 or 2 ROP: zone I	Immature vascularization: zone I, no ROP	Stage 1 ROP: zone II	Immature vascularization: zone II, no ROP
Stage 3 ROP: zone II	Stage 2 ROP: zone II Regressing ROP: zone I	Regressing ROP: zone II	Stage 1 or 2 ROP: zone III Regressing ROP: zone III

NOTE: The presence of plus disease in Zone I or II indicates that peripheral ablation, rather than observation, is appropriate.

From American Academy of Pediatrics: Screening examination of premature infants for retinopathy of prematurity, AAP Policy statement: Pediatrics 2006;117(2):572–576.

E. Management[10]

1. **Type 1 ROP:** Peripheral retinal ablation should be considered. Type 1 ROP classified as:
   a. Zone I, any stage ROP with plus disease
   b. Zone I, stage 3 ROP with or without plus disease
   c. Zone II, stage 2 or 3 ROP with plus disease
2. **Type 2 ROP:** Serial examinations instead of retinal ablation should be considered. Type 2 ROP classified as:
   a. Zone I, stage 1 or 2 ROP without plus disease
   b. Zone II, stage 3 ROP without plus disease
3. **Follow-up** (Table 18-10)

XIV. CONGENITAL INFECTIONS

See Chapter 17

XV. COMMONLY USED MEDICATIONS IN THE NEONATAL INTENSIVE CARE UNIT (NICU) (SEE EXPERT CONSULT, CHAPTER 18, FOR TEXT AND RELATED TABLE 30-10 IN THE FORMULARY ADJUNCT FOR ANTIBIOTIC DOSING IN NEONATES) (HTTP://NEOFAX.THOMSONHC.COM/NEOFAX/INDEX.PHP)

REFERENCES

1. Wiswell TE, Gannon CM, Jacob J, et al. Delivery room management of the apparently vigorous meconium-stained neonate: results of the multicenter, international collaborative trial. *Pediatrics*. 2000;105:1–7.
2. Apgar V. A proposal for new method of evaluation of the newborn infant. *Anesth Analg*. 1953;32:260–267.
3. Ballard JL, Khoury JC, Wedig K, et al. New Ballard Score, expanded to include extremely premature infants. *J Pediatr*. 1991;119:417–423.
4. Cornblath M. Neonatal hypoglycemia. In Donn SM, Fisher CW, eds. *Risk management techniques in perinatal and neonatal practice*. Armonk, NY: Futura; 1996.
5. American Academy of Pediatrics. Clinical practice guideline. *Pediatrics*. 2004;114:297–316.
6. Klaus MH, Fanaroff AA. *Care of the high-risk neonate*, 5th ed. Philadelphia: WB Saunders; 2001.
7. Ohlsson A, Walia R, Shah SS. Ibuprofen for the treatment of PDA in preterm and/or LBW infants. Cochrane Database of Systematic Reviews 2008. Issue 1. Art. No.: CD003481. DOI: 10. 1002/14651858. CD003481.pub3.
8. American Academy of Pediatrics: Subcommittee on Hyperbilirubinemia: Management of hyperbilirubinemia in the newborn infant 35 or more weeks of gestation. *Pediatrics*. 2004;114(1):297–316. Erratum in Pediatrics 2004;114(4):1138.
9. Schmidt B, Davis P, Moddemann D, et al. Long-term effects of indomethacin prophylaxis in ELBW infants. *N Engl J Med*. 2001;344:1966–1972.
10. Good WV. Early Treatment for Retinopathy of Prematurity Cooperative Group. *Arch Ophthalmol*. 2003;121:1684–1694.

Chapter 19

Nephrology

Stacy Cooper, MD

I. WEBSITE

The International Pediatric Hypertension Association: www.pediatrichypertension.org

II. URINALYSIS (UA), URINE DIPSTICK

Best if urine specimen is evaluated within 1 hour after voiding, ideally after the first morning void. Annual screening UAs are no longer recommended by the AAP.

A. Color

Normal urine: Varies in color from almost colorless to amber. In the brick-dust phenomenon, urine appears red or dark due to precipitation of urates.

B. Turbidity

Cloudy urine: Can be normal; is most often the result of crystal formation at room temperature. Uric acid crystals form in acidic urine, and phosphate crystals form in alkaline urine. Cellular material and bacteria can also cause turbidity.

C. Specific Gravity

1. Normal findings: Between 1.003 and 1.030
2. Based on the principle that the refractive index (RI) of a solution is related to the content of dissolved solids. RI varies with, but is not identical to, specific gravity. Glucose, abundant protein, and iodine-containing contrast materials can give falsely high readings. Isosthenuria, the inability to dilute or concentrate urine, will present with a fixed specific gravity of 1.010

D. pH

Estimated using indicator paper or dipstick. To improve accuracy, use a freshly voided specimen and pH meter. Normal pH ranges from 5–8. Levels can be inappropriately high with hypokalemia.

E. Protein

See Section VII.B and related figures.

1. Normal values in a 24-hour urine collection: <4 mg of protein/m^2/hr; significant: 4–40 mg/m^2/hr; nephrotic range: >40 mg/m^2/hr[1]
2. Assess completeness of 24-hour collection by simultaneously measuring urine creatinine: ≥15 mg/kg body weight in a 24-hour collection

F. Sugars

1. Normal urine: Does not contain sugars. Glucosuria is suggestive, but not diagnostic of diabetes mellitus or proximal renal tubular disease (see Section V.B). The presence of other reducing sugars can be confirmed by chromatography
2. Dipstick: Easiest method, but only detects glucose. False-negative results occur with high levels of ascorbic acid (used as preservative in antibiotics) in urine
3. Clinitest tablet (Ames Co.): Nonspecific test; changes color if urine is positive for reducing substances, including reducing sugars (glucose, fructose, galactose, pentoses, lactose), which raises concern for metabolic defects such as galactosemia or fructosemia, but also positive with amino acids, ascorbic acid, chloral hydrate, chloramphenicol, creatinine, cysteine, glucuronates, hippurate, homogentisic acid, isoniazid, acetoacetic acid, acetone, nitrofurantoin, oxalate, total parenteral nutrition, penicillin, salicylates, streptomycin, sulfonamides, tetracycline, and uric acid

G. Ketones

1. Ketouria: Except for trace amounts, ketonuria suggests ketoacidosis, usually from diabetes mellitus or catabolism induced by inadequate intake. Neonatal ketoacidosis may occur with a metabolic defect, such as propionic acidemia, methylmalonic aciduria, or a glycogen storage disease
2. Dipstick: Detects acetoacetic acid best, acetone less well; does not detect β-hydroxybutyrate. False-positive results may occur after phthalein administration or with phenylketonuria
3. Acetest tablet (Ames Co.): Detects only acetoacetic acid and acetone

H. Hemoglobin, Myoglobin

Dipstick reads positive with intact red blood cells (as few as 3–4 red blood cells [RBCs]/high-power field [hpf]), hemoglobin, and myoglobin. False-positive results can occur with the presence of bacterial peroxidases, high ascorbic acid concentrations, and povidone-iodine (Betadine).

I. Bilirubin, Urobilinogen (See Table 19-1)

Dipstick measures each individually.

1. Urine bilirubin: Positive with conjugated hyperbilirubinemia; in this form, bilirubin is water soluble and excreted by the kidney
2. Urobilinogen: Increased in cases of hyperbilirubinemia in which there is no obstruction to enterohepatic circulation

III. URINALYSIS, MICROSCOPY

A. RBCs

1. Normal values: Centrifuged urine usually contains <5 RBCs/hpf. Significant hematuria is 5–10 RBCs/hpf and corresponds to a

TABLE 19-1

URINALYSIS FOR BILIRUBIN/UROBILINOGEN

	Normal	Hemolytic Disease	Hepatic Disease	Biliary Obstruction
Urine urobilinogen	Normal	Increased	Increased	Decreased
Urine bilirubin	Negative	Negative	±	Positive

Chemstrip reading of 50 RBCs/hpf or Labstix reading *trace hemolyzed* or *small*. Microscopy is used to differentiate the presence of hemoglobinuria/myoglobinuria from intact RBCs. Examination of RBC morphology may help to localize source of bleeding, as dysmorphic, small RBCs suggest a glomerular origin, whereas normal RBCs suggest lower tract bleeding

2. Differentiation between hemoglobinuria and myoglobinuria:
   a. Hemoglobinuria is seen with intravascular hemolysis or in hematuric urine that has been standing for extended period
   b. Myoglobinuria is seen in crush injuries, vigorous exercise, major motor seizures, fever, malignant hyperthermia, electrocution, snake bites, ischemia, some muscle and metabolic disorders, and some infections (e.g., influenza)
   c. Clinical laboratories may be able to measure hemoglobin or myoglobin directly
   d. Additionally, in myoglobinuria, the blood urea nitrogen (BUN)/creatinine (Cr) ratio is often low (Cr is released from damaged muscles), and the creatine kinase level is high
3. Suggested evaluation of persistent hematuria: See Section VII.A and related figures

B. Sediment

Using light microscopy, unstained, centrifuged urine can be examined for formed elements, including casts, cells, and crystals.

C. Epithelial Cells

Squamous epithelial cells (>10 per low-power field) are useful as an index of possible contamination by vaginal secretions in females or by foreskin in uncircumcised males.

D. White Blood Cells (WBCs)

>5 WBCs/hpf of properly spun urine specimen is suggestive of a urinary tract infection (UTI). Sterile pyuria is rare in the pediatric population. If present, it is usually transient and accompanies systemic disorder (e.g., Kawasaki disease) or urolithiasis.

E. Urine Gram Stain

Gram stain is used to screen for UTIs. One organism per high-power field in uncentrifuged urine represents at least 10^5 colonies/mL.

IV. EVALUATION AND MANAGEMENT OF UTIS

NOTE: These recommendations are suggestions and vary from institution to institution and physician to physician. Use them together with the routinely practiced guidelines of your institution. At time of publication new UTI management guidelines are currently under consideration. Please see the American Academy of Pediatrics website for the most current recommendations.

American Academy of Pediatrics (AAP) recommendations[1]:

(1) UTI should be considered in those under 2 years with fever
(2) If a child 2 months to 2 years with unexplained fever is sufficiently ill to warrant immediate antibiotics, urine should be obtained by transurethral catheterization
(3) If a child 2 months to 2 years with unexplained fever is not so ill as to require immediate antibiotics, two options exist:
  (a) Obtain urine culture by catheterization
  (b) Obtain urine for urinalysis by most convenient method. If urinalysis suggests UTI, obtain urine culture by catheterization. If urinalysis does not suggest UTI, it is reasonable to follow clinical course without antimicrobial therapy, recognizing that a negative urinalysis does not rule out UTI
(4) Diagnosis of a UTI requires a culture of the urine

A. History

Voiding history (stool, urine), stream characteristics in toilet-trained children, sexual intercourse, sexual abuse, circumcision, masturbation, pinworms, prolonged baths, bubble baths, evaluation of growth curve, recent antibiotic use, and family history of vesicoureteral reflux (VUR), recurrent UTIs, or chronic kidney disease.

B. Physical Examination

Vital signs, especially blood pressure, abdominal examination for flank masses, bowel distention, evidence of impaction; meatal stenosis or circumcision in males; vulvovaginitis or labial adhesions in females; neurologic examination of lower extremities; perineal sensation and reflexes; rectal and sacral examination (for anteriorly placed anus).

C. Laboratory Studies

1. Urinalysis with microscopic examination and urine culture (Table 19-2).

a. Nitrite test: Detects nitrites produced by the reduction of dietary nitrates by urinary gram-negative bacteria (especially *Escherichia coli, Klebsiella,* and *Proteus*). A positive test is virtually diagnostic of UTI. False-negative results can occur with inadequate dietary nitrates, insufficient time for bacterial proliferation, inability of bacteria to reduce nitrates to nitrites (many gram-positive organisms such as *Enterococcus, Mycobacterium* spp. and fungi), and large volumes of dilute urine

TABLE 19-2

URINALYSIS WITH MICROSCOPIC EXAMINATION AND URINE CULTURE

Method of Collection	Colony Count (Pure Culture)	Probability of Infection (%)
Suprapubic aspiration	Gram-negative bacilli: Any number Gram-positive cocci: More than a few thousand	>99
Transurethral catheterization	>100,000	95
	10,000–100,000	Infection likely
	1,000–10,000	Suspicious; repeat
	<1,000	Infection unlikely
Clean-voided (boy)	>10,000	Infection likely
Clean-voided (girl)	3 specimens >100,000	95
	2 specimens >100,000	90
	1 specimen >100,000	80
	50,000–100,000	Suspicious; repeat
	10,000–50,000	Symptomatic, suspicious; repeat
	10,000–50,000	Asymptomatic; infection unlikely
	<10,000	Infection unlikely

b. Leukocyte esterase test: Detects esterases released from broken-down leukocytes, an indirect test for WBCs that may or may not be present with a UTI

2. BUN/Cr ratio

D. Culture-Positive UTI

Treatment: Based on urine culture and sensitivities if possible; for empiric therapy, see Chapter 17.

1. Upper versus lower UTI: Differentiating pyelonephritis (upper UTI) from cystitis (lower UTI) is a clinical diagnosis suggested by the presence of fever, systemic symptoms, and costovertebral angle tenderness. Fever that persists for >48 hours after initiating appropriate antibiotics is also suggestive of pyelonephritis. Although a ^{99m}Tc-dimercaptosuccinic acid (DMSA) scan is the *gold standard* to diagnose pyelonephritis, infants with febrile UTI are assumed to have pyelonephritis and are treated as such
2. Organisms: 75%–90% of pediatric UTIs are caused by *E. coli*. Other common pathogens include *Klebsiella, Proteus* spp., *Staphylococcus saprophyticus,* and *S. aureus*. Group B streptococci and other blood-borne pathogens are important in neonatal UTIs, whereas enterococcus and *Pseudomonas* are more prevalent in abnormal hosts (i.e., recurrent UTI, abnormal anatomy, neurogenic bladder, hospitalized patients, or those with frequent catheterizations)

3. Treatment considerations:
a. Hospitalize all febrile children <4 weeks of age and treat with intravenous (IV) antibiotics due to risk for bacteremia and meningitis
b. AAP recommends parenteral antibiotics for children who are toxic, dehydrated, or unable to tolerate oral medication due to vomiting or noncompliance. Studies comparing duration are inconclusive, but experts traditionally recommend 7–10 days for uncomplicated cases and 14 days for toxic children and those with pyelonephritis. Some recent studies have shown that 2–4 days of oral antibiotics in uncomplicated lower tract UTIs are as effective as 7–10 days of oral treatment[2]
4. Inadequate response to therapy: Repeat urine culture in children with expected response is controversial, but generally thought to be unnecessary. A repeat culture, as well as renal ultrasound to rule out abscess or obstruction, is indicated in children with poor response to therapy. Repeat cultures should also be considered in patients with recurrent UTIs to rule out persistent bacteriuria
5. **Imaging studies (Fig. 19-1):**
a. Abdominal radiograph: If indicated to evaluate stool pattern and for spinal dysraphism
b. Dimercaptosuccinic acid (DMSA): ^{99m}Tc-DMSA scan can detect areas of decreased uptake that may represent acute pyelonephritis or chronic renal scarring; does not differentiate between the two. Routine use not recommended; may be indicated in patients with an abnormal VCUG or renal sonography, in patients with history of asymptomatic bacteriuria and fever or prenatally diagnosed VUR, and in neonates and infants secondary to high incidence of hematologic spread and difficult examination. Repeat in 3–6 months if initial study is positive to evaluate for persistent infection and renal scarring
c. Diethylene triamine pentaacetic acid (DTPA)/Mercaptoacetyl triglycine (MAG-3): May also be used for indications given for DMSA use. Provides quantitative assessment of renal function and drainage of dilated collecting system, as in cases of hydronephrosis in the absence of VUR or ureteropelvic junction obstruction
d. Anatomic Evaluation: Traditionally done to rule out obstructive disease or VUR in all male patients with their first UTI, all female patients <5 years old, and all children with recurrent UTI. Currently studies are ongoing to determine the most appropriate candidates for such screening, therefore please consult the AAP website for up to date recommendations
   (1) Renal sonography: To evaluate for gross structural defects, obstructive lesions, positional abnormalities, and renal size and growth
   (2) VCUG: Performed when asymptomatic and cleared of bacteriuria. May be substituted with RNC, which has 1/100 the radiation exposure of VCUG and increased sensitivity for transient reflux.

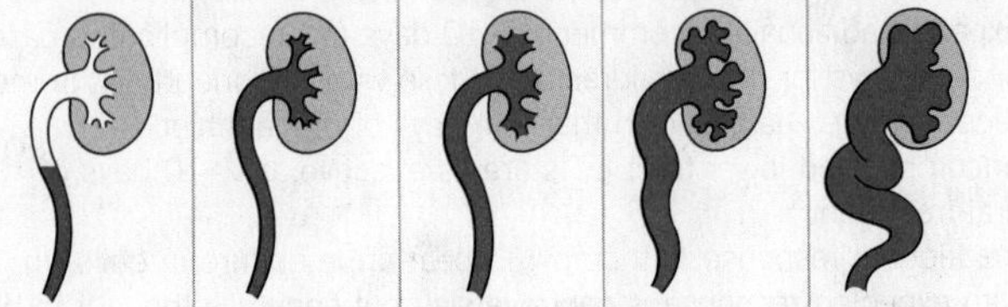

Grade I	Grade II	Grade III	Grade IV	Grade V
Ureter only	Ureter, pelvis, calyces; no dilatation, normal calyceal fornices	Mild or moderate dilatation and/or tortuosity of ureter; mild or moderate dilatation of the pelvis, but no or slight blunting of the fornices	Moderate dilatation and/or tortuosity of the ureter; mild dilatation of renal pelvis and calyces; complete obliteration of sharp angle of fornices, but maintenance of papillary impressions in majority of calyces	Gross dilatation and tortuosity of ureter; gross dilatation of renal pelvis and calyces; papillary impressions are no longer visible in majority of calyces

FIGURE 19-1

International classification of vesicoureteral reflux. *(Modified from Rushton H: Urinary tract infections in children: Epidemiology, evaluation, and management. Pediatr Clin North Am 1997:44:5 and International Reflux Committee: Medical vs. surgical treatment of primary vesicoureteral reflux: report of the International Reflux Study Committee. Pediatrics 1981;67:392.)*

RNC does not visualize urethral anatomy, is not sensitive for low-grade reflux, and cannot grade reflux

(3) Renal ultrasound and VCUG should be done at the earliest convenient time, unless the child fails to demonstrate expected clinical response, which should prompt a renal ultrasound for further evaluation.

6. Antibiotic prophylaxis (Table 19-3): Conventionally, low-dose antibiotic prophylaxis has been recommended in all children with diagnosed VUR and obstructive disease. Prophylaxis in children with recurrent infections, but normal anatomy is controversial and is based on individualized decisions. New data are emerging that calls into question the efficacy of antibiotic prophylaxis, and further studies will be needed to further determine their role[3]

TABLE 19-3

ANTIBIOTIC PROPHYLAXIS FOR VESICOURETERAL REFLUX (VUR)*

Grade	Age (yr)	Scarring	Initial Treatment	Follow-up Treatment Considerations for Refractory Disease
I–II	Any	Yes/no	Antibiotic prophylaxis	No consensus
III–IV	0–5	Yes/no	Antibiotic prophylaxis	Surgery
III–IV	6–10	Yes/no	Unilateral: Antibiotic prophylaxis Bilateral: Surgery	Surgery
V	<1	Yes/no	Antibiotic prophylaxis	Surgery
V	1–5	No	Unilateral: Antibiotic prophylaxis Bilateral: Surgery	Surgery
V	1–5	Yes	Surgery	
V	6–10	Yes/no	Surgery	

***NOTE:** At press time, studies are being conducted to more definitely answer the question of who needs UTI prophylaxis. Refer to the literature for the most recent recommendations.

7. Conventional management of VUR[4]: Prophylaxis with amoxicillin, trimethoprim-sulfamethoxazole or nitrofurantoin for any level of VUR, with surgical correction is indicated in children >2 years of age with high-grade reflux (grades IV or V) and children with breakthrough pyelonephritis (especially with DMSA changes) while on prophylaxis. As above, the consensus on antibiotic prophylaxis is currently evolving, and further research is needed into the effects of renal scarring as well as the efficacy of prophylaxis on the development of renal disease[5–7]
8. Asymptomatic bacteriuria: Defined as bacteria in urine on microscopy and Gram stain in an afebrile, asymptomatic patient without pyuria. Antibiotics not necessary if voiding habits and urinary tract are normal. Prophylaxis may be necessary in patients with bacteriuria and voiding dysfunction. DMSA may be helpful in differentiating pyelonephritis from fever and coincidental bacteriuria
9. Referral to pediatric urology: Consider in children with abnormal voiding function on imaging, neurogenic bladder, abnormal anatomy, recurrent UTI, or poor response to appropriate antibiotics

V. RENAL FUNCTION TESTS

A. Tests of Glomerular Function

1. **Creatinine clearance (Ccr):**

a. Timed urine specimen: Standard measure of glomerular filtration rate (GFR); closely approximates inulin clearance in the normal range of GFR. When GFR is low, Ccr is greater than inulin clearance. Usually inaccurate in children with obstructive uropathy or problems with bladder emptying

$$Ccr\ (mL/min/1.73\ m^2) = (U \times [V/P]) \times 1.73/BSA$$

19

where U (mg/dL) = urinary creatinine concentration; V (mL/min) = total urine volume (mL) divided by the duration of the collection (min) (24 hours = 1440 min); P (mg/dL) = serum creatinine concentration (may average two levels) and BSA (m^2) = body surface area

b. Estimated GFR from plasma creatinine: Useful when a timed specimen cannot be collected; reasonable estimate of GFR for children with relatively normal renal function and body habitus, although does tend to overestimate GFR. If habitus is markedly abnormal or precise measurement of GFR is needed, more standard methods of measuring GFR must be used

$$\text{Estimated GFR (mL/min/1.73 m}^2\text{)} = kL/Pcr$$

where k = proportionality constant; L = height (cm); Pcr = plasma creatinine (mg/dL) (Table 19-4)

2. **Glomerular function as determined by nuclear medicine scans:** Normal values of GFR (measured by inulin clearance) are shown in Table 19-5

TABLE 19-4

PROPORTIONALITY CONSTANT FOR CALCULATING GLOMERULAR FILTRATION RATE

Age	*k* Values
Low birth weight during first year of life	0.33
Term AGA during first year of life	0.45
Children and adolescent girls	0.55
Adolescent boys	0.70

AGA, Appropriate for gestational age.

From Schwartz GJ, Brion LP, Spitzer A: The use of plasma creatinine concentration for estimating glomerular filtration rate in infants, children, and adolescents. Pediatr Clin North Am 1987;34:571.

TABLE 19-5

NORMAL VALUES OF GLOMERULAR FILTRATION RATE

Age	GFR (Mean) (mL/min/1.73 m^2)	Range (mL/min/1.73 m^2)
Neonates <34 wk gestational age		
2–8 days	11	11–15
4–28 days	20	15–28
30–90 days	50	40–65
Neonates >34 wk gestational age		
2–8 days	39	17–60
4–28 days	47	26–68
30–90 days	58	30–86
1–6 mo	77	39–114
6–12 mo	103	49–157
12–19 mo	127	62–191
2 yr–adult	127	89–165

From Holliday MA, Barratt TM: Pediatric nephrology. Baltimore, Williams & Wilkins, 1994, p. 1306.

B. Tests of Tubular Function

1. **Proximal tubule:**

a. Proximal tubule reabsorption: Proximal tubule is responsible for reabsorption of electrolytes, glucose, and amino acids. Studies to determine proximal tubular function compare urine and blood levels of specific compounds, arriving at a percentage of tubular reabsorption (Tx):

$$Tx = 1 - [(Ux/Px)/(Ucr/Pcr)] \times 100\%$$

where Ux = concentration of compound in urine; Px = concentration of compound in plasma; Ucr = concentration of creatinine in urine; Pcr = concentration of creatinine in plasma. This formula can be used for amino acids, electrolytes, calcium, and phosphorus

b. Calculation of fractional excretion of sodium (FENa) is derived from the previous equation:

$$FENa = [(UNa/PNa)/(UCr/PCr)] \times 100\%$$

FENa is usually <1% in prerenal azotemia or glomerulonephritis and >1% (usually >3%) in acute tubular necrosis (ATN) or postrenal azotemia. Recent diuretic use may give inaccurate results

c. Glucose reabsorption: Glucose threshold is plasma glucose concentration at which significant amounts of glucose appear in urine. Glucosuria must be interpreted in relation to simultaneously determined plasma glucose concentration. If plasma glucose concentration is <120 mg/dL, and glucose is present in urine, this implies incompetent tubular reabsorption of glucose and proximal renal tubular disease

d. Bicarbonate reabsorption: Majority occurs in proximal tubule. Abnormalities in reabsorption lead to type 2 renal tubular acidosis (RTA; see Table 19-6)

2. **Distal tubule:**

a. Urine acidification: A urine acidification defect (distal RTA) should be suspected when random urine pH values are >6 in the presence of moderate systemic metabolic acidosis. Confirm acidification defects by simultaneous venous or arterial pH, plasma bicarbonate concentration, and pH meter (not dipstick) determination of the pH of fresh urine

b. Urine concentration occurs in the distal tubule: A random urine specific gravity of ≥1.023 indicates intact concentrating ability within limits of clinical testing; no further tests are indicated. A first-voided specimen after an overnight fast is adequate to test concentrating ability. (For more formal testing, see the water deprivation test in Chapter 10.)

c. Urine calcium: Hypercalciuria is seen usually with distal RTA, vitamin D intoxication, hyperparathyroidism, immobilization, excessive calcium intake, use of steroids or loop diuretics or idiopathic (associated with hematuria and renal calculi). Diagnosis is as follows:

TABLE 19-6

BIOCHEMICAL AND CLINICAL CHARACTERISTICS OF THE VARIOUS TYPES OF RENAL TUBULAR ACIDOSIS

	Type 1	Type 2	Type 4
Etiology	Hereditary Sickle cell Toxins/Drugs Cirrhosis Obstructive uropathy Connective tissue disorder	Hereditary Metabolic disease Fanconi Syndrome Prematurity Toxins/Heavy Metals Amyloidosis PNH	Absolute mineralcorticoid deficiency Adrenal failure CAH DM Pseudohypoaldo Interstitial nephritis
Minimal urine pH	>5.5	<5.5	<5.5
Urinary citrate excretion	↓	↑	?
Plasma K^+ concentration	Normal or ↓	Usually ↓	↑
Urine anion gap†	Positive	Positive or negative	Positive
Nephrocalcinosis/ Nephrolithiasis	Common	Rare	Rare
Treatment	1–3 mEq/kg/day of HCO_3 (5–10 mEq/kg/day if bicarb wasting)	5–20 mEq/kg/day of HCO_3	1–5 mEq/kg/day of HCO_3 May add Fludrocortisone and potassium binders

†Urine anion gap = $[Na^+] + [K^+] - [Cl^-]$ (based on urine electrolytes).

CAH, Congenital adrenal hypoplasia; DM, diabetes mellitus; pseudohypoaldo, pseudohypoaldosteronism.

From Holliday MA et al: Pediatric Nephrology. Baltimore, Williams & Wilkins, 1994, p. 650.

TABLE 19-7

AGE-ADJUSTED CALCIUM/CREATININE RATIOS

Age	Ca^{2+}/Cr Ratio (mg/mg) (95th Percentile for Age)
<7 mo	0.86
7–18 mo	0.60
19 mo–6 yr	0.42
Adults	0.22

Sargent JD, Stukel TA, Kresel J, et al: Normal values for random urinary calcium to creatinine ratios in infancy. J Pediatr 1993;123:393.

(1) 24-hour urine: Calcium >4 mg/kg/24 hr
(2) Spot urine: Determine calcium to creatinine (Ca/Cr) ratio. Follow up abnormally elevated spot urine Ca/Cr ratio with a 24-hr urine calcium determination (Table 19-7)[8]

VI. TUBULAR DISORDERS

A. Renal Tubular Acidosis (Table 19-6)[9]

A group of transport defects resulting in abnormal urine acidification, due to either the reabsorption of bicarbonate (HCO^-_3), the excretion of hydrogen ions (H^+), or both. Results in a persistent nonanion gap metabolic acidosis accompanied by hyperchloremia. The RTA syndromes often do not progress to renal failure but are instead characterized by a normal GFR. Clinical presentation is characterized by failure to thrive, polyuria, constipation, vomiting, and dehydration (see Table 19-6).

B. Type 3 (Combined Proximal and Distal) RTA

Infants with mild type 1 and mild type 2 defects were previously classified as type 3 RTA. Studies have shown that this is not a genetic entity itself, which has resulted in reclassification as a subtype of type 1 RTA that occurs primarily in premature infants.

C. Fanconi Syndrome

A generalized dysfunction of the proximal tubule resulting not only in bicarbonate loss, but also in variable wasting of phosphate, glucose, and amino acids. May be hereditary, as in cystinosis and galactosemia, or acquired through toxin injury and other immunologic factors. Clinically characterized by rickets and impaired growth.

VII. CLINICAL MANIFESTATIONS OF RENAL DISEASE

A. Hematuria[10]

1. Gross hematuria: Bright red blood, clots in urine, or tea-colored urine
2. Microscopic hematuria: >5 RBCs/hpf on more than two occasions
3. Significant or persistent hematuria: Three positive urinalyses, based on dipstick and microscopic examination, over a 2- to 3-week period
4. Etiology: Gross hematuria occurs with kidney stones, trauma, arteriovenous malformations, ATN, and renal vein thrombosis. Asymptomatic hematuria alone, without proteinuria, is often not indicative of significant kidney disease; however, a number of glomerular diseases, including immunoglobulin A (IgA) nephropathy and Alport nephritis, can present with recurrent gross hematuria
5. **Suggested evaluation of persistent hematuria** (Fig. 19-2):
   a. Examination of urine sediment, urine dipstick for protein, urine culture, sickle cell screen, urine Ca/Cr ratio, family history, medication history, and audiology screen if indicated
   b. Serum electrolytes, BUN, serum Cr, serum total protein and albumin, complete blood count (CBC) with smear, immunoglobulins, and hepatitis serologies; consider testing for HIV
   c. ASO titers, C3, C4, and antinuclear antibodies (ANAs)
   d. Renal ultrasonography and other indicated radiologic studies
6. **Management algorithm** (Fig. 19-3)

B. Proteinuria[11]

1. More likely than hematuria to indicate significant renal disease. Protein can be found in the urine of healthy children, with a reasonable upper limit being 150 mg/24 hr (4 mg/m^2/hr)
2. Detection: Commonly detected by dipstick with results of negative, trace, 1+ (~30 mg/dL), 2+ (~100 mg/dL), 3+ (~300 mg/dL), and

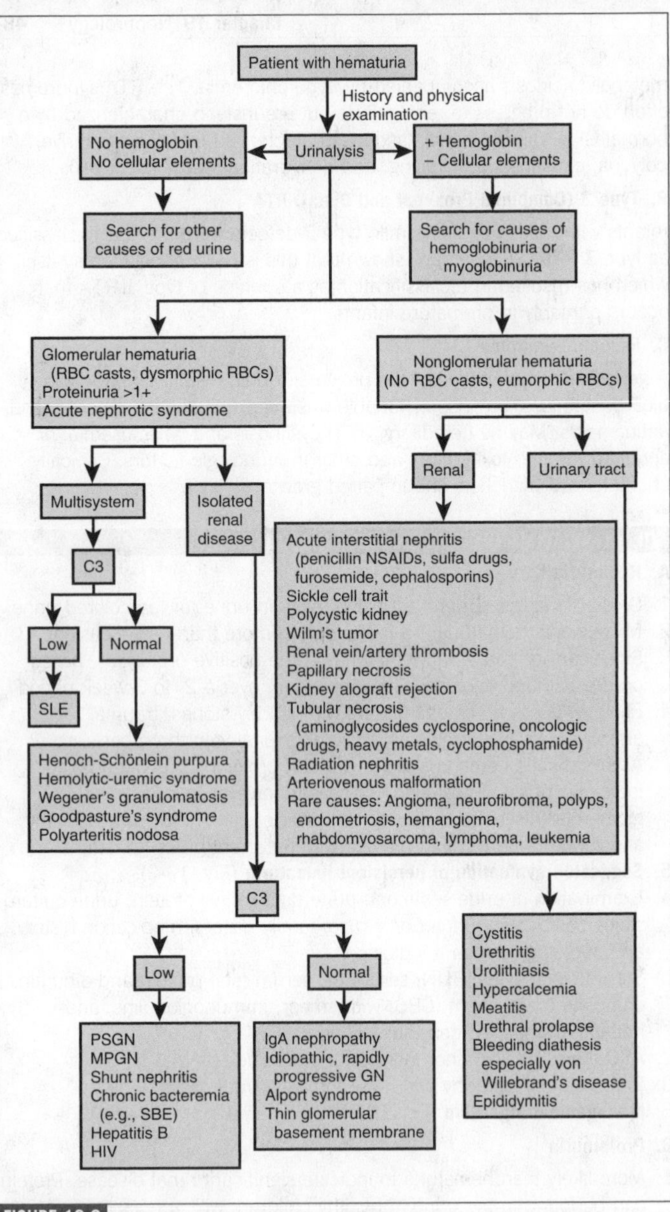

FIGURE 19-2

A diagnostic strategy for hematuria. GN, Glomerulonephritis; HIV, human immunodeficiency virus; MPGN, membranoproliferative glomerulonephritis; NSAIDs, nonsteroidal anti-inflammatory drugs; PSGN, poststreptococcal glomerulonephritis; RBC, red blood cell; SBE, subacute bacterial endocarditis; SLE, systemic lupus erythematosus.

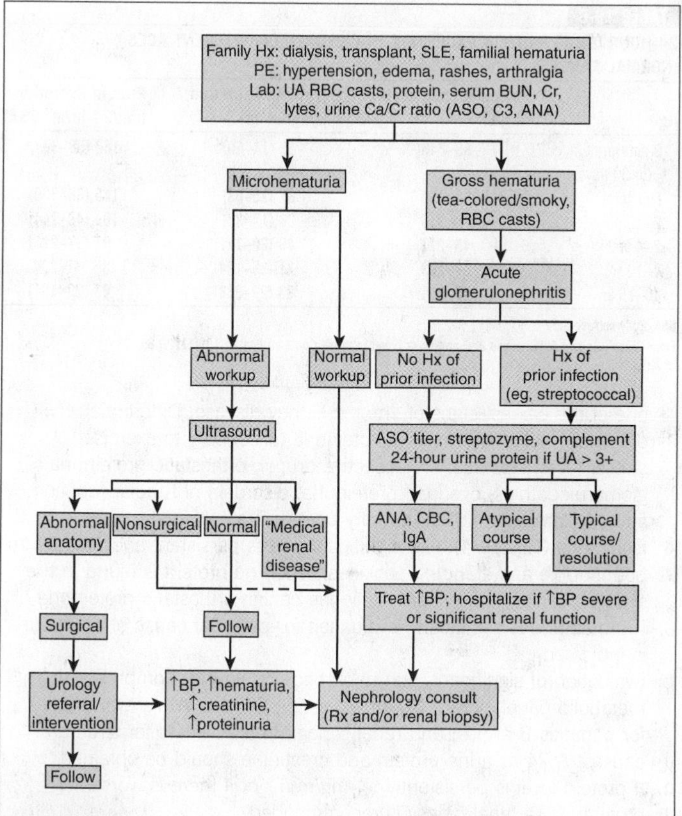

FIGURE 19-3

Management algorithm for hematuria. *(Data from Hay WW et al: Current pediatric diagnosis and treatment, 18th ed. Stamford, CT, Appleton & Lange, 2005, p. 709.)*

4+ (>2000 mg/dL). Dipstick is useful primarily for albuminuria; not an accurate measure of protein excretion. Persistent proteinuria should be precisely quantified by a timed 24-hr urine collection (Table 19-8). If unable to obtain, a timed urine excretion can be estimated by the ratio of urine protein to creatinine concentrations in a first morning voided specimen (or spot urine). Ratios (mg/mg) <0.5 in children <2 years and <0.2 in older children are normal. A ratio >2 suggests nephrotic range proteinuria

3. Etiology: Can be usefully differentiated into nephrotic versus non-nephrotic. Non-nephrotic proteinuria, generally <40 mg/m^2/hr in adults, is rarely associated with edema. Significant non-nephrotic proteinuria is

TABLE 19-8

24-HOUR URINE PROTEIN EXCRETION IN CHILDREN OF DIFFERENT AGES (NORMAL RANGES)

Age	Protein Concentration (mg/L)	Protein Excretion (mg/24 hr)	Protein Excretion (mg/24 hr/m² BSA)
Premature (5–30 days)	88–845	29 (14–60)	182 (88–377)
Full-term	94–455	32 (15–68)	145 (68–309)
2–12 mo	70–315	38 (17–85)	109 (48–244)
2–4 yr	45–217	49 (20–121)	91 (37–223)
4–10 yr	50–223	71 (26–194)	85 (31–234)
10–16 yr	45–391	83 (29–238)	63 (22–181)

BSA, Body surface area.

From Cruz C, Spitzer A: When you find protein or blood in urine. Contemp Pediatr 1998;15(9):89.

one of the earliest signs of chronic kidney disease. Differential diagnosis includes transient proteinuria (secondary to exercise, stress, fever, seizures, or vasoactive drugs), orthostatic proteinuria, glomerulopathies, overload proteinuria, disorders of tubular function, acute inflammation of the urinary tract, or uroepithelial tumors

4. **Evaluation (Fig. 19-4):** Not significant unless persistent and present in both supine and standing positions. When no protein is found in the supine position, the patient likely has benign orthostatic proteinuria
   a. If proteinuria is significant, evaluation for potential cause of proteinuria is indicated
   b. Evaluation of significant, non-nephrotic proteinuria: Comprehensive metabolic panel, serum Cr, albumin, C3, C4, and ANA; evaluation for hepatitis B and C; and renal sonogram to evaluate for structural causes. A 24-hr urine protein and creatinine should be obtained
   c. If protein level is persistently >4 mg/m²/hr or if there is worsening proteinuria, a renal biopsy is recommended

C. Edema

Secondary to excessive accumulation of both Na^+ and water. Causes of generalized edema include the following:

1. Inability to excrete Na^+ with or without water (e.g., glomerular diseases resulting in decreased GFR, excess salt intake)
2. Decreased oncotic pressure (e.g., nephrotic syndrome, protein-losing enteropathy, hepatic failure, congestive heart failure [CHF])
3. Reduced cardiac output (e.g., CHF, pericardial disease)
4. Mineralocorticoid excess (e.g., hyperreninemia, hyperaldosteronism)

D. Oliguria

Urine output <300 mL/m²/24 hr, or <0.5 mL/kg/hr in children and <1.0 mL/kg/hr in infants. May be a normal physiologic response to water with or without salt depletion (prerenal state) or a reflection of renal failure that is associated with azotemia.

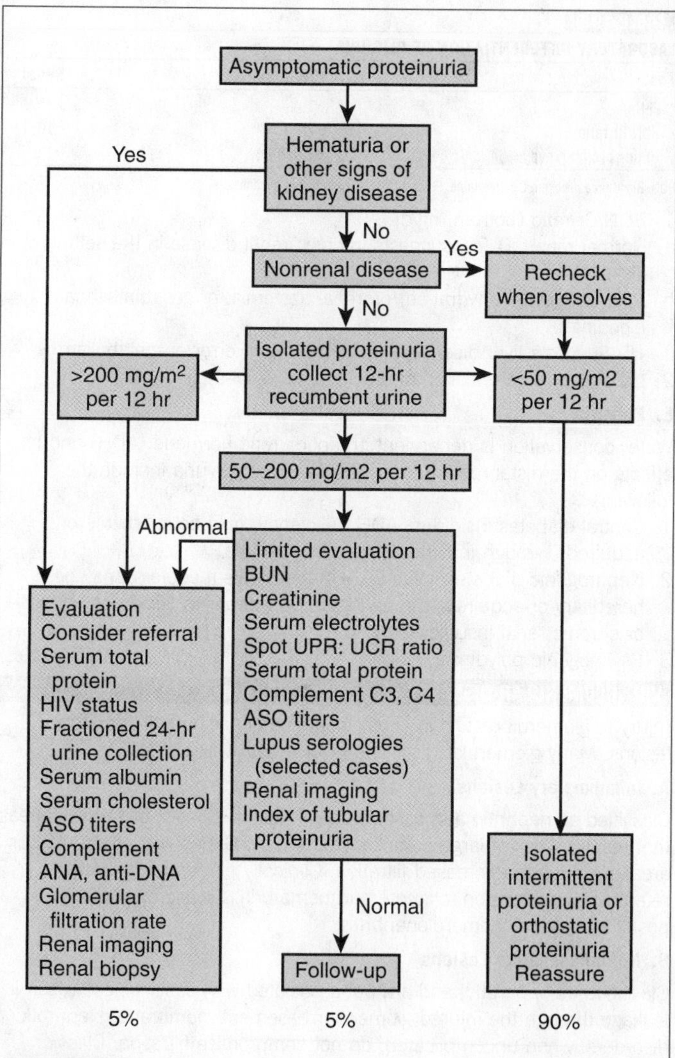

FIGURE 19-4

Suggested evaluation of proteinuria in asymptomatic patients. *(From Cruz C, Spitzer A: When you find protein or blood in the urine. Contemp Pediatr 1998;15[9]:89.)*

19

TABLE 19-9

LABORATORY DIFFERENTIATION OF OLIGURIA

Test	Prerenal	Renal
FENa	<1%	>3%
BUN/Cr ratio	>20:1	<10:1
Urine specific gravity	>1.015	<1.010

BUN, Blood urea nitrogen; Cr, creatinine; FENa, fractional excretion of sodium.

1. BUN/Cr ratio (both in mg/dL):
a. Normal ratio: 10–20; suggests intrinsic renal disease in the setting of oliguria
b. >20: Suggests dehydration, prerenal azotemia, or gastrointestinal bleeding
c. <5: Suggests liver disease, starvation, inborn error of metabolism
2. Laboratory differentiation of oliguria (Table 19-9)

E. Polyuria

Water conservation is dependent on antidiuretic hormone (ADH) and its effects on the distal renal tubules. Etiologies of polyuria include the following:

1. Central diabetes insipidus: ADH deficiency, may be idiopathic or acquired (through infection or pituitary trauma)
2. Nephrogenic diabetes insipidus: Unresponsive receptors; may be hereditary or acquired (through interstitial nephritis, sickle cell disease, or chronic renal insufficiency)
3. Psychogenic polydipsia

VIII. GLOMERULAR DISEASES

Injury to glomeruli results in either inflammatory or noninflammatory lesions. Many glomerular disorders involve both types of lesions.

A. Inflammatory Lesions

Classified as nephritic and associated with casts. Consist of necrotic areas that result in loss of large particles (such as RBCs) as well as edematous areas resulting in decreased filtration. Clinically present with fluid retention, hypertension, oliguria, and hematuria. Classic example is poststreptococcal glomerulonephritis.

B. Noninflammatory Lesions

Classified as nephrotic, and are not associated with casts. These result in leakage through the injured glomerular basement membrane. Nephrotic disorders, when uncomplicated, do not compromise filtration. Classic example is minimal change nephrotic syndrome (MCNS).

C. Nephrotic Syndrome[12]

The most severe form of proteinuria. Classically characterized by proteinuria (>40 mg/m^2/hr), hypercholesterolemia (>200 mg/dL), hypoproteinemia (<2 g/dL), and edema. Clinically, hypoalbuminemia with concomitant decrease in oncotic pressure results in generalized edema.

The initial swelling occurs on the face (especially periorbital) as well as in the pretibial area. Prominent swelling of the scrotum and labia can also be seen. Decreased oncotic pressure also results in compromised splanchnic flow, leading to abdominal pain.

1. Etiology: Exclusively a glomerular disorder that can be primary in the kidney or secondary to other systemic disorder resulting in injury
  a. Primary causes (90%): Idiopathic (most common) and genetic disorders affecting the slit diaphragm. Idiopathic forms divided histologically among MCNS, focal segmental glomerulosclerosis (FSGS), and membranous nephropathy, with MCNS accounting for 85% of idiopathic nephrotic syndrome in children
  b. Secondary causes: Infections (HIV, hepatitis B, hepatitis C), lupus, diabetes mellitus, IgA nephropathy, drugs, and malignancy (leukemias, lymphomas)
2. Factors suggesting a diagnosis other than idiopathic MCNS: Age <1 year or >11 years, positive family history, extrarenal disease (arthritis, rash, anemia), chronic disease, symptoms due to intravascular volume expansion (hypertension, pulmonary edema), renal failure, active urine sediment (RBC casts)
3. Management of MCNS: Aims at restoring intravascular volume and encouraging diuresis to avoid fluid overload. A course of corticosteroid treatment without renal biopsy is recommended for children without atypical features. Hospitalization recommended for children with overwhelming edema or infection
  a. Steroid-responsive: Roughly 95% of patients with MCNS and 20% with focal segmental glomerulosclerosis achieve remission with an 8-wk course of prednisone (60 mg/m^2 daily for 4 weeks followed by 40 mg/m^2 on alternate days for 4 weeks). Response is the best prognostic indicator
  b. Frequently relapsing: Defined as two or more relapses within 6 months of initial response, or four or more relapses in any 12-month period
  c. Steroid-dependent: Defined as two consecutive relapses during tapering or within 14 days of cessation of steroids. Some patients can be managed with low-dose steroids given daily or on alternate days, but many still relapse. Second-line treatments for frequently relapsing and steroid-dependent nephrotic syndrome: Cyclophosphamide, chlorambucil, cyclosporine, or levamisole
  d. Steroid-resistant: Often requires continued high-dose steroid treatment beyond 8 weeks. Second-line agents, including calcineurin inhibitors, are often used, as well as high-dose pulse methylprednisolone, mostly in combination with an alkylating agent
  e. Biopsy is recommended for macroscopic hematuria, severely elevated blood pressure, persistent renal insufficiency, low complement levels, and persistent proteinuria after 4 weeks of adequate steroid treatment
  f. Complications: Acute kidney injury, thromboembolic disease, infection, and side effects of systemic steroids

IX. ACUTE KIDNEY INJURY (FORMERLY ACUTE RENAL FAILURE)[13,14]

Sudden decline in renal function with increasing BUN/Cr ratio, with or without changes in urine output. Causative factors: Impaired renal perfusion, acute renal disease, renal ischemia, or obstructive uropathy.

A. Etiology

Causes are generally subdivided into three categories:

1. Prerenal: Most common etiology in children; usually a result of dehydration, although other forms of impaired perfusion can be a cause
2. Renal:
   a. Parenchymal disease through arterial or glomerular lesions
   b. ATN: Diagnosis of exclusion; when no evidence of renal parenchymal disease is present and prerenal and postrenal causes have been eliminated if possible
3. Postrenal: Obstruction of the urinary tract, found often in neonates with anatomic abnormalities

B. Clinical Presentation

Pallor, decreased urine output, edema, hypertension, vomiting, and lethargy. The hallmark of early renal failure is oliguria.

C. Acute Tubular Necrosis (ATN)

Clinically defined by three phases:

1. Oliguric phase: A period of severe oliguria that lasts about 10 days. If oliguria or anuria persists for longer than 3–6 weeks, renal recovery from ATN is highly unlikely
2. Diuretic phase: Begins with an increase in urine output to passage of large volumes of isosthenuric urine containing sodium levels of 80–150 mEq/L
3. Recovery phase: Signs and symptoms usually resolve rapidly, but polyuria may persist for days to weeks

D. Treatment Considerations

1. Placement of indwelling catheter to monitor urine output
2. Prerenal and postrenal factors should be excluded and intravascular volume maintained with appropriate fluids in consultation with a pediatric nephrologist

E. Complications

Often dependent on clinical severity; usually includes fluid overload (hypertension, CHF, pulmonary edema), electrolyte disturbances (hyperkalemia), metabolic acidosis, hyperphosphatemia, and uremia.

X. ACUTE DIALYSIS

A. Indications

1. Indicated when metabolic or fluid derangements are not controlled by aggressive medical management alone. Generally accepted criteria

include the following, although a nephrologist should always be consulted:

a. Volume overload with evidence of pulmonary edema or hypertension
b. Hyperkalemia >6.5 mEq/L despite conservative measures (>6.0 mEq/L if hypercatabolic)
c. Metabolic acidosis with pH <7.2 or HCO_3^- <10
d. BUN >150 (lower if rising rapidly)
e. Neurologic symptoms secondary to uremia or electrolyte imbalance
f. Calcium and phosphorus imbalance (e.g., hypocalcemia with tetany, seizures in the presence of a very high serum phosphate level)

2. Dialyzable toxin or poison (e.g., lactate, ammonia, alcohol, barbiturates, ethylene glycol, isopropanol, methanol, salicylates, theophylline)

B. Techniques

1. Peritoneal dialysis: Requires catheter to access peritoneal cavity, as well as adequate peritoneal perfusion. May be used acutely or chronically, as in continuous ambulatory or continuous cycling peritoneal dialysis
2. Hemodialysis: Requires placement of special vascular access devices. May be method of choice for certain toxins (e.g., ammonia, uric acid, poisons) or when there are contraindications to peritoneal dialysis
3. Continuous arteriovenous hemofiltration/hemodialysis (CAVH/D) and continuous venovenous hemofiltration/hemodialysis (CVVH/D):

a. Therapies with the primary goal of continuous generation of a plasma ultrafiltrate
b. Indications: Fluid management, renal failure with profound hemodynamic instability, electrolyte disturbances, and intoxication with substances that are freely filtered across the particular ultrafiltration membrane
c. Can be helpful in the management of oliguric patients who are in need of better nutritional support, postoperative cardiac patients, and patients with septicemia
d. Require special vascular access devices

XI. CHRONIC KIDNEY DISEASE ([CKD] FORMERLY CHRONIC RENAL FAILURE)[15]

Kidney damage for >3 months, as defined by structural or functional abnormalities, with or without decreased GFR, or a GFR <60 mL/min/1.73 m^2 for >3 months with or without kidney damage. Classification as below:

Stage I: Kidney injury with normal or increased GFR
Stage II: GFR 60–98 mL/min/1.73 m^2
Stage III: GFR 30–59 mL/min/1.73 m^2
Stage IV: GFR 15–29 mL/min/1.73 m^2
Stage V: GFR <15 mL/min/1.73 m^2 or dialysis

A. Etiology

Close association with age at which renal failure is first detected. Chronic renal failure in children <5 years most commonly a result of anatomic abnormalities (i.e., hypoplasia, dysplasia, malformations), whereas older children predominantly have acquired glomerular diseases (e.g., glomerulonephritis, hemolytic-uremic syndrome) or hereditary disorders (e.g., Alport syndrome, cystic disease).

B. Clinical Manifestations (Table 19-10)

XII. CHRONIC HYPERTENSION[16–18]

NOTE: For management of acute hypertension and normal BP parameters, see Chapters 4 and 7.

A. Definition

For the definition of chronic hypertension, see Chapter 7.

1. Normal blood pressure (BP): Systolic and diastolic BP <90th percentile for age, gender, height, and weight. See Tables 7-1 and 7-2
2. High-normal BP (prehypertension): Average systolic and/or diastolic BP between the 90th and 95th percentiles for age, gender, height, and weight
3. Significant hypertension: Average of three separate systolic and/or diastolic BPs >95th percentile for age, gender, height, and weight
4. Severe hypertension: Average of three systolic and/or diastolic BPs >99th percentile for age, gender, height, and weight
5. Measurement of BP in children
   a. Children ≥3 years should have BP measured at all routine and emergency visits. Children <3 years with risk factors, such as history of prematurity/low birth weight, congenital heart disease, kidney disease or family history of kidney disease, history of malignancy, or solid organ or bone marrow transplant, should have BP measured
   b. BP should be measured at least twice on each occasion at least 3–5 min after resting seated
   c. Appropriate cuff size is two thirds of upper arm length with bladder cuff 80%–100% of arm circumference. Choose the larger size cuff if there is a choice between two cuffs

B. Causes of Hypertension in Neonates, Infants, and Children (Table 19-11)

C. Evaluation of Chronic Hypertension

1. Rule out causes: Rule out factitious causes of hypertension (improper cuff size or measurement technique [i.e., manual versus Dyna map]), nonpathologic causes of hypertension (i.e., fever, pain, anxiety, muscle spasm), and iatrogenic mechanisms (e.g., medications and excessive fluid administration)
2. History: Headache, blurred vision, dyspnea on exertion, edema, obstructive sleep apnea (OSA) symptoms, endocrine symptoms (diaphoresis, flushing, constipation, weakness, etc.), history of neonatal intensive care unit (NICU) stay, last menstrual period (LMP), history of UTIs, history of medications and supplements, illicit drug use, or any family history of renal dysfunction or hypertension

TABLE 19-10

CLINICAL MANIFESTATIONS OF CHRONIC KIDNEY DISEASE

Manifestation	Mechanisms
Azotemia	Decline in GFR
Acidosis	Urinary bicarbonate wasting Decreased excretion of NH_4 and acid
Sodium wasting	Solute diuresis, tubular damage Function tubular adaptation for sodium excretion
Sodium retention	Nephrotic syndrome CHF Anuria
Urinary concentrating defect	Nephron loss, solute diuresis Increased medullary blood flow
Hyperkalemia	Decline in GFR, acidosis Hypoaldosteronism
Renal osteodystrophy	Decreased intestinal calcium absorption Impaired production of 1,25 OH vitamin D Secondary hyperparathyroidism
Growth retardation	Protein-calorie deficiency Renal osteodystrophy Acidosis Anemia Inhibitors of insulin-like growth factors
Anemia	Decreased erythropoietin production Low-grade hemolysis Bleeding Decreased erythrocyte survival Inadequate folic acid intake Inhibitors of erythropoiesis
Bleeding tendency	Thrombocytopenia Defective platelet function
Infection	Defective granulocyte function
Neurologic complaints	Uremic factors Aluminum toxicity
Gastrointestinal ulceration	Gastric acid hypersecretion/gastritis Reflux Decreased motility
Hypertension	Sodium and water overload Excessive renin production
Hypertriglyceridemia	Diminished plasma lipoprotein lipase activity
Pericarditis and cardiomyopathy	Unknown
Glucose intolerance	Tissue insulin resistance

CHF, Congestive heart failure; NH_4, ammonium.

Adapted from Brenner BM: Brenner and Rector's the kidney, 6th ed. Philadelphia, WB Saunders, 2000.

TABLE 19-11

CAUSES OF HYPERTENSION BY AGE GROUP

Age	Cause: Most Common	Cause: Less Common
Neonates/infants	Renal artery thrombosis after umbilical artery catheterization Coarctation of the aorta Renal artery stenosis	Bronchopulmonary dysplasia Medications Patent ductus arteriosus Intraventricular hemorrhage
1–10 yr	Renal parenchymal disease Coarctation of aorta	Renal artery stenosis Hypercalcemia Neurofibromatosis Neurogenic tumors Pheochromocytoma Mineralocorticoid increase Hyperthyroidism Transient hypertension Immobilization-induced Sleep apnea Essential hypertension Medications
11 yr–adolescence	Renal parenchymal disease Essential hypertension	All diagnoses listed in this table

Modified from Sinaiko A: Hypertension in children. N Engl J Med 1996; 335:26.

3. Physical examination: Four extremity pulses and blood pressures, endocrine stigmata, edema, hypertrophied tonsils, skin lesions or rash, abdominal mass or abdominal bruit
4. Clinical evaluation of confirmed hypertension
   a. Laboratory studies: Urinalysis with microscopic evaluation, urine culture, serum electrolytes, CBC, Cr, BUN, calcium, uric acid, cholesterol, and plasma renin level
   b. Imaging: Renal ultrasonography, including renal artery Doppler and other imaging studies as indicated (e.g., echocardiography, renal arteriography)
   c. Consider human chorionic gonadotropin, thyroid function tests, urine catecholamines, and plasma and urinary steroids. Consider polysomnography, fasting lipid profile, fasting glucose, and toxicology screen to evaluate for comorbidity. Consider echocardiogram and retinal examination to evaluate target-organ damage
5. Refer any patient with significant hypertension to a pediatric nephrologist

D. Treatment of Hypertension

1. Nonpharmacologic: Aerobic exercise, salt restriction, smoking cessation, and weight loss, indicated in patients with systolic BP and/or diastolic BP <90th percentile. Reevaluate in 6 months, and begin pharmacologic therapy if persists

TABLE 19-12

CLASSIFICATION OF HYPERTENSION IN CHILDREN AND ADOLESCENTS AND THERAPY RECOMMENDATIONS

	SBP or DBP Percentile	Frequency of BP Measurement	Pharmacologic Therapy (in addition to Lifestyle Modifications)
Normal	<90th percentile	Recheck at next physical examination	None
Prehypertension	90th to <95th percentile or if BP exceeds 120/80 mmHg even if <90th percentile	Recheck in 6 mo	None unless compelling indications: Chronic kidney disease, diabetes mellitus, heart failure, or LVH, exist
Stage 1 hypertension	95th–99th percentile plus 5 mmHg	Recheck in 1–2 wk, sooner if the patient is symptomatic; if persistently elevated on 2 additional occasions, evaluate or refer	Initiate therapy based on symptoms, secondary hypertension, endorgan damage, diabetes, persistent hypertension despite nonpharmacologic measures
Stage 2 hypertension	>99th percentile plus 5 mmHg	Evaluate or refer within 1 wk or immediately if the patient is symptomatic	Initiate therapy

DBP, diastolic blood pressure; LVH, left ventricular hypertrophy; SBP, systolic blood pressure.

Modified from National High Blood Pressure Education Program Working Group on High Blood Pressure in Children and Adolescents: The fourth report on the diagnosis, evaluation and treatment of high blood pressure in children and adolescents. Pediatrics 2004;114(2):555–576.

2. Pharmacologic: Indications include significant hypertension (especially diastolic hypertension), secondary hypertension, symptomatic hypertension, target-organ damage, diabetes mellitus, and persistent hypertension despite nonpharmacologic measures
3. Parenteral: Acute hypertensive crisis

E. Classification of Hypertension in Children and Adolescents, with Measurement Frequency and Therapy Recommendations (Table 19-12)

F. Antihypertensive Drugs for Outpatient Management of Hypertension in Children, Age 1–17 Years (Table 19-13)

XIII. NEPHROLITHIASIS[19]

A. Presentation:

Microscopic hematuria (90%), flank/abdominal pain (50%–75%), gross hematuria (15%–30%), concomitant UTI in up to 20%.

B. Diagnosis:

Noncontrast computed tomography (CT) (96% sensitive), abdominal ultrasound (only 60% sensitive, therefore cannot rule out stone if negative).

TABLE 19-13

ANTIHYPERTENSIVE DRUGS FOR OUTPATIENT MANAGEMENT OF HYPERTENSION IN CHILDREN, 1–17 YEARS OLD

Class	Drug	Comments
Angiotensin-converting enzyme (ACE) inhibitor	Benazepril Captopril Enalapril Fosinopril Lisinopril Quinapril	Blocks angiotensin I to angiotensin II. Decreases proteinuria while preserving renal function. Contraindicated in pregnancy, compromised renal perfusion. Check serum potassium and creatinine periodically to monitor for hyperkalemia and azotemia. Elimination is dependent on creatinine clearance. Cough and angioedema are reportedly less common with newer members of this class than with captopril.
Angiotensin-II receptor blocker (ARB)	Irbesartan Losartan	Contraindicated in pregnancy. Check serum potassium and creatinine periodically to monitor for hyperkalemia and azotemia.
Alpha and beta blocker	Labetalol	Causes decreased peripheral resistance and decreased heart rate. Extremely potent and can be used in hypertensive crisis. Contraindications: Asthma, heart failure, insulin dependent diabetics. Heart rate is dose-limiting. May impair athletic performance.
Beta blocker	Atenolol Bisopropol/HCTZ Metoprolol Propranolol	Decreases heart rate, cardiac output, and renin release. Noncardioselective agents (i.e., propranolol) are contraindicated in asthma and heart failure. Metoprolol and Atenolol are beta-1 selective. Heart rate is dose-limiting. May impair athletic performance. Should not be used in insulin-dependent diabetics. A sustained-release formulation of propranolol is available that is dosed once daily.
Calcium channel blocker	Amlodipine Felodipine Isradipine Extended-release nifedipine	Acts on vascular smooth muscles. Renal perfusion/function is minimally affected. Ideal for post-renal-transplant hypertension and low renin/volume dependent hypertension. Amlodipine and isradipine can be compounded into suspensions. Felodipine and extended-release nifedipine tablets must be swallowed whole. Isradipine is available in both immediate release and sustained-release formulations. May cause tachycardia.

TABLE 19-13

ANTIHYPERTENSIVE DRUGS FOR OUTPATIENT MANAGEMENT OF HYPERTENSION IN CHILDREN, 1–17 YEARS OLD (Continued)

Class	Drug	Comments
Central alpha agonist	Clonidine	Stimulates brainstem α 2 receptors and peripheral adrenergic drive. May cause dry mouth and/or sedation (↓ opiate withdrawal). Effective in renal failure. Transdermal preparation also available. Sudden cessation of therapy can lead to severe rebound hypertension.
Diuretic	HCTZ Budesonide Chlorthalidone Furosemide Spironolactone Triamterene Amiloride	All patients treated with diuretics should have electrolytes monitored shortly after initiating therapy and periodically thereafter. Useful as add-on therapy in patients being treated with drugs from other drug classes. Thiazides are not effective when GFR <50% of normal. Side effects are hypokalemia, hypercalcemia, hyperuricemia, and hyperlipidemia. Furosemide/bumetanide are useful in renal failure. Bumetanide has 40 times more diuretic activity than furosemide but varies with patient/route. Side effects are hyponatremia, hypokalemia, ototoxicity. Potassium-sparing diuretics (i.e., spironolactone, triamterene, amiloride) are modest antihypertensives. They may cause severe hyperkalemia, especially if given with ACE inhibitor or ARB.
Peripheral alpha antagonist	Doxazosin Prazosin Terazosin	May cause hypotension and syncope, especially after first dose.
Vasodilator	Hydralazine Minoxidil	Directly acts on vascular smooth muscle and is very potent. Tachycardia and Na and water retention are common side effects. Used in combination with diuretics or beta blockers. Hydralazine can cause a lupus-like syndrome. Minoxidil is usually reserved for patients with hypertension resistant to multiple drugs.

Modified from National High Blood Pressure Education Program Working Group on High Blood Pressure in Children and Adolescents: The fourth report on the diagnosis, evaluation, and treatment of high blood pressure in children and adolescents. Pediatrics 2004(2);114:568–569; Hospital for Sick Children: The HSC Handbook of Pediatrics, 9th ed. St. Louis, Mosby, 1997; Sinaiko A: Treatment of hypertension in children. Pediatr Nephrol 1994:8:603–609; and Khattak S et al: Efficacy of amlodipine in pediatric bone marrow transplant patients. Clin Pediatr 1998:37:31–35.

C. Treatment:

1. Expectant management if none of the following exist: concurrent infection, intolerable pain, evidence of renal insufficiency, solitary kidney, or stone >5 mm. Expectant management also recommended for neonatal nephrocalcinosis
2. Surgical management: Includes extracorporeal shock wave lithotripsy, ureteroscopy, and percutaneous nephrolithostomy

D. Workup:

Up to 75% of children with a kidney stone will have a metabolic abnormality (i.e., hypercalciuria, hyperoxaluria, hyperuricosuria, cystinuria). Workup should include analysis of the stone (if possible), urinalysis, basic metabolic panel (BMP), phosphate, and uric acid. If evidence of elevated calcium or phosphate, obtain PTH level. 24-hour urine collection should be obtained several weeks after the stone has passed, and measure urine sodium, calcium, urate, oxalate, citrate, creatinine, and cystine.

REFERENCES

1. American Academy of Pediatrics, Committee on Quality Improvement, Subcommittee on Urinary Tract Infection. Practice parameter: the diagnosis, treatment, and evaluation of the initial urinary tract infection in febrile infants and young children. *Pediatrics.* 1999;103(4):843–852.
2. Michael M, Hodson EM, Craig JC, et al. Short versus standard duration oral antibiotic therapy for acute urinary tract infection in children. Cochrane Database of Systematic Reviews 2003, Issue 1. Art. No.: CD003966. DOI: 10.1002/14651858.CD003966.
3. Keren R, Carpenter MA, Hoberman A, et al. Rationale and design issues of the Randomized Intervention for Children With Vesicoureteral Reflux (RIVUR) study. *Pediatrics.* 2008;122(suppl 5):S240–S250.
4. Elder JS, Peters CA, Arant Jr BS, et al. Pediatric Vesicoureteral Reflux Guidelines Panel summary report on the management of primary vesicoureteral reflux in children. *J Urol.* 1997;157(5):1846–1851.
5. Conway PH, Cnaan A, Zaoutis T, et al. Recurrent urinary tract infections in children: risk factors and association with prophylactic antimicrobials. *JAMA.* 2007;298(2):179–186.
6. Craig JC, Irwig LM, Knight JF, et al. Does treatment of vesicoureteric reflux in childhood prevent end-stage renal disease attributable to reflux nephropathy? *Pediatrics.* 2000;105(6):1236–1241.
7. Garin EH, Olavarria F, Garcia Nieto V, et al. Clinical significance of primary vesicoureteral reflux and urinary antibiotic prophylaxis after acute pyelonephritis: a multicenter, randomized, controlled study. *Pediatrics.* 2006;117(3):626–632.
8. Sargent JD, Stukel TA, Kresel J, et al. Normal values for random urinary calcium to creatinine ratios in infancy. *J Pediatr.* 1993;123:393.
9. Soriano JR. Renal tubular acidosis: the clinical entity. *J Am Soc Nephrol.* 2002;13:2160–2170.
10. Massengill SF. Hematuria. *Pediatr Rev.* 2008;29(10):342–348.
11. Cruz C, Spitzer A. When you find protein or blood in urine. *Contemp Pediatr.* 1998;15(9):89.

12. Gordillo R, Spitzer A. The nephrotic syndrome. *Pediatr Rev.* 2009;30(3): 94–104.
13. Whyte DA, Fine RN. Acute renal failure in children. *Pediatr Rev.* 2008;29(9): 299–306.
14. Andreoli SP. Acute kidney injury in children. *Pediatr Nephrol.* 2009;24(2): 253–263.
15. Whyte DA, Fine RN. Chronic kidney disease in children. *Pediatr Rev.* 2008; 29(10):335–341.
16. Sinaiko A. Hypertension in children. *N Engl J Med.* 1996;335:26.
17. National High Blood Pressure Education Program Working Group on High Blood Pressure in Children and Adolescents. The fourth report on the diagnosis, evaluation and treatment of high blood pressure in children and adolescents. *Pediatrics.* 2004;114(2):555–576.
18. Brady TM, Solomon B, Siberry G. Pediatric hypertension: a review of proper screening, diagnosis, evaluation and treatment. *Contemp Pediatr.* 2008;25(11): 46–56.
19. Tanaka ST, Pope 4th JC. Pediatric stone disease. *Curr Urol Rep.* 2009;10(2): 138–143.

GENERAL REFERENCES FOR NEPHROLOGY SOURCES

Kliegman RM, Behrman RE, Jenson HB, et al. *Nelson textbook of pediatrics.* 18th ed. Philadelphia: WB Saunders; 2007.

Brenner BM. *Brenner and Rector's the kidney.* 6th ed. Philadelphia: WB Saunders; 2000.

Hay WW, Levin M, Deterding R, et al. *Current pediatric diagnosis and treatment.* 20th ed. Stamford, CT: Appleton & Lange; 2011.

Chapter 20

Neurology

Delphine Robotham, MD

See additional content on Expert Consult

I. WEBSITES

Child Neurology Society: www.childneurologysociety.org

American Academy of Neurology Practice Guidelines: aan.com/practice/guideline

Royal College of Physicians Clinical Guidelines: www.rcplondon.ac.uk

American Heart Association Statement on Management of Stroke in Infants and Children: stroke.ahajournals.org

II. NEUROLOGIC EXAMINATION[1]

Starts with a thorough history, with emphasis on onset, duration, and progression of symptoms. Must be evaluated relative to developmental norms.

A. Mental Status

Patient should be alert and oriented to time, person, place, and current situation. Assess attentiveness and behavior in infants.

B. Cranial Nerves (Table 20-1)

C. Motor

1. Muscle bulk
2. Tone: High, low
   a. Passive movements: Resting resistance to examiner's movement
   b. Active movements: Regulation of power with defined movements (e.g., posture, gait, pull to stand)
   c. Infants who have low tone or weakness will slip when you hold them under their arms
3. Power, strength: Observe and describe activity (e.g., rising from the floor). Quantify (e.g., distance of standing broad jump, time to run 30 feet, time to climb stairs); see Box 20-1

D. Sensory (Fig. 20-1)

Primary disorders of sensation are rare in children, and reliable examination takes time. Sensory evaluation is most important when there is a specific question of anatomic localization (Table 20-2). Compare side to side, distal to proximal positions within an extremity, and upper to lower extremities as appropriate to the question being asked.

TABLE 20-1
CRANIAL NERVES

Function/Region	Cranial Nerve	Test/Observation
Olfactory	I	Smell (e.g., coffee, vanilla, peppermint)
Vision	II	Acuity, fields, fundus
Pupils	II, III	Sympathetics, size, reaction to light, accommodation
Eye movements and eyelids	III, IV, VI	Range and quality of eye movements, saccades, pursuits, nystagmus, ptosis
Sensation	V	Corneal reflexes, facial sensation
Muscles of mastication	V	Clench teeth
Facial strength	VII	Observe degree of expression of emotions, eye closure strength, smile, puff out cheeks, asymmetry forehead and lower face
Hearing	VIII	Localize sound, attend to finger rub, audiologic testing
Mouth, pharynx	VII, IX, X, XII	Swallowing, speech quality (labial, lingual, or palatal articulation deficits), symmetrical palatal elevation, tongue protrusion
Head control	XI	Lateral head movement, shoulder shrug

BOX 20-1
STRENGTH RATING SCALE

0/5: No movement, i.e., no palpable tension at the tendon
1/5: Flicker of movement or less than full range of movement in a gravity-neutral plane
2/5: Movement in a gravity-neutral plane
3/5: Movement against gravity but not resistance
4/5: Subnormal strength against resistance
5/5: Normal strength against resistance

TABLE 20-2
UPPER AND LOWER MOTOR NEURON FINDINGS

On Exam	Upper	Lower
Power	Decreased	Decreased
Reflexes	Increased	Decreased
Tone	Increased	Normal or decreased
Babinski	Present	Absent

1. Spinal cord level: Best assessed with pinprick and temperature. If concerned about spinal cord impairment, ask about continence. Compare lower to upper, check both anterior and posterior trunk
2. Intraspinal lesions:
a. Anterior pathways: Pinprick and temperature
b. Posterior pathways: Vibratory and joint position sense

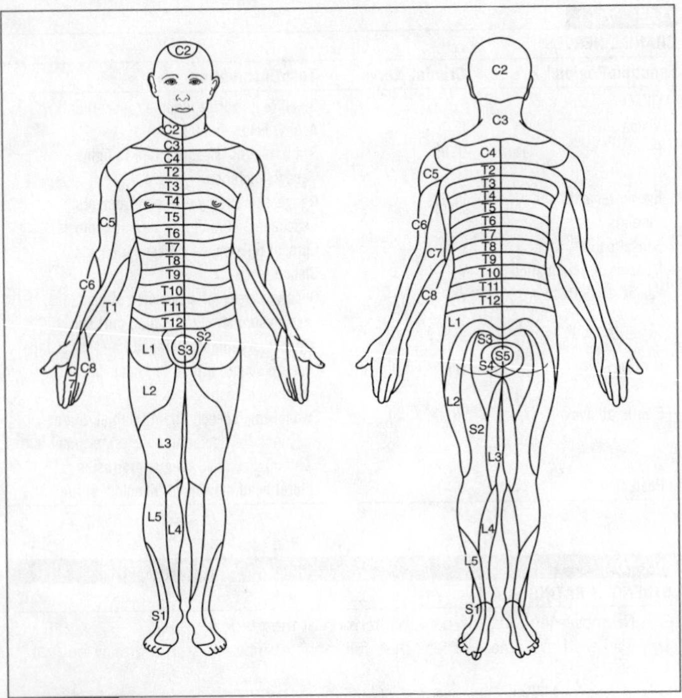

FIGURE 20-1

Dermatomes. *(From Athreya BH, Silverman BK: Pediatric physical diagnosis. Norwalk, CT, Appleton-Century-Crofts, 1985, pp. 238–239.)*

3. Root/plexus/nerve impairment: Pin sensibility, consult dermatomal/nerve maps (see Fig. 20-1)
4. Polyneuropathy: Large fiber (vibration and position sense) versus small fiber (pinprick and temperature). Compare distal to proximal sites in a limb, and lower to upper extremities

E. Tendon Reflexes

This assessment is most helpful in localizing other abnormalities, especially in the presence of weakness or asymmetry (Box 20-2 and Table EC 20-A on Expert Consult).

1. Isolated abnormality of reflexes: Little significance in the setting of normal strength and coordination
2. Brisk reflexes combined with weakness: Indicate upper motor neuron disorder
3. Absent reflexes: Motor neuron, nerve or muscle causes

a. Muscle disease: Reflexes usually diminished commensurate with power

BOX 20-2

REFLEX RATING SCALE

0: None
1+: Diminished (need use of clasped hands/gritting teeth to engage reflex)
2+: Normal
3+: Increased (reflexes cross neighboring joint or cross to other side)
4+: Hyperactive with clonus

BOX 20-3

TESTS FOR CEREBELLAR FUNCTION

1. Rapid alternating and repetitive movements: finger to nose, heel to shin, orbiting, walking, running
2. Note involuntary movements and conditions under which they are enhanced or suppressed: tremor, dystonia, chorea athetosis, tics, myoclonus
3. Note abnormal gait: waddling, wide based, tiptoe

b. Selective reflex dropout: Localize to spinal cord, root, or nerve lesion
c. Compare side to side, upper to lower extremities, distal to proximal reflexes

F. Coordination and Movement

1. Evaluate general coordination while watching activities (e.g., throwing a ball, dressing, writing, or drawing)
2. Test for Cerebellar Function (See Box 20-3)

III. HEADACHES[2]

A. Evaluation of Headaches

1. **Classification:** *The International Classification of Headache Disorders,* 2nd ed., classifies headaches as primary versus secondary.[3] Adults are divided into these broad categories; however, they are not intended to apply to pediatrics
a. Primary headaches: Migraines, tension type, cluster or other trigeminal etiologies
b. Secondary headaches: Caused by other underlying pathologies, such as trauma, substance use or withdrawal, vascular malformations, infection, mass effect, referred pain from teeth, sinuses, and/or eyes, or psychiatric. For the purpose of pediatric headache it is beneficial to differentiate headache based on onset and duration
2. **History and physical examination:** It is important to distinguish those who require specific or immediate treatment vs. those of a more diffuse etiology. See Boxes 20-4, 20-5, 20-6, and 20-7 and Table EC 20-B on Expert Consult.

BOX 20-4

HEADACHE WARNING SIGNS

1. Focal pain that awakens the child from sleep
2. Focal deficits
3. Headache associated with emesis
4. Changes in chronic pattern
5. Altered Mental Status: changes in mood, personality, school performance

BOX 20-5

IMPORTANT HISTORICAL INFORMATION IN EVALUATING HEADACHE

1. Age at onset
2. Associated trauma
3. Presence or absence of aura
4. Change in weight or other constitutional symptoms
5. Change in vision or any other neurologic symptoms
6. Frequency, severity, and duration of headaches (ask about school absences)
7. Quality, site, and radiation of pain (focal occipital pain is concerning for secondary headaches)
8. Associated symptoms, such as weakness or tingling
9. Triggers and relieving and worsening factors (triggers: foods, environmental factors, etc.); presence of photophobia, phonophobia; worsens with activity; relieved by sleep, medications (nonsteroidal anti-inflammatory drugs [NSAIDs], acetaminophen), remaining still
10. Family history of migraine
11. Changes and possible new stressors in school or at home

BOX 20-6

DIFFERENTIAL DIAGNOSIS OF ACUTE HEADACHE

Evaluation of the first acute headache should exclude pathologic causes listed here before consideration of more common etiologies.

1. Increased intracranial pressure (ICP): Trauma, hemorrhage, tumor, hydrocephalus, pseudotumor cerebri, abscess, arachnoid cyst, cerebral edema
2. Decreased ICP: After ventriculoperitoneal shunt, lumbar puncture, cerebrospinal fluid leak from basilar skull fracture
3. Meningeal inflammation: Meningitis, leukemia, subarachnoid or subdural hemorrhage
4. Vascular: Vasculitis, arteriovenous malformation, hypertension, cerebrovascular accident
5. Bone, soft tissue: Referred pain from scalp, eyes, ears, sinuses, nose, teeth, pharynx, cervical spine, temporomandibular joint
6. Infection: Systemic infection, encephalitis, sinusitis, etc.
7. First migraine

BOX 20-7

DIFFERENTIAL DIAGNOSIS OF RECURRENT OR CHRONIC HEADACHES

1. Migraine (with or without aura)
2. Tension
3. Analgesic rebound
4. Caffeine withdrawal
5. Sleep deprivation (e.g., in children with sleep apnea) or chronic hypoxia
6. Tumor
7. Psychogenic: Conversion disorder, malingering
8. Cluster headache

BOX 20-8

LUMBAR PUNCTURE[5]

- Indications: Fever, infection, sudden severe headaches, headache worse when lying down and improves on standing
- Contraindications: Elevated intracranial pressure (ICP) or mass effect due to concern for herniation, computed tomography (CT) before lumbar puncture (LP) if this is a concern
- Standard tests: Cell counts + diff, Gram stain, protein, glucose, consider viral studies
- Special tests: Manometer for opening pressure with legs extended, consider if concern for pseudotumor cerebri
- Correction for white blood cell (WBC): Expected cerebrospinal fluid (CSF) WBC = (RBC CSF/RBC blood)*WBC blood or allow 1 WBC for every 700 (500–1500) RBCs
- Subarachnoid hemorrhage (SAH)/herpes simplex virus (HSV) meningitis: CT preferred initial method but if negative and SAH suspected then LP. Positive test = persistently increased RBCs in tubes 1 + 4 (xanthochromia)

3. **Studies**

a. Neuroimaging: Strongest evidence for the use of neuroimaging is abnormal neurologic examination
   (1) Variables that increase likelihood of a space-occupying lesion causing headache: Headache duration <1 month, absence of family history of migraine, abnormal neurologic examination, gait abnormalities, and occurrence of seizures[4]
   (2) Computed tomography (CT) without contrast or magnetic resonance imaging (MRI): Obtain for focal neurologic findings, suspected increased intracranial pressure (ICP), atypical or progressive pattern, seizures, abrupt-onset severe headache (see Chapter 25 for advantages of each modality.) Note that CT provides poor imaging of the posterior fossa

b. Lumbar Puncture (See Box 20-8)[5]

NOTE: The classic headache secondary to subarachnoid hemorrhage (SAH) is acute, severe, continuous, and generalized—the “worst headache of my life.”

B. Migraine Headache

1. Characteristics as defined by the International Headache Society: Chronic recurrent (at least two attacks with aura and five attacks with no aura); throbbing, pulsatile, or pressure-like in children; usually bifrontal in children, unilateral in adolescents and adults, lasting from 1–72 hours; relieved by sleep; many potential triggers (e.g., stress, caffeine, menses, sleep disruption); hereditary predisposition. Associated symptoms include nausea, vomiting, abdominal pain, motion sickness in smaller children, photophobia, phonophobia, paresthesias, and dizziness; rare associated symptoms include focal weakness, aphasia, ataxia, and confusion
2. **Classification:**
   a. With aura: Classic. Aura is any preceding neurologic abnormality (e.g., visual aberrations, reversible sensory symptoms such as pins and needles or numbness or dysphasia)
   b. Without aura: Common
3. Associated reversible neurologic deficits (rare): Paresthesia, visual-field cuts, aphasia, hemiplegia, ophthalmoplegia, vertigo, ataxia, confusion. These children typically receive neuroimaging due to the complicated nature of their migraines
4. **Treatment[6]:** Includes reassurance and education regarding lifestyle modification (sleep, exercise, stress reduction, fluids, not missing meals). Studies suggest approximately 50% of children improve with reassurance alone. The acute and chronic pharmacologic treatment of migraine headaches in the pediatric population is well studied; however, these recommendations have not yet been incorporated into national guidelines for children
   a. Acute symptomatic:
      (1) For all ages: Dark and quiet room and sleep
      (2) For <12 years of age: Nonsteroidal anti-inflammatory drugs (NSAIDs); i.e., naproxen, ibuprofen, ketorolac and, for some children, acetaminophen. Triptans (Table 20-3) have been reported as useful in children. Caffeine (e.g., Excedrin) can also be used

TABLE 20-3

ABORTIVE TRIPTANS FOR MIGRAINE (SEE FORMULARY FOR SPECIFIC DOSING)

Medication	Dose (Preparation*)	Duration†
Sumatriptan (Imitrex)	6 mg (Im) 5, 20 mg (Ns) 25, 100 mg (T)	Short
Rizatriptan (Maxalt)	5, 10 mg (T) 5, 10 mg (D)	Short
Zolmitriptan (Zomig)	2.5, 5 mg (T) 2.5, 5 mg (D) 5 mg (Ns)	Short
Almotriptan (Axert)	6.25, 12.5 mg (T)	Short
Eletriptan (Relpax)	20, 40 mg (T)	Short
Naratriptan (Amerge)	1, 2.5 mg (T)	Long
Frovatriptan (Frova)	2.5 mg (T)	Long

*D, Dissolvable tablet; Im, intramuscular; Ns, nasal spray; T, tablet.
†Short (4-hr half-life); Long (12–24 hr half-life).

(3) For >12 years of age: Objective data support nasal sumatriptan. If nausea is a factor, antiemetics (metoclopramide). Steroids (e.g., Solu-Medrol) may be useful in intractable cases, although evidence is lacking

(4) Avoid abortive medication overuse (>2–3 doses/wk), which can lead to rebound headache

b. Chronic treatment (if >3 per month and if migraines interfere with daily functioning or school):

(1) Avoid triggers and stress, improve general health with balanced diet restrictive of certain migraine-causing foods, suggest headache journal to help identify potential triggers. Encourage aerobic exercise and regular sleep

(2) Explore issues of secondary gain and role of pain in family's relationships. Offer counseling when appropriate; also consider biofeedback, acupuncture, yoga, massage therapy if parents are interested

(3) Consider medications. See Table 20-4 for summary of preventive therapies, doses, and adverse effects

(4) The natural history of chronic headache includes spontaneous improvement. Delayed treatment may be indicated. No child should be on chronic therapy without re-evaluation. Refer any child with focal deficits to a pediatric neurologist

IV. PAROXYSMAL EVENTS

A. Differential Diagnosis of Recurrent Events that Mimic Epilepsy in Childhood (Table 20-5)

B. Seizures: First and Recurrent[7,8]

1. Seizure: Paroxysmal synchronized discharge of cortical neurons, resulting in alteration of function (motor, sensory, cognitive)
2. Nonepileptic causes of seizure/single seizure

a. Diffuse brain dysfunction: Fever, metabolic compromise, toxin or drugs, hypertension, idiopathic epilepsy

b. Focal brain dysfunction: Stroke, neoplasm, focal cortical dysgenesis, trauma, focal idiopathic epilepsy

3. Evaluation of non-epileptic causes of seizure

a. Febrile-Illness Associated Seizure: Box 20-9

b. Check glucose, Na, K, Ca, Phos, blood urea nitrogen (BUN), creatinine (Cr), complete blood count (CBC), tox screen

c. Blood pressure (BP): Supine and upright

d. Lumbar puncture (LP)

e. Electrocardiogram (ECG) (as clinically indicated)

f. Electroencephalogram (EEG): Recommended in all children with first nonfebrile seizures to classify if there is an epilepsy syndrome.[9] Controversial; routine interictal EEGs are frequently normal. Repeat EEGs, prolonged EEG monitoring with video, or studies done with sleep deprivation or photic stimulation may be more informative

TABLE 20-4

PREVENTATIVE THERAPIES FOR MIGRAINE

Medications	Dose	Adverse Effects	Consider in Patients With the Following Comorbidities
ANTICONVULSANT MEDICATIONS			
Divalproex sodium	<12 yr 10–20 mg/kg/dose qhs >12 yr 250–500 mg/dose qhs	Dizziness, drowsiness, weight gain, GI upset, teratogenicity	Bipolar, epilepsy, underweight
Topiramate	<12 yr 15–30 mg/dose qhs >12 yr 25–50 mg/dose qhs	Cognitive changes, weight loss, sensory changes, paresthesias	Obesity, epilepsy
ANTIDEPRESSANT MEDICATIONS			
Amitriptyline	1 mg/kg/day (10–50 mg/dose) qhs	Sedation, dry mouth, constipation	Depression, insomnia
Nortriptyline	1 mg/kg/day (10–50 mg/dose) qhs	Sedation, dry mouth, constipation	Depression, insomnia
ANTIHISTAMINE MEDICATION			
Cyproheptadine	0.5 mg/kg/day qhs (max 32 mg/day)	Sedation, increased appetite	Seasonal allergies, poor appetite, insomnia
ANTIHYPERTENSIVE MEDICATION			
Propranolol	20 mg BID	Hypotension, exacerbate exercise-induced asthma	Hypertension
CALCIUM CHANNEL BLOCKER			
Flunarizine*	5 mg/day	Drowsiness, weight gain	Hypertension

*Flunarizine-only therapy demonstrated efficacy in prospective randomized, double-blind trials. Other therapies have demonstrated some efficacy in uncontrolled studies.

GI, Gastrointestinal.

BOX 20-9

FEBRILE ILLNESS-ASSOCIATED SEIZURE

Further investigation not required if meeting the following criteria:

1. 6 mo–3 yr (can extend 2 mo–6 yr)
2. Nonfocal motor seizure
3. Short duration (no more than 10 minutes) and rapid recovery (if not meningitis should be high on the differential)
4. Seizure occurs on the first day of illness
5. Sepsis investigation may be warranted based on clinical exam

TABLE 20-5

DIFFERENTIAL DIAGNOSIS OF RECURRENT EVENTS THAT MIMIC EPILEPSY IN CHILDHOOD[7]

Event	Differentiation From Epilepsy
Pseudoseizure (psychogenic seizure)	No EEG changes except movement artifact during event; movements thrashing rather than clonic; brief/absent postictal period; most likely to occur in patient with epilepsy.
Paroxysmal vertigo (toddler)	Patient frightened and crying; no loss of awareness; staggers and falls, vomiting, dysarthria.
GER in infancy, childhood	Paroxysmal dystonic posturing associated with meals (Sandifer syndrome).
Breath-holding spells (18 mo–3 yr)	Loss of consciousness and generalized convulsions, always provoked by an event that makes child cry.
Syncope	Loss of consciousness with onset of dizziness and clouded or tunnel vision; slow collapse to floor; triggered by postural change, heat, emotion, etc.
Cardiogenic syncope	Abnormal ECG/Holter monitor finding (e.g., prolonged QT, atrioventricular block, other arrhythmias); exercise a possible trigger; episodic loss of consciousness without consistent convulsive movement.
Cough syncope	Prolonged cough spasm during sleep in asthmatic, leading to loss of consciousness, often with urinary incontinence.
Paroxysmal dyskinesias	May be precipitated by sudden movement or startle; not accompanied by change in alertness.
Shuddering attacks	Brief shivering spells with continued awareness.
Night terrors (4–6 yr)	Brief nocturnal episodes of terror without typical convulsive movements.
Rages (6–12 yr)	Provoked and goal-directed anger.
Tics/habit spasms	Involuntary, nonrhythmic, repetitive movements not associated with impaired consciousness; suppressible.
Narcolepsy	Sudden loss of tone secondary to cataplexy; emotional trigger; no postictal state or loss of consciousness; EEG with recurrent REM sleep attacks.
Migraine (confusional)	Headache or visual changes that may precede attack; family history of migraine; autonomic or sensory changes that can mimic focal seizure; EEG with regional area of slowing during attack.
Myoclonus	Involuntary muscle jerking or twitch.

ECG, Electrocardiography; EEG, electroencephalography; GER, gastroesophageal reflux; REM, rapid eye movement.

4. **Imaging**

Although not required for diagnosis, MRI and CT can detect focal brain abnormalities that may predispose to focal seizures

a. Head CT without contrast: Can detect mass lesions, acute hemorrhage, hydrocephalus, and calcifications secondary to congenital disease such as cytomegalovirus infection (head ultrasound may be used in early infancy and requires open fontanelles)

BOX 20-10

INTERNATIONAL CLASSIFICATION OF EPILEPTIC SEIZURES[8]

I. Partial seizures (seizures with focal onset)
  A. Simple partial seizures (consciousness unimpaired)
    1. With motor signs
    2. With somatosensory or special sensory symptoms
    3. With autonomic symptoms or signs
    4. With psychic symptoms (higher cerebral functions)
  B. Complex partial seizures (consciousness impaired)
    1. Starting as simple partial seizures
      (a) Without automatisms
      (b) With automatisms (such as lip smacking and drooling, dazed eyes look)
    2. With impairment of consciousness at onset
      (a) Without automatisms
      (b) With automatisms
  C. Partial seizures evolving into secondarily generalized seizures
II. Generalized seizures
  A. Absence seizures: Brief lapse in awareness without postictal impairment (atypical absence seizures may have the following: mild clonic, atonic, tonic, automatism, or autonomic components)
  B. Myoclonic seizures: Brief, repetitive, symmetrical muscle contractions
  C. Clonic seizures: Rhythmic jerking; flexor spasm of extremities
  D. Tonic seizures: Sustained muscle contraction
  E. Tonic-clonic seizures
  F. Atonic seizures: Abrupt loss of muscle tone
III. Unclassified epileptic seizures

b. Brain MRI with contrast: Obtain in infants with epilepsy, children with recurrent partial seizures, focal neurologic deficits, or developmental delay. Not routinely indicated in the evaluation of a first-time seizure
5. **Epilepsy:** (recurrent seizures) requires three levels of assessment
a. Seizure type (Box 20-10)
b. Epilepsy classification (Table 20-6)
c. Severity: How severe the seizures are, how frequently they occur, etc.
6. **Status epilepticus:** Prolonged or recurrent seizures lasting ≥30 min without the patient regaining consciousness. See Chapter 1 for treatment

NOTE: If this is not the first seizure and if patient is receiving antiepileptic therapy, a change in seizure pattern should prompt a drug level (see Table 20-7 for therapeutic drug levels).

7. **Treatment**[9]**:**
a. If patient's first seizure, seizure was nonfocal, and patient has returned to baseline: No antiepileptic medication indicated. Overall recurrence of seizure varies from 14%–65%, with most recurrences occurring in the first 2 years after initial event. EEG is most important indicator for evidence of risk for recurrence

TABLE 20-6

SPECIAL SEIZURE SYNDROMES

Syndrome	Etiology	Evaluation	Treatment	Comment
Neonatal seizures	Underlying brain disorder, hypoxic-ischemic injury, intracranial hemorrhage or metabolic	Screen electrolyte and metabolic abnormalities, pyridoxine deficiency, workup for sepsis, LP, ultrasound, CT or MRI, EEG	Treat underlying abnormality, consider pyridoxine with or without EEG, phenobarbital; may need additional agent topiramate or zonisamide	Occurs within first 28 days of life, may be myoclonic, tonic or subtle Presents as blinking, chewing, bicycling or apnea
Infantile spasms	Symptomatic—67%; CNS malformation (acquired infantile brain injury, tuberous sclerosis, inborn errors of metabolism); Cryptogenic—33%	EEG—hypsarrhythmia, MRI, ketogenic diet	Corticotropin, valproic acid, benzodiazepine, vigabatrin, topiramate, zonisamide, consider ketogenic diet	Usual onset after age 2 mo, peak onset 4–6 mo, initiate treatment as soon as possible Presents as head nodding with flexion and extension of the trunk and extremities
Benign rolandic epilepsy	Autosomal dominant inheritance	EEG—characteristic pattern	No treatment necessary, if frequent seizures may use carbamazepine	Age 3–13 yr, nighttime seizure Presents as clonic activity, grimacing, vocalizations; most outgrow by adulthood
Juvenile myoclonic epilepsy	Unknown genetic predisposition	Clinical history, sleep-deprived EEG	Levetiracetem, other meds for generalized seizure	Adolescent onset, morning myoclonus, generalized bursts on EEG with normal background
Panayiotopoulus syndrome	Benign age-related focal seizure disorder Prolonged seizure with predominately autonomic symptoms	EEG—shifting and/or multiple foci Symptoms: vomiting, pallor, sweating, ± convulsions	Not necessary	Syndrome is specific to childhood

CNS, Central nervous system; CT, computed tomography; EEG, electroencephalography; LP, lumbar puncture; MRI, magnetic resonance imaging.

TABLE 20-7

COMMONLY USED ANTICONVULSANTS, IN ALPHABETICAL ORDER

Anticonvulsant (Trade Name)	Typical Target Dose (mg/kg/day)	Standard Therapeutic Levels (mg/Dl)	Efficacy (Generalized/Partial)	Side Effects
Carbamazepine (Tegretol/Carbatrol)	10–20	8–12	P	Sedation, ataxia, diplopia, Stevens-Johnson syndrome, blood dyscrasias, hepatotoxicity, may worsen generalized seizures
Clonazepam (Klonopin)	0.05–0.2	n/a	G/P	Sedation, drooling, dependence
Ethosuximide (Zarontin)	10–20	40–100	G (absence)	Gastrointestinal upset
Felbamate (Felbatol)	15–45	40–100	G/P	Weight loss, hepatotoxicity, sleep disturbances, aplastic anemia (1:7,900)
Gabapentin (Neurontin)	20–40	3–18	P	Weight gain, leg edema
Lamotrigine (Lamictal)	5–15	3–18	G/P	Rash (increased risk in combination with valproate)
Levetiracetam (Keppra)	10–40	30–60	P	Behavioral changes, irritability, rare psychosis
Oxcarbazepine (Trileptal)	10–30 (3:2 ratio compared with carbamazepine)	MHD level (5–40)	P	Hyponatremia
Phenobarbital (Luminal)	5–10	15–40	G/P	Altered cognition, sedation

Phenytoin (Dilantin)	5–10	10–20	P	Hirsutism, gingival hyperplasia, teratogenicity, rash, purple-glove syndrome with infusion
Pregabalin (Lyrica)	? pediatrics	n/a	P	Peripheral edema, weight gain, constipation, dizziness, ataxia, sedation
Rufinamide (Banzel)	10–45	n/a	G (Lennox-Gastaut)	Shortened QT interval, nausea, dizziness, sedation, headache
Tiagabine (Gabitril)	0.25–1.5	n/a	P	Can worsen generalized seizures
Topiramate (Topomax)	1–9	2–20	G/P	Cognitive side effects, weight loss, renal stones, acidosis, glaucoma
Valproic Acid (Depakote, Depakene)	10–20	75–100	G/P	Weight gain, alopecia, hepatotoxicity, pancreatitis, PCOS, teratogenicity
Vigabatrin (Sabril)	50–150	n/a	G (Infantile spasms)	Rash, weight gain, irritability, dizziness, sedation, visual field defects (requires ophthalmology evaluations)
Zonisamide (Zonegran)	5–10	20–40	G/P	Renal stones, weight loss, rare: Stevens-Johnson syndrome, aplastic anemia

G, Generalized, MHD, 10-Monohydroxy metabolite; n/a, not available; P, partial; PCOS, polycystic ovarian syndrome.
Based on personal communication with Eric Kossoff, MD, Johns Hopkins Pediatric Neurology.

b. Educate parents and patient regarding how to live with epilepsy.[10] Review seizure first aid and cardiopulmonary resuscitation. Recommend that child participate in activities, but have supervision during bathing or swimming. Individualize other restrictions. Know driver's license laws in the state. Advocate teacher and school awareness
c. Pharmacotherapy (Table 20-7): Weigh risk for more seizures without therapy against risk for treatment side effects plus residual seizures despite therapy. Reserve pharmacotherapy for recurrent afebrile seizures. Monotherapy may reduce complications; polytherapy increases risk of complications and side effects more than efficacy
d. Ketogenic diet[11]: High-fat, low-carbohydrate therapy used for intractable seizures. Urine ketones can be monitored, and side effects (e.g., acidosis with bicarbonate value as low as 10–15 mEq/L, kidney stones [6%], constipation) can occur

C. Special Seizure Syndromes[12,13,14]

See Table 20-6 for seizure types, etiologies, evaluations, and treatments of many common seizure syndromes. See Figure 20-2 for febrile seizure evaluation guidelines.

V. HYDROCEPHALUS

A. Diagnosis

Assess increasing head circumference, misshapen skull, frontal bossing, bulging large anterior fontanelle, increased ICP (sunset sign, increased tone/reflexes, vomiting, irritability, papilledema), and developmental delay. Obtain head CT if increase in head circumference crosses more than two percentile lines or if patient is symptomatic. Differentiate hydrocephalus from megalencephaly or hydrocephalus ex vacuo.

B. Treatment[15]

1. Medical:
a. Emergently manage acute increase of ICP (see Chapter 4)
b. Slowly progressive hydrocephalus: Acetazolamide may be effective in children age 2 weeks to 10 months with slowly progressive communicating hydrocephalus (see Formulary for dosing)
2. Surgical: Cerebrospinal fluid (CSF) shunting
a. Shunt types: Ventriculoperitoneal (VP) shunts used most commonly. Ventriculoatrial and pleural shunts are associated with cardiac arrhythmias, pleural effusions, and higher rates of infection
b. Shunt complications: Shunt dysfunction may be caused by infection, obstruction (clogging or kinking), disconnection, and migration of proximal and distal tips. Patient will develop signs of increased ICP with shunt malfunction

C. Evaluation of Shunt Integrity

Obtain head CT to evaluate shunt position, ventricular size, and evidence of increased ICP. Obtain shunt series (skull, neck, chest, and abdominal

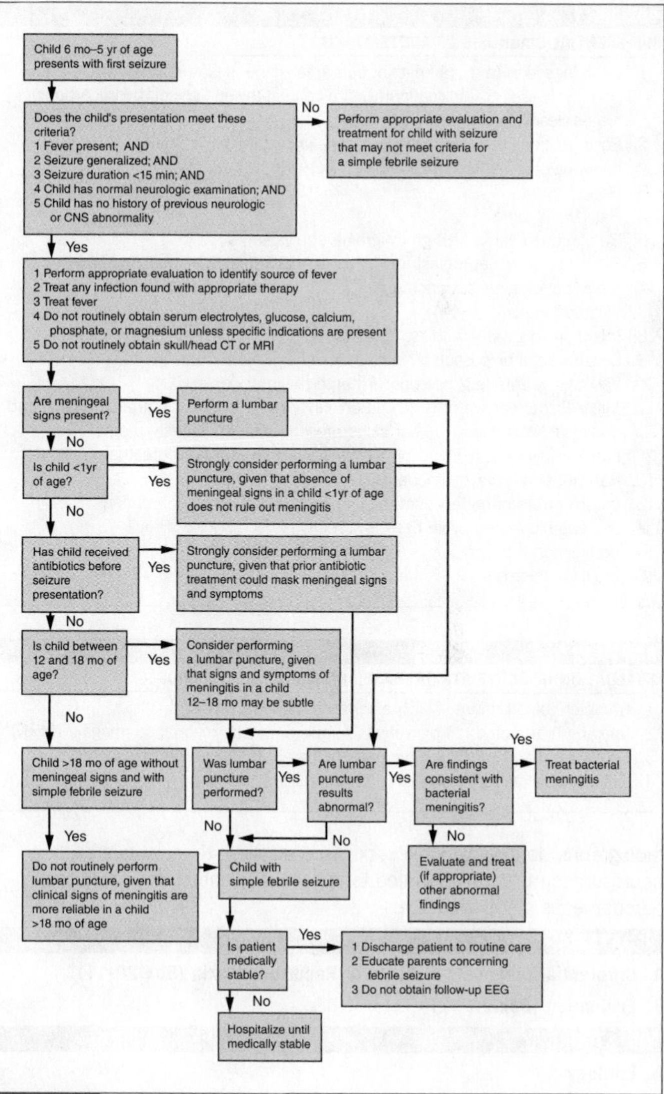

FIGURE 20-2

Guidelines for febrile seizure evaluation.[13]

BOX 20-11

DIFFERENTIAL DIAGNOSIS OF ACUTE ATAXIA

1. Drug ingestion (e.g., phenytoin, carbamazepine, sedatives, hypnotics, and phencyclidine) or intoxication (e.g., alcohol, ethylene glycol, hydrocarbon fumes, lead, mercury, or thallium)
2. Postinfectious (cerebellitis [e.g., varicella], acute disseminated encephalomyelitis)
3. Head trauma
4. Basilar migraine
5. Benign paroxysmal vertigo (migraine equivalent)
6. Brain tumor or neuroblastoma (if accompanied by opsoclonus or myoclonus [i.e., "dancing eyes, dancing feet"])
7. Hydrocephalus
8. Infection (e.g., labyrinthitis, abscess)
9. Seizure (ictal or postictal)
10. Vascular events (e.g., cerebellar hemorrhage or stroke)
11. Miller-Fisher variant of Guillain-Barré syndrome (ataxia, ophthalmoplegia, and areflexia). Warning: If bulbar signs present, disease is likely progressive; patient may lose ability to protect airway and/or ability to breathe
12. Rare inherited paroxysmal ataxias
13. Inborn errors of metabolism (e.g., mitochondrial disorders, amino-acidopathies, urea cycle defects) (See Chapter 13 for workup)
14. Conversion reaction
15. Multiple sclerosis

BOX 20-12

EVALUATION OF ACUTE ATAXIA (BASED ON CLINICAL SCENARIO)

1. Complete blood count (CBC), electrolytes, urine toxicology
2. Imaging (computed tomography [CT] and magnetic resonance imaging [MRI])
3. Lumbar puncture (LP), electroencephalogram (EEG), electromyelography
4. Urine vanillylmandelic acid and homovanillic acid

radiographs) to look for kinking or disconnection. Referral to a neurosurgeon is then warranted to test shunt function and for possible percutaneous shunt drainage.

VI. ATAXIA[16,17]

A. Differential Diagnosis of Acute or Recurrent Ataxia (Box 20-11)

B. Evaluation (Box 20-12)

VII. STROKE[18–21]

A. Etiology

Risk factors for childhood stroke: Include, but are not limited to, congenital heart disease, cerebral arteriopathies, hematologic disorders (most commonly sickle cell disease) including prothrombotic state, serious systemic infection (meningitis, sepsis), head or neck trauma causing arterial dissection, and drugs.

BOX 20-13

DIFFERENTIAL DIAGNOSIS OF ACUTE ONSET HEMIPLEGIA

1. Hemiplegic migraine
2. Focal seizure with postictal (Todd's) paralysis
3. Cervical spinal cord injury (deficits spare the face)
4. Ischemic stroke
5. Hemorrhagic stroke

Based on a personal communication with Lori Jordan, MD, Johns Hopkins Pediatric Neurology.

B. Differential Diagnosis (Box 20-13)

Stroke should be considered in the differential diagnosis for any child who presents with acute-onset focal neurologic deficit, focal seizures with prolonged postictal paralysis, new-onset refractory focal status epilepticus, altered mental status, or unexplained encephalopathy.

C. Initial Workup

1. Acute diagnostic evaluation:
   a. Urgent noncontrast head CT or MRI with susceptibility-weighted image (to exclude hemorrhage) and initial laboratory studies, including CBC, comprehensive metabolic panel, erythrocyte sedimentation rate, prothrombin time, partial thromboplastin time, international normalization ratio, and type and screen (specifically in patients with sickle cell disease) and a urine toxicology screen
   b. MRI with diffusion-weighted imaging and magnetic resonance angiography of the head and neck, may add susceptibility-weighted image to MRI as this sequence identified hemorrhage as well as a head CT
   c. Ideally obtain acutely, but certainly within 24–48 hours
2. Less acute studies:
   a. Echocardiogram and thrombophilia testing
   b. On a case-by-case basis, consider: A fasting lipid panel, rheumatologic and metabolic studies, hemoglobin electrophoresis, and human immunodeficiency virus testing

D. Management

1. There are three published evidence based guidelines that address the evaluation and management of children with stroke. The most comprehensive guidelines are the American Heart Association Guidelines (Roach et al.[20]); this is the only guideline that addresses hemorrhagic stroke
2. Supportive care: Critical and should proceed rapidly and parallel with initial workup. Ensure airway patency, provide supplemental oxygen to maintain SaO_2 >94%, and start maintenance intravenous (IV) fluids
3. Optimize cerebral perfusion pressure: Assure adequate fluid volume and maintenance of median blood pressure for age. Treatment of hypertension is controversial. Unless blood pressure is extremely

elevated, do not use acute antihypertensive therapy because hypertension may be a compensatory reaction to maintain cerebral perfusion

4. Monitoring: Assess neurologic status frequently. Aim for normoglycemia (blood glucose, 60–120 mg/dL). Treat hyperthermia with goal temperature <37°C. Treat seizures aggressively
5. Antiplatelet and anticoagulation therapy: If there is no evidence of hemorrhage, aspirin is typically recommended at a dose of 1–5 mg/kg/day. Anticoagulation with either unfractionated heparin or low molecular weight heparin may be considered on a case-by-case basis, particularly if cardioembolism or arterial dissection is suspected as the etiology of stroke
6. Children with sickle cell disease: Hydration and urgent exchange transfusion to reduce sickle hemoglobin to <30% is recommended. Consult hematology
7. Urgent neurology consultation: Along with transfer to a tertiary care center with expertise in childhood stroke
8. Thrombolytic therapy: Not recommended for children by American Heart Association (AHA) guidelines. Again, neurologic consultation is recommended

REFERENCES

1. Kliegman RM, Behrman RE, Jenson HB, et al. *Nelson textbook of pediatrics,* 18th ed. Philadelphia: Saunders; 2007.
2. Forsyth R, Farrell K. Headache in childhood. *Pediatr Rev.* 1999;20(2):39–45.
3. Olesen J. The international classification of headache disorders, 2nd ed. *J Neurol Neurosurg Psychiatry.* 2004;75(6):808–811.
4. Lewis DW. Practice parameter: evaluation of children and adolescents with recurrent headaches. *Neurology.* 2002;59:490–498.
5. Fishman RA. *Cerebral spinal fluid in diseases of the nervous system.* Philadelphia: WB Saunders; 1992:190.
6. Lewis D. Practice parameter: pharmacological treatment of migraine headache in children and adolescents. *Neurology.* 2004;63:2215–2224.
7. Murphy JV, Dehkharghani F. Diagnosis of childhood seizure disorder. *Epilepsia.* 1994;35(Suppl 2):S7–S17.
8. Committee on Classification and Terminology of the International League against Epilepsy. Classification of epilepsia: its applicability and practical value of different diagnostic categories. *Epilepsia.* 1996;38(11):1051–1059.
9. Hirtz D, Berg A, Bettis D, et al. Practice parameter: treatment of the child with a first unprovoked seizure. *Neurology.* 2003;60:166–175.
10. Freeman JM, Vining EPG, Pillas DJ. *Seizures and epilepsy in childhood: a guide to parents,* 3rd ed. Baltimore: Johns Hopkins University Press; 2000.
11. Freeman J. The ketogenic diet: one decade later. *Pediatrics.* 2007;119: 535–543.
12. American Academy of Pediatrics Subcommittee. Practice parameter: the neurodiagnostic evaluation of the child with a first simple febrile seizure. *Pediatrics.* 1996;97(5):769–772.
13. Baumann RJ, Duffner PK. Treatment of children with simple febrile seizures: the AAP practice parameter. *Pediatr Neurol.* 2000;23(1):11–17.

14. Scher MS. Seizures in the newborn infant: diagnosis, treatment and outcomes. *Clin Perinatol.* 1997;24(4):735–772.
15. Rogers M, ed. *Textbook of pediatric intensive care*, 3rd ed. Baltimore: Williams & Wilkins; 1996.
16. Dinolfo EA. Evaluation of ataxia. *Pediatr Rev.* 2001;22(5):177–178.
17. Ryan M. Acute ataxia in childhood. *J Child Neurol.* 2003;18(5):309–316.
18. Ichord R. Treatment of pediatric neurologic disorders. In: Singer H, et al. eds. *Treatment of pediatric neurologic disorders.* Boca Raton, FL: Taylor & Francis Group; 2005.
19. Monagle P, Chalmers E, Chan AK, et al. Antithrombotic therapy in neonates and children: ACCP evidence-based clinical practice guidelines, 8th ed. *Chest.* 2008;1336(6 Suppl):887S–968S.
20. Roach ES, Golomb M, Adams R, et al. Guidelines on management of stroke in infants and children. *Stroke.* 2008;39(9):2644–2691.
21. United Kingdom Guidelines. Paediatric Stroke Working Group. Stroke in childhood: clinical guidelines for diagnosis, management and rehabilitation, 2004.

Chapter 21

Nutrition and Growth

Brandi Kaye Freeman, MD, and
Jenifer Hampsey, MS, RD, CSP

See additional content on Expert Consult

I. WEBSITES

A. Professional and Government Organizations

Growth Charts and Nutrition Information: http://www.cdc.gov
AAP Children's health topics: Breastfeeding: http://www.aap.org/healthtopics/breastfeeding.cfm
American Dietetic Association: http://www.eatright.org
American Society for Parenteral and Enteral Nutrition: http://www.clinnutr.org
National Institute of Child Health and Human Development: Breastfeeding: http://www.nichd.nih.gov/health/topics/breastfeeding.cfm
U.S. Department of Agriculture healthy eating guidelines: http://www.mypyramid.gov

B. Infant and Pediatric Formula Company Websites for Obtaining Complete and Up-to-Date Product Information

Information regarding more specialized and metabolic formulas can be found using these websites:
Enfamil, EnfaCare, Nutramigen, and Pregestimil: http://www.meadjohnson.com
Carnation, Good Start, Nutren, Peptamen, Vivonex, Boost, and Resource: http://www.nestle-nutrition.com and http://www.nestleinfantnutrition.com
Alimentum, EleCare, Ensure, NeoSure, PediaSure, Pedialyte, and Similac: http://www.abbottnutrition.com
America's Store Brand and Bright Beginnings: http://www.pbmproducts.com
Ketocal, Neocate, and Pepdite: http://www.shsna.com

II. ASSESSMENT OF NUTRITIONAL STATUS

A. Elements of Nutritional Assessment

1. Anthropometric measurements (weight, length/height, head circumference, body mass index [BMI], skin folds): Data are plotted on growth charts according to age and compared with a reference population
2. Clinical assessment (general appearance, including hair, skin, oral mucosa, and gastrointestinal symptoms of nutritional deficiencies)
3. Dietary evaluation (feeding history, current intake)
4. Physical activity and exercise
5. Laboratory findings (comparison with age-based norms)

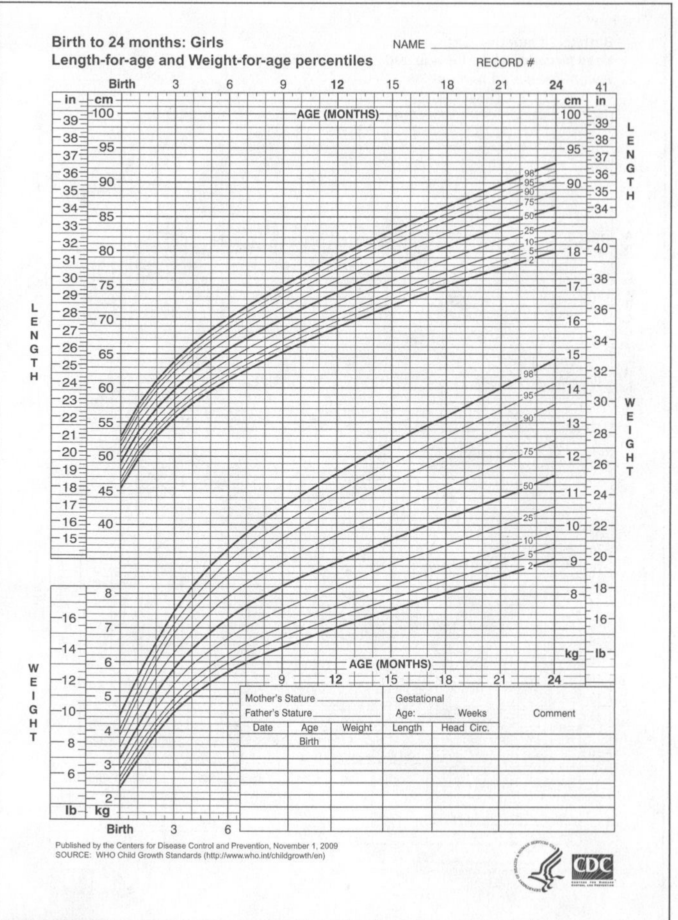

FIGURE 21-1

Length and weight for girls, from birth to age 24 months. *(Published by the Centers for Disease Control and Prevention, November 1, 2009 SOURCE: WHO Child Growth Standards (http://www.who.int/childgrowth/en))*

B. Indicators of Nutritional Status[1] (Growth Charts) (Figs. 21-1, 21-2, 21-3, 21-4, 21-5, 21-6, 21-7, 21-8, and 21-9; Figures EC 21-A to 21-G on Expert Consult)

1. **Growth:** Ideally, should be evaluated over time, but one measurement can be used for screening. Height (or length),

Text continued on page 533

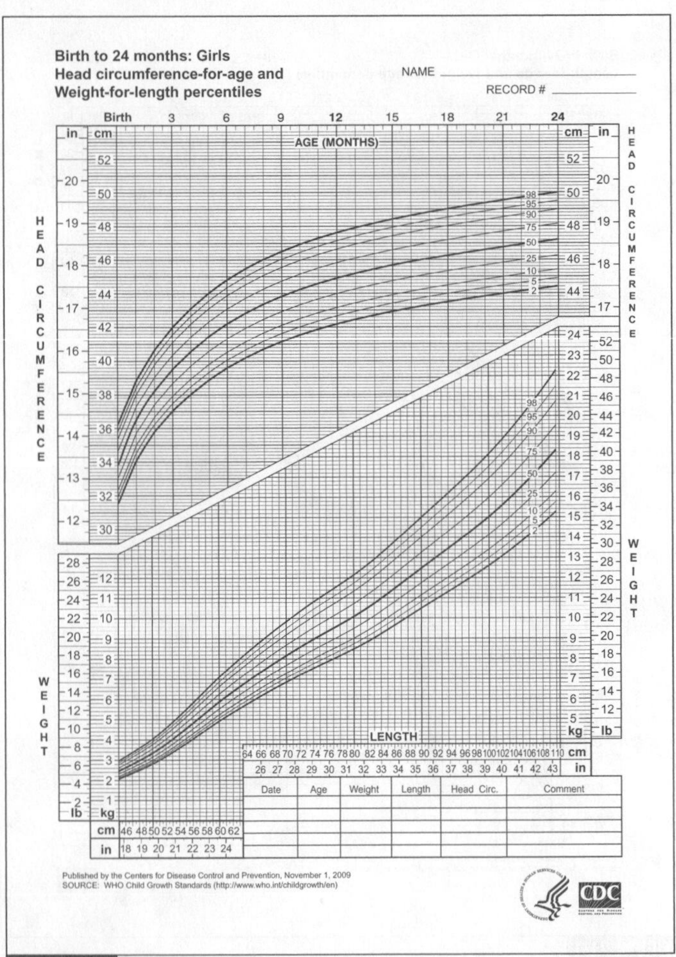

FIGURE 21-2

Head circumference and length-to-weight ratio for girls, from birth to age 24 months. *(Published by the Centers for Disease Control and Prevention, November 1, 2009 SOURCE: WHO Child Growth Standards (http://www.who.int/childgrowth/en))*

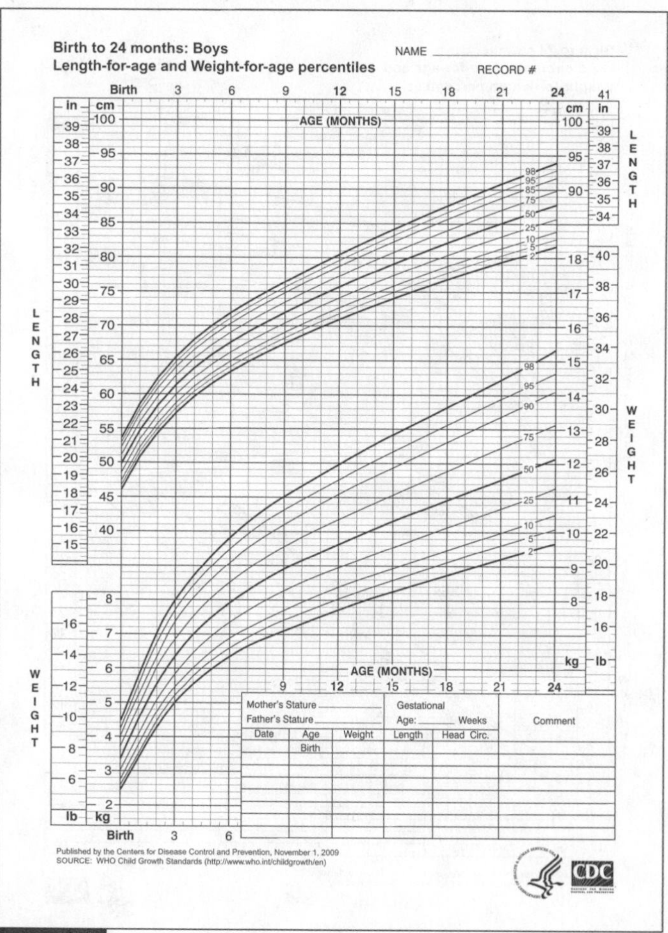

FIGURE 21-3

Length and weight for boys, from birth to age 24 months. *(Published by the Centers for Disease Control and Prevention, November 1, 2009 SOURCE: WHO Child Growth Standards (http://www.who.int/childgrowth/en))*

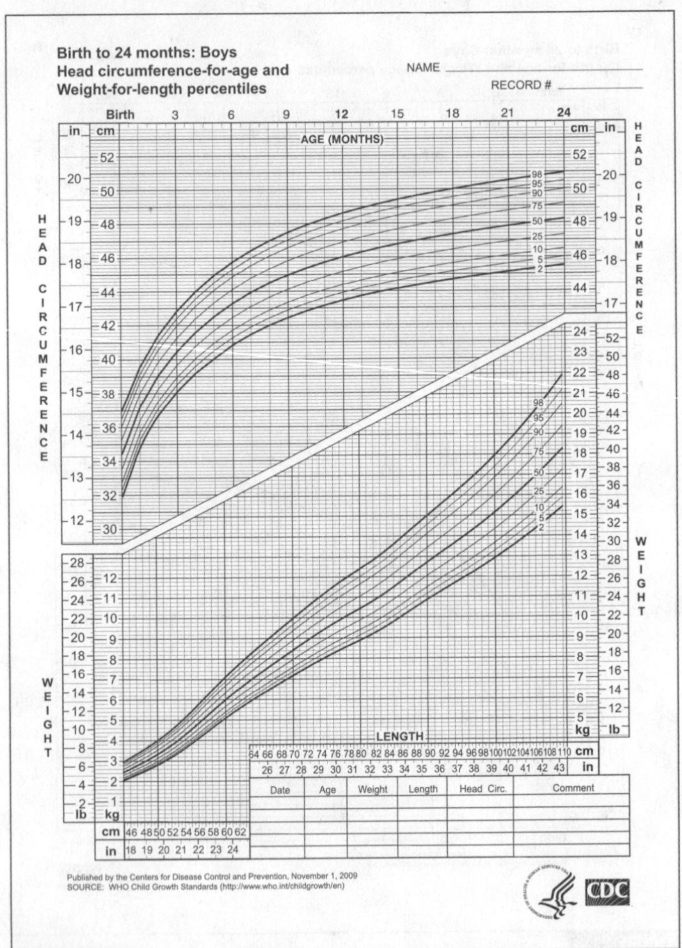

FIGURE 21-4

Head circumference and length-to-weight ratio for boys, from birth to age 24 months. *(Published by the Centers for Disease Control and Prevention, November 1, 2009 SOURCE: WHO Child Growth Standards (http://www.who.int/childgrowth/en))*

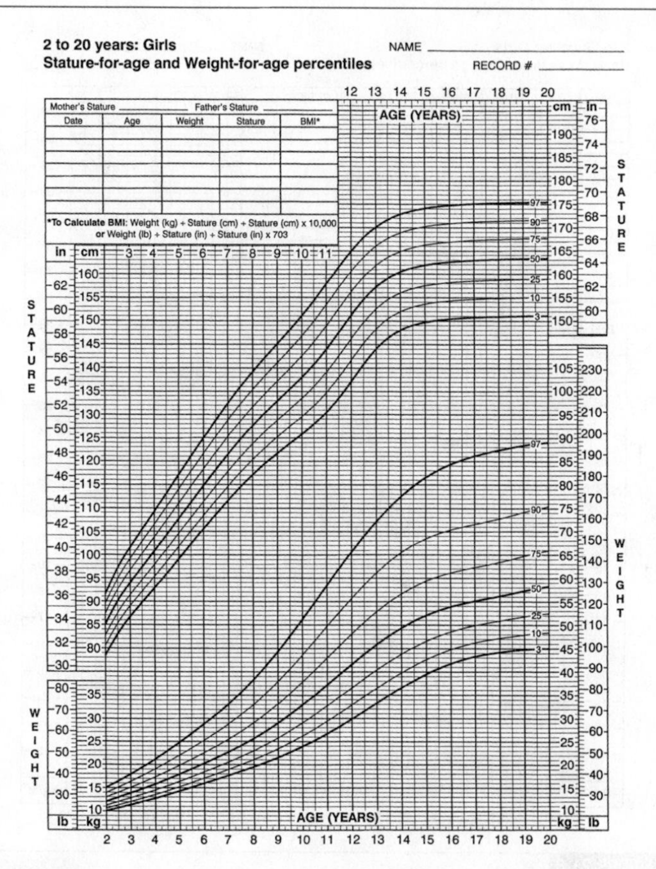

FIGURE 21-5

Stature and weight for girls ages 2–20 years. *(Developed by the National Center for Health Statistics in collaboration with the National Center for Chronic Disease Prevention and Health Promotion, 2000.)*

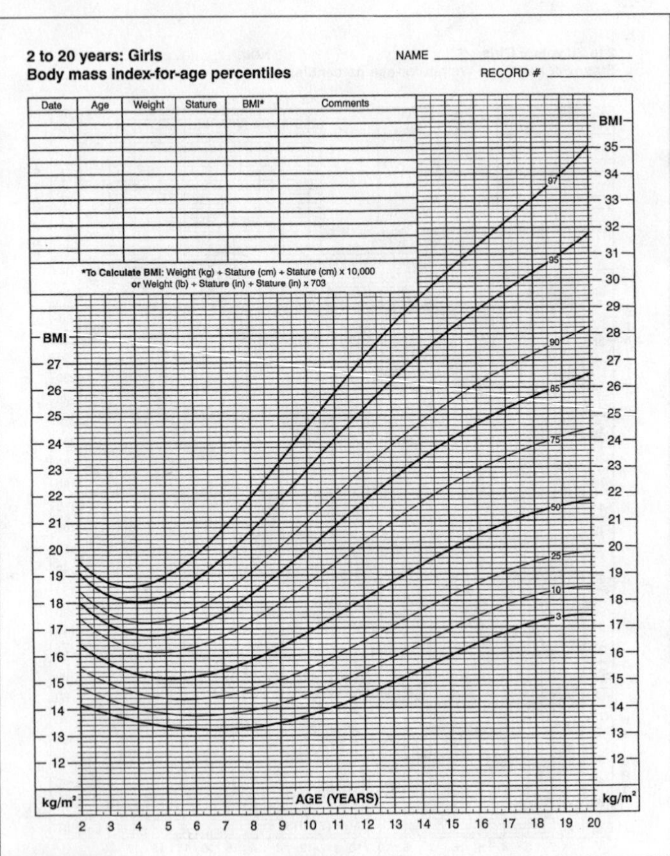

FIGURE 21-6

Body mass index for girls ages 2–20 years. *(Developed by the National Center for Health Statistics in collaboration with the National Center for Chronic Disease Prevention and Health Promotion, 2000.)*

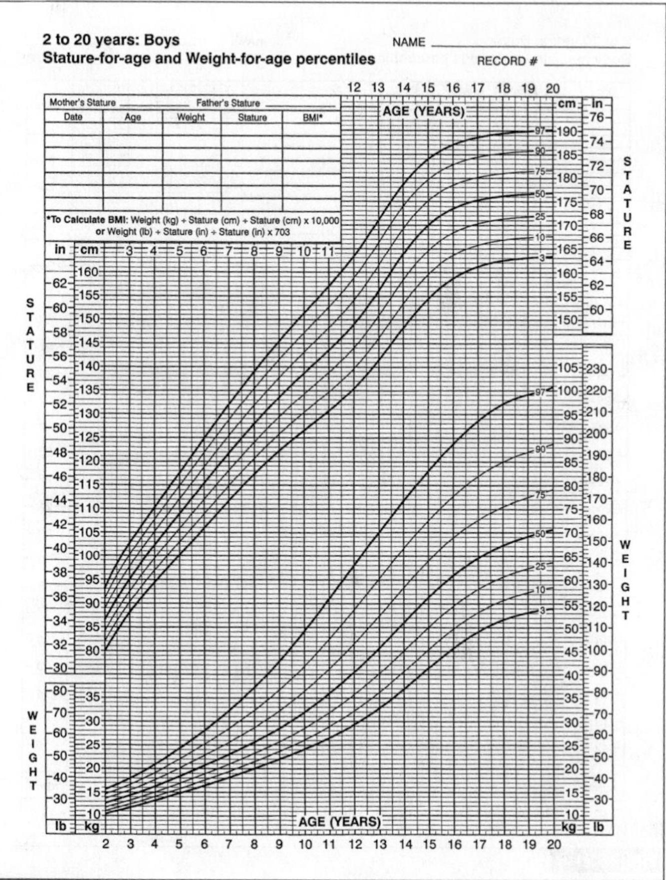

FIGURE 21-7

Stature and weight for boys ages 2–20 years. *(Developed by the National Center for Health Statistics in collaboration with the National Center for Chronic Disease Prevention and Health Promotion, 2000.)*

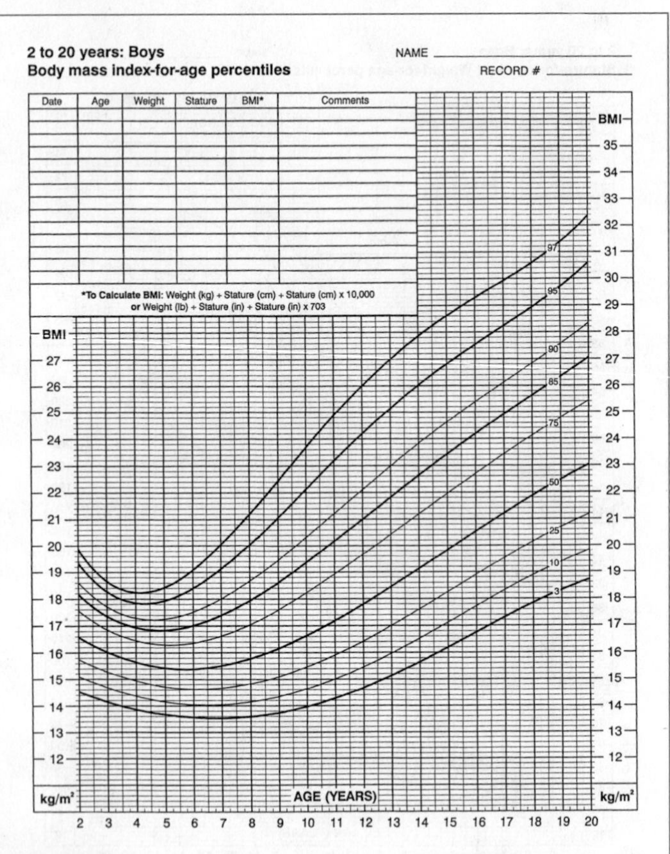

FIGURE 21-8

Body mass index for boys ages 2–20 years. *(Developed by the National Center for Health Statistics in collaboration with the National Center for Chronic Disease Prevention and Health Promotion, 2000.)*

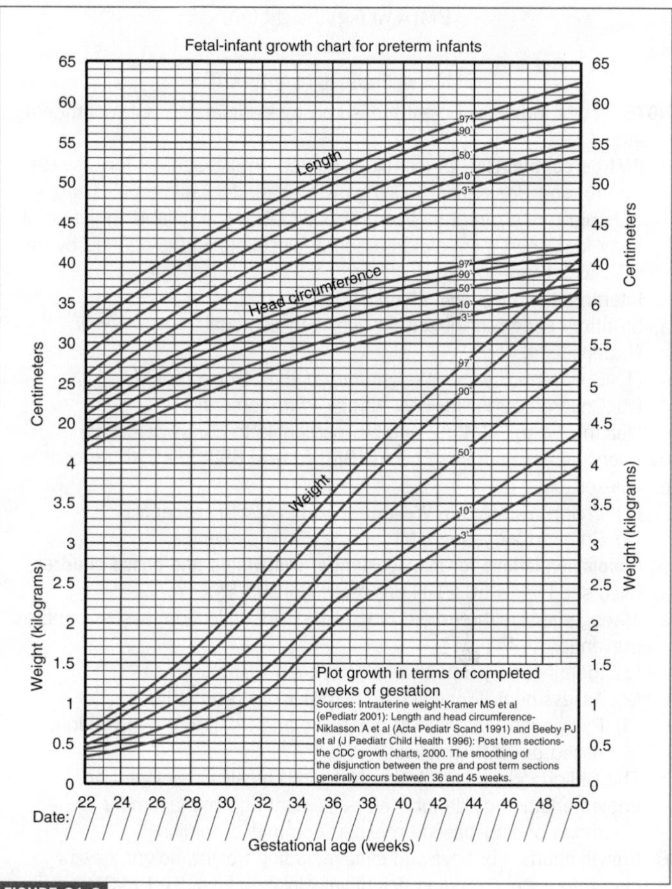

FIGURE 21-9

Length, weight, and head circumference for preterm infants. *(Modified from Fenton TR: A new growth chart for preterm babies: Babson and Benda's chart updated with recent data and new format. BMC Pediatrics 2003;3:13, Fig. 2.)*

weight, and weight for height should be plotted on a growth chart for every patient

2. **BMI:** Defined as an index of healthy weight and as a predictor of morbidity and mortality risk. It is used to classify underweight and overweight individuals.[2] BMI should be determined and plotted for children ≥2 years. Use this formula to calculate BMI:

$$BMI = wt\ (kg)/[height\ (m)]^2$$

or

$$BMI = wt\ (lb)/[height\ (in)]^2 \times 703$$

NOTE: height indicates height measured by stadiometer, not recumbent length

3. **BMI percentile:** BMI percentile is plotted on the Centers for Disease Control and Prevention (CDC) growth charts for children ≥2 years. Although not a direct measure of body fat, it is a reliable indicator of body fatness in most children and adolescents and is defined by the CDC as follows[2]
4. **Interpretation of growth charts:**
   a. Stunting: Length or height for age <5th percentile
   b. Underweight:
      (1) Children <3 years: Weight for length <5th percentile
      (2) Children ≥2 years: BMI for age <5th percentile
   c. Healthy weight: BMI for age 5th percentile to <85th percentile
   d. Overweight: Children >2 years: BMI for age 85th to <95th percentile
   e. Obese:
      (1) Children <3 years: Weight for length >95th percentile
      (2) Children ≥2 years: BMI for age ≥95th percentile
5. **Recommendations for management of overweight and obese children** (also see Figure EC 21-H on Expert Consult)[3,4]
   a. Management is three-tiered focused on identification, assessment, and prevention
      (1) Identification: Calculate BMI at each well-child visit
      (2) Assessment: Medical risk, behavior risk, and attitude
      (3) Prevention: Targeted at behaviors and treatment interventions based on BMI stratification
   b. The Childhood Obesity Action Network has also developed an implementation guide for the assessment and management of childhood obesity based on expert committee opinions[5]
6. **Growth charts:** For boys and girls, including weight, height, head circumference, BMI, and height velocity (see Figs. 21-1 to 21-9 and Figures EC 21-A to 21-G on Expert Consult). CDC recommends that clinicians in the United States use the 2006 WHO international growth charts, rather than the CDC growth charts, for children aged <24 months. Growth charts for children ages 0–20 years including 2000 CDC growth charts for ages 0–36 mo and 2006 WHO growth charts for ages 0–24 mo can be downloaded from http://www.cdc.gov/growthcharts/
7. **Growth charts for special populations:**
   a. Down syndrome: http://www.ndss.org, follow links to healthcare and growth charts (See also Figures EC 21-D to 21-G on Expert Consult)
   b. Turner syndrome: http://aappolicy.aappublications.org/cgi/content/full/pediatrics;111/3/692/F1
   c. Achondroplasia: http://aappolicy.aappublications.org/cgi/content/full/pediatrics;116/3/771

8. **Waist circumference and waist-height ratio:** Both waist circumference (WC) and waist-height ratio are indicators of visceral fat or abdominal obesity in children and adolescents age 2–19 years. Increased visceral adiposity measured by WC increases the risk of obesity-related morbidity and mortality. WC should be measured at the high point of the iliac crest when the individual is standing and at minimal respiration. Waist-height ratio is calculated as a ratio of waist circumference (cm) and height (cm).[6] See CDC waist circumference tables for individuals ages 2–19 years: http://www.cdc.gov/nchs/data/nhsr/nhsr010.pdf, Table 18

III. ESTIMATING ENERGY NEEDS

A. Definitions of Energy Needs[2]

1. **Basal metabolic rate (BMR):** Rate of energy expenditure after an overnight fast, resting comfortably, supine, awake, and motionless in a thermoneutral environment
2. **Basal energy expenditure (BEE):** BMR over 24 hours
3. **Thermic effect of food (TEF):** Increase in energy expenditure elicited by food consumption
4. **Energy deposition:** Energy requirement for growth
5. **Total energy expenditure (TEE):** Sum of BEE, TEF, physical activity, thermoregulation, and the energy expended in depositing new tissues and/or in producing milk
6. **Physical activity level (PAL):** Ratio of total to basal daily energy expenditure (TEE/BEE). Describes and accounts for physical activity habits
7. **Physical activity coefficient (PA):** The physical activity coefficient that correlates with PAL (Table 21-1) can be used to calculate estimated energy requirements (EER; see Section III.B)

B. Estimated Energy Requirements[2]

1. **EER:** Dietary energy intake that is predicted to maintain energy balance in a healthy individual. In children, it includes the needs associated

TABLE 21-1

PHYSICAL ACTIVITY COEFFICIENTS

	Sedentary Activity (Physical Activity Levels Required for Independent Living)	Low Active (30–45 min Sustained Daily Activity)	Active (60 min Sustained Daily Activity)	Very Active (≥90 min Sustained Daily Activity)
PAL	≥1.0 but <1.4	≥1.4 but <1.6	≥1.6 but <1.9	≥1.9 but <2.5
PA (boys ages 3–18)	1.00	1.13	1.26	1.42
PA (girls ages 3–18)	1.00	1.16	1.31	1.56

PA, Physical activity coefficient; PAL, physical activity level.

with growth. For most healthy infants and children, the equations here can be used to determine energy needs.

a. For infants, children, and adolescents, EER (kcal/day) = TEE + energy deposition
b. For most hospitalized patients, it can be assumed PAL = sedentary, PA = 1

2. **EER equations (calculate calories/day):**

a. **Infants and young children:**
   (1) 0–3 months: EER = (89 × weight [kg] – 100) + 175
   (2) 4–6 months: EER = (89 × weight [kg] – 100) + 56
   (3) 7–12 months: EER = (89 × weight [kg] – 100) + 22
   (4) 13–35 months: EER = (89 × weight [kg] – 100) + 20

b. **Boys ages 3–18:**
   (1) 3–8 years: EER = 88.5 – (61.9 × age (yr)) + (PA × 26.7 × weight [kg]) + (903 × height [m]) + 20
   (2) 9–18 years: EER = 88.5 – (61.9 × age (yr)) + (PA × 26.7 × weight [kg]) + (903 × height [m]) + 25

c. **Girls ages 3–18:**
   (1) 3–8 years: EER = 135.3 – (30.8 × age (yr)) + (PA × 10 × weight [kg]) + (934 × height [m]) + 20
   (2) 9–18 years: EER = 135.3 – (30.8 × age (yr)) + (PA × 10 × weight [kg]) + (934 × height [m]) + 25

d. **Pregnancy (14–18 years):** EER = adolescent EER + pregnancy energy deposition:
   (1) First trimester = adolescent EER + 0 kcal
   (2) Second trimester = adolescent EER + 340 kcal
   (3) Third trimester = adolescent EER + 452 kcal

e. **Lactation (14–18 years):** EER = adolescent EER + milk energy output – weight loss:
   (1) First 6 months adolescent EER + 500 – 170
   (2) Second 6 months = adolescent EER + 400 – 0

3. Table 21-2[2] contains the estimated EER for healthy boys and girls of median weight (weight for age at 50th percentile) at both sedentary and active PAL levels

C. EER under Stressed Conditions[7]

Calculation of BEE: In many cases, there is little need to provide critically ill patients with more than their BEE. Ideally, energy expenditure should be measured in critically ill patients, but this requires expensive equipment and may not always be practical. Numerous prediction equations are available. The following equation is from the *Dietary Reference Intakes*[7]:

For boys: BEE (kcal/d) = 68 – (43.3 × age (yr)) + (712 × height (m)) + (19.2 × weight (kg))

For girls: BEE (kcal/d) = 189 – (17.6 × age (yr)) + (625 × height (m)) + (7.9 × weight (kg))

TABLE 21-2

SAMPLE ESTIMATED ENERGY REQUIREMENTS FOR HEALTHY BOYS AND GIRLS OF MEDIAN WEIGHT AND HEIGHT*

Age	Boys EER (kcal/kg/day)	Girls EER (kcal/kg/day)
0–2 mo	107	104
3 mo	95	95
4–35 mo	82	82

	Boys			Girls		
	Median Weight, Boys (kg)	Sedentary† (kcal/kg/d)	Active† (kcal/kg/d)	Median Weight, Girls (kg)	Sedentary† (kcal/kg/d)	Active† (kcal/kg/d)
3 yr	14.3	80	104	13.9	76	100
4 yr	16.2	74	97	15.8	70	93
5 yr	18.4	68	90	17.9	65	87
6 yr	20.7	63	84	20.2	61	81
7 yr	23.1	59	80	22.8	56	75
8 yr	25.6	56	75	25.6	52	71
9 yr	28.6	53	71	29.0	48	65
10 yr	31.9	49	67	32.9	44	60
11 yr	35.9	46	63	37.2	41	56
12 yr	40.5	44	60	41.6	38	52
13 yr	45.6	42	57	45.8	36	50
14 yr	51.0	40	55	49.4	34	47
15 yr	56.3	39	54	52.0	33	45
16 yr	60.9	38	52	53.9	32	44
17 yr	64.6	36	50	55.1	31	43
18 yr	67.2	35	49	56.2	30	42

*Weight and height for age at 50th percentile.

†See definition of sedentary and active PAL for further information.

EER, Estimated energy requirements.

From Otten JJ, Hellwig JP, Meyers LD (eds): Dietary reference intakes: the essential guide to nutrient requirements. Washington, DC, National Academies Press, 2006.

Appropriate changes should be made as indicated by real (not fluid) weight gain and signs and symptoms of overfeeding.

D. Catch-up Growth Requirement for Malnourished Infants and Children (<3 years)[8,9]

1. **Growth failure** (also known as failure to thrive): Condition of undernutrition generally identified in the first 3 years of life. Can be described by the following growth scenarios: weight for age <5th percentile on the CDC growth charts, weight for length (or height) <5th percentile, or decreased growth velocity resulting in weight falling >2 major percentiles over 3–6 months (**NOTE:** WHO growth charts have been very recently recommended by the CDC for children <24 mo and one may consider using these charts to define growth failure)
2. **Catch-up growth:** Time period of accelerated growth as a result of caloric provision in excess of the recommended dietary allowances (RDAs).

BOX 21-1

DETERMINING CATCH-UP GROWTH REQUIREMENTS

1. Plot the child's height and weight on CDC growth charts.
2. Determine recommended calories needed for age (recommended dietary allowances [RDA]).
3. Determine the ideal weight (50th percentile) for child's height.*
4. Multiply the RDA calories by ideal body weight for height (kg).
5. Divide this value by the child's actual weight (kg).

For example, for a 12-month-old boy whose weight is 7 kg and length is 72 cm, RDA for age would be 98 kcal/kg/day and ideal body weight for height is 9 kg (50th percentile weight for height). Thus, his catch-up growth requirement would be as follows:

$$98 \text{ kcal/kg/day} \times (9 \text{ kg}/7 \text{ kg}) = 126 \text{ kcal/kg/day}$$

*The ideal weight can be 10th–85th percentile weight for height, depending on past growth trends; clinical judgment should be used.

Approximately 20%–30% more energy may be required to achieve catch-up growth in children. Protein needs also increase. This should continue until the previous growth percentiles are regained. Catch-up in linear growth may lag several months behind that in weight. Box 21-1 lists the steps for determining catch-up growth requirements

NOTE: Aggressive refeeding in the severely malnourished child can result in metabolic alterations, vomiting, diarrhea, and circulatory decompensation known as refeeding syndrome (hypophosphatemia, hypokalemia, hypomagnesemia, and glucose and/or fluid intolerance).[10]

IV. DIETARY REFERENCE INTAKES FOR INDIVIDUALS[7]

A. Dietary Reference Intakes (DRI)

Reference values that are quantitative estimates of nutrient intakes and are measured in several ways, including the following:

1. **Estimated average requirement (EAR):** Daily nutrient intake level estimated to meet the requirement of half the healthy individuals in a particular life stage and gender group
2. **Recommended dietary allowance (RDA):** EAR ±2 standard deviations. The daily nutrient intake level estimated to meet the requirement of 97%–98% of healthy individuals in a particular life stage and gender group
3. **Adequate intake (AI):** Observed range of intakes in a healthy population used when there are not sufficient data to calculate the EAR and RDA
4. **Tolerable upper intake level (UL):** Highest daily nutrient intake level that is likely to pose no risk for adverse health effects to almost all individuals in the general population

B. Protein Requirements (Table 21-3)[7]

C. Fat Requirements (Table 21-4)[7]

D. Vitamin Requirements (Table 21-5)[7]

TABLE 21-3

PROTEIN REQUIREMENTS

Age	RDA (g/kg/day)
0–6 mo	1.52 (AI)*
7–12 mo	1.2
1–3 yr	1.05
4–8 yr	0.95
9–13 yr	0.95
14–18 yr	0.85
Pregnancy (first half)	Unchanged
Pregnancy (second half)	1.1
Lactation	1.3

*If sufficient scientific evidence is not available to establish an RDA (recommended dietary allowance), an AI (adequate intake) is usually developed. For healthy breast-fed infants, the AI is the mean intake.

From Otten JJ, Hellwig JP, Meyers LD (eds): Dietary reference intakes: the essential guide to nutrient requirements. Washington, DC, National Academies Press, 2006.

TABLE 21-4

FAT REQUIREMENTS: ADEQUATE INTAKE (AI)*

Age	Total Fat (g/day)	Linoleic Acid (g/day)	α-Linolenic Acid (g/day)
0–6 mo	31	4.4 (n-6 PUFA)	0.5 (n-3 PUFA)
7–12 mo	30	4.6 (n-6 PUFA)	0.5 (n-3 PUFA)
1–3 yr	†	7	0.7
4–8 yr	†	10	0.9
9–13 yr, boys	†	12	1.2
9–13 yr, girls	†	10	1.0
14–18 yr, boys	†	16	1.6
14–18 yr, girls	†	11	1.1
Pregnancy	†	13	1.4
Lactation	†	13	1.3

*If sufficient scientific evidence is not available to establish an recommended dietary allowance (RDA), an AI is usually developed. For healthy breast-fed infants, the AI is the mean intake. The AI for other life stage and gender groups is believed to cover the needs of all healthy individuals in the group, but a lack of data or uncertainty in the data prevents being able to specify with confidence the percentage of individuals covered by this intake.

†No AI, estimated average requirement (EAR), or RDA established.

PUFA, polyunsaturated fatty acid.

From Otten JJ, Hellwig JP, Meyers LD (eds): Dietary reference intakes: the essential guide to nutrient requirements. Washington, DC, National Academies Press, 2006.

E. Mineral Requirements (Table 21-6)[7]

F. Fiber Requirements (Table 21-7)[7]

V. VITAMIN-MINERAL SUPPLEMENTATION[11]

A. Vitamin D[8]

1. 400 IU per day recommended for the following: All infants consuming <1,000 mL/day of vitamin D–fortified formula or cow's milk (whether breast or formula-fed)

Text continued on page 544

TABLE 21-5

DIETARY REFERENCE INTAKES: RECOMMENDED INTAKES FOR INDIVIDUALS—VITAMINS

Life Stage	Vit. A[a] (IU)	Vit. C (mg/day)	Vit. D[b,c] (IU)	Vit. E[d] (IU)	Vit. K (mcg/day)	Thiamin (mg/day)	Riboflavin (mg/day)
INFANTS							
0–6 mo	**1,333**	40*	400	4*	2.0*	0.2*	0.3*
7–12 mo	**1,666**	50*	400	5*	2.5*	0.3*	0.4*
CHILDREN							
1–3 yr	**1,000**	**15**	600	**6**	30*	**0.5**	**0.5**
4–8 yr	**1,333**	**25**	600	**7**	55*	**0.6**	**0.6**
MALES							
9–13 yr	**2,000**	**45**	600	**11**	60*	**0.9**	**0.9**
14–18 yr	**3,000**	**75**	600	**15**	75*	**1.2**	**1.3**
19–30 yr	**3,000**	**90**	600	**15**	120*	**1.2**	**1.3**
FEMALES							
9–13 yr	**2,000**	**45**	600	**11**	60*	**0.9**	**0.9**
14–18 yr	**2,333**	**65**	600	**15**	75*	**1.0**	**1.0**
19–30 yr	**2,333**	**75**	600	**15**	90*	**1.1**	**1.1**
PREGNANCY							
<18 yr	**2,500**	**80**	600	**15**	75*	**1.4**	**1.4**
19–30 yr	**2,567**	**85**	600	**15**	90*	**1.4**	**1.4**
LACTATION							
<18 yr	**4,000**	**115**	600	**19**	75*	**1.4**	**1.6**
19–30 yr	**4,333**	**120**	600	**19**	90*	**1.4**	**1.6**

NOTE: This table (taken from the DRI reports; see www.nap.edu) presents recommended dietary allowances (RDAs) in **bold type** and adequate intakes (AIs) in regular type followed by an asterisk (*), RDAs and AIs may both be used as goals for individual intake. RDAs are set to meet the needs of almost all (97%–98%) individuals in a group. For healthy breast-fed infants, the AI is the mean intake. The AI for other life stage and gender groups is believed to cover needs of all individuals in the group, but lack of data or uncertainty in the data prevent being able to specify with confidence the percentage of individuals covered by this intake.

[a]One IU = 0.3 mcg retinol equivalent.

[b]One mcg cholecalciferol = 40 IU vitamin D.

[c]In the absence of adequate exposure to sunlight.

[d]One IU = 1 mg vitamin E.

Niacin[e] (mg/day)	Vit. B_6 (mg/day)	Folate[f] (mcg/day)	Vit. B_{12} (mcg/day)	Pantothenic Acid (mg/day)	Biotin (mcg/day)	Choline[g] (mg/day)
2*	0.1*	65*	0.4*	1.7*	5*	125*
4*	0.3*	80*	0.5*	1.8*	6*	150*
6	**0.5**	**150**	0.9	2*	8*	200*
8	**0.6**	**200**	1.2	3*	12*	250*
12	**1.0**	**300**	1.8	4*	20*	375*
16	**1.3**	**400**	2.4	5*	25*	550*
16	**1.3**	**400**	2.4	5*	30*	550*
12	**1.0**	**300**	1.8	4*	20*	375*
14	**1.2**	**400**	2.4	5*	25*	400*
14	**1.3**	**400**	2.4	5*	30*	425*
18	**1.9**	**600**	2.6	6*	30*	450*
18	**1.9**	**600**	2.6	6*	30*	450*
17	**2.0**	**500**	2.8	7*	35*	550*
17	**2.0**	**500**	2.8	7*	35*	550*

[e]As niacin equivalents (NE). 1 mg of niacin = 60 mg of tryptophan; 0–6 months = preformed niacin (not NE).

[f]As dietary folate equivalents (DFE). 1 DFE = 1 mcg food folate = 0.6 mcg of folic acid from fortified food or as a supplement consumed with food = 0.5 mcg of a supplement taken on an empty stomach. In view of evidence linking folate intake with neural tube defects in the fetus, it is recommended that all women capable of becoming pregnant consume 400 mcg from supplements or fortified foods in addition to intake of food folate from a varied diet. It is assumed that women will continue consuming 400 mcg from supplements or fortified food until their pregnancy is confirmed and they enter prenatal care, which ordinarily occurs after the end of the periconceptual period—the critical time for formation of the neural tube.

[g]Although AIs have been set for choline, there are few data to assess whether a dietary supply of choline is needed at all life stages, and it may be that the choline requirement can be met by endogenous synthesis at some of these stages.

Modified from Otten JJ, Hellwig JP, Meyers LD (eds): Dietary reference intakes: the essential guide to nutrient requirements. Washington, DC, National Academies Press, 2006.

TABLE 21-6

DIETARY REFERENCE INTAKES: RECOMMENDED INTAKES—ELEMENTS

Life Stage	Calcium (mg/day)	Chromium (mcg/day)	Copper (mcg/day)	Fluoride (mg/day)	Iodine (mcg/day)	Iron (mg/day)
INFANTS						
0–6 mo	210*	0.2*	200*	0.01*	110*	0.27*
7–12 mo	270*	5.5*	220*	0.5*	130*	**11**
CHILDREN						
1–3 yr	500*	11*	**340**	0.7*	**90**	**7**
4–8 yr	800*	15*	**440**	1.0*	**90**	**10**
MALES						
9–13 yr	1,300*	25*	**700**	2*	**120**	**8**
14–18 yr	1,300*	35*	**890**	3*	**150**	**11**
19–30 yr	1,000*	35*	**900**	4*	**150**	**8**
FEMALES						
9–13 yr	1,300*	21*	**700**	2*	**120**	**8**
14–18 yr	1,300*	24*	**890**	3*	**150**	**15**
19–30 yr	1,000*	25*	**900**	3*	**150**	**18**
PREGNANCY						
<18 yr	1,300*	29*	**1,000**	3*	**220**	**27**
19–30 yr	1,000*	30*	**1,000**	3*	**220**	**27**
LACTATION						
<18 yr	1,300*	44*	**1,300**	3*	**290**	**10**
19–30 yr	1,000*	45*	1,300	3*	290	9

NOTE: This table presents recommended dietary allowances (RDAs) in **bold type** and adequate intakes (AIs) in ordinary type followed by an asterisk (*). RDAs and AIs may both be used as goals for individual intake. RDAs are set to meet the needs of almost all (97%–98%) individuals in a group. For healthy breast-fed infants, the AI is the mean intake. The AI for other life stage and gender groups is believed to cover needs of all individuals in the group, but lack of data or uncertainty in the data prevent being able to specify with confidence the percentage of individuals covered by this intake.

Modified from Otten JJ, Hellwig JP, Meyers LD (eds): Dietary reference intakes: the essential guide to nutrient requirements. Washington, DC, National Academies Press, 2006.

Magnesium (mg/day)	Manganese (mg/day)	Molybdenum (mcg/day)	Phosphorus (mg/day)	Selenium (mcg/day)	Zinc (mg/day)
30*	0.003*	2*	100*	15*	2*
75*	0.6*	3*	275*	20*	**3**
80	1.2*	**17**	**460**	**20**	**3**
130	1.5*	**22**	**500**	**30**	**5**
240	1.9*	**34**	**1,250**	**40**	**8**
410	2.2*	**43**	**1,250**	**55**	**11**
400	2.3*	**45**	**700**	**55**	**11**
240	1.6*	**34**	**1,250**	**40**	**8**
360	1.6*	**43**	**1,250**	**55**	**9**
310	1.8*	**45**	**700**	**55**	**8**
400	2.0*	**50**	**1,250**	**60**	**13**
350	2.0*	**50**	**700**	**60**	**11**
360	2.6*	**50**	**1,250**	**70**	**14**
310	2.6*	50	700	70	12

TABLE 21-7

FIBER REQUIREMENTS: ADEQUATE INTAKE*

Age	Total Fiber (g/day)
0–12 mo	Not determined
1–3 yr	19
4–8 yr	25
9–13 yr, boys	31
9–13 yr, girls	26
14–18 yr, boys	38
14–18 yr, girls	26
Pregnancy	28
Lactation	29

*Adequate intake (AI). If sufficient scientific evidence is not available to establish a recommended dietary allowance (RDA), an AI is usually developed. For healthy breast-fed infants, the AI is the mean intake. The AI for other life stages and gender groups is believed to cover the needs of all healthy individuals in the group, but a lack of data or uncertainty in the data prevents being able to specify with confidence the percentage of individuals covered by this intake.

Modified from Otten JJ, Hellwig JP, Meyers LD (eds): Dietary reference intakes: the essential guide to nutrient requirements. Washington, DC, National Academies Press, 2006.

2. 600 IU per day recommended for the following: Children and adolescents who do not get regular sunlight exposure, do not ingest 1,000 mL/day of vitamin D–fortified milk, or do not take a daily multivitamin supplement containing at least 600 IU of vitamin D. Generally, an A, D, C multivitamin, such as Tri-Vi-Sol or Poly-Vi-Sol, can be used (Table 21-8)

B. Fluoride

1. Supplementation not needed during the first 6 months of life. Thereafter, 0.5 mg/day is recommended for exclusively breast-fed infants
2. Consider supplementation for those patients who use bottled water and home filtration systems. Most bottled water does not contain adequate amounts of fluoride. Some home water treatment systems can reduce fluoride levels
3. To avoid fluorosis, children should not use fluoridated toothpaste until age 2 years, and then only a small pea-sized amount up to age 6 years. See Formulary for complete fluoride recommendations (i.e., in areas where water is not fluoridated)

C. Iron

1. **Breast-fed infants:**

a. Full-term breast-fed infants: ~1 mg/kg/day is recommended after age 4–6 months, preferably from iron-fortified cereal or alternatively, elemental iron

b. Preterm or low-birth-weight breast-fed infants: Iron supplement of 2 mg/kg/day should be given from age 2–12 months

c. All infants younger than 12 months: Only formula fortified with iron should be used for weaning or supplementing breast milk

TABLE 21-8

INFANT MULTIVITAMIN DROPS ANALYSIS (PER ML)*

Nutrient	Poly-Vi-Sol/ [w/iron], Multivitamin [with iron]	Tri-Vi-Sol[w/iron]	AquADEKs[†‡]	D Vi-Sol	Fer-In-Sol
Vitamin A (IU)	1500	1500	5751	—	—
Vitamin D (IU)	400	400	400	400	—
Vitamin E (IU)	5	—	50	—	—
Vitamin C (mg)	35	35	45	—	—
Thiamin (mg)	0.5	—	0.6	—	—
Riboflavin (mg)	0.6	—	0.6	—	—
Niacin (mg)	8	—	6	—	—
Vitamin B_6 (mg)	0.4	—	0.6	—	—
Vitamin B_{12} (mcg)	2	—	—	—	—
Vitamin K (mcg)	—	—	400	—	—
Iron (mg)	[10]	[10]	—	—	—
Fluoride (mg)	—	—	—	—	15
Zinc (mg)	—	—	5	—	—

*Standard dose = 1 mL.

[†]Also contains biotin 15 mcg; pantothenic acid 3 mg; 87% vitamin A as β-carotene; Coenzyme Q_{10} 2 mg; Selenium 10 mcg.

[‡]Recommended for use in infants with fat malabsorption, such as cystic fibrosis, liver disease.

2. **Formula-fed infants:**
   a. Full-term formula-fed infants: Iron-fortified formula containing 4–12 mg/L of iron from birth to age 12 months
   b. Preterm formula-fed infants: An additional 1 mg/kg/day, administered either as iron drops or in a vitamin preparation with iron

D. Examples of Multivitamins for Infants and Children (Table 21-8 and Table 21-9)

VI. ENTERAL NUTRITION

A. Mixing Instructions for Full-term Standard and Soy-based Infant Formulas (Table 21-10)

B. Common Caloric Modulars

For the child who needs additional protein, carbohydrate, fat, or a combination (Table 21-11)

C. Enteral Formulas, Including Their Main Nutrient Components (Table 21-12)

A comprehensive (but not complete) list. Most of these formulas are cow's milk–based and are designed for normal digestive tracts

D. Clinical Conditions Requiring Special Diets, and Suggested Formula(s) (Table 21-13)

A comprehensive (but not complete) list of special clinical conditions (e.g., cow's milk allergy or intolerance) and the growing number of formulas designed for these conditions

E. Common Oral Rehydration Solutions (Table 21-14)

Text continued on page 560

TABLE 21-9

MULTIVITAMIN TABLETS (ANALYSIS/TABLET)

	Flintstones Sour Gummies	Centrum Kids Complete	Flintstones Complete	Centrum Tablet[+]	ADEK (chewable)	AquADEKs (softgel)	Source CF (chewable)	Vitamax (chewable)	Phlexy-Vits (7g packet)
Vitamin A (IU)	1,000	3,500	3,000	3,500	9,000[a]	18,167	16,000[b]	5,000[c]	2,664
Vitamin D (IU)	100	400	400	400	400	800	1,000	400	400
Vitamin E (IU)	10	30	30	30	150	150	200	200	13.5
Vitamin K (mcg)	—	10	—	25	150	700	800	200	70
Vitamin C (mg)	15	60	60	60	60	75	100	60	50
Thiamin (mg)	—	1.5	1.5	1.5	1.2	1.5	1.5	1.5	1.2
Riboflavin (mg)	—	1.7	1.7	1.7	1.3	1.7	1.7	1.7	1.4
Niacin (mg)	—	20	15	20	10	20	10	20	20
Vitamin B_6 (mg)	0.5	2	2	2	1.5	1.9	1.9	2	1.6
Folate (mcg)	100	400	400	400	200	200	200	200	700
Vitamin B_{12} (mcg)	2.5	6	6	6	12	12	6	6	5
Biotin (mcg)	38	45	40	30	50	100	100	300	150
Pantothenic acid (mg)	2.5	10	10	10	10	12	12	10	5
Calcium (mg)	—	108	100	200	—	—	—	—	1,000
Phosphorus (mg)	—	50	100	20	—	—	—	—	775
Iron (mg)	—	18	18	18	—	—	—	—	15.1
Iodine (mcg)	20	150	150	150	—	—	—	—	150

Magnesium (mg)	—	40	20	50	—	—	—	—	300
Zinc (mg)	1.2	15	12	11	7.5	10	15	7.5	11.1
Copper (mg)	—	2	2	0.5	—	—	—	—	1.5
Manganese (mg)	—	1	—	2.3	—	—	—	—	1.5
Chromium (mcg)	—	20	—	35	—	—	—	—	30
Molybdenum (mcg)	—	20	—	45	—	—	—	—	70
Selenium (mcg)	—	—	—	55	—	75	—	—	75
Fluoride (mg)	—	—	—	—	—	—	—	—	—
Choline (mg)	38	—	38	—		—			—
Sodium (mg)	—	—	10	—		—			8.8
Potassium (mg)	—	—	—	80		—			<1.4
Chloride	—	—	—	72		—			<0.35

[+]Contains boron, nickel, silicon, tin
[a]Vitamin A as palmitate and 60% β-carotene.
[b]Vitamin A: 88% beta-carotene, 12% Palmitate
[c]Vitamin A as acetate and 50% β-carotene.

TABLE 21-10

PREPARATION OF INFANT FORMULAS FOR FULL-TERM STANDARD AND SOY FORMULAS*

Formula Type	Caloric Concentration (kcal/oz)	Amount of Formula	Water (oz)
Liquid concentrates (40 kcal/oz)	20	13 oz	13 oz
	24	13 oz	8.5 oz
	27	13 oz	6.3 oz
	30	13 oz	4.3 oz
Powder (44 kcal/scoop)	20	1 scoop	2 oz
	24	3 scoops	5 oz
	27	3 scoops	4.25 oz
	30	3 scoops	4 oz

*Does not apply to Enfacare LIPIL, Neocate Infant, Neosure Advance, Elecare; Enfamil AR should not be concentrated greater than 24kcal/oz. Use a packed measure for Nutramigen LIPIL and Pregestimil LIPIL; all others unpacked powder.

TABLE 21-12

ENTERAL NUTRITION COMPONENTS (PER LITER)

A. INFANT FORMULAS

	Kcal/oz	Protein (g)	Fat (g)
HUMAN MILK			
Term	20	11	39
Pre-term	20	14	39
HUMAN MILK AND FORTIFIERS ANALYSIS			
Enfamil HMF + Preterm Human Milk (1 pkt/25 mL)	24	25	49
Similac HMF + Preterm Human Milk (1 pkt/25 mL)	24	23	41
PRETERM FORMULAS			
Enfamil Premature LIPIL	20	20	34
Neosure	22	21	41
Enfacare LIPIL	22	21	39
Good Start Premature 24	24	24	42
Similac Special Care 20	20	20	37
Similac Special Care 24 High Protein	24	27	44
Similac Special Care 30	30	30	67

TABLE 21-11

COMMON CALORIC MODULARS*

Component	Calories
PROTEIN	
Resource Beneprotein (powder)	25 kcal/scoop (6 g protein)
Prosource protein powder	30 kcal/scoop (6 g protein)
Complete Amino Acid Mix	3.28 kcal/g (0.82 g protein)
CARBOHYDRATE	
Polycose	Powder: 3.8 kcal/g; 8 kcal/5 mL
FAT	
MCT oil[†]	7.7 kcal/mL
Vegetable oil	8.3 kcal/mL
Microlipid	4.5 kcal/mL
FAT AND CARBOHYDRATE	
Duocal	42 kcal/15 mL; 25 kcal/scoop (59% Carb, 41% Fat, 35% fat as MCT)

*Use these caloric supplements when you want to increase protein or when you have reached the maximum concentration tolerated and wish to further increase caloric density.

[†]MCT oil is unnecessary unless there is fat malabsorption.

Carbs (g)	Na (mEq)	K (mEq)	Ca (mg)	P (mg)	Fe (mg)	Osmolality
72	8	14	279	143	0.3	286
66	11	15	248	128	1.2	290
70	18	23	1,148	628	15.6	325
82	17	30	1,381	777	4.6	N/A
74	17	17	1,100	553	3.4	240
75	11	27	781	461	13.4	250
77	11	20	890	490	13.3	260
84	19	25	1,312	680	14.4	275
70	13	22	1,217	676	12.2	235
81	15	27	1,461	811	14.6	280
78	19	34	1,826	1,014	18.3	325

Continued

TABLE 21-12

ENTERAL NUTRITION COMPONENTS (PER LITER) (Continued)

A. INFANT FORMULAS

	Kcal/oz	Protein (g)	Fat (g)
COW'S MILK BASED FORMULAS			
Enfamil Premium LIPIL	20	14	36
Enfamil LIPIL	20	14	36
Enfamil A.R. LIPIL	20	17	34
Enfamil LactoFree LIPIL	20	14	36
Enfamil RestFull	20	17	34
Enfagrow Premium Next Step	20	18	36
Evap. Milk (13 oz + 19 oz water + 30 mL corn syrup)	20	27	31
Organic Milk Based Infant Formula	20	15	36
Parent's Choice Store Brand (also w/ARA/DHA)	20	14	36
Similac Advance Early Shield	20	14	37
Similac Go and Grow Milk-Based Formula	20	14	37
Similac Sensitive	20	14	37
Similac Organic	20	14	37
Similac PM 60/40	20	15	38
Similac Sensitive RS	20	14	37
SOY BASED			
America's Store Brand Soy (also w/ARA/DHA)	20	17	36
Enfamil Prosobee LIPIL	20	17	36
Enfagrow Soy Next Step	20	22	30
Good Start Soy PLUS	20	17	34
Good Start 2 Soy PLUS	20	19	34
Isomil Advance	20	17	37
Isomil DF	20	18	37
Similac Go and Grow Soy-Based Formula	20	17	37
CASEIN, EXTENSIVELY HYDROLYZED			
Alimentum	20	19	37
Nutramigen LIPIL	20	19	36
Nutramigen with Enflora LGG	20	19	36
Pregestimil LIPIL	20	19	38
WHEY, PARTIALLY HYDROLYZED			
Good Start Gentle PLUS	20	15	34
Good Start Protect PLUS	20	15	34
Good Start 2 Gentle PLUS	20	15	24
Good Start 2 Protect PLUS	20	15	34
WHEY AND CASEIN, PARTIALLY HYDROLYZED			
Enfamil Gentlease	20	15	36

*Liquid formulation.

Carbs (g)	Na (mEq)	K (mEq)	Ca (mg)	P (mg)	Fe (mg)	Osmolality
74	8	19	520	287	12	300
73	8	19	520	287	12	300
74	12	19	520	353	12	230 (240*)
73	9	19	547	307	12	200
74	12	19	520	353	12	230
70	10	23	1,300	867	13.4	270
72	21	32	1,066	832	0.8	N/A
71	7	15	420	280	12	294
72	8	19	520	287	12	295
76	7	18	528	284	12	310
72	7	18	1,014	548	13.5	300
72	9	19	568	379	12.2	200
71	7	18	528	284	12.2	225
69	7	14	379	189	4.7	280
72	9	19	568	379	12.2	180
68	11	21	700	460	12	164
71	11	21	700	460	12	170
79	11	21	1,300	867	13.3	230
75	12	20	704	422	12.1	180
73	12	20	1,273	710	13.4	175
70	13	19	710	507	12.2	200
68	13	19	710	507	12.2	240
70	13	19	1,014	676	13.5	200
69	13	20	710	507	12.2	370
69	14	19	627	347	12	300 (320*)
69	14	19	627	347	12	300
69	14	19	640	350	12.2	250
78	8	19	449	255	10.1	250
75	8	19	449	255	10.1	250
78	8	19	1,273	710	13.4	180
75	8	19	1,273	710	13.4	250
72	10	19	547	307	12	230

Continued

TABLE 21-12

ENTERAL NUTRITION COMPONENTS (PER LITER) (Continued)

A. INFANT FORMULAS

	Kcal/oz	Protein (g)	Fat (g)
AMINO ACID BASED			
Elecare (also w/DHA/ARA)	20	20	32
Neocate Infant (also w/DHA/ARA)	20	21	30
Nutramigen AA Lipil	20	19	36
SPECIALIZED			
3232A	20	19	28
RCF	20	20	36
Enfaport LIPIL	30	35	54

B. TODDLER AND YOUNG CHILD 1–10 YEARS

	Kcal/oz	Protein (g)	Fat (g)
COW'S MILK BASED FORMULAS			
Boost Kid Essentials	30	30	38
Boost Kid Essentials 1.5 (w/fiber)	45	42	75
Carnation Instant Breakfast Lactose Free	30	35	37
Carnation Instant Breakfast Lactose Free Plus	45	52	48
Carnation Instant Breakfast Lactose Free VHC	68	90	123
Carnation Instant Breakfast Essentials	24	43	16
Compleat Pediatric	30	38	39
Cow's Milk, 2%	15	35	20
Cow's Milk, whole	19	34	34
Ketocal 3 : 1	30	22	97
KetoCal 4 : 1	43	30	144
Kindercal TF Vanilla	32	30	44
Monogen	30	27	28
Nutren Junior (also w/fiber)	30	30	50
Pediasure Enteral (w/fiber)	30	30	40
Pediasure 1.5 (w/fiber)	45	59	67
Pediasure Vanilla	30	30	38
Pediasure with Fiber, Vanilla	30	30	38
Portagen	30	32	44
SOY BASED			
Bright Beginnings Soy Pediatric Drink	30	30	50
SEMI-ELEMENTAL, HYDROLYZED			
Peptamen Junior Fiber	30	30	39
Peptamen Junior with Prebio	30	30	39
Peptamen Junior, unflavored (w/fiber, van flavored)	30	30	39
Peptamen Junior 1.5	45	45	68
Vital jr	30	30	41

Carbs (g)	Na (mEq)	K (mEq)	Ca (mg)	P (mg)	Fe (mg)	Osmolality
72	13	26	780	568	10	350
78	11	27	830	624	12.4	375
69	14	19	627	347	12	350
89	13	19	627	420	12.5	250
68	13	19	710	507	12.2	168
102	13	29	940	520	18	280

Carbs (g)	Na (mEq)	K (mEq)	Ca (mg)	P (mg)	Fe (mg)	Osmolality
135	24	30	1,181	886	14	550/600/570
165	30	33	1,300	990	14	390 (405)
133	38	32	500	500	9	480/490
176	51	48	748	748	13.6	620
197	51	46	1,232	1,232	22.4	950
105	24	27	1,539	1,539	13.8	N/A
126	33	42	1,440	1,000	13.2	380
50	22	41	1,258	979	0.5	N/A
48	22	40	1,226	956	0.5	285
10	18	35	1,140	801	16	180
6	26	55	1,600	1,300	22	197
135	16	34	1,010	850	10.6	345
163	21	22	617	480	10.1	370
110	20	34	1,000	800	14	350
133	17	34	972	845	14	335 (345)
160 (165)	17	42	1,476	1,054	11	370 (390)
131	17	34	972	845	14	480
135	17	34	972	845	14	480
104	22	29	850	642	17	350
109	17	40	970	800	14	350
137	20	34	1,000	800	14	390
137	20	34	1,000	800	14	365
138	20	34	1,000	800	14	260 (390)
180	30	51	1,652	1,352	20.8	450
134	31	35	1,055	844	13.9	390

Continued

TABLE 21-12

ENTERAL NUTRITION COMPONENTS (PER LITER) (Continued)

B. TODDLER AND YOUNG CHILD 1–10 YEARS

	Kcal/oz	Protein (g)	Fat (g)
SOY AND PORK, HYDROLYZED			
Pepdite Junior, Unflavored	30	31	50
AMINO ACID BASED			
Elecare, Unflavored and Vanilla	30	31	49
E028 Splash	30	25	35
Neocate Junior Flavored	30	35	47
Neocate Junior Unflavored	30	33	50
Vivonex Pediatric	24	24	24

C. OLDER CHILDREN AND ADULT STANDARD FORMULAS

	Kcal/oz	Protein (g)	Fat (g)
COW'S MILK BASED FORMULAS			
Boost	30	40	17
Boost Glucose Control	32	59	50
Boost High Protein	30	63	25
Boost Plus	45	59	59
Compleat	32	48	40
Crucial	45	94	68
Enlive	31	37	0
Ensure	32	38	25
Ensure Plus	45	55	212
Glucerna 1.0 Cal	30	42	54
Jevity 1 Cal	32	44	35
Jevity 1.2 Cal	36	56	39
Jevity 1.5 Cal	45	64	50
Nepro	54	81	96
Novasource Renal	60	74	100
Nutren 1.0, vanilla (w/fiber)	30	40	38
Nutren 1.5 unflavored	45	60	68
Nutren 2.0	60	80	104
Optimental	30	51	28
Osmolite 1 Cal	32	44	35
Osmolite 1.2 Cal	36	56	39
Osmolite 1.5 Cal	45	63	49
Promote (w/fiber)	30	63	26
Pulmocare	45	63	93

Carbs (g)	Na (mEq)	K (mEq)	Ca (mg)	P (mg)	Fe (mg)	Osmolality
106	18	35	1,130	940	14	430
109	20	39	1,172	852	15	560
146	9	24	620	620	7.7	820
110	19	36	1,200	738	16	690
104	18	35	1,130	697	15	590
130	17	31	970	800	10	360

Carbs (g)	Na (mEq)	K (mEq)	Ca (mg)	P (mg)	Fe (mg)	Osmolality
171	24	43	1,250	1,250	19	625
84	48	29	1,160	928	15	400
138	31	41	1,459	1,250	19	650
188	31	41	1,459	1,250	19	670
128	43	44	760	760	14	340
134	51	48	1,000	1,000	18	490
217	8	5	208	1,166	11	825
173	37	40	1,266	1,055	19	620
47	41	45	1,266	1,266	19	680
96	41	40	705	705	13	355
155	40	40	910	760	14	300
169	59	47	1,200	1,200	18	450
216	61	55	1,200	1,200	18	525
167	46	27	1,060	700	19	585
200	39	21	1,300	650	18	700/960
127	38	32	668	668	12	370 (410)
169	51	48	1,000	1,000	18	430
196	57	49	1,340	1,340	24	745
139	49	44	1,055	1,055	13	585
144	40	40	760	760	14	300
158	58	46	1,200	1,200	18	360
204	61	46	1,000	1,000	18	525
130	44	51	1,200	1,200	18	340 (380)
106	57	50	1,060	1,060	19	475

Continued

TABLE 21-12

ENTERAL NUTRITION COMPONENTS (PER LITER) (Continued)

C. OLDER CHILDREN AND ADULT STANDARD FORMULAS

	Kcal/oz	Protein (g)	Fat (g)
Renalcal	60	35	83
Replete, unflavored	30	63	34
Resource 2.0	60	84	88
Resource Breeze	32	38	0
Suplena	54	45	96
TwoCal HN	60	84	91
SOY BASED			
Fibersource HN	36	53	39
Isosource 1.5 CAL	45	68	65
Isosource HN	36	53	39
SEMI-ELEMENTAL HYDROLYZED			
Peptamen, unflavored	30	40	39
Peptamen with Prebio	30	40	39
Peptamen 1.5, unflavored	45	68	56
Peptamen AF	36	76	55
Perative	39	67	37
Pivot 1.5	45	94	51
Vital 1.0 Cal	30	40	38
Vital HN	30	42	11
AMINO ACID BASED			
Tolerex	30	21	1.5
Vivonex RTF	30	50	12
Vivonex Plus	30	45	7
Vivonex T.E.N.	30	38	3

Carbs (g)	Na (mEq)	K (mEq)	Ca (mg)	P (mg)	Fe (mg)	Osmolality
291	0	0	0	0	0	600
113	39	39	1,000	1,000	18	300/350
217	35	39	1,042	1,042	18.8	790
230	15	1	42	633	11	750
205	35	29	1,055	717	19	600
219	64	63	1,050	1,050	19	725
160	52	51	1,000	1,000	17	490
170	56	58	1,070	1,070	19	650/585
160	48	49	1,200	1,200	15	490
127	25	39	800	700	18	270
127	25	39	800	700	18	300
188	45	48	1,000	1,000	27	550
107	35	41	800	800	14.4	390
180	45	44	870	870	16	460
172	61	51	1,000	1,000	18	595
130	46	36	705	705	13	390
185	25	36	667	667	12	500
230	20	30	560	560	10	550
175	29	31	670	670	12	630
190	27	27	560	560	10	650
210	26	24	500	500	9	630

TABLE 21-13

FORMULAS FOR SPECIAL CLINICAL CIRCUMSTANCES

A. INFANTS

Condition	Formulas
Pre-Term	
Pre-discharge	Enfamil Premature LIPIL Similac Special Care Advance Good Start Premature 24
Post-discharge (through 12 mo)	Enfamil Enfacare LIPIL Similac Neosure
Lactose intolerance	Enfamil LactoFree LIPIL Similac Sensitive Similac Sensitive RS Isomil DF
Vegetarian, lactose intolerance, or galactosemia	America's Store Brand Soy Infant Formula Good Start Soy Plus Good Start Soy 2 Plus (>4 mo) Isomil Advance Similac Go and Grow Soy-Based Formula (9–24 mo) Enfagrow Soy NEXT STEP (9–24 mo) Enfamil Prosobee LIPIL
Protein (e.g., cow's milk) allergy/intolerance and/or fat malabsorption	Alimentum Elecare (and w/ DHA/ARA) Neocate Infant (and w/ DHA and ARA) Nutramigen LIPIL Pregestimil LIPIL
Severe carbohydrate intolerance	3232A RCF
Requiring lower calcium and phosphorus	Similac PM 60/40

B. TODDLERS AND YOUNG CHILDREN AGES 1–10 YR

Condition	Formulas
Vegetarian, lactose intolerance, or milk protein intolerance	Bright Beginnings Soy Pediatric Drink
Protein allergy/intolerance and/or fat malabsorption	Peptide Jr Peptamen Jr (with and without Prebio) Vivonex Pediatric Vital jr Elecare Neocate Junior (Unflavored and Flavored) E028 Splash
Fat malabsorption, intestinal lymphatic obstruction, chylothorax	Portagen Monogen Enfaport LIPIL
Increased caloric needs	Boost Kids Essentials Carnation Instant Breakfast Essentials Nutren Junior (also with fiber) Pediasure (also with fiber)
Requiring clear liquid diet	Resource Breeze Enlive
Intractable epilepsy	KetoCal (3:1 and 4:1)

TABLE 21-13

FORMULAS FOR SPECIAL CLINICAL CIRCUMSTANCES (Continued)

C. OLDER CHILDREN AND ADULTS

Tube feeding	
For malabsorption of protein and/or fat	Peptamen, Peptamen w/ Prebio, Peptamen 1.5 Perative Tolerex Vital HN Vital 1.0 Cal Vivonex Plus and Vivonex T.E.N
For critically ill and/or malabsorption	Crucial Optimental Pulmocare Pivot 1.5 Perative
For impaired glucose tolerance	Glucerna Glytrol Store Brand Diabetic Nutritional Drink
For dialysis patients	Magnacal Renal Nepro NutriRenal
For patients with acute renal failure not on dialysis	Renalcal Suplena
Increased caloric needs (oral)	
With a normal gastrointestinal (GI) tract	Boost, Boost with fiber Boost Plus, Boost High Protein Carnation Instant Breakfast Essentials with whole milk Ensure NUTRA Shake
For clear liquid diet	Resource Breeze Enlive
For patients with cystic fibrosis (CF)	Scandishake with whole milk

TABLE 21-14

ORAL REHYDRATION SOLUTIONS

Solution	Kcal/mL (kcal/oz)	Carbohydrate (g/L)	Na (mEq/L)	K (mEq/L)	Osmolality (mOsm/kg H_2O)
CeraLyte-70	0.16 (4.9)	Rice digest (40)	70	20	N/A
CeraLyte-50	0.16 (4.9)	Rice digest (40)	50	20	N/A
CeraLyte-90	0.16 (4.9)	Rice digest (40)	90	20	N/A
Enfalyte	0.12 (3.7)	Rice syrup solids (30)	50	25	170
Oral Rehydration Salts (WHO)	0.06 (2)	Dextrose (20)	90	20	330
Pedialyte (unflavored)	0.1 (3)	Dextrose (25)	45	20	250

VII. PARENTERAL NUTRITION (PN)[12]

Necessary to adequately support the pediatric patient with insufficient enteral intake.

A. Situations in which PN is Suggested

1. Inability to feed enterally (e.g., extreme prematurity, tracheoesophageal fistulas)
2. When alimentation via gastrointestinal tract needs to be restricted (e.g., chylothorax/chylous ascites, bowel pseudo-obstruction)
3. Gastrointestinal (GI) dysfunction and/or malabsorption (e.g., short-gut syndrome, intestinal atresias, enteric fistulas, gastroschisis)
4. Increased losses or requirements (e.g., severe diarrhea, intractable vomiting, persistent or severe failure to thrive)

B. Suggested Formulations for Initiation and Advancement of PN (Table 21-15)

Suggested glucose, protein, and fat during initiation, as well as recommendations for advancement and maximum allowable amounts

C. Recommended Parenteral Formulations (Table 21-16)

Based on age groups; includes recommendations for electrolytes, elements, and minerals

D. Suggested Monitoring Schedule for Patients Receiving Parenteral Nutrition (Table 21-17)

Important to monitor growth parameters as well as laboratory studies for these patients on periodic basis

TABLE 21-15

INITIATION AND ADVANCEMENT OF PARENTERAL NUTRITION*

Nutrient	Initial Dose	Advancement	Maximum
Glucose	5%–10%	2.5%–5%/day	12.5% peripheral 18 mg/kg/min (maximum rate of infusion)
Protein	1–1.5 g/kg/day	0.5–1 g/kg/day	3–4 g/kg/day 10%–16% of calories
Fat†	0.5–1 g/kg/day	1 g/kg/day	4 g/kg/day 0.17 g/kg/hr (maximum rate of infusion)

*Acceptable osmolarity of parenteral nutrition through a peripheral line varies between 900 and 1,050 osm/L by institution. An estimate of the osmolarity of parenteral nutrition can be obtained with the following formula: Estimated osmolarity = (dextrose concentration × 50) + (amino acid concentration × 100) + (mEq of electrolytes × 2). Consult individual pharmacy for hospital limitations.

†Essential fatty acid deficiency (EFAD) may occur in fat-free parenteral nutrition within 2–4 weeks in infants and children, and as early as 2–14 days in neonates. A minimum of 2%–4% of total caloric intake as linoleic acid and 0.25%–0.5% as linolenic acid is necessary to meet essential fatty acid requirements.

Modified from Baker RD Baker SS, Davis AM: Pediatric parenteral nutrition. New York, Chapman and Hall, 1997; and Cox JH, Melbardis IM: Parenteral nutrition. In Samour PQ, King K (eds): Handbook of pediatric nutrition, 3rd ed. Boston, Jones and Bartlett Publishers, 2005.

TABLE 21-16

PARENTERAL NUTRITION FORMULATION RECOMMENDATIONS

Component	Preterm	Term Infants	1–3 yr	4–6 yr	7–10 yr	11–18 yr
Energy (kcal/kg/day)	85–105	90–108	75–90	65–80	55–70	30–55
Protein (g/kg/day)	2.5–4	2.5–3.5	1.5–2.5	1.5–2.5	1.5–2.5	0.8–2
Sodium (mEq/kg/day)	2–4	2–4	2–4	2–4	2–4	60–150 mEq/day
Potassium (mEq/kg/day)	2–4	2–4	2–4	2–4	2–4	70–180 mEq/day
Calcium (mg/kg/day)	50–60	20–40	10–20	10–20	10–20	200–800 mg/day
Phosphorus (mg/kg/day)	30–45	30–45	15–40	15–40	15–40	280–900 mg/day
Magnesium (mEq/kg/day)	0.5–1	0.25–1	0.25–0.5	0.25–0.5	0.25–0.5	8–24 mEq/day
Zinc (mcg/kg/day)	325–400	100–250	100	100	50	2–5 mg/day
Copper (mcg/kg/day)*	20	20	20	20	5–20	200–300 mcg/day
Manganese (mcg/kg/day)*	1	1	1	1	1	40–50 mcg/day
Selenium (mcg/kg/day)	2	2	2	2	1–2	40–60 mcg/day

*Copper and manganese needs may be lowered in cholestasis.

Modified from Baker RD, Baker SS, Davis AM: Pediatric parenteral nutrition. New York, Chapman and Hall, 1997; Cox JH, Melbardis IM: Parenteral nutrition. In Samour PQ, King K (eds): Handbook of pediatric nutrition, 3rd ed. Boston, Jones and Bartlett Publishers, 2005; and American Society for Parenteral and Enteral Nutrition (ASPEN): Safe practices for parenteral nutrition. JPEN 2004;28(6):S39–S70.

TABLE 21-17

MONITORING SCHEDULE FOR PATIENTS RECEIVING PARENTERAL NUTRITION*

Variable	Initial Period†	Later Period‡
GROWTH		
Weight	Daily	2 times/wk
Height	Weekly (infants)	
	Monthly (children)	Monthly
Head circumference (infants)	Weekly	Monthly§
LABORATORY STUDIES		
Electrolytes and glucose	Daily until stable	Weekly
BUN/creatinine	2 times/wk	Weekly
Albumin or prealbumin	Weekly	Weekly
$Ca2^{+}$, $Mg2^{+}$, P	2 times/wk	Weekly
ALT, AST, ALP	Weekly	Weekly
Total and direct bilirubin	Weekly	Weekly
CBC	Weekly	Weekly
Triglycerides	With each increase	Weekly
Vitamins	—	As indicated
Trace minerals	—	As indicated

*For patients on long-term parenteral nutrition, monitoring every 2–4 weeks is adequate in most cases.
†The period before nutritional goals are reached or during any period of instability.
‡When stability is reached, no changes in nutrient composition.
§Weekly in preterm infants.
ALP, Alkaline phosphatase; ALT, alanine transaminase; AST, aspartate transaminase; BUN, blood urea nitrogen; CBC, complete blood count.

REFERENCES

1. Centers for Disease Control and Prevention (CDC). http://www.cdc.gov/growthcharts/.
2. Centers for Disease Control and Prevention (CDC). http://www.cdc.gov/healthyweight/assessing/bmi/index.html.
3. Barlow SE, Dietz WH. Obesity evaluation and treatment: Expert Committee recommendations. *Pediatrics*. 1998;102(3):e29.
4. Barlow SE; Expert Committee. Expert Committee recommendations regarding the prevention, assessment, and treatment of child and adolescent overweight and obesity: summary report. *Pediatrics*. 2007;120:S164–S192.
5. The Childhood Obesity Action Network Expert Committee recommendation implementation guide. http://www.nichq.org/documents/coan-papers-and-publications/COANImplementationGuide62607FINAL.pdf.
6. Li C, Ford ES, Mokdad AH, et al. Recent trends in waist circumference and waist-height ratio among US children and adolescents. *Pediatrics*. 2006;118:e1390–e1398.
7. Otten JJ, Hellwig JP, Meyers LD, eds. *Dietary reference intakes: the essential guide to nutrient requirements*. Washington, DC: National Academies Press; 2006.
8. Ross AC, Manson JE, Abrams SA. The 2011 Report on Dietary Reference Intakes for Calcium and Vitamin D from the Institute of Medicine: What clinicians need to know. *J Clin Endocrinol Metab*. 2010 Nov 29. [Epub ahead of print]

9. Corrales KM, Utter SL. Growth failure. In: Samour PQ, King K, eds. *Handbook of pediatric nutrition.* Boston: Jones and Bartlett Publishers; 2005:391–406.
10. Solomon SM, Kirby DF. The refeeding syndrome: a review. *J Parenteral Enteral Nutr.* 1990;14:90–96.
11. American Academy of Pediatrics Committee on Nutrition; Kleinman RE, ed. *Pediatric nutrition handbook*, 6th ed. Chicago: American Academy of Pediatrics; 2009.
12. American Society for Parenteral and Enteral Nutrition (ASPEN). Safe practices for parenteral nutrition. *JPEN.* 2004;28(6):S39–S70. http://www.ashp.org/DocLibrary/BestPractices/2004ASPEN.aspx.

Chapter 22

Oncology

Catherine M. Albert, MD

See additional content on Expert Consult

I. WEBSITES

National Cancer Institute (NCI): http://www.cancer.gov/cancertopics/pdq/pediatrictreatment

SEER (Surveillance, epidemiology, and end results) data from the NCI: http://seer.cancer.gov/

Long-term follow-up guidelines for survivors of pediatric cancer: http://www.survivorshipguidelines.org/

II. PRESENTING SIGNS AND SYMPTOMS OF PEDIATRIC MALIGNANCIES (TABLE 22-1)

NOTE: Common presenting signs and symptoms of many malignancies include weight loss, failure to thrive, anorexia, malaise, fever, pallor, and lymphadenopathy.

III. COMMONLY USED CHEMOTHERAPEUTIC DRUGS AND ASSOCIATED ACUTE TOXICITIES (SEE FORMULARY ADJUNCT)

IV. ONCOLOGIC EMERGENCIES[1–3]

A. Hyperleukocytosis

1. **Etiology:** Significantly elevated white blood cell (WBC) count (WBC >100,000/µL), typically seen in leukemia patients. In acute myeloid leukemia (AML) (especially M4 and M5), hyperleukocytosis is more likely to occur with a lower WBC count (100,000/µL and up) versus in acute lymphocytic leukemia (ALL)/chronic myeloid leukemia (CML) where symptoms/complications are more often noted with a WBC count >300,000/µL
2. **Presentation:** Signs and symptoms of hyperviscosity such as hypoxia and dyspnea from pulmonary leukostasis, mental status changes, headaches, seizures, papilledema from leukostasis in cerebral vessels; occasionally, gastrointestinal (GI) bleeding, abdominal pain, renal insufficiency, priapism, intracranial hemorrhage and tumor lysis syndrome
3. **Management:**

a. Transfuse platelets as needed to keep count above 20,000/µL

b. Avoid red blood cell (RBC) transfusions because they will raise viscosity (keep hemoglobin ≤10 g/dL). If RBCs are required, consider partial exchange transfusion

TABLE 22-1

PRESENTING SIGNS AND SYMPTOMS OF PEDIATRIC MALIGNANCIES[1,3,5]

Type of Malignancy	Risk Factors/Patient Characteristics	Signs/Symptoms	Initial Workup
Leukemia	ALL: white race, radiation exposure AML: familial monosomy 7 Both: NF type 1, Down syndrome	Limp, hepatomegaly, splenomegaly, petechiae/bruising, bone pain, anemia, thrombocytopenia	BMA, LP, laboratory studies including morphology and flow cytometry
Lymphoma	HD and Burkitt's lymphoma: EBV, more common in adolescence NHL: immunodeficiency, more common in infants and school-aged children	Night sweats; pruritus; stridor; persistent respiratory symptoms; GI bleeding; back pain; hepatomegaly; splenomegaly; abdominal, head, neck, or chest mass	Imaging (CT chest/abdomen/pelvis), bone scan, LP, BMA, ferritin/LDH/uric acid/ESR
Wilms' tumor	1–5 yr old (peak at 2–3 yr) Associated with some congenital anomalies Aniridia, Beckwith Wiedemann	Hypertension, abdominal distention, hematuria	Imaging (CT chest/abdomen/pelvis), echocardiogram, abdominal ultrasound with Doppler
Neuroblastoma	Peak incidence 1–5 yr old	Emesis; diarrhea; hypertension; opsoclonus-myoclonus; periorbital ecchymoses; Horner syndrome; stridor; persistent respiratory symptoms; abdominal, head, neck or chest mass; limp; blue subcutaneous nodules	Imaging (CT/MRI for staging), BMA, echocardiogram, urine catecholamines (HVA/VMA)
CNS tumors	Optic glioma: NF type I, other genetic syndromes Astrocytoma: full age range Ependymoma and medulloblastoma: more common in infants, school-aged children Craniopharyngioma: peak incidence 8–10 yr old	Irritability, headache, emesis, seizure, cranial nerve palsies, visual changes, proptosis, ataxia	MRI of brain and spine, lumbar puncture (cytopathology)

Continued

TABLE 22-1

PRESENTING SIGNS AND SYMPTOMS OF PEDIATRIC MALIGNANCIES[1,3,5] (Continued)

Type of Malignancy	Risk Factors/Patient Characteristics	Signs/Symptoms	Initial Workup
Testicular tumors	Adolescent age Cryptorchidism	Abdominal pain or tenderness, scrotal swelling or mass	Imaging (CT chest/abdomen/pelvis), serum β-hCG, AFP, LDH, uric acid
Bone tumors	Osteosarcoma: previous treatment with alkylating agents or radiation therapy, Li Fraumeni, hereditary Retinoblastoma Ewing's sarcoma: Caucasian race Both: adolescent age	Limp, back pain, persistent limb pain, fracture	Imaging (CT chest, primary site), x-ray primary site, bone scan; bilateral BMA (Ewing's sarcoma)
Histiocytic disease	Familial disease: infancy	Polyuria, polydipsia, otorrhea, hepatomegaly, splenomegaly, cutaneous lesions, osteolytic lesions, pulmonary infiltrates, anemia, thrombocytopenia	LDH/ferritin/uric acid, skeletal survey, BMA, chest x-ray
Retinoblastoma	<5 yr old, genetic associations	Leukocoria, asymmetrical red reflex, orbital inflammation, hyphema, pupil irregularity	Brain MRI, lumbar puncture for CSF
Rhabdomyosarcoma	More common in children >5 yr and adolescents Li Fraumeni, NF type 1	Symptoms differ based on location of tumor but bone pain, anemia, thrombocytopenia, neutropenia and respiratory symptoms are common with metastatic disease	Laboratory studies including LFTs, imaging based on location of suspected disease (CT, MRI, ultrasound), chest x-ray and bone scan to evaluate for metastatic disease
Hepatoblastoma	Peak incidence <3 yr old Beckwith Wiedemann, FAP	Abdominal pain and distention, anorexia, fatigue, thrombocytosis	Imaging of abdomen, laboratory studies, β-hCG, AFP

AFP, Alpha fetoprotein; ALL, acute lymphocytic leukemia; AML, Acute myeloid leukemia; BMA, bone marrow aspirate; CNS, central nervous system; CSF, cerebrospinal fluid; CT, computed tomography; ESR, erythrocyte sedimentation rate; FAP, familial adenomatous polyposis; GI, gastrointestinal; HD, Hodgkin's disease; β-hCG, beta human chorionic gonadotropin; HVA/VMA, urine catecholamines; LDH, lactic dehydrogenase; LFT, liver function tests; LP, lumbar puncture; MRI, magnetic resonance imaging; NF, neurofibromatosis; NHL, non-Hodgkin's lymphoma.

c. Hydration, alkalinization, and allopurinol should be initiated (as discussed in section IV.B)
d. Administer fresh frozen plasma (FFP) and vitamin K if coagulopathy is present
e. Before cytotoxic therapy, consider leukapheresis or exchange transfusion to lower WBC count if central nervous system (CNS) or pulmonary symptoms exist
f. Start disease treatment as soon as patient is clinically stable

B. Tumor Lysis Syndrome

1. **Etiology:** Lysis of tumor cells before or during early stages of chemotherapy (especially Burkitt lymphoma/leukemia, T-cell ALL); lymphoblasts have four times more intracellular phosphate than lymphocytes
2. **Presentation:** Hyperuricemia, hypocalcemia, hyperkalemia, hyperphosphatemia. Can lead to acute renal failure
3. **Prevention and management:**

a. Hydration and alkalinization: D_5W or D_5 ¼ normal saline + 40 mEq/L $NaHCO_3$ (without K^+) at two times maintenance rate. Keeping urine specific gravity <1.010 and pH 7.0–7.5 reduces risk for urate crystal formation. Risk of calcium phosphate precipitation if pH >7.5 or serum bicarbonate >30 mEq/L
b. Allopurinol (100 mg/m^2/dose) q8hr by mouth (PO), alternative dosing 10 mg/kg/day divided q8hr PO. May also use intravenous (IV) (200–400 mg/m^2/day in three divided doses; max dose = 600 mg/day). Consider rasburicase (recombinant urate oxidase, converts uric acid to allantoin) for higher risk patients, especially those with uric acid >7.5 mg/dL
c. Check K^+, Ca^{2+}, phosphate, uric acid and urinalysis frequently, as often as every 2 hours. Risk for calcium phosphate crystal formation and precipitation when Ca × Phosphate >60
d. Manage abnormal electrolytes as described in Chapter 11. See Chapter 19 for dialysis indications
e. Consider stopping alkalinization soon after starting chemotherapy (if uric acid is normal) to facilitate calcium phosphate excretion

C. Spinal Cord Compression

1. **Etiology:** Intrinsic or extrinsic compression of the spinal cord. Occurs most commonly with brain tumors, sarcomas, leukemia with lymphomatous involvement, lymphoma, and neuroblastoma
2. **Presentation:** Back pain (localized, radicular), weakness, sensory loss, change in bowel or bladder function. Prognosis for recovery based on duration and level of disability at presentation
3. **Diagnosis:** Magnetic resonance imaging (MRI) preferred, or computed tomography (CT) scan of spine. A plain film of the spine has good specificity but detects only two thirds of abnormalities

4. **Management:** (**NOTE:** Steroids may prevent diagnosis of lymphoma; plan diagnostic procedure as soon as possible.)
a. In the presence of neurologic abnormalities, strong history, and rapid progression of symptoms, immediately start bolus dexamethasone 1–2 mg/kg/day IV and obtain an emergent MRI of the spine
b. With back pain but less acute symptoms and no anatomic level of dysfunction, consider lower dose of dexamethasone, 0.25–0.5 mg/kg/day PO divided q6hr; perform MRI of the spine within 24 hours
c. If cause of tumor is known, emergent radiotherapy or chemotherapy indicated for sensitive tumors; otherwise, emergent neurosurgery consultation is warranted
d. If cause of tumor is unknown or debulking may remove most or all of tumor, surgery is indicated to decompress the spine

D. Increased Intracranial Pressure

1. **Etiology:** Ventricular obstruction or impaired cerebrospinal fluid flow
2. **Presentation:** Headaches, irritability, lethargy, emesis (especially if projectile)
3. **Diagnosis:** Obtain CT scan or MRI of the head. MRI more sensitive for diagnosis of posterior fossa tumors. Evaluate vital signs for Cushing's triad, funduscopic examination for papilledema
4. **Management:**
a. See Chapter 4 for basic intracranial pressure (ICP) management
b. If tumor is identified, add dexamethasone, 2 mg/kg/day IV divided q6hr
c. Obtain emergent neurosurgical consultation

E. Cerebrovascular Accident

1. **Etiology:** Hyperleukocytosis, coagulopathy, thrombocytopenia, radiation (fibrosis) or chemotherapy-related (e.g., L-asparaginase-induced hemorrhage or thrombosis, methotrexate). Most common in patients with leukemia
2. **Diagnosis and management:**
a. Platelet transfusions (and likely increase threshold for transfusion), FFP as needed to replace factors (e.g., if depleted by L-asparaginase)
b. Brain CT scan with contrast, MRI, magnetic resonance angiography, or magnetic resonance venography if venous thrombosis is suspected
c. Administer heparin acutely, followed by warfarin, for thromboses (if no venous hemorrhage observed on MRI)
d. Avoid L-asparaginase
e. Leukapheresis for hyperleukocytosis

F. Respiratory Distress and Superior Vena Cava Syndrome

1. **Etiology:** Mediastinal mass, edema, or thrombosis, typically seen with Hodgkin disease, non-Hodgkin lymphoma (e.g., lymphoblastic lymphoma), ALL (T-lineage), germ cell tumors
2. **Presentation:** Orthopnea, headaches, facial swelling, dizziness, plethora

3. **Diagnosis:** Chest radiograph. Consider CT or MRI scan to assess airway. Attempt diagnosis of malignancy (if not known) by least invasive method possible. Avoid sedation or general anesthesia if unstable, high risk
4. **Management:**
   a. Control airway
   b. Biopsy (e.g., bone marrow, pleurocentesis, lymph-node biopsy) before therapy if patient can tolerate sedation or general anesthesia
   c. Empirical therapy: Radiotherapy, steroids, chemotherapy

G. Typhilitis (Neutropenic Enterocolitis)

1. **Etiology:** Inflammation of bowel wall, usually localized to cecum. Occurs most often in association with prolonged neutropenia
2. **Presentation:** Right lower quadrant abdominal pain, nausea, diarrhea, and fever (fever may be absent early in course; neutropenic patient with abdominal pain warrants evaluation for typhlitis and empiric antibacterial coverage). Risk for perforation
3. **Diagnosis:**
   a. Careful serial abdominal examinations
   b. X-ray may show pneumatosis intestinalis, bowel wall edema
   c. CT (non-contrast) most sensitive imaging; may reveal bowel wall thickening, pneumatosis intestinalis
4. **Management:**
   a. Nothing by mouth (NPO), IV fluids; consider nasogastric decompression
   b. Broad anaerobic and gram-negative antibiotic coverage (consider coverage for *Clostridium difficile*)
   c. Follow closely with surgery consult

V. FEVER AND NEUTROPENIA[1,4]

See Figure 22-1.

VI. HEMATOPOIETIC STEM CELL TRANSPLANTATION (HSCT)[1,5]

A. Goal

Administer healthy functioning hematopoietic stem cells from the bone marrow, peripheral blood or umbilical cord blood to a patient whose bone marrow is diseased (from hematologic malignancy) or depleted (after treatment with myeloablative chemotherapy). HSCT is also used for some congenital and acquired hematologic and immunologic diseases

B. Types

1. **Allogeneic**
   a. Recipient is transfused with donor stem cells after a myeloablative preparative regimen that includes chemotherapy and often also radiation. Donors are screened for human leukocyte antigen (HLA) subtype matching to recipient; ideal candidate is an HLA-matched sibling. Matched unrelated donors and haploidentical (*half matched*) related donors are also considered

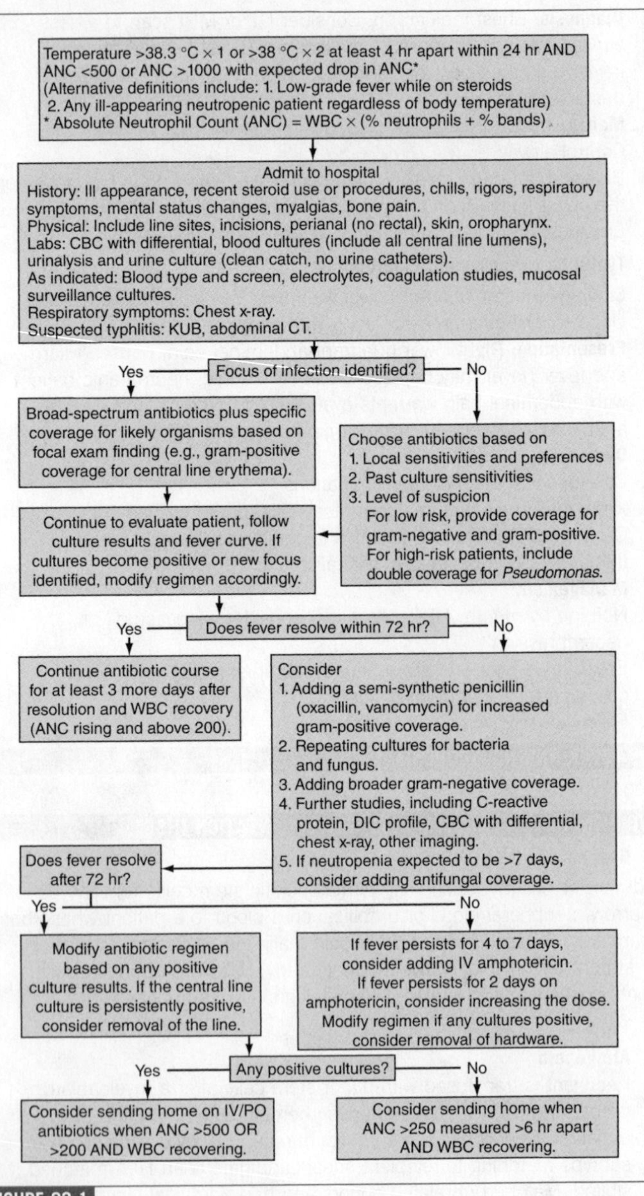

FIGURE 22-1

Fever and neutropenia.[1,4]

b. Provides graft-versus-tumor effect but recipients are also at risk for graft-versus-host complications and rejection
c. Used commonly for ALL (high risk), AML, hemophagocytic lymphohistiocytosis, metastatic neuroblastoma, refractory rhabdomyosarcoma, high-risk Ewing's sarcoma, and a number of nonmalignant hematologic and immunologic diseases

2. **Autologous**
a. Donor is recipient. After several cycles of conventional chemotherapy, stem cells from patient are harvested (often with the assistance of growth factors such as granulocyte colony-stimulating factor [GCSF] to mobilize), stored and given back (*rescue*) after the patient has received what are considered lethal doses of chemotherapy and radiation
b. Avoid the complication of graft-versus-host disease (GVHD)
c. Used commonly for relapsed AML, extramedullary relapse in ALL, Hodgkin's disease, non-Hodgkin's lymphoma, stage IV neuroblastoma, stage IV Ewing's sarcoma, stage IV rhabdomyosarcoma, relapsed brain tumors, some nonmalignant hematologic diseases

3. **Umbilical cord blood**
a. Stem cells are obtained immediately after birth, typed and frozen until use. Used more commonly in children because of the limited number of cells
b. Thought to cause less GVHD but may take longer to engraft

C. Engraftment

1. Recipient's bone marrow is repopulated with donor stem cells that proliferate and mature
2. Usually starts within 2–4 weeks of transplant, but can be significantly delayed with certain conditions, medications, or infection

VII. COMMON COMPLICATIONS OF BONE MARROW TRANSPLANT[1,5]

A. Graft-Versus-Host Disease (GVHD)

1. **Etiology:** Primarily donor T-cell-mediated reaction to foreign antigen; occurs more commonly after allogeneic transplant. Risk factors include HLA disparity, radiation therapy, gender disparity, and increasing age
2. **Presentation:** Usually occurs within 100 days after transplantation, most commonly within 6 weeks
a. Maculopapular skin rash, can progress to bullous lesions and toxic epidermal necrolysis
b. Laboratory findings: Abnormal liver enzymes (direct hyperbilirubinemia and elevated alkaline phosphatase)
c. Upper GI symptoms: Anorexia, dyspepsia, nausea, vomiting
d. Lower GI symptoms: Abdominal cramping, diarrhea
3. **Diagnosis:** Triad of rash, abdominal cramping with diarrhea, hyperbilirubinemia. Tissue biopsy of skin or rectum provides histologic confirmation

4. **Prevention and management:**
a. Prophylaxis: Immunosuppression with cyclosporine or tacrolimus; adjuvants are methotrexate and prednisone
b. First-line treatment: Steroids commonly used
c. Second-line agents: Cyclosporine, tacrolimus, sirolimus, antithymocyte globulin, and mycophenolate mofetil
d. Psoralens plus ultraviolet A photopheresis (PUVA): alternative for skin GVHD
e. Pentostatin: Cutaneous and oral GVHD
5. **Chronic GVHD management:** Acute therapies complemented by monoclonal antibodies, such as infliximab (anti-tumor necrosis factor-α)

B. Veno-Occlusive Disease (Sinusoidal Obstruction Syndrome)

1. **Etiology:** Occlusive fibrosis of terminal intrahepatic venules and sinusoids; occurs as a consequence of hematopoietic cell transplantation, hepatotoxic chemotherapy, and/or high-dose liver radiation. Typically occurs within 3 weeks of the insult, most common at the end of the first week after transplant. Incidence highest with unmatched, unrelated transplants and lowest with autologous transplantation
2. **Presentation:** Tender hepatomegaly, jaundice, edema, ascites, and sudden weight gain
3. **Diagnosis:**
a. Liver ultrasound with Doppler or MRI showing reversal of portal venous flow
b. Elevated bilirubin and aminotransferases (alanine aminotransferase [ALT], aspartate aminotransferase [AST])
c. Prolongation of prothrombin time, decreased factor VII levels (in more severe disease)
d. Portal-hepatic venous gradient of >10 mmHg (invasive but sensitive)
4. **Prevention and management:**
a. Prophylactic measures: Ursodeoxycholic acid, glutamine, and heparin; have not shown consistent benefit
b. Treatment:
   (1) Supportive with fluid and sodium restriction
   (2) Alteplase (tissue plasminogen activator) with or without heparin: risk of hemorrhage
   (3) Defibrotide: Promising results with little toxicity
   (4) Antithrombin infusion for patients with low antithrombin levels
   (5) For severe disease, surgical intervention with transjugular intrahepatic portosystemic stent shunt or liver transplantation

C. Thrombotic Microangiopathy: Thrombotic Thrombocytopenic Purpura (TTP) or Hemolytic Uremic Syndrome (HUS)

1. **Etiology:** Post-HSCT, associated with immunosuppressants (cyclosporine, tacrolimus)

2. **Presentation:** Both TTP and HUS present with microangiopathic hemolytic anemia and thrombocytopenia. HUS completes the triad with renal insufficiency/failure while TTP can be associated with neurologic symptoms
3. **Diagnosis:** Anemia and thrombocytopenia on complete blood count (CBC), schistocytes on peripheral blood smear, hematuria, proteinuria, casts on urinalysis, elevated lactate dehydrogenase (LDH), decreased haptoglobin, impaired renal function, elevated D-dimer on coagulation panel
4. **Prevention and treatment:** Urgent plasma exchange if TTP is suspected, blood products, fluid management, dialysis

D. Hemorrhagic Cystitis

1. **Etiology:** Pretransplant conditioning regimens (specifically those that include cyclophosphamide, pelvic or total body irradiation), viral (adenovirus, BK virus). Allogeneic HSCT from unrelated donor poses high risk
2. **Presentation:** Hematuria, pain with voiding. Acute (within 72 hours of treatment) or delayed
3. **Diagnosis:** Urine studies including viral and bacterial cultures, bladder ultrasound, CBC
4. **Prevention and management:** Hydration and Mesna with preparative regimen. Treatment may include aggressive hydration, administration of blood products, cystoscopy, bladder irrigation, clot evacuation

VIII. HEMATOLOGIC CARE AND COMPLICATIONS[1]

NOTE: Transfuse only irradiated and leukoreduced packed RBC (PRBC) and single donor platelets, cytomegalovirus (CMV)-negative or leukofiltered PRBC/platelets for CMV-negative patients. Use leukofiltered PRBC/platelets for those who may undergo bone marrow transplantation (BMT) in the future to prevent alloimmunization, or for those who have had nonhemolytic febrile transfusion reactions. Many oncology patients have nonhemolytic reactions (temperature elevation, skin rash, hypotension, respiratory distress) to PRBC and/or platelet transfusion and will subsequently be pre-medicated with diphenhydramine and/or acetaminophen for future transfusions

A. Anemia

1. **Etiology:** Blood loss, chemotherapy, marrow infiltration, hemolysis
2. **Management:**
   a. See Chapter 14 for specific details on PRBC transfusions
   b. Hematocrit thresholds for PRBC transfusions in cancer patients are based on clinical status and symptoms, and are not uncommonly less than 30 g/dL

B. Thrombocytopenia

1. **Etiology:** Chemotherapy, marrow infiltration, consumptive coagulopathy, medications

2. **Management:**
   a. See Chapter 14 for specific details on platelet transfusions
   b. Generally, maintain platelet count above 10,000/μL unless patient is actively bleeding or febrile, or before selected procedures (e.g., intramuscular injection). Consider maintaining platelet counts at higher levels for patients who have brain tumors, recent brain surgery, or history of a stroke

C. Neutropenia

1. **Etiology:** Chemotherapy, marrow infiltration, radiation
2. **Management:**
   a. Broad-spectrum antibiotics with concomitant fever (see Fig. 22-1)
   b. GCSF to assist in recovery of neutrophils
   c. Rarely, use of neutrophil transfusion

IX. NAUSEA TREATMENT IN CANCER PATIENTS[1]

A. Etiology

Usual cause is chemotherapy treatment. Also suspect opiate therapy, GI and CNS radiotherapy, obstructive abdominal process, CNS mass, certain antibiotics, or hypercalcemia

B. Presentation

1. **Acute:** Emesis within 24 hours of starting chemotherapy; occurs in one third of patients despite treatment
2. **Delayed:** Emesis occurring 24 hours after chemotherapy; increased risk for females, prior acute emesis, certain agents (e.g., cisplatin)
3. **Anticipatory:** Emesis prior to chemotherapy administration

C. Therapy

Hydration plus one or more antinausea medications (see Formulary for dosing).

1. **Serotonin (5-HT$_3$) antagonists:** Ondansetron, dolasetron, granisetron, or palonosetron. Usually a first-line therapy. Best for acute emesis. Beware of QT prolongation, widening of QRS
2. **Histamine-1 antagonist:** Diphenhydramine; also cyproheptadine (with anticholinergic side effect of appetite stimulation)
3. **Steroids:** Dexamethasone; especially helpful in patients with brain tumor and as prophylaxis for delayed symptoms. Synergy with 5-HT$_3$ antagonists
4. **Benzodiazepines:** Lorazepam; used as an adjunct antiemetic agent
5. **Metoclopramide:** Use diphenhydramine to reduce extrapyramidal symptoms (EPS)
6. **Phenothiazines:** Promethazine, chlorpromazine; use diphenhydramine to reduce EPS
7. **Cannabinoids:** Dronabinol; can be helpful in resistant cases, especially in patients with large tumor burden. May also be used as an appetite stimulant in malnourished patients

TABLE 22-2

ANTIMICROBIAL PROPHYLAXIS IN ONCOLOGY PATIENTS

Organism	Medication	Indication
Pneumocystis jiroveci	TMP-SMX, atovaquone, dapsone, or pentamidine	Chemotherapy and BMT per protocol (usually at least 6 mo after chemotherapy, 12 mo after BMT)
HSV	Acyclovir (dosing is different for zoster, varicella, and mucocutaneous HSV)	After BMT if patient or donor is HSV or CMV positive; recurrent zoster
Candida albicans	Fluconazole or voriconazole	After BMT (usually at least 28 days)
Gram-positive organisms	Penicillin	After BMT (usually at least 1 mo)

BMT, Bone marrow transplantation; CMV, cytomegalovirus; HSV, herpes simplex virus; TMP-SMX, trimethoprim-sulfamethoxazole.

8. **Substance P and neurokinin-1 receptor antagonist:** Aprepitant. Avoid with certain chemotherapy drugs such as ifosphamide, etoposide

X. ANTIMICROBIAL PROPHYLAXIS IN ONCOLOGY PATIENTS (TABLE 22-2)

NOTE: Treatment length and dosage may vary per protocol.

XI. BEYOND CHILDHOOD CANCER: TREATING A CANCER SURVIVOR

A. Understand the Treatment Regimen

1. Identify all components of therapy received: Comprehensive treatment summary from oncologist, summarizing:
a. Diagnosis: Site/stage, date, relapse
b. Chemotherapy: Cumulative doses, *high dose* versus *low dose* for methotrexate and cytarabine
c. Radiation: Locations, cumulative dose
d. Surgeries: Dates, sites, resection
e. BMT: Prep regimen, source of donor cells (including degree of HLA mismatch), GVHD, complications
f. Investigational treatments
g. Adverse drug reactions or allergies
2. Follow-up any investigational treatments used
3. Determine any potential problems by organ system, and devise plan for routine evaluation

B. Common Late Effects[1,5–7] (See Table EC 22-A on Expert Consult)

See also http://www.survivorshipguidelines.org/

1. **Immunocompromise**
a. No utility in *getting vaccinations in* before chemotherapy or HSCT
b. After treatment is finished, time to full recovery of adaptive immune function is variable. Typically takes 3–6 months for patients treated with chemotherapy but no HSCT; for patients treated with HSCT, takes a minimum of several months and often >1 year

c. Chronic GVHD: Functionally asplenic; no live-virus vaccinations, reimmunize against pneumococcus, *Haemophilus influenzae* type b, meningococcus

d. **Patients treated with chemotherapy, but no HSCT:**
   (1) Administer all recommended vaccines prior to starting therapy
   (2) Vaccinations should not have to be repeated and patients can resume receiving all vaccines (including live) 3 months after the cessation of therapy

e. **Patients treated with HSCT:**
   (1) Consider these patients unimmunized and needing a full catch-up immunization schedule
   (2) Do *not* give vaccines from the start of chemotherapy preparation to at least 6 months after HSCT (longer if patient has active GVHD or is taking immunosuppressive medications, such as cyclosporine)

2. **Organ system specific late effects** (See Table EC 22-A on Expert Consult for more specific information)

a. **Endocrine:** Obesity, precocious puberty, growth hormone deficiency, hyperthyroidism/hypothyroidism, ovarian and testicular dysfunction (hypogonadism, infertility)

b. **Neurocognitive/psychosocial:** Cognitive dysfunction, leukoencephalopathy, hearing/vision loss, peripheral neuropathy, seizures, depression/anxiety, post-traumatic stress, limitations in health care and insurance

c. **Skeletal:** Osteopenia/osteoporosis

d. **Cardiac:** Cardiomyopathy (anthracyclines), arrhythmias, atherosclerotic disease/coronary artery disease (radiation), valvular disease, pericardial complications (pericarditis)

e. **Secondary malignancies:** Secondary myelodysplastic syndrome (MDS)/ AML (etoposide, alkylators), brain tumors (cranial x-ray therapy), breast cancer (x-ray therapy for Hodgkin's disease)

REFERENCES

1. Poplack D, Pizzo P. *Principles and practice of pediatric oncology.* 5th ed. Philadelphia: Lippincott Williams and Wilkins; 2006.
2. Kelly KM, Lange B. Oncologic emergencies. *Pediatr Clin North Am.* 1997;44(4):809–830.
3. Fleisher G, Ludwig S, eds. *Textbook of pediatric emergency medicine.* Philadelphia: Lippincott Williams & Wilkins; 2006.
4. Chanock SJ, Pizzo PA. Fever in the neutropenic host. *Infect Dis Clin North Am.* 1996;10(4):777–796.
5. Kliegman RM, Behrman RE, Jenson HB, et al. *Nelson textbook of pediatrics.* 18th ed. Philadelphia: Saunders; 2007.
6. Meck MM, Leary M, Sills RH. Late effects in survivors of childhood cancer. *Pediatr Rev.* 2006;27(7):257–262.
7. Pickering LK, ed. *2009 Red book: report of the Committee on Infectious Diseases.* 28th ed. Elk Grove Village, IL: American Academy of Pediatrics; 2009:72–86.

Chapter 23

Palliative Care

Judson Heugel, MD

23

I. PALLIATIVE CARE

A. Definition[1,2]

Palliative care is the active total care of the child's body, mind, and spirit with the intent to prevent and relieve suffering. It supports the best quality of life for the child and family beginning at diagnosis of a life-limiting condition and continuing regardless of whether or not the child receives treatment. Hospice care is a form of palliative care that focuses on the end of life and bereavement. Effective palliative care requires an interdisciplinary approach that works with child and family to determine goals of care. This is best accomplished when the palliative care team is involved as early in the child's course of illness as possible.

B. Palliative Care Team Composition

1. Child and family
2. Physicians: Primary care physician, specialist attending physician, fellow, resident, intern
3. Nurses: Primary nurse, charge nurse, home care nurse, hospice nurse
4. Pain specialist and hospice palliative care specialist
5. Social worker
6. Child life specialist
7. Pastoral care
8. Patient care coordinator and case manager
9. Bereavement coordinator
10. Community resources: School, faith community, hospice program

II. DECISION MAKING

A. Decision-making Tools (DMT)[3]

1. Provides consistent, reliable format for discussion and formulation of plan of care. Patients, families, and health care providers all participate in the process
2. Four domains of DMT should be updated regularly, especially during "non-crisis" periods

a. Medical indications: Diagnosis, symptoms, risk/benefits of treatment, cure/relapse rate, complications
b. Patient and family preferences: Information, decision making, desire for autonomy and privacy

TABLE 23-1

CONCEPTUALIZATION OF DEATH IN CHILDREN

Age Range	Characteristics	Concepts of Death	Interventions
0–2 yr	Achieve object permanence May sense something is wrong	None	Provide maximal comfort with familiar persons and favorite toys.
2–6 yr	Magical thoughts	Believes death is temporary Does not personalize death Believes death can be caused by thoughts	Minimize separation from parents; correct perceptions that the illness is punishment.
6–12 yr	Concrete thoughts	Understands death can be personal Interested in details of death	Be truthful, evaluate fears, provide concrete details if requested; allow participation in decision making.
12–18 yr	Reality becomes objective Capable of self-reflection	Searches for meaning, hope, purpose, and value of life	Be truthful, allow expression of strong feelings, allow participation in decision making.

c. Quality of life: Important activities of child, important relationships, emotional/spiritual well-being
d. Contextual issues: Identify family unit, home environment, financial barriers, legal issues, cultural and spiritual beliefs

B. Child Participation

1. Development of death concepts in children[4–7] (Table 23-1)
2. Child's capacity to participate in health care decisions. Minor children can participate meaningfully in decision making if they demonstrate all of the following:
a. Communicate understanding of the medical information
b. State his or her preference
c. Communicate understanding of the consequences of decisions

C. Advance Directive

1. Adolescents age 18 years and older can name another adult to make health care decisions if they are unable to speak for themselves
2. Health care team can help patients voice preferences for future health care decisions

III. LEGACY AND MEMORY MAKING

A. Memory Making

1. Provide opportunities for the family to participate in memory making (e.g., create memory boxes/packets, lock of hair, foot/hand molds or prints, videos, photographs)
2. Older children may have specific wishes for funeral, memorial, or for distribution of personal belongings

B. Rituals

Allow for culturally important rituals to be performed by the family (e.g., baptism, bathing, music, faith ceremonies or prayer).

IV. DECISIONS TO LIMIT INTERVENTIONS

A. Do Not Attempt Resuscitation (DNAR)

1. In the event of cardiorespiratory arrest, cardiopulmonary resuscitation (CPR) is automatically initiated in hospitals by health care teams and in community settings by first responders. For patients with life-threatening conditions, CPR may not prolong or enhance quality of life, making it inconsistent with goals of care. The health care team should offer patients and families the option of forgoing CPR and other resuscitative interventions as part of overall care plan that emphasizes comfort and quality of living (Box 23-1)
2. If this option is desired, physician must write a specific order *not* to attempt CPR (e.g., "In the event of cardiopulmonary arrest, do not attempt resuscitation."). Orders must follow local emergency medical services (EMS) policies for patients at home

B. Do Not Escalate Treatment

When escalation of treatment no longer supports goals of care, offer patients and families option to forgo treatment changes even as the patient's condition worsens. Because death is expected, DNAR must also be discussed. Examples of such requests include the following:

1. Do not increase the dose of current medications, such as vasopressors
2. Do not add new medications, such as antibiotics
3. Do not initiate new interventions, such as dialysis or mechanical ventilation
4. Initiate and increase interventions to treat pain and reduce suffering

BOX 23-1

SAMPLE FROM STATE OF MARYLAND EMS/DNAR FORMS AND BRACELET AUTHORIZATION FORM

The physician must sign the *Physician Certification and Order* and initial ONLY ONE of the two options on the form.

Option A:

Maximum Efforts to Prevent Cardiac/Respiratory Arrest

DNAR if Arrest Occurs—No CPR

Option B:

Supportive Care Prior to Cardiac/Respiratory Arrest

DNAR if Arrest Occurs—No CPR

NOTE: If a valid EMS/DNAR Order is located after resuscitation has begun, EMS personnel may withdraw resuscitation.

NOTE: Ambulance personnel cannot honor specific instructions in advance directives that do not conform to the care selections in the *Physician Certification and Order* (e.g., wants intubation but no CPR).

C. Discontinuing Current Interventions

When death is expected regardless of intervention, especially if current interventions are prolonging the dying process, patients and families can be offered the option of discontinuing these interventions (e.g., "Discontinue blood products, monitors, mechanical ventilation, medically provided hydration or nutrition."). Because death is expected, DNAR must also be discussed.

V. BODY, MIND, AND SPIRIT CHANGES AS DEATH APPROACHES[8]

A. Physical Changes

1. Cardiac: Blood pressure decreases, heart rate increases, and pulse becomes weaker
2. Circulation: Cool extremities; cyanosis of fingers, nails, lips; mottling of skin
3. Gastrointestinal: Metabolism slows and gradual decrease in appetite. Liquids are preferred to solids. The body will become naturally dehydrated, and fevers may occur as death approaches. Provide relief with ice chips, moist mouth swabs, antipyretic per rectum
4. Respiratory: Variable pattern of breathing (tachypnea followed by periods of apnea); congestion secondary to secretion build-up; provide relief as follows:
   a. Turn patient every few hours, elevate head of bed, provide frequent mouth care, hyoscyamine as needed
   b. Relief of air hunger: Morphine and lorazepam as needed, oxygen for comfort
   c. **NOTE:** Deep suctioning is not helpful
5. Sensation changes: Senses become overactive with bright lights, noise, or television may be upsetting. Hearing is typically the last sense to diminish. Provide relief by dimming lights, reducing noise, and providing soft background music
6. Sleep: Need for sleep increases as death approaches. Occasionally, the child exhibits a surge of energy to play, eat, or socialize

B. Emotional Changes

Detachment from the outside world: Reduced need to socialize leads to pulling inward of thoughts, emotions, and fears. Listen and reassure family about decreased interactions

C. Mental Changes

Mental status: Confusion, restlessness, agitation, delirium. Provide relief by keeping child oriented to surroundings, surrounding him/her with family as a way to reinforce safety and speaking in calm tones. Use lorazepam and haloperidol as needed.

D. Spiritual Changes

Spiritual: Child may call out or reach out for loved ones who are not physically present. Reassure the family that this is not unusual during the dying process.

VI. LAST HOURS: MEDICATION AND MANAGEMENT[9] (TABLE 23-2)

TABLE 23-2

COMMON MEDICATIONS USED FOR SYMPTOMATIC RELIEF IN PALLIATIVE CARE

Indication	Medication	Initial Regimen
Pain	Morphine	0.3 mg/kg/dose PO, SL, PR q2–4 hr* 0.1–0.2 mg/kg/dose IV q2–4 hr* **NOTE:** Morphine should be titrated to symptomatic relief.
Dyspnea	Morphine	0.1–0.25 mg/kg/dose PO, SL, PR q2–4 hr 0.05–0.1 mg/kg/dose IV q2–4 hr 2.5–5 mg/3 mL normal saline nebulizer q4hr **NOTE:** Nebulized morphine can cause severe bronchospasm and worsen dyspnea. Nebulized fentanyl may be preferred.
Agitation	Lorazepam Haloperidol	0.05 mg/kg/dose PO, IV, SL, PR q4–8 hr 0.01–0.02 mg/kg/dose PO, SL, PR q8–12 hr
Pruritus	Diphenhydramine	0.5–1 mg/kg/dose PO, IV q6–8 hr
Nausea and vomiting	Prochlorperazine Ondansetron	0.1–0.15 mg/kg/dose PO, PR q6–8 hr 0.15 mg/kg/dose PO, IV q6–8 hr
Seizures	Diazepam Lorazepam	0.3–0.5 mg/kg/dose PR q2–4 hr 0.05–0.1 mg/kg/dose IV q2–4 hr
Secretions	Hyoscyamine	0.03–0.06 mg/dose PO, SL q4hr (if <2 yr) 0.06–0.12 mg/dose PO, SL q4hr (if 2–12 yr) 0.12–0.25 mg/dose PO, SL q4hr (if >12 yr)

*Infants <6 mo should receive one third to one half the dose.

IV, intravenous; PO, oral; PR, rectal; SL, sublingual.

Adapted from Himelstein BP, Hilden JM, Boldt AM, et al: Pediatric palliative care. N Engl J Med 2004;350(17): 1752–1762.

VII. DEATH PRONOUNCEMENT[10]

Residents may be called to pronounce the death of a patient in the hospital. This important task should be carried out with competence, compassion, and respect.

A. Preparation

1. **Know the child's name and gender**
2. Be prepared to answer simple pertinent questions from family and friends
3. Consult with nursing for relevant information: Recent events, family response, and family dynamics
4. Determine the need and call for interdisciplinary support: Social work, child life, pastoral care, bereavement coordinator

B. Entering the Room

1. Enter quietly and respectfully along with the primary nurse
2. Introduce yourself and identify your role:

a. "I am Dr. ______, the doctor on call."

b. Determine the relationships of those in the room

c. Inform the family of the purpose ("I am here to examine your child.") and invite them to remain in the room

C. Procedure for Pronouncement

1. Check ID bracelet and pulse
2. Respectfully check response to tactile stimuli
3. Check for spontaneous respirations
4. Check for heart sounds
5. Record the time of death
6. Inform the family of death
7. Offer to contact other family members
8. Remember to convey sympathy: "I am so sorry for your loss."

D. Document Death in the Chart

1. Write date, time of death, and the provider pronouncing the death
2. Document absence of pulse, respirations, and heart sounds
3. Identify family members who were present and informed of death
4. Document notification of attending physician

E. Death Certificate

1. Locate a copy of a sample death certificate for reference
2. Use BLACK INK only and complete *Physician sections*
   a. **NOTE:** Do *NOT* use abbreviations (i.e., spell out the month: January 31 and not 1/31)
   b. **NOTE:** Do *NOT* cross out or use white out; must begin again if mistakes are made
   c. **NOTE:** Cardiopulmonary or respiratory arrest is *NOT* an acceptable primary cause of death

F. Autopsy Consent

1. Obtain family consent if indicated
2. Plan follow-up to contact and review autopsy results

VIII. AFTER DEATH—BEREAVEMENT[10]

A. Etiquette

Families want to know that their children are not forgotten. Sending condolence cards, attending funerals, and contacting the family weeks to months later are all appropriate physician activities that are deeply valued by bereaved families. Respectful listening to families and sharing memories of the child helps provide support during bereavement.

B. Available Services[11]

Be familiar with available services: Pastoral care, social work, bereavement coordinator, community support groups, counseling services, bereavement follow-up programs.

REFERENCES

1. Sepulveda C. Palliative care: World Health's Organization global perspective. *J Pain Symptom Manage.* 2002;24(2):91–96.
2. Nelson R. Palliative care for children: policy statement. *Pediatrics.* 2007;119(2): 351–357.

3. Jonsen A, Siegler M, Winslade W, eds. *Clinical Ethics: A practical approach to ethical decisions in clinical medicine.* 5th ed. New York: McGraw Hill Press; 2002.
4. Sourkes BM. *Armfuls of time: the psychological experience of children with life-threatening illnesses.* Pittsburgh: University of Pittsburgh Press; 1995.
5. Corr CA. Children's understanding of death: striving to understand death. In: Doka KJ, ed. *Children mourning, mourning children.* Washington, DC: Hospice Foundation of America; 1995:8–10.
6. Corr CA, Balk DE, eds. *Handbook of adolescent death and bereavement.* New York: Springer; 1996.
7. Faulkner K. Children's understanding of death. In: Armstrong-Dailey A, Zarbock S, eds. *Hospice care for children.* 2nd ed. New York: Oxford University Press; 2001:9–22.
8. Sigrist D. *Journey's end: a guide to understanding the final stages of the dying process.* Rochester, NY: Genesee Region Home Care; 1995.
9. Himelstein BP, Hilden JM, Boldt AM, et al. Pediatric palliative care. *N Engl J Med.* 2004;350(17):1752–1762.
10. Bailey A. *The palliative response.* Birmingham, AL: Menasha Ridge Press; 2003.
11. AAP Policy Statement. Committee on Bioethics and Committee on Hospital Care: Palliative care for children. *Pediatrics.* 2000;106(2 Pt 1):351–357.

23

Chapter 24

Pulmonology

Allison Kirk, MD

I. WEBSITES

American Lung Association: http://www.lungusa.org
Cystic Fibrosis Foundation: http://www.cff.org
American Academy of Allergy, Asthma and Immunology: http://www.aaaai.org
National Heart Lung and Blood Institute: National Asthma Education and Prevention Program: http://www.nhlbi.nih.gov
American Thoracic Society: http://www.thoracic.org

II. RESPIRATORY PHYSICAL EXAMINATION

A. Normal Respiratory Rates in Children (Table 24-1)

B. Inspection

Evaluate for chest wall abnormalities (barrel chest, pectus excavatum, or pectus carinatum), symmetry, accessory muscle use, cyanosis of lips, skin or nails, or digital clubbing.

C. Palpation and Percussion

D. Auscultation (Table 24-2)

III. EVALUATION OF PULMONARY GAS EXCHANGE

A. Pulse Oximetry[1–5]

1. Pulse oximetry (SpO_2) is an indirect measurement of arterial O_2 saturation (SaO_2) estimated by light absorption characteristics of oxygenated and deoxygenated hemoglobin through the skin in peripheral blood
2. Important uses:
a. Rapid and continuous assessment of oxygenation in acutely ill patients or patients requiring oxygen therapy
b. Assessment of oxygen requirements during feeding, sleep, exercise, or sedation
c. Monitoring of physiologic effects of apnea and bradycardia
3. Limitations:
a. Measures oxygen saturation and not O_2 delivery to tissues. A marginally low saturation may be more significant in an anemic patient due to their reduced O_2-carrying capacity
b. Insensitive to hyperoxia because of the sigmoid shape of the oxyhemoglobin curve (see Fig. 24-1)

TABLE 24-1

NORMAL RESPIRATORY RATES IN CHILDREN

Age (yr)	Respiratory Rate (breaths/min)
0–1*	24–38
1–3	22–30
4–6	20–24
7–9	18–24
10–14	16–22
14–18	14–20

*Slightly higher respiratory rates (i.e., 40–50 breaths/min) in the neonatal period may be normal in the absence of other signs and symptoms.

Data from Bardella IJ: Pediatric advanced life support: a review of the AHA recommendations. Am Fam Phys 1999;60(6):1743–1750.

TABLE 24-2

RESPIRATORY AUSCULTATION

Sound	Description	Possible Causes
Crackles (rales)	Intermittent, scratchy, bubbly noises Heard predominantly on inspiration Produced by reopening of airways closed on previous expiration	Bronchiolitis, pulmonary edema Pneumonia
Wheezes	Continuous, high-pitched, musical sound	Asthma, bronchiolitis, foreign body
Rhonchi	Continuous, low-pitched, nonmusical sound	Pneumonia, cystic fibrosis
Stridor	High-pitched, harsh, blowing sound Heard predominantly on inspiration	Croup, laryngomalacia, subglottic stenosis, allergic reaction, vocal cord dysfunction

c. Artificially increased: Carboxyhemoglobin levels >1%–2% (e.g., in chronic smokers or with smoke inhalation)
d. Artificially decreased: Patient motion, intravenous dyes (methylene blue, indocyanine green), opaque nail polish, and methemoglobin levels >1%
e. Unreliable when pulse signal is poor: Hypothermia, hypovolemia, shock, edema, or movement artifact
f. SpO_2 reading often does not correlate with PaO_2 in sickle cell disease[6]

4. Oxyhemoglobin dissociation curve (Fig. 24-1)

B. Capnography

1. Measures CO_2 concentration of expired gas by infrared spectroscopy or mass spectroscopy
2. End-tidal CO_2 ($ETCO_2$) correlates with $PaCO_2$ (usually within 5 mmHg in healthy subjects)
3. Can be used for demonstrating proper placement of an endotracheal tube, continuous monitoring of CO_2 trends in ventilated patients, and monitoring ventilation during polysomnography

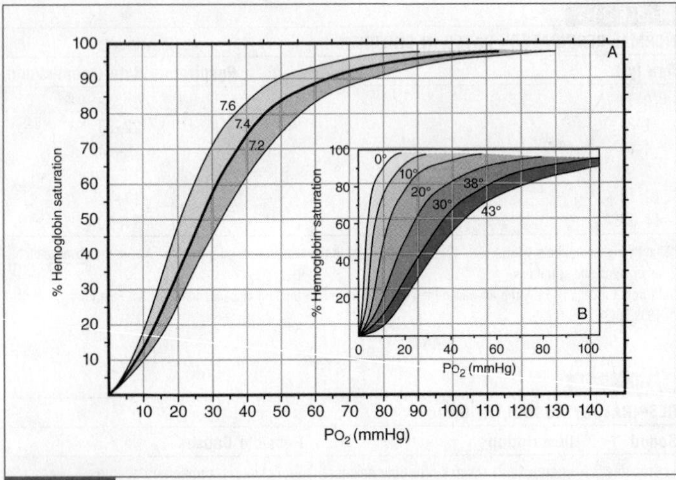

FIGURE 24-1

Oxyhemoglobin dissociation curve. **A,** Curve shifts to the left as pH increases. **B,** Curve shifts to the left as temperature decreases. *(Data from Lanbertsten CJ: Transport of oxygen, CO_2, and inert gases by the blood. In Mountcastle VB [ed]: Medical physiology, 14th ed. St. Louis, Mosby, 1980.)*

C. Blood Gases

1. **Arterial blood gas (ABG):** Most accurate way to assess oxygenation (PaO_2), ventilation ($PaCO_2$), and acid base status (pH and HCO_3^-). See Chapter 27 for normal mean values
2. **Venous blood gas (VBG):** $Pvco_2$ averages 6–8 mmHg higher than $Paco_2$, and venous pH is slightly lower than arterial pH. Measurement is strongly affected by the local circulatory and metabolic environment
3. **Capillary blood gas (CBG):** Correlation with ABG generally best for pH, moderate for PCO_2 and worst for PO_2

D. Analysis of Acid-base Disturbances[7–9]

1. Determine primary disturbance; then assess for mixed disorder by calculating expected compensatory response (see Fig. 24-2 and Table 24-3)

IV. PULMONARY FUNCTION TESTS

Provide objective and reproducible measurements to airway function and lung volumes. Used to characterize disease, assess severity and follow response to therapy.

A. Peak Expiratory Flow Rate (PEFR)

Maximal flow rate generated during a forced expiratory maneuver.

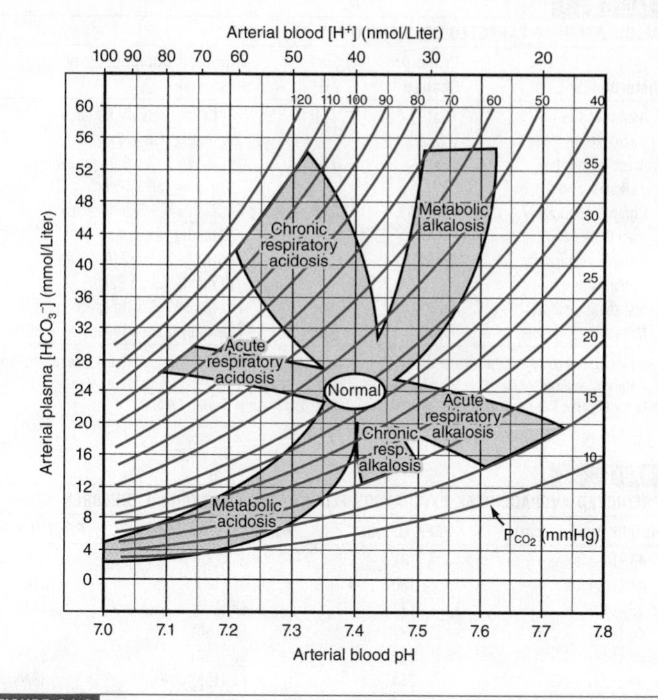

FIGURE 24-2

Interpretation of arterial blood gases. *(Modified from Siggaard-Anderson O: The acid-base status of the blood, 4th ed. Copenhagen, Munksgaard, 1976.)*

1. Often used to follow the course of asthma and response to therapy by comparing a patient's PEFR to the previous "personal best" and the normal predicted value
   a. Limitations: Normal predicted values vary across different racial groups. Measurement is effort dependent and cannot be done reliably by many young children, and PEFR is insensitive to small airway function
2. Normal predicted PEFR values for children (Table 24-4)

B. Maximal Inspiratory and Expiratory Pressures[10,11]

Maximal pressure generated during inhalation and exhalation against a fixed obstruction.

1. Used as a measure of respiratory muscle strength
2. Maximal inspiratory pressure (MIP) is in the range of 80 to 120 cm H_2O at all ages. Maximum expiratory pressure (MEP) increases with age and is greater in males

TABLE 24-3

CALCULATION OF EXPECTED COMPENSATORY RESPONSE

Disturbance	Primary Change	pH*	Expected Compensatory Response
Acute respiratory acidosis	↑$Paco_2$	↓pH	↑HCO_3^- by 1 mEq/L for each 10 mmHg rise in $Paco_2$
Acute respiratory alkalosis	↓$Paco_2$	↑pH	↓HCO_3^- by 1–3 mEq/L for each 10 mmHg fall in $Paco_2$
Chronic respiratory acidosis	↑$Paco_2$	↓pH	↑HCO_3^- by 4 mEq/L for each 10 mmHg rise in $Paco_2$
Chronic respiratory alkalosis	↓$Paco_2$	↑pH	↓HCO_3^- by 2–5 mEq/L for each 10 mmHg fall in $Paco_2$
Metabolic acidosis	↓HCO_3^-	↓pH	↓$Paco_2$ by 1–1.5 times fall in HCO_3^-
Metabolic alkalosis	↑HCO_3^-	↑pH	↑$Paco_2$ by 0.25–1 times rise in HCO_3^-

*Pure respiratory acidosis (or alkalosis): 10 mmHg rise (fall) in $Paco_2$ results in an average 0.08 fall (rise) in pH. Pure metabolic acidosis (or alkalosis): 10 mEq/L fall (rise) in HCO_3^- results in an average 0.15 fall (rise) in pH.

Data from Schrier RW: Renal and electrolyte disorders, 3rd ed. Boston, Little, Brown, 1986.

TABLE 24-4

PREDICTED AVERAGE PEAK EXPIRATORY FLOW RATES FOR NORMAL CHILDREN

Height Inches (cm)	PEFR (L/min)	Height Inches (cm)	PEFR (L/min)
43 (109)	147	56 (142)	320
44 (112)	160	57 (145)	334
45 (114)	173	58 (147)	347
46 (117)	187	59 (150)	360
47 (119)	200	60 (152)	373
48 (122)	214	61 (155)	387
49 (124)	227	62 (157)	400
50 (127)	240	63 (160)	413
51 (130)	254	64 (163)	427
52 (132)	267	65 (165)	440
53 (135)	280	66 (168)	454
54 (137)	293	67 (170)	467
55 (140)	307		

PEFR, Peak expiratory flow rate.

Data from Voter KZ: Diagnostic tests of lung function. Pediatr Rev 1996;17(2):53–63.

3. A low MIP may be an indication for ventilatory support and a low MEP correlates with decreased effectiveness of coughing

C. Spirometry (for Children ≥6 Years)

Plot of airflow versus time during rapid, forceful, and complete expiration from total lung capacity (TLC) to residual volume (RV). Useful to characterize different patterns of airway obstruction (see Fig. 24-3). Usually performed before and after bronchodilation to assess response to therapy or after bronchial challenge to assess airway hyperreactivity.

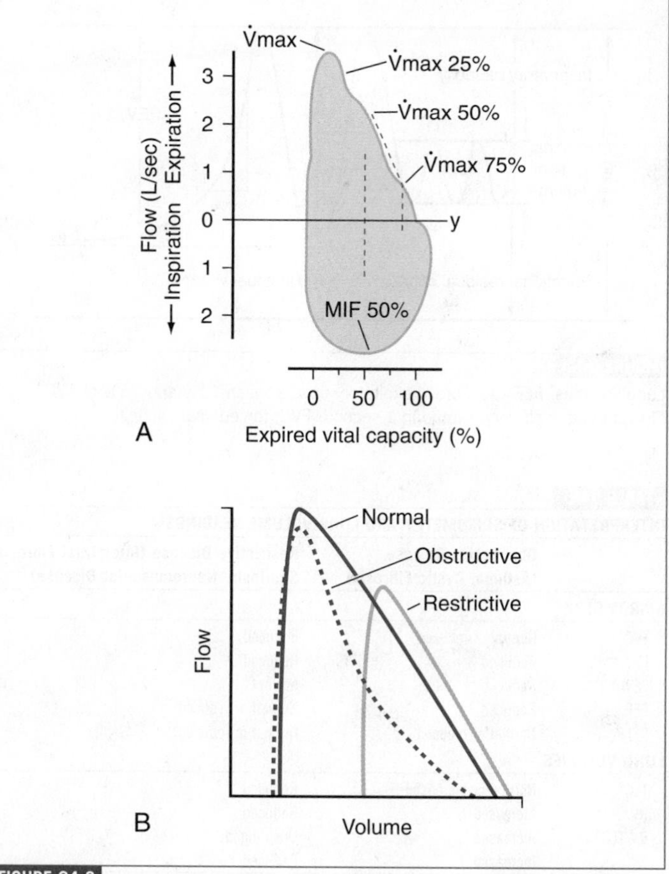

FIGURE 24-3

A, Normal flow-volume curve. **B,** Worsening intrathoracic airway obstruction as in asthma or cystic fibrosis. *(**B,** Data from Baum GL, Wolinsky E: Textbook of pulmonary diseases, 5th ed. Boston, Little, Brown, 1994.)*

1. Important definitions (see Fig. 24-4)

a. Forced vital capacity (FVC): Maximum volume of air exhaled from the lungs after a maximum inspiration. Bedside measurement of vital capacity with a handheld spirometer can be useful in confirming or predicting hypoventilation associated with muscle weakness

b. Forced expiratory volume in 1 second (FEV_1): Volume exhaled during the first second of an FVC maneuver

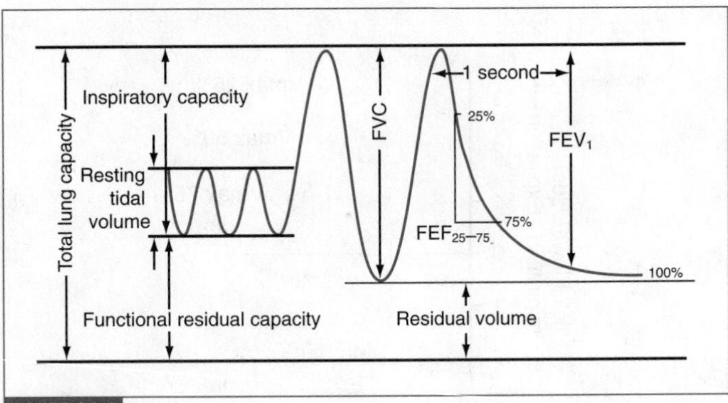

FIGURE 24-4

Lung volumes. FEF_{25-75}, Forced expiratory flow between 25% and 75% of FVC; FEV_1, forced expiratory volume in 1 second; FVC, forced vital capacity.

TABLE 24-5

INTERPRETATION OF SPIROMETRY AND LUNG VOLUME READINGS

	Obstructive Disease (Asthma, Cystic Fibrosis)	Restrictive Disease (Interstitial Fibrosis, Scoliosis, Neuromuscular Disease)
SPIROMETRY		
FVC*	Normal or reduced	Reduced
FEV_1*	Reduced	Reduced§
FEV_1/FVC†	Reduced	Normal
FEF_{25-75}	Reduced	Normal or reduced§
PEFR*	Normal or reduced	Normal or reduced§
LUNG VOLUMES		
TLC*	Normal or increased	Reduced
RV*	Increased	Reduced
RV/TLC‡	Increased	Unchanged
FRC	Increased	Reduced

*Normal range: ± 20% of predicted.

†Normal range: >85%.

‡Normal range: 20 ± 10%.

§Reduced proportional to FVC.

FEF_{25-75}, Forced expiratory flow between 25% and 75% of FVC; FEV_1, forced expiratory volume in 1 second; FRC, functional residual capacity; FVC, forced vital capacity; PEFR, peak expiratory flow rate; RV, residual volume; TLC, total lung capacity.

c. Forced expiratory flow (FEF_{25-75}): Mean rate of airflow over the middle half of the FVC between 25% and 75% of FVC. Sensitive to medium and small airway obstruction

2. Interpretation of spirometry and lung volume readings (Table 24-5)

V. APPARENT LIFE-THREATENING EVENT (ALTE)[12,13]

Definition: Events that are frightening to the observer, and include some combination of obstructive or central apnea, color change (usually cyanosis and/or pallor), a marked change in muscle tone (usually extreme limpness), choking, or gagging. In some cases the observer fears the infant has died or would have died without significant intervention.

A. Differential Diagnosis (Box 24-1)

B. Workup

Clinical story and physical exam guide the workup and treatment tailored to diagnosis and prevention of further events.

1. If history and physical suggest significant event took place consider obtaining a complete blood count (signs of infection or anemia), serum bicarbonate (acid base status), blood glucose (hypoglycemia), electrocardiogram (ECG) (QT interval)

BOX 24-1

DIFFERENTIAL DIAGNOSIS OF APPARENT LIFE-THREATENING EVENT (ALTE)

Gastroenterologic (33%)

Gastroesophageal reflux disease
Gastroenteritis
Esophageal dysfunction
Surgical abdomen
Dysphagias

Neurologic (15%)

Seizure
Central apnea/hypoventilation
Meningitis/encephalitis
Hydrocephalus
Brain tumor
Neuromuscular disorders
Vasovagal reaction

Idiopathic Apnea of Infancy (23%)

Respiratory (11%)

Respiratory syncytial virus
Pertussis
Aspiration
Respiratory tract infection
Reactive airway disease
Foreign body

Otolaryngologic (4%)

Laryngomalacia
Subglottic and/or laryngeal stenosis
Obstructive sleep apnea

Cardiovascular (1%)

Congenital heart disease
Cardiomyopathy
Cardiac arrhythmias/prolonged QT syndrome
Myocarditis

Metabolic/Endocrine

Inborn error of metabolism
Hypoglycemia
Electrolyte disturbance

Infectious

Sepsis
Urinary tract infection

Other Diagnosis

Child maltreatment syndrome
Shaken baby syndrome
Breath-holding spell
Choking
Drug or toxin reaction
Anemia
Unintentional smothering
Periodic breathing
Munchhausen-by-proxy syndrome

Modified from DeWolfe CC: Apparent life-threatening event: a review. Pediatr Clin North Am 2005;52:4.

2. Further evaluations dictated by clinical picture, some common studies listed below:
   a. Chest radiograph: Pneumonia, bronchiolitis, screen for cardiac disease
   b. Cardiopulmonary monitoring and/or polysomnography: Continuous assessment of oxygenation and ventilation (especially for recurrent events or unusual apnea), rule out obstructive apnea
   c. Barium swallow ± pH probe: dysfunctional swallow, upper airway obstruction, gastroesophageal reflux
   d. Electroencephalography (EEG): Seizure disorder
   e. Evaluation for non-accidental trauma if concern from history/physical

VI. ASTHMA[14]

A chronic inflammatory disorder of the airways resulting in recurrent episodes of wheezing, breathlessness, chest tightness, and cough, particularly at night and in the early morning. These episodes are usually associated with lower airway airflow obstruction, reversible either spontaneously or with therapy. The inflammation also causes increased airway hyperreactivity to a variety of stimuli (viral infections, cold air, exercise, emotions, as well as environmental allergens and pollutants).

A. Clinical Manifestations

1. Cough, increased work of breathing (tachypnea, retractions, or accessory muscle use), wheezing, hypoxia, and hypoventilation
2. No audible wheezing may indicate very poor air movement and severe bronchospasm
3. Chest radiographs often show peribronchial thickening, hyperinflation, and patchy atelectasis
   a. If persistent radiographic abnormalities consider right middle lobe syndrome

B. Management

1. Acute management and status asthmaticus; see Chapter 1
2. Initial classification and initiation of treatment for ages 0–4, 5–11, and ≥12 years: Figures 24-5, 24-6, and 24-7
3. Stepwise approach to continued management for ages 0–4, 5–11, and ≥12 years: Figures 24-8, 24-9, and 24-10

C. Prevention of Exacerbations

1. Ensure up to date on immunizations, including influenza
2. Create an asthma action plan (http://www.nhlbi.nih.gov/health/public/lung/index.htm#asthma or http://fha.maryland.gov/pdf/mch/Asthma_Action_Plan.pdf)
3. Attempt to minimize asthma triggers and environmental exposures, including tobacco smoke
4. Assess symptom control, inhaler technique, and medication adherence with regular clinical evaluations
5. Consider specialist referral for formal pulmonary function test (PFT) monitoring and allergy testing

Text continued on page 599

CLASSIFYING ASTHMA SEVERITY AND INITIATING TREATMENT IN CHILDREN 0–4 YEARS OF AGE

Assessing severity and initiating therapy in children who are not currently taking long-term control medication

Components of severity		Classification of asthma severity (0–4 years of age)			
			Persistent		
		Intermittent	Mild	Moderate	Severe
Impairment	Symptoms	≤2 days/week	>2 days/week but not daily	Daily	Throughout the day
	Nighttime awakenings	0	1–2×/month	3–4×/month	>1×/week
	Short-acting $beta_2$-agonist use for symptom control (not prevention of EIB)	≤2 days/week	>2 days/week but not daily	Daily	Several times per day
	Interference with normal activity	None	Minor limitation	Some limitation	Extremely limited
Risk	Exacerbations requiring oral systemic corticosteroids	0–1/year	≥2 exacerbations in 6 months requiring oral systemic corticosteroids, or ≥4 wheezing episodes/1 year lasting >1 day AND risk factors for persistent asthma		
		← Consider severity and interval since last exacerbation. Frequency and severity may fluctuate over time. Exacerbations of any severity may occur in patients in any severity category. →			
Recommended step for initiating therapy (See Fig. 24-8 for treatment steps.)		Step 1	Step 2	Step 3 and consider short course of oral systemic corticosteroids	
		In 2–6 weeks, depending on severity, evaluate level of asthma control that is achieved. If no clear benefit is observed in 4–6 weeks, consider adjusting therapy or alternative diagnoses.			

Key: EIB, exercise-induced bronchospasm

Notes

- The stepwise approach is meant to assist, not replace, the clinical decision making required to meet individual patient needs.
- Level of severity is determined by both impairment and risk. Assess impairment domain by patient's/caregiver's recall of previous 2–4 weeks. Symptom assessment for longer periods should reflect a global assessment such as inquiring whether the patient's asthma is better or worse since the last visit. Assign severity to the most severe category in which any feature occurs.
- At present, there are inadequate data to correspond frequencies of exacerbations with different levels of asthma severity. For treatment purposes, patients who had ≥2 exacerbations requiring oral systemic corticosteroids in the past 6 months, or ≥4 wheezing episodes in the past year, and who have risk factors for persistent asthma may be considered the same as patients who have persistent asthma, even in the absence of impairment levels consistent with persistent asthma.

FIGURE 24-5

Guidelines for classifying asthma severity and initiating treatment in infants and young children (0–4 years of age). *(Adapted from NAEPP—Expert Panel Report 3: Guidelines for the diagnosis and management of asthma, August 2007. http://www.nhlbi.nih.gov/guidelines/asthma/asthgdln.htm.)*

CLASSIFYING ASTHMA SEVERITY AND INITIATING TREATMENT IN CHILDREN 5–11 YEARS OF AGE

Assessing severity and initiating therapy in children who are not currently taking long-term control medication

Components of severity		Classification of asthma severity (5–11 years of age)			
			Persistent		
		Intermittent	Mild	Moderate	Severe
Impairment	Symptoms	≤2 days/week	>2 days/week but not daily	Daily	Throughout the day
	Nighttime awakenings	≤2×/month	3–4×/month	>1×/week but not nightly	Often 7×/week
	Short-acting beta$_2$-agonist use for symptom control (not prevention of EIB)	≤2 days/week	>2 days/week but not daily	Daily	Several times per day
	Interference with normal activity	None	Minor limitation	Some limitation	Extremely limited
	Lung function	• Normal FEV_1 between exacerbations • FEV_1 >80% predicted • FEV_1/FVC >85%	• FEV_1 = >80% predicted • FEV_1/FVC >80%	• FEV_1 = 60%–80% predicted • FEV_1/FVC = 75%–80%	• FEV_1 <60% predicted • FEV_1/FVC <75%
Risk	Exacerbations requiring oral systemic corticosteroids	0–1/year (see note)	≥2/year (see note) →		
		← Consider severity and interval since last exacerbation. Frequency and severity may fluctuate over time for patients in any severity category. →			
		Relative annual risk of exacerbations may be related to FEV_1.			
Recommended step for initiating therapy		Step 1	Step 2	Step 3, medium-dose ICS option	Step 3, medium-dose ICS option, or step 4
				and consider short course of oral systemic corticosteroids	
(See Fig. 24-9 for treatment steps.)		In 2–6 weeks, evaluate level of asthma control that is achieved, and adjust therapy accordingly.			

Key: EIB, exercise-induced bronchospasm; FEV_1, forced expiratory volume in 1 second; FVC, forced vital capacity; ICS, inhaled corticosteroids

Notes

- The stepwise approach is meant to assist, not replace, the clinical decision making required to meet individual patient needs.
- Level of severity is determined by both impairment and risk. Assess impairment domain by patient's/caregiver's recall of previous 2–4 weeks and spirometry. Assign severity to the most severe category in which any feature occurs.
- At present, there are inadequate data to correspond frequencies of exacerbations with different levels of asthma severity. In general, more frequent and intense exacerbations (e.g., requiring urgent, unscheduled care, hospitalization, or ICU admission) indicate greater underlying disease severity. For treatment purposes, patients who had ≥2 exacerbations requiring oral systemic corticosteroids in the past year may be considered the same as patients who have persistent asthma, even in the absence of impairment levels consistent with persistent asthma.

FIGURE 24-6

Guidelines for classifying asthma severity and initiating treatment in children 5–11 years of age. *(Adapted from NAEPP—Expert Panel Report 3: Guidelines for the diagnosis and management of asthma, August 2007. http://www.nhlbi.nih.gov/guidelines/asthma/asthgdln.htm.)*

CLASSIFYING ASTHMA SEVERITY AND INITIATING TREATMENT IN YOUTHS ≥12 YEARS OF AGE

Assessing severity and initiating treatment for patients who are not currently taking long-term control medications

Components of severity		Classification of asthma severity ≥12 years of age			
			Persistent		
		Intermittent	Mild	Moderate	Severe
Impairment **Normal FEV_1/FVC:** 8–19 yr 85% 20–39 yr 80% 40–59 yr 75% 60–80 yr 70%	Symptoms	≤2 days/week	>2 days/week but not daily	Daily	Throughout the day
	Nighttime awakenings	≤2×/month	3–4×/month	>1×/week but not nightly	Often 7×/week
	Short-acting $beta_2$-agonist use for symptom control (not prevention of EIB)	≤2 days/week	>2 days/week but not daily, and not more than 1 time on any day	Daily	Several times per day
	Interference with normal activity	None	Minor limitation	Some limitation	Extremely limited
	Lung function	• Normal FEV_1 between exacerbations • FEV_1 >80% predicted • FEV_1/FVC normal	• FEV_1 >80% predicted • FEV_1/FVC normal	• FEV_1 >60% but <80% predicted • FEV_1/FVC reduced 5%	• FEV_1 <60% predicted • FEV_1/FVC reduced >5%
Risk	Exacerbations requiring oral systemic corticosteroids	0–1/year (see note)	≥2/year (see note) →		
		← Consider severity and interval since last exacerbation. Frequency and severity may fluctuate over time for patients in any severity category. →			
		Relative annual risk of exacerbations may be related to FEV_1.			
Recommended step for initiating treatment **(See Fig. 24-10 for treatment steps.)**		Step 1	Step 2	Step 3 and consider short course of oral systemic corticosteroids	Step 4 or 5 and consider short course of oral systemic corticosteroids
		In 2–6 weeks, evaluate level of asthma control that is achieved and adjust therapy accordingly.			

Key: FEV_1, forced expiratory volume in 1 second; FVC, forced vital capacity; ICU, intensive care unit

Notes

- The stepwise approach is meant to assist, not replace, the clinical decision making required to meet individual patient needs.
- Level of severity is determined by both impairment and risk. Assess impairment domain by patient's/caregiver's recall of previous 2–4 weeks and spirometry. Assign severity to the most severe category in which any feature occurs.
- At present, there are inadequate data to correspond frequencies of exacerbations with different levels of asthma severity. In general, more frequent and intense exacerbations (e.g., requiring urgent, unscheduled care, hospitalization, or ICU admission) indicate greater underlying disease severity. For treatment purposes, patients who had ≥2 exacerbations requiring oral systemic corticosteroids in the past year may be considered the same as patients who have persistent asthma, even in the absence of impairment levels consistent with persistent asthma.

FIGURE 24-7

Guidelines for classifying asthma severity and initiating treatment in youth 12 and older. *(Adapted from NAEPP—Expert Panel Report 3: Guidelines for the diagnosis and management of asthma, August 2007. http://www.nhlbi.nih.gov/guidelines/asthma/asthgdln.htm.)*

STEPWISE APPROACH FOR MANAGING ASTHMA IN CHILDREN 0–4 YEARS OF AGE

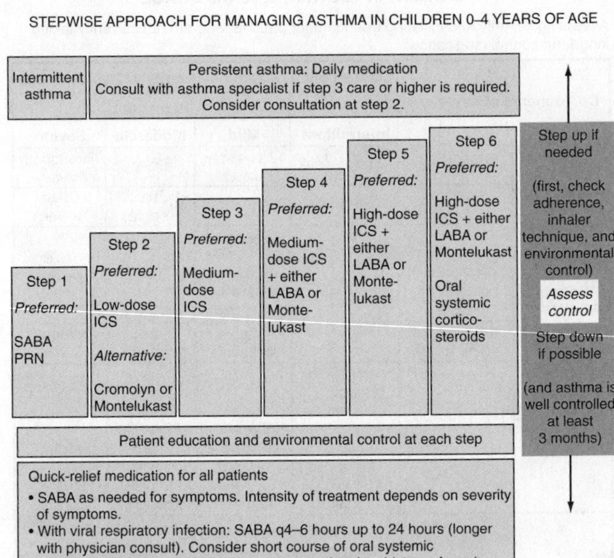

Key: **Alphabetical order is used when more than one treatment option is listed within either preferred or alternative therapy**. ICS, inhaled corticosteroid; LABA, long-acting inhaled beta$_2$-agonist; SABA, short-acting inhaled beta$_2$-agonist

Notes:

- The stepwise approach is meant to assist, not replace, the clinical decision making required to meet individual patient needs.
- If alternative treatment is used and response is inadequate, discontinue it and use the preferred treatment before stepping up.
- If clear benefit is not observed within 4–6 weeks and patient/family medication technique and adherence are satisfactory, consider adjusting therapy or alternative diagnosis.
- Studies on children 0–4 years of age are limited. Step 2 preferred therapy is based on Evidence A. All other recommendations are based on expert opinion and extrapolation from studies in older children.

FIGURE 24-8

Stepwise approach for managing asthma in infants and young children (0–4 years of age). *(Adapted from NAEPP—Expert Panel Report 3: Guidelines for the diagnosis and management of asthma, August 2007. http://www.nhlbi.nih.gov/guidelines/asthma/asthgdln.htm.)*

STEPWISE APPROACH FOR MANAGING ASTHMA IN CHILDREN 5–11 YEARS OF AGE

Intermittent asthma	Persistent asthma: Daily medication Consult with asthma specialist if step 4 care or higher is required. Consider consultation at step 3.					
Step 1 *Preferred:* SABA PRN	**Step 2** *Preferred:* Low-dose ICS *Alternative:* Cromolyn, LTRA, Nedocromil, or Theophylline	**Step 3** *Preferred:* EITHER: Low-dose ICS + either LABA, LTRA, or Theophylline OR Medium-dose ICS	**Step 4** *Preferred:* Medium-dose ICS + LABA *Alternative:* Medium-dose ICS + either LTRA or Theophylline	**Step 5** *Preferred:* High-dose ICS + LABA *Alternative:* High-dose ICS + either LTRA or Theophylline	**Step 6** *Preferred:* High-dose ICS + LABA + oral systemic corticosteroid *Alternative:* High-dose ICS + either LTRA or Theophylline + oral systemic corticosteroid	↑ Step up if needed (first, check adherence, inhaler technique, environmental control, and comorbid conditions) *Assess control* Step down if possible (and asthma is well controlled at least 3 months) ↓

Each step: Patient education, environmental control, and management of comorbidities.
Steps 2–4: Consider subcutaneous allergen immunotherapy for patients who have allergic asthma (see notes).

Quick-relief medication for all patients
- SABA as needed for symptoms. Intensity of treatment depends on severity of symptoms: up to 3 treatments at 20-minute intervals as needed. Short course of oral systemic corticosteroids may be needed.
- Caution: Increasing use of SABA or use >2 days a week for symptom relief (not prevention of EIB) generally indicates inadequate control and the need to step up treatment.

Key: **Alphabetical order is used when more than one treatment option is listed within either preferred or alternative therapy**. ICS, inhaled corticosteroid; LABA, long-acting inhaled beta$_2$-agonist; LTRA, leukotriene receptor antagonist; SABA, short-acting inhaled beta$_2$-agonist

Notes:
- The stepwise approach is meant to assist, not replace, the clinical decision making required to meet individual patient needs.
- If alternative treatment is used and response is inadequate, discontinue it and use the preferred treatment before stepping up.
- Theophylline is a less desirable alternative due to the need to monitor serum concentration levels.
- Step 1 and step 2 medications are based on Evidence A. Step 3 ICS + adjunctive therapy and ICS are based on Evidence B for efficacy of each treatment and extrapolation from comparator trials in older children and adults—comparator trials are not available for this age group; steps 4–6 are based on expert opinion and extrapolation from studies in older children and adults.
- Immunotherapy for steps 2–4 is based on Evidence B for house-dust mites, animal danders, and pollens; evidence is weak or lacking for molds and cockroaches. Evidence is strongest for immunotherapy with single allergens. The role of allergy in asthma is greater in children than in adults. Clinicians who administer immunotherapy should be prepared and equipped to identify and treat anaphylaxis that may occur.

FIGURE 24-9
Stepwise approach for managing asthma in children 5–11. *(Adapted from NAEPP—Expert Panel Report 3: Guidelines for the diagnosis and management of asthma, August 2007. http://www.nhlbi.nih.gov/guidelines/asthma/asthgdln.htm.)*

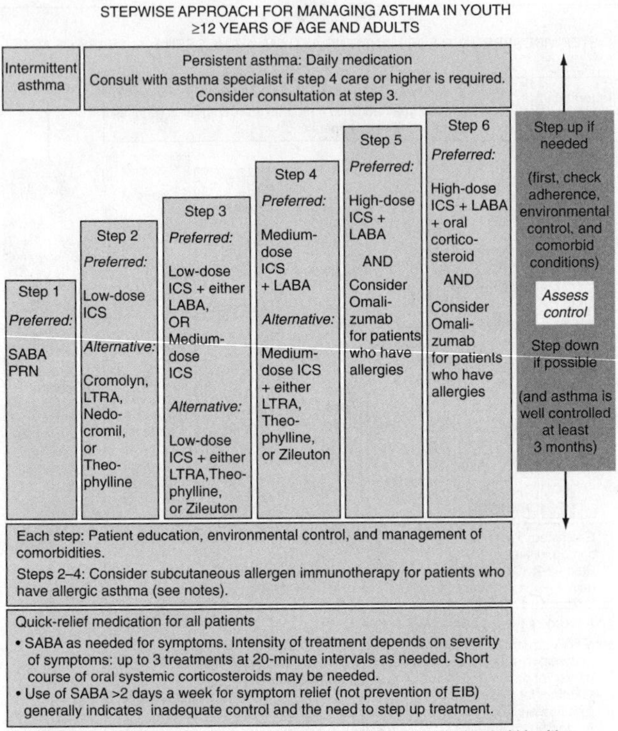

STEPWISE APPROACH FOR MANAGING ASTHMA IN YOUTH ≥12 YEARS OF AGE AND ADULTS

Intermittent asthma	Persistent asthma: Daily medication Consult with asthma specialist if step 4 care or higher is required. Consider consultation at step 3.					
Step 1 *Preferred:* SABA PRN	**Step 2** *Preferred:* Low-dose ICS *Alternative:* Cromolyn, LTRA, Nedocromil, or Theophylline	**Step 3** *Preferred:* Low-dose ICS + either LABA, OR Medium-dose ICS *Alternative:* Low-dose ICS + either LTRA, Theophylline, or Zileuton	**Step 4** *Preferred:* Medium-dose ICS + LABA *Alternative:* Medium-dose ICS + either LTRA, Theophylline, or Zileuton	**Step 5** *Preferred:* High-dose ICS + LABA AND Consider Omalizumab for patients who have allergies	**Step 6** *Preferred:* High-dose ICS + LABA + oral corticosteroid AND Consider Omalizumab for patients who have allergies	Step up if needed (first, check adherence, environmental control, and comorbid conditions) *Assess control* Step down if possible (and asthma is well controlled at least 3 months)

Each step: Patient education, environmental control, and management of comorbidities.

Steps 2–4: Consider subcutaneous allergen immunotherapy for patients who have allergic asthma (see notes).

Quick-relief medication for all patients

- SABA as needed for symptoms. Intensity of treatment depends on severity of symptoms: up to 3 treatments at 20-minute intervals as needed. Short course of oral systemic corticosteroids may be needed.
- Use of SABA >2 days a week for symptom relief (not prevention of EIB) generally indicates inadequate control and the need to step up treatment.

Key: **Alphabetical order is used when more than one treatment option is listed within either preferred or alternative therapy**. EIB, exercise-induced bronchospasm; ICS, inhaled corticosteroid; LABA, long-acting inhaled beta$_2$-agonist; LTRA, leukotriene receptor antagonist; SABA, short-acting inhaled beta$_2$-agonist

Notes:

- The stepwise approach is meant to assist, not replace, the clinical decision making required to meet individual patient needs.
- If alternative treatment is used and response is inadequate, discontinue it and use the preferred treatment before stepping up.
- Zileuton is a less desirable alternative due to limited studies as adjunctive therapy and the need to monitor liver function. Theophylline requires monitoring of serum concentration levels.
- In step 6, before oral systemic corticosteroids are introduced, a trial of high-dose ICS + LABA + either LTRA, theophylline, or zileuton may be considered, although this approach has not been studied in clinical trials.
- Step 1, 2, and 3 preferred therapies are based on Evidence A; step 3 alternative therapy is based on Evidence A for LTRA, Evidence B for theophylline, and Evidence D for zileuton. Step 4 preferred therapy is based on Evidence B, and alternative therapy is based on Evidence B for LTRA and theophylline and Evidence D for zileuton. Step 5 preferred therapy is based on Evidence B. Step 6 preferred therapy is based on Expert Panel Report 2 (1997) and Evidence B for omalizumab.
- Immunotherapy for steps 2–4 is based on Evidence B for house-dust mites, animal danders, and pollens; evidence is weak or lacking for molds and cockroaches. Evidence is strongest for immunotherapy with single allergens. The role of allergy in asthma is greater in children than in adults.
- Clinicians who administer immunotherapy or omalizumab should be prepared and equipped to identify and treat anaphylaxis that may occur.

FIGURE 24-10

Stepwise approach for managing asthma in youth 12 and older. *(Adapted from NAEPP—Expert Panel Report 3: Guidelines for the diagnosis and management of asthma, August 2007. http://www.nhlbi.nih.gov/guidelines/asthma/asthgdln.htm.)*

VII. BRONCHIOLITIS[15]

Lower respiratory tract infection common in infants; characterized by acute inflammation, edema, and necrosis of airway epithelium leading to increased mucus production and bronchospasm.

A. Clinical Manifestations

1. Variable and dynamic course ranging from transient apnea and mucus plugging to progressive lower airway disease
a. Initial symptoms: Clear rhinorrhea, diminished appetite, fever
b. Later symptoms: Tachypnea, wheezing, dyspnea, irritability
2. Radiographic findings: Hyperinflation and patchy atelectasis
3. Most common cause: Respiratory syncytial virus (RSV); also parainfluenza, adenovirus, mycoplasma, human metapneumovirus

B. Treatment

Mainstay is supportive care.

1. Consider hospitalization based on clinical presentation. Should be strongly considered for patients <12 weeks, history of prematurity, underlying cardiopulmonary disease, or immunodeficiency
2. Supplemental oxygen therapy for oxyhemoglobin saturation (SpO_2) consistently low
a. Consider maintaining higher SpO_2 for those with fever, acidosis or hemoglobinopathies due to oxyhemoglobin desaturation curve or for increased work of breathing
3. A trial of bronchodilators is an option, but should be continued only if there is documented improved clinical response
4. Corticosteroids and antibiotics (unless signs of bacterial co-infection) should not be used routinely in bronchiolitis
5. Fluid support is often needed due to increased loses from tachypnea, fever, and poor oral intake
a. Hold oral feedings in hospitalized tachypneic infants to minimize risk of aspiration

C. Clinical Pearls

1. In infants younger than 3 months with RSV, there is an appreciable incidence of co-infection with urinary tract infection (UTI) and/or acute otitis media
2. Infants hospitalized for bronchiolitis are more likely to have recurrent wheezing
3. Ensure RSV immunoprophylaxis for high-risk infants. See Chapter 16

VIII. BRONCHOPULMONARY DYSPLASIA[16,17]

Chronic pulmonary condition that usually evolves after premature birth characterized by need for oxygen supplementation >21% for at least 28 days after birth. Also known as chronic lung disease of prematurity or chronic lung disease of infancy. Thought to be a result of airway inflammation, damage from hyperoxia, hypoxia, or mechanical ventilation, resulting in interference with normal lung alveolar and vascular development.

A. Diagnostic Criteria

1. Severity based on oxygen requirement at time of assessment and characterized as mild if on room air, moderate if requiring <30% oxygen, or severe if requiring >30% oxygen and/or positive pressure
a. If gestational age at birth was <32 weeks: Assess infant at 36 weeks postmenstrual age or at discharge to home, whichever comes first
b. If gestational age at birth >32 weeks: Assess infant at 28–56 days postnatal age or at discharge to home, whichever comes first

B. Clinical Manifestations and Management

1. Persistent respiratory symptoms, airway hyperreactivity, and supplemental oxygen requirements, especially during intercurrent illness
2. Often require interventions such as bronchodilators, anti-inflammatory agents, supplemental oxygen therapy, and diuretics. Severe cases may require tracheostomy and prolonged mechanical ventilation
3. Need close monitoring for complications such as pulmonary or systemic hypertension, electrolyte abnormalities and nephrocalcinosis (from chronic diuretics), neurodevelopmental and growth delay

IX. CYSTIC FIBROSIS (CF)[18–20]

An autosomal recessive disorder in which mutations of the cystic fibrosis transmembrane conductance regulator (*CFTR*) gene changes the function of a chloride channel that usually resides within mucosal epithelial cells in the airways, pancreatic ducts, biliary tree, intestine, vas deference and sweat glands. Most patients have chronic progressive obstructive pulmonary disease, pancreatic exocrine insufficiency with protein and fat malabsorption, and abnormally high sweat electrolyte concentrations.

A. Clinical Manifestations (Table 24-6)

B. Diagnosis

Over half of patients are diagnosed by 6 months old and three-fourths by 2 years old.

1. Quantitative pilocarpine ionoelectrophoresis (sweat chloride) test: Gold standard for diagnosis
a. Positive for CF: >60 mEq/L (mEq/L = mmol/L)
b. Indeterminant:
   (1) Infants <6 months: Indeterminant if 30–60 mEq/L
   (2) Children >6 months: Indeterminant if 40–60 mEq/L
c. Normal:
   (1) Infants <6 months: Normal if <30 mEq/L
   (2) Children >6 months: Normal if <40 mEq/L

TABLE 24-6

MAJOR CLINICAL MANIFESTATIONS OF CYSTIC FIBROSIS BY ORGAN SYSTEM

Respiratory	Chronic productive cough, hemoptysis Bronchiectasis, bronchitis, pneumonia Sinusitis Nasal polyposis
Gastrointestinal	Meconium ileus Rectal prolapse Pancreatic insufficiency Distal intestinal obstruction syndrome (DIOS) Fat-soluble vitamin deficiency (A, D, E, K)
Genitourinary	Infertility (male) and decreased fertility (female) Absence of vas deferens
Miscellaneous	Increased sweat electrolytes Hypokalemic alkalosis Digital clubbing Pulmonary hypertrophic osteoarthropathy Failure to thrive

2. DNA testing becoming increasingly important in diagnosis. Over 1,500 mutations have been described, most common is DeltaF508 (present in 70% of those with CF)
3. Newborn screening (NBS): Many states have adopted universal newborn screening by measuring infants' immunoreactive trypsinogen (IRT) levels and/or DNA testing for most common mutations. A confirmatory sweat chloride test should be performed promptly in those patients who have a positive NBS result
4. Clinical pearl: Elevated sweat chloride levels can be from other disorders including untreated adrenal insufficiency, glycogen storage disease type 1, fucosidosis, hypothyroidism, nephrogenic diabetes insipidus, ectodermal dysplasia, malnutrition, mucopolysaccharidosis, panhypopituitarism, or poor testing technique

C. Pulmonary Therapies

1. Airway clearance therapy (ACT) to mobilize airway secretions and facilitate expectoration: Often manual/mechanical percussion and postural drainage; older children may use high frequency chest wall compression device (vest therapy), mechanical chest percussors, or oscillatory positive expiratory pressure (PEP) handheld devices (e.g., flutter valve and acapella)
2. Aerosolized medications to increase mucociliary clearance: Recombinant human DNAase (dornase alfa) which cleaves nucleic material and hypertonic saline nebs to hydrate airway mucus and stimulate cough
3. Chronic antibiotics: If *Pseudomonas aeruginosa* is persistently present in culture of airways, consider aerosolized tobramycin and/or chronic macrolide therapy

D. Common Complications

1. Pancreatic disease
a. Pancreatic enzyme replacement therapy (PERT) prior to meals to improve digestion and intestinal absorption of dietary protein and fat
b. Nutritional supplementation to maintain body mass index (BMI) ≥50th percentile
c. Monitoring for CF induced diabetes or episodes of pancreatitis
2. Intestinal: Meconium ileus, distal intestinal obstruction syndrome (DIOS), rectal prolapse
3. Infertility:
a. Nearly all males have absence of the vas deferens; however, assisted fertilization is possible using aspiration of viable sperm from the testes
b. Women may have trouble becoming pregnant due to mucus-associated obstruction of the cervix
4. Decreased life expectancy: Survival continues to improve and the median predicted survival age is over 37 years

X. OBSTRUCTIVE SLEEP APNEA SYNDROME (OSAS)[21–23]

Part of the spectrum of sleep-disordered breathing characterized by prolonged partial and/or intermittent partial or complete upper airway obstruction with accompanying hypoxemia, hypercapnia and/or sleep disruption. Alternate names include obstructive hypoventilation, upper airway resistance syndrome.

A. Clinical Manifestations

1. Snoring sometimes accompanied by intermittent pauses in breathing, snorts, or gasps
2. Increased respiratory effort during sleep, disturbed or restless sleep with increased arousals and awakenings
3. Daytime cognitive and/or behavioral problems. Young children rarely present with daytime sleepiness
4. Long-term complications include neurocognitive impairment, behavioral problems, poor growth, and systemic and pulmonary hypertension
5. Risk factors include adenotonsillar hypertrophy, obesity, craniofacial or laryngeal anomalies, central nervous system disease (including brainstem dysfunction or compression), cerebral palsy, and neuromuscular disease

B. Diagnosis

1. Screen for snoring during routine well-child care
2. Refer to specialists for nocturnal polysomnography (sleep study) for patients with history of nightly or near nightly snoring, risk factors, and/or daytime symptoms
a. Polysomnography includes measurement of electroencephalography (EEG), electrooculography (EOG), and electromyography (EMG) to monitor sleep stage and movement, ECG, chest wall and abdominal movement to assess respiratory effort, nasal/oral airflow,

transcutaneous or end tidal CO_2 (ventilation), and pulse oximetry (oxygenation)

b. Diagnosis of OSAS by polysomnography is based on obstructive apnea-hypopnea index (AHI) and gas exchange abnormalities resulting from upper airway obstruction. Polysomnography is used to differentiate OSAS from benign snoring and other disorders that may disrupt sleep including central hypoventilation syndrome, sleep-related respiratory failure related to neuromuscular disease or lung disease, and nocturnal seizures

C. Treatment

1. Tonsillectomy and adenoidectomy are mainstays of treatment
2. Continuous positive airway pressure (CPAP) or bilevel positive airway pressure (BiPAP) for patients who fail surgical therapy or are not candidates for surgery
3. Weight loss in obese children
4. Treatment of upper respiratory allergies

XI. SUDDEN INFANT DEATH SYNDROME[24]

Sudden death of an infant younger than 1 year, which remains unexplained after a thorough case investigation, including performance of complete autopsy, examination of death scene, and review of clinical history. Thought to be caused when a genetically vulnerable infant is exposed to an exogenous stressor during a critical developmental period when there is immaturity of the cardiorespiratory system, autonomic nervous system, immune system, and arousal pathways together with a failure of arousal responsiveness from sleep.

A. Epidemiology

1. Incidence is 0.56 per 1,000 in the United States, 2–3 times higher in African American and Native American populations
2. Peak incidence at 2–4 months of age with male predominance

B. Risk Factors and Protective Factors (Box 24-2)

BOX 24-2

FACTORS ASSOCIATED WITH SUDDEN INFANT DEATH SYNDROME (SIDS)

Risk Factors	Protective Factors
Premature birth	Sleeping in prone position
In utero and postnatal smoke exposure	Sleeping on firm mattress
Side and prone sleeping	Pacifier use during sleep
Sleeping on soft mattress and bedding	Live and sleep in smoke-free zone
Overbundling	Sleep in same room as caregivers
Bed sharing	
Recent infection	
Siblings with SIDS	
Low socioeconomic factors	

REFERENCES

1. Murray CB, Loughlin GM. Making the most of pulse oximetry. *Contemp Pediatr.* 1995;12(7):45–62.
2. Comber JT, Lopez BL. Examination of pulse oximetry in sickle cell anemia patients presenting to the emergency department in acute vasoocclusive crisis. *Am J Emerg Med.* 1996;14(1):16–18.
3. Salyer J. Neonatal and pediatric pulse oximetry. *Respiratory Care.* 2003;48(4): 386–398.
4. AAP Practice Guideline. Apnea, sudden infant death syndrome and home monitoring. *Pediatrics.* 2003;111(4 Pt 1):914–917.
5. Taussig L. *Pediatric respiratory medicine.* 2nd ed. Philadelphia: Mosby; 2008.
6. Blaisdell CJ, Goodman S, Clark K, et al. Pulse oximetry is a poor predictor of hypoxemia in stable children with sickle cell disease. *Arch Pediatr Adolesc Med.* 2000;154(9):900–903.
7. Schrier RW: *Renal and electrolyte disorders.* 6th ed. Philadelphia: Lippincott Williams and Wilkins; 2002.
8. Brenner BM, Rector FC, eds. *The kidney.* Vol. 1, 7th ed. Philadelphia: WB Saunders; 2003.
9. Lanbertsten CJ. Transport of oxygen, CO2, and inert gases by the blood. In Mountcastle VB, ed. *Medical physiology.* 14th ed. St. Louis: Mosby; 1980.
10. Panitch HB. The pathophysiology of respiratory impairment in pediatric neuromuscular diseases. *Pediatrics.* 2009;123:S215–S218.
11. Domènech-Clar R, López-Andreu JA, Compte-Torrero L, et al. Maximal static respiratory pressures in children and adolescents. *Pediatr Pulmonol.* 2003;35: 126–132.
12. DeWolfe C. Apparent life-threatening event: a review. *Pediatr Clin North Am.* 2005;52:1127–1146.
13. McMillan JA, Feigin RD, DeAngelis CD, et al. *Oski's pediatrics: principles and practice.* 4th ed. Philadelphia: Lippincott Williams and Wilkins; 2006.
14. NAEPP–Expert Panel Report 3. Guidelines for the diagnosis and management of asthma. August 2007. Accessed 27 July 2009. http://www.nhlbi.nih.gov/guidelines/asthma/asthgdln.htm.
15. AAP Clinical Practice Guideline. Diagnosis and management of bronchiolitis. *Pediatrics.* 2006;118(4):1774–1793.
16. Jobe A, Bancalari E. Bronchopulmonary dysplasia. *Am J Respir Crit Care Med.* 2001;163:1723–1729.
17. Allen J, Zwerdling R, Ehrenkranz R, et al. American Thoracic Society. Statement on the care of the child with chronic lung disease of infancy and childhood. *Am J Respir Crit Care Med.* 2003;168:356–396.
18. Montgomery G, Howenstine M. Cystic fibrosis. *Pediatr Rev.* 2009;30: 302–310.
19. Farrell P. Guidelines for diagnosis of cystic fibrosis in newborns through older adults: Cystic Fibrosis Foundation Consensus Report. *J Pediatr.* 2008;153: S4–S14.
20. Flume PA, O'Sullivan BP, Robinson KA, et al. Cystic fibrosis pulmonary guidelines: chronic medicines for maintenance of lung health. *Am J Resp Crit Care Med.* 2007;176:957–969.
21. AAP Clinical Practice Guideline. Diagnosis and management of childhood obstructive sleep apnea. *Pediatrics.* 2002;109(4):704–712.

22. Carroll JL. Obstructive sleep-disordered breathing in children: new controversies, new directions. *Clin Chest Med.* 2003;24(2):261–282.
23. Wagner M, Torrez D. Interpretation of the polysomnogram in children. *Otolaryngol Clin North Am.* 2007;40:745–759.
24. Moon R, Horne R, Hauck F. Sudden infant death syndrome. *Lancet.* 2007;370: 1578–1587.

Chapter 25

Radiology

Judson Heugel, MD

I. GENERAL PEDIATRIC PRINCIPLES

Children are receiving an increasing amount of radiation from medical sources. Considerations unique to the pediatric population include an increased radiosensitivity of the thyroid gland, breast tissue and gonads. They also have a longer lifespan in which to manifest radiation-related cancer compared with adults. A computed tomography (CT) scan of the chest is approximately equivalent to 68 chest x-rays.[1]

A. Employ Judicious Use of CT

Consider ultrasound (US) or magnetic resonance imaging (MRI) whenever possible. If CT is indicated, remember the following to help minimize radiation exposure[2]:

1. Adjust your technique to limit exposure: *Child size* the kVp and mA
2. One scan (single phase) is often enough
3. Scan only the indicated areas (e.g., do not include pelvis if only abdomen is needed)
4. Body CT scans *without* IV contrast are helpful in delineating fine bony detail, calcifications and lung parenchyma, but almost nothing else. If your clinical question concerns something other than these areas, and you cannot use IV contrast, then consider ultrasound as a substitute for CT

II. HEAD[3]

Most intracranial processes, malformations, and tumors are best imaged with MRI. MRI is useful for neurodegenerative and demyelination disorders, diffuse axonal injury, neurocutaneous syndromes, structural lesions in focal seizure disorders, and vascular lesions. Compared with CT, MRI is more useful in detecting lesions in the posterior fossa.

A. Germinal Matrix Hemorrhage

Premature infants should undergo head US to detect intraventricular hemorrhage and periventricular leukomalacia and to screen for hydrocephalus and congenital abnormalities.

B. Congenital Malformations

Once detected on US, malformations are best further defined with MRI.

C. Congenital Infections

1. Congenital infections such as herpes simplex virus (HSV): Best imaged with MRI

2. Calcifications consistent with toxoplasmosis and cytomegalovirus (CMV) infection: May be best detected with CT
a. Calcifications in toxoplasmosis have a predilection for the basal ganglia and tend to be more diffuse than those of CMV, which primarily affects the periventricular region

D. Head Trauma

1. Best imaged by non-contrast CT to reveal skull fractures and subdural and epidural hematomas. A head CT should be part of a physical abuse workup
2. Skull radiography: Of limited value
3. Multiple hemorrhages of various ages: Best detected with MRI

E. Ventriculoperitoneal (VP) Shunt Malfunction

Initial imaging includes head CT to determine ventricle size. If signs of shunt malfunction are noted, radiographs of the length of the shunt (a shunt series) should follow to look for kinks or disconnections.

F. Craniosynostosis

Suture examination is best done initially with radiographs of the skull. If there are changes consistent with craniosynostosis, three-dimensional CT reconstructions should be obtained.

III. EYES: ORBITAL CELLULITIS

Best imaged with contrast CT with orbital cuts. To determine whether an infection is preseptal or postseptal, a line is drawn from the medial to the lateral bony walls of the orbit on transverse cuts.

IV. SPINE

A. Cervical Spine Trauma[4,5]

1. After immobilization in a collar, lateral and anteroposterior (AP) radiographs of the cervical spine (C-spine) should be performed in all children who have sustained significant head trauma, deceleration injury or undergone unwitnessed trauma. The seventh cervical vertebral body and the C7–T1 junction must be visualized. C-spine injuries are most common from the occiput to C3 in children (especially subluxation at the atlanto-occipital joint or atlantoaxial joint in infants and toddlers) and in the lower C-spine in older children and adults
2. Flexion-extension films may be helpful, especially in patients with Down syndrome, who are at risk for atlantoaxial subluxation
3. Odontoid views may be helpful in older children with suspected occipitocervical injury (e.g., whiplash)

B. Reading C-spine Films[4,5]

The following ABCDDS (or ABCDs) mnemonic is useful:

1. **Alignment:** The anterior vertebral body line, posterior vertebral body line, facet line, and spinous process line should each form a continuous line with smooth contour and no step-offs

2. **Bones:** Assess each bone looking for chips or fractures
3. **Count:** Must see C7 body in its entirety
4. **Dens:** Examine for chips or fractures
5. **Disk spaces:** Should see consistent distance between each vertebral body
6. **Soft tissue:** Assess for swelling, particularly in the prevertebral area

C. Spinal Cord Injury without Radiographic Abnormality (SCIWORA)[4,5]

1. Definition: A functional C-spine injury that cannot be excluded by abnormality on a radiograph. It is thought to be attributable to the increased mobility of a child's spine
2. Should be suspected in the setting of normal C-spine images when clinical signs or symptoms (e.g., point tenderness, focal neurologic symptoms) suggest C-spine injury
3. If neurologic symptoms persist despite normal C-spine and flexion-extension views, MRI is indicated to rule out swelling, contusion, or intramedullary hemorrhage of the cord

D. Spinal Dysraphism (e.g., Myelocele, Myelomeningocele)

Initial imaging: Radiographs. Most often screened for with US. Complications are followed by MRI.

E. Scoliosis

Best evaluated by erect AP spine radiograph. Posteroanterior (PA) views can be used in postpubertal girls to decrease breast radiation dose.

V. AIRWAY[4]

A. Lateral Radiograph

1. Lateral radiograph of the upper airway is the most useful film for evaluating a child with stridor. If possible, should be obtained on inspiration
2. A radiologic workup should always include AP and lateral radiographs of the chest, with inclusion of the upper airway on the AP chest radiograph. Diagnosis is based on airway radiologic examination in conjunction with clinical presentation (Table 25-1; Figs. 25-1 and 25-2)

TABLE 25-1

DIAGNOSIS OF DISEASES BASED ON AIRWAY RADIOLOGIC EXAMINATION

Diagnosis	Findings on Airway Films
Croup	AP and lateral films with subglottic narrowing (*steeple sign*)
Epiglottitis	Enlarged, indistinct epiglottis on lateral film (*thumb print sign*)
Vascular ring	AP and lateral films with narrowing; double or right aortic arch
Retropharyngeal abscess or pharyngeal mass	Soft tissue air or persistent enlargement of prevertebral soft tissues; more than half of a vertebral body above C3 and one vertebral body below C3
Immunodeficiency	Absence of adenoidal and tonsillar tissue after age 6 mo

AP, Anteroposterior.

B. Vascular Rings

1. Vascular rings and other masses that extrinsically obstruct the lower airways can be imaged with contrast-enhanced CT or MRI
2. Tracheomalacia and intrinsic masses can be studied with bronchoscopy

C. Foreign Bodies

1. **Lower airway foreign bodies:** In the absence of a radiopaque foreign body, radiologic findings include air trapping, hyperinflation, atelectasis, consolidation, pneumothorax, and pneumomediastinum. Further studies should include expiratory films (in a cooperative patient), bilateral decubitus chest films (in an uncooperative patient), or airway fluoroscopy
2. **Esophageal foreign bodies:** Usually lodged at one of three locations: the thoracic inlet, the level of the aortic arch and left mainstem bronchus, or the gastroesophageal junction. Evaluation should include the following:
   a. Lateral airway film (include nasopharynx)
   b. AP film of the chest and abdomen (including the supraclavicular region)
   c. Contrast study of the esophagus if other films are normal. If perforation is suspected, use nonionic, water-soluble contrast

VI. CHEST[4,5]

A. Posteroanterior and Lateral Radiographs

First images obtained when studying the chest (Figs. 25-3 and 25-4).

B. Pneumonia

1. Lobar or segmental consolidation: More typical of bacterial infections
2. Hyperinflation, bilateral patchy or streaky densities, and peribronchial thickening: More typical of nonbacterial disease

C. Atelectasis Versus Infiltrate

1. **Atelectasis:** When air is removed from the lung, the tissue collapses, resulting in volume loss on chest radiographs. If severe enough, the mediastinum and/or diaphragm are pulled toward the lesion. Air may still remain in larger bronchi, creating air bronchograms on radiograph. Collapse and re-expansion can occur quickly
2. **Infiltrate:** A fluid (blood, pus, edema) that invades one of the compartments of the lung (bronchoalveolar air space or peribronchial interstitial space) is seen as a density on a radiograph. When alveolar air is displaced by fluid, but air remains in the bronchi, the classic pneumonic infiltrate with air bronchograms is seen. When infiltrate is interstitial, its borders can be vague, and bronchial walls may be thickened. Typically, infiltrates resolve in 2–6 weeks

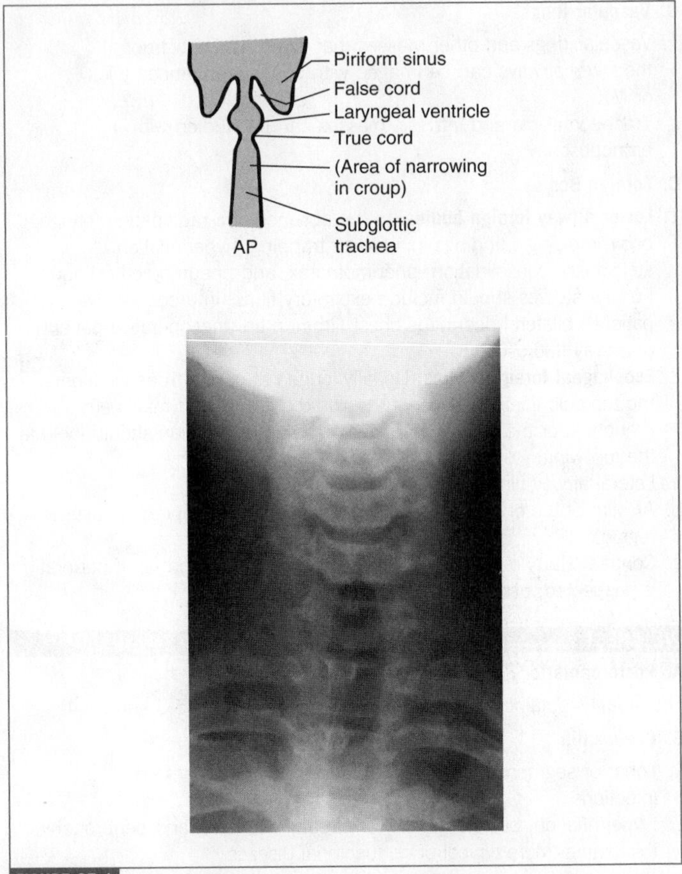

FIGURE 25-1
Anteroposterior (AP) neck film with normal anatomy on AP airway view.

D. Parapneumonic Effusions and Empyema

Initially, PA and lateral radiographs are obtained. Lateral decubitus radiographs may also be helpful. Ultrasound is often the best modality for early identification of loculation, however a contrast-enhanced CT may be needed to further delineate loculation or differentiate between pleural fluid and collapsed or consolidated tissue.

E. Parenchymal Findings

1. Lung abscess, cavitary necrosis, and lung contusions: Best imaged with contrast-enhanced CT

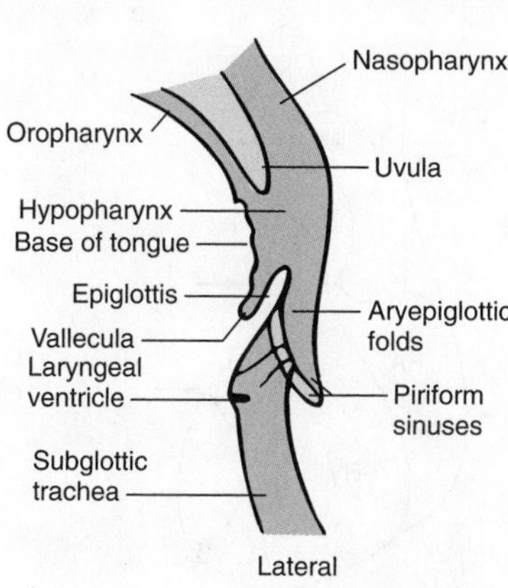

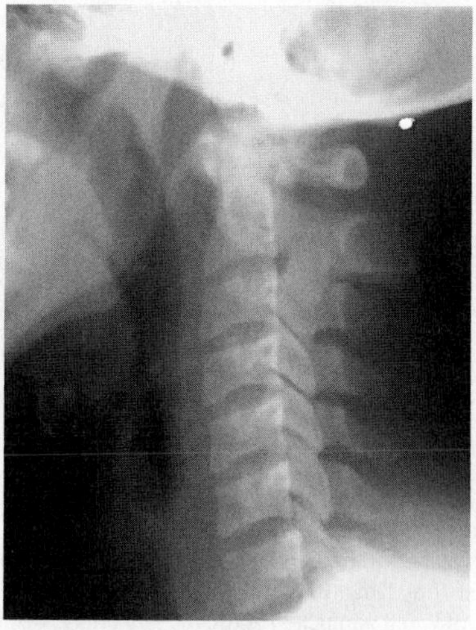

FIGURE 25-2

Lateral neck film with normal anatomy on lateral airway view.

2. Pneumatocele, fungal infections and interstitial lung disease: Use non-contrast CT

F. Mediastinal Masses

Mediastinal masses (thymus, lymphoma, bronchogenic cyst, neuroblastoma, neurofibroma) are initially imaged with plain films, followed by contrast-enhanced CT or MRI.

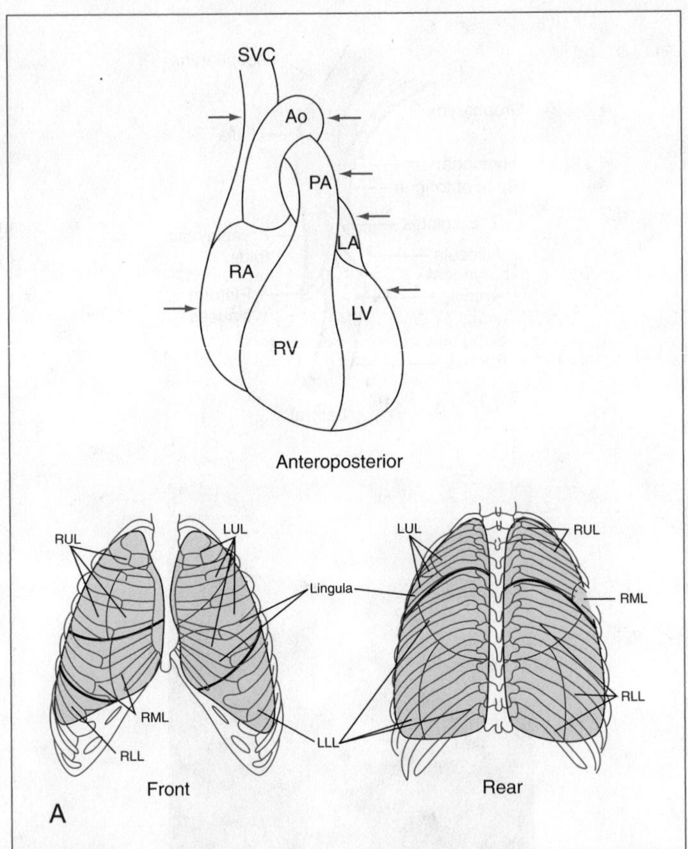

FIGURE 25-3

A, Lung and cardiac anatomy on an AP chest radiograph. Divisions within lobes indicate segments matched with x-rays. *Arrows* indicate contours seen on anteroposterior chest x-ray films (**B**). Ao, Aorta; LA, left atrium; LLL, left lower lobe; LUL, left upper lobe; LV, left ventricle; PA, pulmonary artery; RA, right atrium; RLL, right lower lobe; RML, right middle lobe; RUL, right upper lobe; RV, right ventricle; SVC, superior vena cava. *(Heart diagram modified from Kirks DR, Griscom NT: Practical pediatric imaging: diagnostic radiology of infants and children, 3rd ed. Philadelphia, Lippincott-Raven, 1998.)*

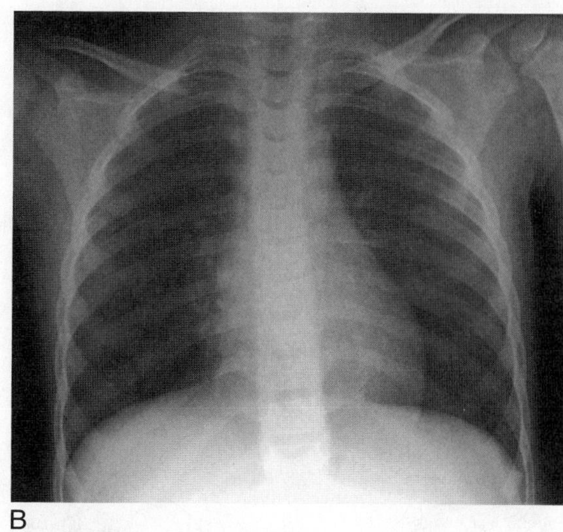

FIGURE 25-3 (Continued)

G. Central Line Placement

On chest radiograph, central venous catheters entering from the neck or arm are ideally placed with catheter tip at the junction of the superior vena cava and the right atrium. Some extension into the right atrium is acceptable, but if the catheter is noted to curve to the patient's left on PA film, the catheter may be positioned in the right ventricle. Catheters inserted below the diaphragm should be placed with tip at the level of the diaphragm.

H. Endotracheal Tube (ETT) Placement

On chest radiograph, the end of the ETT should rest approximately midway between the thoracic inlet and the carina. The lung fields should show symmetrical aeration.

VII. HEART AND VESSELS[4]

A. Congenital Heart Disease

Most clearly defined by echocardiography, but initial PA and lateral chest radiograph may yield important clues:

1. Position of the aortic arch: Left or right
2. Situs: Noting the position of the apex, stomach bubble, and liver
3. Heart size: With particular attention paid to the lateral chest radiograph

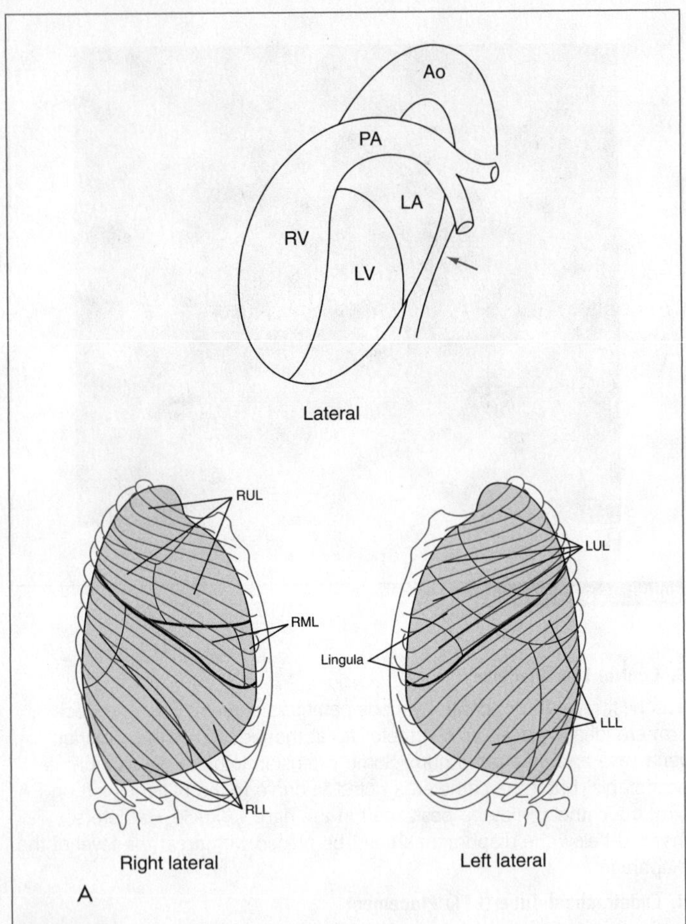

FIGURE 25-4

A, Lung and cardiac anatomy on lateral chest radiograph. Divisions within lobes indicate segments matched with x-rays. *Arrow* indicates contours seen on lateral chest x-ray films (**B**). Ao, Aorta; LA, left atrium; LLL, left lower lobe; LUL, left upper lobe; LV, left ventricle; PA, pulmonary artery; RLL, right lower lobe; RML, right middle lobe; RUL, right upper lobe; RV, right ventricle. *(Heart diagram modified from Kirks DR, Griscom NT: Practical pediatric imaging: diagnostic radiology of infants and children, 3rd ed. Philadelphia, Lippincott-Raven, 1998.)*

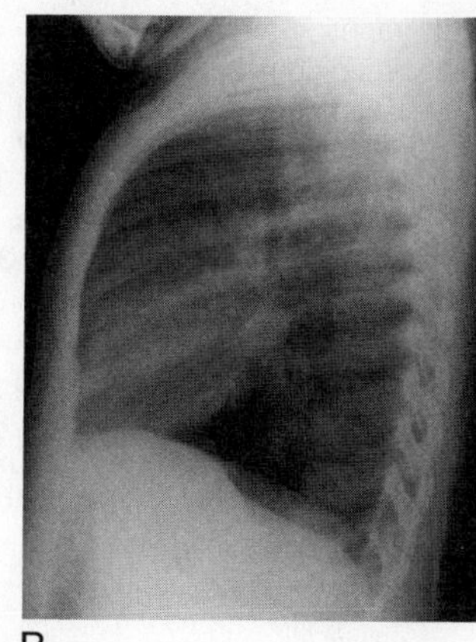

FIGURE 25-4 (Continued)

4. Pulmonary vascularity: Increased or decreased flow in arteries and veins

B. Vessels

1. Moving blood is detected by ultrasonographic frequency shifts
2. Color Doppler flow imaging: Can be used to evaluate deep vein thrombosis (DVT), vascular patency, intracranial blood flow (including Transcranial Doppler (TCD) to screen for ischemic brain injury risk in sickle cell disease), cardiac shunt flow, transplant vascularity, veno-occlusive disease of the liver, and testicular perfusion in testicular torsion
3. Power Doppler is particularly sensitive in detecting slow flow in small vessels (e.g., infant testes)

C. Vessel Abnormalities

Can be studied with echocardiography/US, CT, and MRI. Use these modalities to detect coarctation of the aorta, aortic stenosis, pulmonary artery and vein abnormalities, vascular rings, arteriovenous (AV) malformations and hemangiomas, aneurysms, and postoperative complications such as thrombosis and stenosis.

VIII. ABDOMEN[4,5]

A. Neonatal Enterocolitis

Clinically diagnosed and followed by abdominal radiographs, which may show focal dilation, featureless loops, pneumatosis, and portal venous gas.

B. Esophageal Atresia and Tracheoesophageal Fistula (TEF)

Studied initially with radiographs of the chest, which may reveal the air-distended esophageal atretic pouch, the nasogastric tube curled up in this pouch, or excessive dilation of stomach as a result of fistula communication.

C. High Intestinal Obstruction

1. Diagnosed with upper gastrointestinal (UGI) series: Contrast is ingested, and esophagus, stomach, and duodenum are visualized
   a. Causes: Esophageal webs and rings, masses, duodenal atresia or webs, annular pancreas, midgut volvulus, and Ladd bands
2. UGI can also help evaluate hiatal hernias, varices, gastric outlet obstruction, motility problems, ulcerations, and reflux
3. During UGI, identification of the duodenojejunal junction (the ligament of Treitz) helps to diagnose malrotation. Normally, the junction is to the left of spine, at or above level of duodenal bulb

D. Pyloric Stenosis

1. US is the preferred examination because it directly visualizes the pyloric muscle. Normally, the pylorus is <17 mm in length and its muscular wall <4 mm in width
2. Radiographs: Show gastric distention
3. UGI: Delayed gastric emptying and a narrow pyloric channel will be evident

E. Bowel Obstruction

1. Determination of large or small bowel obstruction: Often aided by supine radiograph, prone radiograph, and either upright, supine cross-table lateral, or left lateral decubitus film to look for free air and air-fluid levels
   a. Causes of obstruction: Adhesions, appendicitis, incarcerated inguinal hernias, Meckel diverticulum, and intussusception
2. US: Can be helpful in thin patients as well as in female patients who have ovarian pathology in their differential for abdominal pain
3. CT with intravenous, oral, or rectal contrast is more useful with an obese patient or when looking for perforated appendicitis or abscess
4. Contrast enemas with dilute, water-soluble agents can also be useful in lower intestinal obstruction in the newborn

F. Intussusception

1. On abdominal radiographs, particularly the prone view, findings include minimal gas in right abdomen and ascending colon
2. Ultrasound will show alternating rings. Doppler will show flow in the intussuscepted mesentery, which will allow confirmation of the diagnosis as well as assessment of the viability of the intussusceptum

3. For fluoroscopy-guided therapeutic enema, air insufflation is preferred, but other contrast agents may also be used. Reducing an intussusception with air or contrast is contraindicated if perforation is suspected

G. Meckel Diverticulum

Suggested by painless lower GI bleeding; diagnosed by nuclear scintigraphy using ^{99m}Tc-pertechnetate.

H. Abdominal Trauma

CT of abdomen and pelvis to detect solid organ injury, vascular extravasation, free fluid, bowel wall thickening, and organ laceration.

I. Biliary Atresia

1. In neonates with jaundice, US initially to distinguish biliary atresia from hepatitis. The gallbladder will be small or absent with biliary atresia
2. Hepatobiliary scintigraphy with ^{99m}Tc-iminodiacetate (HIDA) reveals the absence of radionuclide in the GI tract with biliary atresia

J. Nasoduodenal Tube Placement

Visualize tube on a plain abdominal AP film passing through the stomach, crossing the midline and passing into the duodenal bulb (where tip of tube will just begin to point inferiorly). If it remains unclear if tube is in duodenum or coiled in stomach, a lateral film is indicated (a properly placed ND tube tip will lie posterior, near the spine).

IX. GENITOURINARY TRACT[4]

A. Urinary Tract Infection (UTI)

1. Initial febrile UTIs in children <5 years require imaging to look for congenital anomalies (e.g., posterior urethral valves, ureterocele), vesicoureteral reflux, baseline renal measurements, and damage to the cortex of the kidneys
2. Workup first includes US to diagnose hydronephrosis, ureteropelvic junction obstruction, posterior urethral valves, multicystic dysplastic kidneys, chronic pyelonephritis, renal fusion (horseshoe kidney), and renal cysts
3. Voiding cystourethrogram (VCUG) can then be performed to diagnose vesicoureteral reflux, abnormalities of bladder or urethral function and anatomy, including ureterocele, and posterior urethral valves
4. Occasionally, dimercaptosuccinic acid (DMSA) scan is useful in following renal cortical scarring and pyelonephritis

B. Uterine and Ovarian Pathology

Transvaginal or transabdominal US should be performed if the clinical picture is suspicious for ovarian torsion, tubo-ovarian abscess (TOA), or ectopic pregnancy.

X. EXTREMITIES[4]

A. Trauma

1. Adequate evaluation requires AP and lateral radiographs. Restricting the film to include only the area of interest improves the resolution (i.e., for a thumb injury, ask for an image of the thumb, not the hand)
2. Comparison films of the uninvolved extremity not necessary, but may be helpful, such as in evaluation of joint effusions (particularly the hip), suspected osteomyelitis, or pyarthrosis and/or the evaluation of subtle fractures, especially in areas of multiple ossification centers such as the elbow
3. Salter Harris Classification of growth-plate injury—See Chapter 4
4. Avulsion injuries tend to occur at the knee and pelvis

B. Stress Fractures

1. Occur most often at the tibia, fibula, metatarsals, and calcaneus
2. Radiography will show a band of sclerosis and new bone formation
3. Skeletal scintigraphy is a sensitive method for making the diagnosis

C. Osteomyelitis

1. Tends to occur at the metaphysis of long bones and within flat bones
2. Radiography will show deep soft-tissue swelling and bony changes (may take 10 days to appear)
3. Skeletal scintigraphy and MRI will often be positive before radiographic changes are noticeable

D. Hip Disorders

1. Developmental dysplasia of the hip (congenital hip dislocation) is imaged initially with US. Once the femoral heads ossify, radiographs are more helpful
2. Legg-Calvé-Perthes disease (avascular necrosis of the femoral head) can be imaged with AP and frog-leg lateral hip films as well as MRI and bone scintigraphy
3. Slipped capital femoral epiphysis (SCFE) will show displacement of the femoral head on frog-leg lateral and AP radiographs

E. Bone Age

Obtain a PA view of the left hand and wrist.

F. Skeletal Survey

1. In cases of suspected child abuse, should include lateral skull film with C-spine film, AP chest film (bone technique), oblique views of the ribs, AP view of the pelvis, abdominal film (bone technique) with the lateral thoracic and lumbar spine, and AP long-bone films
2. Classic findings: Multiple metaphyseal injuries (especially corner and bucket-handle fractures) and other fractures of various ages. Suspicion should also be raised by fracture at unusual sites, such as posterior rib fractures or solitary spiral and transverse fractures of the long bones with an inconsistent history of trauma

REFERENCES

1. Frush DP, Donnelly LF, Rosen NS. Computed tomography and radiation risks: what pediatric health care providers should know. *Pediatrics.* 2003;112:951–957.
2. The Alliance for Radiation Safety in Pediatric Imaging. http://www.imagegently.org.
3. Kirks DR, Griscom NT. *Practical pediatric imaging: diagnostic radiology of infants and children.* 3rd ed. Philadelphia: Lippincott-Raven; 1998.
4. Kuhn JP, Slovis T, Haller J. *Caffey's pediatric diagnostic imaging.* 10th ed. St. Louis: Mosby; 2003.
5. Donnelly LF. *Fundamentals of pediatric radiology.* Philadelphia: WB Saunders; 2001.

Chapter 26

Rheumatology

Marc A. Callender, MD

See additional content on Expert Consult

I. WEBSITE

American College of Rheumatology: http://www.rheumatology.org/

II. LABORATORY STUDIES

Most laboratory studies used in diagnosis of rheumatic diseases are nonspecific for rheumatic diseases; they must be put into the context of the full clinical picture. However, once a diagnosis is established, they can be used to follow the clinical course of rheumatic diseases, indicating flares or remission of disease state. Sensitivities and specificities of rheumatologic tests must be considered with any clinical decision (see Chapter 28).

A. Acute Phase Reactants

1. **Overview:**
   a. Indicate presence of inflammation when elevated
   b. Elevation is nonspecific: Can result from trauma, infection, rheumatic diseases, or malignancy[1]
   c. Markers include erythrocyte sedimentation rate (ESR), C-reactive protein (CRP), platelet count, ferritin, haptoglobin, fibrinogen, serum amyloid A, and complement[1,2]
2. **ESR:**
   a. Measure of the rate of fall of red blood cells in anticoagulated blood within a vertical tube; reflects level of rouleaux formation caused by acute phase reactants[1]
   b. Can be falsely lowered in afibrinogenemia, anemia, and sickle cell disease; these states interfere with rouleaux formation[2]
   c. Levels vary depending on age, ethnicity, gender, and freshness of blood sample[1]
   d. Serial measurements may help in monitoring disease severity/activity in diseases such as systemic lupus erythematosus (SLE) and juvenile rheumatoid arthritis (JRA)
3. **CRP[1,3]**
   a. Synthesized by the liver; assists in the clearance of pathologic bacteria and damaged cells via activation of complement-mediated phagocytosis, mediates acute inflammation by alteration of cytokine release, and is thought to prevent autoimmunity by binding to and masking autoantigens

TABLE 26-1

AUTOANTIBODIES ASSOCIATED WITH COMMON RHEUMATOLOGIC DISEASES

Systemic Lupus Erythematosus (SLE)	Juvenile Rheumatoid Arthritis	Vasculitis	Polymyositis/ Dermatomyositis
• ANA • Anti-double stranded DNA • Anti-Smith • Anti-RNP • Anti-microsomal • Anti-phospholipids*	• Rheumatoid Factor • Anti-cyclic citrullinated peptide (CCP)	• ANCA-cytoplasmic/PR3 • ANCA-perinuclear/MPO	• ANA • Anti-Jo-1
Mixed Connective Tissue Disease	**Drug–Induced SLE**	**Sjögren Syndrome**	**Scleroderma**
• ANA • Anti-RNP	• Anti-histone	• ANA • Anti-Ro • Anti-La	• ANA • Anti-centromere • Anti-RNP

*Anti-phospholipids: anticardiolipin, lupus anticoagulant, and anti-glycoprotein I.

Adapted from Kliegman RM, Behrman RE, Jenson HB, et al: Nelson textbook of pediatrics, 18th ed. Philadelphia, Saunders Elsevier, 2007.

b. Increases and decreases rapidly due to its short half-life (~18 hours)
c. Elevation is nonspecific, indicating only inflammation
   (1) Most active phases of rheumatic disease result in elevation to 1–10 mg/dL
   (2) Level >10 mg/dL raises concern for bacterial infection or systemic vasculitis

B. Autoantibodies (Table 26-1)

The positive predictive value of any autoantibody assay depends on clinical context. These studies can prove valuable in confirming clinical suspicion. However, in the absence of suspicion, they have low yield and may be misleading.

1. **Antinuclear antibody (ANA):**
a. Nonspecific test for rheumatic disease[1]
b. Positive in approximately 60%–70% of children with an autoimmune disease, but can be seen in about 15%–35% of normal persons
c. If positive, consider ordering individual autoantibodies (see Table 26-1)
d. Can be positive in non-rheumatic diseases:
   (1) Neoplasm
   (2) Infections (transiently positive): mononucleosis, endocarditis, hepatitis, malaria.
e. If positive in pauciarticular JRA, there is increased risk of uveitis
2. **Rheumatoid factor (RF)**[1]
a. Immunoglobulin M antibodies to the Fc portion of immunoglobulin G

b. Positive in rheumatic and non-rheumatic disease:
   (1) Rheumatic diseases: SLE, mixed cryoglobulinemia, JRA, mixed connective tissue disease, and Henoch-Schönlein purpura
   (2) Numerous infections such as hepatitis B, bacterial endocarditis, tuberculosis, and congenital TORCH infections
c. Negative RF: Does not rule out rheumatic disease
d. Prognostic importance in polyarticular JRA: Positive RF suggests more progressive disease (see Section III)

3. **Anti-cyclic citrullinated peptide (anti-CCP) antibodies:**
a. Currently being explored as an RF adjunct.[4–6] (Routine use in the pediatric setting not indicated until the full clinical significance in this population has been established.)
b. Although pediatric studies are few, anti-CCP has been shown to have a high sensitivity and specificity for adult rheumatoid arthritis (RA)
c. May predict future development of RA in RF-negative patients who have undifferentiated arthritis, and a more progressive disease in established RA patients, thus allowing for earlier and/or aggressive treatment
d. Anti-CCP positive JRA patients are usually also RF positive; thus are females with late-onset polyarthritis[6]
e. Anti-CCP positivity has been shown to correlate with erosive joint disease in JRA

C. Complement[1,7]

The complement system is composed of a series of plasma proteins and cellular receptors that function together to mediate host defense and inflammation. Inflammatory processes may increase complement protein synthesis or increase their consumption.

1. **Total hemolytic complement level (CH_{50}):**
a. General measure of complement; also an acute phase reactant
b. Increased in the acute phase response of numerous inflammatory states
c. Useful screening test for homozygous complement deficiency states
d. Typically decreased in SLE

2. **C3 and C4:**
a. Most common complement proteins assayed
b. May be increased or decreased in rheumatic diseases, depending upon stage of disease or severity
c. Trends are more instructive than isolated results

3. **Decreased levels of complement proteins:**
a. Indicator of immune complex formation:
   (1) Can occur in active SLE as well as some vasculitides, and in multiple infections, including gram-negative sepsis, hepatitis, and pneumococcal infections
   (2) Decreased levels typically signify more severe SLE, particularly with regard to renal disease

b. Severe hepatic failure: Synthesis of complement proteins occurs primarily in the liver
c. Congenital complement deficiency, which may predispose to the development of autoimmune disease
4. **Increased levels of complement proteins:**
a. Indicates the active phase of most rheumatic diseases, including SLE, JRA, dermatomyositis
b. May be seen in multiple infections as part of the acute phase response, including hepatitis and pneumococcal pneumonia

D. Other Laboratory Studies

1. **Urinalysis**
a. Renal involvement occurs in many rheumatic diseases
b. Findings may include proteinuria, hematuria, or casts. (see Chapter 19)
2. **Serum muscle enzymes**[2]
a. Including aspartate aminotransferase (AST), lactate dehydrogenase (LDH), aldolase, and creatine kinase (CK)
b. Can be elevated in certain rheumatic diseases that cause muscle inflammation or destruction, such as dermatomyositis

NOTE: Patients with chronic, ongoing myositis may have an elevated CK-MB fraction (that is noncardiac in origin) when measuring serum CK levels.

3. **Joint fluid analysis** (Fig. 26-1)[8]
a. Important study in the presence of an effusion, especially in monoarticular disease
b. Effusion can be seen in rheumatic and other disease processes such as septic arthritis

III. ARTHRITIDES

A. JRA[1,2,7] or Juvenile Idiopathic Arthritis (JIA)[9]

1. **Definition of arthritis:** Joint swelling or limitation/tenderness upon range of motion lasting ≥6 weeks and not due to other identifiable cause[9]
2. **Diagnosis**
a. Challenge of diagnosis: Children may not present with joint pain/swelling, but with other symptoms: morning stiffness, limp, refusal to walk, irritability, poor growth, or limb discrepancy
b. Classical divisions: Based on clinical course over the first 6 months of illness in children <16 years with arthritis present for at least 6 weeks.[1,2] Multiple classification systems exist, of which the American College of Rheumatology (ACR) and the International League of Associations for Rheumatology (ILAR) are the most widely used.[9] The divisions used here are based on the ACR (Table 26-2)

NOTE: When evaluating a child with a history of constant extremity pain (including nighttime awakenings due to pain), low white blood cell count, and low-normal platelets, consider in the differential malignancy such as acute lymphocytic leukemia (even without blasts seen on peripheral smear). Bone marrow studies may be indicated.[10]

26

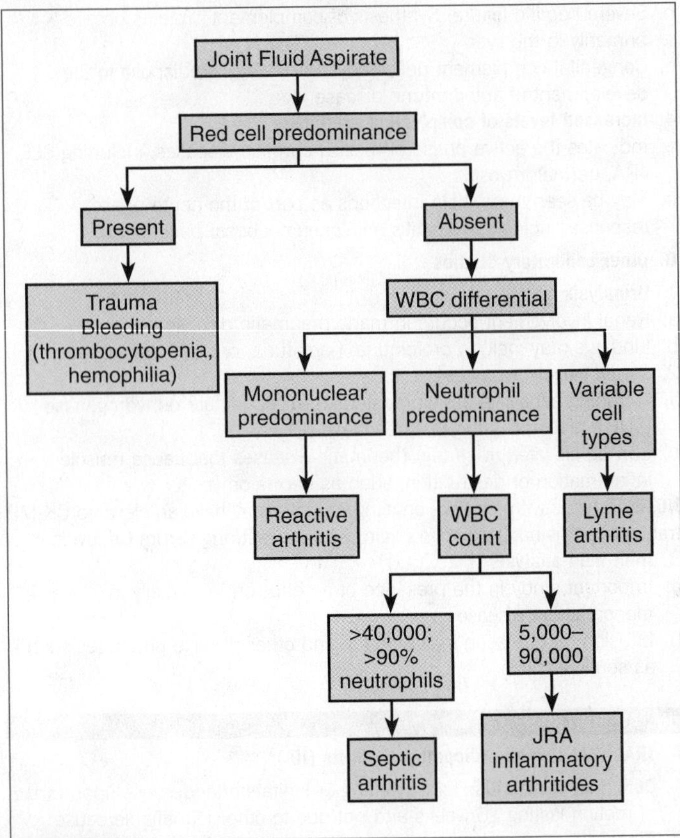

FIGURE 26-1

Joint fluid analysis algorithm. *(Data from Hay W, Levin M, Sondheimer J, et al: Current pediatric diagnosis & treatment, 17th ed. New York, Lange Medical/ McGraw-Hill, 2005.)*

B. Psoriatic Arthritis (PsA)[11,12]

1. **Classification:** Traditionally referred to as a seronegative spondyloarthropathy; ILAR classification considers PsA to be a subtype of JIA[9]
2. **History of psoriasis:** Not required for diagnosis (*psoriatic arthritis sine psoriasis*)
   a. Patients often have a first-degree relative with psoriasis or
   b. Patients may develop skin findings months or years after arthritis onset

TABLE 26-2

CLASSICAL DIVISIONS OF JUVENILE RHEUMATOID ARTHRITIS[30]

	Pauciarticular	Polyarticular	Systemic-Onset
Frequency of cases	60%	30%	10%
Number of joints involved (in first 6 mo)	≤4	≥5	Variable
Age predominance	Type I: preschool age Type II: 9–11 yr	2–5 yr and 10–18 yr	None
Gender ratio (female : male)	Type I: 4 : 1 Type II: 1 : 20	3 : 1	1 : 1
Involved joints	Knees and ankles	Larger joints, symmetric involvement	Any, including hips
Chronic uveitis	20% (higher with (+) ANA)	5%	Rare
Extra-articular manifestations	Uveitis	Mild fever, hepatosplenomegaly, lymphadenopathy, subcutaneous nodules	Once to twice daily high-spiking fevers, hepatosplenomegaly, lymphadenopathy, polyserositis, pericarditis, and characteristic macular rash
Seropositivity			
ANA	75%–85%	40%–50%	10%
RF	10% (increases with age)	75%–85%	10%
Destructive Arthritis	Rare	>50%	>50%
Major Morbidities	Uveitis, leg length discrepancy		Pericarditis, pleuropericarditis, secondary amyloidosis, macrophage activation syndrome*
Prognosis	Excellent apart from eyesight	Poorer prognosis with RF seropositivity and later onset	Moderate to poor

ANA, Antinuclear antibody; RF, Rheumatoid factor.

*Macrophage activation syndrome (MAS) or reactive hematophagocytic lymphohistiocytosis: uncontrolled activation of T cells and macrophages leading to rapid hepatic failure, encephalopathy, pancytopenia, purpura, mucosal bleeding, and renal failure. Paradoxically low erythrocyte sedimentation rate (ESR) with hypofibrinogenemia, elevated ferritin, and triglycerides, with disseminated intravascular coagulation (DIC).

Adapted from McMillan JA, Feigin RD, DeAngelis CD, et al: Oski's pediatrics, 4th ed. Philadelphia, Lippincott Williams & Wilkins, 2006.

3. **Presentation:**
a. Mostly an oligoarthritis, but may be a polyarthritis or an axial arthritis
b. ± sacroiliitis, inflammatory spinal pain/stiffness, synovitis, enthesitis, or dactylitis (swelling beyond joint margins, producing a *sausage digit*) of toes or fingers
c. Fingernails may show onycholysis or pitting
4. **Laboratory studies:** No specific laboratory findings that suggest a diagnosis of psoriatic arthritis, although markers of inflammation (CRP, ESR) may be helpful in tracking activity of disease. RF is usually negative
5. **Radiographic findings:** Blend of destruction and proliferation on plain films
6. **Prognosis:** If left untreated, will result in a deforming combination of erosions and ankylosis within joints of digits
7. **Major morbidities:** Chronic uveitis may develop. Regular screening by an ophthalmologist is recommended

C. Reactive Arthritis[2]

1. **Definition:** A diverse group of inflammatory arthritides that follow a bacterial or viral infection, particularly involving the respiratory, gastrointestinal, and genitourinary tracts
2. **Onset:** Infection typically precedes development of arthritis by 1–4 weeks; approximately 80% of cases are preceded by gastroenteritis
3. **Common precipitating organisms:** *Mycoplasma, Chlamydia, Yersinia, Salmonella, Shigella, Campylobacter,* Epstein-Barr virus (EBV), parvovirus B19, and enteroviruses
4. **Presentation:** Sometimes accompanied by constitutional signs and symptoms, including fever, weight loss, and fatigue, as well as dermatologic and ophthalmologic findings
5. **HLA-B27:**
a. Strong association between HLA-B27 and susceptibility to developing reactive arthritis following an infection with a bacterial arthritogenic organism
b. Approximately 50%–65% frequency seen in reactive arthritis
6. **Laboratory studies:**
a. ± evidence of systemic inflammation (leukocytosis, thrombocytosis, and elevated ESR and CRP)
b. Autoantibodies are typically absent
c. Stool cultures, serum *Chlamydia pneumoniae* and *Mycoplasma* titers, and urinary *Chlamydia* DNA probe can be helpful. Negative stool culture does not exclude diagnosis of reactive arthritis secondary to an enteric organism
d. Consider enterovirus, EBV, and parvovirus B19 antibody titers
e. Joint fluid analysis may be helpful to distinguish a septic arthritis from a reactive arthritis, especially because, in the case of *Salmonella,* either a septic or reactive arthritis may develop

7. **Prognosis:** Arthritis can last weeks to months, with eventual remission or development of recurrent episodes

D. Management of Arthritis

1. **Pharmacologic agents**[1,2,7,13]**:** (Please see Formulary for dosing guidelines, and Table EC 26-A on Expert Consult for related side effects and lab surveillance)

a. Nonsteroidal anti-inflammatory drugs (NSAIDs): First-line treatment; e.g., naproxen and ibuprofen

b. Disease-modifying antirheumatic drugs (DMARDs): Slow disease progression; e.g., methotrexate, sulfasalazine, and hydroxychloroquine

c. Biologic immunomodulators: Tumor necrosis factor (TNF) inhibitors (etanercept, infliximab, and adalimumab); rituximab (anti-CD20); and anakinra (IL-1 receptor antagonist)

d. Cytotoxic and immunosuppressive drugs: Cyclosporine

e. Corticosteroids: Can be systemic or intra-articular

2. **Health maintenance**[1,7,13]**:**

a. Vaccines: Generally, follow regular immunization schedule. Special considerations should be made for immunocompromised hosts, i.e., patients on biologic or immunosuppressive therapy (see Chapter 16)

b. Prevention or minimization of osteopenia: Adequate calcium and vitamin D intake and weight-bearing activities

c. Physical and occupational therapy: Important in maintaining range of motion of a joint and strength of associated muscle groups as well as decreasing pain and preventing joint deformity and contractures

d. Orthopedic surgery: Necessary in some cases for pain control, improvement in function, or contractures

E. Uveitis

Due to insidious and asymptomatic development of uveitis, routine pediatric ophthalmology screening is required for children with JRA.

1. **At diagnosis:** First ophthalmologic exam should be within 1 month
2. **Inactive disease:** Frequency of examination varies based on ANA status, disease duration and age at diagnosis[14]
3. **Active disease:** Ophthalmologic examination every 3 months, regardless of ANA status

IV. SYSTEMIC LUPUS ERYTHEMATOSUS (SLE)

An episodic, multisystem autoimmune disease characterized by inflammation of blood vessels and connective tissue. Apart from drug-induced SLE, the etiology remains unknown.

A. American College or Rheumatology Classification Criteria (Table 26-3)

These are not strict *diagnostic* criteria, but *classification* criteria for research purposes. Use caution when applying them to pediatric and international/multiethnic patients; there are few studies that validate the ACR criteria for these populations.[15,16]

TABLE 26-3

THE 1997 UPDATE OF THE 1982 AMERICAN COLLEGE OF RHEUMATOLOGY REVISED CRITERIA FOR CLASSIFICATION OF SYSTEMIC LUPUS ERYTHEMATOSUS

Criterion	
1. Malar rash	Fixed erythema, flat or raised, over the malar eminences, tending to spare the nasolabial folds; telangiectasias
2. Discoid rash	Erythematous raised patches with adherent keratotic scaling and follicular plugging; atrophic scarring may occur in older lesions
3. Photosensitivity	Skin rash as a result of unusual reaction to sunlight, by patient history or physician observation
4. Oral ulcers	Oral or nasopharyngeal ulceration, usually painless, observed by physician
5. Nonerosive arthritis	Involving 2 or more peripheral joints, characterized by tenderness, swelling, or effusion
6. Pleuritis or pericarditis	a. Pleuritis: history of pleuritic pain or rubbing heard by a physician or evidence of pleural effusion AND/OR b. Pericarditis: documented by electrocardiogram or rub or evidence of pericardial effusion
7. Renal disorder	a. Persistent proteinuria >0.5 g/day or >3+ if quantitation not performed AND/OR b. Cellular casts—may be red cell, hemoglobin, granular, tubular, or mixed
8. Neurologic disorder	Seizures or psychosis: in the absence of offending drugs, hypertension or known metabolic derangements
9. Hematologic disorder	a. Hemolytic anemia—with reticulocytosis AND/OR b. Leukopenia—<4,000/μL on ≥2 occasions AND/OR c. Thrombocytopenia—<100,000/μL in the absence of offending drugs
10. Autoimmune Markers	a. Anti-DNA: antibody to native DNA in abnormal titer AND/OR b. Anti-Sm: presence of antibody to Sm nuclear antigen
11. Positive antinuclear antibody	An abnormal titer of antinuclear antibody by immunofluorescence or an equivalent assay at any point in time in the absence of drugs

Data from http://www.rheumatology.org/, which was adapted from Tan E, Cohen AS, Fries JF, et al: The 1982 revised criteria for the classification of systemic lupus erythematosus. Arthritis Rheum 1982;25:1271–1277.

B. Clinical Features and Management of SLE

1. **Diagnosis:**
   a. Most often based on meeting 4 or more of the 11 classification criteria
   b. Do not exclude the possibility of an SLE diagnosis for a pediatric patient who does not fully meet these criteria
   c. The majority of pediatric patients with *incomplete* SLE (<4 criteria) will likely completely fulfill these criteria in subsequent years

2. **Epidemiology:**
a. Females more commonly affected; onset usually at age 9–15 years (median age, 12 years)[15]
b. African Americans more commonly affected than whites[1]
3. **Laboratory studies and surveillance**[1,15]
a. Complete blood count (CBC) with differential and direct Coombs
b. Urinalysis and serum creatinine: May reveal renal involvement. Of note, renal disease is the leading cause of death in lupus patients. See Table EC 26-B on Expert Consult for WHO Classification of SLE nephritis[17]
c. ESR or CRP: May be increased with active disease; CRP levels may not correlate with disease activity[18]
d. Complement levels (C3 and C4): Serial levels most useful; congenital complement deficiencies may also be seen in SLE, especially in males with SLE. Decreasing complement levels may indicate renal disease
e. Autoantibodies (see Table 26-1)[1]
 (1) ANA: Most patients with positive ANA do not have SLE, but almost all patients with SLE have positive ANA[4]
 (2) Anti-dsDNA: Highly specific for SLE, seen in about 60% of patients; titers rise/fall depending on disease activity and usually increase during development of lupus nephritis. Not associated with discoid or sub acute cutaneous lupus[4]
 (3) Anti-Sm: Highly specific for SLE; seen in about 10%–30% of patients
4. **Treatment**[1]**:**
a. NSAIDs: Targeted to treat arthralgia and arthritis (used with caution, as lupus patients are more susceptible to renal toxicity with these agents)
b. Hydroxychloroquine: Treats milder manifestations such as skin lesions, arthritis, and also may lower lipid levels, decreasing the risk for thromboembolic disease
c. Corticosteroids: Used to treat symptoms and decrease autoantibody production
d. Cytotoxic therapy: Reserved for more severe cases. Cyclophosphamide is used in patients with lupus nephritis, vasculitis, pulmonary hemorrhage or central nervous system involvement
e. DMARDs: Methotrexate, cyclosporine, and mycophenolate mofetil
f. Biologic agents: Target cytokine production, and include anti CD20/22 monoclonal antibodies (i.e., rituximab)

C. Drug-induced SLE[1,2]

1. **Pathogenesis:**
a. Inciting drugs (including but not limited to): Hydralazine, minocycline, ethosuximide, doxycycline, procainamide, isoniazid, chlorpromazine, phenytoin, and carbamazepine
b. Usually resolves with discontinuation of drug

2. **Clinical and laboratory features:**
a. The most frequent clinical manifestations are cutaneous and pleuropericardial involvement
b. Often associated with anti-histone antibodies

D. Neonatal SLE[1,17]

1. **Pathogenesis:** Neonates born to mothers with active SLE can develop a transient lupus-like syndrome in the perinatal period. Transplacental passage of anti-Ro (anti-SS-A) and anti-La (anti-SS-B) (also seen in Sjögren syndrome), mediate the disease process
2. **Clinical and laboratory features:**
a. Thrombocytopenia, hemolytic anemia
b. Inflammatory features of neonatal lupus will resolve within 6 months as maternal autoantibodies are cleared
c. Congenital heart block (associated with anti-Ro): *Permanent* condition, usually requires placement of a pacemaker

V. VASCULITIS (TABLE 26-4)

A. General

1. **Definition:** Inflammation of a blood vessel wall. Systemic vasculitis syndromes, although rare, are a concern in childhood
2. **Clinical presentation:** Variable, ranging from rash or fever of unknown origin to progressive multisystem failure[19]
3. **Initial laboratory tests:** CBC, basic metabolic panel, liver function tests, acute phase reactants, stool guaiac, and complete urinalysis
4. **Diagnosis:**
a. Small vessel vasculitis: Confirmed by biopsy. (Magnetic resonance angiography may also be helpful but a negative test does not rule out disease.)
b. Medium-large vessel vasculitis: Magnetic resonance angiography

B. Henoch-Schönlein Purpura (HSP)[1,2,20]

1. **Epidemiology:**
a. Most common small-vessel vasculitis in children
b. More frequent in males than females
c. Typical age of onset 2–7 years
d. History of viral upper respiratory infection several weeks preceding onset of illness in ½ to ⅔ of cases
2. **Presentation**[2,19–21]**:**
a. Non-thrombocytopenic palpable purpura:
   (1) Most common and frequently presenting feature
   (2) Evolution of rash: Urticarial lesions progress to a maculopapular rash followed by purpuric lesions, involving the ankles, buttocks, and elbows, beginning on lower extremities but can involve the entire body
   (3) New lesions can appear over 2–4 weeks, leaving a mixed-stage appearance

TABLE 26-4

CHILDHOOD VASCULITIS SYNDROMES

Vessel Size	Vasculitis Syndrome	Clinical and Distinguishing Features
Large arteries	Takayasu arteritis	Aortic arch involvement, leading to aneurysms, thrombosis, and stenosis Predominantly seen in young women Hypertension is the most common sign
Aorta and large branches directed toward major body regions	Giant cell (temporal arteritis)	Granulomatous inflammation of aorta and major branches, with predilection for extracranial branches of the carotid artery
Medium-sized arteries	Kawasaki disease	Arteritis including large, medium and small arteries; associated with mucocutaneous lymph node syndrome (see Chapter 7)
Renal, hepatic, coronary, and mesenteric arteries	Polyarteritis nodosa	Cutaneous lesions include livedo reticularis, tender nodules and purpura Hypertension, renal failure, abdominal pain, intestinal infarction, and cerebrovascular accidents are common complications
Small arterioles and venules	Microscopic polyangiitis	Rare in pediatrics p-ANCA or myeloperoxidase (MPO) positive Glomerulonephritis and pulmonary capillaritis Associated with streptococcal infection or URIs
Venules, capillaries, arterioles, and intraparenchymal distal arteries	Henoch-Schönlein purpura	Most common pediatric vasculitis IgA-dominant immune deposits; palpable purpura involving buttocks and lower extremity; colicky abdominal pain, arthralgias/arthritis
	Wegener granulomatosis	Necrotizing granulomatous vasculitis of small and medium-sized vessels Presents with respiratory tract and kidney involvement c-ANCA or proteinase 3 (PR3) positive May also involve medium-sized vessels
	Churg-Strauss syndrome	Eosinophil-rich and granulomatous inflammation involving respiratory tract; associated with asthma

URI, Upper respiratory infection.

Adapted from Kliegman RM, Behrman, RE, Jenson HB, et al: Nelson textbook of pediatrics, 18th ed. Philadelphia, Saunders Elsevier, 2007; Cassidy J, Petty R: Textbook of pediatric rheumatology, 5th ed. Philadelphia, WB Saunders, 2005; Kim S, Dedeoglu F: Update on pediatric vasculitis. Curr Opin Pediatr 2005;17:695–702; Dillon M, Ozen S: A new international classification of childhood vasculitis. Pediatr Nephrol 2006;21:1219–1222.

b. Migratory polyarthritis and/or polyarthralgias:
   (1) Presenting feature in 25% of cases: Very tender and painful periarticular joint swelling of the ankles and knees (most often), without effusion
   (2) Joint involvement is transient with no permanent deformities

c. Abdominal pain:
   (1) Colicky in nature, secondary to hemorrhage and edema of the small intestine
   (2) Intussusception results in about 2% of cases (usually ileoileal)
   (3) Stool can be guaiac positive without obvious signs of intestinal bleeding
d. Glomerulonephritis:
   (1) Occurs in 20%–60% of patients, may develop months after onset or prior to development of rash
   (2) Renal biopsy: Typically consistent with IgA nephropathy, but crescentic glomerulonephritis may also be seen
   (3) More common in male patients, those with gastrointestinal (GI) bleeding, factor VIII activity <80%, and in patients younger than 4 years[22]
e. Other features: Acute scrotal inflammation (2%–38% of male patients), dorsal edema of the feet, occult pulmonary involvement

3. **Diagnosis:** Based on clinical characteristics[2,19,20]
4. **Laboratory findings:** Can help to exclude other diagnoses and illuminate specific organ involvement
   a. Hematologic: Normal to elevated platelet count, normal platelet function tests and bleeding time, normal coagulation studies
   b. Urinalysis: ± proteinuria and hematuria, but casts are uncommon
   c. Antibodies: IgA levels may be elevated, especially in the acute phase of the disease
   d. Stool guaiac: May be positive
   e. ASO titer: May be elevated
   f. Throat culture may be positive for group A β-hemolytic streptococcus, warranting antibiotic treatment
5. **Treatment[23,24]:**
   a. Supportive care: Adequate hydration, analgesia for joint pain
   b. Monitoring vital signs due to GI bleeding and renal involvement
   c. Serial urinalyses at routine office visits
   d. Consider steroids, especially if GI and renal systems involved (minimal supporting evidence)
   e. Prolonged immunosuppression may be needed for renal disease (cyclophosphamide or azathioprine)
6. **Prognosis:** Typically self-limited course, but may recur in a minority (10%–20%) of cases

VI. GRANULOMATOUS DISEASE

A. Differential Diagnosis[25,26]

1. **Infectious causes:** Tuberculosis, atypical mycobacterium including leprosy, histoplasmosis, coccidioidomycosis, brucellosis, chlamydia, tularemia, treponemal organisms, leishmaniasis, and toxoplasmosis
2. **Environmental exposures:** Hypersensitivity pneumonitis, berylliosis, silicosis, other metals (aluminum and titanium), and talc

3. **Immune dysregulation:** Wegener's granulomatosis, primary biliary cirrhosis, Churg-Strauss syndrome, sarcoidosis, Takayasu arteritis, Crohn's disease, and chronic granulomatous disease
4. **Other:** Malignancy, foreign bodies, medications

B. Sarcoidosis[2,26–29]

1. **Pathophysiology:** Multisystem infiltrative noncaseating granulomatous disease of unknown etiology
2. **Epidemiology:**
   a. Before puberty (very rare): Primarily affects Caucasians
   b. During and after puberty: African Americans predominate
   c. Incidence increases with age, peaking between ages 20 and 40 years
   d. Males and females affected equally
3. **Two forms of pediatric sarcoidosis:**
   a. Before puberty (usually <4 years): May be familial. Dominated by skin, musculoskeletal, and eye involvement
   b. During or after puberty: Very similar to adult disease. Dominated by lung, lymphatic, eye, and systemic involvement
4. **Presentation:** Lymphadenopathy is most common initial manifestation
   a. General: Weight loss, fever, anorexia, and fatigue
   b. Musculoskeletal: Usually only seen in young children. Tenosynovitis and polyarthritis, mostly of wrists, knees, and ankles[27]
   c. Pulmonary: Dyspnea on exertion, chest pain, chronic dry cough, wheezing or stridor, bilateral hilar lymphadenopathy with or without parenchymal disease on chest x-ray or computed tomography (CT), and restrictive pattern with impaired gas exchange on pulmonary function tests
   d. Ophthalmologic: Bilateral uveitis (anterior, posterior, or pan-uveitis), band keratopathy, synechiae, iris nodules, cataracts, glaucoma, chorioretinitis, conjunctivitis, papilledema
   e. Dermatologic: Erythema nodosum, plaques, maculopapules, and subcutaneous nodules
   f. Lymphatic: Hilar, mediastinal, and mobile, nontender peripheral lymphadenopathy
   g. Neurologic: Headache, seizures, CN (VI, VII, VIII) palsies, pseudotumor cerebri, obstructive hydrocephalus, hemiparesis
      (1) CN VII palsy: Most common neurologic manifestation in adolescent/adult form[28]
      (2) Magnetic resonance imaging (MRI) may show mass lesion(s), periventricular white matter lesions, nodular or diffuse leptomeningeal enhancement[29]
   h. Cardiovascular: Arrhythmia, valvular disease, vasculitis of any size vessel
   i. Renal: Renal failure (due to hypercalcemia or parenchymal infiltration) and nephrolithiasis

j. GI: Hepatosplenomegaly, elevated transaminases, hyperbilirubinemia due to parenchymal and biliary tree infiltration, parotitis. Intestinal obstruction with rectal prolapse (rare)
k. Endocrine: Pituitary dysfunction (e.g., diabetes insipidus, hypercalcemia)
5. **Laboratory studies:** Nonspecific
a. Hypercalcemia (due to pulmonary alveolar macrophage hydroxylation of vitamin D to active 1,25 dihydroxy form)
b. Elevated serum angiotensin-converting enzyme (produced by epithelial cells in granulomata)
c. Leukopenia, increased immunoglobulins, and eosinophilia are common
6. **Initial evaluation:** Thorough history and physical examination, chest x-ray or CT, complete metabolic panel, pulmonary function testing, electrocardiogram, and ophthalmologic (slit-lamp) examination
7. **Diagnosis:** Biopsy demonstrating noncaseating granulomas in absence of other known cause
8. **Treatment:** Glucocorticoids are standard. Methotrexate, azathioprine are secondary alternatives

VII. OTHER RHEUMATIC DISEASES

A. Juvenile Dermatomyositis[1,2,7,30–32]

1. **Pathogenesis:**
a. Nonsuppurative inflammation of the skin, GI tract, and striated muscle
b. Unlike adult-onset form, juvenile dermatomyositis is not related to malignancy
2. **Epidemiology:**
a. One study found the incidence to be 3.2 cases per million children per year; female-to-male ratio of 2.3:1
b. Peak age of onset for juvenile form is 5–14 years
3. **Presentation**
a. Constitutional: Fever, fatigue, and weight loss
b. Musculoskeletal: Symmetrical proximal muscle pain or weakness involving shoulder and pelvic girdles
c. Dermatologic: Heliotropic rash involving upper eyelids (or malar rash); Gottron papules (thickened, erythematous, scaly rash on extensor surfaces of elbows, knees, metacarpophalangeal and proximal interphalangeal joints). Dystrophic cutaneous calcifications or photosensitivity may be present
d. Respiratory: Dyspnea/tachypnea may be present (restrictive lung disease due to respiratory muscle weakness) indicating more severe disease and poorer prognosis
e. Other: Dysphagia, periorbital edema, nail-fold or eyelid rim capillary abnormalities, including dilation, aneurysms, and dropout
4. **Laboratory studies:**
a. Elevated muscle enzymes: AST, alanine aminotransferase (ALT), CK, LDH, and aldolase; may be normal at initial diagnosis[32]

b. ANA may be positive, acute phase reactants (ESR and CRP) are frequently not elevated[31]

5. **Diagnosis:**

a. Muscle biopsy: Gold standard for definitive diagnosis

b. MRI: Often used to demonstrate affected areas: T1-weighted images may show fibrosis, atrophy, and fatty infiltration; T2-weighted images may demonstrate active myositis

See additional rheumatology information on Expert Consult, Chapter 26:

B. Scleroderma[2,21]

C. Sjögren's Syndrome[2]

REFERENCES

1. Kliegman RM, Behrman, RE, Jenson HB, et al. *Nelson textbook of pediatrics.* 18th ed. Philadelphia: Saunders Elsevier; 2007.
2. Cassidy J, Petty R. *Textbook of pediatric rheumatology.* 5th ed. Philadelphia: WB Saunders; 2005.
3. Marnell L, Mold C, Du Clos TW, et al. C-reactive protein: ligands, receptors and role in inflammation. *Clin Immunol.* 2005;117:104–111.
4. Bosch X, Guilabert A, Font J. Antineutrophil cytoplasmic antibodies. *Lancet.* 2006;368:404–418.
5. van Venrooij W, Zendman, AJ. Anti-CCP2 antibodies: an overview and perspective of the diagnostic abilities of this serological marker for early rheumatoid arthritis. *Clin Rev Allergy Immunol.* 2008;34(1):36–39.
6. Habib HM, Mosaad YM, Youssef HM, et al. Anti-cyclic citrullinated peptide antibodies in patients with juvenile idiopathic arthritis. *Immunol Invest.* 2008;37:849–857.
7. Harris ED, Budd RC, Genovese MC, et al. *Kelley's textbook of rheumatology.* 7th ed. Philadelphia: WB Saunders; 2005.
8. Hay W, Levin M, Sondheimer J, et al. *Current pediatric diagnosis & treatment.* 17th ed. New York: Lange Medical/McGraw-Hill; 2005.
9. Petty RE, Southwood TR, Manners P, et al. International League of Associations for Rheumatology classification of juvenile idiopathic arthritis: Second revision, Edmonton, 2001. *J Rheum.* 2004;31:390–392.
10. Jones OY, Spender CH, Bowyer SL, et al. A multicenter case-control study on predictive factors distinguishing childhood leukemia from juvenile rheumatoid arthritis. *Pediatrics.* 2006;117:840–844.
11. Helliwell P, Taylor WJ. Classification and diagnostic criteria for psoriatic arthritis. *Ann Rheum Dis.* 2005;64:3–8.
12. Stoll ML, Zurakowski D, Nigrovic LE, et al. Patients with juvenile psoriatic arthritis comprise two distinct populations. *Arthritis Rheum.* 2006;54:3564–3572.
13. Milojevic D, Ilowite N. Treatment of rheumatic diseases in children: Special considerations. *Rheum Dis Clin North Am.* 2002;28:461–482.
14. Cassidy J, Kivlin J, Lindsley C, et al. Ophthalmologic examinations in children with juvenile rheumatoid arthritis. *Pediatrics.* 2006;117(5):1843–1845.
15. Tan EM, Cohen AS, Fries JF, et al. The 1982 revised criteria for the classification of systemic lupus erythematosus. *Arthritis Rheum.* 1982;25:1271–1277.
16. Bader-Meunier B, Armengaud JB, Haddad E. Initial presentation of childhood-onset systemic lupus erythematosus: a French multicenter study. *J Pediatr.* 2005;146:648–653.

17. Petri M, Magder L. Classification criteria for systemic lupus erythematosus: a review. *Lupus.* 2004;13:829–837.
18. Williams RC, Harmon ME, Burlingame R. Studies of serum C-reactive protein in systemic lupus erythematosus. *J Rheumatol.* 2005;32:454–461.
19. Gross WL, Trabandt A, Reinhold-Keller T, et al. Diagnosis and evaluation of vasculitis. *Rheumatology.* 2000;39:245–252.
20. Sundel R, Szer I. Vasculitis in childhood. *Rheum Dis Clin North Am.* 2002;28(3):625–654.
21. McMillan JA, Feigin RD, DeAngelis CD, et al. *Oski's pediatrics.* 4th ed. Philadelphia: Lippincott Williams & Wilkins; 2006.
22. Sano H, Izumida M, Ogawa Y, et al. Risk factors of renal involvement and significant proteinuria in Henoch-Schönlein purpura. *Eur J Pediatr.* 2002;161: 196–201.
23. Kim S, Dedeoglu F. Update on pediatric vasculitis. *Curr Opin Pediatr.* 2005;17: 695–702.
24. Dillon M, Ozen S. A new international classification of childhood vasculitis. *Pediatr Nephrol.* 2006;21:1219–1222.
25. Frosch M, Foell D. Wegener granulomatosis in childhood and adolescence. *Eur J Pediatr.* 2004;163:425–434.
26. Newman LS, Rose CS, Maier LA, et al. Sarcoidosis. *N Engl J Med.* 1997;336: 1224–1234.
27. Lindsley C, Petty R. Overview and report on international registry of sarcoid arthritis in children. *Curr Rheumatol Rep.* 2000;2:343–348.
28. Baumann R, Robertson W. Neurosarcoid presents differently in children than in adults. *Pediatrics.* 2003;112:e480–e486.
29. Nowak D, Widenka D. Neurosarcoidosis: a review of its intracranial manifestation. *J Neurol.* 2001;248:363–372.
30. Mendez EP, Lipton R, Ramsey-Goldman R. US incidence of juvenile dermatomyositis, 1995–1998: results from the National Institute of Arthritis and Musculoskeletal and Skin Diseases Registry. *Arthritis Rheum.* 2003;49: 300–305.
31. McCann LJ, Juggins AD, Maillard SM, et al. The Juvenile Dermatomyositis National Registry and Repository (UK and Ireland)—clinical characteristics of children recruited within the first 5 years. *Rheumatology.* 2006;45:1255–1260.
32. Ravelli A, Ruperto N, Trail L. Clinical assessment in juvenile dermatomyositis. *Autoimmunity.* 2006;39(3):197–203.

PART III

REFERENCE

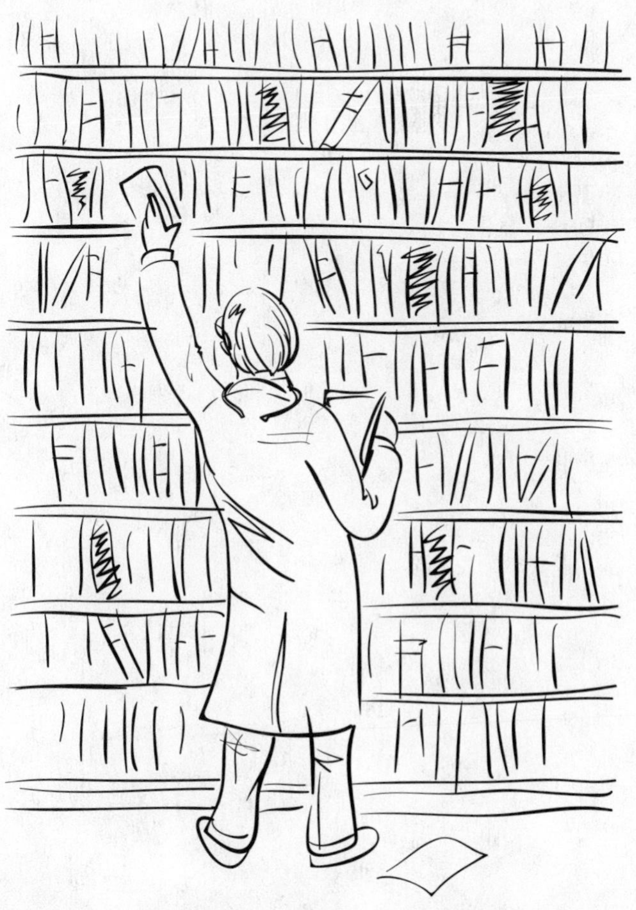

Chapter 27

Blood Chemistries and Body Fluids

Kristin M. Arcara, MD

27

The determination of normal reference ranges of laboratory studies in pediatric patients poses some major challenges. The available literature is often limited due to the small sample sizes of patients in many studies that have been used to derive these suggested normal ranges. **Please use great caution and be aware of this limitation when interpreting pediatric laboratory studies.**

The following values are compiled from the published literature and from the Johns Hopkins Hospital Department of Laboratory Medicine. Normal values vary with analytic method used. Consult your laboratory for its analytic method and range of normal values and for less commonly used parameters, which are beyond the scope of this text. Additional normal laboratory values may be found in Chapters 10, 14, and 15.

A special thanks to Lori Sokoll, Ph. D., for her guidance in preparing this chapter.

I. REFERENCE VALUES (TABLE 27-1)

Text continued on page 647

TABLE 27-1
REFERENCE VALUES

	Conventional Units	SI Units
ACID PHOSPHATASE		
(Major sources: Prostate and erythrocytes)		
Newborn	7.4–19.4 U/L	7.4–19.4 U/L
2–13 yr	6.4–15.2 U/L	6.4–15.2 U/L
Adult male	0.5–11.0 U/L	0.5–11.0 U/L
Adult female	0.2–9.5 U/L	0.2–9.5 U/L
ALANINE AMINOTRANSFERASE (ALT)[1,2]		
(Major sources: Liver, skeletal muscle, and myocardium)		
Infant <5 days	6–50 U/L	6–50 U/L
Infant <12 mo	13–45 U/L	13–45 U/L
1–3 yr	5–45 U/L	5–45 U/L
4–6 yr	10–25 U/L	10–25 U/L
7–9 yr	10–35 U/L	10–35 U/L
10–11 yr		
Female	10–30 U/L	10–30 U/L
Male	10–35 U/L	10–35 U/L

Continued

TABLE 27-1

REFERENCE VALUES (Continued)

	Conventional Units	SI Units
ALANINE AMINOTRANSFERASE (ALT)[1,2]		
(Major sources: Liver, skeletal muscle, and myocardium)		
12–13 yr		
Female	10–30 U/L	10–30 U/L
Male	10–55 U/L	10–55 U/L
14–15 yr		
Female	5–30 U/L	5–30 U/L
Male	10–45 U/L	10–45 U/L
>16 yr		
Female	5–35 U/L	5–35 U/L
Male	10–40 U/L	10–40 U/L
ALBUMIN		
(See Proteins)		
ALDOLASE[3]		
(Major sources: Skeletal muscle and myocardium)		
10–24 mo	3.4–11.8 U/L	3.4–11.8 U/L
2–16 yr	1.2–8.8 U/L	1.2–8.8 U/L
Adult	1.7–4.9 U/L	1.7–4.9 U/L
ALKALINE PHOSPHATASE[4]		
(Major sources: Liver, bone, intestinal mucosa, placenta, and kidney)		
Infant	150–420 U/L	150–420 U/L
2–10 yr	100–320 U/L	100–320 U/L
Adolescent male	100–390 U/L	100–390 U/L
Adolescent female	100–320 U/L	100–320 U/L
Adult	30–120 U/L	30–120 U/L
AMMONIA[2]		
(Heparinized venous specimen on ice analyzed within 30 min)		
Newborn	90–150 mcg/dL	64–107 μmol/L
0–2 wk	79–129 mcg/dL	56–92 μmol/L
Infant/child	29–70 mcg/dL	21–50 μmol/L
Adult	15–45 mcg/dL	11–32 μmol/L
AMYLASE[3]		
(Major sources: Pancreas, salivary glands, and ovaries)		
0–3 mo	0–30 U/L	0–30 U/L
3–6 mo	0–50 U/L	0–50 U/L
6–12 mo	0–80 U/L	0–80 U/L
>1 yr	30–100 U/L	30–100 U/L
ANTINUCLEAR ANTIBODY (ANA)[2]		
Negative	<1:40	
Patterns with clinical correlation:		
Centromere: CREST		
Nucleolar: Scleroderma		
Homogeneous: Systemic lupus erythematosus (SLE)		

TABLE 27-1

REFERENCE VALUES (Continued)

	Conventional Units	SI Units
ANTISTREPTOLYSIN O TITER[5]		
(Fourfold rise in paired serial specimens is significant)		
Newborn	Similar to mother's value	
6–24 mo	≤50 Todd units/mL	
2–4 yr	≤160 Todd units/mL	
≥5 yr	≤330 Todd units/mL	
ASPARTATE AMINOTRANSFERASE (AST)[2]		
(Major sources: Liver, skeletal muscle, kidney, myocardium, and erythrocytes)		
0–10 days	47–150 U/L	47–150 U/L
10 day–24 mo	9–80 U/L	9–80 U/L
>24 mo		
Female	13–35 U/L	13–35 U/L
Male	15–40 U/L	15–40 U/L
BICARBONATE[2,4]		
Newborn	17–24 mEq/L	17–24 mmol/L
Infant	19–24 mEq/L	19–24 mmol/L
2 mo–2 yr	16–24 mEq/L	16–24 mmol/L
>2 yr	22–26 mEq/L	22–26 mmol/L
BILIRUBIN (TOTAL)[4,6]		
(Please see Chapter 18 for more complete information about neonatal hyperbilirubinemia and acceptable bilirubin values)		
Cord:		
Term and preterm	<2 mg/dL	<34 μmol/L
0–1 days:		
Term and preterm	<8 mg/dL	<137 μmol/L
1–2 days:		
Preterm	<12 mg/dL	<205 μmol/L
Term	<11.5 mg/dL	<197 μmol/L
3–5 days:		
Preterm	<16 mg/dL	<274 μmol/L
Term	<12 mg/dL	<205 μmol/L
Older infant:		
Preterm	<2 mg/dL	<34 μmol/L
Term	<1.2 mg/dL	<21 μmol/L
Adult	<1.5 mg/dL	<20.5 μmol/L
BILIRUBIN (CONJUGATED)[2–4]		
Neonate	<0.6 mg/dL	<10 μmol/L
Infants/children	<0.2 mg/dL	<3.4 μmol/L

BLOOD GAS, ARTERIAL (BREATHING ROOM AIR)[2]

	pH	Pa_{O_2} (mmHg)	Pa_{CO_2} (mmHg)	HCO_3^- (mEq/L)
Cord blood	7.28 ± 0.05	18.0 ± 6.2	49.2 ± 8.4	14–22
Newborn (birth)	7.11–7.36	8–24	27–40	13–22
5–10 min	7.09–7.30	33–75	27–40	13–22
30 min	7.21–7.38	31–85	27–40	13–22

Continued

TABLE 27-1

REFERENCE VALUES (Continued)

BLOOD GAS, ARTERIAL (BREATHING ROOM AIR)[2]

	pH	Pa_{O_2} (mmHg)	Pa_{CO_2} (mmHg)	HCO_3^- (mEq/L)
60 min	7.26–7.49	55–80	27–40	13–22
1 day	7.29–7.45	54–95	27–40	13–22
Child/adult	7.35–7.45	83–108	32–48	20–28

NOTE: Venous blood gases can be used to assess acid-base status, not oxygenation. P_{CO_2} averages 6–8 mmHg higher than Pa_{CO_2}, and pH is slightly lower. Peripheral venous samples are strongly affected by the local circulatory and metabolic environment. Capillary blood gases correlate best with arterial pH and moderately well with Pa_{CO_2}.

	Conventional Units	SI Units
C-REACTIVE PROTEIN[4]	0–0.5 mg/dL	
CALCIUM (TOTAL)[2]		
Premature neonate	6.2–11 mg/dL	1.55–2.75 mmol/L
0–10 days	7.6–10.4 mg/dL	1.9–2.6 mmol/L
10 d–24 mo	9–11 mg/dL	2.25–2.75 mmol/L
24 mo–12 yr	8.8–10.8 mg/dL	2.2–2.7 mmol/L
12–18 yr	8.4–10.2 mg/dL	2.1–2.55 mmol/L
CALCIUM (IONIZED)[3]		
0–1 mo	3.9–6.0 mg/dL	1.0–1.5 mmol/L
1–6 mo	3.7–5.9 mg/dL	0.95–1.5 mmol/L
1–18 yr	4.9–5.5 mg/dL	1.22–1.37 mmol/L
Adult	4.75–5.3 mg/dL	1.18–1.32 mmol/L
CARBON DIOXIDE (CO_2 CONTENT)[2] (See Blood Gas, Arterial)		
CARBON MONOXIDE (CARBOXYHEMOGLOBIN)		
Nonsmoker	0.5%–1.5% of total hemoglobin	
Smoker	4%–9% of total hemoglobin	
Toxic	20%–50% of total hemoglobin	
Lethal	>50% of total hemoglobin	

	Conventional Units	Si Units
CHLORIDE (SERUM)[3]		
0–6 mo	97–108 mEq/L	97–108 mmol/L
6–12 mo	97–106 mEq/L	97–106 mmol/L
Child/adult	97–107 mEq/L	97–107 mmol/L
CHOLESTEROL (See Lipids)		
CREATINE KINASE (CREATINE PHOSPHOKINASE)[2] (Major sources: Myocardium, skeletal muscle, smooth muscle, and brain)		
Newborn	145–1,578 U/L	145–1,578 U/L
>6 wk–Adult male	20–200 U/L	20–200 U/L
>6 wk–Adult female	20–180 U/L	20–180 U/L
CREATININE (SERUM)[2]		
Cord	0.6–1.2 mg/dL	53–106 μmol/L
Newborn	0.3–1.0 mg/dL	27–88 μmol/L
Infant	0.2–0.4 mg/dL	18–35 μmol/L
Child	0.3–0.7 mg/dL	27–62 μmol/L

TABLE 27-1

REFERENCE VALUES (Continued)

	Conventional Units	SI Units
Adolescent	0.5–1.0 mg/dL	44–88 μmol/L
Adult male	0.9–1.3 mg/dL	80–115 μmol/L
Adult female	0.6–1.1 mg/dL	53–97 μmol/L
ERYTHROCYTE SEDIMENTATION RATE (ESR)[2]		
Child	0–10 mm/hr	
Adult male	0–15 mm/hr	
Adult female	0–20 mm/hr	
FERRITIN[2]		
Newborn	25–200 ng/mL	56–450 pmol/L
1 mo	200–600 ng/mL	450–1,350 pmol/L
2–5 mo	50–200 ng/mL	112–450 pmol/L
6 mo–15 yr	7–140 ng/mL	16–315 pmol/L
Adult male	20–250 ng/mL	45–562 pmol/L
Adult female	10–120 ng/mL	22–270 pmol/L
FIBRINOGEN		
(See Chapter 14)		
FOLATE (SERUM)[3]		
Newborn	16–72 ng/mL	16–72 nmol/L
Child	4–20 ng/mL	4–20 nmol/L
Adult	10–63 ng/mL	10–63 nmol/L
FOLATE (RBC)[2]		
Newborn	150–200 ng/mL	340–453 nmol/L
Infant	74–995 ng/mL	168–2,254 nmol/L
2–16 yr	>160 ng/mL	>362 nmol/L
>16 yr	140–628 ng/mL	317–1,422 nmol/L
GALACTOSE[2]		
Newborn	0–20 mg/dL	0–1.11 mmol/L
Older child	<5 mg/dL	<0.28 mmol/L
GAMMA-GLUTAMYL TRANSFERASE (GGT)[2,5]		
(Major sources: Liver [biliary tree] and kidney)		
Cord	37–193 U/L	37–193 U/L
0–1 mo	13–147 U/L	13–147 U/L
1–2 mo	12–123 U/L	12–123 U/L
2–4 mo	8–90 U/L	8–90 U/L
4 mo–10 yr	5–32 U/L	5–32 U/L
10–15 yr	5–24 U/L	5–24 U/L
Adult male	11–49 U/L	11–49 U/L
Adult female	7–32 U/L	7–32 U/L
GLUCOSE (SERUM)[2,5]		
Preterm	20–60 mg/dL	1.1–3.3 mmol/L
Newborn, <1 day	40–60 mg/dL	2.2–3.3 mmol/L
Newborn, >1 day	50–90 mg/dL	2.8–5.0 mmol/L
Child	60–100 mg/dL	3.3–5.5 mmol/L
>16 yr	70–105 mg/dL	3.9–5.8 mmol/L

Continued

TABLE 27-1

REFERENCE VALUES (Continued)

	Conventional Units	SI Units
HAPTOGLOBIN[2]		
Newborn	5–48 mg/dL	50–480 mg/L
>30 days	26–185 mg/dL	260–1,850 mg/L
HEMOGLOBIN A_{1C}[7]		
Normal	4.5%–5.6%	
At risk for diabetes	5.7%–6.4%	
Diabetes mellitus	≥6.5%	
HEMOGLOBIN F, % TOTAL HEMOGLOBIN [MEAN (SD)][2]		
1 day	77.0 (7.3)	
5 days	76.8 (5.8)	
3 wk	70.0 (7.3)	
6–9 wk	52.9 (11)	
3–4 mo	23.2 (16)	
6 mo	4.7 (2.2)	
8–11 mo	1.6 (1.0)	
Adult	<2.0	
IRON[2]		
Newborn	100–250 mcg/dL	17.9–44.8 μmol/L
Infant	40–100 mcg/dL	7.2–17.9 μmol/L
Child	50–120 mcg/dL	9.0–21.5 μmol/L
Adult male	65–175 mcg/dL	11.6–31.3 μmol/L
Adult female	50–170 mcg/dL	9.0–30.4 μmol/L
LACTATE[2,3]		
Capillary blood:		
0–90 days	9–32 mg/dL	1.1–3.5 mmol/L
3–24 mo	9–30 mg/dL	1.0–3.3 mmol/L
2–18 yr	9–22 mg/dL	1.0–2.4 mmol/L
Venous	4.5–19.8 mg/dL	0.5–2.2 mmol/L
Arterial	4.5–14.4 mg/dL	0.5–1.6 mmol/L
LACTATE DEHYDROGENASE (AT 37°C)[2] (Major sources: Myocardium, liver, skeletal muscle, erythrocytes, platelets, and lymph nodes)		
0–4 days	290–775 U/L	290–775 U/L
4–10 days	545–2,000 U/L	545–2,000 U/L
10 days–24 mo	180–430 U/L	180–430 U/L
24 mo–12 yr	110–295 U/L	110–295 U/L
>12 yr	100–190 U/L	100–190 U/L
LEAD[2]		
Child	<10 mcg/dL	<0.48 μmol/L
LIPASE[3]		
0–30 days	6–55 U/L	6–55 U/L
1–6 mo	4–29 U/L	4–29 U/L
6–12 mo	4–23 U/L	4–23 U/L
>1 yr	3–32 U/L	3–32 U/L

TABLE 27-1

REFERENCE VALUES (Continued)

	Cholesterol (mg/dL)			LDL (mg/dL)				HDL (mg/dL)
	Desirable	**Borderline**	**High**	**Optimal**	**Near/Above optimal**	**Borderline**	**High**	**Desirable**
LIPIDS[8,9]								
Child/adolescent	<170	170–199	>200	<110		110–129	>130	>35
Adult	<200	200–239	<240	<100	100–129	130–159	>160	40–60

	Conventional Units	SI Units
MAGNESIUM[2]	1.26–2.1 mEq/L	0.63–1.05 mmol/L
METHEMOGLOBIN[2]	0.78% (± 0.37%) of total hemoglobin	
OSMOLALITY[2]	275–295 mOsm/kg	275–295 mmol/kg
PHENYLALANINE[2]		
Preterm	2.0–7.5 mg/dL	121–454 μmol/L
Newborn	1.2–3.4 mg/dL	73–206 μmol/L
Adult	0.8–1.8 mg/dL	48–109 μmol/L
PHOSPHORUS[2]		
0–9 days	4.5–9.0 mg/dL	1.45–2.91 mmol/L
10 days–24 mo	4–6.5 mg/dL	1.29–2.10 mmol/L
3–9 yr	3.2–5.8 mg/dL	1.03–1.87 mmol/L
10–15 yr	3.3–5.4 mg/dL	1.07–1.74 mmol/L
>15 yr	2.4–4.4 mg/dL	0.78–1.42 mmol/L
PORCELAIN[10]	9.0–25.04 mg/dL	5.0–31.03 mmol/L
POTASSIUM[2]		
Preterm	3.0–6.0 mEq/L	3.0–6.0 mmol/L
Newborn	3.7–5.9 mEq/L	3.7–5.9 mmol/L
Infant	4.1–5.3 mEq/L	4.1–5.3 mmol/L
Child	3.4–4.7 mEq/L	3.4–4.7 mmol/L
Adult	3.5–5.1 mEq/L	3.5–5.1 mmol/L
PREALBUMIN[3]		
Newborn	7–39 mg/dL	
1–6 mo	8–34 mg/dL	
6 mo–4 yr	12–36 mg/dL	
4–6 yr	12–30 mg/dL	
6–19 yr	12–42 mg/dL	

PROTEIN ELECTROPHORESIS (g/dL)[2]

Age	Total Protein	Albumin	α-1	α-2	β	γ
Cord	4.8–8.0					
Premature	3.6–6.0					
Newborn	4.6–7.0					
0–15 day	4.4–7.6	3.0–3.9	0.1–0.3	0.3–0.6	0.4–0.6	0.7–1.4
15 day–1 yr	5.1–7.3	2.2–4.8	0.1–0.3	0.5–0.9	0.5–0.9	0.5–1.3

Continued

TABLE 27-1

REFERENCE VALUES (Continued)

PROTEIN ELECTROPHORESIS (g/dL)[2]

Age	Total Protein	Albumin	α-1	α-2	β	γ
1–2 yr	5.6–7.5	3.6–5.2	0.1–0.4	0.5–1.2	0.5–1.1	0.5–1.7
3–16 yr	6.0–8.0	3.6–5.2	0.1–0.4	0.5–1.2	0.5–1.1	0.5–1.7
≥16 yr	6.0–8.3	3.9–5.1	0.2–0.4	0.4–0.8	0.5–1.0	0.6–1.2

	Conventional Units	SI Units
PYRUVATE[3]	0.7–1.32 mg/dL	0.08–0.15 mmol/L
RHEUMATOID FACTOR[2]	<30 U/mL	
SODIUM[1]		
<1 yr	130–145 mEq/L	130–145 mmol/L
>1 yr	135–147 mEq/L	135–147 mmol/L
TOTAL IRON-BINDING CAPACITY (TIBC)[2]		
Infant	100–400 mcg/dL	17.9–71.6 μmol/L
Adult	250–425 mcg/dL	44.8–76.1 μmol/L
TOTAL PROTEIN (See Proteins)		
TRANSAMINASE (SGOT) (See Aspartate aminotransferase [AST])		
TRANSAMINASE (SGPT) (See Alanine aminotransferase [ALT])		
TRANSFERRIN[2]		
Newborn	130–275 mg/dL	1.30–2.75 g/L
3 mo–16 yr	203–360 mg/dL	2.03–3.6 g/L
Adult	215–380 mg/dL	2.15–3.8 g/L

TOTAL TRIGLYCERIDE[3]

	Conventional Units (mg/dL)		SI Units (mmol/L)	
	Male	Female	Male	Female
0–7 day	21–182	28–166	0.24–2.06	0.32–1.88
8–30 day	30–184	30–165	0.34–2.08	0.34–1.86
31–90 day	40–175	35–282	0.45–1.98	0.4–3.19
91–180 day	45–291	50–355	0.51–3.29	0.57–4.01
181–365 day	45–501	36–431	0.51–5.66	0.41–4.87
1–3 yr	27–125	27–125	0.31–1.41	0.31–1.41
4–6 yr	32–116	32–116	0.36–1.31	0.36–1.31
7–9 yr	28–129	28–129	0.32–1.46	0.32–1.46
10–19 yr	24–145	37–140	0.27–1.64	0.42–1.58

	Conventional Units	SI Units
TROPONIN-I[3]		
0–30 day	<4.8 mcg/L	
31–90 day	<0.4 mcg/L	
3–6 mo	<0.3 mcg/L	
7–12 mo	<0.2 mcg/L	
1–18 yr	<0.1 mcg/L	

TABLE 27-1
REFERENCE VALUES (Continued)

	Conventional Units	SI Units
UREA NITROGEN[1,2]		
Premature (<1 wk)	3–25 mg/dL	1.1–8.9 mmol/L
Newborn	2–19 mg/dL	0.7–6.7 mmol/L
Infant/child	5–18 mg/dL	1.8–6.4 mmol/L
Adult	6–20 mg/dL	2.1–7.1 mmol/L
URIC ACID[3,5]		
0–30 day	1.0–4.6 mg/dL	0.059–0.271 mmol/L
1–12 mo	1.1–5.6 mg/dL	0.065–0.33 mmol/L
1–5 yr	1.7–5.8 mg/dL	0.1–0.35 mmol/L
6–11 yr	2.2–6.6 mg/dL	0.13–0.39 mmol/L
Male 12–19 yr	3.0–7.7 mg/dL	0.18–0.46 mmol/L
Female 12–19 yr	2.7–5.7 mg/dL	0.16–0.34 mmol/L
VITAMIN A (RETINOL)[2,3]		
Preterm	13–46 mcg/dL	0.46–1.61 μmol/L
Full term	18–50 mcg/dL	0.63–1.75 μmol/L
1–6 yr	20–43 mcg/dL	0.7–1.5 μmol/L
7–12 yr	20–49 mcg/dL	0.9–1.7 μmol/L
13–19 yr	26–72 mcg/dL	0.9–2.5 μmol/L
VITAMIN B_1 (THIAMINE)[2]	4.5–10.3 mcg/dL	106–242 μmol/L
VITAMIN B_2 (RIBOFLAVIN)	4–24 mcg/dL	106–638 nmol/L
VITAMIN B_{12} (COBALAMIN)[2]		
Newborn	160–1,300 pg/mL	118–959 pmol/L
Child/adult	200–835 pg/mL	148–616 pmol/L
VITAMIN C (ASCORBIC ACID)[2]	0.4–2.0 mg/dL	23–114 μmol/L
VITAMIN D_3 (1,25-dIhYDROXY-VITAMIN D)[2]	16–65 pg/mL	42–169 pmol/L
VITAMIN E[1,2,3]		
Preterm	0.5–3.5 mg/L	1–8 μmol/L
Full term	1.0–3.5 mg/L	2–8 μmol/L
1–12 yr	3.0–9.0 mg/L	7–21 μmol/L
13–19 yr	6.0–10.0 mg/L	14–23 μmol/L
ZINC[2]	70–120 mcg/dL	10.7–18.4 mmol/L

CREST: **C**alcinosis, **R**aynaud's syndrome, **E**sophageal dysmotility, **S**clerodactyly, **T**elangiectasia

II. EVALUATION OF BODY FLUIDS

A. Evaluation of Transudate Versus Exudate (Table 27-2)

B. Evaluation of Cerebrospinal Fluid (Table 27-3)

C. Evaluation of Synovial Fluid (Table 27-4)

TABLE 27-2

EVALUATION OF TRANSUDATE VS. EXUDATE (PLEURAL, PERICARDIAL, OR PERITONEAL FLUID)

Measurement*	Transudate	Exudate†
Protein (g/dL)	<3.0	>3.0
Fluid : serum ratio	<0.5	≥0.5
LDH (IU)	<200	≥200
Fluid : serum ratio (isoenzymes not useful)	<0.6	≥0.6
WBCs‡	<10,000/μL	>10,000/μL
RBCs	<5,000	>5,000
Glucose	>40	<40
pH§	>7.2	<7.2

NOTE: Amylase >5,000 U/mL or pleural fluid:serum ratio > 1 suggests pancreatitis.

*Always obtain serum for glucose, LDH, protein, amylase, and so forth.

†All of the following criteria do not have to be met for consideration as an exudate.

‡In peritoneal fluid, WBC count >800/μL suggests peritonitis.

§Collect anaerobically in a heparinized syringe.

LDH, Lactate dehydrogenase; RBCs, red blood cells; WBCs, white blood cells.

Data from Nichols DG, Ackerman AD, Carcillo JA, et al: Rogers textbook of pediatric intensive care, 4th ed. Baltimore, Williams & Wilkins, 2008.

TABLE 27-3

EVALUATION OF CEREBROSPINAL FLUID

Age[4,11]	WBC count/μL (median)	95th percentile
0–28 d	0–12* (3)	19
29–56 d	0–6* (2)	9
Child	0–7	
	Conventional Units	**SI Units**
GLUCOSE[4,12]		
Preterm	24–63 mg/dL	1.3–3.5 mmol/L
Term	34–119 mg/dL	1.9–6.6 mmol/L
Child	40–80 mg/dL	2.2–4.4 mmol/L
PROTEIN[4,12,13]		
Preterm	65–150 mg/dL	0.65–1.5 g/L
0–14d	79 (±23) mg/dL†	0.79 (±0.23) g/L†
15–28d	69 (±20) mg/dL†	0.69 (±0.20) g/L†
29–42d	58 (±17) mg/dL†	0.58 (±0.17) g/L†
43–56d	53 (±17) mg/dL†	0.53 (±0.17) g/L†
Child	5–40 mg/dL	5–40 mg/dL
OPENING PRESSURE (LATERAL RECUMBENT POSITION[4,14])		
Newborn	8–11 cm H_2O	
1–18 years	11.5–28 cm H_2O*	
Respiratory variations	0.5–1 cm H_2O	

CSF, Cerebrospinal fluid; PMNs, polymorphonuclear lymphocytes; WBC, white blood cell.

*Up to 90th percentile

†Mean (±SD)

TABLE 27-4

CHARACTERISTICS OF SYNOVIAL FLUID IN THE RHEUMATIC DISEASES

Group	Condition	Synovial Complement	Color/Clarity	Viscosity	Mucin Clot	WBC Count	PMN (%)	Miscellaneous Findings
Noninflammatory	Normal	N	Yellow Clear	↑↑	G	<200	<25	
	Traumatic arthritis	N	Xanthochromic Turbid	↑	F–G	<2,000	<25	Debris
	Osteoarthritis	N	Yellow Clear	↑	F–G	1,000	<25	
Inflammatory	Systemic lupus erythematosus	↓	Yellow Clear	N	N	5,000	10	Lupus cells
	Rheumatic fever	N–↑	Yellow Cloudy	↓	F	5,000	10–50	
	Juvenile rheumatoid arthritis	N–↓	Yellow Cloudy	↓	Poor	15,000–20,000	75	
	Reiter's syndrome	↑	Yellow Opaque	↓	Poor	20,000	80	Reiter's cells
Pyogenic	Tuberculous arthritis	N–↑	Yellow-white Cloudy	↓	Poor	25,000	50–60	Acid-fast bacteria
	Septic arthritis	↑	Serosanguinous Turbid	↓	Poor	50,000–300,000	>75	Low glucose, bacteria

F, Fair; G, good; H, high; N, normal; PMN, polymorphonuclear leukocyte; VH, very high; WBC, white blood cell; ↓, decreased; ↑, increased.
From Cassidy JT, Petty RE: Textbook of pediatric rheumatology, 5th ed. Philadelphia, WB Saunders, 2005.

III. CONVERSION FORMULAS

A. Temperature

1. **To convert degrees Celsius to degrees Fahrenheit:**

$$([9/5] \times \text{Temperature}) + 32$$

2. **To convert degrees Fahrenheit to degrees Celsius:**

$$(\text{Temperature} - 32) \times (5/9)$$

B. Length and Weight

1. **Length:** To convert inches to centimeters, multiply by 2.54.
2. **Weight:** To convert pounds to kilograms, divide by 2.2.

REFERENCES

1. Meites S, ed. *Pediatric clinical chemistry*. 3rd ed. Washington, DC: American Association for Clinical Chemistry; 1989.
2. Wu Alan HB. *Tietz guide to laboratory tests*. 4th ed. Philadelphia: WB Saunders; 2006.
3. Soldin SJ, Brugnara C, Wong EC. *Pediatric reference intervals*. 6th ed. Washington, DC: AACC Press; 2007.
4. McMillan JA. *Oski's pediatrics: principles and practice*. 4th ed. Philadelphia: JB Lippincott; 2006.
5. Kleigman RM, Behrman RE, Jenson HB, et al. *Nelson textbook of pediatrics*. 18th ed. Philadelphia: WB Saunders; 2007.
6. Chernecky CC, Berger BJ. *Laboratory tests and diagnostic procedures*. 5th ed. St. Louis: Elsevier; 2008.
7. American Diabetes Association. Diagnosis and classification of diabetes mellitus—2010. *Diabetes Care*. 2010;33:S62–S69.
8. National Cholesterol Education Program (NCEP). Highlights of the Report of the Expert Panel on Blood Cholesterol Levels in Children and Adolescents. NCEP Expert Panel on Blood Cholesterol Levels in Children and Adolescents. *Pediatrics*. 1992;89:495–501.
9. Executive Summary of the Third Report of the National Cholesterol Education Program (NCEP) Expert Panel on Detection, Evaluation, and Treatment of High Blood Cholesterol in Adults (Adult Treatment Panel III). *JAMA*. 2001;285: 2486–2497.
10. Arcara KM, Tschudy MM. *Surviving pediatric chief residency at Hopkins: yin and yang*. Baltimore: Johns Hopkins University Press; 2010–2011.
11. Kestenbaum LA, Ebberson J, Zorc JJ, et al. Defining cerebrospinal fluid white blood cell count reference values in neonates and young infants. *Pediatrics*. 2010 Feb;125(2):257–264.
12. Sarff LD, Platt LH, McCracken GH. Cerebrospinal fluid evaluation in neonates: Comparison of high-risk infants with and without meningitis. *The Journal of Pediatrics*. 1976;883:473–477.
13. Shah SS, Ebberson J, Kestenbaum LA, et al. Age-specific reference values for cerebrospinal fluid protein concentration in neonates and young infants. *J Hosp Med*. 2011 Jan;6(1):22–27.
14. Avery RA, Shah SS, Licht DJ, et al. Reference range for cerebrospinal fluid opening pressure in children. *N Engl J Med*. 2010 Aug 26;363(9):891–893.

Chapter 28

Biostatistics and Evidence-Based Medicine

Karsten Lunze, MD, MPH

I. WEBSITES

BMJ Statistics at Square One: http://www.bmj.com/collections/statsbk/index.dtl

Centre for Evidence Based Medicine: http://www.cebm.net

JAMAevidence: www.jamaevidence.com

Johns Hopkins University Welch Medical Library: Evidence Based Medicine Resources: http://www.welch.jhu.edu/internet/ebr.html

University of Washington Healthlinks: Evidence-Based Practice: http://healthlinks.washington.edu/ebp

II. EVIDENCE-BASED MEDICINE

A. Evidence-Based Medicine:

Refers to the method of integrating individual clinical expertise with the best available evidence from systematic research. It typically involves the following framework[1]:

1. **Formulate the clinical question**
   a. Precisely describe the patient or problem, deciding whether the evidence you seek is on therapy, diagnosis or screening, prognosis, etiology or causation, cost effectiveness, or a qualitative study
   b. Specifically describe the intervention under consideration
   c. Compare the intervention to an alternative, if applicable
   d. Formulate a specific outcome of interest
2. **Search for the evidence to answer that question**
   a. Define search terms that fit the clinical question
   b. Develop your search strategy using PubMed or other primary search sources
   c. Scan your results and apply methodological filters to target the right type of study
3. **How to read a study**

Critically appraise the evidence: Decide whether the study findings are valid, and whether they are important to your question.

a. Therapy:
   (1) Were patient groups randomized for treatment?
   (2) Were groups comparable and treated equally, aside from the allocated treatment?
   (3) Were study subjects and investigators blinded?

(4) Were all patients entering the trial accounted for, in the groups they were randomized (intention to treat)?
(5) How large was the treatment effect (see Section III C. 5–7), and how precise was the estimate of the treatment effect?

b. Diagnosis:
(1) Was the test compared to an independent, blind reference (gold) standard of diagnosis?
(2) Was the test evaluated in an appropriate spectrum of patients?

c. Prognosis:
(1) Were study patients defined early in their course and followed-up over a sufficient time?
(2) How likely are these outcomes over a defined time period and how precise are estimates of prognosis?

For more comprehensive criteria or other types of studies, use appropriate appraisal frameworks[1]

4. **Apply the evidence to the clinical question:**

If the evidence is valid and important, integrate it with your clinical expertise. Decide whether patients in the study were similar to your individual patient and whether the:

a. Patient will benefit from the therapy and accept its regimen and consequences
b. Test is available, affordable, accurate, and precise
c. Study findings will impact what to tell or offer the patient

III. BIOSTATISTICS FOR MEDICAL LITERATURE

A. Statistical Tests: Table 28-1

1. Different statistics apply to test a hypothesis of whether observed differences are statistically significant:

a. Parametric statistical tests are more powerful and used when data follow a normal distribution. Nonparametric tests are used when a normal distribution cannot be assumed; they rank data rather than taking absolute differences into account
b. Paired tests are performed on paired data, e.g., when the same parameter or observation is measured twice on each study subject, often before and after an intervention. Unpaired tests compare values from independent samples
c. A two-tailed test has to be performed whenever an intervention could potentially lead to either an increase or decrease of the parameter. When the difference can only go in one direction, a one-tailed test can be used, which has greater statistical power

2. *Correlation* and *regression* describe the degree of linear association between two quantitative variables; however, they do not imply causation

a. Correlation measures the strength of association between two values, expressed by the correlation coefficient r, also termed Pearson's correlation coefficient

TABLE 28-1

SOME COMMONLY USED STATISTICAL TESTS

Parametric Test	Nonparametric Test	Purpose of Test	Example
Two sample (unpaired) *t* test	Mann-Whitney U test	Compares two independent samples drawn from the same population	To compare girls' heights with boys' heights
One sample (paired) *t* test	Wilcoxon matched pairs test	Compares two sets of observations on a single sample	To compare weight of infants before and after a feed
One way analysis of variance (*F* test) using total sum of squares	Kruskall-Wallis analysis of variance by ranks	Effectively, a generalization of the paired *t* or Wilcoxon matched pairs test where three or more sets of observations are made on a single sample	To determine whether plasma glucose level is higher 1 hour, 2 hours, or 3 hours after a meal
Two-way analysis of variance	Two-way analysis of variance by ranks	As above, but tests the influence (and interaction) of two different covariates	In the above example, to determine if the results differ in male and female subjects
χ^2 test	Fisher's exact test	Tests the null hypothesis that the distribution of a discontinuous variable is the same in two (or more) independent samples	To assess whether male or female adolescents are more likely to smoke
Product moment correlation coefficient (Pearson's *r*)	Spearman's rank correlation coefficient (r_σ)	Assesses the strength of the straight-line association between two continuous variables	To assess whether and to what extent plasma HbA1 concentration is related to plasma triglyceride concentration in diabetic patients
Regression by least squares method	Nonparametric regression (various tests)	Describes the numerical relation between two quantitative variables, allowing one value to be predicted from the other	To see how peak expiratory flow rate varies with height
Multiple regression by least squares method	Nonparametric regression (various tests)	Describes the numerical relation between a dependent variable and several predictor variables (covariates)	To determine whether and to what extent a person's age, body fat, and sodium intake determine his or her blood pressure

Adapted from: Greenhalgh, T. How to read a paper. Statistics for the non-statistician. I: different types of data need different statistical tests. BMJ 1997 9, 315(7104):364–366.

28

b. As a next step of describing association, the regression equation constructs the optimal straight line illustrating the correlation and allows the prediction of a (dependent) variable from a known (independent) variable. The method of multiple regression is used when there are multiple independent variables. Multiple regression accounts for influences of various factors on the outcome

3. **α (Significance level of statistical test):**
   a. Definition: Probability of finding a statistical association by chance alone when in reality there is no association (type I error)
   b. α typically set at of 0.05, which allows interpretation with 95% certainty that a detected association is true
   c. p value (probability of a difference occurring by chance) is complementary to α: If p is under the significance level (typically set at 0.05), then the detected association is unlikely to be due to chance alone
4. **Power (of a statistical test):**
   a. β = Probability of finding no statistical association when there truly is one (type II error)
   b. Power = $1 - \beta$ = Probability of finding a statistical association when there truly is one
   c. Power typically set at 0.80, which allows interpretation with 80% certainty that a detected lack of association is true
5. **Sample size:** Number of subjects required in a study to detect a certain (expected) effect magnitude with a sufficiently high power and sufficiently low α
6. **Confidence interval (95%):** Describes the 95% certainty that the reported interval contains the true value. When confidence intervals for groups overlap, then they do not differ in a statistically significant manner

B. Study Design Comparison (Table 28-2)

C. Measurements of Disease Occurrence and Treatment Effects (Table 28-3)

1. **Prevalence:**
   a. Proportion of study population who have a disease (at one point or period in time)
   b. Number of old cases and new cases divided by total population
   c. In cross-sectional studies (see Table 28-3):

$$\mathbf{(A + B)/(A + B + C + D)}$$

2. **Incidence:**
   a. Number of people in study population who newly develop an outcome (disease) per total study population per given time period
   b. Number of new cases divided by the total population over a given time period
   c. For cohort studies and clinical trials (see Table 28-3):

$$\mathbf{(A + B)/(A + B + C + D)}$$

TABLE 28-2

STUDY DESIGN COMPARISON

Design Type	Definition	Advantages	Disadvantages
Case-control (often called retrospective)	Define diseased subjects (cases) and nondiseased subjects (controls); compare proportion of cases with exposure (risk factor) with proportion of controls with exposure (risk factor).	Good for rare diseases Small sample size Shorter study times (not followed over time) Less expensive	Highest potential for biases (recall, selection, and others) Weak evidence for causality No prevalence, PPV, NPV
Cohort (usually prospective; occasionally retrospective)	In study population, define exposed group (with risk factor) and nonexposed group (without risk factor). Over time, compare proportion of exposed group with outcome (disease) with proportion of nonexposed group with outcome (disease).	Defines incidence Stronger evidence for causality Decreases biases (sampling, measurement, reporting)	Expensive Long study times May not be feasible for rare diseases/outcomes Factors related to exposure and outcome may falsely alter effect of exposure on outcome (confounding)
Cross-sectional	In study population, concurrently measure outcome (disease) and risk factor. Compare proportion of diseased group with risk factor with proportion of nondiseased group with risk factor.	Defines prevalence Short time to complete	Selection bias Weak evidence for causality
Clinical trial (experiment)	In study population, assign (randomly) subjects to receive treatment or receive no treatment. Compare rate of outcome (e.g., disease cure) between treatment and nontreatment groups.	Randomized, blinded trial is gold standard Randomization reduces confounding Best evidence for causality	Expensive Risks of experimental treatments in humans Longer study time Bad for rare outcomes/ diseases

NPV, Negative predictive value; PPV, positive predictive value.

TABLE 28-3

GRID FOR CALCULATIONS IN CLINICAL STUDIES

	Exposure or Risk Factor or Treatment	
Disease or Outcome	**Positive**	**Negative**
Positive	A	B
Negative	C	D

3. **Relative risk (RR):**

a. Ratio of incidence of disease among people with risk factor to incidence of disease among people without risk factor

b. For cohort studies or clinical trials (see Table 28-3):

$$[A/(A + C)]/[B/(B + D)]$$

c. Values:

(1) RR = 1: No effect of exposure (or treatment) on outcome (or disease)

(2) RR <1: Exposure or treatment protective against outcome

(3) RR >1: Exposure or treatment increases probability of outcome

4. **Odds ratio (OR):**

a. For case-control studies, ratio of [odds of having risk factor in people with disease (A/B)] to [odds of having risk factor in people without disease (C/D)] (see Table 28-3):

$$(A/B)/(C/D) = (A \times D)/(B \times C)$$

b. OR is a good estimate of RR if disease is rare:

(1) OR = 1: No association between risk factor and disease

(2) OR <1: Suggests that risk factor is protective against disease

(3) OR >1: Suggests association between risk factor and disease

5. **Absolute risk reduction (ARR), absolute risk difference:**

Definition: Absolute difference the treatment makes, expressed as difference between (risk of the outcome in the control group) minus (risk of the outcome in the treatment group)

6. **Relative risk reduction (RRR):**

Definition: Clinical significance of treatment effect, expressed as (absolute risk reduction) divided by (risk of the outcome in the control group), or 1 – RR

7. **Number needed to treat (NNT):**

Definition: patients to be treated with treatment under question to prevent one undesirable outcome as the inverse of the ARR, or 1 divided by ARR

D. Measurements of Test Validity and Reliability (Table 28-4)

1. **Sensitivity (Sens):**

a. Proportion of all diseased who have positive test (see Table 28-4):

$$A/(A + C)$$

TABLE 28-4

GRID FOR EVALUATING A CLINICAL TEST

	Disease Status	
Test Result	**Positive**	**Negative**
Positive	A (true positive)	B (false positive)
Negative	C (false negative)	D (true negative)

b. Use highly sensitive test to help exclude a disease. (Low false-negative rate. Desirable for screening tests.)

2. **Specificity (Spec):**

a. Proportion of all nondiseased who have a negative test (see Table 28-4):

$$D/(B + D)$$

b. Use highly specific test to help confirm a disease. (Low false-positive rate.)

3. **Positive predictive value (PPV):**

a. Proportion of all those with positive tests who truly have disease (see Table 28-4):

$$A/(A + B)$$

b. Increased PPV with higher disease prevalence and higher specificity (and, to a lesser degree, higher sensitivity)

4. **Negative predictive value (NPV):**

a. Proportion of all those with negative tests who truly do not have disease (see Table 28-4):

$$D/(C + D)$$

b. Increased NPV with lower prevalence (rarer disease) and higher sensitivity

5. **Likelihood ratio (LR):**

a. LR positive: Ability of positive test result to confirm diseased status:

$$\text{LR positive} = (\text{Sens})/(1 - \text{Spec})$$

b. LR negative: Ability of negative test result to confirm non-diseased status:

$$\text{LR negative} = (\text{Spec})/(1 - \text{Sens})$$

$$[\text{Alternative LR negative} = (1 - \text{Sens})/\text{Spec}]$$

c. Good tests have LR ≥10. (Good tests have LR ≤0.1 if using alternative LR-negative formula.) Physical examination findings often have LR of about 2

d. LR should not be affected by disease prevalence. Can be used to calculate increase in probability of disease from baseline prevalence with positive test (LR positive) and decrease in probability of disease from baseline prevalence with negative test (using alternative LR negative) for any level of disease prevalence (Fig. 28-1)

28

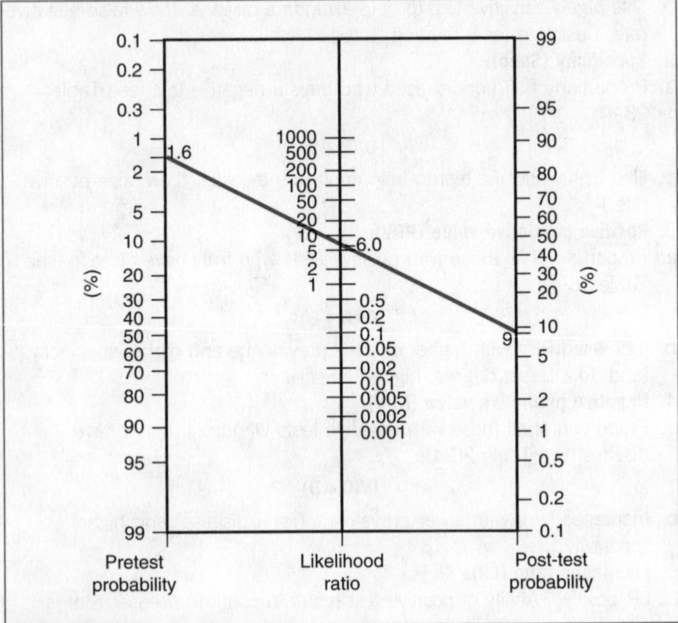

FIGURE 28-1

Nomogram for calculating the change in probability by applying tests with known likelihood ratios (LRs). For example, the prevalence (i.e., pretest probability) of occult bacteremia in a well-appearing 3- to 36-month-old with temperature ≥39°C without source is 1.6%. LR positive for white blood cell (WBC) count >20 × 10^9/L is 6.0. For infants, then, with a WBC count >20 × 10^9/L, you can use the nomogram to determine the increased probability from the positive test. Anchor a straight edge at 1.6% on the left pretest probability column and direct the straight edge through the central column at the LR of 6.0. The straight edge will intersect the right column with your answer to give a post-test probability of about 9%. It is then up to you to decide the clinical importance of a 9% probability of bacteremia. *(Data from Fagan TJ: Letter: nomogram for Bayes theorem. N Engl J Med 1975;293:257; Lee GM, Harper MB: Risk of bacteremia for febrile young children in the post-Haemophilus influenzae type b era. Arch Pediatr Adolesc Med 1998;152:624–628.)*

REFERENCES

1. Straus SE, Richardson WS, Glasziou P, et al. *Evidence-based medicine.* 3rd ed. Edinburgh: Churchill Livingstone; 2005.
2. Greenhalgh T. How to read a paper. Statistics for the non-statistician. I: different types of data need different statistical tests. *BMJ.* 1997;315(7104):364–366.

Further Reading

3. Gordis L. Epidemiology. 4th ed. Philadelphia: Saunders; 2009.

PART IV

FORMULARY

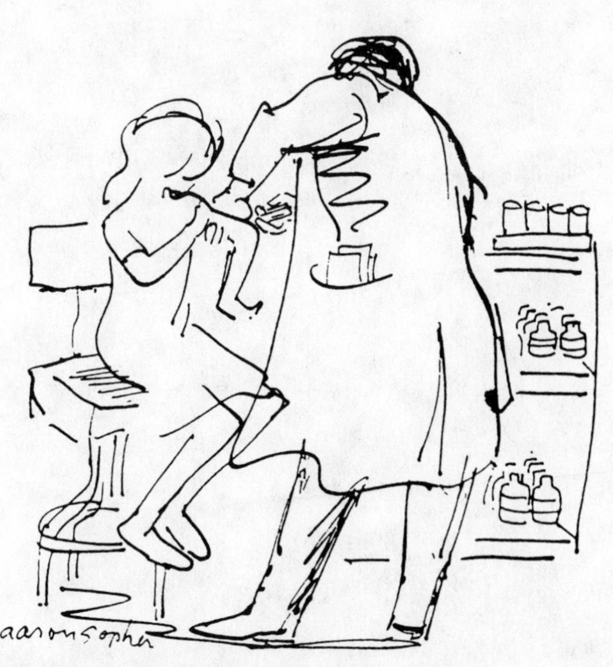

Chapter 29

Drug Doses

Carlton K. K. Lee, PharmD, MPH; Megan M. Tschudy, MD; and Kristin M. Arcara, MD

I. NOTE TO READER

The authors have made every attempt to check dosages and medical content for accuracy. Because of the incomplete data on pediatric dosing, many drug dosages will be modified after the publication of this text. We recommend that the reader check product information and published literature for changes in dosing, especially for newer medicines.

In our efforts to prevent prescribing errors, the use of abbreviations has been greatly discouraged. The following is a list of abbreviations from The Joint Commission that is and should be considered prohibited for use.

THE JOINT COMMISSION

Official "Do Not Use" List[1]

Do Not Use	Potential Problem	Use Instead
U (unit)	Mistaken for "0" (zero), the number "4" (four) or "cc"	Write "unit"
IU (International Unit)	Mistaken for IV (intravenous) or the number 10 (ten)	Write "International Unit"
Q.D., QD, q.d., qd (daily)	Mistaken for each other	Write "daily"
Q.O.D., QOD, q.o.d, qod (every other day)	Period after the Q mistaken for "I" and the "O" mistaken for "I"	Write "every other day"
Trailing zero (X.0 mg)*	Decimal point is missed	Write X mg
Lack of leading zero (.X mg)		Write 0.X mg
MS	Can mean morphine sulfate or magnesium sulfate	Write "morphine sulfate" Write "magnesium sulfate"
MSO_4 and $MgSO_4$	Confused for one another	

[1]Applies to all orders and all medication-related documentation that is handwritten (including free-text computer entry) or on pre-printed forms.

***Exception:** A "trailing zero" may be used only where required to demonstrate the level of precision of the value being reported, such as for laboratory results, imaging studies that report size of lesions, or catheter/tube sizes. It may not be used in medication orders or other medication-related documentation.

Additional Abbreviations, Acronyms and Symbols
(For <u>possible</u> future inclusion in the Official "Do Not Use" List)

Do Not Use	Potential Problem	Use Instead
> (greater than) < (less than)	Misinterpreted as the number "7" (seven) or the letter "L" Confused for one another	Write "greater than" Write "less than"
Abbreviations for drug names	Misinterpreted due to similar abbreviations for multiple drugs	Write drug names in full
Apothecary units	Unfamiliar to many practitioners Confused with metric units	Use metric units
@	Mistaken for the number "2" (two)	Write "at"
cc	Mistaken for U (units) when poorly written	Write "mL" or "ml" or "milliliters" ("mL" is preferred)
μg	Mistaken for mg (milligrams) resulting in one thousand-fold overdose	Write "mcg" or "micrograms"

II. SAMPLE ENTRY

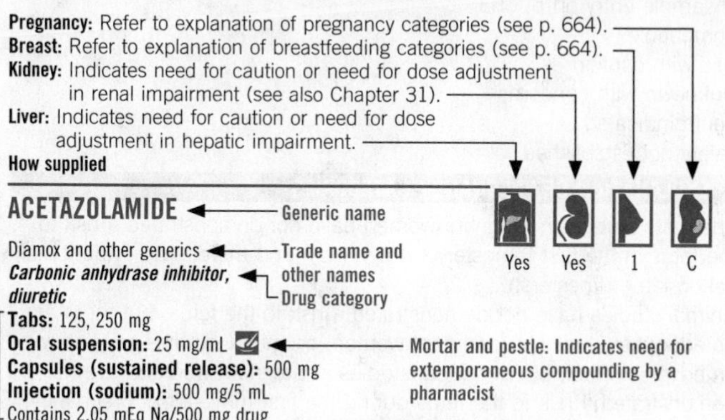

Diuretic (PO, IV)

Child: 5 mg/kg/dose once daily or every other day

Adult: 250–375 mg/dose once daily or every other day

Glaucoma

Child:

PO: 8–30 mg/kg/24 hr ÷ Q6–8 hr

IM/IV: 20–40 mg/kg/24 hr ÷ Q6 hr

Adult:

PO (simple chronic; open-angle): 1000 mg/24 hr ÷ Q6 hr

IV (acute secondary; closed-angle): For rapid decrease in intraocular pressure, administer 500 mg/dose IV

Seizures: 8–30 mg/kg/24 hr ÷ Q6–12 hr PO

Max. dose: 1 g/24 hr

Urine alkalinization: 5 mg/kg/dose PO repeated BID–TID over 24 hr.

Management of hydrocephalus (see remarks): Start with 20 mg/kg/24 hr ÷ Q8 hr PO/IV; may increase to 100 mg/kg/24 hr up to a **max. dose** of 2 g/24 hr.

Pseudotumor cerebri (PO; see remarks):

Child: Start with 25 mg/kg/24 hr ÷ once daily–QID, increase by 25 mg/kg/24 hr until clinical response or as tolerated up to a maximum of 100 mg/kg/24 hr.

Adolescent: Start with 1 g/24 hr ÷ once daily-QID, increase by 250 mg/24 hr until clinical response or as tolerated up to a maximum of 4 g/24 hr.

Drug dosing

Contraindicated in hepatic failure, severe renal failure (GFR <10 mL/min), and hypersensitivity to sulfonamides.

$T_{1/2}$: 2–6 hr; **do not use** sustained release capsules in seizures; IM injection may be painful; bicarbonate replacement therapy may be required during long-term use (see *Citrate or Sodium Bicarbonate*). For use in pseudotumor cerebri, doses of 60 mg/kg/24 hr may be required.

Possible side effects (more likely with long-term therapy) include GI irritation, paresthesias, sedation, hypokalemia, acidosis, reduced urate secretion, aplastic anemia, polyuria, and development of renal calculi.

May increase toxicity of cyclosporine. Aspirin may increase toxicity of acetazolamide. May decrease the effects of salicylates, lithium, and phenobarbital. False-positive urinary protein may occur with several assays. **Adjust dose in renal failure (see Chapter 31).**

Brief remarks about side effects, drug interactions, precautions, therapeutic monitoring, and other relevant information

III. EXPLANATION OF BREASTFEEDING CATEGORIES

See sample entry on p. 663.

1 Compatible
2 Use with caution
3 Unknown with concerns
X Contraindicated
? Safety not established

IV. EXPLANATION OF PREGNANCY CATEGORIES

A Adequate studies in pregnant women have not demonstrated a risk to the fetus in the first trimester of pregnancy, and there is no evidence of risk in later trimesters.

B Animal studies have not demonstrated a risk to the fetus, but there are no adequate studies in pregnant women; or animal studies have shown an adverse effect, but adequate studies in pregnant women have not demonstrated a risk to the fetus during the first trimester of pregnancy, and there is no evidence of risk in later trimesters.

C Animal studies have shown an adverse effect on the fetus, but there are no adequate studies in humans; or there are no animal reproduction studies and no adequate studies in humans.

D There is evidence of human fetal risk, but the potential benefits from the use of the drug in pregnant women may be acceptable despite its potential risks.

X Studies in animals or humans demonstrate fetal abnormalities or adverse reaction; reports indicate evidence of fetal risk. The risk of use in pregnant women clearly outweighs any possible benefit.

V. DRUG INDEX

Trade Names	Generic Name
1,25-dihydroxycholecalciferol	Calcitriol
2-PAM*	Pralidoxime Chloride
3TC*	Lamivudine
5-aminosalicylic acid	Mesalamine
5-ASA	Mesalamine
5-FC*	Flucytosine
5-Fluorocytosine*	Flucytosine
8-Arginine Vasopressin*	Vasopressin
9-Fluorohydrocortisone*	Fludrocortisone Acetate
27% Elemental Ca	Calcium Chloride
A-200	Pyrethrins
Abelcet	Amphotericin B Lipid Complex
Accolate	Zafirlukast
AccuNeb (prediluted nebulized solution)	Albuterol
Accutane	Isotretinoin
Acetadote	Acetylcysteine
Acticin	Permethrin
Actigall	Ursodiol

*Common abbreviation or other name (not recommended for use when writing a prescription).

Trade Names	Generic Name
Actiq	Fentanyl
Activase	Alteplase
Acular, Acular LS, Acular PF	Ketorolac
Aczone	Dapsone
Adalat CC	Nifedipine
Adderall, Adderall XR	Dextroamphetamine + Amphetamine
Adenocard	Adenosine
Adrenaline	Epinephrine HCl
Advair Diskus, Advair HFA	Fluticasone Propionate and Salmeterol
Advil, Children's Advil	Ibuprofen
Aerobid, Aerobid-M	Flunisolide
Aerospan	Flunisolide
Afrin	Oxymetazoline
Aftate	Tolnaftate
Akarpine	Pilocarpine HCl
AK-Poly-Bac Ophthalmic	Bacitracin + Polymyxin B
AK-Spore H.C. Otic	Polymyxin B Sulfate, Neomycin Sulfate, Hydrocortisone
AK-Sulf	Sulfacetamide Sodium Ophthalmic
AKTob	Tobramycin
AK-Tracin Ophthalmic	Bacitracin
Albuminar	Albumin, Human
Albutein	Albumin, Human
Aldactone	Spironolactone
Aleve [OTC]	Naproxen/Naproxen Sodium
Allegra, Allegra ODT	Fexofenadine
Allegra-D 12 Hour, Allegra-D 24 Hour	Fexofenadine + Pseudoephedrine
Allergen Ear Drops	Antipyrine and Benzocaine
Alloprim	Allopurinol
Almacone, Almacone II Double Strength	Aluminum Hydroxide with Magnesium Hydroxide
AlternaGEL	Aluminum Hydroxide
Alu-Tab	Aluminum Hydroxide
Alvesco	Ciclesonide
AmBisome	Amphotericin B, Liposomal
Amicar	Aminocaproic Acid
Amikin	Amikacin Sulfate
Aminoxin, Vitamin B_6	Pyridoxine
Amnesteem	Isotretinoin
Amoxil	Amoxicillin
Amphadase	Hyaluronidase
Amphocin	Amphotericin B
Amphojel	Aluminum Hydroxide
Anacin	Aspirin
Anaprox	Naproxen/Naproxen Sodium
Ancef	Cefazolin
Ancobon	Flucytosine
Anectine	Succinylcholine
Antilirium	Physostigmine Salicylate

*Common abbreviation or other name (not recommended for use when writing a prescription).

Trade Names	Generic Name
Antiminth	Pyrantel Pamoate
Antipyrine and Benzocaine Otic	Antipyrine and Benzocaine
Antizol	Fomepizole
Anzemet	Dolasetron
Apresoline	Hydralazine Hydrochloride
Aquachloral Supprettes	Chloral Hydrate
Aquasol A	Vitamin A
Aquasol E	Vitamin E
Aquavit-E	Vitamin E
Aralen	Chloroquine HCl/Phosphate
Aranesp	Darbepoetin Alfa
Arestin	Minocycline
Aristospan	Triamcinolone
ASA*	Aspirin
Asacol, Asacol HD	Mesalamine
Asmanex Twisthaler	Mometasone Furoate
Asprin Free Anacin	Acetaminophen
Astelin	Azelastine
Ativan	Lorazepam
AtroPen	Atropine Sulfate
Atrovent	Ipratropium Bromide
Augmentin, Augmentin ES-600, Augmentin XR	Amoxicillin-Clavulanic Acid
Auralgan (available in Canada)	Antipyrine and Benzocaine
Auro Ear Drops	Carbamide Peroxide
Aventyl	Nortriptyline Hydrochloride
Avita	Tretinoin
Ayr Saline	Sodium Chloride—Inhaled Preparations
Azactam	Aztreonam
Azasan	Azathioprine
Azasite	Azithromycin
Azmacort	Triamcinolone
Azo-Standard [OTC]	Phenazopyridine HCl
Azulfidine, Azulfidine EN-tabs	Sulfasalazine
Baciguent Topical	Bacitracin
Bactrim	Sulfamethoxazole and Trimethoprim
Bactroban, Bactroban Nasal	Mupirocin
BAL*	Dimercaprol
Beconase AQ	Beclomethasone Dipropionate
Benadryl	Diphenhydramine
Benzac AC Wash 2 1/2, 5, 10; Benzac 5, 10	Benzoyl Peroxide
Beta-Val	Betamethasone
Biaxin, Biaxin XL	Clarithromycin
Bicillin C-R, Bicillin C-R 900/300	Penicillin G Preparations—Penicillin G Benzathine and Penicillin G Procaine
Bicillin L-A	Penicillin G Preparations—Benzathine
Biocef	Cephalexin
Bleph 10	Sulfacetamide Sodium Ophthalmic

*Common abbreviation or other name (not recommended for use when writing a prescription).

Trade Names	Generic Name
Brethine	Terbutaline
Brevibloc	Esmolol HCl
Brevoxyl Creamy Wash	Benzoyl Peroxide
British anti-Lewisite	Dimercaprol
Bufferin	Aspirin
Bumex	Bumetanide
Buminate	Albumin, Human
Cafcit	Caffeine Citrate
Cafergot	Ergotamine Tartrate + Caffeine
Caldolor	Ibuprofen
Calan, Calan SR	Verapamil
Calciferol	Ergocalciferol
Calcijex	Calcitriol
Calcionate	Calcium Glubionate
Calciquid	Calcium Glubionate
Cal-Citrate	Calcium Citrate
Calcium disodium versenate	Edetate (EDTA) Calcium Disodium
Cal-G	Calcium Glubionate
Cal-Lac	Calcium Lactate
Camphorated opium tincture	Paregoric
Canasa	Mesalamine
Cancidas	Caspofungin
Cankaid	Carbamide Peroxide
Capoten	Captopril
Carafate	Sucralfate
Carbatrol	Carbamazepine
Cardene, Cardene SR	Nicardipine
Cardizem, Cardizem SR, Cardizem CD, Cardizem LA	Diltiazem
Carnitor	Carnitine
Catapres, Catapres TTS	Clonidine
Cathflo Activase	Alteplase
Caysten	Aztreonam
Ceclor, Ceclor CD	Cefaclor
Cecon	Ascorbic Acid
Cedax	Ceftibuten
Cefizox	Ceftizoxime
Cefotan	Cefotetan
Ceftin	Cefuroxime Axetil
Cefzil	Cefprozil
Celestone	Betamethasone
CellCept	Mycophenolate Mofetil
Cephulac	Lactulose
Ceptaz	Ceftazidime
Cerebyx	Fosphenytoin
Chemet	Succimer
Chibroxin	Norfloxacin
Chloromycetin	Chloramphenicol
Chlor-Trimeton	Chlorpheniramine Maleate

*Common abbreviation or other name (not recommended for use when writing a prescription).

Trade Names	Generic Name
Cholestyramine Light	Cholestyramine
Chronulac	Lactulose
Ciloxan ophthalmic	Ciprofloxacin
Cipro, Cipro XR, Ciprodex, Cipro HC Otic	Ciprofloxacin
Citracel	Calcium Citrate
Claforan	Cefotaxime
Claravis	Isotretinoin
Claritin, Claritin Children's Allergy, Claritin RediTabs	Loratadine
Claritin-D 12 Hour, Claritin-D 24 Hour	Loratadine + Pseudoephedrine
Cleocin-T, Cleocin	Clindamycin
Cogentin	Benztropine Mesylate
Colace	Docusate
Colocort	Hydrocortisone
CoLyte	Polyethylene Glycol—Electrolyte Solution
Compazine	Prochlorperazine
Concerta	Methylphenidate HCl
Copegus	Ribavirin
Cordarone	Amiodarone HCl
Cordron-D NR, Cordron-D	Carbinoxamine + Pseudoephedrine
Cortef	Hydrocortisone
Cortenema	Hydrocortisone
Cortifoam	Hydrocortisone
Cortisporin Otic	Polymyxin B Sulfate, Neomycin Sulfate, Hydrocortisone
Co-Trimoxazole	Sulfamethoxazole and Trimethoprim
Coumadin	Warfarin
Covera-HS	Verapamil
Cozaar	Losartan
Crolom	Cromolyn
Cruex	Clotrimazole
Cuprimine	Penicillamine
Curosurf	Surfactant, Pulmonary/Poractant Alfa
Cutivate	Fluticasone Propionate
Cyanoject	Cyanocobalamin/Vitamin B_{12}
Cyclogyl	Cyclopentolate
Cyclomydril	Cyclopentolate with Phenylephrine
Cyomin	Cyanocobalamin/Vitamin B_{12}
Cytovene	Ganciclovir
D-3, D3-5, D3-50	Cholecalciferol
Dantrium	Dantrolene
Daraprim	Pyrimethamine
Daytrana	Methylphenidate HCl
DDAVP*	Desmopressin Acetate
DDS*	Dapsone
D Drops	Cholecalciferol
Debrox	Carbamide Peroxide
Decadron	Dexamethasone
Deltasone	Prednisone

*Common abbreviation or other name (not recommended for use when writing a prescription).

Trade Names	Generic Name
Deodorized tincture of opium	Opium Tincture
Depacon	Valproic Acid
Depakene	Valproic Acid
Depakote, Depakote ER	Divalproex Sodium
Depen	Penicillamine
Depo-Medrol	Methylprednisolone
Depo-Provera	Medroxyprogesterone
Depo-Sub Q Provera 104	Medroxyprogesterone
Desquam-E 5, Desquam-E 10	Benzoyl Peroxide
Desyrel (previously available as)	Trazodone
Dexedrine Spansules	Dextroamphetamine
DexFerrum	Iron—Injectable Preparations (iron dextran)
Dexpak Taperpak	Dexamethasone
DextroStat	Dextroamphetamine ± Amphetamine
Di-5-ASA*	Olsalazine
Dialume	Aluminum Hydroxide
Diaminodiphenylsulfone	Dapsone
Diamox	Acetazolamide
Diastat, Diastat AcuDial	Diazepam
Diflucan and others	Fluconazole
Digibind, DigiFab	Digoxin Immune Fab (Ovine)
Digitek	Digoxin
Dilacor XR	Diltiazem
Dilantin, Dilantin Infatab	Phenytoin
Dilaudid, Dilaudid-HP	Hydromorphone HCl
Di-mesalazine	Olsalazine
Dimetapp Children's Cold and Allergy	Brompheniramine with Phenylephrine
Dipentum	Olsalazine
Diprolene, Diprolene AF	Betamethasone
Diprosone	Betamethasone
DisperMox	Amoxicillin
Ditropan, Ditropan XL	Oxybutynin Chloride
Diurigen	Chlorothiazide
Diuril	Chlorothiazide
DMSA [dimercaptosuccinic acid]*	Succimer
Dobutrex (previously available as)	Dobutamine
Dolophine	Methadone HCl
Dopram	Doxapram HCl
Doxidan	Bisacodyl
Dramamine, Children's Dramamine	Dimenhydrinate
Drisdol	Ergocalciferol
Dulcolax	Bisacodyl
Dulera	Mometasone Furoate + Formoterol Fumarate
Duraclon	Clonidine
Duragesic	Fentanyl
Duramist 12-Hr Nasal	Oxymetazoline
Duricef	Cefadroxil
Dycill	Dicloxacillin Sodium
Dynacin	Minocycline

*Common abbreviation or other name (not recommended for use when writing a prescription).

29

Trade Names	Generic Name
Dyrenium	Triamterene
EC-Naprosyn	Naproxen
Efidac 24	Chlorpheniramine Maleate
Efidac/24-Pseudoephedrine	Pseudoephedrine
Elavil	Amitriptyline
Elidel	Pimecrolimus
Elimite	Permethrin
Elitek	Rasburicase
Elixophyllin	Theophylline
Elocon	Mometasone Furoate
Emfamil D-Vi-Sol	Cholecalciferol
EMLA, Eutectic mixture of lidocaine and prilocaine	Lidocaine and Prilocaine
E-Mycin	Erythromycin Preparations
Enbrel	Etanercept
Endocet	Oxycodone and Acetaminophen
Enemeez	Docusate
Enlon	Edrophonium Chloride
Entocort EC	Budesonide
Enuloase	Lactulose
EpiPen	Epinephrine HCl
Epitol	Carbamazepine
Epivir, Epivir-HBV	Lamivudine
Epogen	Epoetin Alfa
Epsom salts	Magnesium Sulfate
Ergomar	Ergotamine Tartrate
Ery-Ped	Erythromycin
Erythrocin, Pediamycin, E-Mycin, Ery-Ped	Erythromycin
Erythropoietin	Epoetin Alfa
Eryzole	Erythromycin Ethylsuccinate and Acetylsulfisoxazole
Famvir	Famciclovir
Fansidar	Pyrimethamine + Sulfadoxine
Felbatol	Felbamate
Fentora	Fentanyl
Feosol	Iron—Oral Preparations (Ferrous sulfate)
Fergon	Iron—Oral Preparations (Ferrous sulfate)
Fer-In-Sol	Iron—Oral Preparations (Ferrous gluconate)
Ferrlecit	Iron—Injectable Preparations (Ferric gluconate)
Feverall	Acetaminophen
Fiberall	Psyllium
FIV-ASA	Mesalamine
FK506	Tacrolimus
Flagyl, Flagyl ER	Metronidazole
Fleet Babylax	Glycerin
Fleet Laxative, Fleet Bisacodyl	Bisacodyl
Fleet Mineral Oil	Mineral Oil
Fleet, Fleet Phospho-Soda	Sodium Phosphate

*Common abbreviation or other name (not recommended for use when writing a prescription).

Trade Names	Generic Name
Fletcher's Castoria	Senna/Sennosides
Flonase HFA	Fluticasone Propionate
Florinef acetate	Fludrocortisone Acetate
Flovent Diskus	Fluticasone Propionate
Floxin, Floxin Otic	Ofloxacin
Flumadine	Rimantadine
Fluohydrisone	Fludrocortisone Acetate
Fluoritab	Fluoride
Folvite	Folic Acid
Foradil Aerolizer	Formoterol
Fortamet	Metformin
Fortaz	Ceftazidime
Fortical Nasal Spray	Calcitonin—Salmon
Foscavir	Foscarnet
Fulvicin U/F, Fulvicin P/G	Griseofulvin
Fungizone	Amphotericin B
Furadantin	Nitrofurantoin
Gabarone	Gabapentin
Gabitril	Tiagabine
Galzin	Zinc Salts, Systemic
Gamma benzene hexachloride*	Lindane
Garamycin	Gentamicin
Gastrocrom	Cromolyn
Gas-X	Simethicone
Gengraf	Cyclosporine Modified
GlucaGen, Glucagon Emergency Kit	Glucagon HCl
Glucophage, Glucophage XR	Metformin
Gly-Oxide	Carbamide Peroxide
GoLYTELY	Polyethylene Glycol—Electrolyte Solution
Grifulvin V	Griseofulvin
Grisactin	Griseofulvin
Gris-PEG	Griseofulvin
Gyne-Lotrimin 3, Gyne-Lotrimin	Clotrimazole
H.P. Acthar Gel	Corticotropin
Haldol, Haldol Decanoate 50, Haldol Decanoate 100	Haloperidol
Hexadrol	Dexamethasone
Humatin	Paromomycin Sulfate
Hydase	Hyaluronidase
Hydrodiuril	Hydrochlorothiazide
Hydro-Tussin CBX	Carbinoxamine + Pseudoephedrine
Hylenex	Hyaluronidase
Hypersal	Sodium Chloride—Inhaled Preparations
Imitrex	Sumatriptan Succinate
Imodium, Imodium AD	Loperamide
Imuran	Azathioprine
Inapsine	Droperidol
Inderal	Propranolol
Indocin, Indocin SR, Indocin I.V.	Indomethacin

*Common abbreviation or other name (not recommended for use when writing a prescription).

29

Trade Names	Generic Name
Infasurf	Surfactant, Pulmonary/Calfactant
INFeD	Iron—Injectable Preparations (iron dextran)
INH*	Isoniazid
Intal (previously available as)	Cromolyn
Intropin (previously available as)	Dopamine
Invanz	Ertapenem
Iosat	Potassium Iodide
Iquix	Levofloxacin
IsonaRif	Isoniazid
Isoptin, Isoptin SR	Verapamil
Isopto Carpine	Pilocarpine HCl
Isopto Hyoscine	Scopolamine Hydrobromide
Isuprel	Isoproterenol
Kantrex	Kanamycin
Kaopectate, Kaopectate Children's	Bismuth Subsalicylate
Kayexalate	Sodium Polystyrene Sulfonate
Keflex	Cephalexin
Kemstro	Baclofen
Kenalog	Triamcinolone
Keppra, Keppra XR	Levetiracetam
Ketalar	Ketamine
Kionex	Sodium Polystyrene Sulfonate
Klonopin	Clonazepam
Kondremul	Mineral Oil
Konsyl	Psyllium
K-PHOS Neutral	Phosphorus Supplements
Kytril	Granisetron
Lamictal, Lamictal ODT, Lamictal XR	Lamotrigine
Laniazid	Isoniazid
Lanoxin, Lanoxicaps	Digoxin
Lariam	Mefloquine HCl
Lasix	Furosemide
Lax-Pills	Senna/Sennosides
L-Carnitine	Carnitine
Levaquin, Quixin, Iquix	Levofloxacin
Levocarnitine	Carnitine
Levophed and others	Norepinephrine Bitartrate
Levothroid	Levothyroxine (T_4)
Levoxyl	Levothyroxine (T_4)
Lialda	Mesalamine
Lidoderm	Lidocaine
Lioresal	Baclofen
Liquid Pred	Prednisone
Lithobid	Lithium
L-M-X	Lidocaine
Loniten (previously available as)	Minoxidil
Lopressor, Toprol-XL	Metoprolol
Lotrimin AF	Clotrimazole
Lotrimin AF	Miconazole

*Common abbreviation or other name (not recommended for use when writing a prescription).

Trade Names	Generic Name
Lovenox	Enoxaparin
Luminal	Phenobarbital
Luride	Fluoride
Maalox	Aluminum Hydroxide with Magnesium Hydroxide
Maalox Total Relief	Bismuth Subsalicylate
Macrobid	Nitrofurantoin
Macrodantin	Nitrofurantoin
Mag-200, Mag-Ox 400, Uro-Mag	Magnesium Oxide
Marinol	Dronabinol
Maxidex	Dexamethasone
Maxipime	Cefepime
Maxivate	Betamethasone
Maxolon	Metoclopramide
Medrol, Medrol Dosepack	Methylprednisolone
Mefoxin	Cefoxitin
Mephyton	Phytonadione/Vitamin K_1
Mepron	Atovaquone
Merrem	Meropenem
Mestinon	Pyridostigmine Bromide
Metadate ER	Methylphenidate HCl
Metamucil	Psyllium
Methadose	Methadone HCl
Methylin, Methylin ER	Methylphenidate HCl
Metozolv	Metoclopramide
MetroCream	Metronidazole
MetroGel, MetroGel-Vaginal	Metronidazole
MetroLotion	Metronidazole
Miacalcin, Miacalcin Nasal Spray	Calcitonin—Salmon
Micatin	Miconazole
Milk of Magnesia	Magnesium Hydroxide
Minocin	Minocycline
Mintezol	Thiabendazole
Mintox	Aluminum Hydroxide with Magnesium Hydroxide
MiraLax	Polyethylene Glycol—Electrolyte Solution
Monistat	Miconazole
Motrin, Children's Motrin	Ibuprofen
MS Contin	Morphine Sulfate
Mucomyst	Acetylcysteine
Mucosol	Acetylcysteine
Murine Ear	Carbamide Peroxide
Myambutol	Ethambutol HCl
Mycamine	Micafungin Sodium
Mycelex, Mycelex-7	Clotrimazole
Mycifradin	Neomycin Sulfate
Mycobutin	Rifabutin
Mycostatin	Nystatin
Myfortic	Mycophenolate Sodium
Mylanta Gas	Simethicone
Mylanta, Mylanta Extra Strength	Aluminum Hydroxide with Magnesium Hydroxide

*Common abbreviation or other name (not recommended for use when writing a prescription).

Trade Names	Generic Name
Mylicon	Simethicone
Mysoline	Primidone
Nallpen	Nafcillin
Naprelan	Naproxen/Naproxen Sodium
Naprosyn	Naproxen/Naproxen Sodium
Narcan	Naloxone
Nasacort HFA, Nasacort AQ	Triamcinolone
Nasalcrom	Cromolyn
Nasarel	Flunisolide
Nascobal	Cyanocobalamin/Vitamin B_{12}
Nasonex	Mometasone Furoate
Nebcin	Tobramycin
NebuPent	Pentamidine Isethionate
Nembutal	Pentobarbital
NeoBenz Micro	Benzoyl Peroxide
Neo-fradin	Neomycin Sulfate
NeoProfen (IV)	Ibuprofen
Neoral	Cyclosporine
Neosporin, Neosporin Ophthalmic	Neomycin/Polymyxin B/Bacitracin
Neosporin GU Irrigant	Neomycin/Polymyxin B
Neo-Synephrine	Phenylephrine HCl
Neo-Synephrine 12-Hr Nasal	Oxymetazoline
Neo-Tabs	Neomycin Sulfate
Nephron	Epinephrine, Racemic
Neupogen, G-CSF	Filgrastim
Neurontin	Gabapentin
Neut	Sodium Bicarbonate
Nexium	Esomeprazole
Niacor	Niacin (Vitamin B_3)
Niaspan	Niacin (Vitamin B_3)
Nicotinic acid	Niacin (Vitamin B_3)
Nifediac CC	Nifedipine
Niferex	Iron—Oral Preparations
Nilstat	Nystatin
Nipride (previously available as)	Nitroprusside
Nitro-Bid	Nitroglycerin
Nitro-Dur	Nitroglycerin
Nitro-Mist	Nitroglycerin
Nitropress	Nitroprusside
Nitrostat	Nitroglycerin
Nitro-Time	Nitroglycerin
Nix	Permethrin
Nizoral, Nizoral A-D	Ketoconazole
Norcuron	Vecuronium Bromide
Noriate	Metronidazole
Normal Serum Albumin (Human)	Albumin, Human
Normodyne	Labetalol
Noroxin	Norfloxacin

*Common abbreviation or other name (not recommended for use when writing a prescription).

Trade Names	Generic Name
Norvasc	Amlodipine
Nostrilla	Oxymetazoline
NuLYTELY	Polyethylene Glycol—Electrolyte Solution
Nutr-E-sol	Vitamin E/Alpha-Tocopherol
NVP*	Nevirapine
Nydrazid	Isoniazid
OCL*	Polyethylene Glycol—Electrolyte Solution
Ocean	Sodium Chloride—Inhaled Preparations
Ocuflox	Ofloxacin
Ocusulf-10	Sulfacetamide Sodium Ophthalmic
Omnaris	Ciclesonide
Ofirmev	Acetaminophen
Omnicef	Cefdinir
Omnipaque 140, Omnipaque 240, Omnipaque 300, and Omnipaque 350	Iohexol
Omnipen	Ampicillin
Opticrom	Cromolyn
Optivar	Azelastine
Orajel Perioseptic	Carbamide Peroxide
Oramorph SR	Morphine Sulfate
Orapred, Orapred ODT	Prednisolone
Orasone	Prednisone
Orazinc	Zinc Salts, Systemic
Os-Cal	Calcium Carbonate
Osmitrol	Mannitol
OsmoPrep	Sodium Phosphate
Oxy-5, Oxy-10	Benzoyl Peroxide
OxyContin	Oxycodone
Oxytrol	Oxybutynin Chloride
Pacerone	Amiodarone HCl
Palasbumin	Albumin, Human
Palgic	Carbinoxamine
Palmitate-A 5000	Vitamin A
Pamelor	Nortriptyline Hydrochloride
Pamix	Pyrantel Pamoate
Panadol	Acetaminophen
Paracetamol	Acetaminophen
Pataday	Olopatadine
Patanase	Olopatadine
Patanol	Olopatadine
Pathocil	Dicloxacillin Sodium
Paxil, Paxil CR	Paroxetine
Pediaflor	Fluoride
Pediamycin	Erythromycin Preparations
Pediapred	Prednisolone
Pediazole	Erythromycin Ethylsuccinate and Acetylsulfisoxazole
PediOtic	Polymyxin B Sulfate, Neomycin Sulfate, Hydrocortisone

*Common abbreviation or other name (not recommended for use when writing a prescription).

Trade Names	Generic Name
Pentam 300	Pentamidine Isethionate
Pentasa	Mesalamine
Pepcid, Pepcid AC [OTC], Pepcid Complete [OTC], Pepcid RPD	Famotidine
Pepto-Bismol	Bismuth Subsalicylate
Percocet	Oxycodone and Acetaminophen
Percodan	Oxycodone and Aspirin
Perdiem Fiber Therapy	Psyllium
Perforomist	Formoterol
Periactin (previously available as)	Cyproheptadine
Periostat	Doxycycline
Pexeva	Paroxetine
Pfizerpen	Penicillin G Preparations—Aqueous Potassium and Sodium
PGE_1*	Alprostadil
Phazyme	Simethicone
Phenergan	Promethazine
Phenytek	Phenytoin
PhosLo	Calcium Acetate
Pilocar	Pilocarpine HCl
Pilopine HS	Pilocarpine HCl
Pima	Potassium Iodide
Pin-Rid	Pyrantel Pamoate
Pin-X	Pyrantel Pamoate
Pipracil	Piperacillin
Pitressin	Vasopressin
Plaquenil	Hydroxychloroquine
Polymox	Amoxicillin
Polysporin Ophthalmic	Bacitracin + Polymyxin B
Polysporin Topical	Bacitracin + Polymyxin B
Polytrim Ophthalmic Solution	Polymyxin B Sulfate and Trimethoprim Sulfate
Posture	Calcium Phosphate, Tribasic
Potassium Phosphate	Phosphorus Supplements
Prelone	Prednisolone
Prevacid	Lansoprazole
Prevalite	Cholestyramine
Prilosec, Prilosec OTC	Omeprazole
Primacor	Milrinone
Primaxin IV	Imipenem and Cilastatin
Principen	Ampicillin
Prinivil	Lisinopril
Procanbid	Procainamide
Procardia, Procardia XL	Nifedipine
Procrit	Epoetin Alfa
Proglycem	Diazoxide
Prograf	Tacrolimus
Pronestyl	Procainamide
Pronto	Pyrethrins
Prostaglandin E_1	Alprostadil

*Common abbreviation or other name (not recommended for use when writing a prescription).

Trade Names	Generic Name
Prostigmin	Neostigmine
Prostin VR Pediatric	Alprostadil
Protonix	Pantoprazole
Protopam	Pralidoxime Chloride
Protopic	Tacrolimus
Protostat	Metronidazole
Proventil, Proventil HFA (aerosol inhaler)	Albuterol
Provera	Medroxyprogesterone
Prozac, Prozac Weekly	Fluoxetine Hydrochloride
Pseudo Carb Pediatric	Carbinoxamine + Pseudoephedrine
PTU*	Propylthiouracil
Pulmicort Respules, Pulmicort Turbuhaler, Pulmicort Flexhaler	Budesonide
Pulmozyme	Dornase Alfa/Dnase
Pyrazinoic acid amide	Pyrazinamide
Pyridium	Phenazopyridine HCl
Pyrinyl	Pyrethrins
Quelicin	Succinylcholine
Questran, Questran Light	Cholestyramine
Quineprox	Hydroxychloroquine
Quinidex	Quinidine
Quixin	Levofloxacin
QVAR*	Beclomethasone Dipropionate
Raniclor	Cefaclor
Rapamune	Sirolimus
Rebetol	Ribavirin
Reese's Pinworm	Pyrantel Pamoate
Regitine	Phentolamine Mesylate
Reglan	Metoclopramide
Renova	Tretinoin
Resectisol	Mannitol
Restasis	Cyclosporine, Cyclosporine Microemulsion, Cyclosporine Modified
Retin-A, Retin-A Micro	Tretinoin
Retrovir, AZT	Zidovudine
Revatio	Sildenafil
Reversol	Edrophonium Chloride
Revonto	Dantrolene
R-Gene 10	Arginine Chloride
Rhinaris	Sodium Chloride—Inhaled Preparations
Rhinocort Aqua Nasal Spray	Budesonide
Ribaspheres	Ribavirin
RID	Pyrethrins
Rifadin	Rifampin
Rifamate	Isoniazid + Rifampin
Rifater	Pyrazinamide + Isoniazid + Rifampin
Rimactane	Rifampin
Riomet	Metformin

*Common abbreviation or other name (not recommended for use when writing a prescription).

Trade Names	Generic Name
Risperdal, Risperdal M-Tab, Risperdal Consta	Risperidone
Ritalin, Ritalin SR, Ritalin LA	Methylphenidate HCl
Robinul	Glycopyrrolate
Rocaltrol	Calcitriol
Rocephin	Ceftriaxone
Rogaine, Men's Rogaine Extra Strength	Minoxidil
Romazicon	Flumazenil
Rowasa	Mesalamine
Roxanol	Morphine Sulfate
Roxicet	Oxycodone and Acetaminophen
Roxicodone	Oxycodone
Roxilox	Oxycodone and Acetaminophen
Roxiprin	Oxycodone and Aspirin
RuLox Plus	Aluminum Hydroxide with Magnesium Hydroxide
S-2 Inhalant	Epinephrine, Racemic
Sabril	Vigabatrin
Salagen	Pilocarpine HCl
Salicylazosulfapyridine	Sulfasalazine
Sal-Tropine	Atropine Sulfate
Sandimmune	Cyclosporine
Sandostatin, Sandostatin LAR Depot	Octreotide Acetate
Sani-Supp	Glycerin
Sarafem	Fluoxetine Hydrochloride
SAS*	Sulfasalazine
Scopace	Scopolamine Hydrobromide
Selsun and others	Selenium Sulfide
Senna-Gen	Senna/Sennosides
Senokot	Senna/Sennosides
Septra	Sulfamethoxazole and Trimethoprim
Serevent Diskus	Salmeterol
Serutan	Psyllium
Sildec	Carbinoxamine + Pseudoephedrine
Silvadene	Silver Sulfadiazine
Simply Saline	Sodium Chloride—Inhaled Preparations
Singulair	Montelukast
Slo-Niacin	Niacin (Vitamin B_3)
Slow FE	Iron—Oral Preparations
Sodium Phosphate	Phosphorus Supplements
Solodyn	Minocycline
Solu-cortef	Hydrocortisone
Solu-Medrol	Methylprednisolone
Soluspan	Betamethasone
Sotret	Isotretinoin
Sporanox	Itraconazole
SPS*	Sodium Polystyrene Sulfonate
SSD Cream, SSD AF Cream	Silver Sulfadiazine
SSKI*	Potassium Iodide
Stimate	Desmopressin Acetate

*Common abbreviation or other name (not recommended for use when writing a prescription).

Trade Names	Generic Name
Strattera	Atomoxetine
Streptase	Streptokinase
Sublimaze	Fentanyl
Sudafed	Pseudoephedrine
Sulfatrim	Sulfamethoxazole and Trimethoprim
Sumycin	Tetracycline HCl
Sunkist Vitamin C	Ascorbic Acid
Suprax	Cefixime
Surfak	Docusate
Survanta	Surfactant, Pulmonary/Beractant
Symbicort	Budesonide and Formoterol
Symmetrel	Amantadine Hydrochloride
Synagis	Palivizumab
Synercid	Quinupristin and Dalfopristin
Synthroid	Levothyroxine T_4
Tagamet, Tagamet HB [OTC]	Cimetidine
Tambocor	Flecainide Acetate
Tamiflu	Oseltamivir Phosphate
Tapazole	Methimazole
Tazicef	Ceftazidime
Tazidime	Ceftazidime
Tegretol, Tegretol-XR	Carbamazepine
Tempra	Acetaminophen
Tenormin	Atenolol
Tensilon	Edrophonium Chloride
Tetrahydrocannabinol	Dronabinol
THC*	Dronabinol
Theo-24	Theophylline
TheoCap	Theophylline
Theochron	Theophylline
Therazene	Silver Sulfadiazine
Thiamilate	Thiamine
Thorazine	Chlorpromazine
ThyroSave	Potassium Iodide
ThyroShield	Potassium Iodide
Tiazac	Diltiazem
Tigan	Trimethobenzamide HCl
Timentin	Ticarcillin and Clavulanate
Tinactin	Tolnaftate
Tisit	Pyrethrins
TMP-SMX*	Sulfamethoxazole and Trimethoprim
TOBI	Tobramycin
Tobrex	Tobramycin
Tofranil, Tofranil-PM	Imipramine
Topamax	Topiramate
Toprol-XL	Metoprolol
Totacillin	Ampicillin
tPA*	Alteplase
Trandate	Labetalol

*Common abbreviation or other name (not recommended for use when writing a prescription).

Trade Names	Generic Name
Transderm Scop	Scopolamine Hydrobromide
Triaz	Benzoyl Peroxide
Trileptal	Oxcarbazepine
Trilisate and others	Choline Magnesium Trisalicylate
TriLyte	Polyethylene Glycol—Electrolyte Solution
Trimethoprim-sulfamethoxazole	Sulfamethoxazole and Trimethoprim
Trimox	Amoxicillin
Tums	Calcium Carbonate
Tylenol	Acetaminophen
Tylenol #1, #2, #3, #4	Codeine and Acetaminophen
Tylox	Oxycodone and Acetaminophen
Unasyn	Ampicillin/Sulbactam
Unipen	Nafcillin
Uniphyl	Theophylline
Urecholine	Bethanechol Chloride
Uro-KP-Neutral	Phosphorus Supplements
Urolene Blue	Methylene Blue
Urso 250, Urso Forte	Ursodiol
Vagistat-3	Miconazole
Valcyte	Valganciclovir
Valium	Diazepam
Valtrex	Valacyclovir
Vancocin	Vancomycin
Vantin	Cefpodoxime Proxetil
VariZig	Varicella-Zoster Immune Globulin (Human)
Vasotec	Enalapril Maleate
Vasotec IV	Enalaprilat
Veetids	Penicillin V Potassium
Venofer	Iron—Injectable Preparations (iron sucrose)
Ventolin HFA	Albuterol
Veramyst	Fluticasone Propionate
Verelan, Verelan PM	Verapamil
Vermox	Mebendazole
Versed (previously available as)	Midazolam
VFEND	Voriconazole
Viagra	Sildenafil
Vibramycin	Doxycycline
Viramune	Nevirapine
Virazole	Ribavirin
Visicol	Sodium Phosphate
Visine LR	Oxymetazoline
Vistaril	Hydroxyzine
Vistide	Cidofovir
Vitamin B_1	Thiamine
Vitamin B_2	Riboflavin
Vitamin B_{12}	Cyanocobalamin/Vitamin B_{12}
Vitamin B_3	Niacin/Vitamin B_3
Vitamin B_6	Pyridoxine
Vitamin C	Ascorbic Acid

*Common abbreviation or other name (not recommended for use when writing a prescription).

Trade Names	Generic Name
Vitrase	Hyaluronidase
VoSpire ER	Albuterol
Vyvanse	Lisdexamfetamine
VZIG	Varicella-Zoster Immune Globulin (Human)
WinRho-SDF	Rh_0 (D) Immune Globulin Intravenous (Human)
Wycillin	Penicillin G Preparations—Procaine
Wymox	Amoxicillin
Xopenex, Xopenex HFA	Levalbuterol
Xylocaine	Lidocaine
Zantac, Zantac 75 [OTC], Zantac 150 Maximum Strength [OTC]	Ranitidine HCl
Zarontin	Ethosuximide
Zaroxolyn	Metolazone
Zegerid	Omeprazole
Zemuron	Rocuronium
Zestril	Lisinopril
Zinacef	Cefuroxime
Zincate	Zinc Salts, Systemic
Zithromax, Zithromax TRI-PAK, Zithromax Z-PAK, Zmax	Azithromycin
Zoderm	Benzoyl Peroxide
Zofran	Ondansetron
Zolicef	Cefazolin
Zoloft	Sertraline HCl
Zonegran	Zonisamide
ZORprin	Aspirin
Zosyn	Piperacillin with Tazobactam
Zovirax	Acyclovir
Zyloprim	Allopurinol
Zyrtec, Children's Zyrtec	Cetirizine
Zyrtec-D 12 Hour	Cetirizine + Pseudoephedrine
Zyvox	Linezolid

*Common abbreviation or other name (not recommended for use when writing a prescription).

ACETAMINOPHEN

Tylenol, Tempra, Panadol, Feverall, Asprin Free Anacin, Paracetamol, Ofirmev, and many other generics

Analgesic, antipyretic

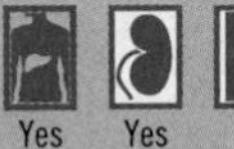
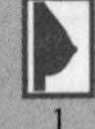
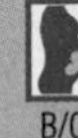

Yes Yes 1 B/C

Tabs [OTC]: 325, 500, 650 mg
Chewable tabs [OTC]: 80, 160 mg; some may contain phenylalanine
Infant drops, solution/suspension [OTC]: 80 mg/0.8 mL
Child suspension/syrup [OTC]: 160 mg/5 mL
Oral liquid [OTC]: 160, 166.7 mg/5 mL; may contain 7% alcohol
Elixir [OTC]: 160 mg/5 mL
Caplet [OTC]: 160, 500, 650 mg
Extended release caplet/geltab [OTC]: 650 mg
Gelcap [OTC]: 500 mg
Capsules [OTC]: 500 mg
Dispersible tabs (Tylenol Children's Meltaways) [OTC]: 80 mg
Suppositories [OTC]: 80, 120, 325, 650 mg
(Combination product with Codeine, see *Codeine and Acetaminophen*)
Injection (Ofirmev): 10 mg/mL (100 mL)

PO/PR

Neonate: 10–15 mg/kg/dose PO/PR Q6–8 hr. Some advocate loading doses of 20–25 mg/kg/dose for PO dosing or 30 mg/kg/dose for PR dosing.

Pediatric: 10–15 mg/kg/dose PO/PR Q4–6 hr; **max. dose:** 90 mg/kg/24 hr. For rectal dosing, some may advocate a 40–45 mg/kg/dose loading dose.

Dosing by weight (preferred) or age (PO/PR Q4–6 hr):

Weight (lbs)	Weight (kg)	Age	Dosage (mg)
6–11	2.7–5	0–3 mo	40
12–17	5.1–7.7	4–11 mo	80
18–23	7.8–10.5	1–2 yr	120
24–35	10.6–15.9	2–3 yr	160
36–47	16–21.4	4–5 yr	240
48–59	21.5–26.8	6–8 yr	320
60–71	26.9–32.3	9–10 yr	400
72–95	32.4–43.2	11 yr	480

Adult: 325–650 mg/dose

Max. dose: 4 g/24 hr, 5 doses/24 hr

IV (minimum dosing interval of 4 hr):

Child (age >2–12 yr) and adolescent/adult <50 kg: 15 mg/kg/dose Q6 hr, OR 12.5 mg/kg/dose Q4 hr IV up to a maximum of 75 mg/kg/24 hr.

Adolescent and adult (>50 kg): 1000 mg Q6 hr, OR 650 mg Q4 hr up to a **maximum** of 4000 mg/24 hr.

Does not possess anti-inflammatory activity. **Use with caution** in patients with known G6PD deficiency.

$T_{1/2}$: 1–3 hr, 2–5 hr in neonates; metabolized in the liver; see Chapter 2 and acetylcysteine for management of overdosage.

Some preparations contain alcohol (7%–10%) and/or phenylalanine; all suspensions should be shaken before use.

Continued

ACETAMINOPHEN *continued*

May decrease the activity of lamotrigine and increase the activity of zidovudine. Rifampin and anticholinergic agents (e.g., scopolamine) may decrease the effect of acetaminophen. Increased risk for hepatotoxicity may occur with barbiturates, carbamazepine, phenytoin, carmustine (with high acetaminophen doses), and chronic alcohol use. **Adjust dose in renal failure (see Chapter 31).**

FOR IV USE: Administer dose undiluted over 15 min. Most common side effects with IV use include nausea, vomiting, constipation, pruritus, agitation, and atelectrasis in children; and nausea, vomiting, headache, and insomnia in adults. IV route has not been studied in children <2 yr.

Pregnancy category "B" for PO and PR routes and "C" for IV route.

ACETAZOLAMIDE
Diamox and other generics
Carbonic anhydrase inhibitor, diuretic

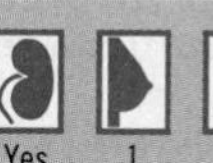
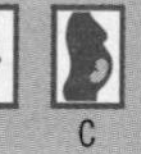

Yes Yes 1 C

Tabs: 125, 250 mg
Oral suspension: 25 mg/mL
Capsules (sustained release): 500 mg
Injection (sodium): 500 mg/5 mL
Contains 2.05 mEq Na/500 mg drug

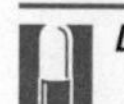

Diuretic (PO, IV)
Child: 5 mg/kg/dose once daily or every other day
Adult: 250–375 mg/dose once daily or every other day

Glaucoma
Child:
PO: 8–30 mg/kg/24 hr ÷ Q6–8 hr
IM/IV: 20–40 mg/kg/24 hr ÷ Q6 hr
Adult:
PO (simple chronic; open-angle): 1000 mg/24 hr ÷ Q6 hr
IV (acute secondary; closed-angle): For rapid decrease in intraocular pressure, administer 500 mg/dose IV

Seizures: 8–30 mg/kg/24 hr ÷ Q6–12 hr PO
Max. dose: 1 g/24 hr
Urine alkalinization: 5 mg/kg/dose PO repeated BID–TID over 24 hr.
Management of hydrocephalus (see remarks): Start with 20 mg/kg/24 hr ÷ Q8 hr PO/IV; may increase to 100 mg/kg/24 hr up to a **max. dose** of 2 g/24 hr.
Pseudotumor cerebri (PO; see remarks):
Child: Start with 25 mg/kg/24 hr ÷ once daily–QID, increase by 25 mg/kg/24 hr until clinical response or as tolerated up to a maximum of 100 mg/kg/24 hr.
Adolescent: Start with 1 g/24 hr ÷ once daily–QID, increase by 250 mg/24 hr until clinical response or as tolerated up to a maximum of 4 g/24 hr.

Contraindicated in hepatic failure, severe renal failure (GFR <10 mL/min), and hypersensitivity to sulfonamides.

$T_{1/2}$: 2–6 hr; **do not use** sustained release capsules in seizures; IM injection may be painful; bicarbonate replacement therapy may be required during long-term use (see *Citrate* or *Sodium Bicarbonate*). For use in pseudotumor cerebri, doses of 60 mg/kg/24 hr may be required.

Possible side effects (more likely with long-term therapy) include GI irritation, paresthesias, sedation, hypokalemia, acidosis, reduced urate secretion, aplastic anemia, polyuria, and development of renal calculi.

May increase toxicity of cyclosporine. Aspirin may increase toxicity of acetazolamide. May decrease the effects of salicylates, lithium, and phenobarbital. False-positive urinary protein may occur with several assays. **Adjust dose in renal failure (see Chapter 31).**

For explanation of icons, see p. 663.

ACETYLCYSTEINE

Mucomyst, Mucosol, Acetadote

Mucolytic, antidote for acetaminophen toxicity

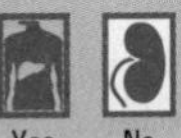
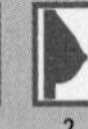
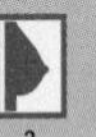
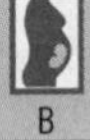

Solution: 100 mg/mL (10%) or 200 mg/mL (20%) (4, 10, 30 mL); contains EDTA
Injectable (Acetadote): 200 mg/mL (20%) (30 mL); contains EDTA 0.5 mg/mL

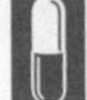

Acetaminophen poisoning (see Chapter 2 for additional information).

PO: 140 mg/kg × 1, followed by 70 mg/kg/dose Q4 hr for a total of 17 doses. Repeat dose if vomiting occurs with 1 hr of administration.

IV: 150 mg/kg × 1 diluted in D_5W or $D_5W1/2NS$ administered over 60 min, followed by 50 mg/kg diluted in D_5W administered over 4 hr, then 100 mg/kg diluted in D_5W administered over 16 hr.

Recommended weight-based drug dilution volumes:

Weight (kg)	Volume of D5W or D5W1/2NS for 150 mg/kg Loading Dose Administered Over 60 Minutes	Volume of D5W for 50 mg/kg Second Dose Administered Over 4 Hours	Volume of D5W for 100 mg/kg Third Dose Administered Over 16 Hours
≤20	3 mL/kg	7 mL/kg	14 mL/kg
>20–<40	100 mL	250 mL	500 mL
≥40	200 mL	500 mL	1000 mL

Nebulizer:

Infant: 1–2 mL of 20% solution (diluted with equal volume of H_2O, or sterile saline to equal 10%), or 2–4 mL of 10% solution; administered TID–QID

Child: 3–5 mL of 20% solution (diluted with equal volume of H_2O, or sterile saline to equal 10%), or 6–10 mL of 10% solution; administer TID–QID

Adolescent: 5–10 mL of 10% or 20% solution; administer TID–QID

Distal intestinal obstruction syndrome in Cystic Fibrosis:

Adolescent and adult: 10 mL of 20% solution (diluted in a sweet drink) PO QID with 100 mL of 10% solution PR as an enema once daily–QID

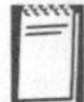

Use with caution in asthma. For nebulized use, give inhaled bronchodilator 10–15 min before use and follow with postural drainage and/or suctioning after acetylcysteine administration. Prior hydration is essential for distal intestinal obstruction syndrome treatment.

May induce bronchospasm, stomatitis, drowsiness, rhinorrhea, nausea, vomiting, and hemoptysis. Anaphylactoid reactions have been reported with IV use.

For IV use, elimination $T_{1/2}$ is longer in newborns (11 hr) than in adults (5.6 hr). $T_{1/2}$ is increased by 80% in patients with severe liver damage (Child-Pugh score of 7–13) and biliary cirrhosis (Child-Pugh score of 5–7).

For oral administration, chilling the solution and mixing with carbonated beverages, orange juice, or sweet drinks may enhance palatability.

ACTH

See Corticotropin

ACYCLOVIR
Zovirax and other generics
Antiviral

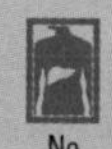 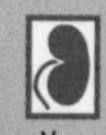  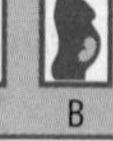
No Yes 1 B

Capsules: 200 mg
Tabs: 400, 800 mg
Oral suspension: 200 mg/5 mL; may contain parabens
Ointment: 5% (15 g)
Cream: 5% (2 g)
Injection in powder (with sodium): 500, 1000 mg
Injection in solution (with sodium): 50 mg/mL
Contains 4.2 mEq Na/1 g drug
Oral therapy for HSV suppression and neurodevelopment following treatment with IV acyclovir for 14-21 days: 300 mg/m²/dose Q8 hr PO × 6 mo

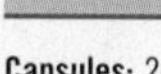

IMMUNOCOMPETENT:
Neonatal (HSV and HSV encephalitis; birth–3 mo):
<35 wk postconceptional age: 40 mg/kg/24 hr ÷ Q12 hr IV × 14–21 days
≥35 wk postconceptional age: 60 mg/kg/24 hr ÷ Q8 hr IV × 14–21 days
HSV encephalitis (duration of therapy: 14–21 days):
Birth–3 mo: use above dosage.
3 mo–12 yr: 60 mg/kg/24 hr ÷ Q8 hr IV; some experts recommend 45 mg/kg/24 hr ÷ Q8 hr IV
≥12 yr: 30 mg/kg/24 hr ÷ Q8 hr IV
Mucocutaneous HSV (including genital, ≥12 yr):
Initial infection:
IV: 15 mg/kg/24 hr or 750 mg/m²/24 hr ÷ Q8 hr × 5–7 days
PO: 1000–1200 mg/24 hr ÷ 3–5 doses per 24 hr × 7–10 days. For pediatric dosing, use 40–80 mg/kg/24 hr ÷ Q6–8 hr × 5–10 days (**max. pediatric dose:** 1000 mg/24 hr)
Recurrence (≥12 yr):
PO: 1000 mg/24 hr ÷ 5 doses per 24 hr × 5 days, or 1600 mg/24 hr ÷ Q12 hr × 5 days, or 2400 mg/24 hr ÷ Q8 hr × 2 days
Chronic suppressive therapy (≥12 yr):
PO: 800 mg/24 hr ÷ Q12 hr for up to 1 year
Zoster:
IV (all ages): 30 mg/kg/24 hr or 1500 mg/m²/24 hr ÷ Q8 hr × 7–10 days
PO (≥12 yr): 4000 mg/24 hr ÷ 5×/24 hr × 5–7 days
Varicella:
IV (≥2 yr): 30 mg/kg/24 hr or 1500 mg/m²/24 hr ÷ Q8 hr × 7–10 days
PO (≥2 yr): 80 mg/kg/24 hr ÷ QID × 5 days (begin treatment at earliest signs/symptoms); **max. dose:** 3200 mg/24 hr

Max. dose of oral acyclovir in children = 80 mg/kg/24 hr
IMMUNOCOMPROMISED:
HSV:
IV (all ages): 750–1500 mg/m²/24 hr ÷ Q8 hr × 7–14 days
PO (≥2 yr): 1000 mg/24 hr ÷ 3–5 times/24 hr × 7–14 days; **max. dose** for child: 80 mg/kg/24 hr
HSV prophylaxis:
IV (all ages): 750 mg/m²/24 hr ÷ Q8 hr during risk period
PO (≥2 yr): 600–1000 mg/24 hr ÷ 3–5 times/24 hr during risk period; **max. dose** for child: 80 mg/kg/24 hr
Varicella or zoster:
IV (all ages): 1500 mg/m²/24 hr ÷ Q8 hr × 7–10 days

Continued

For explanation of icons, see p. 663.

ACYCLOVIR *continued*

PO (consider using valacyclovir or famciclovir for better absorption):
Infant and child: 20 mg/kg/dose (max. 800 mg) Q6 hr × 7–10 days
Adolescent and adult: 20 mg/kg/dose (max. 800 mg) 5 times daily × 7–10 days
Max. dose of oral acyclovir in children = 80 mg/kg/24 hr.
TOPICAL: Apply 0.5 inch ribbon of 5% ointment for 4-inch square surface area 6 times a day × 7 days.

See most recent edition of the AAP *Red Book* for further details. **Use with caution** in patients with pre-existing neurologic or **renal impairment (adjust dose; see Chapter 31)** or dehydration. Adequate hydration and slow (1 hr) IV administration are essential to prevent crystallization in renal tubules. **Do not use** topical product on the eye or for the prevention of recurrent HSV infections. Oral absorption is unpredictable (15%–30%); consider using valacyclovir or famciclovir for better absorption. Use ideal body weight for obese patients when calculating dosages. Resistant strains of HSV and VZV have been reported in immunocompromised patients (e.g., advanced HIV infection).

Can cause renal impairment; has been infrequently associated with headache, vertigo, insomnia, encephalopathy, GI tract irritation, elevated liver function tests, rash, urticaria, arthralgia, fever, and adverse hematologic effects. Probenecid decreases acyclovir renal clearance. Acyclovir may increase the concentration of tenofovir, and meperidine and its metabolite (normeperidine).

ADDERALL

See Dextroamphetamine ± Amphetamine

ADENOSINE
Adenocard
Antiarrhythmic

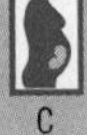

No No ? C

Injection: 3 mg/mL (2, 4 mL); preservative-free

Supraventricular tachycardia:
Neonate: 0.05 mg/kg by rapid IV push over 1–2 seconds; may increase dose by 0.05 mg/kg increments every 2 min to **max** of 0.25 mg/kg.
Child: 0.1–0.2 mg/kg (**initial max. dose:** 6 mg) by rapid IV push over 1–2 seconds; may increase dose by 0.05 mg/kg increments every 2 min to max. of 0.25 mg/kg (up to 12 mg), or until termination of SVT. **Max. subsequent single dose:** 12 mg.
Adolescent and adult ≥50 kg: 6 mg rapid IV push over 1–2 seconds; if no response after 1–2 min, give 12 mg rapid IV push. May repeat a second 12 mg dose after 1–2 min if required. **Max. single dose:** 12 mg.

Contraindicated in 2nd and 3rd degree AV block or sick-sinus syndrome unless pacemaker placed. **Use with caution** in combination with digoxin (enhanced depressant effects on SA and AV nodes).

Follow each dose with NS flush. $T_{1/2}$: <10 seconds.

May precipitate bronchoconstriction, especially in asthmatics. Side effects include transient asystole, facial flushing, headache, shortness of breath, dyspnea, nausea, chest pain, and lightheadedness.

Carbamazepine and dipyridamole may increase the effects/toxicity of adenosine. Methylxanthines (e.g., caffeine and theophylline) may decrease the effects of adenosine.

ALBUMIN, HUMAN
Albuminar, Albutein, Buminate, Plasbumin, Normal Serum Albumin (Human), and others
Blood product derivative, plasma volume expander

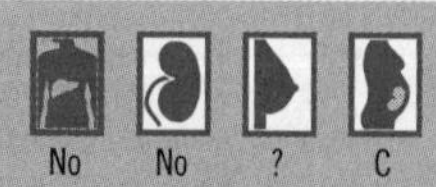

Injection: 5% (50 mg/mL) (50, 250, 500, mL); 25% (250 mg/mL) (20, 50, 100 mL); both concentrations contain 130–160 mEq Na/L

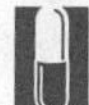

Hypoalbuminemia:
Child: 0.5–1 g/kg/dose IV over 30–120 min; repeat Q1–2 days PRN
Adult: 25 g/dose IV over 30–120 min; repeat Q1–2 days PRN
Max. dose: 2 g/kg/24 hr

Hypovolemia:
Child: 0.5–1 g/kg/dose IV rapid infusion
Adult: 25 g/dose IV rapid infusion; may repeat PRN
Max. dose: 6 g/kg/24 hr or 250 g/48 hr

Contraindicated in cases of CHF or severe anemia; rapid infusion may cause fluid overload; hypersensitivity reactions may occur; may cause rapid increase in serum sodium levels.

Caution: 25% concentration **contraindicated** in preterm infants due to risk of IVH.

For infusion, use 5-micron filter or larger. Both 5% and 25% products are isotonic but differ in oncotic effects. Dilutions of the 25% product should be made with D5W or NS; **avoid using sterile water.**

ALBUTEROL
Proventil, VoSpire ER (sustained release tabs), Proventil HFA (aerosol inhaler), Ventolin HFA (aerosol inhaler), AccuNeb (prediluted nebulized solution), and many other nebulized solutions
Beta-2-adrenergic agonist

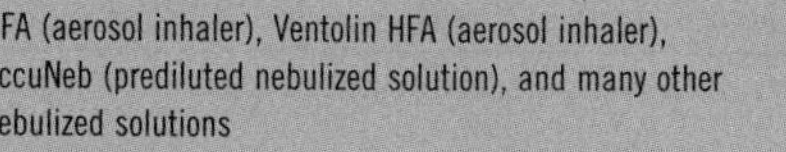

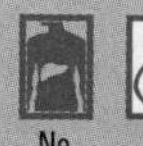
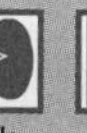
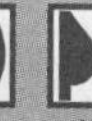
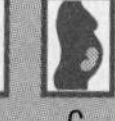

Tabs: 2, 4 mg
Sustained release tabs: 4, 8 mg
Oral solution: 2 mg/5 mL (473 mL)
Aerosol inhaler (HFA): 90 mcg/actuation (60 actuations/inhaler) (8.5 g)
Nebulization solution: 0.5% (5 mg/mL) (20 mL)
Prediluted nebulized solution: 0.63 mg in 3 mL NS, 1.25 mg in 3 mL NS, and 2.5 mg in 3 mL NS (0.083%)

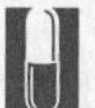

Inhalations (non-acute use):
Aerosol (HFA): 2 puffs (90 mcg) Q4–6 hr PRN
Nebulization:
<1 yr: 0.05–0.15 mg/kg/dose Q4–6 hr
1–5 yr: 1.25–2.5 mg/dose Q4–6 hr
5–12 yr: 2.5 mg/dose Q4–6 hr
>12 yr: 2.5–5 mg/dose Q4–8 hr

For use in acute exacerbations more aggressive dosing may be employed.

Oral (discouraged—see remarks):
2–6 yr: 0.3 mg/kg/24 hr PO ÷ TID; **max. dose:** 12 mg/24 hr
6–12 yr: 6 mg/24 hr PO ÷ TID; **max. dose:** 24 mg/24 hr
>12 yr and adult: 2–4 mg/dose PO TID-QID; **max. dose:** 32 mg/24 hr

Continued

FORMULARY

For explanation of icons, see p. 663.

ALBUTEROL *continued*

Inhaled doses may be given more frequently than indicated. In such cases, consider cardiac monitoring and monitoring of serum potassium (hypokalemia). Systemic effects are dose related. Please verify the concentration of the nebulization solution used.

Use of oral dosage form is discouraged due to increased side effects and decreased efficacy compared to inhaled formulations.

Possible side effects include tachycardia, palpitations, tremor, insomnia, nervousness, nausea, and headache.

The use of tube spacers or chambers may enhance efficacy of the metered dose inhalers and have been proven to be just as effective and sometimes safer than nebulizers.

ALLOPURINOL

Zyloprim, Alloprim, and others

Uric acid lowering agent, xanthine oxidase inhibitor

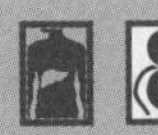 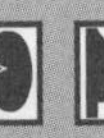 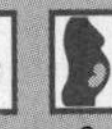

Yes Yes 1 C

Tabs: 100, 300 mg
Oral suspension: 20 mg/mL
Injection (Alloprim): 500 mg
Contains ~1.45 mEq Na/500 mg drug

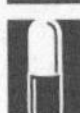

For use in tumor lysis syndrome, see Chapter 22.

Child:

Oral: 10 mg/kg/24 hr PO ÷ BID–QID; **max. dose:** 800 mg/24 hr
Injectable: 200 mg/m²/24 hr IV ÷ Q 6–12 hr; **max. dose:** 600 mg/24 hr

Adult:

Oral: 200–800 mg/24 hr PO ÷ BID–TID
Injectable: 200–400 mg/m²/24 hr IV ÷ Q 6–12 hr; **max. dose:** 600 mg/24 hr

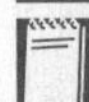

Adjust dose in renal insufficiency (see Chapter 31). Must maintain adequate urine output and alkaline urine.

Drug interactions: increases serum theophylline level; may increase the incidence of rash with ampicillin and amoxicillin; increased risk of toxicity with azathioprine, didanosine, and mercaptopurine; and increased risk of hypersensitivity reactions with ACE inhibitors and thiazide diuretics. Use with didanosine is **contraindicated** due to increased risk for didanosine toxicity.

Side effects include rash, neuritis, hepatotoxicity, GI disturbance, bone marrow suppression, and drowsiness.

IV dosage form is very alkaline and must be **diluted to a minimum concentration** of 6 mg/mL and infused over 30 min.

ALPROSTADIL

Prostin VR Pediatric, Prostaglandin E_1, PGE_1

Prostaglandin E_1, vasodilator

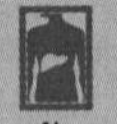 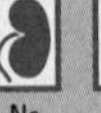 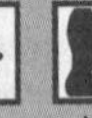 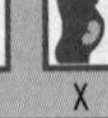

No No ? X

Injection: 500 mcg/mL (1 mL); contains dehydrated alcohol

Neonate:

Initial: 0.05–0.1 mcg/kg/min. Advance to 0.2 mcg/kg/min if necessary.
Maintenance: When increase in PaO_2 is noted, decrease immediately to lowest effective dose. Usual dosage range: 0.01–0.4 mcg/kg/min; doses above 0.4 mcg/kg/min not likely to produce additional benefit.

To prepare infusion: see IV Infusions on page i.

Continued

ALPROSTADIL *continued*

For palliation only. Continuous vital sign monitoring essential. May cause apnea (10%–12%), fever, seizures, flushing, bradycardia, hypotension, diarrhea, gastric outlet obstruction, and reversible cortical proliferation of long bones (with prolonged use). Decreases platelet aggregation.

ALTEPLASE
Activase, Cathflo Activase, tPA
Thrombolytic agent, tissue plasminogen activator

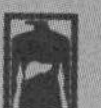
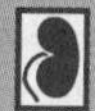
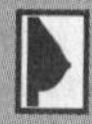
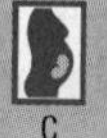

Yes Yes ? C

Injection:
Cathflo Activase: 2 mg
Activase: 50 mg (29 million unit), 100 mg (58 million unit)
Contains: L-arginine and polysorbate 80

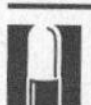

Occluded IV catheter:
Aspiration method: Use 1 mg/1 mL concentration as follows:

Age/Weight	Single-Lumen CVL	Double-Lumen CVL	Subcutaneous Port
<10 kg	0.5 mg, dilute with normal saline to required volume to fill line	0.5 mg each lumen, dilute with normal saline to required volume to fill line and treat one lumen at a time	0.5 mg, dilute with normal saline to 3 mL
≥10 kg	1–2 mg, use required amount to fill lumen (**max:** 2 mg)	1–2 mg each lumen, use required amount to fill lumen (**max:** 2 mg per lumen) and treat one lumen at a time	2 mg, dilute with normal saline to 3 mL

CVL, central venous line.

Instill into catheter over 1–2 min and leave in place for 2 hr before attempting blood withdrawal. After 2 hr, attempts to withdraw blood may be made every 2 hr for 3 attempts. Dose may be repeated once in 24 hr using a longer catheter dwell time of 3–4 hr. After 3–4 hr (repeat dose), attempts to withdrawal blood may be made every 2 hr for 3 attempts. **DO NOT** infuse into patient.

Systemic thrombolytic therapy (use in consultation with a hematologist; see remarks): dosage regimens ranging from lower dosages (0.01 mg/kg/hr) to higher dosages (0.1–0.6 mg/kg/hr) have been reported (*Chest* 2008;133:887–968S). The length of continuous infusion is variable as patients may respond to longer or shorter courses of therapy.

Current use in the pediatric population is limited. May cause bleeding, rash, and increase prothrombin time.

THROMBOLYTIC USE: History of stroke, transient ischemic attacks, other neurologic disease, and hypertension are **contraindications** for adults but considered relative **contraindications** for children. Monitor fibrinogen, thrombin clotting time, PT, and aPTT when used as a thrombolytic. For systemic thrombosis therapy, efficacy has been reported at 40%–97% with the risk for bleeding at 3%–27%. Poor efficacy in VTE in children has been recently reported. **Use with caution** in severe hepatic or renal dysfunction (systemic use only).

Newborns have reduced plasminogen levels (~50% of adult values), which decrease the thrombolytic effects of alteplase. Plasminogen supplementation may be necessary.

For explanation of icons, see p. 663.

ALUMINUM HYDROXIDE
Amphojel, Alu-Tab, Dialume, AlternaGEL, and various generics
Antacid, phosphate binder

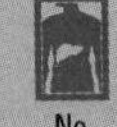
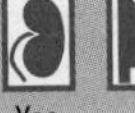
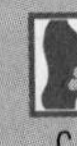

No Yes ? C

Oral suspension [OTC]: 320 mg/5 mL and 600 mg/5 mL (30, 360, 480 mL)
Each 5 mL suspension contains <0.13 mEq Na.

(mL volume dosages are based on the 320 mg/5 mL oral suspension concentration):
Peptic ulcer:
Child: 5–15 mL PO Q3–6 hr or 1–3 hr PC and HS
Adult: 15–45 mL PO Q3–6 hr or 1–3 hr PC and HS
Prophylaxis against GI bleeding:
Neonate: 1 mL/kg/dose PO Q4 hr PRN
Infant: 2–5 mL PO Q1–2 hr
Child: 5–15 mL PO Q1–2 hr
Adult: 30–60 mL PO Q1–2 hr
Hyperphosphatemia:
Child: 50–150 mg/kg/24 hr ÷ Q4–6 hr PO
Adult: 30–40 mL TID–QID PO between meals and QHS

Use with caution in patients with renal failure and upper GI hemorrhage.
Interferes with the absorption of several orally administered medications, including digoxin, ethambutol, indomethacin, isoniazid, naproxen, mycophenolate, tetracyclines, fluoroquinolones (e.g., Ciprofloxacin), and iron. Generally, **do not** take oral medications within 1–2 hours of taking aluminum dose unless specified.
May cause constipation, decreased bowel motility, encephalopathy, and phosphorus depletion.

ALUMINUM HYDROXIDE WITH MAGNESIUM HYDROXIDE
Maalox, Mylanta, Mylanta Extra Strength, Almacone, Almacone II Double Strength, RuLox Plus, Mintox, and many others (see remarks)
Antacid

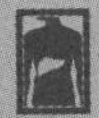
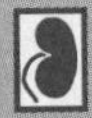
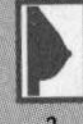
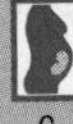

No Yes ? C

Chewable tabs [OTC]: (Al $(OH)_3$: Mg $(OH)_2$)
Mintox: 200 mg: 200 mg; contains saccharin
Each tablet contains 0.03–0.06 mEq Na
Oral suspension [OTC] (see remarks):
Maalox, Mylanta, and Almacone: each 5 mL contains 200 mg ALOH, 200 mg MgOH, and 20 mg simethicone (150, 360, 720 mL)
Mylanta Extra Strength, and Almacone II Double Strength: each 5 mL contains 400 mg ALOH, 400 mg MgOH, and 40 mg simethicone (360, 480 mL)
RuLox Plus: each 5 mL contains 500 mg ALOH, 450 mg MgOH, and 40 mg simethicone (355 mL)
Many other combinations exist.
Contains 0.03–0.06 mEq Na/5 mL

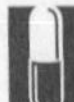

Same as for aluminum hydroxide preparations. **Do not use** combination product for hyperphosphatemia.

Continued

ALUMINUM HYDROXIDE WITH MAGNESIUM HYDROXIDE *continued*

May have laxative effect. May cause hypokalemia. **Use with caution** in patients with renal insufficiency (magnesium), gastric outlet obstruction.

Interferes with the absorption of the benzodiazepines, chloroquine, digoxin, naproxen, mycophenolate, phenytoin, quinolones (e.g., ciprofloxacin), tetracyclines, and iron. Generally, **do not** take oral medications within 1–2 hr of taking antacid dose unless specified.

DO NOT use Maalox Total Relief (bismuth subsalicylate), Mylanta Supreme or Ultimate Strength Chewables (calcium carbonate + magnesium hydroxide), Children's Mylanta Chewable Tablets (calcium carbonate) as these products do not contain aluminum hydroxide and magnesium hydroxide.

AMANTADINE HYDROCHLORIDE
Symmetrel and others
Antiviral agent

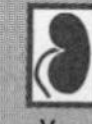
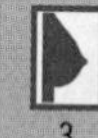
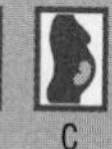

Yes Yes 3 C

Capsule: 100 mg
Tabs: 100 mg
Syrup: 50 mg/5 mL (480 mL); may contain parabens

Influenza A prophylaxis and treatment (for treatment, it is best to initiate therapy immediately after the onset of symptoms; within 2 days; see remarks):
1–9 yr: 5 mg/kg/24 hr PO ÷ once daily–BID; **max. dose:** 150 mg/24 hr
>9 yr:
<40 kg: 5 mg/kg/24 hr PO ÷ once daily–BID; **max. dose:** 200 mg/24 hr
≥40 kg: 200 mg/24 hr ÷ once daily–BID

Alternative dosing for influenza A prophylaxis:
Child >20 kg and adult: 100 mg/24 hr PO ÷ once daily–BID

Prophylaxis (duration of therapy):
Single exposure: at least 10 days
Repeated/uncontrolled exposure: up to 90 days
Use with influenza A vaccine when possible.

Symptomatic treatment (duration of therapy):
Continue for 24–48 hr after disappearance of symptoms.

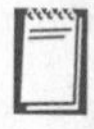

Do not use in the first trimester of pregnancy. **Use with caution** in patients with liver disease, seizures, renal disease, congestive heart failure, peripheral edema, orthostatic hypotension, history of recurrent eczematoid rash, and in those receiving CNS stimulants. **Adjust dose in patients with renal insufficiency (see Chapter 31).**

Resistance to influenza A and recommendations against the use for treatment and prophylaxis have been reported by the CDC. Check with local microbiology laboratories and the CDC for seasonal susceptibility/resistance. Individuals immunized with live attenuated influenza vaccine should not receive amantadine prophylaxis for 14 days after the vaccine.

May cause dizziness, anxiety, depression, mental status change, rash (livedo reticularis), nausea, orthostatic hypotension, edema, CHF, and urinary retention. Neuroleptic malignant syndrome has been reported with abrupt dose reduction or discontinuation (especially if patient is receiving neuroleptics).

For explanation of icons, see p. 663.

AMIKACIN SULFATE
Amikin
Antibiotic, aminoglycoside

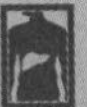 No 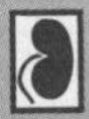 Yes 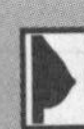 1 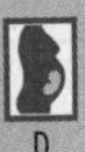 D

Injection: 250 mg/mL; may contain sodium bisulfite

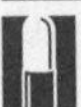

Initial empiric dosage; patient-specific dosage defined by therapeutic drug monitoring (see remarks).

Neonate: See the following table.

Post-conceptional Age (wk)	Postnatal Age (days)	Dose (mg/kg/dose)	Interval (hr)
≤29*	0–7	18	48
	8–28	15	36
	>28	15	24
30–33	0–7	18	36
	>7	15	24
34–37	0–7	15	24
	>7	15	18–24
≥38	0–7	15	24
	>7	15	12–18

*Or significant asphyxia, PDA, indomethacin use, poor cardiac output, reduced renal function.

Infant and child: 15–22.5 mg/kg/24 hr ÷ Q8 hr IV/IM; infants and patients requiring higher doses (e.g., Cystic Fibrosis) may receive initial doses of 30 mg/kg/24 hr ÷ Q8 hr IV/IM

Adult: 15 mg/kg/24 hr ÷ Q8–12 hr IV/IM

Initial max. dose: 1.5 g/24 hr, then monitor levels

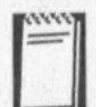

Use with caution in pre-existing renal, vestibular, or auditory impairment; concomitant anesthesia or neuromuscular blockers, neurotoxic; concomitant neurotoxic, ototoxic, or nephrotoxic drugs; sulfite sensitivity; and dehydration. **Adjust dose in renal failure (see Chapter 31).** Rapidly eliminated in patients with Cystic Fibrosis, burns, and in febrile neutropenic patients. CNS penetration is poor beyond early infancy.

Therapeutic levels: peak, 20–30 mg/L; trough 5–10 mg/L. Recommended serum sampling time at steady-state: trough within 30 min prior to the third consecutive dose and peak 30–60 minutes after the administration of the third consecutive dose.

Peak levels of 25–30 mg/L have been recommended for CNS, pulmonary, bone, life-threatening, *Pseudomonas* infections and in febrile neutropenic patients. Longer dosing intervals may be necessary for neonates receiving indomethacin for PDAs and for all patients with poor cardiac output.

For initial dosing in obese patients, use an adjusted body weight (ABW). ABW = Ideal Body Weight + 0.4 (Total Body Weight – Ideal Body Weight).

May cause ototoxicity, nephrotoxicity, neuromuscular blockade, and rash. Loop diuretics may potentiate the ototoxicity of all aminoglycoside antibiotics.

AMINOCAPROIC ACID
Amicar and other generics
Hemostatic agent

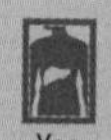 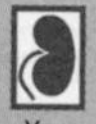 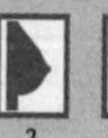 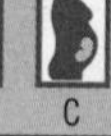 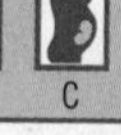
Yes Yes ? C

Tabs: 500, 1000 mg
Oral liquid/syrup: 250 mg/mL (240, 480 mL); may contain 0.2% methylparaben and 0.05% propylparaben
Injection: 250 mg/mL (20 mL); contains 0.9% benzyl alcohol

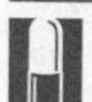

Child:

Loading dose: 100–200 mg/kg IV/PO
Maintenance: 100 mg/kg/dose Q4–6 hr; **max. dose:** 30 g/24 hr

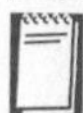

Contraindications: DIC, hematuria. **Use with caution** in patients with cardiac, renal, or hepatic disease. Should not be given with Factor IX Complex concentrates or Anti-Inhibitor Coagulant concentrates because of risk for thrombosis. Dose should be reduced by 75% in oliguria or end-stage renal disease. Hypercoagulation may be produced when given in conjunction with oral contraceptives.

May cause nausea, diarrhea, malaise, weakness, headache, decreased platelet function, hypotension, and false increase in urine amino acids. Elevation of serum potassium may occur, especially in patients with renal impairment.

AMINOPHYLLINE
Various generic products
Bronchodilator, methylxanthine

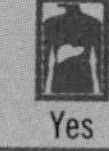 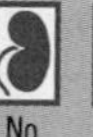 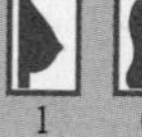 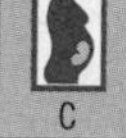
Yes No 1 C

Tabs: 100, 200 mg (79% theophylline)
Injection: 25 mg/mL (79% theophylline)
NOTE: Pharmacy may dilute IV dosage forms to enhance accuracy of neonatal dosing.

PO:

Infant: (see *Theophylline* and convert to mg of Aminophylline)
1–9 yr: 27 mg/kg/24 hr ÷ Q4–6 hr
9–12 yr: 20 mg/kg/24 hr ÷ Q6 hr
12–16 yr: 16 mg/kg/24 hr ÷ Q6 hr
Adult: 12.5 mg/kg/24 hr ÷ Q6 hr

Neonatal apnea:

Loading dose: 5–6 mg/kg IV or PO
Maintenance dose: 1–2 mg/kg/dose Q6–8 hr, IV or PO

IV loading: 6 mg/kg IV over 20 min (each 1.2 mg/kg dose raises the serum theophylline concentration 2 mg/L)

IV maintenance: Continuous IV drip:

Neonate: 0.2 mg/kg/hr
6 wk–6 mo: 0.5 mg/kg/hr
6 mo–1 yr: 0.6–0.7 mg/kg/hr
1–9 yr: 1–1.2 mg/kg/hr
9–12 yr and young adult smoker: 0.9 mg/kg/hr
>12 yr healthy nonsmoker: 0.7 mg/kg/hr

The above total daily doses may also be administered IV ÷ Q4–6 hr.

Continued

For explanation of icons, see p. 663.

AMINOPHYLLINE *continued*

Consider mg of theophylline available when dosing aminophylline.

Monitoring serum levels is essential especially in infants and young children. Intermittent dosing for infants and children 1–5 yr may require Q4 hr dosing regimen due to enhanced metabolism. Side effects: restlessness, GI upset, headache, tachycardia, seizures (may occur in absence of other side effects with toxic levels).

Therapeutic level (theophylline): for asthma, 10–20 mg/L; for neonatal apnea, 6–13 mg/L.

Recommended Guidelines for obtaining levels:

- IV bolus: 30 min after infusion
- IV continuous; 12–24 hr after initiation of infusion
- PO liquid, immediate-release tab:
  - *Peak:* 1 hr post dose
  - *Trough:* just before dose
- PO sustained-release:
  - *Peak:* 4 hr post dose
  - *Trough:* just before dose

Ideally, obtain levels after steady state has been achieved (after at least 1 day of therapy). Liver impairment, cardiac failure, and sustained high fever may increase theophylline levels. See *Theophylline* for drug interactions.

Use in breastfeeding may cause irritability in infant.

AMIODARONE HCL

Cordarone, Pacerone, and various generics

Antiarrhythmic, Class III

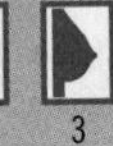 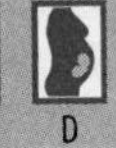

Yes No 3 D

Tabs: 100, 200, 400 mg

Oral suspension: 5 mg/mL

Injection: 50 mg/mL (3, 9, 18 mL) (contains 20.2 mg/mL benzyl alcohol and 100 mg/mL polysorbate 80 or Tween 80)

Contains 37% iodine by weight.

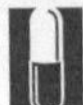

See Resuscitation Medications on page ii for arrest dosing.

Child PO:

<1 yr: 600–800 mg/1.73 m^2/24 hr ÷ Q12–24 hr × 4–14 days and/or until adequate control achieved, then reduce to 200–400 mg/1.73 m^2/24 hr.

≥1 yr: 10–15 mg/kg/24 hr ÷ Q12–24 hr × 4–14 days and/or until adequate control achieved, then reduce to 5 mg/kg/24 hr ÷ Q12–24 hr if effective.

Child IV (limited data):

5 mg/kg over 30 min followed by a continuous infusion starting at 5 micrograms (mcg)/kg/min; infusion may be increased up to a **max. dose** of 15 mcg/kg/min or 20 mg/kg/24 hr.

Adult PO:

Loading dose: 800–1600 mg/24 hr ÷ Q12–24 hr for 1–3 wk

Maintenance: 600–800 mg/24 hr ÷ Q12–24 hr × 1 mo, then 200 mg Q12–24 hr

Use lowest effective dose to minimize adverse reactions.

Adult IV:

Loading dose: 150 mg over 10 min (15 mg/min) followed by 360 mg over 6 hr (1 mg/min); followed by a maintenance dose of 0.5 mg/min. Supplemental boluses of 150 mg over 10 min may be given for breakthrough VF or hemodynamically unstable VT, and the maintenance infusion may be increased to suppress the arrhythmia. **Max. dose:** 2.1 g/24 hr.

Continued

AMIODARONE HCL *continued*

Used in the resuscitation algorithm for ventricular fibrillation/pulseless ventricular tachycardia (see Resuscitation Medications on page ii for arrest dosing and Pediatric Cardiac Arrest algorithm in back of book). Overall use of this drug may be limited to its potentially life-threatening side effects and the difficulties associated with managing its use.

Contraindicated in severe sinus node dysfunction, marked sinus bradycardia, second- and third-degree AV block. **Use with caution** in hepatic impairment.

Long elimination half-life (40–55 days). Major metabolite is active.

Increases cyclosporine, digoxin, phenytoin, tacrolimus, warfarin, calcium channel blockers, theophylline, and quinidine levels. Amiodarone is a CYP P450 3A3/4 substrate and inhibits CYP 3A3/4, 2C9, and 2D6. Risk of rhabdomyolysis is increased when used with simvastatin at doses greater than 20 mg/24hr.

Proposed therapeutic level with chronic oral use: 1–2.5 mg/L.

Asymptomatic corneal microdeposits should appear in all patients. Alters liver enzymes, thyroid function. Pulmonary fibrosis reported in adults. May cause worsening of preexisting arrhythmias with bradycardia and AV block. May also cause hypotension, anorexia, nausea, vomiting, dizziness, paresthesias, ataxia, tremor, SIADH, and hypothyroidism or hyperthyroidism.

Intravenous continuous infusion concentration for peripheral administration **should not exceed** 2 mg/mL and **must be** diluted with D_5W. The intravenous dosage form can leach out plasticizers such as DEHP. It is recommended to reduce the potential exposure to plasticizers in pregnant women and children at the toddler stages of development and younger by using alternative methods of IV drug administration. The preservative-free intravenous product is available as an orphan/compassionate use drug from Academic Pharmaceuticals, Inc. at (847) 735-1170.

Oral administration should be consistent with regards to meals because food increases the rate and extent of oral absorption.

AMITRIPTYLINE

Elavil and others

Antidepressant, tricyclic

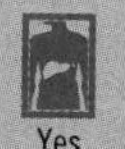
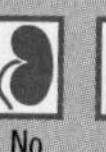
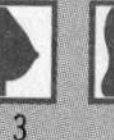
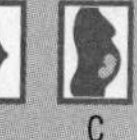

Yes No 3 C

Tabs: 10, 25, 50, 75, 100, 150 mg

Oral suspension: 1 mg/mL 

Antidepressant:

Child: Start with 1 mg/kg/24 hr ÷ TID PO for 3 days; then increase to 1.5 mg/kg/24 hr. Dose may be gradually increased to a **max. dose** of 5 mg/kg/24 hr if needed. Monitor ECG, BP, and heart rate for doses >3 mg/kg/24 hr.

Adolescent: 10 mg TID PO and 20 mg QHS; dose may be gradually increased up to a **max. dose** of 200 mg/24 hr if needed.

Adult: 40–100 mg/24 hr ÷ QHS–BID PO; dose may be gradually increased up to 300 mg/24 hr if needed; gradually decrease dose to lowest effective dose when symptoms are controlled.

Augment analgesia for chronic pain:

Initial: 0.1 mg/kg/dose QHS PO; increase as needed and tolerated over 2–3 wk to 0.5–2 mg/kg/dose QHS

Migraine prophylaxis:

Child: Initial 0.1–0.25 mg/kg/dose QHS PO; increase as needed and tolerated every 2 wk by 0.1–0.25 mg/kg/dose up to a **max. dose** of 2 mg/kg/24 hr or 75 mg/24 hr. For doses >1 mg/kg/24 hr, divide daily dose BID and monitor ECG.

Adult: 25–50 mg/dose QHS PO

Continued

For explanation of icons, see p. 663.

AMITRIPTYLINE *continued*

Contraindicated in narrow-angle glaucoma, seizures, severe cardiac disorders, and patients who received MAO inhibitors within 14 days. **See Chapter 2 for management of toxic ingestion.**

$T_{1/2}$ = 9–25 hr in adults. Maximum antidepressant effects may not occur for 2 wk or more after initiation of therapy. **Do not abruptly discontinue therapy in patients receiving high doses for prolonged periods.**

Therapeutic levels (sum of amitriptyline and nortriptyline): 100–250 ng/mL. Recommended serum sampling time: obtain a single level 8 hr or more after an oral dose (following 4–5 days of continuous dosing). Amitriptyline is a substrate for CYP 450 1A2, 2C9, 2C19, 2D6, and 3A3/4.

Side effects include sedation, urinary retention, constipation, dry mouth, dizziness, drowsiness, liver enzyme elevation and arrhythmia. May discolor urine (blue/green). QHS dosing during first weeks of therapy will reduce sedation. Monitor ECG, BP, CBC at start of therapy and with dose changes. Decrease dose if PR interval reaches 0.22 sec, QRS reaches 130% of baseline, HR rises above 140/min, or if BP is more than 140/90. Tricyclics may cause mania. For antidepressant use, monitor for clinical worsening of depression and suicidal ideation/behavior following the initiation of therapy or after dose changes.

AMLODIPINE

Norvasc

Calcium channel blocker, antihypertensive

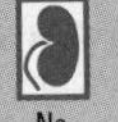
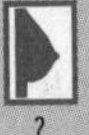
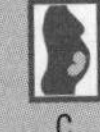

Yes No ? C

Tabs: 2.5, 5, 10 mg

Oral suspension: 1 mg/mL 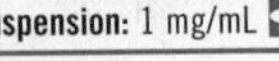

Child:

Hypertension: Start with 0.1 mg/kg/dose (**max. dose:** 5 mg) PO once daily–BID; dosage may be gradually increased to a **max. dose** of 0.6 mg/kg/24 hr up to 20 mg/24 hr.

Adult:

Hypertension: 5–10 mg/dose once daily PO; use 2.5 mg/dose once daily PO in patients with hepatic insufficiency.

Max. dose: 10 mg/24 hr

Use with caution in combination with other antihypertensive agents. Younger children may require higher mg/kg doses than older children and adults. A BID dosing regimen may provide better efficacy in children.

Reduce dose in hepatic insufficiency. Allow 5–7 days of continuous initial dose therapy before making dosage adjustments because of the drug's gradual onset of action and lengthy elimination half-life. Amlodipine is a substrate for CYP 450 3A4 and should be used with **caution** with 3A4 inhibitors such as protease inhibitors and azole antifungals (e.g., fluconazole and ketoconazole).

Dose-related side effects include edema, dizziness, flushing, fatigue, and palpitations. Other side effects include headache, nausea, abdominal pain, and somnolence.

AMMONIUM CHLORIDE

Diuretic, urinary acidifying agent

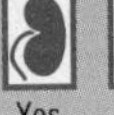

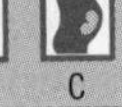

Yes Yes ? C

Injection: 5 mEq/mL (26.75%) (20 mL); contains EDTA

1 mEq = 53 mg

Continued

AMMONIUM CHLORIDE *continued*

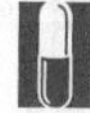

Urinary acidification:

Child: 75 mg/kg/24 hr ÷ Q6 hr IV; **max. dose:** 6 g/24 hr

Adult: 1.5 g/dose Q6 hr IV

Drug administration: Dilute to concentration ≤0.4 mEq/mL. Infusion **not to exceed** 50 mg/kg/hr or 1 mEq/kg/hr.

Contraindicated in hepatic or renal insufficiency and primary respiratory acidosis. **Use with caution** in infants.

May produce acidosis, hyperammonemia, and GI irritation. Monitor serum chloride level, acid/base status, and serum ammonia.

AMOXICILLIN
Amoxil, Trimox, Wymox, Polymox, DisperMox, Moxatag, and others
Antibiotic, aminopenicillin

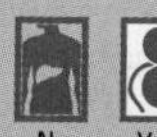
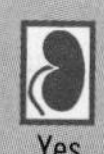
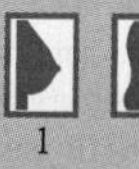

No Yes 1 B

Oral suspension: 125, 250 mg/5 mL (80, 100, 150 mL); and 200, 400 mg/5 mL (50, 75, 100 mL)
Caps: 250, 500 mg
Tablets: 500, 875 mg
Chewable tabs: 125, 250 mg
Extended-release tabs (Moxatag; see remarks): 775 mg
Tablets for oral suspension (DisperMox): 200, 400 mg; contains phenylalanine

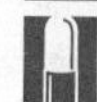

Neonate– ≤3 mo: 20–30 mg/kg/24 hr ÷ Q12 hr PO

Child:

Standard dose: 25–50 mg/kg/24 hr ÷ Q8–12 hr PO

High dose (resistant* S. pneumoniae*): 80–90 mg/kg/24 hr ÷ BID PO

Adult:

Mild/moderate infections: 250 mg/dose Q8 hr PO OR 500 mg/dose Q12 hr PO

Severe infections: 500 mg/dose Q8 hr PO OR 875 mg/dose Q12 hr PO

Max. dose: 2–3 g/24 hr

Recurrent otitis media prophylaxis: 20 mg/kg/dose QHS PO

SBE prophylaxis: see Chapter 7.

Early Lyme disease:

Child: 50 mg/kg/24 hr ÷ Q8 hr PO × 14–21 days; **max. dose:** 1.5 g/24 hr

Adult: 500 mg/dose Q8 hr PO × 14–21 days

Renal elimination. **Adjust dose in renal failure (see Chapter 31).** Serum levels about twice those achieved with equal dose of ampicillin. Less GI effects, but otherwise similar to ampicillin. Side effects: rash and diarrhea. Rash may develop with concurrent EBV infection.

High dose regimen increasingly useful is recommended in respiratory infections, acute otitis media, and sinusitis, owing to increasing incidence of penicillin-resistant pneumococci. Chewable tablets and DisperMox may contain phenylalanine and **should not be used** by phenylketonurics.

Extended-release tablets (Moxatag) 775 mg once daily PO × 10 days is indicated for children ≥12 yr and adults for the treatment of tonsillitis/pharyngitis due to *S. pyogenes.*

DisperMox oral suspension is prepared by swirling/stirring each tablet thoroughly in approximately 10 mL of water only. **Do not** chew or swallow (whole tablets) DisperMox.

For explanation of icons, see p. 663.

AMOXICILLIN-CLAVULANIC ACID
Augmentin, Augmentin ES-600, Augmentin XR, and various generic products
Antibiotic, aminopenicillin with beta-lactamase inhibitor

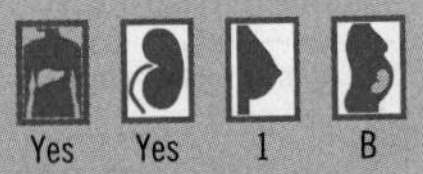

Tabs:

For TID dosing: 250, 500 mg (with 125 mg clavulanate)

For BID dosing: 875 mg amoxicillin (with 125 mg clavulanate); Augmentin XR: 1 g amoxicillin (with 62.5 mg clavulanate)

Chewable tabs:

For TID dosing: 125, 250 mg amoxicillin (31.25 and 62.5 mg clavulanate, respectively); contains saccharin

For BID dosing: 200, 400 mg amoxicillin (28.5 and 57 mg clavulanate, respectively); contains saccharin and aspartame

Oral suspension:

For TID dosing: 125, 250 mg amoxicillin/5mL (31.25 and 62.5 mg clavulanate/5 mL, respectively) (75, 100, 150 mL); contains saccharin

For BID dosing: 200, 400 mg amoxicillin/5 mL (28.5 and 57 mg clavulanate/5 mL, respectively) (50, 75, 100 mL); 600 mg amoxicillin/5 mL (Augmentin ES-600; contains 42.9 mg clavulanate/5 mL) (50, 75, 100, 150 mL); contains saccharin and/or aspartame

Contains 0.63 mEq K^+ per 125 mg clavulanate (Augmentin ES-600 contains 0.23 mEq K^+ per 42.9 mg clavulanate)

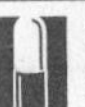

Dosage based on amoxicillin component.

Child <3 mo: 30 mg/kg/24 hr ÷ Q12 hr PO (recommended dosage form is 125 mg/5 mL suspension)

Child ≥3 mo:

TID dosing (see remarks):

20–40 mg/kg/24 hr ÷ Q8 hr PO

BID dosing (see remarks):

25–45 mg/kg/24 hr ÷ Q12 hr PO

Augmentin ES-600:

≥3 mo and <40 kg: 90 mg/kg/24 hr ÷ Q12 hr PO × 10 days

Adult: 250–500 mg/dose Q8 hr PO or 875 mg/dose Q12 hr PO for more severe and respiratory infections

Augmentin XR:

≥16 yr and adult: 2 g Q12 hr PO × 10 days for acute bacterial sinusitis or × 7–10 days for community-acquired pneumonia

Clavulanic acid extends the activity of amoxicillin to include beta-lactamase producing strains of *H. influenzae, M. catarrhalis, N. gonorrhoeae,* some *S. aureus* and may increase the risk for diarrhea. See *Amoxicillin* for additional comments. **Adjust dose in renal failure (see Chapter 31). Contraindicated** in patients with a history of cholestatic jaundice/hepatic dysfunction associated with amoxicillin-clavulanic acid. Augmentin XR is **contraindicated** in patients with CrCl <30 mL/min.

The BID dosing schedule is associated with less diarrhea. For BID dosing, the 875 mg, 1 g tablets, the 200 mg, 400 mg chewable tablets or the 200 mg/5 mL, 400 mg/5 mL, 600 mg/5 mL suspensions should be used. These BID dosage forms contain phenylalanine and **should not be used** by phenylketonurics. For TID dosing, the 250 mg, 500 mg tablets, the 125 mg, 250 mg chewable tablets or the 125mg/5mL, 250mg/5mL suspensions should be used.

Continued

AMOXICILLIN-CLAVULANIC ACID *continued*

Higher doses of 80–90 mg/kg/24 hr (amoxicillin component) have been recommended for resistant strains of *S. pneumoniae* in acute otitis media (use BID formulations containing 7:1 ratio of amoxicillin to clavulanic acid or Augmentin ES-600).

The 250 or 500 mg tablets **cannot** be substituted for Augmentin XR.

AMPHOTERICIN B
Fungizone, Amphocin
Antifungal, polyene

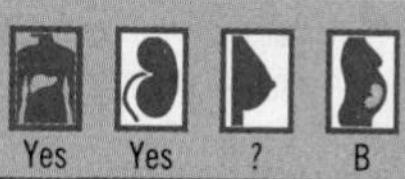

Injection: 50 mg vials

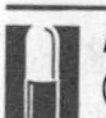

IV: mix with D_5W to concentration 0.1 mg/mL (peripheral administration) or 0.25 mg/mL (central line only). pH >4.2. Infuse over 2–6 hr.

Optional test dose: 0.1 mg/kg/dose IV up to **max. dose** of 1 mg (followed by remaining initial dose).

Initial dose: 0.5–1 mg/kg/24 hr; if test dose NOT used infuse first dose over 6 hr and monitor frequently during the first several hr.

Increment: Increase as tolerated by 0.25–0.5 mg/kg/24 hr once daily or every other day. Use larger dosage increment (0.5 mg once daily) for critically ill patients.

Usual maintenance:

Once daily dosing: 0.5–1 mg/kg/24 hr once daily

Every other day dosing: 1.5 mg/kg/dose every other day

Max. dose: 1.5 mg/kg/24 hr

Intrathecal: 25–100 mcg Q48–72 hr. Increase to 500 mcg as tolerated.

Bladder irrigation for urinary tract mycosis: 5–15 mg in 100 mL sterile water for irrigation at 100–300 mL/24 hr. Instill solution into bladder, clamp catheter for 1–2 hr then drain; repeat TID–QID for 2–5 days.

Monitor renal, hepatic, electrolyte, and hematologic status closely. Hypercalciuria, hypokalemia, hypomagnesemia, RTA, renal failure, acute hepatic failure, hypotension, and phlebitis may occur. **For dosing information in renal failure, see Chapter 31.**

Common infusion-related reactions include fever, chills, headache, hypotension, nausea, vomiting; may premedicate with acetaminophen and diphenhydramine 30 min before and 4 hr after infusion. Meperidine useful for chills. Hydrocortisone, 1 mg/mg ampho (**max.:** 25 mg) added to bottle may help prevent immediate adverse reactions. Use total body weight for obese patients when calculating dosages.

Salt loading with 10–15 mL/kg of NS infused prior to each dose may minimize the risk of nephrotoxicity.

AMPHOTERICIN B LIPID COMPLEX
Abelcet
Antifungal, polyene

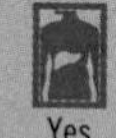
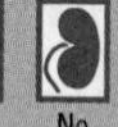
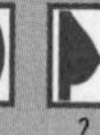
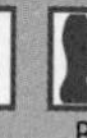

Injection: 5 mg/mL (10, 20 mL)
(formulated as a 1:1 molar ratio of amphotericin B to lipid complex comprised of dimyristoylphosphatidylcholine and dimyristoylphosphatidylglycerol)

IV: 2.5–5 mg/kg/24 hr once daily

For visceral leishmaniasis that failed to respond to or relapsed after treatment with antimony compound, a dosage of 1–3 mg/kg/24 hr once daily × 5 days has been used.

Continued

For explanation of icons, see p. 663.

AMPHOTERICIN B LIPID COMPLEX *continued*

Mix with D_5W to concentration 1 mg/mL or 2 mg/mL for fluid restricted patients.
Infusion rate: 2.5 mg/kg/hr; shake the infusion bag every 2 hr if total infusion time exceeds 2 hr. **Do not use** an in-line filter.

Monitor renal, hepatic, electrolyte, and hematologic status closely. Thrombocytopenia, anemia, leukopenia, hypokalemia, hypomagnesemia, diarrhea, respiratory failure, skin rash, and increases in liver enzymes and bilirubin may occur.

Highest concentrations achieved in spleen, lung, and liver from human autopsy data from one heart transplant patient. CNS/CSF levels are lower than amphotericin B, liposomal (AmBisome). In animal models, concentrations are higher in the liver, spleen, and lungs but the same in the kidneys when compared to conventional amphotericin B. Pharmacokinetics in renal and hepatic impairment have not been studied.

Common infusion-related reactions include fever, chills, rigors, nausea, vomiting, hypotension, and headache; may premedicate with acetaminophen, diphenhydramine, and meperidine (see *Amphotericin B* remarks).

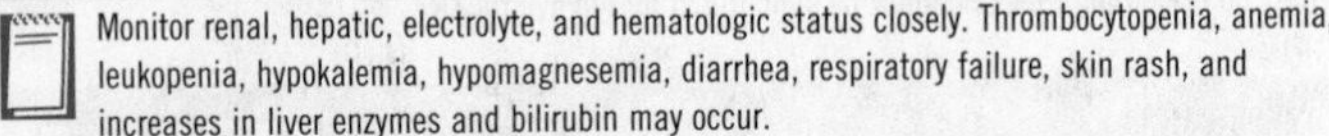

AMPHOTERICIN B, LIPOSOMAL
AmBisome
Antifungal, polyene

Injection: 50 mg (vials); contains soy, sucrose
(formulated in liposomes composed of hydrogenated soy phosphatidylcholine, cholesterol, distearoylphosphatidylglycerol, and alpha-tocopherol)

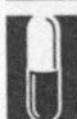

Systemic fungal infections: 3–5 mg/kg/24 hr IV once daily; an upper dosage limit of 10 mg/kg/24 hr has been suggested based on pharmacokinetic endpoints and risk for hypokalemia. However, dosages as high as 15 mg/kg/24 hr have been used. Dosages as high as 10 mg/kg/24 hr have been used in patients with aspergillus.
Empiric therapy for febrile neutropenia: 3 mg/kg/24 hr IV once daily
Cryptococcal meningitis in HIV: 6 mg/kg/24 hr IV once daily
Mix with D_5W to concentration 1–2 mg/mL (0.2–0.5 mg/mL may be used for infants and small children).
Infusion rate: Administer dose over 2 hr; infusion may be reduced to 1 hr if well tolerated.

Monitor renal, hepatic, electrolyte, and hematologic status closely. Thrombocytopenia, tachycardia, hypokalemia, hypomagnesemia, hypocalcemia, hyperglycemia, diarrhea, dyspnea, skin rash, low back pain, and increases in liver enzymes and bilirubin may occur. Safety and effectiveness in neonates have not been established.

When compared to conventional amphotericin B, higher concentrations found in the liver and spleen; and similar concentrations found in the lungs and kidney. CNS/CSF concentrations are higher than other amphotericin B products. Pharmacokinetics in renal and hepatic impairment have not been studied.

Common infusion-related reactions include fever, chills, rigors, nausea, vomiting, hypotension, and headache; may premedicate with acetaminophen, diphenhydramine, and meperidine (see *Amphotericin B* remarks).

AMPICILLIN
Omnipen, Principen, Totacillin, and others
Antibiotic, aminopenicillin

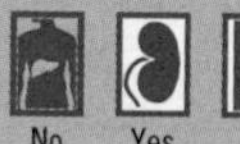
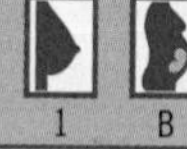
No Yes 1 B

Oral suspension: 125 mg/5 mL (100 mL), 250 mg/5 mL (100, 200 mL)
Caps: 250, 500 mg
Injection: 250, 500 mg; 1, 2, 10 g
Contains 3 mEq Na/1 g IV drug

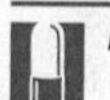

Neonate (IM/IV):
- *<7 days:*
  - ***<2 kg:*** 50–100 mg/kg/24 hr ÷ Q12 hr
  - ***≥2 kg:*** 75–150 mg/kg/24 hr ÷ Q8 hr
  - ***Group B streptococcal meningitis:*** 200–300 mg/kg/24 hr ÷ Q8 hr
- *≥7 days:*
  - ***<1.2 kg:*** 50–100 mg/kg/24 hr ÷ Q12 hr
  - ***1.2–2 kg:*** 75–150 mg/kg/24 hr ÷ Q8 hr
  - ***>2 kg:*** 100–200 mg/kg/24 hr ÷ Q6 hr
  - ***Group B streptococcal meningitis:*** 300 mg/kg/24 hr ÷ Q4–6 hr

Infant/child:
- ***Mild-moderate infections:***
  - ***IM/IV:*** 100–200 mg/kg/24 hr ÷ Q6 hr
  - ***PO:*** 50–100 mg/kg/24 hr ÷ Q6 hr; **max. PO dose:** 2–3 g/24 hr
- ***Severe infections:*** 200–400 mg/kg/24 hr ÷ Q4–6 hr IM/IV

Adult:
- ***IM/IV:*** 500–3000 mg Q4–6 hr
- ***PO:*** 250–500 mg Q6 hr

Max. IV/IM dose: 12 g/24 hr
SBE prophylaxis: see Chapter 7.

Use higher doses with shorter dosing intervals to treat CNS disease and severe infection. CSF penetration occurs only with inflamed meninges. **Adjust dose in renal failure (see Chapter 31).**

Produces the same side effects as penicillin, with cross-reactivity. Rash commonly seen at 5–10 days and rash may occur with concurrent EBV infection or allopurinol use. May cause interstitial nephritis, diarrhea, and pseudomembranous enterocolitis. Chloroquine reduces ampicillin's absorption.

AMPICILLIN/SULBACTAM
Unasyn
Antibiotic, aminopenicillin with beta-lactamase inhibitor

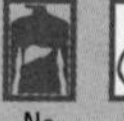
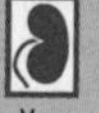
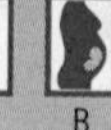
No Yes 1 B

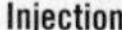

Injection:
1.5 g = ampicillin 1 g + sulbactam 0.5 g
3 g = ampicillin 2 g + sulbactam 1 g
Contains 5 mEq Na per 1.5 g drug combination

Dosage based on ampicillin component:
Infant ≥1 mo:
- ***Mild/moderate infections:*** 100–150 mg/kg/24 hr ÷ Q6 hr IM/IV
- ***Meningitis/severe infections:*** 200–300 mg/kg/24 hr ÷ Q6 hr IM/IV

Continued

For explanation of icons, see p. 663.

AMPICILLIN/SULBACTAM *continued*

Child:

Mild/moderate infections: 100–200 mg/kg/24 hr ÷ Q6 hr IM/IV

Meningitis/severe infections: 200–400 mg/kg/24 hr ÷ Q4–6 hr IM/IV

Adult: 1–2 g Q6–8 hr IM/IV

Max. dose: 8 g ampicillin/24 hr

Similar spectrum of antibacterial activity to ampicillin with the added coverage of beta-lactamase producing organisms. Total sulbactam dose **should not exceed** 4 g/24 hr.

Use higher doses with shorter dosing intervals to treat CNS disease and severe infection. **Adjust dose in renal failure (see Chapter 31).** Similar CSF distribution and side effects to ampicillin.

ANTIPYRINE AND BENZOCAINE

Allergen Ear Drops, Antipyrine and Benzocaine Otic, Autoguard Otic, Auralgan (available in Canada), and others

Otic analgesic, ceruminolytic

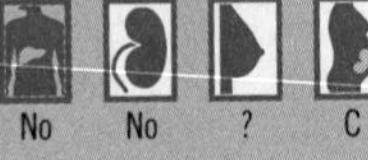

Otic solution: antipyrine 5.4%, benzocaine 1.4% (15 mL); may contain oxyquinoline sulfate

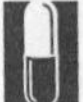

Otic analgesia: Fill external ear canal (2–4 drops) Q1–2 hr PRN. After instillation of the solution, a cotton pledget should be moistened with the solution and inserted into the meatus.

Ceruminolytic: Fill external ear canal (2–4 drops) TID–QID for 2–3 days.

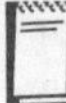

Benzocaine sensitivity may develop and not intended for prolonged use. **Contraindicated** if tympanic membrane perforated or PE tubes in place. Local reactions (e.g., burning, stinging) and hypersensitivity reactions may occur. Risk of benzocaine-induced methemoglobinemia may be increased in infants ≤3 mo of age.

ARGININE CHLORIDE

R-Gene 10

Metabolic alkalosis agent, urea cycle disorder treatment agent, growth hormone diagnostic agent

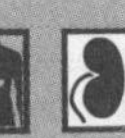

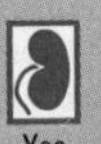

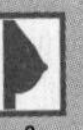

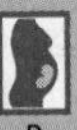

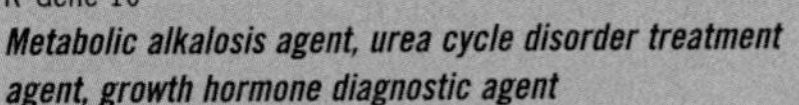

Injection: 10% (100 mg/mL) arginine hydrochloride, contains 47.5 mEq chloride per 100 mL (300 mL)

Osmolality: 950 mOsmol/L

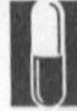

Used as a secondary alternative agent for patients that are unresponsive or unable to receive sodium chloride and potassium chloride.

Correction of hypochloremia: Arginine chloride dose in milliequivalents (mEq) = 0.2 × patient's weight (kg) × [103 – patient's serum chloride in mEq/L]. Administer ½ to ⅔ of the calculated dose and re-assess.

Drug administration: **Do not exceed** an IV infusion rate of 1 g/kg/hr (4.75 mEq/kg/hr). Drug may be administered without further dilution but should be diluted to reduce risk of tissue irritation.

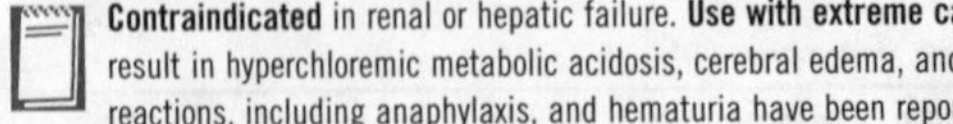

Contraindicated in renal or hepatic failure. **Use with extreme caution** as overdosages may result in hyperchloremic metabolic acidosis, cerebral edema, and death. Hypersensitivity reactions, including anaphylaxis, and hematuria have been reported.

Arginine hydrochloride is metabolized to nitrogen-containing products for renal excretion. Excess arginine increases the production of nitric oxide (NO) to cause vasodilation/hypotension.

Continued

ARGININE CHLORIDE *continued*

Monitor acid/base status closely. Hyperglycemia, hyperkalemia, GI disturbances, IV extravasation, headache, and flushing may occur.

In addition to its use for chloride supplementation, arginine in urea cycle disorder therapy (increase arginine levels and prevent breakdown of endogenous proteins) and as a diagnostic agent for growth hormone (stimulates pituitary release of growth hormone).

ASCORBIC ACID
Vitamin C, Cecon, Sunkist Vitamin C, and many others
Water soluble vitamin

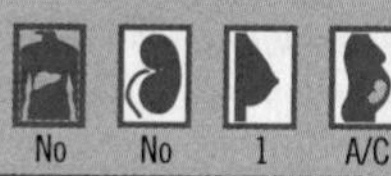

Tabs [OTC]: 250, 500 mg, 1, 1.5 g
Chewable tabs (Sunkist Vitamin C) [OTC]: 500 mg; some may contain aspartame
Tabs (timed release) [OTC]: 0.5, 1, 1.5 g
Caps [OTC]: 500 mg
Extended release caps [OTC]: 500 mg, 1 g
Injection: 500 mg/mL; may contain sodium hydrosulfite
Oral solution (Cecon) [OTC]: 100 mg/mL (50 mL with dropper)
Oral liquid [OTC]: 500 mg/5 mL (120, 480 mL)
Lozenges [OTC]: 25 mg (20s); contains 5 mg Na
Crystals [OTC]: 1 g per 1/4 teaspoonful (170 g, 1000 g)
Some products may contain approximately 5 mEq Na/1 g drug and/or calcium.

Scurvy (PO/IM/IV/SC):
Child: 100–300 mg/24 hr ÷ once daily–BID for at least 2 wk
Adult: 100–250 mg once daily–BID for at least 2 wk

U.S. Recommended Daily Allowance (RDA):
See Chapter 21.

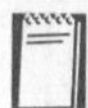

Adverse reactions: nausea, vomiting, heartburn, flushing, headache, faintness, dizziness, hyperoxaluria. Use high doses with **caution** in G6PD patients. May cause false-negative and false-positive urine glucose determinations with glucose oxidase and cupric sulfate tests, respectively.

May increase the absorption of aluminum hydroxide and increase the adverse/toxic effects of deferoxamine. May reduce the effects of amphetamines.

Oral dosing is preferred with or without food. IM route is the preferred parenteral route. Protect the injectable dosage form from light.

Pregnancy category changes to "C" if used in doses above the RDA.

ASPIRIN
ASA, Anacin, Bufferin, ZORprin, and various trade names
Nonsteroidal antiinflammatory agent, antiplatelet agent, analgesic

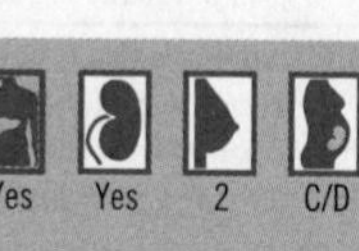

Tabs [OTC]: 325, 500 mg
Tabs, enteric-coated [OTC]: 81, 325 mg
Tabs, time-release:
OTC: 81, 650 mg
Prescription (ZORprin): 800 mg

Continued

For explanation of icons, see p. 663.

ASPIRIN *continued*

Tabs, buffered [OTC]: 325, 500 mg; may contain magnesium, aluminum, and/or calcium
Tabs, chewable [OTC]: 81 mg
Gum [OTC]: 227.5 mg
Suppository [OTC]: 120, 200, 300, 600 mg

Analgesic/antipyretic: 10–15 mg/kg/dose PO/PR Q4–6 hr up to total of 60–80 mg/kg/24 hr
Max. dose: 4 g/24 hr
Anti-inflammatory: 60–100 mg/kg/24 hr PO ÷ Q6–8 hr
Kawasaki disease: 80–100 mg/kg/24 hr PO ÷ QID during febrile phase until defervesces then decrease to 3–5 mg/kg/24 hr PO QAM. Continue for at least 8 wk or until both platelet count and ESR are normal.

Do not use in children <16 yr for treatment of varicella or flu-like symptoms (risk for Reye's syndrome), in combination with other nonsteroidal anti-inflammatory drugs, or in severe renal failure. **Use with caution** in bleeding disorders, renal dysfunction, gastritis, and gout. May cause GI upset, allergic reactions, liver toxicity, and decreased platelet aggregation. **See Chapter 2 for management of overdose.**

Drug interactions: may increase effects of methotrexate, valproic acid, and warfarin, which may lead to toxicity (protein displacement). Buffered dosage forms may decrease absorption of ketoconazole and tetracycline. GI bleeds have been reported with concurrent use of SSRIs (e.g., fluoxetine, paroxetine, sertraline).

Therapeutic levels: antipyretic/analgesic: 30–50 mg/L, anti-inflammatory: 150–300 mg/L. Tinnitus may occur at levels of 200–400 mg/L. Recommended serum sampling time at steady state: obtain trough level just prior to dose following 1–2 days of continuous dosing. Peak levels obtained 2 hr (for non-sustained release dosage forms) after a dose may be useful for monitoring toxicity.

Pregnancy category changes to "D" if full-dose aspirin is used during the third trimester. **Adjust dose in renal failure (see Chapter 31).**

ATENOLOL

Tenormin and various generics
Beta-1 selective adrenergic blocker

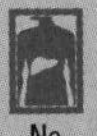
No

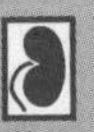
Yes

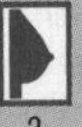
2

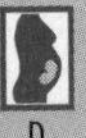
D

Tab: 25, 50, 100 mg
Oral suspension: 2 mg/mL 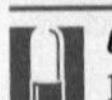

Child and adolescent: 0.5–1 mg/kg/dose PO once daily–BID; **max. dose:** 2 mg/kg/24 hr up to 100 mg/24 hr.
Adult:
PO: 25–100 mg/dose PO once daily; **max. dose:** 100 mg/24 hr

Contraindicated in pulmonary edema, cardiogenic shock. May cause bradycardia, hypotension, second- or third-degree AV block, dizziness, fatigue, lethargy, and headache. **Use with caution** in diabetes and asthma. Wheezing and dyspnea have occurred when daily dosage exceeds 100 mg/24 hr. Postmarketing evaluation reports a temporal relationship for causing elevated LFTs and/or bilirubin, hallucinations, psoriatic rash, thrombocytopenia, visual disturbances, and dry mouth. **Avoid** abrupt withdrawal of the drug. Does not cross the blood-brain barrier; lower incidence of CNS side effects compared to propranolol. Neonates born to mothers receiving atenolol during labor or while breastfeeding may be at risk for hypoglycemia.

Use with disopyramide, amiodarone, or digoxin may enhance bradycardic effects. **Adjust dose in renal impairment (see Chapter 31).**

ATOMOXETINE
Strattera
Norepinephrine reuptake inhibitor, attention deficit hyperactivity disorder agent

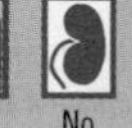
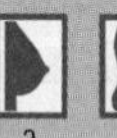
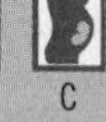

Yes No 3 C

Capsules: 10, 18, 25, 40, 60, 80, 100 mg

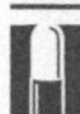

≤70 kg (child ≥6 yr and adolescent; see remarks):
Start with 0.5 mg/kg/24 hr PO QAM and increase after a minimum of 3 days to approximately 1.2 mg/kg/24 hr PO ÷ QAM or BID (morning and late afternoon/early evening). **Max. daily dose:** 1.4 mg/kg/24 hr or 100 mg, whichever is less.
If used with a strong CYP 450 2D6 inhibitor (e.g., fluoxetine, paroxetine, quinidine) or in patients with reduced CYP 450 2D6 activity: Maintain above initial dose for 4 wk and increase to a max. of 1.2 mg/kg/24 hr if symptoms do not improve and initial dose is tolerated.

>70 kg (child, adolescent, and adult; see remarks):
Start with 40 mg PO QAM and increase after a minimum of 3 days to about 80 mg/24 hr PO ÷ QAM or BID (morning and late afternoon/early evening). After 2–4 wk, dose may be increased to a max. of 100 mg/24 hr.
If used with a strong CYP 450 2D6 inhibitor (e.g., fluoxetine, paroxetine, quinidine) or in patients with reduced CYP 450 2D6 activity: Maintain above initial dose for 4 wk and increase to 80 mg/24 hr if symptoms do not improve and initial dose is tolerated.

Contraindicated in patients with narrow angle glaucoma and pheochromocytoma. **Do not** administer with or within 2 wk after discontinuing an MAO inhibitor; fatal reactions have been reported. **Use with caution** in hypertension, tachycardia, cardiovascular or cerebrovascular diseases, or with concurrent albuterol therapy. Increased risk of suicidal thinking has been reported; closely monitor for clinical worsening, agitation, irritability, suicidal thinking or behaviors, and unusual changes in behavior when initiating (first few months) or at times of dose changes (increases or decreases).

Atomoxetine is a CYP 450 2D6 substrate.

Doses >1.2 mg/kg/24 hr in patients ≤70 kg have not been shown to be of additional benefit. Reduce dose (initial and target doses) by 50% and 75% for patients with moderate (Child-Pugh Class B) and severe (Child-Pugh Class C) hepatic insufficiency, respectively.

Major side effects include GI discomfort, vomiting, fatigue, anorexia, dizziness, and mood swings. Hypersensitivity reactions, aggression, irritability, and severe liver injury have also been reported. Consider interrupting therapy in patients who are not growing or gaining weight satisfactorily.

Doses may be administered with or without food. Atomoxetine can be discontinued without tapering.

ATOVAQUONE
Mepron
Antiprotozoal

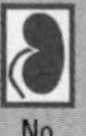
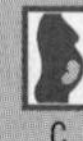
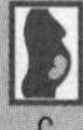

Yes No 3 C

Oral suspension: 750 mg/5 mL (210 mL); contains benzyl alcohol

Pneumocystis jiroveci (formerly carinii) pneumonia (PCP):
Treatment (21 day course):
Child: 30–40 mg/kg/24 hr PO ÷ BID with fatty foods; **max. dose:** 1500 mg/24 hr. Infants 3–24 mo may require higher doses of 45 mg/kg/24 hr.
≥13 yr and adult: 750 mg/dose PO BID

Continued

For explanation of icons, see p. 663.

ATOVAQUONE *continued*

Pneumocystis jiroveci (formerly carinii) pneumonia (PCP) (cont'd):
Prophylaxis (1st episode and recurrence):

Child 1–3 mo or >24 mo: 30 mg/kg/24 hr PO once daily; **max. dose:** 1500 mg/24 hr
Child 4–24 mo: 45 mg/kg/24 hr PO once daily; **max. dose:** 1500 mg/24 hr
≥13 yr and adult: 1500 mg/dose PO once daily

Toxoplasma gondii:

Child:

First episode prophylaxis: Use PCP prophylaxis dosages.

Adult:

Treatment: 1500 mg/dose PO BID ± sulfadiazine 1000–1500 mg PO Q6 hr.
First episode prophylaxis: 1500 mg/dose PO once daily ± pyrimethamine 25 mg PO once daily PLUS leucovorin 10 mg PO once daily.
Recurrence prophylaxis: 750 mg/dose PO Q6–12 hr ± pyrimethamine 25 mg PO once daily PLUS leucovorin 10 mg PO once daily.

Not recommended in the treatment of severe PCP due to the lack of clinical data. Patients with GI disorders or severe vomiting and who cannot tolerate oral therapy should consider alternative IV therapies. Rash, pruritus, sweating, GI symptoms, LFT elevation, dizziness, headache, insomnia, anxiety, cough, and fever are common. Anemia and pancreatitis have been reported.

Metoclopramide, rifampin, rifabutin, and tetracycline may decrease atovaquone levels. Shake oral suspension well before dispensing all doses. Take all doses with high fat foods to maximize absorption.

ATROPINE SULFATE
Sal-Tropine, AtroPen, and many other generic products
Anticholinergic agent

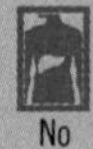
No
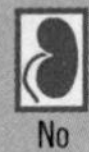
No
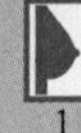
1
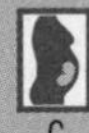
C

Tabs (Sal-Tropine): 0.4 mg
Injection: 0.4, 1 mg/mL
Injection (auto-injector):

AtroPen 0.5 mg: delivers a single 0.5 mg (0.7 mL) dose (blue colored pen)
AtroPen 1 mg: delivers a single 1 mg (0.7 mL) dose (dark red colored pen)
AtroPen 2 mg: delivers a single 2 mg (0.7 mL) dose (green colored pen)

Ointment (ophthalmic): 1% (1, 3.5 g)
Solution (ophthalmic): 1% (2, 5, 15 mL)

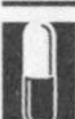

Pre-anesthesia dose (30–60 min pre operation):

Child: 0.01 mg/kg/dose SC/IV/IM, **max. dose:** 0.4 mg/dose; **min. dose:** 0.1 mg/dose; may repeat Q4–6 hr
Adult: 0.5 mg/dose SC/IV/IM

Cardiopulmonary resuscitation (see remarks):

Child: 0.02 mg/kg/dose IV Q5 min × 2–3 doses PRN; **min. dose:** 0.1 mg; **max. single dose:** 0.5 mg in children, 1 mg in adolescents; **max. total dose:** 1 mg children, 2 mg adolescents
Adult: 0.5–1 mg/dose IV Q5 min; **max. total dose:** 2 mg

Bronchospasm: 0.025–0.05 mg/kg/dose (**max. dose:** 2.5 mg/dose) in 2.5 mL NS Q6–8 hr via nebulizer

Nerve agent and insecticide poisoning for muscarinic symptoms (organophosphate or carbamate poisoning) (IV/IM/ET; dilute in 1–2 mL NS for ET administration):

Child: 0.05–0.1 mg/kg Q 5–10 min until bronchial or oral secretions terminate.
Adult: 2–5 mg/dose Q5–10 min until bronchial or oral secretions terminate.

Continued

ATROPINE SULFATE *continued*

AtroPen device (IM route): Inject as soon as exposure is known or suspected. Give one dose for mild symptoms and two additional doses (total 3 doses) in rapid succession 10 min after the first dose for severe symptoms as follows:

Child 6 mo–4 yr (15–40 lbs): 0.5 mg
Child 4–10 yr (40–90 lbs): 1 mg
Child >10 yr and adult (≥90 lbs): 2 mg

Ophthalmic (uveitis):

Child: (0.5% solution; prepared by diluting equal volume of the 1% atropine ophthalmic solution with artificial tears) 1–2 drops in each eye once daily–TID
Adult: (1% solution) 1–2 drops in each eye once daily–QID

Contraindicated in glaucoma, obstructive uropathy, tachycardia, and thyrotoxicosis. **Use with caution** in patients sensitive to sulfites.

Doses <0.1 mg have been associated with paradoxical bradycardia. Side effects include dry mouth, blurred vision, fever, tachycardia, constipation, urinary retention, CNS signs (dizziness, hallucinations, restlessness, fatigue, headache).

In case of bradycardia, may give via endotracheal tube (dilute with NS to volume of 1–2 mL) or intraosseous (IO) route. Use injectable solution for nebulized use; can be mixed with albuterol for simultaneous administration.

AURALGAN

See Antipyrine and Benzocaine

AZATHIOPRINE

Imuran, Azasan, and others
Immunosuppressant

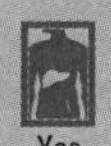
Yes
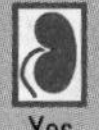
Yes

3
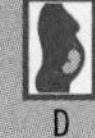
D

Oral suspension: 50 mg/mL
Tabs:
Imuran: 50 mg
Azasan: 75, 100 mg
Injection: 100 mg (20 mL)

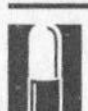

Immunosuppression:
Child and adult:
Initial: 3–5 mg/kg/24 hr IV/PO once daily
Maintenance: 1–3 mg/kg/24 hr IV/PO once daily

Toxicity: bone marrow suppression, rash, stomatitis, hepatotoxicity, alopecia, arthralgias, and GI disturbances. Use ¼–⅓ dose when given with allopurinol. Increased risk for hepatosplenic T-cell lymphoma has been reported in adolescents and young adults. Toxicity: bone marrow suppression, rash, stomatitis, hepatotoxicity, alopecia, arthralgias, and GI disturbances. Use ¼–⅓ dose when given with allopurinol. Dose reduction or discontinuance is recommended in patients with low or absent thiopurine methyl transferase (TPMT) activity. Severe anemia has been reported when used in combination with captopril or enalapril. Monitor CBC, platelets, total bilirubin, alkaline phosphatase, BUN, and creatinine. **Adjust dose in renal failure (see Chapter 31).**

Administer oral doses with food to minimize GI discomfort.

For explanation of icons, see p. 663.

AZELASTINE
Astelin, Opitvar
Antihistamine

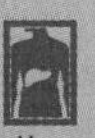
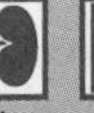
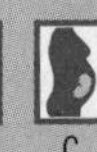

Yes Yes ? C

Nasal spray (Astelin): 1% (137 mcg/spray), 200 actuations (30 mL)
Ophthalmic drops (Opitvar): 0.05% (0.5 mg/mL) (6 mL)

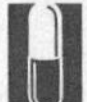

Seasonal allergic rhinitis:

Child 5–11 yr: 1 spray each nostril BID
≥12 yr and adult: 2 sprays each nostril BID

Ophthalmic:

≥3 yr and adult: Instill 1 drop into each affected eye BID

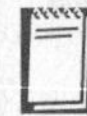

Use with caution in asthmatics. Reduced dosages have been recommended in patients with renal and hepatic dysfunction. Optivar **should not be used** to treat contact lens related irritation. Soft contact lens users should wait at least 10 min after dose instillation before they insert their lenses.

Drowsiness may occur despite the nasal route of administration (**avoid** concurrent use of alcohol or CNS depressants). Bitter taste, nasal burning, pharyngitis, weight gain, fatigue, and epistaxis may also occur with nasal route. Eye burning and stinging have been reported in about 30% of patients receiving the ophthalmic dosage form.

AZITHROMYCIN
Zithromax, Zithromax TRI-PAK, Zithromax Z-PAK,
Zmax (extended release oral suspension), Azasite
Antibiotic, macrolide

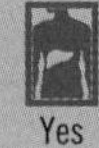
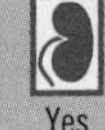
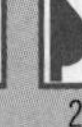
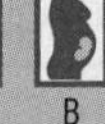

Yes Yes 2 B

Tablets: 250, 500, 600 mg
TRI-PAK: 500 mg (3s as unit dose pack)
Z-PAK: 250 mg (6s as unit dose pack)
Oral suspension: 100 mg/5 mL (15 mL), 200 mg/5 mL (15, 22.5, 30 mL)
Oral Powder (Sachet): 1 g (3s, 10s)
Extended release oral suspension (microspheres):
Zmax: 2 g reconstituted with 60 mL of water
Injection: 500 mg; contains 9.92 mEq Na/1 g drug
Ophthalmic solution (Azasite): 1% (2.5 mL)

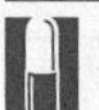

Child:
Otitis media (≥6 mo):

5 day regimen: 10 mg/kg PO day 1 (**max. dose:** 500 mg), followed by 5 mg/kg/24 hr PO once daily (**max. dose:** 250 mg/24 hr) on days 2–5
3 day regimen: 10 mg/kg/24 hr PO once daily × 3 days (**max. dose:** 500 mg/24 hr)
1 day regimen: 30 mg/kg/24 hr PO ×1 (**max. dose:** 1500 mg/24 hr)

Community acquired pneumonia (≥6 mo):

Tablet or oral suspension: Use otitis media 5 day regimen from above.
Extended release oral suspension (Zmax): 60 mg/kg (**max. dose:** 2 g) PO × 1.

Pharyngitis/tonsillitis (2–15 yr): 12 mg/kg/24 hr PO once daily × 5 days (**max. dose:** 500 mg/24 hr)
Acute sinusitis (≥6 mo): 10 mg/kg/dose (**max. dose:** 500 mg) PO once daily × 3 days

Continued

AZITHROMYCIN *continued*

Pertussis:

Infant <6 mo: 10 mg/kg/dose PO once daily × 5 days.

≥6 mo: 10 mg/kg/dose (**max. dose:** 500 mg) PO × 1, followed by 5 mg/kg (**max. dose:** 250 mg) PO once daily on days 2–5.

M. avium complex in HIV (see www.aidsinfo.nih.gov/guidelines for most current recommendations):

Prophylaxis for first episode: 20 mg/kg/dose PO Q 7 days (**max. dose:** 1200 mg/dose); alternatively, 5 mg/kg/24 hr PO once daily (**max. dose:** 250 mg/dose) with or without rifabutin.

Prophylaxis for recurrence: 5 mg/kg/24 hr PO once daily (**max. dose:** 250 mg/dose), plus ethambutol 15 mg/kg/24 hr (**max. dose:** 900 mg/24 hr) PO once daily with or without rifabutin 5 mg/kg/24 hr (**max. dose:** 300 mg/24 hr).

Treatment: 10–12 mg/kg/24 hr PO once daily (**max. dose:** 500 mg/24 hr) × 1 month or longer, plus ethambutol 15–25 mg/kg/24 hr (**max. dose:** 1 g/24 hr) PO once daily with or without rifabutin 10–20 mg/kg/24 hr (**max. dose:** 300 mg/24 hr).

Anti-inflammatory agent in Cystic Fibrosis:

25–39 kg: 250 mg PO every Mondays, Wednesdays, and Fridays.

≥40 kg: 500 mg PO every Mondays, Wednesdays, and Fridays.

Adolescent and adult:

Pharyngitis, tonsillitis, skin, and soft tissue infection: 500 mg PO day 1, then 250 mg/24 hr PO on days 2–5

Mild/moderate bacterial COPD exacerbation: above 5 day dosing regimen OR 500 mg PO once daily × 3 days

Community acquired pneumonia:

Tablets: 500 mg PO day 1, then 250 mg/24 hr PO on days 2–5

Extended release oral suspension (Zmax): Single dose 2 g PO

IV and tablet regimen: 500 mg IV once daily × 2 days followed by 500 mg PO once daily to complete a 7- to 10-day regimen (IV and PO)

Sinusitis:

Tablets: 500 mg PO once daily × 3 days

Extended release oral suspension (Zmax): Single dose 2 g PO

Uncomplicated chlamydial cervicitis or urethritis: Single 1 g dose PO

Gonococcal cervicitis or urethritis: Single 2 g dose PO

Acute PID (chlamydia): 500 mg IV once daily × 1–2 days followed by 250 mg PO once daily to complete a 7 day regimen (IV and PO).

M. avium complex in HIV (see www.aidsinfo.nih.gov/guidelines for most recent recommendations):

Prophylaxis for first episode: 1200 mg PO Q 7 days with or without rifabutin 300 mg PO once daily

Prophylaxis for recurrence: 500 mg PO once daily, plus ethambutol 15 mg/kg/dose PO QD, with or without rifabutin 300 mg PO once daily

Treatment: 500–600 mg PO once daily with ethambutol 15 mg/kg/dose PO once daily with or without rifabutin 300 mg PO once daily.

Anti-inflammatory agent in Cystic Fibrosis: use same dosing in children.

Ophthalmic:

≥1 yr and adult: Instill one drop into the affected eye(s) BID, 8–12 hr apart, × 2 days, followed by one drop once daily for the next 5 days.

Contraindicated in hypersensitivity to macrolides and history of cholestatic jaundice/hepatic dysfuction associated with prior use. **Use with caution** in impaired hepatic function, GFR <10 mL/min (limited data), and prolonged QT intervals. Can cause increase in hepatic

Continued

For explanation of icons, see p. 663.

AZITHROMYCIN *continued*

hepatic enzymes, cholestatic jaundice, GI discomfort, and pain at injection site (IV use). Compared to other macrolides, less risk for drug interactions. Nelfinavir may increase azithromycin levels; monitor for liver enzyme abnormalities and hearing impairment. Vomiting, diarrhea, and nausea have been reported at higher frequency in otitis media with 1 day dosing regimen. Exacerbations of myasthenia gravis/syndrome have been reported. CNS penetration is poor.

Aluminum- and magnesium-containing antacids decrease absorption. Tablet and oral suspension dosage forms may be administered with or without food. Extended release oral suspension should be taken on an empty stomach (at least 1 hr before or 2 hr following a meal). Intravenous administration is over 1–3 hr; **do not** give as a bolus or IM injection.

Ophthalmic use: **Do not** wear contact lenses. Eye irritation is the most common side effect.

AZTREONAM

Azactam, Caysten

Antibiotic, monobactam

No Yes 1 B

Injection: 1, 2 g

Frozen injection: 1 g/50 mL 3.4% dextrose, 2 g/50 mL 1.4% dextrose (iso-osmotic solutions)

Each 1 g drug contains approximately 780 mg L-Arginine

Nebulizer solution (Caysten): 75 mg powder to be reconstituted with the supplied diluent of 1 mL 0.17% sodium chloride (28 day course kit contains 84 sterile vials of Caysten and 88 ampules of diluent)

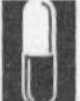

Neonate:

30 mg/kg/dose:

<1.2 kg and 0–4 wk age: Q12 hr IV/IM

1.2–2 kg and 0–7 days: Q12 hr IV/IM

1.2–2 kg and >7 days: Q8 hr IV/IM

>2 kg and 0–7 days: Q8 hr IV/IM

>2 kg and >7 days: Q6 hr IV/IM

Child: 90–120 mg/kg/24 hr ÷ Q6–8 hr IV/IM

Cystic Fibrosis: 150–200 mg/kg/24 hr ÷ Q6–8 hr IV/IM

Adult:

Moderate infections: 1–2 g/dose Q8–12 hr IV/IM

Severe infections: 2 g/dose Q6–8 hr IV/IM

Max. dose: 8 g/24 hr

Inhalation:

Cystic Fibrosis prophylaxis therapy:

≥7 yr and adult: 75 mg TID (minimum 4 hr between doses) administered in repeated cycles of 28 days on drug followed by 28 days off drug. Administer each dose with the Altera Nebulizer System.

Typically indicated in multidrug resistant aerobic gram-negative infections when beta-lactam therapy is **contraindicated**. Well-absorbed IM. **Use with caution** in arginase deficiency. Low cross-allergenicity between aztreonam and other beta-lactams. Adverse reactions: thrombophlebitis, eosinophilia, leukopenia, neutropenia, thrombocytopenia, elevation of liver enzymes, hypotension, seizures, and confusion. Good CNS penetration. **Adjust dose in renal failure (see Chapter 31).**

INHALATIONAL USE: Cough, nasal congestion, wheezing, pharyngolaryngeal pain, pyrexia, chest discomfort, abdominal pain, and vomiting may occur. Bronchospasm has been reported. Use the following order of administration: bronchodilator first, chest physiotherapy, other inhaled medications (if indicated), and aztreonam last.

BACITRACIN ± POLYMYXIN B
AK-Tracin Ophthalmic, Baciguent Topical, and others; in combination with polymyxin b: AK-Poly-Bac Ophthalmic, Polysporin Ophthalmic, Polysporin Topical, and others
Antibiotic, topical

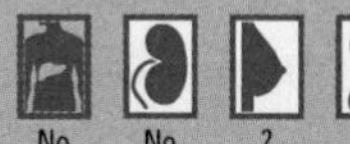

BACITRACIN:
Ophthalmic ointment: 500 units/g (3.5 g)
Topical ointment: 500 units/g (15, 30 g)
BACITRACIN IN COMBINATION WITH POLYMYXIN B:
Ophthalmic ointment: 500 units bacitracin + 10,000 units polymyxin B/g (3.5 g)
Topical ointment: 500 units bacitracin + 10,000 units polymyxin B/g (15, 30 g)

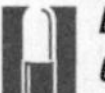

BACITRACIN
Child and adult:
Topical: Apply to affected area 1–5 times/24 hr.
Ophthalmic: Apply 0.25–0.5 inch ribbon into the conjunctival sac of the infected eye(s) Q 3–12 hr; frequency depends on severity of infection. Administer Q3–4 hr × 7–10 days for mild/moderate infections.
BACITRACIN + POLYMYXIN B
Child and adult:
Topical: Apply ointment or powder to affected area once daily–TID
Ophthalmic: Apply 0.25–0.5 inch ribbon into the conjunctival sac of the infected eye(s) Q 3–12 hr; frequency depends on severity of infection. Administer Q3–4 hr × 7–10 days for mild/moderate infections.

Hypersensitivity reactions to bacitracin and/or polymyxin B can occur. **Do not use** topical ointment for the eyes. Side effects may include rash, itching, burning, and edema. Ophthalmic dosage form may cause temporary blurred vision and retard corneal healing. For neomycin containing products, see *Neomycin/Polymyxin B/± Bacitracin.*

BACLOFEN
Lioresal, Kemstro, and various
Centrally acting skeletal muscle relaxant

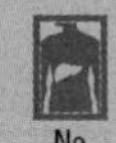
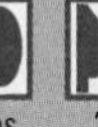
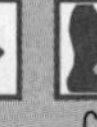
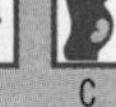

Tabs: 10, 20 mg
Disintegrating oral tabs (Kemstro): 10, 20 mg; contains phenylalanine
Oral suspension: 5, 10 mg/mL
Intrathecal injection: 50 mcg/mL (1 mL), 0.5 mg/mL (20 mL), 2 mg/mL (5 mL); preservative-free

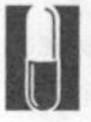

Oral: Dosage increments, if tolerated, are made at 3-day intervals until desired effect or* max. dose *is achieved. Initiate first dosage level at QHS, followed by Q12 hr and then Q8 hr. Dosage increments are made by first increasing the QHS dosage, followed by the morning dosage and then the remaining mid-day dosage.
Child (PO, see remarks):
<20 kg: Start at 2.5 mg QHS, increase in 2.5-mg increments if needed up to the recommended **max. dose** below.
≥20–50 kg: Start at 5 mg QHS, increase in 5-mg increments if needed up to the recommended **max. dose** below.
>50 kg: Start at 10 mg QHS, increase in 10-mg increments if needed up to the recommended **max. dose** below.

Continued

For explanation of icons, see p. 663.

BACLOFEN *continued*

Recommended max. PO dose:

<8 yr: 60 mg/24 hr

8–16 yr: 80 mg/24 hr

>16 yr: 120 mg//24 hr

Adult (PO):

Start at 5 mg TID, increase in 5-mg increments if needed up to a maximum of 80 mg/24 hr.

Intrathecal continuous infusion maintenance therapy (not well established):

<12 yr: average dose of 274 mcg/24 hr (range: 24–1199 mcg/24 hr) has been reported.

≥12 yr and adult: most required 300–800 mcg/24 hr (range: 12–2003 mcg/24 hr with limited experience at doses >1000 mcg/24 hr)

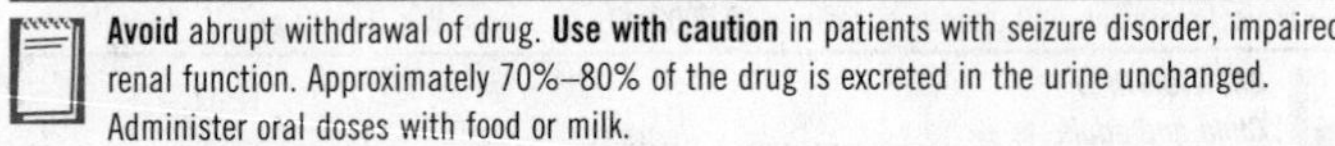

Avoid abrupt withdrawal of drug. **Use with caution** in patients with seizure disorder, impaired renal function. Approximately 70%–80% of the drug is excreted in the urine unchanged. Administer oral doses with food or milk.

Adverse effects: Drowsiness, fatigue, nausea, vertigo, psychiatric disturbances, rash, urinary frequency, and hypotonia. **Avoid** abrupt withdrawal of intrathecal therapy to prevent potential life-threatening events (rhabdomyolysis, multiple organ-system failure, and death).

Usual ranges observed from a single institution retrospective review in 87 patients include the following:

2 yr: 10–20 mg/24 hr

2–7 yr: 20–30 mg/24 hr

≥8 yr: 30–40 mg/24 hr

BECLOMETHASONE DIPROPIONATE

QVAR, Beconase AQ

Corticosteroid

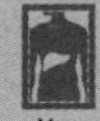
Yes
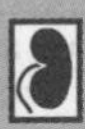
No
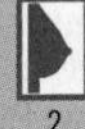
2
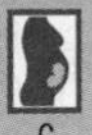
C

Inhalation, oral:

QVAR: 40 mcg/inhalation (100 inhalations, 7.3 g), 80 mcg/inhalation (100 inhalations, 7.3 g); CFC-free product (HFA)

Inhalation, nasal:

Beconase AQ: 42 mcg/inhalation (200 metered doses, 25 g)

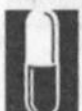

Oral inhalation (QVAR):

5–11 yr: 40 mcg BID; **max. dose:** 80 mcg BID

≥12 yr and adult:

Corticosteroid naïve: 40–80 mcg BID; **max. dose:** 320 mcg BID

Previous corticosteroid use: 40–160 mcg BID; **max. dose:** 320 mcg BID

Nasal inhalation (Beconase AQ):

6–12 yr: Start with 1 spray each nostril BID, may increase to 2 sprays each nostril BID if needed. Once symptoms are controlled, decrease dose to 1 spray each nostril BID.

>12 yr and adult: 1–2 spray(s) each nostril BID

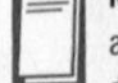

Not recommended for children <5 yr with oral inhalation and <6 yr with the nasal administration due to unknown safety and efficacy. Dose should be titrated to lowest effective dose. **Avoid** using higher than recommended doses.

CYP 450 3A4 inhibitors (e.g., ketoconazole, erythromycin, and protease inhibitors) or significant hepatic impairment may increase systemic exposure of beclomethasone.

Monitor for hypothalamic, pituitary, adrenal, or growth suppression, and hypercorticism. Rinse mouth and gargle with water after oral inhalation; may cause thrush. Consider using with tube spacers for oral inhalation.

BENZOYL PEROXIDE
Benzac AC Wash 2 1/2, 5, 10; Benzac 5,10; Brevoxyl Creamy Wash, Desquam-E 5, Desquam-E 10, NeoBenz Micro, Oxy-5, Oxy-10, Triaz, Zoderm, and many other names
Topical acne product

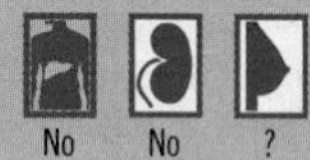

Liquid wash: 2.5% (240 mL), 5% (120, 150, 240 mL), 10% (120, 150, 240 mL)
Liquid cream wash: 4% (180 g), 8% (10 g)
Bar: 5% [OTC] (113 g), 10% [OTC] (106, 113 g)
Lotion: 3% (170, 340 g), 4% (297 g), 5% [OTC] (30 mL), 6% (170, 340 g), 8% (297 g), 10% [OTC] (30 mL, 85, 170, 340 g)
Cleanser: 4.5% (400 mL), 6.5% (400 mL), 8.5% (400 mL)
Cleanser/Mask: [OTC] 3.5% (125 mL)
Cream: 3.5% (45 g), 4.5% (125 mL), 5% [OTC] (18 g), 5.5% (45 g), 6.5% (125 mL), 8.5% (45 g, 125 mL), 10% [OTC] (30 g)
Gel: 2.5% (60 g), 3% (42.5 g), 4% (42.5, 90 g), 4.5% (125 mL), 5% [OTC] (42.5, 60, 90 g), 6% (42.5%), 7% (45, 90 g), 8% (42.5, 90 g), 8.5% (125 mL), 9% (42.5 g), 10% (45, 60, 90, 113.4 g)
NOTE: Some preparations may contain alcohol.
Combination product with erythromycin (Benzamycin and others):
Gel: 30 mg erythromycin and 50 mg benzoyl peroxide per g (0.8, 23.3, 46 g); some preparations may contain 20% alcohol
Combination product with clindamycin:
Gel:
BenzaClin and generics: 10 mg clindamycin and 50 mg benzoyl peroxide per g (25, 50 g); some preparations may contain methylparaben.
Duac: 10 mg clindamycin and 50 mg benzoyl peroxide per g (45 g); Duac CS is packaged with a bottle of soap-free cleanser lotion containing PEG 75, sodium cocoyl isethionate steraryl alcohol, and parabens.
Acanya: 12 mg clindamycin and 25 mg benzoyl peroxide per g (50 g).

Child ≥12 yr and adult:
Cleansers (liquid wash, or bar): Wet affected area prior to application. Apply and wash once daily–BID; rinse thoroughly and pat dry. Modify dose frequency or concentration to control the amount of drying or peeling.
Lotion, cream, or gel: Cleanse skin and apply small amounts over affected areas once daily initially; increase frequency to BID–TID if needed. Modify dose frequency or concentration to control drying or peeling.
Combination products:
Benzamycin, BenzaClin, and generics: Apply BID (morning and evening) to affected areas after washing and drying skin.
Duac: Apply QHS to affected areas after washing and drying skin.
Acanya: Apply pea-sized amount once daily.

Contraindicated in known history of hypersensitivity to product's components (benzoyl peroxide, clindamycin, or erythromycin). **Avoid** contact with mucous membranes and eyes. May cause skin irritation, stinging, dryness, peeling, erythema, edema, and contact dermatitis. Anaphylaxis have been reported with products containing clindamycin and benzoyl peroxide.

Concurrent use with tretinoin (Retin-A) will increase risk of skin irritation. Products containing clindamycin and erythromycin should not be used in combination.

Any single application resulting in excessive stinging or burning may be removed with mild soap and water. Lotion, cream, and gel dosage forms should be applied to dry skin.

For explanation of icons, see p. 663.

BENZTROPINE MESYLATE
Cogentin and various generics
Anticholinergic agent, drug induced dystonic reaction antidote, anti-Parkinson's agent

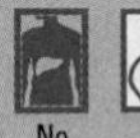 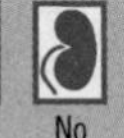  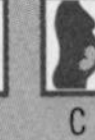
No No ? C

Injection: 1 mg/mL (2 mL)
Tabs: 0.5, 1, 2 mg

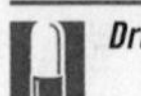

Drug-induced extrapyramidal symptoms:
>3 yr: 0.02–0.05 mg/kg/dose once daily–BID PO/IM/IV
Adult: 1–4 mg/dose once daily–BID PO/IM/IV

Acute dystonic reaction (phenothiazines):
Child: 0.02 mg/kg/dose (**max. dose:** 1 mg) × 1 IM/IV
Adult: 1–2 mg/dose ×1 IM/IV

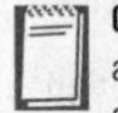

Contraindicated in myasthenia gravis, GI/GU obstruction, untreated narrow-angle glaucoma, and peptic ulcer. Use IV route **only** when PO and IM routes are not feasible. May cause anti-cholinergic side effects, especially constipation and dry mouth. Drug interactions include potentiation of CNS depressant effects when used with CNS depressants; enhance CNS side effects of amantadine; and inhibit the response of neuroleptics.

Onset of action: 15 min for IV/IM and 1 hr for PO.
Oral doses should be administered with food to decrease GI upset.

BERACTANT

See Surfactant, pulmonary

BETAMETHASONE
Beta-Val, Celestone, Celestone Soluspan, Diprolene, Diprolene AF, Diprosone, Maxivate, and others
Corticosteroid

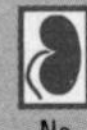 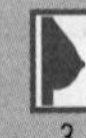 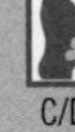
No No 3 C/D

Betamethasone base (Celestone):
Oral solution: 0.6 mg/5 mL (120 mL); contains alcohol

Na Phosphate and Acetate (Celestone Soluspan):
Injection suspension: 6 mg/mL (3 mg/mL Na phosphate + 3 mg/mL betamethasone acetate) (5 mL)

Dipropionate (Diprosone, Maxivate, and others):
Topical aerosol: 0.1% (85g) with 10% isopropyl alcohol
Topical cream: 0.05% (15, 45 g)
Topical lotion: 0.05% (20, 30, 60 mL); may contain 46.8% alcohol
Topical ointment: 0.05% (15, 45 g)

Valerate (Beta-Val and others):
Topical cream: 0.05%, 0.1% (15, 45 g)
Topical foam: 1.2 mg/g (50, 100 g); may contain 60.4% ethanol, cetyl alcohol, stearyl alcohol
Topical lotion: 0.1% (30, 60 mL); may contain 47.5% isopropyl alcohol
Topical ointment: 0.1% (15, 45 g)

Continued

BETAMETHASONE *continued*

Dipropionate augmented (Diprolene, Diprolene AF, and others):

Topical cream: 0.05% (15, 45, 50 g); contains propylene glycol
Topical gel: 0.05% (15, 50 g); contains propylene glycol
Topical lotion: 0.05% (30, 60 mL); contains 30% isopropyl alcohol
Topical ointment: 0.05% (15, 45, 50 g); contains propylene glycol

All dosages should be adjusted based on patient response and severity of condition (see remarks).

Anti-inflammatory:

Child:

Oral: 0.0175–0.25 mg/kg/24 hr or 0.5–7.5 mg/m²/24 hr ÷ Q6–8 hr
IM: 0.0175–0.125 mg/kg/24 hr or 0.5–7.5 mg/m²/24 hr ÷ Q6–12 hr

Adolescent and adult:

Oral: 2.4–4.8 mg/24 hr ÷ Q6–12 hr; may range from 0.6–7.2 mg/24 hr depending on disease being treated
IM: 0.6–9 mg/24 hr ÷ Q12–24 hr

Topical (use smallest amount for shortest period of time to avoid adrenal suppression and reassess diagnosis if no improvement is achieved after 2 weeks; see remarks):

Valerate and dipropionate forms:

Child and adult: Apply to affected areas once daily–BID

Dipropionate augmented forms:

≥13 yr–adult: Apply to affected areas once daily–BID
Max. dose: 14 days and
Cream and ointment: 45 g/week
Gel: 50 g/week
Lotion: 50 mL/week

Use with caution in hypothyroidism, cirrhosis, and ulcerative colitis. See Chapter 30 for relative steroid potencies and doses based on body surface area. Betamethasone is inadequate when used alone for adrenocortical insufficiency because of its minimal mineralocorticoid properties. Like all steroids, may cause hypertension, pseudotumor cerebri, acne, Cushing's syndrome, adrenal axis suppression, GI bleeding, hyperglycemia, and osteoporosis.

Na phosphate and acetate injectable suspension recommended for IM, intraarticular, intrasynovial, intralesional, soft tissue use only; but not for IV use. **Topical betamethasone dipropionate augmented (Diprolene and Diprolene AF) is not recommended in children ≤12 yr owing to the higher risk for adrenal suppression.**

Used in premature labor to stimulate fetal lung maturation. Pregnancy category changes to "D" if used in first trimester.

BETHANECHOL CHLORIDE

Urecholine and other brand names
Cholinergic agent

No No ? C

Tabs: 5, 10, 25, 50 mg
Oral suspension: 1, 5 mg/mL 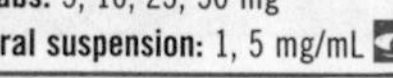

Child:

Abdominal distention/urinary retention: 0.6 mg/kg/24 hr ÷ Q6–8 hr PO
Gastroesophageal reflux: 0.1–0.2 mg/kg/dose 30 min–1 hr before meals and QHS PO; **max. dose:** 4 doses/24 hr

Continued

For explanation of icons, see p. 663.

BETHANECHOL CHLORIDE *continued*

Adult:

Urinary retention: 10–50 mg Q6–12 hr PO

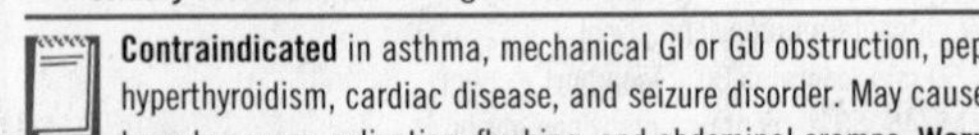

Contraindicated in asthma, mechanical GI or GU obstruction, peptic ulcer disease, hyperthyroidism, cardiac disease, and seizure disorder. May cause hypotension, nausea, bronchospasm, salivation, flushing, and abdominal cramps. **Warning: severe hypotension may occur when given with ganglionic blockers (e.g., trimethaphan). Atropine is the antidote.**

BICITRA

See Citrate Mixtures

BISACODYL

Dulcolax, Fleet Laxative, Fleet Bisacodyl, Doxidan, and various other names

Laxative, stimulant

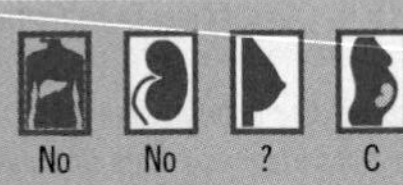

Tabs (enteric-coated): 5 mg
Suppository: 10 mg
Enema (Fleet Bisacodyl): 10 mg/30 mL (37.5 mL)
Delayed released tabs (Doxidan): 5 mg

Oral:

Child (3–12 yr): 0.3 mg/kg/24 hr or 5–10 mg to be given 6 hr before desired effect; **max. dose:** 30 mg/24 hr

Adolescent and adult (>12 yr): 5–15 mg to be given 6 hr before desired effect; **max. dose:** 30 mg/24 hr

Rectal suppository (as a single dose):

<2 yr: 5 mg
2–11 yr: 5–10 mg
>11 yr and adult: 10 mg

Rectal enema (as a single dose):

≥12 yr and adult: 30 mL

Do not use in newborn period. **Do not** chew or crush tablets (shallow whole); **do not** give within 1 hr of antacids or milk. May cause abdominal cramps, nausea, vomiting, and rectal irritation. Oral usually effective within 6–10 hr; rectal usually effective within 15–60 min.

BISMUTH SUBSALICYLATE

Pepto-Bismol, Kaopectate, Kaopectate Children's, Maalox Total Relief, and others (see remarks)

Antidiarrheal, gastrointestinal ulcer agent

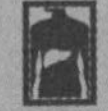

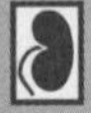

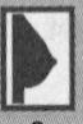

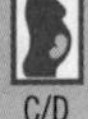

Liquid [OTC]: 262 mg/15 mL (120, 240, 360, 480 mL), 524 mg/15mL (120, 240, 360 mL)

Kaopectate Children's [OTC]: 87 mg/5 mL (180 mL)

Maalox Total Relief [OTC]: 525 mg/15 mL (355 mL)

Caplet [OTC]: 262 mg
Chewable tabs [OTC]: 262 mg

Continued

B

FORMULARY

BISMUTH SUBSALICYLATE *continued*

Contains 102 mg salicylate per 262 mg tablet; or 129 mg salicylate per 15 mL of the 262 mg/15 mL suspension.

Diarrhea:

Child: 100 mg/kg/24 hr ÷ 5 equal doses for 5 days; **max. dose:** 4.19 g/24 hr

Dosage by age: Give following dose Q 30 min to 1 hr PRN up to a **max. dose** of 8 doses/24 hr:

3–5 yr: 87.3 mg (1/3 tablet or 5 mL of 262 mg/15 mL)
6–8 yr: 174.7 mg (2/3 tablet or 10 mL of 262 mg/15 mL)
9–11 yr: 262 mg (1 tablet or 15 mL of 262 mg/15 mL)
≥12 yr–adult: 524 mg (2 tablets or 30 mL of 262 mg/15 mL)

H. pylori gastric infection (in combination with ampicillin and metronidazole or with tetracycline and metronidazole for adults; doses not well established for children):

<10 yr: 262 mg PO QID × 6 wk
≥10 yr–adult: 524 mg PO QID × 6 wk

Generally **not recommended** in children <16 yr with chicken pox or flu-like symptoms (risk for Reye's syndrome), in combination with other nonsteroidal anti-inflammatory drugs, anticoagulants or oral antidiabetic agents, or in severe renal failure. **Use with caution** in bleeding disorders, renal dysfunction, gastritis, and gout. May cause darkening of tongue and/or black stools, GI upset, impaction, and decreased platelet aggregation.

Drug combination appears to have antisecretory and antimicrobial effects with some anti-inflammatory effects. Absorption of bismuth is negligible, whereas approximately 80% of the salicylate is absorbed. Decreases absorption of tetracycline. Pregnancy category changes to "D" if used during the third trimester.

DO NOT use Children's Pepto (calcium carbonate) because it does not contain bismuth subsalicylate. **Avoid use in renal failure (see Chapter 31).**

BROMPHENIRAMINE WITH PHENYLEPHRINE
Dimetapp Children's Cold and Allergy, and many others
Antihistamine + decongestant

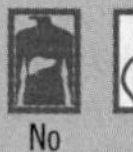
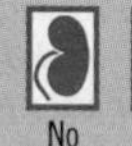
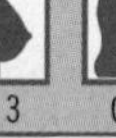
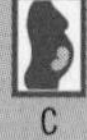

No No 3 C

Elixir (Dimetapp Children's Cold and Allergy) [OTC]: Brompheniramine 1 mg + phenylephrine 2.5 mg/5 mL (237 mL)
Chewable tab (Dimetapp Children's Cold and Allergy) [OTC]: Brompheniramine 1 mg + phenylephrine 2.5 mg

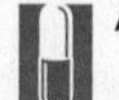

All doses based on brompheniramine component.

2–<6 yr: 1 mg Q4 hr PO up to a **max. dose** of 6 mg/24 hr
6–12 yr: 2 mg Q4 hr PO up to a **max. dose** of 12 mg/24 hr
≥12 yr: 4 mg Q4 hr PO up to a **max. dose** of 24 mg/24 hr

Alternatively, dosing based on specific dosage forms/products. CAUTION: These products are available in different concentrations.

Oral, elixir (Dimetapp Children's Cold and Allergy):

6–<12 yr: 10 mL Q4 hr PO up to a **max. dose** of 60 mL/24 hr
≥12 yr: 20 mL Q4 hr PO up to a **max. dose** of 120 mL/24 hr

Oral, chewable tab (Dimetapp Children's Cold and Allergy):

6–<12 yr: Chew 2 tablets Q4 hr PO; **max. dose:** 6 doses/24 hr
≥12 yr: Chew 4 tablets Q4 hr PO; **max. dose:** 6 doses/24 hr

Continued

For explanation of icons, see p. 663.

BROMPHENIRAMINE WITH PHENYLEPHRINE *continued*

Generally **not recommended** for treating URIs for infants. No proven benefit for infants and young children with URIs. Over the counter (OTC or non-prescription) use of this product is **not recommended** for children younger than 6 yr due to reports of serious adverse effects (cardiac and respiratory distress, convulsions, and hallucinations) and fatalities (from unintentional overdosages, including combined use of other OTC products containing the same active ingredients).

Contraindicated with use of MAO inhibitors; concurrent use and within 14 days after discontinuing MAO inhibitor. **Use with caution** in narrow-angle glaucoma, bladder neck obstruction, asthma, pyloroduodenal obstruction, symptomatic prostatic hypertrophy, hypertension, coronary artery disease, diabetes mellitus, and thyroid disease. Discontinue use 48 hours prior to allergy skin testing. May cause drowsiness, fatigue, CNS excitation, xerostomia, blurred vision, and wheezing.

BUDESONIDE
Pulmicort Respules, Pulmicort Turbuhaler, Pulmicort Flexhaler, Rhinocort Aqua Nasal Spray, Entocort EC
Corticosteroid

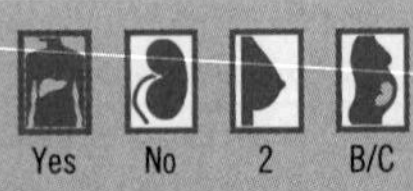

Nasal spray (Rhinocort Aqua): 32 mcg/actuation (8.6 g, delivers approx. 120 sprays)
Nebulized inhalation suspension (Pulmicort Respules): 0.25 mg/2 mL, 0.5 mg/2 mL (30s)
Oral inhaler:
- **Pulmicort Turbohaler inhalation powder:** 200 mcg/metered dose (104 mg, delivers approx. 200 doses)
- **Pulmicort Flexhaler inhalation powder:** 90 mcg/metered dose (165 mg, delivers 60 doses), 180 mcg/metered dose (225 mg, delivers 120 doses); contains lactose

Enteric coated caps (Entocort EC): 3 mg

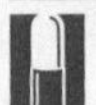

Nebulized inhalation suspension:

Child 1–8 yr:
- ***No prior steroid use:*** 0.5 mg/24 hr ÷ once daily–BID; **max. dose:** 0.5 mg/24 hr
- ***Prior inhaled steroid use:*** 0.5 mg/24 hr ÷ once daily–BID; **max. dose:** 1 mg/24 hr
- ***Prior oral steroid use:*** 1 mg/24 hr ÷ once daily–BID; **max. dose:** 1 mg/24 hr

NIH Asthma Guideline 2007 recommendations (divide doses once daily–TID):

Child 0–4 yr:
- ***Low dose:*** 0.25–0.5 mg/24 hr
- ***Medium dose:*** >0.5–1 mg/24 hr
- ***High dose:*** >1 mg/24 hr

Child 5–11 yr:
- ***Low dose:*** 0.5 mg/24 hr
- ***Medium dose:*** 1 mg/24 hr
- ***High dose:*** 2 mg/24 hr

Oral inhalation:

Pulmicort Turbuhaler:

Child ≥6 yr: Start at 1 inhalation (200 mcg) BID and increase, as needed, up to a **max. dose** of 4 inhalations/24 hr.

Continued

BUDESONIDE *continued*

Adult:

No prior steroid use: 1–2 inhalations (200–400 mcg) BID; **max. dose:** 4 inhalations/24 hr

Prior inhaled steroid use: Start at 1–2 inhalations (200–400 mcg) BID and increase, as needed, up to a **max. dose** of 8 inhalations/24 hr

Prior oral steroid use: Start at 2–4 (400–800 mcg) inhalations BID; **max. dose:** 8 inhalations/24 hr

Pulmicort Flexhaler:

Child ≥6 yr: Start at 180 mcg BID; **max. dose:** 720 mcg/24 hr.

Adult: Start at 180–360 mcg BID; **max. dose:** 1440 mcg/24 hr.

Nasal inhalation (≥6 yr and adult):

Rhinocort Aqua: (initial): 1 spray in each nostril once daily. Increase dose as needed up to **max. dose.**

Max. nasal dose: 6–11 yr: 128 mcg/24 hr (4 sprays/24 hr); ≥ 12 yr and adult: 256 mcg/24 hr (8 sprays/24 hr)

Oral administration for Crohn's disease (Encort EC):

Child ≥6 yr: Data is limited as the following dosages have been reported. Additional studies are needed.

Active disease: 9 mg once daily × 7–8 wks

Maintenance of remission: 6 mg once daily × 3–4 wks

Additionally, a report in 10–19 yr old children demonstrated higher remission rates with an induction dose of 12 mg once daily × 4 wks, followed by 9 mg once daily × 3 wks, followed by 6 mg once daily × 3 wks.

Adult:

Active disease: 9 mg QAM × 8 wks; if remission is not achieved, a second 8-week course may be given.

Maintenance of remission: 6 mg once daily for up to 3 mo. If symptom control is maintained at 3 mo, taper dosage to compete cessation. Remission therapy beyond 3 mo has not shown to provide substantial clinical benefit.

Reduce maintenance dose to as low as possible to control symptoms. May cause pharyngitis, cough, epistaxis, nasal irritation, and HPA-axis suppression. Rinse mouth after each use via the oral inhalation route. Nebulized budesonide has been shown effective in mild to moderate croup at doses of 2 mg × 1. Ref: *N Engl J Med* 331(5):285.

Hypersensitivity reactions, including anaphylaxis, has been reported with the inhaled route. Anaphylactic reactions and benign intracranial hypertension have been reported with oral route of administration.

CYP 450 3A4 inhibitors (e.g., ketoconazole, erythromycin, and protease inhibitors) or significant hepatic impairment may increase systemic exposure of budesonide (inhalation and PO routes).

Onset of action for oral inhalation and nebulized suspension is within 1 day and 2–8 days, respectively, with peak effects at 1–2 wk and 4–6 wk, respectively. The therapeutic ratio between the Flexhaler and Turbohaler product has not been established.

For nasal use, onset of action is seen after 1 day with peak effects after 3–7 days of therapy. Discontinue therapy if no improvement in nasal symptoms after 3 wk of continuous therapy.

Pregnancy category is "B" for inhalation routes of administration and "C" for the oral route. **Do not** crush or chew the oral capsule dosage form.

For explanation of icons, see p. 663.

BUDESONIDE AND FORMOTEROL
Symbicort
Corticosteroid and long-acting beta-2-adrenergic agonist

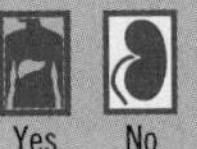 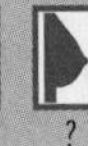 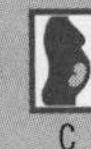 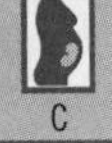
Yes No ? C

Aerosol inhaler:
80 mcg budesonide + 4.5 mcg formoterol fumarate dihydrate (6.9 g delivers 60 inhalations, 10.2 g delivers about 120 inhalations)
160 mcg budesonide + 4.5 mcg formoterol fumarate dihydrate (6 g delivers 60 inhalations, 10.2 g delivers about 120 inhalations)

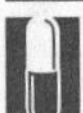

5–11 yr (NIH Asthma Guideline 2007 recommendations): Two inhalations BID of 80 mcg budesonide + 4.5 mcg formoterol; **max. dose:** 4 inhalations/24 hr.
≥12 yr and adult:
No prior inhaled steroid use: Start with two inhalations BID of 80 mcg budesonide + 4.5 mcg fomoterol OR 160 mcg budesonide + 4.5 mcg fomoterol, depending on severity.
Prior low to medium doses of inhaled steroid use: Start with two inhalations BID of 80 mcg budesonide + 4.5 mcg fomoterol.
Prior medium to high doses of inhaled steroid use: Start with two inhalations BID of 160 mcg budesonide + 4.5 mcg fomoterol.
Max. dose: 2 inhalations of 160 mcg budesonide + 4.5 mcg formoterol BID

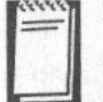

See *Budesonide and Fomoterol* for remarks. Should only be used for patients not adequately controlled on other asthma-controller medications (e.g., low-to-medium dose inhaled corticosteroids) or whose disease severity requires the use of two maintenance therapies.

Titrate to the lowest effective strength after asthma is adequately controlled. Proper patient education including dosage administration technique is essential; see patient package insert for detailed instructions. Rinse mouth after each use.

BUMETANIDE
Bumex and other generic injectable dosage forms
Loop diuretic

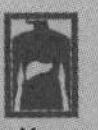 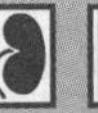 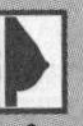 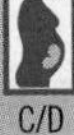 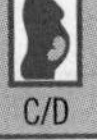
Yes No ? C/D

Tabs: 0.5, 1, 2 mg
Injection: 0.25 mg/mL (some preparations may contain 1% benzyl alcohol)

Neonate and infant (see remarks): PO/IM/IV
≤6 mo: 0.01–0.05 mg/kg/dose once daily or every other day
Infant and child: PO/IM/IV
>6 mo: 0.015–0.1 mg/kg/dose once daily or every other day; **max. dose:** 10 mg/24 hr

Adult:
PO: 0.5–2 mg/dose once daily–BID
IM/IV: 0.5–1 mg over 1–2 min. May give additional doses Q2–3 hr PRN

Usual max. dose (PO/IM/IV): 10 mg/24 hr

Cross-allergenicity may occur in patients allergic to sulfonamides. Dosage reduction may be necessary in patients with hepatic dysfunction. Administer oral doses with food.

Side effects include cramps, dizziness, hypotension, headache, electrolyte losses (hypokalemia, hypocalcemia, hyponatremia, hypochloremia), and encephalopathy. May also lead to metabolic alkalosis. Serious skin reactions (e.g., Stevens Johnson, TEN) have been reported.

Continued

BUMETANIDE *continued*

Drug elimination has been reported to be slower in neonates with respiratory disorders compared to neonates without. May displace bilirubin in critically ill neonates. **Maximal** diuretic effect for infants ≤6 mo has been reported at 0.04 mg/kg/dose with greater efficacy seen at lower dosages.

Pregnancy category changes to "D" if used in pregnancy-induced hypertension.

CAFFEINE CITRATE
Cafcit and others
Methylxanthine, respiratory stimulant

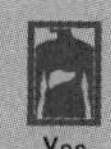 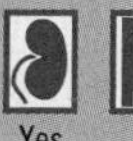 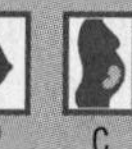 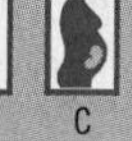

Yes Yes 2 C

Injection: 20 mg/mL (3 mL)
Oral liquid: 20 mg/mL (3 mL), also available as powder for compounding 10, 20 mg/mL
20 mg/mL caffeine citrate salt = 10 mg/mL caffeine base

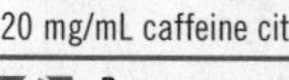

Doses expressed in mg of caffeine citrate.
Neonatal apnea:
Loading dose: 20–25 mg/kg IV/PO × 1
Maintenance dose: 5–10 mg/kg/dose PO/IV Q24 hr, to begin 24 hr after loading dose

Avoid use in symptomatic cardiac arrhythmias. **Do not use** caffeine benzoate formulation since it has been associated with kernicterus in neonates. **Use with caution** in impaired renal or hepatic function.

Therapeutic levels: 5–25 mg/L. Cardiovascular, neurologic, or GI toxicity reported at serum levels >50 mg/L. Recommended serum sampling time: obtain trough level within 30 min prior to a dose. Steady-state is typically achieved 3 wk after the initiation of therapy. Levels obtained prior to steady-state are useful for preventing toxicity.

For IV administration, give loading dose over 30 min and maintenance dose over 10 min.

CALCITONIN—SALMON
Miacalcin, Miacalcin Nasal Spray, Fortical Nasal Spray
Hypercalcemia antidote, antiosteoporotic

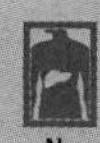 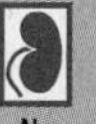  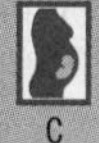

No No ? C

Injection: 200 U/mL (2 mL); contains phenol
Nasal spray: 200 U/metered dose (3.7 mL, provides at least 30 doses); may contain benzyl alcohol

Hypercalcemia (see remarks):
Adult: Start with 4 U/kg/dose IM/SC Q12 hr; if response is unsatisfactory after 1 or 2 days, increase dose to 8 U/kg/dose Q12 hr. If response remains unsatisfactory after 2 more days, increase to a **max. dose** of 8 U/kg/dose Q6 hr.

Paget's disease (see remarks):
Adult: Start with 100 U IM/SC once daily initially, followed by a usual maintenance dose of 50 U once daily **or** 50–100 U Q 1–3 days.

Contraindicated in patients sensitive to salmon protein or gelatin. A skin test is recommended prior to starting IM/SC therapy due to hypersensitivity risk (e.g., bronchospasm, airway swelling, anaphylaxis). Prepare a 10 U/mL dilution with normal saline and administer 0.1 mL intradermally as a skin test (observe for 15 min for wheal or significant erythemia).

Tachyphylaxis has been reported in 2–3 days of use for the treatment of hypercalcemia of malignancy.

Continued

For explanation of icons, see p. 663.

CALCITONIN—SALMON *continued*

Nausea, abdominal pain, diarrhea, flushing, and inflammation at the injection site has been reported with IM/SC route of administration.

Intranasal use currently indicated for postmenopausal osteoporosis in adults. Nasal irritation (alternate nostrils to reduce risk), rhinitis, epistaxis may occur with the intranasal product.

If the injection volume exceeds 2 mL, use IM route and multiple sites of injection.

CALCITRIOL

1,25-dihydroxycholecalciferol, Rocaltrol, Calcijex, and others

Active form vitamin D, fat soluble

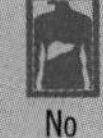
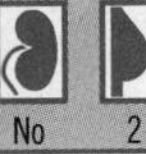
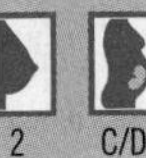

No No 2 C/D

Caps: 0.25, 0.5 mcg
Oral solution: 1 mcg/mL (15 mL)
Injection: (Calcijex and others) 1, 2 mcg/mL (1 mL); contains EDTA

Hypoparathyroidism (evaluate dosage at 2–4 week intervals):

Child >1 yr and adult: Initial dose of 0.25 mcg/dose PO once daily. May increase daily dosage by 0.25 mcg at 2- to 4-week intervals. Usual maintenance dosage as follows:

<1 yr: 0.04–0.08 mcg/kg/dose PO once daily
1–5 yr: 0.25–0.75 mcg/dose PO once daily
>6 yr and adult: 0.5–2 mcg/dose PO once daily

Renal failure: See the National Kidney Foundation guidelines at www.kidney.org/professionals/dkoqi/guidelines_pedbone/guide9.htm.

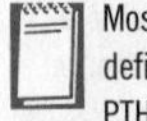

Most potent vitamin D metabolite available. Should not be used to treat 25-OH vitamin D deficiency; use cholecalciferol or ergocalciferol. Monitor serum calcium and phosphorus; and PTH in dialysis patients. **Avoid** concomitant use of Mg^{2+}-containing antacids. IV dosing applies if patient undergoing hemodialysis.

Contraindicated in patients with hypercalcemia, vitamin D toxicity. Side effects include weakness, headache, vomiting, constipation, hypotonia, polydipsia, polyuria, myalgia, metastatic calcification, etc. Allergic reactions, including anaphylaxis, have been reported.

Pregnancy category changes to "D" if used in doses above the recommended daily allowance.

CALCIUM ACETATE

PhosLo; 25% Elemental Ca

Calcium supplement, phosphorous lowering agent

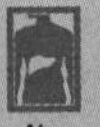
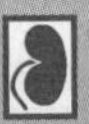
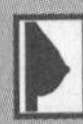
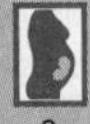

No Yes ? C

Tabs: 667 mg (169 mg elemental Ca)
Capsules: 333.5 mg (84.5 mg elemental Ca), 667 mg (169 mg elemental Ca)
Gelcaps: 667 mg (169 mg elemental Ca)
Contains polyethylene glycol 8000
Each 1 g of salt contains 12.7 mEq (250 mg) elemental Ca.

Doses expressed in mg of calcium acetate.

Hyperphosphatemia:

Adult: Start with 1334 mg PO with each meal. Dosage may be increased gradually to bring serum phosphorous levels below 6 mg/dL, as long as hypercalcemia does not occur. Most patients require 2001–2668 mg PO with each meal.

Continued

CALCIUM ACETATE *continued*

Contraindicated in ventricular fibrillation. **Use with caution** in renal impairement as hypercalcemia may develop in end-stage renal failure. Nausea and hypercalcemia may occur. Approximately 40% of dose is systemically absorbed under fasting conditions and up to 30% in nonfasting conditions. May reduce absorption of tetracyclines, iron, and effectiveness of polystyrene sulfonate. May potentiate effects of digoxin.

Administer with meals and plenty of fluids for use as a phosphorus lowering agent.

CALCIUM CARBONATE

Tums, Os-Cal, Children's Pepto, Children's Mylanta, and many others; 40% Elemental Ca

Calcium supplement, antacid

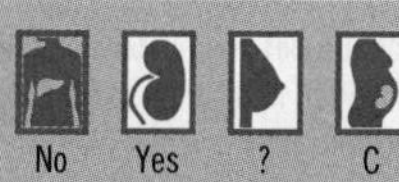

Tab, chewable [OTC]: 400, 500, 750, 1000, 1250 mg

Children's Pepto, Children's Mylanta [OTC]: 400 mg

Tab [OTC]: 500, 600, 650, 1250 mg

Oral suspension [OTC]: 1250 mg/5 mL

Caps [OTC]: 1250 mg

Gum [OTC]: 100, 500 mg; may contain phenylalanine

Powder [OTC]: 454 g

Each 1 g of salt contains 20 mEq elemental Ca (400 mg elemental Ca).

Hypocalcemia (Doses expressed in mg of elemental calcium. To convert to mg of salt, divide elemental dose by 0.4):

Neonate: 50–150 mg/kg/24 hr ÷ Q4–6 hr PO; **max. dose**: 1 g/24 hr

Child: 45–65 mg/kg/24 hr PO ÷ QID

Adult: 1–2 g/24 hr PO ÷ TID–QID

Antacid (Doses expressed in mg of calcium carbonate):

2–5 yr: 400 mg PO as symptoms occur; **max. dose**: 1200 mg/24 hr

>6–11 yr: 800 mg PO as symptoms occur; **max. dose**: 2400 mg/24 hr

>11 yr and adult: 1000-3000 mg PO as symptoms occur; **max. dose**: 7500 mg/24 hr.

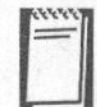

See *Calcium acetate* for **contraindications, precautions,** and drug interactions. Side effects: Constipation, hypercalcemia, hypophosphatemia, hypomagnesemia, nausea, vomiting, headache, and confusion. Some products may contain trace amounts of sodium. Administer with plenty of fluids. For use as a phosphorus lowering agent, administer with meals.

CALCIUM CHLORIDE

Various generics; 27% Elemental Ca

Calcium supplement

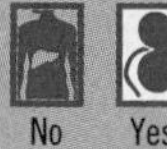
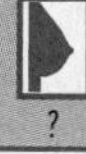
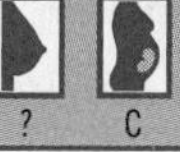

Injection: 100 mg/mL (10%) (1.36 mEq Ca/mL); 1 g of salt contains 13.6 mEq (273 mg) elemental Ca

Each 1 g of salt contains 13.5 mEq (270 mg) elemental Ca.

Doses expressed in mg of CaCl.

Cardiac arrest or calcium channel blocker toxicity:

Infant/child: 20 mg/kg/dose IV Q10 min PRN, if effective, an infusion of 20–50 mg/kg/hr may be used

Adult: 500–1000 mg/dose IV Q10 min PRN or 2–4 mg/kg/dose Q10 min PRN

Continued

FORMULARY

For explanation of icons, see p. 663.

CALCIUM CHLORIDE *continued*

MAXIMUM IV ADMINISTRATION RATES:

IV push: **Do not exceed** 100 mg/min (over 10–20 sec in cardiac arrest).

IV infusion: **Do not exceed** 45–90 mg/kg/hr with a **max.** concentration of 20 mg/mL.

Contraindicated in ventricular fibrillation. **Not recommended** for asystole and electromechanical dissociation. **Use with caution** in renal impairment as hypercalcemia may develop in end-stage renal failure. May potentiate effects of digoxin.

Use IV with **extreme caution**. Extravasation may lead to necrosis. Hyaluronidase may be helpful for extravasation. Central-line administration is preferred IV route of administration. **Do not use** scalp veins. **Do not administer** IM or SC route.

Rapid IV infusion associated with bradycardia, hypotension, and peripheral vasodilation. May cause hyperchloremic acidosis.

CALCIUM CITRATE

Cal-Citrate, Citracal, and others; 21% Elemental Ca

Calcium supplement

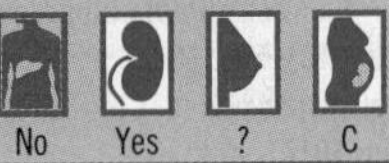

No Yes ? C

Tabs [OTC]: 950 mg (200 mg elemental), 1150 mg calcium citrate (250 mg elemental Ca)

Effervescent tabs [OTC]:

As elemental calcium: 500 mg; contains phenylalanine

Caps [OTC]:

As elemental calcium: 180, 225 mg

Granules [OTC]:

As elemental calcium: 760 mg/teaspoonful (454 g)

Each 1 g of salt contains 10.6 mEq (211 mg) elemental Ca.

Doses expressed as mg of elemental calcium. To convert to mg of salt, divide elemental dose by 0.21.

Hypocalcemia:

Neonate: 50–150 mg/kg/24 hr ÷ Q4–6 hr PO; **max. dose:** 1 g/24 hr

Child: 45–65 mg/kg/24 hr PO ÷ QID

Adult: 1–2 g/24 hr PO ÷ TID–QID

See *Calcium Acetate* for **contraindications, precautions,** and drug interactions. Side effects: Constipation, hypercalcemia, hypophosphatemia, hypomagnesemia, nausea, vomiting, headache, and confusion.

Administer with meals for use as a phosphorus lowering agent or with use of the granule dosage form. For hypocalcemia, do not administer with or before meals/food and take plenty of fluids.

CALCIUM GLUBIONATE

Calcionate, Calciquid, and others; 6.4% Elemental Ca

Calcium supplement

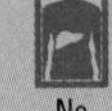 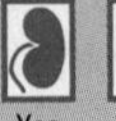 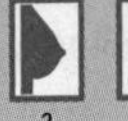 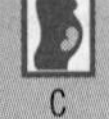

No Yes ? C

Syrup [OTC]: 1.8 g/5 mL (480 mL) (1.2 mEq Ca/mL)

Each 1 g of salt contains 3.2 mEq (64 mg) elemental Ca.

Continued

CALCIUM GLUBIONATE *continued*

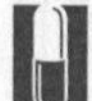

Doses expressed in mg calcium glubionate.
Hypocalcemia:
Neonate: 1200 mg/kg/24 hr PO ÷ Q4–6 hr
Infant/child: 600–2000 mg/kg/24 hr PO ÷ QID; **max. dose**: 9 g/24 hr
Adult: 6–18 g/24 hr PO ÷ QID

See *Calcium Acetate* for **contraindications, precautions,** and drug interactions. Side effects include GI irritation, dizziness, and headache. High osmotic load of syrup (20% sucrose) may cause diarrhea.

Best absorbed when given before meals. Absorption inhibited by high phosphate load.

CALCIUM GLUCONATE
Cal-G and various generics; 9% Elemental Ca
Calcium supplement

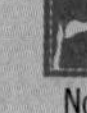 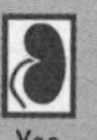 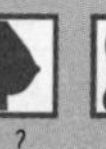 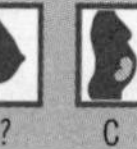

No Yes ? C

Tabs [OTC]: 500, 650 mg
Powder for oral suspension [OTC]: 3852.2 mg (346.7 mg elemental Ca)/15 mL (454 g)
Caps (Cal-G) [OTC]: 700 mg
Injection: 100 mg/mL (10%) (0.45 mEq Ca^{2+}/mL)
Each 1 g of salt contains 4.5 mEq (90 mg) elemental Ca.

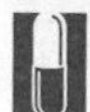

Doses expressed in mg calcium gluconate.
Maintenance/hypocalcemia:
Neonate: IV: 200–800 mg/kg/24 hr ÷ Q6 hr
Infant:
IV: 200–500 mg/kg/24 hr ÷ Q6 hr
PO: 400–800 mg/kg/24 hr ÷ Q6 hr
Child: 200–500 mg/kg/24 hr IV or PO ÷ Q6 hr
Adult: 2–15 g/24 hr IV or PO ÷ Q6 hr

For cardiac arrest:
Infant and child: 100 mg/kg/dose IV Q10 min
Adult: 500–800 mg/dose IV Q10 min
Max. dose: 3 g/dose

For tetany:
Neonate, infant, child: 100–200 mg/kg dose IV over 5–10 min, repeat dose 6 hr later if needed; **max. dose**: 500 mg/kg/24 hr
Adult: 1–3 IV over 10–30 min, repeat dose 6 hr later if needed.

MAXIMUM IV ADMINISTRATION RATES:
IV push: **Do not exceed** 100 mg/min (over 10–20 sec in cardiac arrest)
IV infusion: **Do not exceed** 120–240 mg/kg/hr with a **maximum concentration** of 50 mg/mL

Contraindicated in ventricular fibrillation. **Use with caution** in renal impairment as hypercalcemia may develop in end-stage renal failure. **Avoid** peripheral infusion as extravasation may cause tissue necrosis. IV infusion associated with hypotension and bradycardia. Also associated with arrhythmias in digitalized patients. May reduce absorption of tetracycline, iron, and effectiveness of polystyrene sulfonate with oral route of administration.

May precipitate when used with bicarbonate. **Do not use** scalp veins. **Do not administer** IM or SC.

For explanation of icons, see p. 663.

CALCIUM LACTATE
Cal-Lac and various generics; 13% Elemental Ca
Calcium supplement

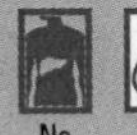 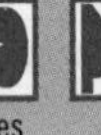 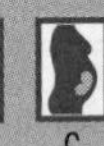 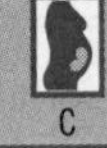
No Yes ? C

Tabs [OTC]: 650 mg
Caps (Cal-Lac) [OTC]: 500 mg
Each 1 g salt contains 6.5 mEq (130 mg) elemental Ca.

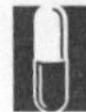

Doses expressed in mg of calcium lactate.
Hypocalcemia:
Infant: 400–500 mg/kg/24 hr PO ÷ Q4–6 hr
Child: 500 mg/kg/24 hr PO ÷ Q6–8 hr
Adult: 1.5–3 g PO Q8 hr
Max. dose: 9 g/24 hr

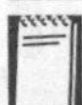

See *Calcium Acetate* for **contraindications, precautions**, and drug interactions. May cause constipation, headache, and hypercalcemia.

Give with or following meals and with plenty of fluids. **Do not** dissolve tablets in milk.

CALCIUM PHOSPHATE, TRIBASIC
Posture; 39% Elemental Ca
Calcium supplement

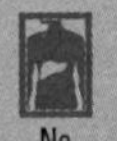 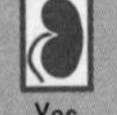 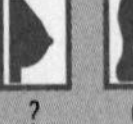 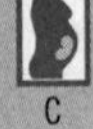
No Yes ? C

Tabs [OTC]: 600 mg elemental calcium
NOTE: Pharmacy may crush tablets into a powder to enhance drug delivery for children unable to swallow tablets and to accommodate smaller doses.
Each 1 g of salt contains 19.3 mEq (390 mg) elemental Ca and 280 mg elemental phosphorus.

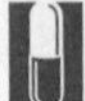

Doses expressed as mg of elemental calcium.
Hypocalcemia:
Neonate: 20–80 mg/kg/24 hr ÷ Q4–6 hr PO; **max. dose:** 1 g/24 hr
Child: 45–65 mg/kg/24 hr PO ÷ Q6 hr
Adult: 1–2 g/24 hr PO ÷ Q6–8 hr

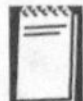

Contraindicated in ventricular fibrillation. **Use with caution** in renal impairment as hypercalcemia may develop in end-stage renal failure (avoid use in dialysis with hypercalcemia), history of kidney stones, and parathyroid disorders. May cause constipation, GI disturbances, and hypercalcemia. See *Calcium Acetate* for drug interactions.

Give with or following meals and with plenty of fluids.

CALFACTANT

See *Surfactant, pulmonary*

CAPTOPRIL
Capoten and various generics
Angiotensin converting enzyme inhibitor, anti-hypertensive

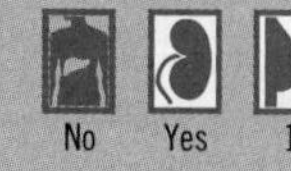

Tabs: 12.5, 25, 50, 100 mg
Oral suspension: 0.75, 1 mg/mL

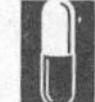

Neonate: 0.01–0.05 mg/kg/dose PO Q8–12 hr.
Infant <6 mo: Initially 0.01–0.5 mg/kg/dose PO BID–TID; titrate upward if needed; **max. dose:** 6 mg/kg/24 hr.
Child: Initially 0.3–0.5 mg/kg/dose PO BID–TID; titrate upward if needed; **max. dose:** 6 mg/kg/24 hr up to 450 mg/24 hr.
Adolescent and adult: Initially 12.5–25 mg/dose PO BID–TID; increase weekly if necessary by 25 mg/dose to **max. dose:** 450 mg/24 hr. Usual dosage range: 25–100 mg/24 hr ÷ BID.

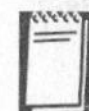

Onset within 15–30 min of administration. Peak effect within 1–2 hr. **Adjust dose with renal failure (see Chapter 31).** Should be administered on an empty stomach 1 hr before or 2 hr after meals. Titrate to minimal effective dose. Lower doses should be used in patients with sodium and water depletion due to diuretic therapy.

Use with caution in collagen vascular disease and concomitant potassium sparing diuretics. **Avoid use** with dialysis with high-flux membranes since anaphylactoid reactions have been reported. May cause rash, proteinuria, neutropenia, cough, angioedema (head, neck and intestinal), hyperkalemia, hypotension, or diminution of taste perception (with long term use). Known to decrease aldosterone and increase renin production. Captopril is a CYP P450 2D6 substrate.

Pregnancy category is a "C" during the first trimester but changes to a "D" for the second and third trimester (fetal injury and death have been reported). Despite the pregnancy category, an increased risk for major congenital malformations has been reported with use of ACE inhibitors during the first trimester. Captopril should be discontinued as soon as possible when pregnancy is detected.

CARBAMAZEPINE
Epitol, Tegretol, Tegretol-XR, Carbatrol, and various generics
Anticonvulsant

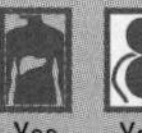
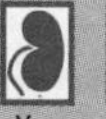
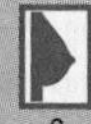
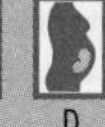
Yes Yes 2 D

Tabs: 200 mg
Chewable tabs: 100 mg
Extended-release tabs (Tegretol-XR): 100, 200, 400 mg
Extended-release caps (Carbatrol): 100, 200, 300 mg
Oral suspension: 100 mg/5 mL (10, 450 mL)

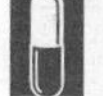

See remarks regarding dosing intervals and dosage forms:
<6 yr:
Initial: 10–20 mg/kg/24 hr PO ÷ BID–TID (QID for suspension)
Increment: Q5–7 days up to **max. dose** of 35 mg/kg/24 hr PO

6–12 yr:
Initial: 10 mg/kg/24 hr PO ÷ BID up to **max. dose:** 100 mg/dose BID
Increment: 100 mg/24 hr at 1 wk intervals (÷ TID–QID) until desired response is obtained
Maintenance: 20–30 mg/kg/24 hr PO ÷ BID–QID; usual maintenance dose is 400–800 mg/24 hr; **max. dose:** 1000 mg/24 hr

Continued

For explanation of icons, see p. 663.

CARBAMAZEPINE *continued*

>12 yr and adult:

Initial: 200 mg PO BID

Increment: 200 mg/24 hr at 1-wk intervals (÷ BID–QID) until desired response is obtained

Maintenance: 800–1200 mg/24 hr PO ÷ BID–QID

Max. dose:

Child 12–15 yr: 1000 mg/24 hr

Child >15 yr: 1200 mg/24 hr

Adult: 1.6–2.4 g/24 hr

Contraindicated for patients taking MAO inhibitors or who are sensitive to tricyclic antidepressants. Should **not** be used in combination with clozapine due to increased risk for bone marrow suppression and agranulocytosis. Increased risk for severe dermatological reactions (e.g., SJS and TEN) has been associated with the HLA-B*1502 alle (prevalent among Asian descent).

Erythromycin, diltiazem, verapamil, cefixime, cimetidine, itraconazole, and INH may increase serum levels. Carbamazepine may decrease activity of warfarin, doxycycline, oral contraceptives, cyclosporine, theophylline, phenytoin, benzodiazepines, ethosuximide, and valproic acid. Carbamazepine is a CYP 450 3A3/4 substrate and inducer of CYP 450 1A2, 2C, and 3A3/4.

Suggested dosing intervals for specific dosage forms: extended-release tabs or caps (BID); chewable and immediate-release tablets (BID–TID); suspension (QID). Doses may be administered with food. **Do not** crush or chew extended-release dosage forms. Shake bottle well prior to dispensing oral suspension dosage form and **do not** administer simultaneously with other liquid medicines or diluents.

Drug metabolism typically increases after the first month of therapy due to hepatic autoinduction.

Therapeutic blood levels: 4–12 mg/L. Recommended serum sampling time: obtain trough level within 30 min prior to an oral dose. Steady-state is typically achieved 1 month following the initiation of therapy (following enzymatic autoinduction). Levels obtained prior to steady-state are useful for preventing toxicity. Blood levels of 7–10 mg/L have been recommended for bipolar disorders.

Side effects include sedation, dizziness, diplopia, aplastic anemia, neutropenia, urinary retention, nausea, SIADH, and Stevens-Johnson syndrome. Suicidal behavior or ideation have been reported. Pretreatment CBCs and LFTs are suggested. Patient should be monitored for hematologic and hepatic toxicity. **Adjust dose in renal impairment (see Chapter 31).**

See Chapter 2 for management of ingestions.

CARBAMIDE PEROXIDE

Debrox, Murine Ear, Auro Ear Drops, Cankaid, Gly-Oxide, Orajel Perioseptic, and others

Cerumenolytic, topical oral analgesic

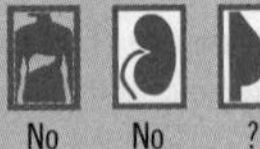
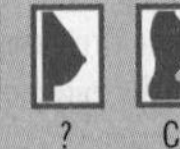

No No ? C

Otic solution (OTC): 6.5% (15, 30 mL); may contain propylene glycol or alcohol

Oral liquid (OTC): 10% (Cankaid, Gly-Oxide) (15, 60 mL), 15% (Orajel Perioseptic) (240 mL)

Cerumenolytic:

<12 yr: Tilt head sideways and instill 1–5 drops (according to patient size) into affected ear and keep drops in ear for several min. Remove wax by gently flushing the ear with warm water, using a soft rubber bulb ear syringe. Dose may be repeated BID PRN for **up to** 4 days.

≥12 yr: Following the same instructions from above, instill 5–10 drops into affected ear BID PRN for **up to** 4 days.

Continued

CARBAMIDE PEROXIDE *continued*

Oral analgesic (see remarks):

Liquid:

≥3 yr (able to follow instructions): Instill several drops to affected area and expectorate after 2–3 min OR place 10 drops on tongue and mix with saliva, swish for several min, and expectorate. Administer QID, after meals and QHS, for **up to** 7 days.

Contraindicated if tympanic membrane perforated; following otic surgery; ear discharge, drainage, pain, irritation or rash; or PE tubes in place. Tip of applicator should not enter ear canal when used as a cerumenolytic.

Prolonged use of the oral product may result in fungal overgrowth. **Do not** rinse the mouth or drink for at least 5 min when using oral preparation.

CARBINOXAMINE ± PSEUDOEPHEDRINE
Palgic and other generics
In combination with pseudoephedrine: Sildec, Cordron-D NR, Pseudo Carb Pediatric, Cordron-DL, and Hydro-Tussin CBX
Antihistamine with/without decongestant

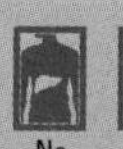
No
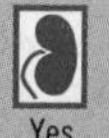
Yes

?
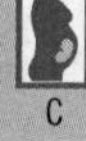
C

CARBINOXAMINE:

Liquid: 4 mg/5 mL (473 mL); may contain propylene glycol
Tabs: 4 mg

CARBINOXAMINE + PSEUDOEPHEDRINE:

Oral drops (Sildec): Carbinoxamine 1 mg + pseudoephedrine 15 mg/1 mL (30 mL); contains saccharin and sorbitol

Oral liquid:

Cordron-D NR and Pseudo Carb Pediatric: Carbinoxamine 2 mg + pseudoephedrine 12.5 mg/5 mL (118, 473 mL); may contain saccharin and sorbitol (alcohol and dye free)
Cordron-DL: Carbinoxamine 2 mg + pseudoephedrine 17.5 mg/5 mL (473 mL); contains saccharin and sorbitol (alcohol and dye free)
Hydro-Tussin CBX: Carbinoxamine 2 mg + pseudoephedrine 25 mg/5 mL (473 mL)

NOTE: alternative decongestant combination product, carbinoxamine and phenylephrine (Histamax D and XiraHist drops), is available by prescription.

CARBINOXAMINE:

Child (PO; see remarks): 0.2–0.4 mg/kg/24 hr PO ÷ TID–QID; alternative dosing by age (**do not exceed** 0.4 mg/kg/24 hr):
2–3 yr: 2 mg TID–QID
3–6 yr: 2–4 mg TID–QID
≥6 yr: 4–6 mg TID–QID
Adult: 4–8 mg TID–QID

CARBINOXAMINE + PSEUDOEPHEDRINE (PE):

Child (PO; see remarks): carbinoxamine at 0.2–0.4 mg/kg/24 hr and pseudoephedrine at 4 mg/kg/24 hr ÷ TID–QID. Alternative dosing information for combination products:

Continued

For explanation of icons, see p. 663.

CARBINOXAMINE ± PSEUDOEPHEDRINE *continued*

Age	*Oral Drops	#Oral Syrup
1–3 mo	0.25 mL QID	
>3–6 mo	0.5 mL QID	
>6–9 mo	0.75 mL QID	
>9–18 mo	1 mL QID	
>18 mo–6 yr		2.5 mL QID
≥6 yr and adult		5 mL QID

*1 mg carbinoxamine + 15 mg pseudoephedrine/1 mL
#2 mg carbinoxamine + 15 mg pseudoephedrine/5 mL

Also see specific combination product package insert for additional dosing information.

Generally not recommended for treating URIs for infants. No proven benefit for infants and young children with URIs. **The FDA does not recommend use for URIs in children <2 yr because of reports of increased fatalities.**

Contraindicated in acute asthma, hypersensitivity with other ethanolamine antihistamines, MAO inhibitors, severe hypertension, narrow-angle glaucoma, severe coronary artery disease, and urinary retention. **Be aware of the corresponding amount of pseudoephedrine** if using combination product (see *Pseudoephedrine* for additional remarks).

May cause drowsiness, vertigo, dry mucus membranes, and headache. Contact dermatitis and CNS excitation have been reported.

Pregnancy category is "C" for both carbinoxamine and pseudoephedrine. Use of pseudoephedrine during the first trimester may be associated with gastroschisis, small intestinal atresia, and hemifacial microsomia.

CARNITINE

Levocarnitine, Carnitor, L-Carnitine
Nutritional supplement, amino acid

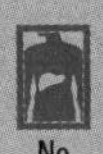
No

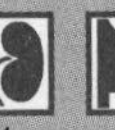
Yes

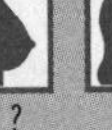
?

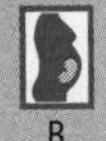
B

Tabs: 330, 500 mg
Caps: 250 mg
Oral solution: 100 mg/mL (118 mL)
Injection: 200 mg/mL (5mL) (preservative free)

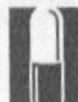

Primary carnitine deficiency:

Oral:

Child: 50–100 mg/kg/24 hr PO ÷ Q8–12 hr; increase slowly as needed and tolerated to **max. dose** of 3 g/24 hr

Adult: 330 mg to 1 g/dose BID–TID PO; **max. dose**: 3 g/24 hr

IV:

Child and adult: 50 mg/kg as loading dose; may follow with 50 mg/kg/24 hr IV infusion (for severe cases); maintenance: 50 mg/kg/24 hr ÷ Q4–6 hr; increase to **max. dose** of 300 mg/kg/24 hr if needed.

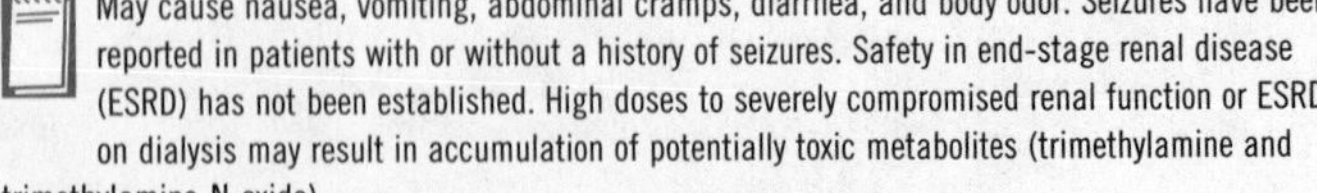

May cause nausea, vomiting, abdominal cramps, diarrhea, and body odor. Seizures have been reported in patients with or without a history of seizures. Safety in end-stage renal disease (ESRD) has not been established. High doses to severely compromised renal function or ESRD on dialysis may result in accumulation of potentially toxic metabolites (trimethylamine and trimethylamine-N-oxide).

Give bolus IV infusion over 2–3 min.

C

CASPOFUNGIN
Cancidas
Antifungal, echinocandin

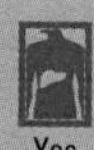 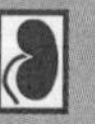 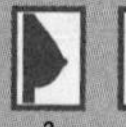 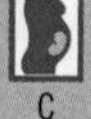 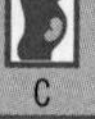
Yes No ? C

Injection: 50, 70 mg; contains sucrose (39 mg in 50 mg vial and 54 mg in 70 mg vial)

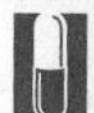

Preterm neonate– <3 mo infant (based on a small pharmacokinetic study, achieving similar plasma exposure as seen in adults receiving 50 mg/24 hr): 25 mg/m²/dose IV once daily. Alternatively, 1 mg/kg/dose IV once daily × 2 days followed by 2 mg/kg/dose IV once daily has been reported in a case series with excellent microbiological results.

3 mo infant – 17 yr (see remarks): 70 mg/m²/dose IV loading dose on day 1 followed by 50 mg/m²/dose IV once daily maintenance dose. Increase the maintenance dose to 70 mg/m²/dose if response is inadequate or if the patient is receiving an enzyme inducing medication (see remarks).

Maximum loading and maintenance dose: 70 mg/dose.

Adolescent and adult (see remarks):

Loading dose: 70 mg IV × 1

Maintenance dose:

Usual: 50 mg IV once daily. If tolerated and response is inadequate or if patient is receiving an enzyme inducing medication (see remarks), increase to 70 mg IV once daily.

Hepatic insufficiency (Child-Pugh score 7 to 9): 35 mg IV once daily.

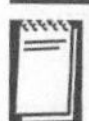

Use with caution in hepatic impairment and concomitant enzyme inducing drugs. Higher maintenance doses (70 mg/m²/dose in children and 70 mg in adults) are recommended for concomitant use of enzyme inducers such as carbamazepime, dexamethasone, phenytoin, nevirapine, efavirenz, or rifampin. Use Mosteller formula for calculating BSA.

Most common adverse effects (>10%) in children include fever, diarrhea, rash, elevated ALT/AST, hypokalemia, hypotension, and chills. May also cause facial swelling, nausea/vomiting, headache, infusion site phlebitis, and LFT elevation. Hepatobiliary adverse effects have been reported in pediatric patients with serious underlying medical conditions.

Reduce daily dose by 30% in moderate hepatic impairment (Child-Pugh score 7 to 9).

Use with cyclosporine may cause transient increase in LFTs and caspofungin level elevations. May decrease tacrolimus levels.

Administer doses by slow IV infusion over 1 hr. **Do not** mix or co-infuse with other medications and **avoid** using dextrose-containing diluents (e.g., D5W).

CEFACLOR
Ceclor, Ceclor CD, Raniclor, and others
Antibiotic, cephalosporin (second generation)

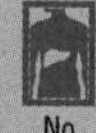 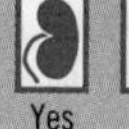 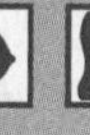 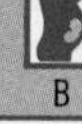
No Yes 1 B

Caps: 250, 500 mg
Extended-release tabs (Ceclor CD): 375, 500 mg
Chewable tabs (Raniclor): 125, 187, 250, 375 mg; contains phenylalanine
Oral suspension: 125 mg/5 mL (150 mL); 187 mg/5 mL (100 mL); 250 mg/5 mL (75, 150 mL); 375 mg/5 mL (100 mL)

Child >1 mo old (use regular-release dosage forms): 20–40 mg/kg/24 hr PO ÷ Q8 hr; **max. dose:** 2 g/24 hr (Q12 hr dosage interval optional in otitis media or pharyngitis)

Adult: 250–500 mg/dose PO Q8 hr; **max. dose:** 4 g/24 hr

Extended-release tablets: 375–500 mg/dose PO Q12 hr

Continued

FORMULARY

For explanation of icons, see p. 663.

CEFACLOR *continued*

Use with caution in patients with penicillin allergy or renal impairment. Side effects include elevated liver function tests, bone marrow suppression, and moniliasis. Probenecid may increase cefaclor concentrations. May cause positive Coomb's test or false-positive test for urinary glucose. Serum sickness reactions have been reported in patients receiving multiple courses of cefaclor.

Do not crush, cut, or chew extended-release tablets. Doses should be given on an empty stomach. Extended-release tablets **not recommended** for children. **Adjust dose in renal failure (see Chapter 31).**

CEFADROXIL

Duricef and others

Antibiotic, cephalosporin (first generation)

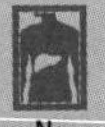
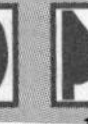
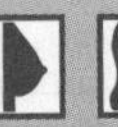
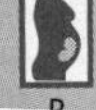

No Yes 1 B

Oral suspension: 250, 500 mg/5 mL (75, 100 mL)
Tabs: 1 g
Caps: 500 mg

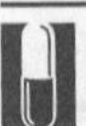

Infant and child: 30 mg/kg/24 hr PO ÷ Q12 hr (daily dose may be administered once daily for group A beta-hemolytic streptococci pharyngitis/tonsillitis); **max. dose:** 2 g/24 hr
Adolescent and adult: 1–2 g/24 hr PO ÷ Q12–24 hr (administer Q12 hr for complicated UTIs); **max.dose:** 2 g/24 hr

See *Cephalexin* for **precautions** and interactions. Rash, nausea, vomiting, and diarrhea are common. Transient neutropenia, and vaginitis have been reported. **Adjust dose in renal failure (see Chapter 31).**

CEFAZOLIN

Ancef, Zolicef, and others

Antibiotic, cephalosporin (first generation)

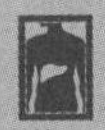
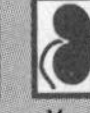
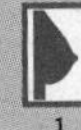
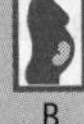

Yes Yes 1 B

Injection: 0.5, 1, 5, 10, 20 g
Frozen injection: 1 g/50 mL 5% dextrose (iso-osmotic solutions)
Contains 2.1 mEq Na/g drug

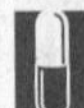

Neonate IM, IV:
- ***Postnatal age ≤7 days:*** 40 mg/kg/24 hr ÷ Q12 hr
- ***Postnatal age >7 days:***
  - ***≤2000 g:*** 40 mg/kg/24 hr ÷ Q12 hr
  - ***>2000 g:*** 60 mg/kg/24 hr ÷ Q8 hr

Infant >1 mo/child: 50–100 mg/kg/24 hr ÷ Q6–8 hr IV/IM; **max. dose:** 6 g/24 hr
Adult: 2–6 g/24 hr ÷ Q6–8 hr IV/IM; **max. dose:** 12 g/24 hr
Bacterial endocarditis prophylaxis for dental and upper respiratory procedures:
- ***Infant and child:*** 50 mg/kg IV/IM (**max. dose:** 1 g) 30 min before procedure
- ***Adult:*** 1 g IV/IM 30 min before procedure

Use with caution in renal impairment or in penicillin-allergic patients. Does not penetrate well into CSF. May cause phlebitis, leukopenia, thrombocytopenia, transient liver enzyme elevation, false-positive urine reducing substance (Clinitest) and Coombs' test.

For dosing in obese patients, use higher end of the dosing recommendation. **Adjust dose in renal failure (see Chapter 31).**

CEFDINIR
Omnicef
Antibiotic, cephalosporin (third generation)

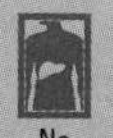 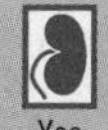  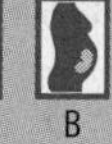 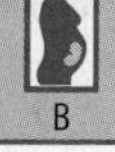
No Yes 1 B

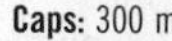

Caps: 300 mg
Oral suspension: 125 mg/5 mL (60, 100 mL)

6 mo-12 yr:

Otitis media, sinusitis, pharyngitis/tonsillitis: 14 mg/kg/24 hr PO ÷ Q12–24 hr; **max. dose:** 600 mg/24 hr

Uncomplicated skin infections (see remarks): 14 mg/kg/24 hr PO ÷ Q12 hr; **max. dose:** 600 mg/24 hr

≥13 yr and adult:

Bronchitis, sinusitis, pharyngitis/tonsillitis: 600 mg/24 hr PO ÷ Q12–24 hr

Community-acquired pneumonia, uncomplicated skin infections (see remarks): 600 mg/24 hr PO ÷ Q12 hr

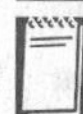

Use with caution in penicillin-allergic patients or in presence of renal impairment. Good gram-positive cocci activity. May cause diarrhea and false-positive urine reducing substance (Clinitest) and Coombs' test. Eosinophilia and abnormal liver function tests have been reported with higher than usual doses.

Once daily dosing has not been evaluated in pneumonia and skin infections. Probenecid increases serum cefdinir levels. Avoid concomitant administration with iron and iron-containing vitamins and antacids containing aluminum or magnesium (space by 2 hr apart) to reduce the risk for decreasing antibiotic's absorption. Doses may be taken without regard to food. **Adjust dose in renal failure (see Chapter 31).**

CEFEPIME
Maxipime
Antibiotic, cephalosporin (fourth generation)

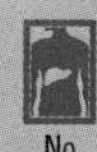 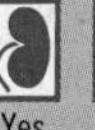 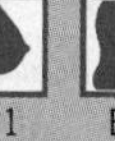 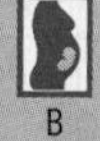
No Yes 1 B

Injection: 1, 2 g
Each 1 g drug contains 725 mg L-Arginine.

Neonate:

<14 days: 60 mg/kg/24 hr ÷ Q12 hr IV/IM

≥14 days: 100 mg/kg/24 hr ÷ Q12 hr IV/IM. For meningitis or *Pseudomonas* infections, use 150 mg/kg/24 hr ÷ Q8 hr IV/IM

Child ≥2 mo: 100 mg/kg/24 hr ÷ Q12 hr IV/IM; **max. dose:** 4 g/24 hr

Meningitis, fever, and neutropenia, or serious infections: 150 mg/kg/24 hr ÷ Q8 hr IV/IM; **max. dose:** 6 g/24 hr

Cystic Fibrosis: 150 mg/kg/24 hr ÷ Q8 hr IV/IM, up to a **max. dose** of 6 g/24 hr.

Adult: 1–4 g/24 hr ÷ Q12 hr IV/IM

Severe infections: 6 g/24 hr ÷ Q8 hr IV/IM

Max. dose: 6 g/24 hr

Use with caution in patients with penicillin allergy or renal impairment. Good activity against *P. aeruginosa* and other gram-negative bacteria plus most gram-positives (*S. aureus*). May cause thrombophlebitis, gastrointestinal discomfort, transient increases in liver enzymes, false-positive urine reducing substance (Clinitest) and Coombs' test. Probenecid increases serum cefepime levels. Encephalopathy, myoclonus, seizures, transient leukopenia, neutropenia, agranulocytosis, and thrombocytopenia have been reported. **Adjust dose in renal failure (see Chapter 31).**

For explanation of icons, see p. 663.

CEFIXIME
Suprax
Antibiotic, cephalosporin (third generation)

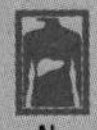
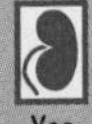

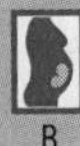
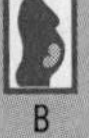

No Yes 1 B

Oral suspension: 100 mg/5 mL (50, 75 mL)
Tabs: 400 mg

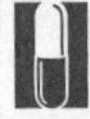

Infant (>6 mo) and child: 8 mg/kg/24 hr ÷ Q12–24 hr PO; **max. dose:** 400 mg/24 hr

Acute UTI: 16 mg/kg/24 hr ÷ Q12 hr on day 1, followed by 8 mg/kg/24 hr Q24 hr PO × 13 days. **Max. dose:** 400 mg/24 hr

Adolescent and adult: 400 mg/24 hr ÷ Q12–24 hr PO

Uncomplicated cervical, urethral, or rectal infections due to N. gonorrhoeae: 400 mg × 1 PO plus azithromycin 1 g PO × 1 or doxycycline 100 mg PO BID × 7 days

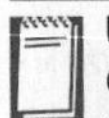

Use with caution in patients with penicillin allergy or renal failure. Adverse reactions include diarrhea, abdominal pain, nausea, and headaches. Do not use tablets for the treatment of otitis media due to reduced bioavailability. Probenecid increases serum cefixime levels. May increase carbamazepine serum concentrations. May cause false-positive urine reducing substance (Clinitest), Coombs' test, and nitroprusside test for ketones. **Adjust dose in renal failure (see Chapter 31).**

CEFOTAXIME
Claforan
Antibiotic, cephalosporin (third generation)

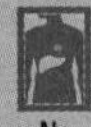
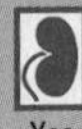

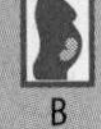

No Yes 1 B

Injection: 0.5, 1, 2, 10 g
Frozen injection: 1 g/50 mL 3.4% dextrose, 2 g/50 mL 1.4% dextrose (iso-osmotic solutions)
Contains 2.2 mEq Na/g drug

Neonate: IV/IM:

Postnatal age ≤7 days:
- ***<2000 g:*** 100 mg/kg/24 hr ÷ Q12 hr
- ***≥2000 g:*** 100–150 mg/kg/24 hr ÷ Q8–12 hr

Postnatal age >7 days:
- ***<1200 g:*** 100 mg/kg/24 hr ÷ Q12 hr
- ***1200–2000 g:*** 150 mg/kg/24 hr ÷ Q8 hr
- ***>2000 g:*** 150–200 mg/kg/24 hr ÷ Q6–8 hr

Infant and child (1 mo–12 yr and <50 kg): 100–200 mg/kg/24 hr ÷ Q6–8 hr IV/IM. Higher doses of 150–225 mg/kg/24 hr ÷ Q6–8 hr have been recommended for infections outside the CSF due to penicillin-resistant pneumococci.

Meningitis: 200 mg/kg/24 hr ÷ Q6 hr IV/IM. Higher doses of 225–300 mg/kg/24 hr ÷ Q6–8 hr, in combination with vancomycin (dosed at CNS target levels), have been recommended for meningitis due to penicillin-resistant pneumococci.

Max. dose: 12 g/24 hr

Child (>12 yr or ≥50 kg) and adult: 1–2 g/dose Q6–8 hr IV/IM

Severe infection: 2 g/dose Q4–6 hr IV/IM

Max. dose: 12 g/24 hr

Uncomplicated gonorrhea: 0.5–1 g × 1 IM

Continued

CEFOTAXIME *continued*

Use with caution in penicillin allergy and renal impairment (reduce dosage). Toxicities similar to other cephalosporins: allergy, neutropenia, thrombocytopenia, eosinophilia, false-positive urine reducing substance (Clinitest) and Coombs' test, elevated BUN, creatinine, and liver enzymes. Probenecid increases serum cefotaxime levels.

Good CNS penetration. **Adjust dose in renal failure (see Chapter 31).**

CEFOTETAN
Cefotan
Antibiotic, cephalosporin (second generation)

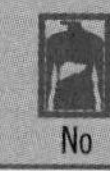
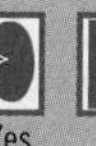
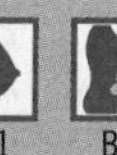
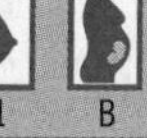

No Yes 1 B

Injection: 1, 2, 10 g
Frozen injection: 1 g/50 mL 3.8% dextrose, 2 g/50 mL 2.2% dextrose (iso-osmotic solutions)
Contains 3.5 mEq Na/g drug

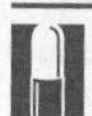

Infant and child (limited data): 40–80 mg/kg/24 hr ÷ Q12 hr IV/IM
Adolescent and adult: 2–4 g/24 hr ÷ Q12 hr IV/IM
PID: 2 g Q12 hr IV × 24–48 hr after clinical improvement with doxycycline 100 mg Q12 hr PO/IV × 14 days

Max. dose (all ages): 6 g/24 hr

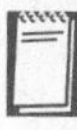

Use with caution in penicillin-allergic patients or in presence of renal impairment. Has good anaerobic activity. May cause disulfiram-like reaction with ethanol, increase effects/toxicities of anticoagulants, false-positive urine reducing substance (Clinitest), and false elevations of serum and urine creatinine (Jaffe method). Hemolytic anemia has been reported. CSF penetration is poor. **Adjust dose in renal failure (see Chapter 31).**

CEFOXITIN
Mefoxin
Antibiotic, cephalosporin (second generation)

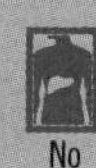
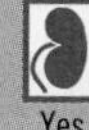
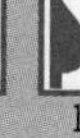
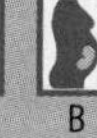

No Yes 1 B

Injection: 1, 2, 10 g
Frozen injection: 1 g/50 mL 4% dextrose, 2 g/50 mL 2.2% dextrose (iso-osmotic solutions)
Contains 2.3 mEq Na/g drug

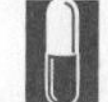

Neonate: 90–100 mg/kg/24 hr ÷ Q8 hr IM/IV
Infant (>3 mo) and child:
Mild/moderate infections: 80–100 mg/kg/24 hr ÷ Q6–8 hr IM/IV
Severe infections: 100–160 mg/kg/24 hr ÷ Q4–6 hr IM/IV
Adult: 1–2 g/dose Q6–8 hr IM/IV
PID: 2 g IV Q6h × 24–48 hr after clinical improvement. Doxycycline 100 mg Q12 hr PO/IV × 14 days is also initiated at the same time.

Max. dose (all ages): 12 g/24 hr

Use with caution in penicillin-allergic patients or in presence of renal impairment. Has good anaerobic activity but poor CSF penetration. Probenecid increases serum cefoxitin levels. May cause false-positive urine reducing substance (Clinitest and other copper reduction method tests), and false elevations of serum and urine creatinine (Jaffe and KDA methods).

Adjust dose in renal failure (see Chapter 31).

For explanation of icons, see p. 663.

CEFPODOXIME PROXETIL
Vantin
Antibiotic, cephalosporin (third generation)

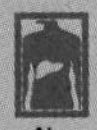 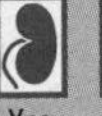 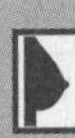 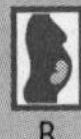
No Yes 1 B

Tabs: 100, 200 mg
Oral suspension: 50, 100 mg/5 mL (50, 75, 100 mL)

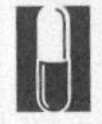

2 mo–12 yr:
Otitis media: 10 mg/kg/24 hr PO ÷ Q12–24 hr; **max. dose:** 400 mg/24 hr
Pharyngitis/tonsillitis: 10 mg/kg/24 hr PO ÷ Q12 hr; **max. dose:** 200 mg/24 hr
Acute maxillary sinusitis: 10 mg/kg/24 hr PO ÷ Q12 hr; **max. dose:** 400 mg/24 hr

≥13 yr–adult:
Exacerbation of chronic bronchitis, community acquired pneumonia, and sinusitis: 400 mg/24 hr PO ÷ Q12 hr
Pharyngitis/tonsillitis: 200 mg/24 hr PO ÷ Q12 hr
Skin/skin structure infection: 800 mg/24 hr PO ÷ Q12 hr
Uncomplicated gonorrhea: 200 mg PO × 1

Use with caution in penicillin-allergic patients or in presence of renal impairment. May cause diarrhea, nausea, vomiting, vaginal candidiasis, and false-positive Coombs' test.

Tablets should be administered with food to enhance absorption. Suspension may be administered without regard to food. High doses of antacids or H_2 blockers may reduce absorption. Probenecid increases serum cefpodoxime levels.

Adjust dose in renal failure (see Chapter 31).

CEFPROZIL
Cefzil and others
Antibiotic, cephalosporin (second generation)

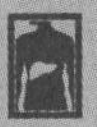 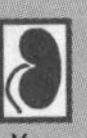 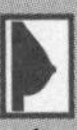 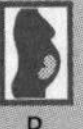
No Yes 1 B

Tabs: 250, 500 mg
Oral suspension: 125 mg/5 mL, 250 mg/5 mL (50, 75, 100 mL) (contains aspartame and phenylalanine)

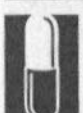

Otitis media:
6 mo–12 yr: 30 mg/kg/24 hr PO ÷ Q12 hr

Pharyngitis/tonsillitis:
2–12 yr: 15 mg/kg/24 hr PO ÷ Q12 hr

Acute sinusitis:
6 mo–12 yr: 15–30 mg/kg/24 hr PO ÷ Q12–24 hr

Uncomplicated skin infections:
2–12 yr: 20 mg/kg/24 hr PO Q24 hr

Other:
≥13 yr and adult: 500–1000 mg/24 hr PO ÷ Q12–24 hr

Max. dose (all ages): 1 g/24 hr

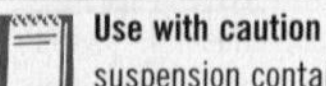

Use with caution in penicillin-allergic patients or in presence of renal impairment. Oral suspension contains aspartame and phenylalanine and should not be used by phenyketonurics. May cause nausea, vomiting, diarrhea, liver enzyme elevations, false-positive urine reducing substance (Clinitest and other copper reduction method tests) and Coombs' test. Probenecid increases serum cefprozil levels. Absorption is not affected by food. **Adjust dose in renal failure (see Chapter 31).**

CEFTAZIDIME
Fortaz, Tazidime, Tazicef, Ceptaz (arginine salt)
Antibiotic, cephalosporin (third generation)

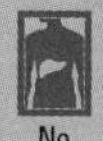
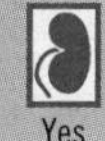

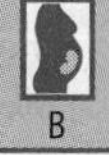
No Yes 1 B

Injection: 0.5, 1, 2, 6, 10 g
Frozen injection: 1 g/50 mL 4.4% dextrose, 2 g/50 mL 3.2% dextrose (iso-osmotic solutions)
(Fortaz, Tazicef, Tazidime contains 2.3 mEq Na/g drug)
(Ceptaz contains 349 mg L-arginine/g drug)

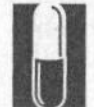

Neonate: IV/IM:
Postnatal age ≤7 days:
<2000 kg: 100 mg/kg/24 hr ÷ Q12 hr
≥2000 kg: 100–150 mg/kg/24 hr ÷ Q8–12 hr
Postnatal age >7 days:
<1200 g: 100 mg/kg/24 hr ÷ Q12 hr
≥1200 g: 150 mg/kg/24 hr ÷ Q8 hr

Infant (>1 mo) and child: 90–150 mg/kg/24 hr ÷ Q8 hr IV/IM; **max. dose:** 6 g/24 hr
Cystic Fibrosis and meningitis: 150 mg/kg/24 hr ÷ Q8 hr IV/IM; **max. dose:** 6 g/24 hr
Adult: 2–6 g/24 hr ÷ Q8–12 hr IV/IM; **max. dose:** 6 g/24 hr

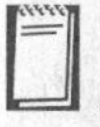

Use with caution in penicillin-allergic patients or in presence of renal impairment. Good *Pseudomonas* coverage and CSF penetration. May cause rash, liver enzyme elevations, false-positive urine reducing substance (Clinitest and other copper reduction method tests) and Coombs' test. Probenecid increases serum ceftazidime levels. **Adjust dose in renal failure (see Chapter 31).**

CEFTIBUTEN
Cedax
Antibiotic, cephalosporin (third generation)

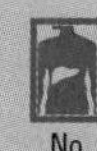
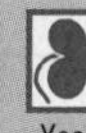
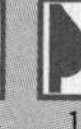
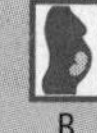
No Yes 1 B

Oral suspension: 90 mg/5 mL (30, 60, 90, 120 mL)
Caps: 400 mg

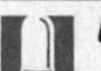

Child:
Otitis media and pharyngitis/tonsillitis: 9 mg/kg/24 hr PO once daily; **max. dose:** 400 mg/24 hr
≥12 yr and adult: 400 mg PO once daily; **max. dose:** 400 mg/24 hr

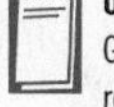

Use with caution in penicillin-allergic patients or in presence of renal impairment. May cause GI symptoms and elevations in eosinophils and BUN. Stevens Johnson Syndrome has been reported. Gastric acid lowering medications (e.g., ranitidine and omeprazole) may enhance bioavailability of ceftibutin.

Oral suspension should be administered 2 hr before or 1 hr after a meal. **Adjust dose in renal failure (see Chapter 31).**

For explanation of icons, see p. 663.

CEFTIZOXIME
Cefizox
Antibiotic, cephalosporin (third generation)

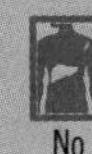
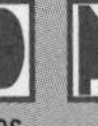
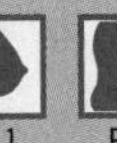
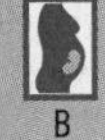
No Yes 1 B

Injection: 0.5, 1, 2, 10 g
Frozen injection: 1 g/50 mL 3.8% dextrose, 2 g/50 mL 1.9% dextrose (iso-osmotic solutions)
Contains 2.6 mEq Na/g drug

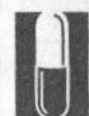

Infant >1 mo and <6 mo: 100–200 mg/kg/24 hr ÷ Q6–8 hr IV/IM
Infant ≥6 mo and child: 150–200 mg/kg/24 hr ÷ Q6–8 hr IV/IM; **max. dose:** 12 g/24 hr
Adult: 2–12 g/24 hr ÷ Q8–12 hr IV/IM; **max. dose:** 12 g/24 hr
Uncomplicated gonorrhea: 1 g IM × 1

Use with caution in penicillin-allergic patients or in presence of renal impairment. May cause liver enzyme elevation, false-positive urine reducing substances (Clinitest, Benedict's solution) and interfere with serum and urine creatinine assays (Jaffe method). Good CNS penetration. Probenecid increases serum ceftizoxime levels. **Adjust dose in renal failure (see Chapter 31).**

CEFTRIAXONE
Rocephin
Antibiotic, cephalosporin (third generation)

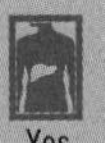
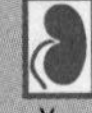
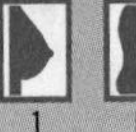
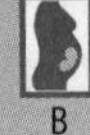
Yes Yes 1 B

Injection: 0.25, 0.5, 1, 2, 10 g
Frozen injection: 1 g/50 mL 3.8% dextrose, 2 g/50 mL 2.4% dextrose (iso-osmotic solutions)
Intramuscular kit with 1% lidocaine diluent: 0.5, 1 g
Contains 3.6 mEq Na/gm drug

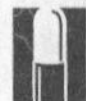

Neonate:
Gonococcal ophthalmia or prophylaxis: 25–50 mg/kg/dose IM/IV × 1; **max. dose:** 125 mg/dose
Infant (>1 mo) and child: 50–75 mg/kg/24 hr ÷ Q12–24 hr IM/IV; **max. dose:** 2 g/24 hr. Higher doses of 80–100 mg/kg/24 hr ÷ Q12–24 hr (**max. dose:** 2 g/dose and 4 g/24 hr) has been recommended for infections outside the CSF due to penicillin-resistant pneumococci.
Meningitis (including penicillin resistant pneumococci): 100 mg/kg/24 hr IM/IV ÷ Q12 hr; **max. dose:** 2 g/dose and 4 g/24 hr
Acute otitis media: 50 mg/kg IM × 1; **max. dose:** 1 g
Adult: 1–2 g/dose Q12–24 hr IV/IM; **max. dose:** 2 g/dose and 4 g/24 hr
Uncomplicated gonorrhea or chancroid: 250 mg IM × 1
Bacterial endocarditis prophylaxis for dental and upper respiratory procedures:
Infant and child: 50 mg/kg IV/IM (**max. dose:** 1 g) 30 min before procedure
Adult: 1 g IV/IM 30 min before procedure

Contraindicated in neonates with hyperbilirubinemia. **Do not** administer with calcium-containing solutions or products (mixed or administered simultaneously via different lines) in neonates (<28 days old) because of risk of precipitation of ceftriaxone-calcium salt. Cases of fatal reactions with calcium-ceftriaxone precipitates in lung and kidneys in term and pre-term neonates have been reported. Do not administer simultaneously with IV calcium-containing solutions via a Y-site for any age group. IV calcium-containing products may be administered sequentially (for patients >28 days old) only when the infusion lines are thoroughly flushed between infusions with a compatible fluid.

Continued

CEFTRIAXONE *continued*

Use with caution in penicillin-allergy; patients with gallbladder, biliary tract, liver, or pancreatic disease; presence of renal impairment; or in neonates with continuous dosing (risk for hyperbilirubinemia). In neonates, consider using an alternative third-generation cephalosporin with similar activity. Unlike other cephalosporins, ceftriaxone is significantly cleared by the biliary route (35%–45%).

Rash, injection site pain, diarrhea, and transient increase in liver enzymes are common. May cause reversible cholelithiasis, sludging in gallbladder, and jaundice. May interfere with serum and urine creatinine assays (Jaffe method) and cause false-positive urinary protein and urinary reducing substances (Clinitest).

For IM injections, dilute drug with either sterile water for injection or 1% lidocaine to a concentration of 250 or 350 mg/mL (250 mg/mL has lower incidence of injection site reactions). See *Lidocaine* for additional remarks.

CEFUROXIME (IV, IM)/CEFUROXIME AXETIL (PO)
CEFUROXIME AXETIL (PO)
IV: Zinacef; PO: Ceftin
Antibiotic, cephalosporin (second generation)

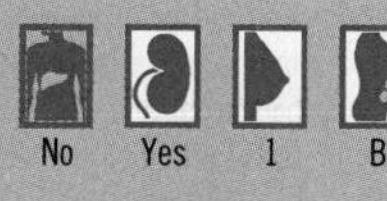

Injection: 0.75, 1.5, 7.5 g
Frozen injection: 750 mg/50 mL 2.8% dextrose, 1.5 g/50 mL water (iso-osmotic solutions)
Injectable dosage forms contain 2.4 mEq Na/g drug
Tabs: 125, 250, 500 mg
Oral suspension: 125, 250 mg/5 mL (50, 100 mL)

IM/IV:
- ***Neonate:*** 50–100 mg/kg/24 hr ÷ Q12 hr
- ***Infant (>3 mo)/child:*** 75–150 mg/kg/24 hr ÷ Q8 hr
- ***Adult:*** 750–1500 mg/dose Q8 hr

Max. dose: 9 g/24 hr

PO (see remarks):

Child (3 mo–12 yr):

Pharyngitis and tonsillitis:
- ***Oral suspension:*** 20 mg/kg/24 hr ÷ Q12 hr; **max. dose:** 500 mg/24 hr

Otitis media, impetigo, and maxillary sinusitis:
- ***Oral suspension:*** 30 mg/kg/24 hr ÷ Q12 hr; **max. dose:** 1 g/24 hr
- ***Tab:*** 250 mg Q12 hr

Child (≥13 yr):

Sinusitis, otitis media, pharyngitis and tonsillitis:
- ***Tab:*** 250 mg Q12 hr

Adult: 250–500 mg BID

Max. dose: 1 g/24 hr

Use with caution in penicillin-allergic patients or in presence of renal impairment. May cause GI discomfort; thrombophlebitis at the infusion site; false-positive urine reducing substance (Clinitest and other copper reduction method tests) and Coombs' test; and may interfere with serum and urine creatinine determinations by the alkaline picrate method. **Not recommended** for meningitis.

Tablets and oral suspension are **NOT** bioequivalent and are **NOT** substitutable on a mg/mg basis. Administer suspension with food. Concurrent use of antacids, H_2 blockers, and proton pump inhibitors may decrease oral absorption. **Adjust dose in renal failure (see Chapter 31).**

For explanation of icons, see p. 663.

CEPHALEXIN
Keflex, Biocef, and others
Antibiotic, cephalosporin (first generation)

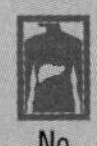 No 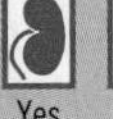 Yes 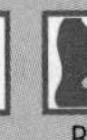 1 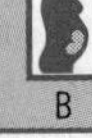 B

Caps and tabs: 250, 500 mg
Oral suspension: 125 mg/5 mL, 250 mg/5 mL (100, 200 mL)

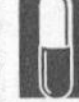

Infant and child: 25–100 mg/kg/24 hr PO ÷ Q6 hr. Less frequent dosing (Q8–12 hr) can be used for uncomplicated infections. Total daily dose may be divided Q12 hr for streptococcal pharyngitis (>1 yr) and skin/skin structure infections.
Adult: 1–4 g/24 hr PO ÷ Q6 hr
Max. dose (all ages): 4 g/24 hr
Bacterial endocarditis prophylaxis for dental and upper respiratory procedures:
Infant and child: 50 mg/kg PO (**max. dose:** 2 g) 1 hr before procedure
Adult: 2 g PO 1 hr before procedure

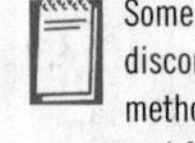

Some cross-reactivity with penicillins. **Use with caution** in renal insufficiency. May cause GI discomfort, false-positive urine reducing substance (Clinitest and other copper reduction method tests) and Coombs' test; false elevation of serum theophylline levels (HPLC method); and false urinary protein test. Probenecid increases serum cephalexin levels and concomitant administration with cholestyramine may reduce cephalexin absorption. May increase the effects of metformin.

Administer doses on an empty stomach; 2 hr prior or 1 hr after meals. **Adjust dose in renal failure (see Chapter 31).**

CETIRIZINE ± PSEUDOEPHEDRINE
Zyrtec, Children's Zyrtec
In combination with pseudoephedrine:
Zyrtec-D 12 Hour
Antihistamine, less-sedating

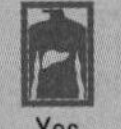 Yes 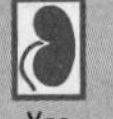 Yes 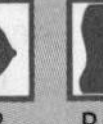 ?  B/C

Syrup (OTC): 5 mg/5 mL (120, 473 mL)
Tabs: 5 mg, 10 mg (OTC)
Chewable tabs (OTC): 5, 10 mg
In combination with pseudoephedrine (PE):
Extended release tabs (Zyrtec-D 12 Hour; OTC): 5 mg cetirizine + 120 mg PE

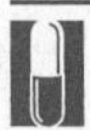

Cetirizine (see remarks for dosing in hepatic impairment):
6 mo and <2 yr: 2.5 mg PO once daily; dose may be increased for children 12–23 mo to a **max. dose** of 2.5 mg PO Q12 hr.
2–5 yr: Initial dose: 2.5 mg PO once daily; if needed, may increase dose to a **max. dose** of 5 mg/24 hr once daily or divided BID.
≥6 yr–adult: 5–10 mg PO once daily
Cetirizine in combination with pseudoephedrine (PE) (see remarks for dosing in hepatic impairment):
≥12 yr and adult:
Zyrtec-D 12 Hour: 1 tablet PO BID

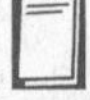

Generally not recommended for treating URIs for infants. No proven benefit for infants and young children with URIs. **The FDA does not recommend use for URIs in children <2 yr because of reports of increased fatalities.**

Continued

CETIRIZINE ± PSEUDOEPHEDRINE *continued*

May cause headache, pharyngitis, GI symptoms, dry mouth, and sedation. Aggressive reactions and convulsions have been reported. Has **NOT** been implicated in causing cardiac arrhythmias when used with other drugs that are metabolized by hepatic microsomal enzymes (e.g., ketoconazole, erythromycin).

In hepatic impairment, the following doses have been recommended:

Cetirizine:

- **<6 yr:** use is **not recommended**
- **6–11 yr:** <2.5 mg PO once daily
- **≥12 yr–adult:** 5 mg PO once daily

Cetirizine in combination with pseudoephedrine:

- **≥12 yr–adult:** 1 tablet PO once daily

Doses may be administered regardless to food. For Zyrtec-D 12 Hour, see *Pseudoephedrine* for additional remarks. **Dosage adjustment is recommended in renal impairment (see Chapter 31).**

CHARCOAL, ACTIVATED

See Chapter 2

CHLORAL HYDRATE

Aquachloral Supprettes and others

Sedative, hypnotic

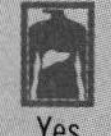
Yes
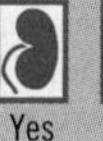
Yes
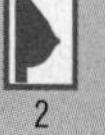
2
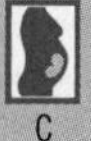
C

Caps: 500 mg
Syrup: 250, 500 mg/5 mL
Suppository (Aquachloral Supprettes): 325, 500, 650 mg; may contain tartrazine

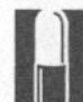

Infant and child:

Sedative: 25–50 mg/kg/24 hr PO/PR ÷ Q6–8 hr; **max. dose:** 500 mg/dose

Sedation for procedures: 50–75 mg/kg/dose PO/PR 30–60 min prior to procedure; may repeat in 30 min if needed to up to a total **max. dose** of 120 mg/kg or 1 g total for infants and 2 g total for children

Adult:

Sedative: 250 mg/dose TID PO/PR

Hypnotic: 500–1000 mg/dose PO/PR; **max. dose:** 2 g/24 hr

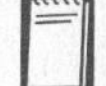

Contraindicated in patients with hepatic or renal disease. **Avoid** use if GFR <50 mL/min (see Chapter 31). **Use with caution** in combination with IV furosemide (vasodilation) or warfarin (potentiates warfarin). May cause GI irritation, paradoxical excitement, hypotension, and myocardial/respiratory depression. Chronic administration in neonates can lead to accumulation of active metabolites. Requires same monitoring as other sedatives.

Not analgesic. Peak effects occur within 30–60 min. **Do not exceed** 2 wk of chronic use. **Avoid** use in moderate/severe renal failure. Sudden withdrawal may cause delirium tremens.

For additional information see Chapter 6.

For explanation of icons, see p. 663.

CHLORAMPHENICOL
Chloromycetin and others
Antibiotic

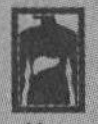 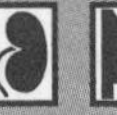 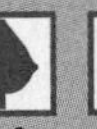 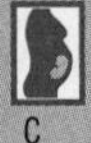
Yes Yes 3 C

Injection: 1 g
Contains 2.25 mEq Na/g drug

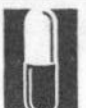

Neonate IV:
Loading dose: 20 mg/kg
Maintenance dose (first dose should be given 12 hours after loading dose):
≤7 days: 25 mg/kg/24 hr Q24 hr
>7 days:
≤2 kg: 25 mg/kg/24 hr Q24 hr
>2 kg: 50 mg/kg/24 hr ÷ Q12 hr
Infant/child/adult: 50–75 mg/kg/24 hr IV ÷ Q6 hr
Meningitis: 75–100 mg/kg/24 hr IV ÷ Q6 hr
Max. dose (all ages): 4 g/24 hr

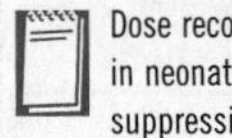

Dose recommendations are just guidelines for therapy; monitoring of blood levels is essential in neonates and infants. Follow hematologic status for dose related or idiosyncratic marrow suppression. "Gray baby" syndrome may be seen with levels >50 mg/L. **Use with caution** in G6PD deficiency, renal or hepatic dysfunction, and neonates.

Concomitant use of phenobarbital and rifampin may lower chloramphenicol serum levels. Phenytoin may increase chloramphenicol serum levels. Chloramphenicol may increase the effects/toxicity of phenytoin, chlorpropamide, cyclosporine, tacrolimus, and oral anticoagulants; and decrease absorption of vitamin B_{12}. Chloramphenicol is an inhibitor of CYP 450 2C9.

Therapeutic levels: Peak: 15–25 mg/L for meningitis, and 10–20 mg/L for other infections. Trough: 5–15 mg/L for meningitis, and 5–10 mg/L for other infections. Recommended serum sampling time: trough (IV/PO) within 30 min prior to next dose; peak (IV) 30 min after the end of infusion; peak (PO) 2 hr after oral administration. Time to achieve steady-state: 2–3 days for newborns; 12–24 hr for children and adults. **NOTE:** higher serum levels may be achieved using the oral, rather than the IV route.

CHLOROQUINE HCL/PHOSPHATE
Aralen and others
Amebicide, antimalarial

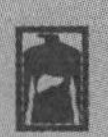 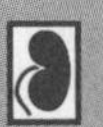  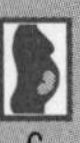
Yes Yes 2 C

Tabs: 250, 500 mg as phosphate (150, 300 mg base, respectively)
Oral suspension: 16.67 mg/mL as phosphate (10 mg/mL base), 15 mg/mL as phosphate (9 mg/mL base)
Injection: 50 mg/mL as HCl (40 mg/mL base) (5 mL)

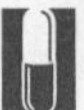

Doses expressed in mg of chloroquine base:
Malaria prophylaxis (start 1 wk prior to exposure and continue for 4 wk after leaving endemic area):
Infant and child: 5 mg/kg/dose PO Q wk; **max. dose:** 300 mg/dose
Adult: 300 mg/dose PO Q wk

Continued

C FORMULARY

CHLOROQUINE HCL/PHOSPHATE *continued*

Malaria treatment (chloroquine sensitive strains):
For treatment for malaria, consult with ID specialist or see the latest edition of the AAP Red Book.
For IV use, consider safer alternatives such as quinidine or quinine.

Infant and child: 10 mg/kg/dose (**max. dose:** 600 mg/dose) PO × 1; followed by 5 mg/kg/dose (**max. dose:** 300 mg/dose) 6 hr later and then once daily for 2 days.

Adult: 600 mg/dose PO × 1; followed by 300 mg/dose 6 hr later and then once daily for 2 days.

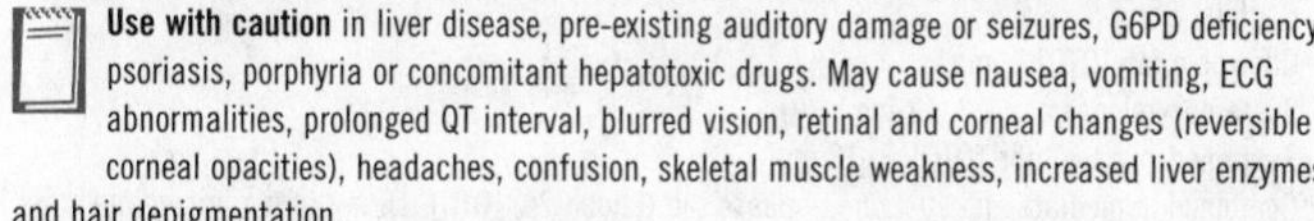

Use with caution in liver disease, pre-existing auditory damage or seizures, G6PD deficiency, psoriasis, porphyria or concomitant hepatotoxic drugs. May cause nausea, vomiting, ECG abnormalities, prolonged QT interval, blurred vision, retinal and corneal changes (reversible corneal opacities), headaches, confusion, skeletal muscle weakness, increased liver enzymes, and hair depigmentation.

Antacids, ampicillin, and kaolin may decrease the absorption of chloroquine (allow 4 hr interval between these drugs and chloroquine). Cimetidine may increase effects/toxicity of chloroquine. May increase serum cyclosporine levels. Co-administration with mefloquine may increase risk of convulsions. May reduce the antibody response to intradermal human diploid-cell rabies vaccine.

Adjust dose in renal failure (see Chapter 31).

CHLOROTHIAZIDE
Diuril, Diurigen, and others
Thiazide diuretic

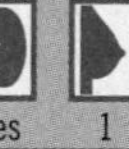 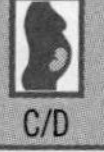

Yes Yes 1 C/D

Tabs: 250, 500 mg
Oral suspension: 250 mg/5 mL (237 mL); contains 0.5% alcohol, 0.12% methylparaben, 0.02% propylparaben, and 0.1% benzoic acid
Injection: 500 mg; contains 5 mEq Na/1 g drug

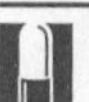

<6 mo:

PO: 20–40 mg/kg/24 hr ÷ Q12 hr

IV: Start at 2–8 mg/kg/24 hr ÷ Q12 hr, may increase to 20–40 mg/kg/24 hr ÷ Q12 hr if needed.

≥6 mo:

PO: 20 mg/kg/24 hr ÷ Q12 hr; **maximum PO dose** by age:

6 mo–2 yr: 375 mg/24 hr
2–12 yr: 1 g/24 hr
>12 yr: 2 g/24 hr

IV: Start at 4 mg/kg/24 hr ÷ Q12–24 hr, may increase to 20 mg/kg/24 hr ÷ Q12 hr if needed.

Adult: 500–2000 mg/24 hr ÷ Q12–24 hr PO/IV; alternative IV dosing, some may respond to intermittent dosing on alternate days or on 3–5 days each week.

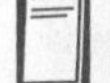

Use with caution in liver and severe renal disease. May increase serum calcium, bilirubin, glucose, and uric acid. May cause alkalosis, pancreatitis, dizziness, hypokalemia, and hypomagnesemia.

Avoid IM or subcutaneous administration.

Pregnancy category changes to "D" if used in pregnancy-induced hypertension.

For explanation of icons, see p. 663.

CHLORPHENIRAMINE MALEATE/DEXCHLORPHENIRAMINE MALEATE
Chlorpheniramine: Chlor-Trimeton, Efidac 24, and others
Dexchlorpheniramine: various generics
Antihistamine

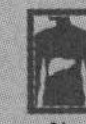
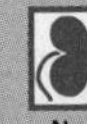
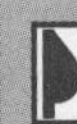
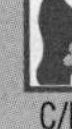

No No ? C/B

CHLORPHENIRAMINE MALEATE:

Tabs [OTC]: 4 mg
Caplets: 8 mg
Chewable tab [OTC]: 2 mg
Sustained-release caps: 8, 12 mg
Sustained-release tabs [OTC]: 8, 12 mg
Combined immediate and sustained-release tab (Efidac 24) [OTC]: 16 mg (4 mg immediate and 12 mg sustained)
Syrup [OTC]: 2 mg/5 mL (473 mL); contains 5% alcohol
Oral suspension: 4 mg/5 mL (118 mL), 8 mg/5 mL (473 mL); contains methylparaben

DEXCHLORPHENIRAMINE MALEATE:

Sustained-release tabs: 4, 6 mg
Syrup: 2 mg/5 Ml (473 Ml); contains alcohol

CHLORPHENIRAMINE MALEATE DOSING:

Child <12 yr: 0.35 mg/kg/24 hr PO ÷ Q4–6 hr or dose based on age as follows:
2–5 yr: 1 mg/dose PO Q4–6 hr; **max. dose:** 6 mg/24 hr
6–11 yr: 2 mg/dose PO Q4–6 hr; **max. dose:** 12 mg/24 hr
Sustained-release (6–12 yr): 8 mg/dose PO Q12 hr
≥12 yr–adult: 4 mg/dose Q4–6 hr PO; **max. dose:** 24 mg/24 hr
Sustained-release: 8 or 12 mg PO Q 12 hr
Efidac 24: 16 mg PO Q24 hr; **max. dose:** 16 mg/24 hr

DEXCHLORPHENIRAMINE MALEATE DOSING:

2–5 yr: 0.5 mg/dose PO Q4–6hr; **max. dose:** 3 mg/24 hr
6–11 yr: 1 mg/dose PO Q4–6 hr; **max. dose:** 6 mg/24 hr
Sustained-release: 4 mg PO QHS
≥12 yr–adult: 2 mg/dose PO Q4–6hr; **max. dose**: 12 mg/24 hr
Sustained-release: 4 or 6 mg PO QHS or Q8–10 hr; **max. dose:** 12 mg/24 hr

Use with caution in asthma. May cause sedation, dry mouth, blurred vision, urinary retention, polyuria, and disturbed coordination. Young children may be paradoxically excited.

Combination over the counter (OTC or nonprescription) cough and cold products are not recommended for children <6 yr old due to reports of serious adverse effects (cardiac and respiratory distress, convulsions, and hallucinations) and fatalities (from unintentional overdosages, including combined use of other OTC products containing the same active ingredients).

NOTE: Dexchlorpheniramine maleate doses are 50% of chlorpheniramine maleate and do not possess any significant advantages over other antihistamines.

Doses may be administered PRN. Administer doses with food. Sustained-release forms are **NOT recommended** in children <6 yr and should **NOT** be crushed, chewed, or dissolved.

Pregnancy category is "C" for chlorpheniramine and "B" for dexchlorpheniramine.

CHLORPROMAZINE
Thorazine and others
Antiemetic, antipsychotic, phenothiazine derivative

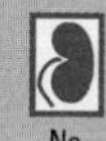  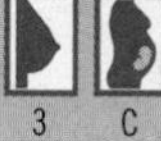

No No 3 C

Tabs: 10, 25, 50, 100, 200 mg
Extended-release caps: 30, 75, 150 mg
Suppository: 100 mg
Injection: 25 mg/mL (contains 2% benzyl alcohol)

Psychosis:
Child >6 mo:
PO: 2.5–6 mg/kg/24 hr ÷ Q4–6 hr
PR: 1 mg/kg/dose Q6–8 hr
IM/IV: 2.5–4 mg/kg/24 hr ÷ Q6–8 hr
Max. IM/IV dose:
<5 yr: 40 mg/24 hr
5–12 yr: 75 mg/24 hr
Adult:
PO: 10–25 mg/dose Q4–6 hr; **max. dose:** 2 g/24 hr
IM/IV: Initial: 25 mg; repeat with 25–50 mg/dose, if needed, Q1–4 hr up to a **max. dose** of 400 mg/dose Q4–6 hr

Antiemetic:
Child (≥6 mo):
IV/IM: 0.5–1 mg/kg/dose Q6–8 hr PRN
Max. IM/IV dose:
<5 yr: 40 mg/24 hr
5–12 yr: 75 mg/24 hr
PO: 0.5–1 mg/kg/dose Q4–6 hr PRN
PR: 1.1 mg/kg/dose Q6–8 hr PRN
Adult:
IV/IM: 25–50 mg/dose Q4–6 hr PRN
PO: 10–25 mg/dose Q4–6 hr PRN
PR: 50–100 mg/dose Q6–8 hr PRN

Adverse effects include drowsiness, jaundice, lowered seizure threshold, extrapyramidal/anticholinergic symptoms, hypotension (more with IV), arrhythmias, agranulocytosis, and neuroleptic malignant syndrome. May potentiate effect of narcotics, sedatives, and other drugs. Monitor BP closely. ECG changes include prolonged PR interval, flattened T waves, and ST depression. **Do not administer** oral liquid dosage form **simultaneously** with carbamazepine oral suspension because an orange rubbery precipitate may form.

CHOLECALCIFEROL
D-3, D3-5, D3-50, D Drops, Emfamil D-Vi-Sol, and many others
Vitamin D_3

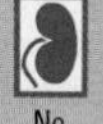 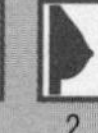 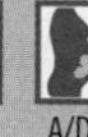

No No 2 A/D

Tablet (OTC): 400, 1000, 2000, 5000 IU
Softgel caps (OTC): 2000, 4000, 5000 IU
Caps: 1000 IU

Continued

For explanation of icons, see p. 663.

CHOLECALCIFEROL *continued*

Caps:

D3-5: 5000 IU
Maximum D3: 10,000 IU
D3-50: 50,000 IU

Oral drops (D Drops) [OTC]: 400, 1000, 2000 IU/drop (10 mL)
Oral liquid: (Emfamil D-Vi-Sol): 400 IU/mL (50 mL)

Dietary supplementation (see Chapter 21 for additional information):

Preterm: 400–800 IU/24 hr PO
Infant (<1 yr): 400 IU/24 hr PO
Child (≥1 yr) and adolescent: 600 IU/24 hr PO

Vitamin D deficiency and/or rickets (with calcium and phosphorus supplementation; decrease dose (all ages) to 400 IU once daily when radiologic proven healing is achieved):

<1 mo: 1000 IU/24 hr PO × 2–3 mo
1-12 mo: 1000–5000 IU/24 hr PO × 2–3 mo
>12 mo: 5000–10,000 IU/24 hr PO × 2–3 mo

Renal failure (CKD stages 2–5) and 25-OH vitamin D levels <30 ng/mL (monitor serum 25-OH vitamin D and corrected calcium/phosphorus one month after initiation and Q 3 mo thereafter):

Child (PO):

25-OH vitamin D <5 ng/mL: 8000 IU/24 hr × 4 wk followed by 4000 IU/24 hr × 2 mo; or 50,000 IU weekly × 4 wk followed by 50,000 IU twice monthly for 2 mo
25-OH vitamin D 5–15 ng/mL: 4000 IU/24 hr × 12 wks; or 50,000 IU every other week × 12 wk
25-OH vitamin D 16-30 ng/mL: 2000 IU/24 hr × 3 mo; or 50,000 IU monthly × 3 mo
Maintenance dose (following repletion): 200–1000 IU once daily

Biological potency and oral absorption may be greater than ergocalciferol (vitamin D_2). Requires activation by the liver (25-hydroxylation) and kidney (1-hydroxylation) to the active form, calcitriol.

Monitor serum Ca^{2+}, PO_4, 25-OH vitamin D (goal level for infant and child: ≥20 ng/mL) and alkaline phosphate. Serum Ca^{2+}, PO_4 product should be <70 mg/dL to avoid ectopic calcification. Serum 25-OH vitamin D level of ≥35 ng/mL has been suggested in Cystic Fibrosis patients to decrease the risk of hyperparathyroidism and bone loss.

Toxic effects in infants may result in nausea, vomiting, constipation, abdominal pain, loss of appetite, polydipsia, polyuria, muscle weakness, muscle/joint pain, confusion, and fatigue; renal damage may also occur.

Pregnancy category changes to "D" if used in doses above the U.S. RDA.

CHOLESTYRAMINE
Questran, Questran Light, Cholestyramine Light, Prevalite, and others
Antilipemic, binding resin

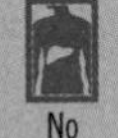
No
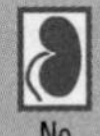
No
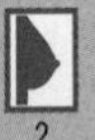
2
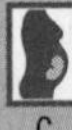
C

Powder for oral suspension:

Questran and others: 4 g anhydrous resin per 9 g powder (9, 378 g)
Questran Light: 4 g anhydrous resin per 6.4 g powder with aspartame (210, 239 g)
Cholestyramine Light: 4 g anhydrous resin per 5.7 g powder with aspartame (210, 239 g)
Prevalite: 4 g anhydrous resin per 5.5 g powder with aspartame (5.5, 231 g)

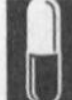

All doses based in terms of anhydrous resin. Titrate dose based on response and tolerance.
Child: 240 mg/kg/24 hr ÷ TID; doses normally **do not exceed** 8 g/24 hr (higher doses do not provide additional benefit). Give PO as slurry in water, juice, or milk before meals.

Continued

CHOLESTYRAMINE *continued*

Adult: 3–4 g of cholestyramine BID–QID
Max. dose: 32 g/24 hr

In addition to the use for managing hypercholesterolemia, drug may be used for itching associated with elevated bile acids, and diarrheal disorders associated with excess fecal bile acids or *Clostridium difficile* (pseudomembranous colitis). May cause constipation, abdominal distention, vomiting, vitamin deficiencies (A, D, E, K), and rash. Hyperchloremic acidosis may occur with prolonged use.

Give other oral medications 4–6 hr after cholestyramine or 1 hr before dose to avoid decreased absorption.

CHOLINE MAGNESIUM TRISALICYLATE
Trilisate and others
Nonsteroidal anti-inflammatory agent

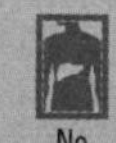
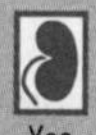
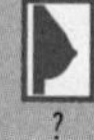
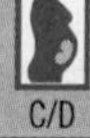

No Yes ? C/D

Combination of choline salicylate and magnesium salicylate (1 : 1.24 ratio, respectively); strengths expressed in terms of mg salicylate:

Tabs: 750 mg
Oral liquid: 500 mg/5 mL (237 mL)

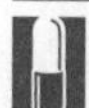

Dose based on total salicylate content.
Child: 30–60 mg/kg/24 hr PO ÷ TID–QID
Adult: 500 mg–1.5 g/dose PO once daily–TID

Avoid use in patients with suspected varicella or influenza due to concerns of Reye's Syndrome. **Use with caution** in severe renal failure because of risk for hypermagnesemia, or in peptic ulcer disease. Less GI irritation than aspirin and other NSAIDs. No antiplatelet effects.

Pregnancy category changes to "D" if used during the third trimester.

Therapeutic salicylate levels, see *Aspirin.* 500 mg choline magnesium trisalicylate is equivalent to 650 mg aspirin.

CICLESONIDE
Alvesco, Omnaris
Corticosteroid

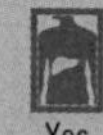
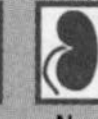
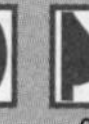
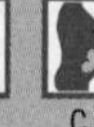

Yes No 2 C

Aerosol inhaler (Alvesco): 80 mcg/actuation (6.1 g = 60 doses), 160 mcg/actuation (6.1 g = 60 doses)
Nasal spray (Omnaris): 50 mcg/actuation (12.5 g = 120 doses)

Intranasal (allergic rhinitis):
≥6 yr and adult: 2 sprays (100 mcg) per nostril once daily. **Max. dose:** 200 mcg/24 hr.
Oral inhalation (asthma):
6–11 yr: see remarks
≥12 yr and adult (see remarks):
Prior use with bronchodilator only: 80 mcg/dose BID; **max. dose:** 320 mcg/24 hr
Prior use with inhaled corticosteroid: 80 mcg/dose BID; **max. dose:** 640 mcg/24 hr
Prior use with oral corticosteroid: 320 mcg/dose BID; **max. dose:** 640 mcg/24 hr

Ciclesonide is a prodrug hydrolyzed to an active metabolite, des-ciclesonide via esterases in nasal mucosa and lungs; further metabolism via hepatic CYP3A4 and 2D6. Concurrent use with ketoconazole and other CYP 450 3A4 inhibitors may increase des-ciclesonide levels. **Use with caution** and monitor in hepatic impairment.

Continued

For explanation of icons, see p. 663.

CICLESONIDE *continued*

Oral inhalation (asthma): Rinse mouth after each use. May cause headache, arthralgia, nasal congestion, nasopharyngitis, and URIs. Maximum benefit may not be achieved until 4 wk after initiation; consider dose increase if response is inadequate after 4 wk after initial dosage. In Canada, the aerosol inhaler is available in 50, 100, and 200 mcg/actuation strengths and is labeled for use as follows:

6–11 yr: 100–200 mcg once daily (1–2 puffs once daily).

≥12 yr and adult: Start with 400 mcg once daily; maintenance 100–800 mcg/24 hr (1–2 puffs once daily–BID).

Intranasal (allergic rhinitis): Clear nasal passages prior to use. May cause otalgia, epistaxis, nasaopharyngitis and headache. Onset of action: 24–48 hours; further improvement observed over 1–2 wk in seasonal allergic rhinitis or 5 wk in perennial allergic rhinitis.

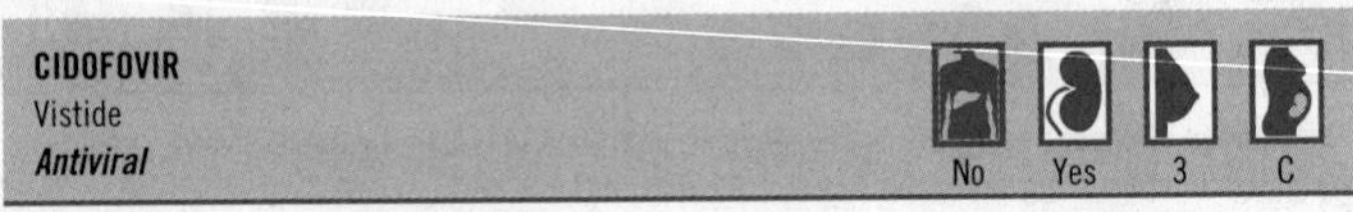

CIDOFOVIR
Vistide
Antiviral

Injection: 75 mg/mL (5 mL); preservative free

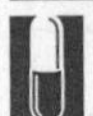

Safety and efficacy has not been established in children.

CMV retinitis:

Adult:

Induction: 5 mg/kg IV once weekly × 2 with probenecid and hydration

Maintenance: 5 mg/kg IV Q2 weeks with probenecid and hydration

Adenovirus infection in immunocompromised oncology patients (limited data; see remarks):

Child: 5 mg/kg/dose IV once weekly until PCR negative. Administer oral probenecid 1–1.25 g/m^2/dose (rounded to the nearest 250 mg interval) 3 hr prior to and 1 hr and 8 hr after each dose of cidofovir. Also give IV normal saline at three times maintenance fluid 1 hr prior to and 1 hr after cidofovir, followed by 2 times maintenance fluid for an additional 2 hr. For patients with renal dysfunction (see remarks), give 1 mg/kg/dose IV three times weekly until PCR negative.

BK virus hemorrhagic cystitis (limited data): 1 mg/kg/dose IV once weekly without probenecid.

Contraindicated in hypersensitivity to probenecid or sulfa-containing drugs; sCr >1.5 mg/dL, CrCl ≤55 mL/min, urine protein ≥100 mg/dL (2+ proteinuria), direct intraocular injection of cidofovir, and concomitant nephrotoxic drugs. **Renal impairment is the major dose-limiting toxicity.** IV NS prehydration and probencid must be used (unless not indicated) to reduce risk of nephrotoxicity. May also cause nausea, vomiting, headache, rash, metabolic acidosis, uveitis, decreased intraocular pressure, and neutropenia.

A reported criteria for defining renal dysfunction in children included a sCr >1.5 mg/dL, GFR <90 mL/min/1.73 m^2 and >2+ proteinuria. For adults, reduce dose to 3 mg/kg if sCr increases 0.3–0.4 mg/dL from baseline. Discontinue therapy if sCr increases ≥0.5 mg/dL from baseline or development of ≥3+ proteinuria.

Administer doses via IV infusion over 1 hr at a concentration ≤8 mg/mL.

CIMETIDINE
Tagamet, Tagamet HB [OTC], and many others
Histamine-2-antagonist

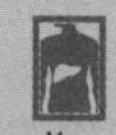 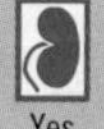  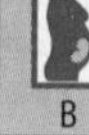 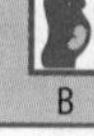

Yes Yes 2 B

Tabs: 200 (OTC), 300, 400, 800 mg
Oral solution: 300 mg/5 mL (240, 480 mL); may contain 2.8% alcohol
Injection: 150 mg/mL; may contain benzyl alcohol
Pre-mixed injection: 300 mg in 50 mL normal saline

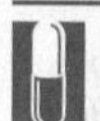

Neonate: 5–20 mg/kg/24 hr IM/PO/IV ÷ Q6–12 hr
Infant: 10–20 mg/kg/24 hr IM/PO/IV ÷ Q6–12 hr
Child: 20–40 mg/kg/24 hr IM/PO/IV ÷ Q6 hr
Adult:
- ***PO:*** 300 mg/dose QID or 400 mg/dose BID or 800 mg/dose QHS
- ***IV/IM:*** 300 mg/dose Q6 hr; **max. dose:** 2400 mg/24 hr
- ***Continuous IV infusion:*** 150 mg IV × 1 followed by 37.5 mg/hr; infusions have ranged from 40–600 mg/hr with a mean rate of 160 mg/hr
- ***Ulcer prophylaxis:*** 400–800 mg PO QHS

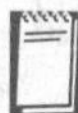

Diarrhea, rash, myalgia, confusion, neutropenia, gynecomastia, elevated liver function tests, or dizziness may occur. **Use with caution** in hepatic and renal impairment **(adjust dose in renal failure; see Chapter 31).**

Inhibits CYP 450 1A2, 2C9, 2C19, 2D6, 2E1, and 3A4 isoenzymes, therefore increases levels and effects of many hepatically metabolized drugs (i.e., theophylline, phenytoin, lidocaine, diazepam, warfarin). Cimetidine may decrease the absorption of iron, ketoconazole, and tetracyclines.

CIPROFLOXACIN
Cipro, Cipro XR, Ciloxan ophthalmic, Cetraxal, Ciprodex, Cipro HC Otic, and others
Antibiotic, quinolone

 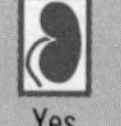  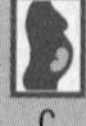

No Yes 2 C

Tabs: 100, 250, 500, 750 mg
Extended-release tabs (Cipro XR): 500, 1000 mg
Oral suspension: 500 mg/5 mL (100 mL)
Injection: 10 mg/mL (40 mL)
Pre-mixed injection: 200 mg/100 mL 5% dextrose, 400 mg/100 mL 5% dextrose (iso-osmotic solutions)
Ophthalmic solution: 3.5 mg/mL (2.5, 5, 10 mL)
Ophthalmic ointment: 3.3 mg/g (3.5 g)
Otic suspension:
- **Cetraxal:** 0.5 mg/0.25 mL (14s)
- **With dexamethasone (Ciprodex):** 3 mg/mL ciprofloxacin + 1 mg/mL dexamethasone (7.5 mL); contains benzalkonium chloride
- **With hydrocortisone (Cipro HC Otic):** 2 mg/mL ciprofloxacin + 10 mg/mL hydrocortisone (10 mL); contains benzyl alcohol

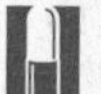

Child:
- ***PO:*** 20–30 mg/kg/24 hr ÷ Q12 hr; **max. dose:** 1.5 g/24 hr
- ***IV:*** 20–30 mg/kg/24 hr ÷ Q12 hr; **max. dose:** 800 mg/24 hr

Continued

For explanation of icons, see p. 663.

CIPROFLOXACIN *continued*

Child (cont'd):

Complicated UTI or pyelonephritis (×10–21 days):

PO: 20–40 mg/kg/24 hr ÷ Q12 hr; **max. dose:** 1.5 g/24 hr

IV: 18–30 mg/kg/24 hr ÷ Q8 hr; **max. dose:** 1.2 g/24 hr

Cystic Fibrosis:

PO: 40 mg/kg/24 hr ÷ Q12 hr; **max. dose:** 2 g/24 hr

IV: 30 mg/kg/24 hr ÷ Q8 hr; **max. dose:** 1.2 g/24 hr

Anthrax (see remarks):

Inhalational/systemic/cutaneous: Start with 20–30 mg/kg/24 hr ÷ Q12 hr IV (**max. dose:** 800 mg/24 hr) and convert to oral dosing with clinical improvement at 20–30 mg/kg/24 hr ÷ Q12 hr PO (**max. dose:** 1 g/24 hr). Duration of therapy: 60 days (IV and PO combined)

Post exposure prophylaxis: 20–30 mg/kg/24 hr ÷ Q12 hr PO × 60 days; **max. dose:** 1 g/24 hr

Adult:

PO

Immediate release: 250–750 mg/dose Q12 hr

Extended release (Cipro XR):

Uncomplicated UTI/Cystitis: 500 mg/dose Q24 hr

Complicated UTI/Uncomplicated pyelonephritis: 1000 mg/dose Q24 hr

IV: 200–400 mg/dose Q12 hr; 400 mg/dose Q8 hr for more severe/complicated infections

Anthrax (see remarks):

Inhalational/systemic/cutaneous: Start with 400 mg/dose Q12 hr IV and convert to oral dosing with clinical improvement at 500 mg/dose Q12 hr PO. Duration of therapy: 60 days (IV and PO combined)

Post exposure prophylaxis: 500 mg/dose Q12 hr PO × 60 days.

Ophthalmic solution: 1–2 drops Q2 hr while awake × 2 days, then 1–2 gtts Q4 hr while awake × 5 days

Ophthalmic ointment: Apply 0.5 inch ribbon TID × 2, then BID × 5 days

Otic:

Cetraxal:

Acute otitis externa, ≥1 yr and adult: 0.25 mL to affected ear(s) BID × 7 days

Ciprodex:

Acute otitis media with tympanostomy tubes or acute otitis externa, ≥ 6 mo and adult: 4 drops to affected ear(s) BID × 7 days

Cipro HC Otic:

Otitis externa, >1 yr and adult: 3 drops to affected ear(s) BID × 7 days

---

Can cause GI upset, renal failure, and seizures. GI symptoms, headache, restlessness, and rash are common side effects. Photosensitivity has been reported. **Use with caution** in children <18 yr. Like other quinolones, tendon rupture can occur during or after therapy. **Do not use** otic suspension with perforated tympanic membranes and with viral infections of the external ear canal.

For dosing in obese patients, use an adjusted body weight (ABW). ABW = Ideal Body Weight + 0.45 (Total Body Weight − Ideal Body Weight).

Combinational antimicrobial therapy is recommended for anthrax. For penicillin-susceptible strains, consider changing to high-dose amoxicillin (25–35 mg/kg/dose TID PO). See www.bt.cdc.gov for the latest information.

Inhibits CYP 450 1A2. Ciprofloxacin can increase effects and/or toxicity of theophylline, warfarin, tizanidine (excessive sedation and dangerous hypotension), and cyclosporine.

Do not administer antacids or other divalent salts with or within 2–4 hr of oral ciprofloxacin dose. **Adjust dose in renal failure (see Chapter 31).**

CITRATE MIXTURES
Alkalinizing agent, electrolyte supplement

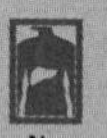
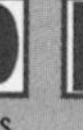
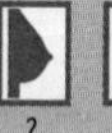
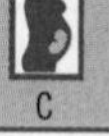
No Yes ? C

Each mL contains the following mEq of electrolyte:

	Na	K	Citrate or HCO_3
Polycitra or Cytra-3 (120, 480 mL)	1	1	2
Polycitra-LC* or Cytra-LC* (120, 480 mL)	1	1	2
Polycitra-K or Cytra-K (120, 480 mL)	0	2	2
Bicitra^, Cytra-2, or Sodium Citrate/Citric Acid^ (15, 30, 120, 480 mL)	1	0	1
Oracit (15, 30, 500 mL)	1	0	1

*LC = low calorie (contains no sucrose, sorbitol, glycerin).
^Sugar-free.

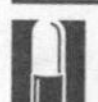

Dilute dose in water or juice.
All mEq doses based on citrate.
Infant and child (PO): 2–3 mEq/kg/24 hr ÷ Q6–8 hr or 5–15 mL/dose Q6–8 hr (after meals and before bedtime)
Adult (PO): 100–200 mEq/24 hr ÷ Q6–8 hr or 15–30 mL/dose Q6–8 hr (after meals and before bedtime)

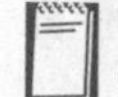

Contraindicated in severe renal impairment and acute dehydration. **Use with caution** in patients already receiving potassium supplements or who are sodium restricted. May have laxative effect and cause hypocalemia and metabolic alkalosis.

Adjust dose to maintain desired pH. 1 mEq of citrate is equivalent to 1 mEq HCO_3 in patients with normal hepatic function.

CLARITHROMYCIN
Biaxin, Biaxin XL
Antibiotic, macrolide

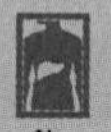
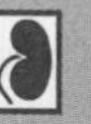
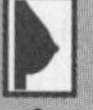
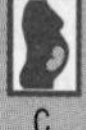
No Yes 2 C

Film tablets: 250, 500 mg
Extended-release tablets (Biaxin XL): 500 mg
Granules for oral suspension: 125, 250 mg/5 mL (50, 100 mL)

Infant and child:

Acute otitis media, pharyngitis/tonsillitis, pneumonia, acute maxillary sinusitis, or uncomplicated skin infections: 15 mg/kg/24 hr PO ÷ Q12 hr

M. avium complex (MAC):

Prophylaxis (1st episode and recurrence): 15 mg/kg/24 hr PO ÷ Q12 hr
Treatment: 15 mg/kg/24 hr PO ÷ Q12 hr with other antimycobacterial drugs
Max. dose: 1 g/24 hr

Adolescent and adult:

Pharyngitis/tonsillitis, acute maxillary sinusitis, bronchitis, pneumonia, or uncomplicated skin infections:

Immediate release: 250–500 mg/dose Q12 hr PO
Extended release (Biaxin XL): 1000 mg Q24 hr PO (currently not indicated for pharyngitis/tonsillitis or uncomplicated skin infections)

Continued

For explanation of icons, see p. 663.

CLARITHROMYCIN *continued*

Adult:

M. avium complex:

Prophylaxis (1st episode and recurrence): 500 mg/dose Q12 hr PO

Treatment: 500 mg Q12 hr PO with other antimycobacterial drugs

Bacterial endocarditis prophylaxis for dental and upper respiratory procedures:

Infant and child: 15 mg/kg PO (max. dose: 500 mg) 1 hr before procedure

Adult: 500 mg PO 1 hr before procedure

Contraindicated in patients allergic to erythromycin and history of cholestatic jaundice/hepatic dysfunction with prior use. As with other macrolides, clarithromycin has been associated with QT prolongation and ventricular arrhythmias, including ventricular tachycardia and torsades de pointes. May cause cardiac arrhythmias in patients also receiving cisapride. Side effects: diarrhea, nausea, abnormal taste, dyspepsia, abdominal discomfort (less than erythromycin but greater than azithromycin), and headache. Rare cases of anaphylaxis, Stevens-Johnson, and toxic epidermal necrolysis have been reported. Hepatic dysfunction has been reported. May increase effects/toxicity of carbamazepine, theophylline, cyclosporine, digoxin, ergot alkaloids, fluconazole, tacrolimus, triazolam, and warfarin. Substrate and inhibitor of CYP 450 3A4, and inhibits CYP 1A2.

Adjust dose in renal failure (see Chapter 31). Doses, regardless of dosage form, may be administered with food.

CLINDAMYCIN
Cleocin-T, Cleocin, and others
Antibiotic, lincomycin derivative

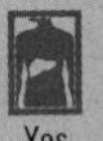
Yes
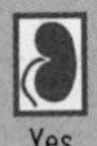
Yes
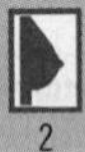
2
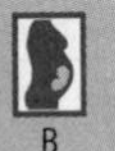
B

Caps: 75, 150, 300 mg
Oral solution: 75 mg/5 mL (100 mL)
Injection: 150 mg/mL (contains 9.45 mg/mL benzyl alcohol)
Solution, topical (Cleocin-T): 1% (30, 60 mL); may contain 50% isopropyl alcohol
Gel, topical (Cleocin-T): 1% (30, 60 g); may contain methylparaben
Lotion, topical (Cleocin-T): 1% (60 mL); may contain methylparaben
Foam, topical: 1% (50, 100 g); contains 58% ethanol
See *Benzoyl Peroxide* for combination topical product (clindamycin and benzoyl peroxide)
Vaginal cream: 2% (40 g); may contain benzyl alcohol
Vaginal suppository: 100 mg (3s)

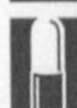

Neonate: IV/IM: 5 mg/kg/dose

≤7 days:

≤2 kg: Q12 hr

>2 kg: Q8 hr

>7 days:

<1.2 kg: Q12 hr

1.2–2 kg: Q8 hr

>2 kg: Q6 hr

Child:

PO: 10–30 mg/kg/24 hr ÷ Q6–8 hr; **max. dose:** 1.8 g/24 hr

IM/IV: 25–40 mg/kg/24 hr ÷ Q6–8 hr

Adult:

PO: 150–450 mg/dose Q6–8 hr; **max. dose:** 1.8 g/24 hr

IM/IV: 1200–1800 mg/24 hr IM/IV ÷ Q6–12 hr; **max. dose:** 4.8 g/24 hr

Continued

CLINDAMYCIN *continued*

Bacterial endocarditis prophylaxis for dental and upper respiratory procedures:
Infant and child: 20 mg/kg PO (**max. dose:** 600 mg) 1 hr before procedure
Adult: 600 mg PO (1 hr before procedure) or IV (30 min before procedure).
Topical (≥12 yr and adult): apply to affected area BID.
Bacterial vaginosis (adolescent and adult):
Suppositories: 100 mg/dose QHS × 3 days
Vaginal cream (2%): 1 applicator dose (5 g) QHS for 3 or 7 days in non-pregnant patients and for 7 days in pregnant patients in second and third trimester.

Not indicated in meningitis; CSF penetration is poor.

Pseudomembranous colitis may occur up to several wk after cessation of therapy. May cause diarrhea, rash, Stevens-Johnson syndrome, granulocytopenia, thrombocytopenia, or sterile abscess at injection site.

Clindamycin may increase the neuromuscular blocking effects of tubocurarine, pancuronium. **Do not exceed** IV infusion rate of 30 mg/min because hypotension, cardiac arrest has been reported with rapid infusions.

Dosage reduction may be required in severe renal or hepatic disease but not necessary in mild/moderate conditions. Oral liquid preparation is not palatable; consider use of oral capsules as a sprinkle onto applesauce or pudding.

CLONAZEPAM
Klonopin and others
Benzodiazepine

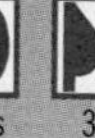 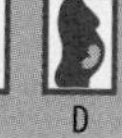

Yes | Yes | 3 | D

Tabs: 0.5, 1, 2 mg
Disintegrating oral tabs: 0.125, 0.25, 0.5, 1, 2 mg; contains phenylalanine
Oral suspension: 100 mcg/mL

Infant and child: <10 yr or <30 kg:
Initial: 0.01–0.03 mg/kg/24 hr ÷ Q8 hr PO
Increment: 0.25–0.5 mg/24 hr Q3 days, up to **maximum maintenance dose** of 0.1–0.2 mg/kg/24 hr ÷ Q8 hr
Child ≥10 yr or ≥30 kg and adult:
Initial: 1.5 mg/24 hr PO ÷ TID
Increment: 0.5–1 mg/24 hr Q3 days; **max. dose:** 20 mg/24 hr

Contraindicated in severe liver disease and acute narrow-angle glaucoma. Drowsiness, behavior changes, increased bronchial secretions, GI, CV, GU, and hematopoietic toxicity (thrombocytopenia, leukopenia) may occur. Monitor for depression, suicidal behavior/ideation, and unusual changes in behavior/mood. **Use with caution** in patients with renal impairment. **Do not** discontinue abruptly. $T_{1/2}$ = 24–36 hr.

Proposed therapeutic levels (not well established): 20–80 ng/mL. Recommended serum sampling time: Obtain trough level within 30 min prior to an oral dose. Steady-state is typically achieved after 5–8 days continuous therapy using the same dose.

Carbamazepine, phenytoin, and phenobarbital may decrease clonazepam levels and effect. Drugs that inhibit CYP-450 3A4 isoenzymes (e.g., erythromycin) may increase clonazepam levels and effects/toxicity.

For explanation of icons, see p. 663.

CLONIDINE
Catapres, Catapres TTS, Duraclon, and others
Central alpha-adrenergic agonist, antihypertensive

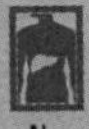 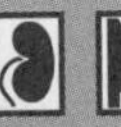  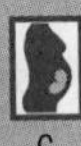 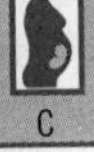

No No 3 C

Tabs: 0.1, 0.2, 0.3 mg
Oral suspension: 0.1 mg/mL
Transdermal patch (Catapres TTS): 0.1, 0.2, 0.3 mg/24 hr (7 day patch); contains metalic components (see remarks)
Injection, epidural (Duraclon): 100, 500 mcg/mL (10 mL); preservative free

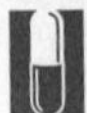

Hypertension:

Child (PO): 5–10 mcg/kg/24 hr ÷ Q8–12 hr initially; if needed, increase at 5–7 day intervals to 5–25 mcg/kg/24 hr ÷ Q6 hr; **max. dose:** 25 mcg/kg/24 hr up to 0.9 mg/24 hr.

≥12 yr and adult (PO): 0.1 mg BID initially; increase in 0.1 mg/24 hr increments at weekly intervals until desired response is achieved (usual range: adolescent: 0.2–0.6 mg/24 hr ÷ BID; adult: 0.1–0.8 mg/24 hr ÷ BID), **max. dose:** 2.4 mg/24 hr

Transdermal patch:

Child: conversion to patch only after establishing an optimal oral dose first. Use a transdermal dosage closest to the established total oral daily dose.

Adult: Initial 0.1 mg/24 hr patch for first wk. May increase dose by 0.1 mg/24 hr at 1–2 wk intervals PRN. Usual range: 0.10.3 mg/24 hr. Each patch lasts for 7 days. Doses >0.6 mg/24 hr do not provide additional benefit.

ADHD:

Child (PO): Start with 0.05 mg QHS; if needed, increase by 0.05 mg every 3–7 days up to a **max. dose** of 0.4 mg/24 hr. Titrated doses may be divided TID–QID.

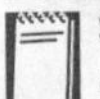

Side effects: Dry mouth, dizziness, drowsiness, fatigue, constipation, anorexia, arrhythmias, and local skin reactions with patch. **Do not abruptly discontinue;** signs of sympathetic overactivity may occur; taper gradually over >1 wk.

Beta-blockers may exacerbate rebound hypertension during and following the withdrawal of clonidine. If patient is receiving both clonidine and a beta-blocker and clonidine is to be discontinued, the beta-blocker should be withdrawn several days prior to tapering the clonidine. If converting from clonidine over to a beta-blocker, introduce the beta-blocker several days after discontinuing clonidine (following taper).

Monitor heart rate when used with digitalis, calcium channel blockers, and beta-blockers. Use with diltiazem or verapamil may result in sinus bradycardia.

$T_{1/2}$: 44–72 hr (neonate), 6–20 hr (adult). Onset of action (antihypertensive): 0.5–1 hr for oral route, 2–3 days for transdermal route. Do not use transdermal route while patient is undergoing a MRI procedure; these transdermal patches contains metals and may result in serious patient burns when undergoing MRI.

CLOTRIMAZOLE
Lotrimin AF, Cruex, Gyne-Lotrimin 3, Gyne-Lotrimin 7, Mycelex, Mycelex-7, and others
Antifungal, imidazole

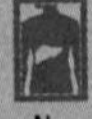 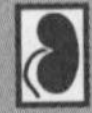  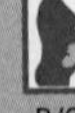 

No No ? B/C

Oral troche: 10 mg
Cream, topical (OTC): 1% (15, 30, 45 g); contains benzyl alcohol
Solution, topical (OTC): 1% (10, 30 mL)

Continued

CLOTRIMAZOLE *continued*

Lotion, topical (OTC): 1% (20 mL); contains benzyl alcohol
Vaginal suppository (OTC): 200 mg
Vaginal cream (OTC): 1% (45 g), 2% (21 g)
Combination packs:
Mycelex-7 Combination Pack (OTC): Vaginal suppository 100 mg (7) and vaginal cream 1% (7 g)
Gyne-Lotrimin 3 Combination Pack (OTC): Vaginal suppository 200 mg (3) and vaginal cream 1% (21 g)

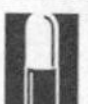

Topical: Apply to affected skin areas BID × 4–8 wk
Vaginal candidiasis (>12 yr and adult):
Vaginal suppositories (may be used as a part of a combination pack where a 1% cream is also applied onto the vulva once daily or BID):
100 mg/dose intravaginally QHS × 7 days, or
200 mg/dose intravaginally QHS × 3 days
Vaginal cream:
1 applicator dose (5 g) of 1% cream intravaginally QHS × 7–14 days, or
1 applicator dose of 2% cream intravaginally QHS × 3 days
Thrush:
>3 yr–adult: Dissolve slowly (15–30 min) one troche in the mouth 5 times/24 hr × 14 days

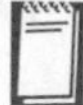

May cause erythema, blistering, or urticaria with topical use. Liver enzyme elevation, nausea and vomiting may occur with troches. **Avoid use** of condoms and diaphragms with vaginal cream or suppository as latex can be weakened. **Do not use** troches for systemic infections.

Pregnancy code is a "B" for topical and vaginal dosage forms and "C" for troches.

CODEINE
Various generics
Narcotic, analgesic, antitussive

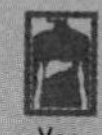 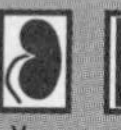 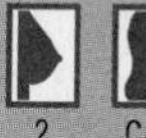 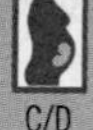

Yes	Yes	2	C/D

Tabs: 15, 30, 60 mg; as sulfate

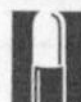

Analgesic (all doses PO PRN):
Child: 0.5–1 mg/kg/dose Q4–6 hr; **max. dose:** 60 mg/dose
Adult: 15–60 mg/dose Q4–6 hr
Antitussive (all doses PO PRN): 1–1.5 mg/kg/24 hr ÷ Q4–6 hr; alternatively dose by age:
2–5 yr: 2.5–5 mg/dose Q4–6 hr; **max. dose:** 30 mg/24 hr
6–12 yr: 5–10 mg/dose Q4–6 hr; **max. dose:** 60 mg/24 hr
≥12 yr and adult: 10–20 mg/dose Q4–6 hr; **max. dose:** 120 mg/24 hr

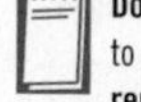

Do not use in children <2 yr old as antitussive. **Use with caution** in hypersensitivity reactions to other opoids, respiratory disorders, and severe liver or renal insufficiency **(adjust dose in renal failure; see Chapter 31).** Side effects: CNS and respiratory depression, constipation, cramping, hypotension, and pruritis. May be habit forming.

Codeine's analgesic effect is due to its metabolism to morphine. For analgesia, use with acetaminophen orally. **See Chapter 6 for equianalgesic dosing.**

Pregnancy risk factor changes to a "D" if used for prolonged periods or in high doses at term. Nursing infants whose mothers are taking codeine and are "ultra-rapid" metabolizers (CYP 450 2D6) of codeine may have a more rapid and complete conversion to morphine. This may increase the risk for morphine overdose to the nursing infant.

For explanation of icons, see p. 663.

CODEINE AND ACETAMINOPHEN
Tylenol #1, #2, #3, #4, and various generics
Narcotic analgesic combination product

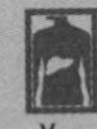 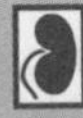 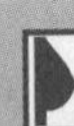 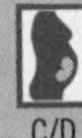
Yes Yes 2 C/D

Elixir (7% alcohol and saccharin), oral suspension, oral solution: acetaminophen 120 mg and codeine phosphate 12 mg/5 mL (120, 473 mL)
Tabs: (all containing 300 mg acetaminophen per tab and may contain metabisulfite)

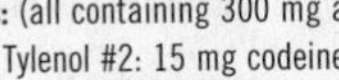

Tylenol #2: 15 mg codeine
Tylenol #3: 30 mg codeine
Tylenol #4: 60 mg codeine

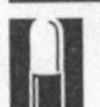

See *Acetaminophen and Codeine* for additional dosing information:
Analgesic:
Child: 0.5–1 mg codeine/kg/dose PO Q4–6 hr PRN; **max. dose:** 60 mg/dose
Using elixir, oral suspension, or oral solution:
- ***3–6 yr:*** 5 mL (12 mg codeine and 120 mg acetaminophen) PO Q6–8 hr PRN
- ***7–12 yr:*** 10 mL (24 mg codeine and 240 mg acetaminophen) PO Q6–8 hr PRN
- ***≥12 yr:*** 15 mL (36 mg codeine and 360 mg acetaminophen) PO Q4 hr PRN

Adult: 0.5–2 tablets (15–60 mg codeine; check tablet strength) PO Q4–6 hr PRN; **max. codeine dose:** 360 mg/24 hr, **max. acetaminophen dose:** 4 g/24 hr

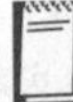

See *Acetaminophen and Codeine*. Pregnancy category is a "C" (changing to "D" if used for prolonged periods or in high doses at term) for codeine. **Do not use** combination product in renal impairment because codeine requires dosage adjustment; consider using each drug separately with proper dose adjustments.

CORTICOTROPIN
H.P. Acthar Gel
Adrenocorticotropic hormone

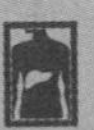 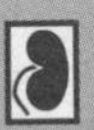 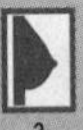 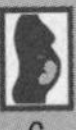
No No ? C

Injection, repository gel: 80 U/mL (5 mL)
1 unit = 1 mg

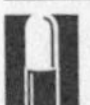

Anti-inflammatory:
0.8 U/kg/24 hr ÷ Q12–24 hr IM
Infantile spasms: many regimens exist
20–40 U/24 hr IM once daily × 6 wk or 150 U/m²/24 hr ÷ BID for 2 wk; followed by a gradual taper.

Contraindicated in acute psychoses, CHF, Cushing's disease, TB, peptic ulcer, ocular herpes, fungal infections, recent surgery, and sensitivity to porcine products. **Repository gel dosage form is only for IM route.**

Hypersensitivity reactions may occur. Similar adverse effects as corticosteroids.

CORTISONE ACETATE

Various generics

Corticosteroid

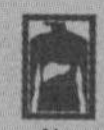
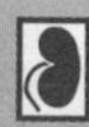

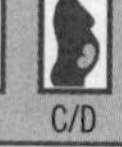

No No ? C/D

Tabs: 25 mg

Anti-inflammatory/immunosuppressive:

PO: 2.5–10 mg/kg/24 hr ÷ Q6–8 hr

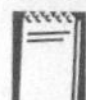

May produce glucose intolerance, Cushing's syndrome, edema, hypertension, adrenal suppression, cataracts, hypokalemia, skin atrophy, peptic ulcer, osteoporosis, and growth suppression.

Pregnancy category changes to "D" if used in the first trimester.

CO-TRIMOXAZOLE

See *Sulfamethoxazole and Trimethoprim*

CROMOLYN

Nasalcrom, Gastrocrom, Crolom, Opticrom, and various generics; previously available as Intal

Anti-allergic agent, mast cell stabilizer

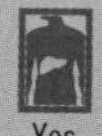
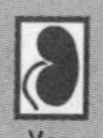

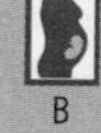

Yes Yes ? B

Nebulized solution: 10 mg/mL (2 mL)
Oral concentrate (Gastrocrom): 100 mg/5 mL
Ophthalmic solution (Crolom, Opticrom): 4% (10 mL)
Nasal spray (Nasalcrom) [OTC]: 4% (5.2 mg/spray) (100 sprays, 13 mL; 200 sprays, 26 mL); contains benzalkonium chloride and EDTA

Nebulization:

Child ≥2 yr and adult: 20 mg Q6–8 hr

Nasal:

Child ≥2 yr and adult: 1 spray each nostril TID–QID

Ophthalmic:

Child >4 yr and adult: 1–2 gtts 4–6 times/24 hr

Food allergy/inflammatory bowel disease:

2–12 yr: 100 mg PO QID; give 15–20 min AC and QHS; **max. dose:** 40 mg/kg/24 hr

>12 yr and adult: 200–400 mg PO QID; give 15–20 min AC and QHS

Systemic mastocytosis:

Infant and child <2 yr: 20 mg/kg/24 hr ÷ QID PO; **max. dose:** 30 mg/kg/24 hr

2–12 yr: 100 mg PO QID; give 30 min AC and QHS; **max. dose:** 40 mg/kg/24 hr

>12 yr and adult: 200 mg PO QID; give 30 min AC and QHS; **max. dose:** 40 mg/kg/24 hr

May cause rash, cough, bronchospasm, and nasal congestion. May cause headache, diarrhea with oral use. **Use with caution** in patients with renal or hepatic dysfunction.

Therapeutic response often occurs within 2 wk, however, a 4- to 6-wk trial may be needed to determine maximum benefit. For exercise-induced asthma, give no longer than 1 hr before activity. Oral concentrate can only be diluted in water. Nebulized solution can be mixed with albuterol nebs.

For explanation of icons, see p. 663.

CYANOCOBALAMIN/VITAMIN B_{12}
Cyanoject, Cyomin, Nascobal, Vitamin B_{12} and others
Vitamin (synthetic), water soluble

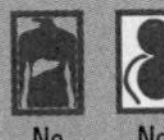 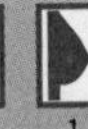 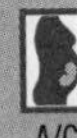 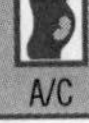
No No 1 A/C

Tabs (OTC): 100, 250, 500, 1000, 5000 mcg
Sublingual tabs: 2500 mcg
Lozenges (OTC): 50, 100, 250, 500 mcg
Nasal spray (Nascobal): 500 mcg/spray (2.3 mL delivers 8 doses); contains benzalkonium chloride
Injection (Cyanoject, Cyomin): 1000 mcg/mL (1, 10, 30 ml); some preparations may contain benzyl alcohol
Contains cobalt (4.35%)

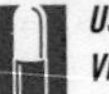

US RDA: See Chapter 21.
Vitamin B_{12} deficiency, treatment:
Child (IM or deep SC): 100 mcg/24 hr × 10–15 days
Maintenance: At least 60 mcg/mo
Adult (IM or deep SC): 30–100 mcg/24 hr × 5–10 days
Maintenance: 100–200 mcg/mo
Pernicious anemia:
Child (IM or deep SC): 30–50 mcg/24 hr for at least 14 days to total dose of 1000 mcg
Maintenance: 100 mcg/month
Adult (IM or deep SC): 100 mcg/24 hr × 7 days, followed by 100 mcg/dose every other day × 14 days, then 100 mcg/dose Q 3–4 days until remission is complete.
Maintenance:
IM/deep SC: 100–1000 mcg/mo
Intranasal: 500 mcg in one nostril once weekly
Sublingual: 1000–2000 mcg/24 hr

Contraindicated in optic nerve atrophy. May cause hypokalemia, hypersensitivity, pruritis, and vascular thrombosis. Pregnancy category changes to "C" if used in doses above the RDA or if administered by the intranasal route.

Prolonged use of acid-suppressing medications may reduce cyanocobalamin oral absorption. Protect product from light. Oral route of administration is generally **not recommended** for pernicious anemia and B_{12} deficiency due to poor absorption. IV route of administration is not recommended because of a more rapid elimination. **See Chapter 21 for multivitamin preparations.**

CYCLOPENTOLATE
Cyclogyl and others
Anticholinergic, mydriatic agent

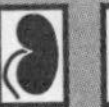  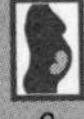
No No ? C

Ophthalmic solution: 0.5%, 1%, 2% (2, 5, 15 mL); may contain benzalkonium chloride

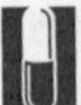

Administer dose approximately 40–50 min prior to examination/procedure.
Infant: Use of cyclopentolate/phenylephrine (Cyclomydril) due to lower cyclopentolate concentration and reduced risk of systemic side effects.
Child: 1 drop of 0.5–1% OU, followed by repeat drop, if necessary, in 5 min.
Adult: 1 drop of 1% OU followed by another drop OU in 5 min; use 2% solution for heavily pigmented iris.

Continued

CYCLOPENTOLATE *continued*

Do not use in narrow-angle glaucoma. May cause a burning sensation, behavioral disturbance, tachycardia, and loss of visual accommodation. Psychotic reactions and behavioral disturbances have been reported in children. To minimize absorption, apply pressure over nasolacrimal sac for at least 2 min. CNS and cardiovascular side effects are common with the 2% solution in children. **Avoid** feeding infants within 4 hr of dosing to prevent potential feeding intolerance.

Onset of action: 15–60 min. Duration of action: 6–24 hr; complete recovery of accommodation may take several days for some patients. Observe patient closely for at least 30 min after dose.

CYCLOPENTOLATE WITH PHENYLEPHRINE
Cyclomydril
Anticholinergic/sympathomimetic, mydriatic agent

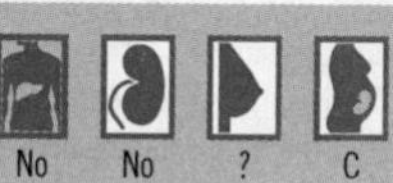

Ophthalmic solution: 0.2% cyclopentolate and 1% phenylephrine (2, 5 mL); contains 0.1% benzalkonium chloride, EDTA and boric acid

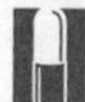

Administer dose approximately 40–50 min prior to examination/procedure.
Neonate–adult: 1 drop OU Q5–10 min; **max. dose:** 3 drops per eye

Used to induce mydriasis. See *Cyclopentolate* for additional remarks.
Onset of action: 15–60 min. Duration of action: 4–12 hr.

CYCLOSPORINE, CYCLOSPORINE MICROEMULSION, CYCLOSPORINE MODIFIED
Sandimmune, Gengraf, Neoral, Restasis, and others
Immunosuppressant

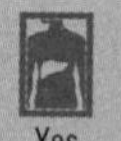
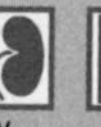
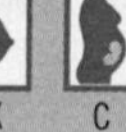

CYCLOSPORINE (Sandimmune and others):
- **Injection:** 50 mg/mL; contains 32.9% alcohol and 650 mg/mL polyoxyethylated castor oil
- **Oral solution:** 100 mg/mL (50 mL); contains 12.5% alcohol
- **Caps:** 25, 50, 100 mg; contains 12.8% alcohol

CYCLOSPORINE MICROEMULSION (Neoral):
- **Caps:** 25, 100 mg
- **Oral solution:** 100 mg/mL (50 mL)
- Neoral products contain 11.9% alcohol

CYCLOSPORINE MODIFIED (Gengraf):
- **Caps:** 25, 100 mg; contains 12.8% alcohol
- **Oral solution:** 100 mg/mL (50 mL): contains caster oil
- **Ophthalmic emulsion (Restasis):** 0.05% (0.4 mL as 30 single-use vials/box); preservative-free

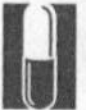

Neoral manufacturer recommends a 1 : 1 conversion ratio with Sandimmune. Due to its better absorption, however, lower doses of Neoral and Gengraf may be required. Exact dosing will vary depending on transplant type.
Oral: 15 mg/kg/24 hr as a single dose given 4–12 hr pretransplantation; give same daily dose for 1–2 wk posttransplantation, then reduce by 5% per wk to 3–10 mg/kg/24 hr ÷ Q12–24 hr

Continued

For explanation of icons, see p. 663.

CYCLOSPORINE, CYCLOSPORINE MICROEMULSION, CYCLOSPORINE MODIFIED *continued*

IV: 5–6 mg/kg/24 hr as a single dose given 4–12 hr pretransplantation; administer over 2–6 hr; give same daily dose posttransplantation until patient able to tolerate oral form

Ophthalmic:

≥16 yr and adult: Instill one drop onto affected eye(s) Q12 hr.

May cause nephrotoxicity, hepatotoxicity, hypomagnesemia, hyperkalemia, hyperuricemia, hypertension, hirsutism, acne, GI symptoms, tremor, leukopenia, sinusitis, gingival hyperplasia, and headache. Encephalopathy, convulsions, vision and movement disturbances, and impaired consciousness have been reported, especially in liver transplant patients. Psoriasis patients previously treated with PUVA and, to a lesser extent, methotrexate or other immunosuppressive agents, UVB, coal tar, or radiation therapy, are at increased risk for skin malignancies when taking Neoral or Gengraf.

Opportunistic infections and activation of latent viral infections have been reported.

BK virus-associated nephropathy has been observed in renal transplant patients.

Use caution with concomitant use of other nephrotoxic drugs (e.g., amphotericin B, aminoglycosides, nonsteroidal anti-inflammatory drugs, and tacrolimus).

Plasma concentrations increased with the use of fluconazole, ketoconazole, itraconazole, erythromycin, clarithromycin, voriconazole, nefazodone, diltiazem, verapamil, nicardipine, carvedilol, and corticosteroids. Plasma concentrations decreased with the use of carbamazepine, nafcillin, rifampin, oxcarbazepine, bosentin, phenobarbital, octreotide, and phenytoin. May increase methotrexate and repaglinide levels. Cyclosporine is a substrate for CYP 450 3A4.

Children may require dosages 2–3 times higher than adults. Plasma half-life 6–24 hrs.

Monitor trough levels (just prior to a dose at steady-state). Steady-state is generally achieved after 3–5 days of continuous dosing. Interpretation will vary based on treatment protocol and assay methodology (RIA monoclonal vs. RIA polyclonal vs. HPLC) as well as whole blood vs. serum sample. Additional monitoring and dosage adjustments may be necessary in renal and hepatic impairment or when changing dosage forms.

For ophthalmic use: Remove contact lens prior to use; lens may be inserted 15 min after dose administration. May be used with artificial tears but need to be separated by 15 min for one another.

CYPROHEPTADINE

Various generics; previously available as Periactin

Antihistamine

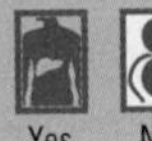
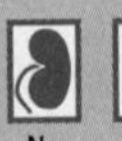

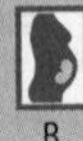

Yes No 3 B

Tabs: 4 mg

Syrup: 2 mg/5 ml (473 mL); may contain alcohol

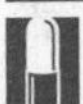

Antihistaminic uses:

Child: 0.25 mg/kg/24 hr or 8 mg/m²/24 hr ÷ Q8–12 hr PO or by age:

2–6 yr: 2 mg Q8–12 hr PO; **max. dose:** 12 mg/24 hr

7–14 yr: 4 mg Q8–12 hr PO; **max. dose:** 16 mg/24 hr

Adult: Start with 12 mg/24 hr ÷ TID PO; dosage range: 12–32 mg/24 hr ÷ TID PO; **max. dose:** 0.5 mg/kg/24 hr

Migrane prophylaxis: 0.25–0.4 mg/kg/24 hr ÷ BID–TID PO up to following **max. doses:**

2–6 yr: 12 mg/24 hr

7–14 yr: 16 mg/24 hr

Adult: 0.5 mg/kg/24 hr or 32 mg/24 hr

Continued

CYPROHEPTADINE *continued*

Appetite stimulation:

4–8 yr (limited data): 2 mg Q8 hr PO

>13 yr and adult: Start with 2 mg Q6 hr PO; dose may be gradually increased to 8 mg Q6 hr over a 3-wk period.

Contraindicated in neonates, patients currently on MAO inhibitors, and patients suffering from asthma, glaucoma, or GI/GU obstruction. May produce anti-cholinergic side effects including sedation and appetite stimulation. Consider reducing dosage with hepatic insufficiency.

Allow 4 to 8 wk of continuous therapy for assessing efficacy in migrane propylaxis.

DANTROLENE
Dantrium, Revonto, and many generics
Skeletal muscle relaxant

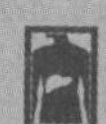 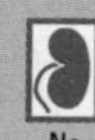 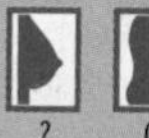 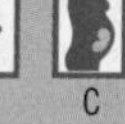

Yes No ? C

Cap: 25, 50, 100 mg
Oral suspension: 5 mg/mL
Injection (Dantrium, Revonto): 20 mg; contains 3 gm mannitol/20 mg drug

Chronic spasticity:

Child (<5 yr):

Initial: 0.5 mg/kg/dose PO BID

Increment: Increase frequency to TID–QID at 4- to 7-day intervals, then increase doses by 0.5 mg/kg/dose

Max. dose: 3 mg/kg/dose PO BID–QID, up to 400 mg/24 hr

Malignant hyperthermia:

Prevention:

PO: 4–8 mg/kg/24 hr ÷ Q6 hr × 1–2 days before surgery with last dose administered 3–4 hr prior to surgery.

IV: 2.5 mg/kg over 1 hr beginning 1.25 hr before anesthesia, additional doses PRN

Treatment: 1 mg/kg IV, repeat PRN to **maximum cumulative dose** of 10 mg/kg, followed by a post-crisis regimen of 4–8 mg/kg/24 hr PO ÷ Q6 hr for 1–3 days

Contraindicated in active hepatic disease. Monitor transaminases for hepatotoxicity. **Use with caution** in children with cardiac or pulmonary impairment. May cause change in sensorium, weakness, diarrhea, constipation, incontinence, and enuresis.

Avoid unnecessary exposure of medication to sunlight. **Avoid** extravasation into tissues.

A decrease in spasticity sufficient to allow daily function should be therapeutic goal. Discontinue if benefits are not evident in 45 days.

DAPSONE
Aczone, Diaminodiphenylsulfone, DDS
Antibiotic, sulfone derivative

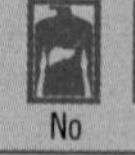 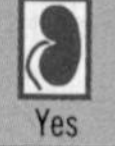 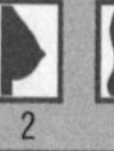 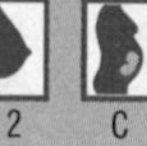

No Yes 2 C

Tabs: 25, 100 mg
Oral suspension: 2 mg/mL
Topical gel (Aczone): 5% (30, 60 g)

Pneumocystis jiroveci (formerly carinii) prophylaxis:

Child ≥1 mo: 2 mg/kg/24 hr PO once daily; **max. dose:** 100 mg/24 hr. Alternative weekly dosing, 4 mg/kg/dose PO Q7 days; **max. dose:** 200 mg/dose

Continued

For explanation of icons, see p. 663.

DAPSONE *continued*

Adult: 100 mg/24 hr PO ÷ once daily–BID with pyrimethamine 50 mg PO Q7 days and leucovorin 25 mg PO Q7 days; other combination regimens with pyrimethamine and leucovorin can be used (see http://www.hivatis.org/trtgdlns.html#Opportunistic).

Toxoplasma gondii prophylaxis:

Child ≥1 mo: 2 mg/kg/24 hr PO once daily (**max. dose:** 25 mg/24 hr) with pyrimethamine 1 mg/kg/24 hr (**max.** 25 mg/dose) PO once daily and leucovorin 5 mg PO Q3 days.

Adult: 50 mg PO once daily with pyrimethamine 50 mg PO Q7 days and leucovorin 25 mg PO Q7 days; other combination regimens with pyrimethamine and leucovorin can be used (see http://www.hivatis.org/trtgdlns.html#Opportunistic).

Leprosy (See www.who.int/lep/disease/disease.htm for latest recommendations including combination regimens such as rifampin ± clofazimine):

Child: 1–2 mg/kg/24 hr PO once daily; **max. dose:** 100 mg/24 hr

Adult: 50–100 mg PO once daily

Acne vulgaris:

≥12 yr: Apply small amount of topical gel onto clean, acne affected areas BID.

Patients with HIV, glutathione deficiency, or G6PD deficiency may be at increased risk for developing methemoglobinemia. Side effects include hemolytic anemia (dose related), agranulocytosis, methemoglobinemia, aplastic anemia, nausea, vomiting, hyperbilirubinemia, headache, nephrotic syndrome, and hypersensitivity reaction (sulfone syndrome). Peripheral neuropathy has been reported with systemic use.

Didanosine, rifabutin, and rifampin decreases dapsone levels. Trimethoprim increases dapsone levels. Pyrimethamine, nitrofurantoin, and primaquine increases risk for hematological side effects.

Oral suspension may not be absorbed as well as tablets.

TOPICAL USE: Dry skin, erythema, and peeling of the skin may occur. Use of topical gel followed by benzoyl peroxide for acne has resulted in temporary local discoloration (yellow/orange) of the skin and facial hair.

DARBEPOETIN ALFA

Aranesp

Erythropoiesis stimulating protein

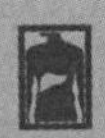
Yes

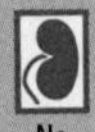
No

?

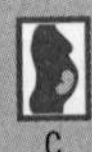
C

Injection: 25, 40, 60, 100, 200, 300 mcg/1 mL (1 mL), 150 mcg/0.75 mL (0.75 mL)

Single dose pre-filled injection syringe (27 gauge 1/2-inch needle): 25 mcg/0.42 mL, 40 mcg/0.4 mL, 60 mcg/0.3 mL, 100 mcg/0.5 mL, 150 mcg/0.3 mL, 200 mcg/0.4 mL, 300 mcg/0.6 mL, 500 mcg/1 mL

Both dosage forms contain either albumin (2.5 mg/mL) or polysorbate (0.05 mg/mL).

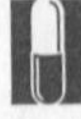

Anemia in chronic renal failure (see remarks):

Child (>1 yr) and adult: Start with 0.45 mcg/kg/dose IV/SC once weekly and adjust dose according to the table that follows.

Continued

DARBEPOETIN ALFA *continued*

DARBEPOETIN ALFA DOSE ADJUSTMENT IN ANEMIA ASSOCIATED WITH CHRONIC RENAL FAILURE (RECOMMENDED HEMOGLOBIN TARGET LEVEL 10–12 g/dL)

Response to Dose	Dose Adjustment
<1 g/dL increase in hemoglobin and below target range after 4 wk of therapy	Increase dose by 25% not more frequently than once monthly. Further increases, if needed, may be done at 4-wk intervals.
>1 g/dL increase in hemoglobin in any 2-wk period, or if hemoglobin exceeds and approaches 12 g/dL	Decrease dose by 25%
Hemoglobin continues to increase despite dosage reduction	Discontinue therapy; reinitiate therapy at a 25% lower dose of the previous dose after the hemoglobin starts to decrease

Anemia associated with chemotherapy (patients with nonmyeloid malignancies):

Child (limited data) and adult (see remarks): Start with 2.25 mcg/kg/dose SC once weekly and adjust dose according to the table that follows (discontinue use after completing chemotherapy course):

DARBEPOETIN ALFA DOSE ADJUSTMENT IN ANEMIA ASSOCIATED WITH CHEMOTHERAPY

Response to Dose	Dose Adjustment
<1 g/dL increase in hemoglobin and below target range after 6 wk of therapy	Increase dose to 4.5 mcg/kg/dose once weekly SC/IV
>1 g/dL increase in hemoglobin in any 2-wk period, or when hemoglobin reaches a level needed to avoid transfusion	Decrease dose by 40%
If hemoglobin exceeds a level needed to avoid transfusion	Hold therapy until hemoglobin approaches a level where transfusions may be required and restart at a reduced dose by 40%

Conversion from epoetin alfa to darbepoetin alfa (see table that follows):

Previous Weekly Epoetin Alfa Dose (Units/week)[1]	PEDIATRIC Weekly Darbepoetin Alfa Dose (mcg/week) Administered SC/IV Once Weekly[2]	ADULT Weekly Darbepoetin Alfa Dose (mcg/week) Administered SC/IV Once Weekly[2]	ADULT Once every 2 weeks Darbepoetin Alfa Dose (mcg every 2 weeks) Administered SC/IV Once Every 2 Weeks[3]
<1500	Insufficient data	6.25	12.5
1500–2499	6.25	6.25	12.5
2500–4999	10	12.5	25
5000–10,999	20	25	50
11,000–17,999	40	40	80
18,000–33,999	60	60	120
34,000–89,000	100	100	200
≥90,000	200	200	400

1. 200 units of epoetin alfa is equivalent to 1 mcg darbepoetin alfa.
2. If patient was receiving epoetin alfa 2–3 times weekly, darbepoetin alfa should be administered once weekly.
3. If patient was receiving epoetin alfa once weekly, darbepoetin alfa should be administered once every 2 wk.

Continued

For explanation of icons, see p. 663.

DARBEPOETIN ALFA *continued*

Contraindicated in uncontrolled hypertension and patients hypersensitive to albumin/polysorbate 80 or epoetin alfa. Darbepoetin alfa is not intended for patients requiring acute correction of anemia. **Use with caution** in seizures and liver disease. Evaluate serum iron, feritin, and TIBC; concurrent iron supplementation may be necessary. Red cell aplasia and severe anemia associated with neutralizing antibodies to erythropoietin have been reported.

USE IN CHRONIC RENAL FAILURE: In pediatric patients, higher doses may be needed for individuals being switched from epoetin alfa compared to naïve patients. May cause edema, fatigue, GI disturbances, headache, blood pressure changes, fever, cardiac arrhythmia/arrest, infections and myalgia. Higher risk for mortality and serious cardiovascular events have been reported with higher targeted hemoglobin levels (13.5–14 g/dL). If hemoglobin levels do not increase or reach targeted levels despite appropriate dose titrations over a 12-wk period: (1) **do not** administer higher doses and use the lowest dose that will maintain hemoglobin levels to avoid the need for recurrent blood transfusions; (2) evaluate and treat other causes of anemia; (3) always follow the dose adjustment instructions; and (4) discontinue use if patient remains transfusion dependent.

USE IN CANCER: Use only for anemia due to myelosuppressive chemotherapy; not effective in reducing the need for transfusions in patients with anemia not due to chemotherapy. May cause fatigue, fever, edema, dizziness, headache, GI disturbances, arthralgia/myalgia and rash. Use lowest dose to avoid transfusions and **do not exceed** hemoglobin levels >12 g/dL; increased frequency of adverse events, including mortality and thrombotic vascular events, have been reported. Shortened survival and time to tumor progression have also been reported in patients with various cancers.

Targeted hemoglobin in adults is 9–12 g/dL; **do not exceed 12 g/dL** (all ages). Monitor hemoglobin, BP, serum chemistries, and reticulocyte count. Increases in dose should **not** be made more frequently than once a mo. For IV administration, infuse over 1–3 min.

DEFEROXAMINE MESYLATE

Desferal

Chelating agent

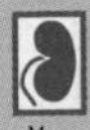 Yes
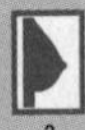 Yes
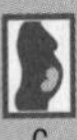 ?
C

Injection: 500, 2000 mg

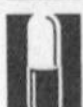

Acute iron poisoning (if using IV route, convert to IM as soon as the patient's clinical condition permits; see remarks):

Child:

IV: 15 mg/kg/hr or
IM: 50 mg/kg/dose Q6 hr
Max. dose: 6 g/24 hr

Adult:

IV: 15 mg/kg/hr
IM: 1 g × 1, then 0.5 g Q4 hr × 2; may repeat 0.5 g Q4–12 hr
Max. dose: 6 g/24 hr

Chronic iron overload (see remarks):

Child:

IV: 15 mg/kg/hr; **max. dose:** 6 g/24 hr
SC: 20–40 mg/kg/dose once daily as infusion over 8–12 hr; **max. dose:** 2 g/24 hr

Adult:

IV: 15 mg/kg/hr; **max. dose:** 6 g/24 hr
IM: 0.5–1 g/dose once daily
SC: 1–2 g/dose once daily as infusion over 8–24 hr

Continued

DEFEROXAMINE MESYLATE *continued*

Contraindicated in severe renal disease or anuria. Not approved for use in primary hemochromatosis. May cause flushing, erythema, urticaria, hypotension, tachycardia, diarrhea, leg cramps, fever, cataracts, hearing loss, nausea, and vomiting. Iron mobilization may be poor in children <3 yr. Serum creatinine elevation, acute renal failure, renal tubular disorders, and hepatic dysfunction have been reported.

High doses and concomitant low ferritin levels have also been associated with growth retardation. Growth velocity may resume to pretreatment levels by reducing the dosage. Acute respiratory distress syndrome has been reported following treatment with excessively high intravenous doses in patients with acute iron intoxication or thalassemia. Toxicity risk has been reported with infusions >8 mg/kg/hr for >4 days for thalassemia; and with infusions of 15 mg/kg/hr for >1 day for acute iron toxicity. Pulmonary toxicity was not seen in 193 courses.

For IV infusion, **maximum rate:** 15 mg/kg/hr. Infuse IV infusion over 6–12 hr for mild/moderate iron intoxication and over 24 hr for severe cases, then reassess. SC route is via a portable controlled-infusion device and is **not recommended** in acute iron poisoning.

DESMOPRESSIN ACETATE
DDAVP, Stimate, and others
Vasopressin analog, synthetic; hemostatic agent

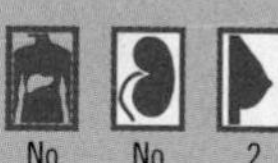
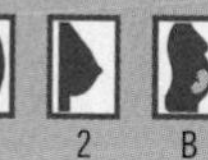

Tabs: 0.1, 0.2 mg
Nasal solution (with rhinal tube): DDAVP, 100 mcg/mL (2.5 mL); contains 9 mg NaCl/mL
Injection: 4 mcg/mL (1, 10 mL); contains 9 mg NaCl/mL
Nasal spray:
100 mcg/mL, 10 mcg/spray (50 sprays, 5 mL); contains 7.5 mg NaCl/mL
Stimate: 1500 mcg/mL, 150 mcg/spray (25 sprays, 2.5 mL); contains 9 mg NaCl/mL
Conversion: 100 mcg = 400 IU arginine vasopressin

Diabetes insipidus (see remarks):
Oral:
Child ≤12 yr: Start with 0.05 mg/dose BID; titrate to effect; usual dose range: 0.1–0.8 mg/24 hr.
Child >12 yr and adult: Start with 0.05 mg/dose BID; titrate dose to effect; usual dose range: 0.1–1.2 mg/24 hr ÷ BID–TID.
Intranasal:
3 mo–12 yr: 5–30 mcg/24 hr ÷ once daily–BID
>12 yr and adult: 10–40 mcg/24 hr ÷ once daily–TID; titrate dose to achieve control of excessive thirst and urination. Morning and evening doses should be adjusted separately for diurnal rhythm of water turnover.
IV/SC:
<12 yr (limited data): 0.1–1 mcg/24 hr ÷ once daily–BID; start with lower dose and increase as needed.
≥12 yr and adult: 2–4 mcg/24 hr ÷ BID
Hemophilia A and von Willebrand's disease (see remarks):
Intranasal: 2–4 mcg/kg/dose
IV: 0.2–0.4 mcg/kg/dose over 15–30 min
Nocturnal enuresis (≥6 yr; see remarks):
Oral: 0.2 mg at bedtime, titrated to a max. dose of 0.6 mg to achieve desired effect.

Continued

For explanation of icons, see p. 663.

DESMOPRESSIN ACETATE *continued*

Use with caution in hypertension, patients at risk for water intoxication with hyponatremia, and coronary artery disease. May cause headache, nausea, seizures, blood pressure changes, hyponatremia, nasal congestion, abdominal cramps, and hypertension.

NOCTURNAL ENURESIS: Intranasal formulations are no longer indicated by the FDA for primary nocturnal enuresis (children are susceptible for severe hyponatremia and seizures) or in patients with a history of hyponatremia. Patients using tablets should have their therapy interrupted during acute illnesses that may lead to fluid and/or electrolyte imbalance.

Injection may be used SC or IV at approximately 10% of intranasal dose. Adjust fluid intake to decrease risk of water intoxication and monitor serum sodium.

If switching stablized patient from intranasal route to IV/SC route, use 10% of intranasal dose. Peak effects: 1–5 hr with intranasal route; 1.5–3 hr with IV route; and 2–7 hr with PO route.

For hemophilia A and von Willebrand's disease, administer dose intranasally, 2 hr before procedure; IV, 30 min before procedure.

DEXAMETHASONE

Decadron, Dexpak Taperpak, Hexadrol, Maxidex, and many generics

Corticosteroid

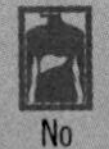

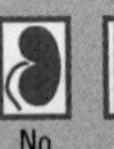

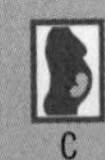

No No 3 C

Tabs (Decadron and other generics): 0.25, 0.5, 0.75, 1, 1.5, 2, 4, 6 mg
Dexpak Taperpak: 1.5mg [21 tabs (6 day), 35 tabs (10 day), 51 tabs (13 day)]
Injection (sodium phosphate salt): 4, 10, 20 mg/mL (some preparations contain benzyl alcohol or methyl/propyl parabens)
Elixir: 0.5 mg/5 mL (some preparations contain 5% alcohol)
Oral solution: 0.1, 1 mg/mL (some preparations contain 30% alcohol)
Ophthalmic solution: 0.1% (5 mL)
Ophthalmic suspension (Maxidex): 0.1% (5 mL)

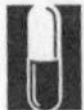

Airway edema: 0.5–2 mg/kg/24 hr IV/IM ÷ Q6 hr (begin 24 hr before extubation and continue for 4–6 doses after extubation)
Croup: 0.6 mg/kg/dose PO/IV/IM × 1
Antiemetic (chemotherapy induced):
- ***Initial:*** 10 mg/m²/dose IV; **max. dose:** 20 mg
- ***Subsequent:*** 5 mg/m²/dose Q6 hr IV

Anti-inflammatory:
- ***Child:*** 0.08–0.3 mg/kg/24 hr PO, IV, IM ÷ Q6–12 hr
- ***Adult:*** 0.75–9 mg/24 hr PO, IV, IM ÷ Q6–12 hr

Brain tumor associated cerebral edema:
- ***Loading dose:*** 1–2 mg/kg/dose IV/IM × 1
- ***Maintenance:*** 1–1.5 mg/kg/24 hr ÷ Q4–6 hr; **max. dose:** 16 mg/24 hr

Spinal cord compression with neurological abnormalities:
- ***Child:*** 2 mg/kg/24 hr IV ÷ Q6 hr

Ophthalmic use (child and adult):
- ***Ointment:*** Apply a thin coating of ointment to the conjunctival sac of the affected eye(s) TID–QID. When a favorable response is achieved, reduce daily dosage to BID and later to once daily as a maintenance dose sufficient to control symptoms.
- ***Solution:*** Instill 1 to 2 drops into the conjunctival sac of the affected eye(s) Q1 hr during the day and Q2 hr during the night as initial therapy. When a favorable response is achieved, reduce dosage to 1 drop Q4 hr. Further dose reduction to 1 drop TID–QID may be sufficient to control symptoms.

Continued

DEXAMETHASONE *continued*

Suspension: Shake well before using. Instill 1–2 drops in the conjunctival sacs of the affected eye(s). For severe disease, drops may be Q1 hr, being tapered to discontinuation as inflammation subsides. For mild disease, drops may be used ≤4 to 6 times/24 hr.

Not recommended for systemic therapy in the prevention or treatment of chronic lung disease in infants with very low birth weight because of increase risk for adverse events (*Pediatrics* 2002;109(2):330–338). Dexamethasone is a substrate of CYP P450 3A3/4 and P-glycoprotein.

Toxicity: same as for prednisone without mineralcorticoid effects. **Contraindicated** in active untreated infections and fungal, viral, and mycobacterial ocular infections.

OPHTHALMIC USE: Use ophthalmic preparation only in consultation with an ophthalmologist. **Use with caution** in corneal/scleral thinning and glaucoma. Consider the possibility of persistent fungal infections of the cornea after prolonged use. Ophthalmic solution/suspension may be used in otitis externa.

Oral peak serum levels occur 1–2 hr and within 8 hr following IM administration. **For other uses, doses based on body surface area, and dose equivalence to other steroids, see Chapter 30; Table 30-1.**

DEXTROAMPHETAMINE ± AMPHETAMINE
DextroStat, Dexedrine Spansules, and many other generics
In combination with amphetamine: Adderall, Adderall XR
CNS stimulant

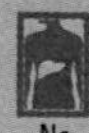
No
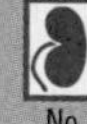
No
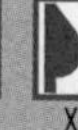
X
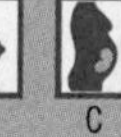
C

Tabs: 5, 10 mg
Sustained-release caps (Dexedrine Spansules): 5, 10, 15 mg
In combination with amphetamine (Adderall): Available as 1 : 1:1 : 1 mixture of dextroamphetamine sulfate, dextroamphetamine saccharate, amphetamine aspartate, and amphetamine sulfate salts; for example, the 5 mg tablet contains 1.25 mg dextroamphetamine sulfate, 1.25 mg dextroamphetamine saccharate, 1.25 mg amphetamine aspartate, and 1.25 mg amphetamine sulfate:
Tabs: 5, 7.5, 10, 12.5, 15, 20, 30 mg
Caps, extended-release (Adderal XR): 5, 10, 15, 20, 25, 30 mg
Oral suspension: 1 mg/mL

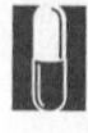

Dosages are in terms of mg of dextroamphetamine when using dextroamphetamine alone OR in terms of mg of the total dextroamphetamine and amphetamine salts when using Adderall. Non-extended release dosage forms are usually given BID–TID (first dose on awakening and subsequent doses at intervals of 4–6 hr later). Extended/sustained-released dosage forms are usually given PO once daily, sometimes BID.

Attention deficit hyperactivity disorder:
3–5 yr: 2.5 mg/24 hr QAM; increase by 2.5 mg/24 hr at weekly intervals to a **max. dose** of 40 mg/24 hr ÷ once daily–TID.
≥6 yr: 5 mg/24 hr QAM; increase by 5 mg/24 hr at weekly intervals to a **max. dose** of 40 mg/24 hr ÷ once daily–TID.

Narcolepsy:
6–12 yr: 5 mg/24 hr ÷ once daily–TID; increase by 5 mg/24 hr at weekly intervals to a **max. dose** of 60 mg/24 hr
>12 yr and adult: 10 mg/24 hr ÷ once daily–TID; increase by 10 mg/24 hr at weekly intervals to a **max. dose** of 60 mg/24 hr

Continued

For explanation of icons, see p. 663.

DEXTROAMPHETAMINE ± AMPHETAMINE *continued*

Use with caution in presence of hypertension or cardiovascular disease. **Avoid** use in known serious structural cardiac abnormalities, cardiomyopathy, serious heart rhythm abonormalities, coronary artery disease, or other serious cardiac problems that may increase risk of sympathomimetic effects of amphetamines (sudden death, stroke, and MI have been reported). **Do not give** with MAO inhibitors or general anesthetics.

Not recommended for <3 yr. Medication should generally not be used in children <5 yr old as diagnosis of ADHD in this age group is extremely difficult (use in consultation with a specialist). Interrupt administration occasionally to determine need for continued therapy. Many side effects, including insomnia (**avoid** dose administration within 6 hr of bedtime), restlessness, anorexia, psychosis, visual disturbances, headache, vomiting, abdominal cramps, dry mouth, and growth failure. Paranoia, mania, and auditory hallucination have been reported. Tolerance develops. Same guidelines as for methylphenidate apply.

DIAZEPAM

Valium, Diastat, Diastat AcuDial, and various generics
Benzodiazepine; anxiolytic, anticonvulsant

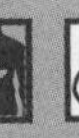 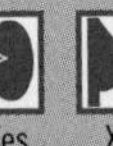 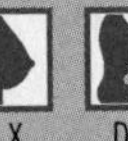 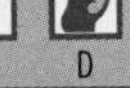

Yes Yes X D

Tabs: 2, 5, 10 mg
Oral solution: 1 mg/mL, 5 mg/mL (contains 19% alcohol)
Injection: 5 mg/mL (contains 40% propylene glycol, 10% alcohol, 5% sodium benzoate, and 1.5% benzyl alcohol)
Pediatric rectal gel (Diastat): 2.5 mg (5 mg/mL concentration with 4.4 cm rectal tip delivery system; contains 10% alcohol, 1.5% benzyl alcohol, and propylene glycol); in twin packs.
Pediatric/Adult rectal gel (Diastat AcuDial):
- **4.4 cm rectal tip delivery system (Pediatric/Adult):** 10 mg (5 mg/mL, delivers set doses of either 5, 7.5, or 10 mg); contains 10% alcohol, and 1.5% benzyl alcohol; in twin packs.
- **6 cm rectal tip delivery system (Adult):** 20 mg (5 mg/mL, delivers set doses of either 10, 12.5, 15, 17.5, 20 mg); contains 10% alcohol, and 1.5% benzyl alcohol; in twin packs.

Sedative/muscle relaxant:
- ***Child:***
  - ***IM or IV:*** 0.04–0.2 mg/kg/dose Q2–4 hr; **max. dose:** 0.6 mg/kg within an 8-hr period.
  - ***PO:*** 0.12–0.8 mg/kg/24 hr ÷ Q6–8 hr
- ***Adult:***
  - ***IM or IV:*** 2–10 mg/dose Q3–4 hr PRN
  - ***PO:*** 2–10 mg/dose Q6–12 hr PRN

Status epilepticus:
- ***Neonate:*** 0.3–0.75 mg/kg/dose IV Q15–30 min × 2–3 doses; **max. total dose:** 2 mg.
- ***Child >1 mo:*** 0.2–0.5 mg/kg/dose IV Q15–30 min; **max. total dose:** <5 yr: 5 mg; ≥5 yr: 10 mg. May repeat dosing in 2–4 hr as needed.
- ***Adult:*** 5–10 mg/dose IV Q10–15 min; **max. total dose:** 30 mg in an 8-hr period. May repeat dosing in 2–4 hr as needed.
- ***Rectal dose (using IV dosage form):*** 0.5 mg/kg/dose followed by 0.25 mg/kg/dose in 10 min PRN.
- ***Rectal gel:*** all doses rounded to the nearest available dosage strength; repeat dose in 4–12 hr PRN
  - ***2–5 yr:*** 0.5 mg/kg/dose
  - ***6–11 yr:*** 0.3 mg/kg/dose
  - ***≥12 yr: and adult:*** 0.2 mg/kg/dose

Continued

DIAZEPAM *continued*

Contraindicated in myasthenia gravis, severe respiratory insufficiency, severe hepatic failure and sleep apnea syndrome. Hypotension and respiratory depression may occur. **Use with caution** in hepatic and renal dysfunction, glaucoma, shock, and depression. **Do not use** in combination with protease inhibitors. Concurrent use with CNS depressants, cimetidine, erythromycin, itraconazole, and valproic acid may enhance the effects of diazepam. Diazepam is a substrate for CYP P450 2B6, 2C8, 2C9, and 3A5-7; and minor substrate and inhibitor for CYP P450 2C19 and 3A3/4. The active desmethyldiazepam metabolite is a CYP P450 2C19 substrate.

Administer the conventional IV product undiluted no faster than 2 mg/min. **Do not mix** with IV fluids.

In status epilepticus, diazepam must be followed by long-acting anticonvulsants. Onset of anticonvulsant effect: 1–3 min with IV route; 2–10 min with rectal route. **For management of status epilepticus, see Chapter 1, Table 1-5. For additional information, see Chapter 20 (Table 20-7).**

DIAZOXIDE
Proglycem
Antihypertensive agent, antihypoglycemic agent

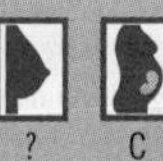

No Yes ? C

Oral suspension: 50 mg/mL (30 mL); contains 7.25% alcohol

Hyperinsulinemic hypoglycemia (due to insulin-producing tumors; start at the lowest dose):
Newborn and infant: 8–15 mg/kg/24 hr ÷ Q8–12 hr PO
Child and adult: 3–8 mg/kg/24 hr ÷ Q8–12 hr PO

Hypoglycemia should be treated initially with IV glucose; diazoxide should be introduced only if refractory to glucose infusion. Should not be used in patients hypersensitive to thiazides unless benefit outweighs risk. **Use with caution** in renal impairment (clearance of drug is reduced); consider dosage reduction.

Sodium and fluid retention is common in young infants and adults and may precipitate CHF in patients with compromised cardiac reserve (usually responsive to diuretics). Hirsutism (reversible), GI disturbances, transient loss of taste, tachycardia, ketoacidosis, palpitations, rash, headache, weakness, and hyperuricemia may occur. Monitor BP closely for hypotension.

Hyperglycemic effect with PO administration occurs within 1 hr, with a duration of 8 hr.

DICLOXACILLIN SODIUM
Dycill, Pathocil, and others
Antibiotic, penicillin (penicillinase-resistant)

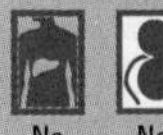
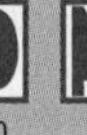
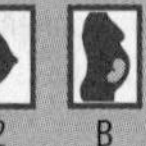

No No 2 B

Caps: 250, 500 mg; contains 0.6 mEq Na/250 mg

Child (<40 kg) (see remarks):
Mild/moderate infections: 12.5–50 mg/kg/24 hr PO ÷ Q6 hr
Severe infections: 50–100 mg/kg/24 hr PO ÷ Q6 hr
Child (≥40 kg) and adult: 125–500 mg/dose PO Q6 hr; **max. dose:** 2 g/24 hr

Contraindicated in patients with a history of penicillin allergy. **Use with caution** in cephalosporin hypersensitivity. May cause nausea, vomiting, and diarrhea.

Limited experience in neonates and very young infants. Higher doses (50–100 mg/kg/24 hr) are indicated following IV therapy for osteomyelitis.

Administer 1 hr before meals or 2 hr after meals.

For explanation of icons, see p. 663.

DIGOXIN
Lanoxin, Digitek, Lanoxicaps
Antiarrhythmic agent, inotrope

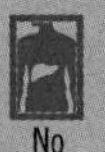
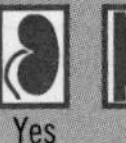

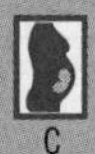
No Yes 2 C

Caps (Lanoxicaps): 100, 200 mcg
Tabs: 125, 250 mcg
Elixir: 50 mcg/mL (60 mL); may contain 10% alcohol
Injection: 100, 250 mcg/mL; may contain propylene glycol and alcohol

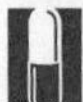

Digitalizing: Total digitalizing dose (TDD) and maintenance doses in mcg/kg/24 hr (see the table that follows):

DIGOXIN DIGITALIZING AND MAINTENANCE DOSES

	TDD		Daily Maintenance	
Age	**PO**	**IV/IM**	**PO**	**IV/IM**
Premature neonate	20	15	5	3–4
Full term neonate	30	20	8–10	6–8
1 mo – <2 yr	40–50	30–40	10–12	7.5–9
2–10 yr	30–40	20–30	8–10	6–8
>10 yr and <100 kg	10–15	8–12	2.5–5	2–3

Initial: ½ TDD, then ¼ TDD Q8–18 hr × 2 doses; obtain ECG 6 hr after dose to assess for toxicity
Maintenance:

<10 yr: Give maintenance dose ÷ BID
≥10 yr: Give maintenance dose once daily

Contraindicated in patients with ventricular dysrhythmias. **Use with caution** in renal failure and with adenosine (enhanced depressant effects on SA and AV nodes). May cause AV block or dysrhythmias. In the patient treated with digoxin, cardioversion, or calcium infusion may lead to ventricular fibrillation (pretreatment with lidocaine may prevent this). Decreased serum potassium and magnesium, or increased magnesium and calcium may increase risk for digoxin toxicity. For signs and symptoms of toxicity, see Chapter 2.

Excreted via the kidney; **adjust dose in renal failure (see Chapter 31).** Therapeutic concentration: 0.8–2 ng/mL. Higher doses may be required for supraventricular tachycardia. Neonates, pregnant women, and patients with renal, hepatic, or heart failure may have falsely elevated digoxin levels, due to the presence of digoxin-like substances.

Digoxin is a CYP450 3A4 and P-glycoprotein substrate. Calcium channel blocker, amiodarone, quinidine, cyclosporine, itraconazole, and macrolide antibiotics may increase digoxin levels.

$T_{1/2}$: Premature infants, 61–170 hr; full-term neonates, 35–45 hr; infants, 18–25 hr; and children, 35 hr.

Recommended serum sampling at steady-state: Obtain a single level from 6 hr postdose to just before the next scheduled dose following 5–8 days of continuous dosing. Levels obtained prior to steady-state may be useful in preventing toxicity.

DIGOXIN IMMUNE FAB (OVINE)
Digibind, DigiFab
Antidigoxin antibody

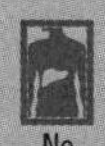 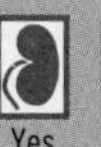 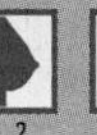 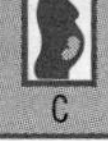
No Yes ? C

Injection:
Digibind: 38 mg
DigiFab: 40 mg

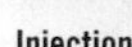

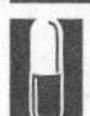

First, determine total body digoxin load (TBL):
TBL (mg) = serum digoxin level (ng/mL) × 5.6 × wt (kg) ÷ 1000, **OR** TBL (mg) = mg digoxin ingested × 0.8

Then, calculate digoxin immune Fab dose:
Dose in number of digoxin immune Fab vials (Digibind or DigiFab): vials = TBL ÷ 0.5

Infuse IV over 15–30 min; administer through 0.22-micron filter only if using Digibind.

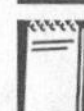

Contraindicated if hypersensitive to sheep products. **Use with caution** in renal or cardiac failure. May cause rapidly developing severe hypokalemia, decreased cardiac output, rash, and edema. Digoxin therapy may be reinstituted in 3–7 days, when toxicity has been corrected.

Digoxin immune FAB will intefere with digitalis immunoassay measurements to result in misleading concentrations. **See Chapter 2 for additional information.**

DILTIAZEM
Cardizem, Cardizem SR, Cardizem CD, Cardizem LA, Dilacor XR, Tiazac, and many others
Calcium channel blocker, antihypertensive

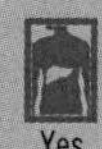 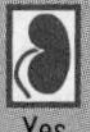  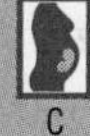
Yes Yes 1 C

Tabs: 30, 60, 90, 120 mg
Extended-release tabs:
Cardizem LA: 120, 180, 240, 300, 360, 420 mg
Extended-release caps:
Various generics: 60, 90, 120, 180, 240, 300, 360, 420 mg
Cardizem CD: 120, 180, 240, 300, 360 mg
Dilacor XR: 120, 180, 240 mg
Tiazac: 120, 180, 240, 300, 360, 420 mg
Oral liquid: 12 mg/mL
Injection: 5 mg/mL (5, 10, 25 mL)

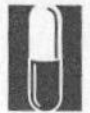

Child: 1.5–2 mg/kg/24 hr PO ÷ TID–QID; max. dose: 3.5 mg/kg/24 hr, alternative **max. dose** of 6 mg/kg/24 hr up to 360 mg/24 hr have been recommended.

Adolescent and adult:
Immediate release: 30–120 mg/dose PO TID–QID; usual range 180–360 mg/24 hr.
Extended release: 120–300 mg/24 hr PO ÷ once daily–BID (BID dosing with Cardizem SR; once daily dosing with Cardizem CD, Cardizem LA, Dilacor XR, Tiazac); **max. dose:** 540 mg/24 hr.

Contraindicated in acute MI with pulmonary congestion, second- or third-degree heart block, and sick sinus syndrome. **Use with caution** in CHF or renal and hepatic impairment. Dizziness, headache, edema, nausea, vomiting, heart block, and arrhythmias may occur.

Diltiazem is a substrate and inhibitor of the CYP 450 3A4 enzyme system. May increase levels and/or effect of buspirone, cyclosporine, carbamazepine, fentanyl, digoxin, quinidine, tacrolimus, benzodiazepines, and beta-blockers. Cimetidine may increase diltiazem serum levels. Rifampin may decrease diltiazem serum levels.

Maximal antihypertensive effect seen within 2 wk.

For explanation of icons, see p. 663.

DIMENHYDRINATE
Dramamine, Children's Dramamine and other brand names
Antiemetic, antihistamine

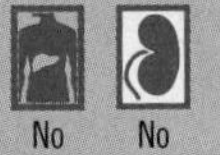  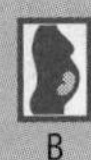
No No ? B

Tabs (OTC): 50 mg
Chewable tabs (OTC): 50 mg; contains 1.5 mg phenylalanine
Oral liquid: 12.5 mg/4 mL (OTC), 12.5 mg/5 mL (OTC), 15.62 mg/5 mL; some preparations may contain 5% alcohol
Injection: 50 mg/mL; contains benzyl alcohol and propylene glycol

Child (<12 yr): 5 mg/kg/24 hr ÷ Q6 hr PO/IM/IV; alternative oral dosing by age:
2–5 yr: 12.5–25 mg/dose Q6–8 hr PRN PO with the **max. dosage** in the subsequent list
6–12 yr: 25–50 mg/dose Q6–8 hr PRN PO with the **max. dosage** in the subsequent list
≥12 yr and adult: 50–100 mg/dose Q4–6 hr PRN PO/IM/IV
MAXIMUM PO DOSE:
2–5 yr: 75 mg/24 hr
6–12 yr: 150 mg/24 hr
≥12 yr and adult: 400 mg/24 hr
MAXIMUM IM DOSE:
Child: 300 mg/24 hr

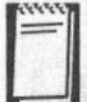

Causes drowsiness and anticholinergic side effects. May mask vestibular symptoms and cause CNS excitation in young children. **Caution** when taken with ototoxic agents or history of seizures. **Use should be limited to management of prolonged vomiting of known etiology. Not recommended** in children <2 yr. Toxicity resembles anticholinergic poisoning.

DIMERCAPROL
BAL, British Anti-Lewisite
Heavy metal chelator (arsenic, gold, mercury, lead)

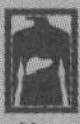 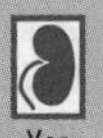  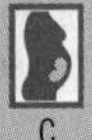
Yes Yes ? C

Injection (in oil): 100 mg/mL; contains 20% benzyl benzoate and peanut oil (3 mL)

Give all injections deep IM.
Lead poisoning:
Acute severe encephalopathy (lead level >70 mcg/dL): 4 mg/kg/dose Q4 hr × 2–7 days with the addition of Ca-EDTA (given at separate site) at the time of the second dose.
Less severe poisoning: 4 mg/kg × 1, then 3 mg/kg/dose Q4 hr × 2–7 days.
Arsenic or gold poisoning (see table below):

	Mild Cases	Severe Cases
Days 1 and 2	2.5 mg/kg/dose Q6 hr	3 mg/kg/dose Q4 hr
Day 3	2.5 mg/kg/dose Q12 hr	3 mg/kg/dose Q6 hr
Days 4–13	2.5 mg/kg/dose Q24 hr	3 mg/kg/dose Q12 hr

Mercury poisoning: 5 mg/kg × 1, then 2.5 mg/kg/dose once daily–BID × 10 days

Contraindicated in hepatic or renal insufficiency. May cause hypertension, tachycardia, GI disturbance, headache, fever (30% of children), nephrotoxicity, transient neutropenia. Symptoms are usually relieved by antihistamines. Urine should be kept alkaline to protect the kidneys. **Use with caution** with G6PD deficiency and peanut-sensitive patients. **Do not use** concomitantly with iron.

DIPHENHYDRAMINE
Benadryl and many other brand names
Antihistamine

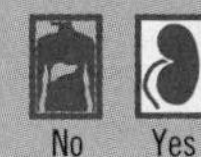

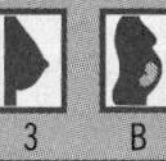

No Yes 3 B

Elixir (OTC): 12.5 mg/5 mL; may contain 5.6% alcohol
Syrup: 12.5 mg/5 mL; some may contain 5% alcohol
Oral suspension: 25 mg/5 mL; may contain phenylalanine
Oral liquid/solution (OTC): 12.5 mg/5 mL
Caps/Tabs (OTC): 25, 50 mg
Tabs, orally disintegrating (OTC): 12.5 mg; contains aspartame, phenylalanine
Strips, orally disintegrating (OTC): 12.5, 25 mg; may contain <5% alcohol
Chewable tabs: 12.5 mg (OTC), 25 mg; contains aspartame, phenylalanine
Injection: 50 mg/mL
Cream (OTC): 1, 2% (30 g)
Topical gel (OTC): 1% (37.5 g), 2% (120 g)
Topical spray (OTC): 1, 2% (60 mL)

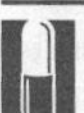

Severe allergic reaction (anaphylaxis) and dystonic reactions (including phenothiazine toxicity) (PO/IM/IV):

Child: 1–2 mg/kg/dose Q6 hr; usual dose: 5 mg/kg/24 hr ÷ Q6 hr. **Maximum dose:** 50 mg/dose and 300 mg/24 hr.

Adult: 25–50 mg/dose Q4–8 hr; **max. dose:** 400 mg/24 hr

Sleep aid (PO/IM/IV): Administer dose 30 min before bedtime.

2–11 yr: 1 mg/kg/dose; **max. dose:** 50 mg/dose
≥12 yr: 50 mg

Contraindicated with concurrent MAO inhibitor use, acute attacks of asthma, GI or urinary obstruction. **Use with caution** in infants and young children, and **do not use** in neonates due to potential CNS effects. Side effects include sedation, nausea, vomiting, xerostoma, blurred vision and other reactions common to antihistamines. CNS side effects more common than GI disturbances. May cause paradoxical excitement in children. **Adjust dose in renal failure (see Chapter 31).**

DIVALPROEX SODIUM
Depakote, Depakote ER
Anticonvulsant

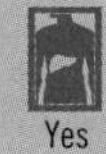
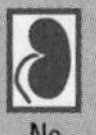
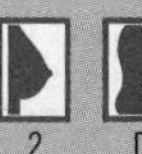

Yes No 2 D

Delayed-release tabs: 125, 250, 500 mg
Extended-release tabs (Depakote ER): 250, 500 mg
Sprinkle caps: 125 mg

Dose: see *Valproic Acid*

See *Valproic Acid.* Preferred over valproic acid for patients on ketogenic diet. Depakote ER is prescribed by a once daily interval; whereas Depakote is typically prescribed BID. Depakote and Depakote ER are not bioequivalent; see package insert for dose conversion.

For explanation of icons, see p. 663.

DOBUTAMINE

Various generics; previously available as Dobutrex
Sympathomimetic agent

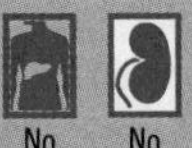 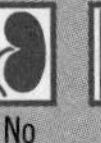 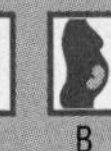

No No ? B

Injection: 12.5 mg/mL (20 mL); contains sulfites
Prediluted injection in D_5W: 1 mg/mL (250, 500 mL), 2 mg/mL (250 mL), 4 mg/mL (250 mL)

Continuous IV infusion (all ages): 2.5–15 mcg/kg/min;
Max. dose: 40 mcg/kg/min.
To prepare infusion: see IV Infusions on page i.

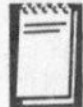

Contraindicated in idiopathic hypertrophic subaortic stenosis (IHSS). Tachycardia, arrhythmias (PVCs), and hypertension may occasionally occur (especially at higher infusion rates). Correct hypovolemic states before use. Increases AV conduction, may precipitate ventricular ectopic activity.

Dobutamine has been shown to increase cardiac output and systemic pressure in pediatric patients of every age group. However, in premature neonates, dobutamine is less effective than dopamine in raising systemic blood pressure without causing undue tachycardia, and dobutamine has not been shown to provide any added benefit when given to such infants already receiving optimal infusions of dopamine.

Monitor BP and vital signs. $T_{1/2}$: 2 min. Peak effects in 10–20 min. Use with linezolid may potentially increase blood pressure.

DOCUSATE

Colace, Surfak, Enemeez and many other brands
Stool softener, laxative

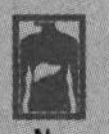 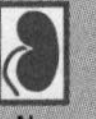 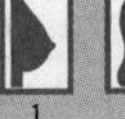 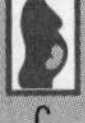

No No 1 C

Available as docusate sodium:

Caps (OTC): 50, 100, 250 mg; sodium content (50 mg cap: 3 mg; 100 mg cap: ~5 mg)
Tabs (OTC): 100 mg
Syrup (OTC): 16.7 mg/5 mL, 20 mg/5 mL; may contain alcohol
Oral liquid (OTC): 10 mg/mL; contains 1 mg/mL sodium
Rectal enema (Enemeez; OTC): 283 mg/5 mL (5 mL); Enemeez Plus product contains benzocaine

Available as docusate calcium:

Caps (Surfak; OTC): 240 mg

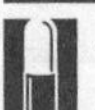

PO: (take with liquids)
<3 yr: 10–40 mg/24 hr ÷ once daily–QID
3–6 yr: 20–60 mg/24 hr ÷ once daily–QID
6–12 yr: 40–150 mg/24 hr ÷ once daily–QID
>12 yr and adult: 50–400 mg/24 hr ÷ once daily–QID

Rectal:
Older child and adult: add 50–100 mg of oral liquid (not syrup) to enema fluid (saline or oil retention enemas).

Oral dosage effective only after 1–3 days of therapy. Incidence of side effects is exceedingly low. Rash, nausea, and throat irritation have been reported. Oral liquid is bitter; give with milk, fruit juice, or formula to mask taste.

A few drops of the 10 mg/mL oral liquid may be used in the ear as a cerumenolytic. Effect is usually seen within 15 min.

DOLASETRON
Anzemet and generics
Antiemetic agent, 5-HT$_3$ antagonist

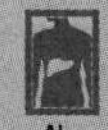 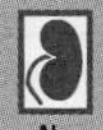  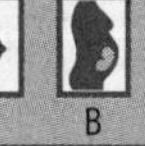
No No ? B

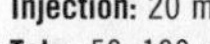

Injection: 20 mg/mL (0.625, 5, 25 mL)
Tabs: 50, 100 mg
Oral suspension: 10 mg/mL

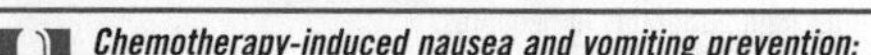

Chemotherapy-induced nausea and vomiting prevention:
2 yr–adult: 1.8 mg/kg/dose IV/PO up to a max. dose of 100 mg. Administer IV doses 30 min prior to chemotherapy and administer PO doses 60 min prior to chemotherapy.

Postoperative nausea and vomiting prevention: Administer IV doses 15 min prior to cessation of anesthesia and PO doses 2 hr prior to surgery.

2–16 yr:
- ***IV:*** 0.35 mg/kg/dose (**max. dose:** 12.5 mg) × 1
- ***PO:*** 1.2 mg/kg/dose × 1 (**max. dose:** 100 mg) × 1

Adult:
- ***IV:*** 12.5 mg/dose × 1
- ***PO:*** 100 mg/dose × 1

Postoperative nausea and vomiting treatment: Administer IV at onset of nausea and vomiting.
2–16 yr: 0.35 mg/kg/dose (**max. dose:** 12.5 mg)
Adult: 12.5 mg/dose

May cause hypotension and prolongation of cardiac conduction intervals; particularly QTc interval (dose dependent effect). Common side effects include dizziness, headache, sedation, blurred vision, fever, chills, and sleep disorders. Rare cases sustained supraventricular and ventricular arrhythmias, fatal cardiac arrest and MI have been reported in children and adolescents.

Avoid use in patients with congenital long QTc syndrome, hypomagnesemia, hypokalemia, or with concurrent use with other drugs that increase QTc interval (eg., erythromycin, cisapride). Drug's active metabolite (hydrodolasetron) is a substrate for CYP 450 2D6 and 3A3/4 isoenzymes; concomitant use of enzyme inhibitors (e.g., cimetidine) may increase risk for side effects and use of enzyme inducers (e.g., rifampin) may decrease dolasetron's efficacy. Although no dosage adjustments are necessary, hyrdrodolasetron's clearance decreases 42% with severe hepatic impairment and 44% with severe renal impairment.

IV doses may be administered undiluted over 30 sec.

DOPAMINE
Various generics; previously available as Intropin
Sympathomimetic agent

 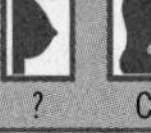
No No ? C

Injection: 40, 80, 160 mg/mL (5, 10 mL)
Prediluted injection in D$_5$W: 0.8, 1.6, 3.2 mg/mL (250, 500 mL)

All ages:
Low dose: 2–5 mcg/kg/min IV; increases renal blood flow; minimal effect on heart rate and cardiac output
Intermediate dose: 5–15 mcg/kg/min IV; increases heart rate, cardiac contractility, cardiac output, and to a lesser extent, renal blood flow.
High dose: >20 mcg/kg/min IV; alpha adrenergic effects are prominent; decreases renal perfusion.
Max. dose recommended: 20–50 mcg/kg/min IV

To prepare infusion: see IV Infusions on page i.

Continued

For explanation of icons, see p. 663.

DOPAMINE *continued*

Do not use in pheochromocytoma, tachyarrhythmias, or hypovolemia. Monitor vital signs and blood pressure continuously. Correct hypovolemic states. Tachyarrhythmias, ectopic beats, hypertension, vasoconstriction, and vomiting may occur. **Use with caution** with phenytoin because hypotension and bradycardia may be exacerbated. Use with linezolid may potentially increase blood pressure.

Newborn infants may be more sensitive to the vasoconstrictive effects of dopamine. Children <2 yr of age clear dopamine faster and exhibit high variability in neonates.

Should be administered through a central line or large vein. Extravasation may cause tissue necrosis; treat with phentolamine. **Do not administer** into an umbilical arterial catheter.

DORNASE ALFA/DNASE

Pulmozyme

Inhaled mucolytic

No No ? B

Inhalation solution: 1 mg/mL (2.5 mL)

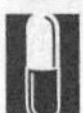

Child >5 yr and adult: 2.5 mg via nebulizer once daily. Some patients may benefit from 2.5 mg BID.

Contraindicated in patients with hypersensitivity to epoetin alfa. Voice alteration, pharyngitis, laryngitis may result. These are generally reversible without dose adjustment. Safety and efficacy has not been demonstrated in patients >1 year of continuous use.

Do not mix with other nebulized drugs. A beta-agonist may be useful before administration to enhance drug distribution. Chest physiotherapy should be incorporated into treatment regimen. The following nebulizer compressor systems have been recommended for use: Pulmo-Aide, Pari-Proneb, Mobilaire, Porta-Neb, or PariBaby. Use of the "Sidestream" nebulizer cup can significantly reduce the medication administration time.

DOXAPRAM HCL

Dopram

CNS stimulant

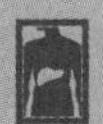
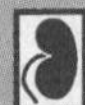
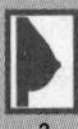
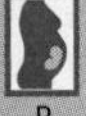

No No ? B

Injection: 20 mg/mL (20 mL); contains 0.9% benzyl alcohol

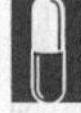

Methylxanthine-refractory neonatal apnea: Load with 2.5–3 mg/kg over 15 min, followed by a continuous infusion of 1 mg/kg/hr titrated to the lowest effective dose; **max. dose:** 2.5 mg/kg/hr

Contraindicated in seizures, proven or suspected pulmonary embolism, head injuries, cerebral vascular accident, cerebral edema, cardiovascular or coronary artery disease, severe hypertension, pheochromocytoma, hyperthyroidism, and in patients with mechanical disorders of ventilation. **Do not use** with general anesthetic agents that can sensitize the heart to catecholamines (e.g., halothane, cyclopropane, and enflurane) to reduce the risk of cardiac

Continued

DOXAPRAM HCL *continued*

arrhythmias, including ventricular tachycardia and ventricular fibrillation. **Do not** initiate doxapram until the general anesthetic agent has been completely excreted.

Hypertension occurs with higher doses (>1.5 mg/kg/hr). May also cause tachycardia, arrhythmias, seizure, hyperreflexia, hyperpyrexia, abdominal distension, bloody stools, and sweating. **Avoid** extravasation into tissues.

DOXYCYCLINE

Vibramycin, Periostat, and others

Antibiotic, tetracycline derivative

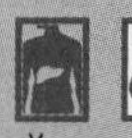
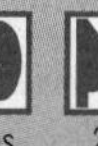
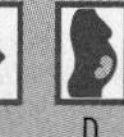

Yes Yes 2 D

Caps: 20 (Periostat), 50, 75, 100 mg
Tabs: 20 (Periostat), 50, 75, 100 mg
Syrup: 50 mg/5 mL (60 mL)
Oral suspension: 25 mg/5 mL (60 mL)
Injection: 100, 200 mg

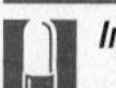

Initial:

≤45 kg: 2.2 mg/kg/dose BID PO/IV × 1 day to **max. dose:** of 200 mg/24 hr
>45 kg: 100 mg/dose BID PO/IV × 1 day

Maintenance:

≤45 kg: 2.2–4.4 mg/kg/24 hr once daily–BID PO/IV
>45 kg: 100–200 mg/24 hr ÷ once daily–BID PO/IV

Max. dose: 200 mg/24 hr

PID: 100 mg Q12 hr PO/IV × 14 day in combination with other antibiotics.

Anthrax (inhalation/systemic/cutaneous; see remarks): Initiate therapy with IV route and convert to PO route when clinically appropriate. Duration of therapy is 60 days (IV and PO combined):

≤8 yr or ≤45 kg: 2.2 mg/kg/dose BID IV/PO; **max. dose:** 200 mg/24 hr
>8 yr and >45 kg: 100 mg/dose BID IV/PO

Malaria prophylaxis (start 1–2 days prior to exposure and continue for 4 wk after leaving endemic area):

>8 yr: 2 mg/kg/24 hr PO once daily; **max. dose:** 100 mg/24 hr and max. duration of 4 mo.
Adult: 100 mg PO once daily

Periodontitis:

Adult: 20 mg BID PO × ≤9 mo

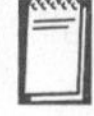

Use with caution in hepatic and renal disease. May cause increased intracranial pressure. Generally **not recommended** for use in children <8 yr due to risk for tooth enamel hypoplasia and discoloration. However, the AAP *Red Book* recommends doxycycline as the drug of choice for rickettsial disease regardless of age. May cause GI symptoms, photosensitivity, hemolytic anemia, rash, and hypersensitivity reactions.

Doxycycline is approved for the treatment of anthrax (*Bacillus anthracis*) in combination with one or two other antimicrobials. If meningitis is suspected, consider using an alternative agent because of poor CNS penetration. Consider changing to high-dose amoxicillin (25–35 mg/kg/dose TID PO) for penicillin-susceptible strains. See www.bt.cdc.gov for the latest information.

Rifampin, barbiturates, phenytoin, and carbamazepine may increase clearance of doxycycline. Doxycycline may enhance the hypoprothrombinemic effect of warfarin. See *Tetracycline* for additional drug/food interactions and remarks.

Infuse IV over 1–4 hr. **Avoid** prolonged exposure to direct sunlight.

For periodontitis, take capsules ≥1 hr prior to meals; and take tablets ≥1 hr prior or 2 hr after meals.

For explanation of icons, see p. 663.

DRONABINOL
Tetrahydrocannabinol, THC, Marinol
Antiemetic

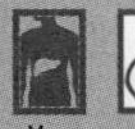 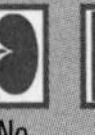 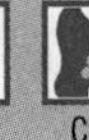

Yes No X C

Caps: 2.5, 5, 10 mg; contains sesame oil

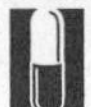

Antiemetic:

Child and adult (PO): 5 mg/m^2/dose 1–3 hr prior to chemotherapy, then Q2–4 hr up to a **max. dose** of 6 doses/24 hr; doses may be gradually increased by 2.5 mg/m^2/dose increments up to a **max. dose** of 15 mg/m^2/dose if needed and tolerated

Appetite stimulant:

Adult (PO): 2.5 mg BID 1 hr before lunch and dinner; if not tolerated, reduce dose to 2.5 mg QHS. **Max. dose:** 20 mg/24 hr (**use caution** when increasing doses because of increased risk of dose-related adverse reactions at higher dosages)

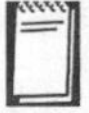

Contraindicated in patients with history of substance abuse and mental illness, allergy to sesame oil. **Use with caution** in heart disease, seizures, hepatic disease (reduce dose if severe). Side effects: euphoria, dizziness, difficulty concentrating, anxiety, mood change, sedation, hallucinations, ataxia, paresthesia, hypotension, excessively increased appetite, and habit forming potential.

Onset of action: 0.5–1 hr. Duration of psychoactive effects 4–6 hr, appetite stimulation, 24 hr.

DROPERIDOL
Inapsine and others
Sedative, antiemetic

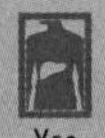 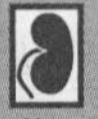 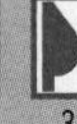 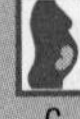

Yes Yes 3 C

Injection: 2.5 mg/mL (1, 2 mL)

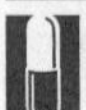

Antiemetic/sedation:

Child: 0.03–0.07 mg/kg/dose IM or IV over 2–5 min; if needed, may give 0.1–0.15 mg/kg/dose; **initial max. dose:** 0.1 mg/kg/dose and subsequent **max. dose:** 2.5 mg/dose.

Dosage interval:

Antiemetic: PRN Q4–6 hr

Sedation: Repeat dose in 15–30 min if necessary

Adult: 2.5–5 mg IM or IV over 2–5 min; **initial max. dose** is 2.5 mg.

Dosage interval:

Antiemetic: PRN Q3–4 hr

Sedation: Repeat dose in 15–30 min if necessary.

Use with caution in renal and hepatic impairment; 75% of metabolites are excreted renally and drug is extensively metabolized in the liver. Side effects include hypotension, tachycardia, extrapyramidal side effects such as dystonia, feeling of motor restlessness, laryngospasm, bronchospasm. May lower seizure threshold. **Fatal arrhythmias and QT interval prolongation has been associated with use.**

Onset in 3–10 min. Peak effects within 10–30 min. Duration of 2–4 hr. Often given as adjunct to other agents.

EDETATE (EDTA) CALCIUM DISODIUM

Calcium disodium versenate

Chelating agent, antidote for lead toxicity

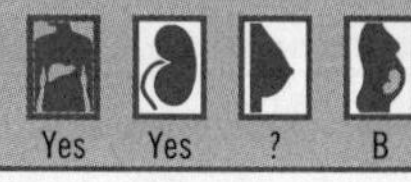

Injection: 200 mg/mL (2.5 mL)

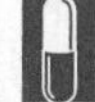

Lead poisoning:

Lead level >70 mcg/dL (use with dimercaprol): Initiate at the time of the second dimercaprol dose and treat for 3–5 days. May repeat a course as needed after 2–4 days of no EDTA.

IM: 1000–1500 mg/m²/24 hr ÷ Q4 hr

IV: 1000–1500 mg/m²/24 hr as an 8–24 hour infusion or divided Q12 hr.

Use 1500 mg/m²/24 hr for 5 days in the presence of encephalopathy.

Lead level 20–70 mcg/dL: 1000 mg/m²/24 hr IV as an 8–24 hr infusion OR intermittent dosing divided Q12 hr × 5 days. May repeat course as needed after 2–4 days of no EDTA.

Max. daily dose: 75 mg/kg/24 hr.

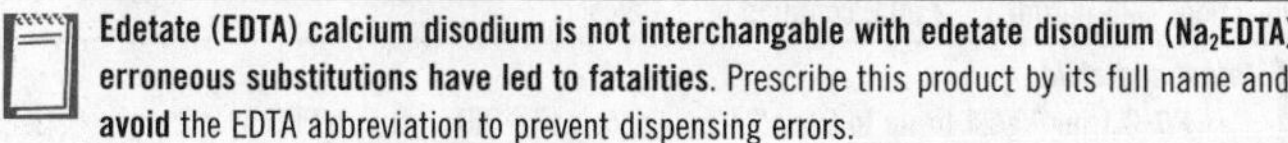

Edetate (EDTA) calcium disodium is not interchangable with edetate disodium (Na_2EDTA); erroneous substitutions have led to fatalities. Prescribe this product by its full name and **avoid** the EDTA abbreviation to prevent dispensing errors.

May cause renal tubular necrosis. **Do not use** in the presence of anuria, hepatitis, and active renal disease. Dosage reduction is recommended with mild renal disease. Follow urinalysis and renal function. Monitor ECG continuously for arrhythmia when giving IV. Rapid IV infusion may cause sudden increase in intracranial pressure in patients with cerebral edema. May cause zinc and copper deficiency. Monitor Ca^{2+} and PO_4.

IM route preferred. Give IM with 0.5% procaine.

EDROPHONIUM CHLORIDE

Tensilon, Enlon, Reversol

Anticholinesterase agent, antidote for neuromuscular blockade

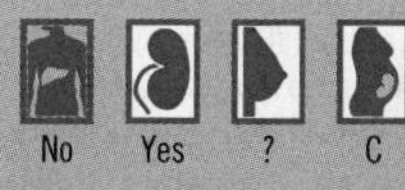

Injection: 10 mg/mL (15 mL) (contains 0.45% phenol and 0.2% sulfite)

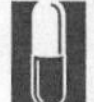

Diagnosis for myasthenia gravis (IV):

Neonate: 0.1 mg single dose

Infant and child:

Initial: 0.04 mg/kg/dose × 1

Max. dose: 1 mg for <34 kg, 2 mg for ≥34 kg

If no response after 1 min, may give 0.16 mg/kg/dose for a total of 0.2 mg/kg

Total max. dose: 5 mg for <34 kg, 10 mg for ≥34 kg

Adult: 2 mg test dose IV; if no reaction, give 8 mg after 45 sec.

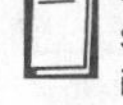

May precipitate cholinergic crisis, arrhythmias, and bronchospasm. Keep atropine available in syringe and have resuscitation equipment ready. Hypersensitivity to test dose (fasciculations or intestinal cramping) is indication to stop giving drug. **Contraindicated** in GI or GU obstruction, or arrhythmias. Dose may need to be reduced in chronic renal failure.

Reported doses for reversing neuromuscular blockade in children have ranged from 0.1–1.43 mg/kg/dose. Antagonism of nondepolarizing neuromuscular blocking drugs in children is more rapid than in adults.

Short duration of action with IV route (5–10 min). **Antidote:** atropine 0.01–0.04 mg/kg/dose.

For explanation of icons, see p. 663.

EMLA

See *Lidocaine and Prilocaine*

ENALAPRIL MALEATE (PO), ENALAPRILAT (IV)

Enalapril: Vasotec and others
Enalaprilat: Vasotec IV and others
Angiotensin converting enzyme inhibitor, antihypertensive

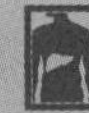
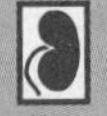
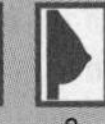
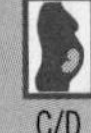
No Yes 2 C/D

Enalapril:
Tabs: 2.5, 5, 10, 20 mg
Oral suspension: 0.1, 1 mg/mL

Enalaprilat:
Injection: 1.25 mg/mL (1, 2 mL); contains benzyl alcohol

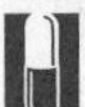

Infant and child:
PO: 0.1 mg/kg/24 hr up to 5 mg/24 hr ÷ once daily–BID; increase PRN over 2 wk.
Max. dose: 0.6 mg/kg/24 hr up to 40 mg/24 hr
IV: 0.005–0.01 mg/kg/dose Q8–24 hr

Adolescent and adult:
PO: 2.5–5 mg/24 hr once daily initially to **max. dose** of 40 mg/24 hr ÷ once daily–BID
IV: 0.625–1.25 mg/dose IV Q6 hr; doses as high as 5 mg Q6 hr is reported to be tolerated for up to 36 hr.

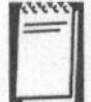

Use with caution in bilateral renal artery stenosis. **Avoid** use with dialysis with high-flux membranes since anaphylactoid reactions have been reported. Side effects: nausea, diarrhea, headache, dizziness, hyperkalemia, hypoglycemia, hypotension, and hypersensitivity. Cough is a reported side effect of ACE inhibitors.

Enalapril (PO) is converted to its active form (Enalaprilat) by the liver. Administer IV over 5 min.

Adjust dose in renal impairment (see Chapter 31).

Nitritoid reactions have been in patients receiving concomitent IV gold therapy.

Pregnancy category is "C" during the first trimester but changes to "D" during the second and third trimester (fetal injury and death have been reported). Despite the pregnancy category, enalapril/enalaprilat should be discontinued as soon as possible when pregnancy is detected.

ENOXAPARIN

Lovenox
Anticoagulant, low molecular weight heparin

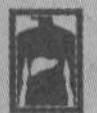
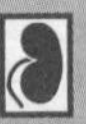
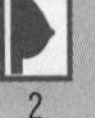
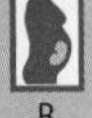
No Yes 2 B

Injection: 100 mg/mL (3 mL); contains 15 mg/mL benzyl alcohol
Injection (pre-filled syringes with 27-gauge × ½ needle): 30 mg/0.3 mL, 40 mg/0.4 mL, 60 mg/0.6 mL, 80 mg/0.8 mL, 100 mg/1 mL, 120 mg/0.8 mL, 150 mg/1 mL
Approximate anti-factor Xa activity: 100 IU per 1 mg

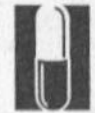

Initial empiric dosage; patient specific dosage defined by therapeutic drug monitoring when indicated (see remarks).

DVT treatment:
Infant <2 mo: 1.5 mg/kg/dose Q12 hr SC
Infant ≥2 mo–adult: 1 mg/kg/dose Q12 hr SC; alternatively, 1.5 mg/kg/dose Q24 hr SC can be used in adults.

Continued

ENOXAPARIN *continued*

Dosage adjustment for DVT treatment to achieve target anti-factor Xa low molecular weight heparin (LMWH) levels of 0.5–1 units/mL (see the following table).

Anti-factor Xa LMWH Level (units/mL)	Hold Next Dose?	Dose Change	Repeat Anti-factor Xa LMWH Level ?
<0.35	No	Increase by 25%	4 hr post next new dose
0.35–0.49	No	Increase by 10%	4 hr post next new dose
0.5–1	No	No	1 week later at 4 hr post dose
1.1–1.5	No	Decrease by 20%	4 hr post next new dose
1.6–2	3 hr	Decrease by 30%	4 hr post next new dose
>2	Until anti-factor Xa LMWH reaches 0.5 units/mL (levels can be measured Q12 hr until it reaches ≤0.5 units/mL).	When anti-factor Xa LMWH reaches 0.5 units/mL, dose may be restarted at a dose 40% less than originally prescribed.	4 hr post next new dose

DVT prophylaxis:

Infant <2 mo: 0.75 mg/kg/dose Q12 hr SC

Infant ≥2 mo–child 18 yr: 0.5 mg/kg/dose Q12 hr SC; **max. dose:** 30 mg/dose

Patients with indwelling epidural catheters/neuraxial anesthesia (≥2 mo–child 18 yr): 1 mg/kg/dose Q24 hr SC; **max. dose:** 40 mg/dose. Twice daily dosing is **contraindicated** for these patients. See remarks.

Adjust dosage for DVT prophylaxis to achieve target anti-factor Xa LMWH levels of 0.1–0.3 units/mL for all children.

Adult:

Knee or hip replacement surgery: 30 mg BID SC × 7–14 days; initiate therapy 12–24 hr after surgery provided hemostasis is established. Alternatively for hip replacement surgery, 40 mg once daily SC × 7–14 days initially up to 3 wk thereafter; initiate therapy 9–15 hr prior to surgery.

Abdominal surgery: 40 mg once daily SC × 7–12 days initiated 2 hr prior to surgery.

Patients at risk due to severe restricted mobility during an acute illness: 40 mg once daily SC × 6–14 days.

Inhibits thrombosis by inactivating factor Xa without significantly affecting bleeding time, platelet function, PT, or aPTT at recommended doses. Dosages of enoxaparin, heparin, or other low molecular weight heparins **cannot** be used interchangeably on a unit-for-unit (or mg-for-mg) basis because of differences in pharmacokinetics and activity. Peak anti-factor Xa LMWH activity is achieved 4 hr after a dose. **Anti-factor Xa LMWH is NOT THE SAME as unfractionated heparin anti-Xa level (used for monitoring heparin therapy).**

Contraindicated in major bleeding and drug-induced thrombocytopenia. **Use with caution** in uncontrolled arterial hypertension, bleeding diathesis, history of recurrent GI ulcers, diabetic retinopathy, and severe renal dysfunction (reduce dose by increasing the dosage interval from Q12 hr to Q24 hr if GFR <30 mL/min). Prophylactic use is **not recommended** in patients with prosthetic heart valves (especially in pregnant women) due to reports of fatalities in patients and fetuses. **Concurrent use with spinal or epidural anesthesia, or spinal puncture has resulted in long-term or permanent paralysis; potential benefits must be weighed against the risks.** May cause fever, confusion, edema,

Continued

For explanation of icons, see p. 663.

ENOXAPARIN *continued*

nausea, hemorrhage, thrombocytopenia, hypochromic anemia, and pain/erythema at injection site. **Protamine sulfate is the antidote;** 1 mg protamine sulfate neutralizes 1 mg enoxaparin.

DVT prophylaxis for patients with epidural catheters/neuaxial anesthesia: If placing needle, hold anticoagulation for 12 hr and restart dosing no sooner than 4 hrs after needle insertion. If removing catheter, hold anticoagulation for 12 hr and restart dosing no sooner than 2 hr after catheter removal.

Recommended anti-factor Xa LMWH levels obtained 4 hr after subcutaneous dose after the third consecutive dose:

DVT treatment: 0.5–1 units/mL
DVT prophylaxis: 0.1–0.3 units/mL

Administer by deep SC injection by having the patient lie down. Alternate administration between the left and right anterolateral and left and right posterolateral abdominal wall. See package insert for detailed SC administration recommendations. To minimize bruising, **do not** rub the injection site. IV or IM route of administration is **not recommended.**

For additional information, see *Chest* 2008;133:887–968 and *Regional Anesth Pain Med* 2003;28(3):172–197.

EPINEPHRINE HCL
Adrenalin, EpiPen, and others
Sympathomimetic agent

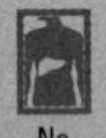
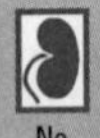
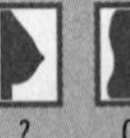
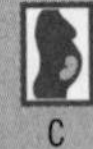

No No ? C

Injection:
1:1000 (aqueous): 1 mg/mL (1, 30 mL)
1:10,000 (aqueous): 0.1 mg/mL (10 mL pre-filled syringes with either 18-G 3.5-inch or 21-G 1.5-inch needles or 10 mL vials)

Autoinjector:
EpiPen: Delivers a single 0.3 mg (0.3 mL) dose (1 or 2 pack)
EpiPen Jr: Delivers a single 0.15 mg (0.3 mL) dose (1 or 2 pack)

Aerosol: 0.22 mg epinephrine base/spray (15, 22.5 mL); may contain alcohol
Oral inhalation solution: 1% (10 mg/mL or 1:100) (7.5 mL)
Some preparations may contain sulfites.

Cardiac uses:
Neonate:
Asystole and bradycardia: 0.01–0.03 mg/kg of 1:10,000 solution (0.1–0.3 mL/kg) IV/ET Q3–5 min PRN.

Infant and child:
Bradycardia/asystole and pulseless arrest: See page ii and PALS algorithms in back of book.

Bradycardia, asystole, and pulseless arrest (see remarks):
First dose: 0.01 mg/kg of 1:10,000 solution (0.1 mL/kg) IO/IV; **max. dose:** 1 mg (10 mL). Subsequent doses Q3–5 min PRN should be the same. High-dose epinephrine after failure of standard dose has not been shown to be effective (see remarks). Must circulate drug with CPR. For ET route see below.
All ET doses: 0.1 mg/kg of 1:1000 solution (0.1 mL/kg) ET Q3–5 min.

Adult:
Asystole: 1–5 mg IV/ET Q3–5 min.

IV drip (all ages): 0.1–1 mcg/kg/min; titrate to effect; to prepare infusion, see IV Infusions on page i.

Continued

EPINEPHRINE HCL *continued*

Respiratory uses:

Bronchodilator: 1 : 1000 (aqueous):

Infant and child: 0.01 mL/kg/dose SC (**max. single dose** 0.5 mL); repeat Q15 min × 3–4 doses or Q4 hr PRN

Adult: 0.3–0.5 mg (0.3–0.5 mL)/dose SC Q20 min × 3 doses.

Inhalation: 1–2 puffs Q4 hr PRN

Nebulization (alternative to racemic epinephrine): 0.5 mL/kg of 1 : 1000 solution diluted in 3 mL NS; **max. doses**: ≤4 yr: 2.5 mL/dose; >4 yr: 5 mL/dose

Hypersensitivity reactions (see remarks for IV dosing):

Child: 0.01 mg/kg/dose IM/SC up to a **max. dose** of 0.5 mg/dose Q20 min–4 hr PRN. If using EpiPen or EpiPen Jr, administer only via the IM route using the following dosage:

<30 kg: 0.15 mg

≥30 kg: 0.3 mg

Adult: Start with 0.1–0.5 mg IM/SC Q20 min–4 hr PRN; doses may be increased if necessary to a single **max. dose** of 1 mg.

High-dose rescue therapy for in-hospital cardiac arrest in children after failure of an initial standard dose has been reported to be of no benefit compared to standard dose (*N Engl J Med* 2004;350:1722–1730).

Hypersensitivity reactions: For bronchial asthma and certain allergic manifestations (e.g., angioedema, urticaria, serum sickness, anaphylactic shock) use epinephrine SC. Patients with anaphylaxis may benefit from IM administration. The adult IV dose for hypersensitivity reactions or to relieve bronchospasm usually ranges from 0.1 to 0.25 mg injected slowly over 5–10 min Q5–15 min as needed. Neonates may be given a dose of 0.01 mg/kg body weight; for infants, 0.05 mg is an adequate initial dose and this may be repeated at 20- to 30-min intervals in the management of asthma attacks.

May produce arrhythmias, tachycardia, hypertension, headaches, nervousness, nausea, vomiting. Necrosis may occur at site of repeated local injection.

Concomitant use of noncardiac selective beta-blockers or tricyclic antidepressants may enhance epinephrine's pressor response. Chlorpromazine may reverse the pressor response.

ETT doses should be diluted with NS to a volume of 3–5 mL before administration. Follow with several positive pressure ventilations.

EpiPen and EpiPen Jr should be administered IM into the anterolateral aspect of the thigh.

EPINEPHRINE, RACEMIC
S-2 Inhalant
Sympathomimetic agent

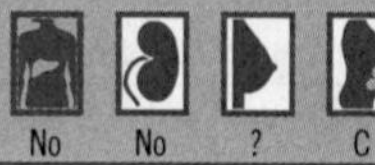

Solution for inhalation: 2.25% (1.25% epinephrine base) (0.5 mL)
Contains sulfites

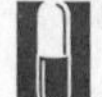

<4 yr:

Croup (using 2.25% solution): 0.05 mL/kg/dose up to a **max. dose** of 0.5 mL/dose diluted to 3 mL with NS. Given via nebulizer over 15 min PRN but **not** more frequently than Q1–2 hr.

≥4 yrs: 0.5 mL/dose diluted to 3 mL with NS via nebulizer over 15 min Q3–4 hr PRN

Tachyarrhythmias, headache, nausea, palpitations reported. Rebound symptoms may occur. Cardiorespiratory monitoring should be considered if administered more frequently than Q1–2 hr.

For explanation of icons, see p. 663.

EPOETIN ALFA
Erythropoietin, Epogen, Procrit
Recombinant human erythropoietin

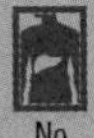 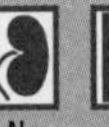 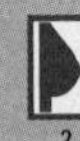 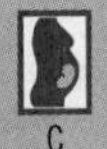
No No ? C

Injection (single-dose, preservative-free vials): 2000, 3000, 4000, 10,000, 40,000 U/mL (1 mL)
Injection (multi-dose vials): 10,000 U/mL (2 mL), 20,000 U/mL (1 mL); contains 1% benzyl alcohol
All dosage forms contains 2.5 mg albumin per 1 mL.

Anemia in chronic renal failure (see remarks for dosage adjustment): SC/IV

Inital dose:

Child: Start at 50 U/kg/dose 3 times per week. Reported dosage range for children (3 mo–20 yr) not requiring dialysis, 50–250 U/kg/dose 3 times per week. Reported dosage range for children receiving hemodialysis, 50–450 U/kg/dose 2–3 times per week.

Adult: Start at 50–100 U/kg/dose 3 times per week

Maintenance dose: Dose is individualized to achieve and maintain the lowest Hgb level sufficient to avoid transfusions and **not to exceed** 12 g/dL.

Anemia in cancer (see remarks for dosage reduction and withholding therapy):

Initial dose:

Child (5–18 yr): Start at 600 U/kg (**max. dose:** 40,000 U) IV once weekly.

Adult: Start at 150 U/kg/dose SC 3 times per week or 40,000 U SC once every week.

Increasing doses (if needed):

3 times a week dosing: If no reduction in transfusion requirements or rise in Hgb after 8 weeks, increase dosage to 300 U/kg/dose 3 times per week.

Weekly dosing: If no increase in Hgb >1 g/dL after 8 wk of therapy, in the absence of a transfusion:

Child: increase dose to 900 U/kg/dose IV (**max. dose:** 60,000 U) once weekly.

Adult: 60,000 U SC once weekly.

AZT treated HIV patients (see remarks for dosage adjustment): SC/IV

Child: Reported dosage range in children (8 mo–17 yr), 50–400 U/kg/dose 2–3 times per wk.

Adult (with serum erythropoietin ≤500 milliunits/mL and receiving ≤4200 mg AZT per week): Start at 100 U/kg/dose 3 times per wk × 8 wk.

Dose increments, if needed: If response is not satisfactory in reducing transfusion requirements or increasing Hgb levels after 8 wk of therapy, dose may be increased by 50–100 U/kg/dose given 3 times per wk and reevaluate every 4–8 wk thereafter. Patients are unlikely to respond to doses >300 U/kg/dose 3 times per wk.

Anemia of prematurity (many regimens exist):

25–100 U/kg/dose SC 3 times per wk; alternatively, 200–400 U/kg/dose IV/SC 3–5 times per wk for 2–6 wk (**total dose per wk** is 600–1400 U/kg).

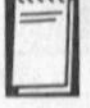

Use the lowest dose to avoid transfusions and **do not exceed** hemoglobin levels >12 g/dL. Increased risk for death, serious cardiovascular events, and thrombosis in cancer patients with Hgb levels >12 g/dL have been reported with epoetin alfa and other erythropoiesis-stimulating agents. Shortened survival and time to tumor progression have also been reported in patients with various cancers.

Evaluate serum iron, ferritin, TIBC before therapy. Iron supplementation recommended during therapy unless iron stores are already in excess. Monitor Hct, BP, clotting times, platelets, BUN, serum creatinine. Peak effect in 2–3 wk.

Recommended Hgb treatment goals:

Anemia in chronic renal failure 10–12 g/dL.

Cancer: lowest Hgb level sufficient to avoid transfusion and ≤12 g/dL.

Continued

EPOETIN ALFA *continued*

DOSAGE ADJUSTMENTS:

Reduce dose by 25%: when target Hgb is reached, OR when Hgb increases >1 g/dL in any 2-wk period.

Increase dose: when Hgb does not increase by 2 g/dL after 8 wk of therapy and Hgb remains at a level not sufficient to avoid the need for transfusion. Dosage increments should **not be** made more frequently than once per mo.

Withholding therapy: when Hgb >12 g/dL; restart therapy at a 25% lower dose after Hgb decreases to target levels or <11 g/dL.

May cause hypertension, seizure, hypersensitivity reactions, headache, edema, dizziness. SC route provides sustained serum levels compared to IV route.

ERGOCALCIFEROL
Drisdol, Calciferol
Vitamin D_2

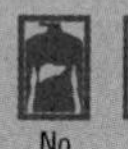
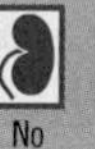
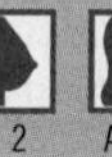

No No 2 A/C

Caps: 50,000 IU (1.25 mg)
Drops (OTC): 8000 IU/mL (200 mcg/mL) (60 mL); contains propylene glycol
1 mg = 40,000 IU vitamin D activity

Dietary supplementation (see Chapter 21 for additional information):

Preterm: 400–800 IU/24 hr PO
Infant (<1 yr): 400 IU/24 hr PO
Child (≥1 yr) and adolescent: 600 IU/24 hr PO

Renal failure (CKD stages 2-5) and 25-OH vitamin D levels <30 ng/mL (monitor serum 25-OH vitamin D and corrected calcium/phosphorus one month after initiation and Q3 mo thereafter):

25-OH vitamin D <5 ng/mL:
Child: 8000 IU/24 hr × 4 wk followed by 4000 IU/24 hr × 2 mo; or 50,000 IU weekly × 4 wk followed by 50,000 IU twice monthly for 2 mo

25-OH vitamin D 5–15 ng/mL:
Child: 4000 IU/24 hr PO × 12 wk or 50,000 IU every other wk × 12 wk

25-OH vitamin D 16–30 ng/mL:
Child: 2000 IU/24 hr PO × 3 mo or 50,000 IU every mo × 3 mo.

Vitamin D dependent rickets:
Child: 3000–5000 IU/24 hr PO; max. dose: 60,000 IU/24 hr

Nutritional rickets:
Child and adult with normal GI absorption: 2000–5000 IU/24 hr PO × 6–12 week
Malabsorption:
Child: 10,000–25,000 IU/24 hr PO
Adult: 10,000–300,000 IU/24 hr PO

Vitamin D resistant rickets (with phosphate supplementation):
Child: initial dose 40,000–80,000 IU/24 hr PO; increase daily dose by 10,000–20,000 IU PO Q3–4 mo if needed
Adult: 10,000–60,000 IU/24 hr PO

Hypoparathyroidism (with calcium supplementation):
Child: 50,000–200,000 IU/24 hr PO
Adult: 25,000–200,000 IU/24 hr PO

Continued

For explanation of icons, see p. 663.

ERGOCALCIFEROL *continued*

Monitor serum Ca^{2+}, PO_4, 25-OH vitamin D (goal level for infant and child: ≥20 ng/mL) and alkaline phosphate. Serum Ca^{2+}, PO_4 product should be <70 mg/dl to avoid ectopic calcification. Titrate dosage to patient response. Watch for symptoms of hypercalcemia: weakness, diarrhea, polyuria, metastatic calcification, nephrocalcinosis. Vitamin D_2 is activated by 25-hydroxylation in liver and 1-hydroxylation in kidney.

Serum 25-OH vitamin D level of ≥35 ng/mL has been suggested in Cystic Fibrosis patients to decrease the risk of hyperparathyroidism and bone loss.

Injectable dosage form is no longer available.

Pregnancy category changes to "C" if used in doses above the US RDA.

ERGOTAMINE TARTRATE ± CAFFEINE

Ergomar

In combination with caffeine: Cafergot and others

Ergot alkaloid

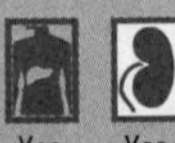

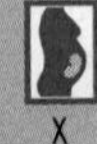

Yes Yes X X

Sublingual tabs (Ergomar): 2 mg

In combination with caffeine:

Tabs: 1 mg and 100 mg caffeine

Suppository: 2 mg and 100 mg caffeine

Drug also available in combinations with belladonna alkaloids and/or phenobarbital.

Doses based on mg of ergotamine.

Older child and adolescent:

PO/SL: 1 mg at onset of migraine attack, then 1 mg Q30 min PRN up to **max. dose** of 3 mg per attack.

Adult:

PO/SL: 2 mg at onset of migraine attack, then 1–2 mg Q30 min up to 6 mg per attack; **do not exceed** 10 mg per wk.

Suppository: 2 mg at first sign of attack; follow with second 2 mg dose after 1 hr; **max. dose** 4 mg per attack, **not to exceed** 10 mg/wk.

Use with caution in renal or hepatic disease. May cause paresthesias, GI disturbance, angina-like pain, rebound headache with abrupt withdrawal, or muscle cramps. **Contraindicated** in pregnancy and has **not been recommended** in breastfeeding. Concurrent administration with protease inhibitors, clarithromycin, erythromycin, or other CYP 450 3A4 inhibitors is **contraindicated** owing to risk of ergotism (nausea, vomiting, vasospastic ischemia leading to cerebral and peripheral ischemia).

ERTAPENEM

Invanz

Antibiotic, carbapenem

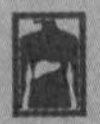
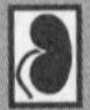
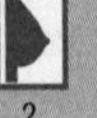
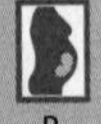

No Yes 2 B

Injection: 1 g

Contains ~6 mEq Na/g drug

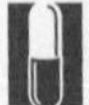

3 mo–12 yr: 15 mg/kg/dose IV/IM Q12 hr; **max. dose:** 1 g/24 hr

Adolescent and adult: 1 g IV/IM Q24 hr

Recommended duration of therapy (all ages):

Complicated intra-abdominal infection: 5–14 days

Complicated skin/subcutaneous tissue infections, diabetic foot infection without osteomyelitis: 7–14 days

Continued

ERTAPENEM *continued*

Community acquired pneumonia, complicated UTI/pyelonephritis: 10–14 days
Acute pelvic infection: 3–10 days

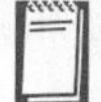

Ertapenem has poor activity against *P. aeruginosa, Acinetobacter,* MRSA, and *Enterococcus.* **Do not use** in meningitis due to poor CSF penetration. **Use with caution** with CNS disorders including seizures. Adjust dosage in renal impairment by decreasing dose by 50% when GFR <30 mL/min.

Diarrhea, infusion complications, nausea, headache, vaginitis, phlebitis/thrombophlebitis, and vomiting are common. Seizures and DRESS syndrome have been reported primarily in renal insufficiency and/or CNS disorders such as brain lessions or seizures. Increased ALT, AST, and neutropenia have been reported in pediatric clinical trials. Decreases valproic acid levels. Probenecid may increase ertapenem levels.

IM route requires reconstitution with 1% lidocaine and **should not** be administered by IV. **Do not** reconstitute or co-infuse with dextrose containing solutions.

ERYTHROMYCIN ETHYLSUCCINATE AND ACETYLSULFISOXAZOLE

Pediazole, Eryzole, and others
Antibiotic, macrolide + sulfonamide derivative

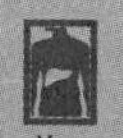 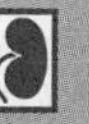 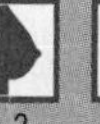 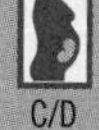

Yes Yes 2 C/D

Oral suspension: 200 mg erythromycin and 600 mg sulfisoxazole/5 mL (100, 200 mL)

Otitis media:

≥2 mo: 50 mg/kg/24 hr (as erythromycin) and 150 mg/kg/24 hr (as sulfisoxazole) ÷ Q6–8 hr PO, or give 1.25 mL/kg/24 hr ÷ Q6–8 hr PO.
Max. dose: 2 g erythromycin, 6 g sulfisoxasole/24 hr

Contraindicated in liver dysfunction or porphyria. See adverse effects of *Erythromycin* and *Sulfisoxazole.* **Not recommended** in infants <2 mo. **Do not use** in renal impairment because dosage adjustments are inconsistent for sulfisoxazole and erythromycin.

Pregnancy category changes to "D" if administered near term.

ERYTHROMYCIN PREPARATIONS

Erythrocin, Pediamycin, E-Mycin, Ery-Ped, and others
Antibiotic, macrolide

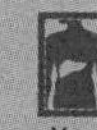 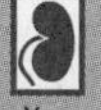  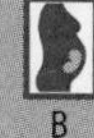

Yes Yes 2 B

Erythromycin base:
- Tabs: 250, 500 mg
- Delayed release tabs: 250, 333, 500 mg
- Delayed release caps: 250 mg
- Topical ointment: 2% (25 g)
- Topical gel: 2% (30, 60 g); contains alcohol 92%
- Topical solution: 1.5%, 2% (60 mL); may contain 44%–66% alcohol
- Topical swab: 2% (60s)
- Ophthalmic ointment: 0.5% (1, 3.5 g)

Erythromycin ethyl succinate (EES):
- Oral suspension: 200, 400 mg/5 mL (100, 480 mL)
- Oral drops: 100 mg/2.5 mL (100 mL)
- Chewable tabs: 200 mg
- Tabs: 400 mg

Continued

For explanation of icons, see p. 663.

ERYTHROMYCIN PREPARATIONS *continued*

Erythromycin estolate:
Suspension: 125, 250 mg/5 mL (480 mL)
Erythromycin stearate:
Tabs: 250 mg
Erythromycin lactobionate:
Injection: 500, 1000 mg; may contain benzyl alcohol

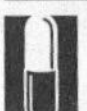

Oral:
Neonate (use EES preparation):
<1.2 kg: 20 mg/kg/24 hr ÷ Q12 hr PO
≥1.2 kg:
0–7 days: 20 mg/kg/24 hr ÷ Q12 hr PO
>7 days:
1.2–2 kg: 30 mg/kg/24 hr ÷ Q8 hr PO
>2 kg: 30–40 mg/kg/24 hr ÷ Q6–8 hr PO
Chlamydial conjunctivitis and pneumonia: 50 mg/kg/24 hr ÷ Q6 hr PO × 14 days
Child (use base or EES preparation): 30–50 mg/kg/24 hr ÷ Q6–8 hr; **max. dose:** 2 g/24 hr
Adult: 1–4 g/24 hr ÷ Q6 hr; max. dose: 4 g/24 hr
Parenteral:
Child: 20–50 mg/kg/24 hr ÷ Q6 hr IV
Adult: 15–20 mg/kg/24 hr ÷ Q6 hr IV
Max. dose: 4 g/24 hr
Rheumatic fever prophylaxis: 500 mg/24 hr ÷ Q12 hr PO
Ophthalmic: Apply 0.5 inch ribbon to affected eye BID–QID. Apply as a one time dose for prophylaxis of neonatal gonococcal ophthalmia
Pertussis: Estolate salt: 50 mg/kg/24 hr ÷ Q6 hr PO × 14 days; use azithromycin for infants <1 mo.
Preoperative bowel prep: 20 mg/kg/dose PO erythromycin base × 3 doses, with neomycin, 1 day before surgery
Prokinetic agent:
Infant and child: 10–20 mg/kg/24 hr PO ÷ TID–QID (QAC or QAC and QHS)

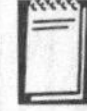

Avoid IM route (pain, necrosis). GI side effects common (nausea, vomiting, abdominal cramps). **Use with caution** in liver disease. Estolate may cause cholestatic jaundice, although hepatotoxicity is uncommon (2% of reported cases). Inhibits CYP 450 1A2, 3A3/4 isoenzymes. May produce elevated digoxin, theophylline, carbamazepine, clozapine, cyclosporine, and methylprednisolone levels. **Avoid** use with astemizole, cisapride, pimozide, or terfenadine. Hypertrophic pyloric stenosis in neonates receiving prophylactic therapy for pertussis; life-threatening episodes of ventricular tachycardia associated with prolonged QTc interval; and exacerbation of myasthenia gravis have been reported.

Oral therapy should replace IV as soon as possible. Give oral doses after meals. Because of different absorption characteristics, higher oral doses of EES are needed to achieve therapeutic effects. Use ideal body weight for obese patients when calculating doses. May produce false-positive urinary catecholamines.

Adjust dose in renal failure (see Chapter 31).

ERYTHROPOIETIN

See *Epoetin Alfa*

ESMOLOL HCL
Brevibloc
Beta-1-selective adrenergic blocking agent, antihypertensive agent, class II antiarrhythmic

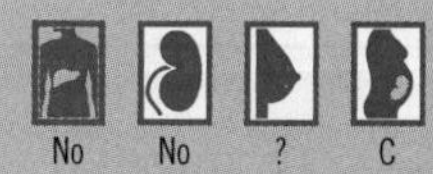

Injection: 10 mg/mL (10 mL)
Injection, premixed infusion in iso-osmotic sodium chloride: 10 mg/mL (250 mL), 20 mg/mL (100 mL)

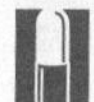

Postoperative hypertension: Titrate to response (limited information):
Loading dose: 500 mcg/kg IV over 1 min.
Maintenance dose: 50–250 mcg/kg/min IV as infusion. Titrate doses upward 50–100 mcg/kg/min Q 5–10 min as needed. Dosages as high as 1000 mcg/kg/min have be administered to children 1–12 yr.
SVT: Titrate to response (limited information).
Loading dose: 100–500 mcg/kg IV over 1 min.
Maintenance dose: 25–100 mcg/kg/min IV as infusion. Titrate doses upward 50–100 mcg/kg/min Q5–10 min as needed. Dosages as high as 1000 mcg/kg/min have been administered.

Contraindicated in sinus bradycardia, >1st degree heart block, and cardiogenic shock or heart failure. Short duration of action; $T_{1/2}$ = 2.9–4.7 min for children and 9 min for adults. May cause bronchospasm, congestive heart failure, hypotension (at doses > 200 mcg/kg/min), nausea, and vomiting. May increase digoxin (by 10%–20%) and theophylline levels. Morphine may increase esmolol level by 46%. Theophylline may decrease esmolol's effects.

Administer only in a monitored setting. Concentration for administration is typically ≤10 mg/mL; however, 20 mg/mL has been administered in pediatric patients.

ESOMEPRAZOLE
Nexium
Gastric acid proton pump inhibitor

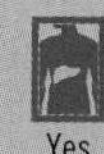
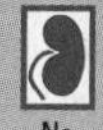

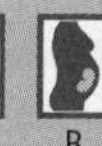

Caps, delayed-released: 20, 40 mg; contains magnesium
Powder for oral suspension: 10, 20, 40 mg packets (30s); contains magnesium
Injection: 20, 40 mg; contains EDTA

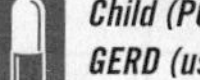

Child (PO):
GERD (use for up to 8 weeks):
1–11 yr: 10 mg once daily
≥12 yr: 20–40 mg once daily
Erosive esophagitis in GERD:
1–11 yr:
<20 kg: 10 mg once daily
≥20 kg: 10 or 20 mg once daily

Adult (PO/IV):
GERD: 20 or 40 mg once daily × 4–8 wk
Prevention of NSAID-induced gastric ulcers: 20 or 40 mg once daily for up to 6 mo
Pathological hypersecretory conditions (e.g., Zollinger-Ellison Syndrome): 40 mg BID; doses up to 240 mg/24 hr have been used
Hepatic impairment: Patients with severe hepatic function impairment (Child-Pugh class C) **should not exceed** 20 mg/24 hr

Continued

For explanation of icons, see p. 663.

ESOMEPRAZOLE *continued*

Cross-allergic reactions with other proton pump inhibitors (e.g., lansoprazole, pantoprazole, rabeprazole). **Use with caution** in liver impairment (see dosage adjustment recommendation in dosing section). GI disturbances and headache are common. Hypomagnesemia may occur with continuous use. Erythema multiforme, Stevens-Johnson syndrome, TEN, pancreatitis, and fractures of the hip, wrist, and spine (in adults >50 yrs old receiving high doses or prolonged therapy >1 yr) have been reported. Drug is a substrate and inhibitor of CYP 450 2C19 and substrate of CYP 450 3A4. May decrease the absorption of atazanavir, ketoconazole, itraconazole, and iron salts. May increase the effect/toxicity of diazepam, midazolam, digoxin, carbamazepine, and warfarin. Voriconazole may increase the effects of esomeprazole. May be used in combination with clarithromycin and amoxicillin for *H. pylori* infections.

Administer all doses before meals. Administer 30 min before sucralfate. **Do not** crush or chew capsules. IV doses may be given as fast as 3 min or infused over 10–30 min.

ETANERCEPT
Enbrel
Antireheumatic, immuno-modulatory agent, tumor necrosis factor receptor p75 Fc fusion protein

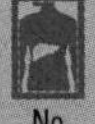
No
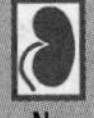
No
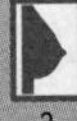
3
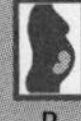
B

Pre-filled injection: 25 mg (0.51 mL of 50 mg/mL solution), 50 mg (0.98 mL of 50 mg/mL solution); contains sucose, L-arginine
Injection (powder): 25 mg with diluent (1 mL bacteriostatic water containing 0.9% benzyl alcohol); contains mannitol, sucrose, tromethamine

Juvenile idiopathic arthritis:
Child 2–17 yrs: 0.4 mg/kg/dose SC twice weekly administered 72–96 hr apart; **max. dose:** 25 mg. Alternative once weekly dose of 0.8 mg/kg/dose SC (**max. dose:** 50 mg/wk and **max. single injection site dose** of 25 mg) may be used.

Rheumatoid arthritis, psoriatic arthritis, ankylosing spondylitis:
Adult: 25 mg SC twice weekly administered 72–96 hr apart. Alternative once weekly dose of 50 mg SC (**max. single injection site dose** of 25 mg) may be used.

Plaque psoriasis:
Adult: Start with 50 mg SC twice weekly administered 72–96 hr apart × 3 mo, followed by a reduced maintenance dose of 50 mg SC per wk. Starting doses of 25 mg or 50 mg per wk have also been shown to be effective.
Max. single injection site dose: 25 mg.

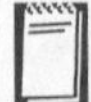

Contraindicated in serious infections, sepsis, or hypersensitivity to any of medication components. **Use with caution** in patients with history of recurrent infections or underlying conditions that may predispose them to infections (including concomitant immunosuppressive therapy), CNS demyelinating disorders, malignancies, immune-related diseases, and latex allergy. Common adverse effects in children include headache, abdominal pain, vomiting, and nausea. Injection site reactions (e.g., discomfort, itching, swelling), rhinitis, dizziness, rash, depression, infections (varicella, aseptic meningitis, rare cases of TB, and fatal/serious infections and sepsis), bone marrow suppression (e.g., aplastic anemia), vertigo, and CNS demyelinating disorder have also been reported. Malignancies (some fatal and ~50% were lymphomas) have been reported in children and adolescents.

Do not administer live vaccines concurrently with this drug. In JRA, it is recommended that the patient be brought up to date with all immunizations in agreement with current immunization guidelines prior to initiating therapy.

Onset of action is 1–4 wk, with peak effects usually within 3 mo.

Continued

ETANERCEPT *continued*

Patients must be properly instructed on preparing and administering the medication. Drug requires reconstitution by gently swirling its contents with the supplied diluent (**do not** shake or vigorously agitate) as some foaming will occur. Reconstituted solutions should be clear and colorless and used within 6 hr.

Drug is administered subcutaneously by rotating injection sites (thigh, abdomen, or upper arm) with a **max. single injection site dose** of 25 mg. Administer new injections ≥1 inch from an old site and **never** where the skin is tender, bruised, red, or hard.

ETHAMBUTOL HCL
Myambutol
Antituberculosis drug

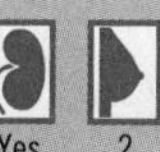
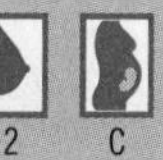

No Yes 2 C

Tabs: 100, 400 mg

Tuberculosis:

Infant, child, adolescent, and adult: 20–25 mg/kg/dose PO once daily or 50 mg/kg/dose PO twice weekly; **max. dose:** 2.5 g/24 hr

Nontuberculous mycobacterial infection; and M. avium complex in AIDS (recurrence prophylaxis or treatment; use in combination with other medications):

Infant, child, adolescent, and adult: 15–25 mg/kg/24 hr PO once daily; **max. dose:** 2.5 g/24 hr

May cause reversible optic neuritis, especially with larger doses. Obtain baseline ophthalmologic studies before beginning therapy and then monthly. Follow visual acuity, visual fields, and (red-green) color vision. **Do not use** in optic neuritis and in children whose visual acuity cannot be assessed. **Discontinue** if any visual deterioration occurs. Monitor uric acid, liver function, heme status, and renal function. Hyperuricemia, GI disturbances, and mania are common. Erythema multiforme has been reported. Coadministration with aluminum hydroxide can reduce ethambutol's absorption; space administration by 4 hr. Give with food. **Adjust dose with renal failure (see Chapter 31).**

ETHOSUXIMIDE
Zarontin
Anticonvulsant

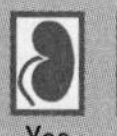
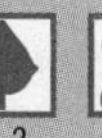

Yes Yes 2 D

Caps: 250 mg
Syrup: 250 mg/5 mL

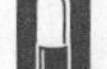

Oral:

≤6 yr: Initial: 15 mg/kg/24 hr ÷ BID; **max. dose:** 500 mg/24 hr; increase as needed Q4–7 days. Usual maintenance dose: 15–40 mg/kg/24 hr ÷ BID

>6 yr and adult: 250 mg BID; increase by 250 mg/24 hr as needed Q4–7 days; usual maintenance dose: 20–40 mg/kg/24 hr ÷ BID

Max. dose (all ages): 1500 mg/24 hr

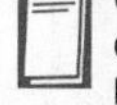

Use with caution in hepatic and renal disease. Ataxia, anorexia, drowsiness, sleep disturbances, rashes, and blood dyscrasias are rare idiosyncratic reactions. May cause lupus-like syndrome; may increase frequency of grand mal seizures in patients with mixed type seizures. May increase risk of suicidal thoughts/behavior. Cases of birth defects have been reported; ethosuximide crosses the placenta. Drug of choice for absence seizures.

Continued

For explanation of icons, see p. 663.

ETHOSUXIMIDE *continued*

Carbamazepine, phenytoin, primidone, phenobarbital, valproic acid, nevirapine, and ritonavir may decrease ethosuximide levels.

Therapeutic levels: 40–100 mg/L. $T_{1/2}$ = 24–42 hr. Recommended serum sampling time at steady-state: obtain trough level within 30 min prior to the next scheduled dose after 5–10 days of continuous dosing.

To minimize GI distress, may administer with food or milk. Abrupt withdrawal of drug may precipitate absence status.

FAMCICLOVIR
Famvir and generics
Antiviral

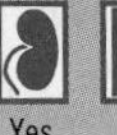
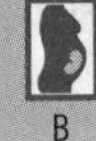

No Yes ? B

Tabs: 125, 250, 500 mg

Adult:

Herpes zoster: 500 mg Q8 hr PO × 7 days; initiate therapy promptly as soon as diagnosis is made (initiation within 48 hr after rash onset is ideal; currently no data for starting treatment >72 hr after rash onset).

Genital herpes (first episode): 250 mg Q8 hr PO × 7–10 days.

Recurrent genital herpes:

Immunocompetent: 1000 mg Q12 hr PO × 1 day or 125 mg Q12 hr PO × 5 days; initiate therapy at first sign or symptom. Efficacy has not been established when treatment is initiated >6 hr after onset of symptoms or lessions.

Immunocompromised: 500 mg Q8 hr PO × 7 days.

Suppression of recurrent genital herpes (immunocompetent): 250 mg Q12 hr PO up to 1 year, then reassess for HSV infection recurrence.

Recurrent herpes labialis:

Immunocompetent: 1500 mg PO × 1.

Immunocompromised: 500 mg Q8 hr PO × 7 days.

Recurrent mucocutaneous herpes in HIV: 500 mg Q12 hr PO × 7 days.

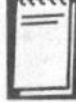

Drug is converted to its active form (penciclovir). Better absorption than PO acyclovir. May cause headache, diarrhea, nausea, and abdominal pain. Serious skin reactions (e.g., TEN and Stevens-Johnson), cholestatic jaundice, and abnormal LFTs have been reported. Concomitant use with probenecid and other drugs eliminated by active tubular secretion may result in decreased penciclovir clearance. **Reduce dose in renal impairment (see Chapter 31).**

Safety and efficacy in suppression of recurrent genital herpes have not been established beyond 1 year. May be administered with or without food.

FAMOTIDINE
Pepcid, Pepcid AC [OTC], Pepcid Complete [OTC], Pepcid RPD, and others
Histamine-2-receptor antagonist

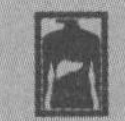
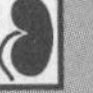
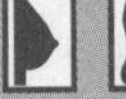
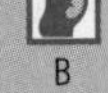

No Yes 1 B

Injection: 10 mg/mL (2, 4, 20, 50 mL); multidose vials contain 0.9% benzyl alcohol
Premixed injection: 20 mg/50 mL in iso-osmotic sodium chloride
Oral suspension: 40 mg/5 mL (contains parabens)
Tabs: 10 (OTC), 20 (OTC), 40 mg
Gel caps: 10 mg (OTC)

Continued

FAMOTIDINE *continued*

Disintegrating oral tabs (Pepcid RPD): 20, 40 mg; contains aspartame
Chewable tabs: 10 mg (OTC); contains aspartame
Pepcid Complete (OTC): 10 mg famotidine with 800 mg calcium carbonate and 165 mg magnesium hydroxide

Neonate and <3 mo:
IV: 0.25–0.5 mg/kg/dose Q24 hr
PO: 0.5–1 mg/kg/dose Q24 hr
≥3 mo–1 yr (GERD): 0.5 mg/kg/dose PO Q12 hr
Child (1–12 yr):
IV: initial: 0.6–0.8 mg/kg/24 hr ÷Q8–12 hr up to a **max.** of 40 mg/24 hr
PO: initial: 1–1.2 mg/kg/24 hr ÷Q8–12 hr up to a **max.** of 40 mg/24 hr
Peptic ulcer: 0.5 mg/kg/24 hr PO QHS or ÷ Q12 hr up to a **max. dose** of 40 mg/24 hr
GERD: 1–2 mg/kg/24 hr PO ÷Q 12 hr up to a **max. dose** of 80 mg/24 hr
Adolescent and adult:
Duodenal ulcer:
PO: 20 mg BID or 40 mg QHS × 4–8 wk, then maintenance therapy at 20 mg QHS
IV: 20 mg BID
GERD: 20 mg BID PO × 6 wk
Esophagitis: 20–40 mg BID PO × 12 wk

A Q12 hr dosage interval is generally recommended; however, infants and young children may require a Q8 hr interval because of enhanced drug clearance. Headaches, dizziness, constipation, diarrhea, and drowsiness have occurred. **Dosage adjustment is required in severe renal failure (see Chapter 31).**

Shake oral suspension well prior to each use. Disintegrating oral tablets should be placed on the tongue to be disintegrated and subsequently swallowed. Doses may be administered with or without food.

FELBAMATE
Felbatol
Anticonvulsant

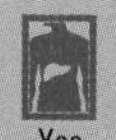
Yes
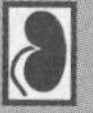
Yes
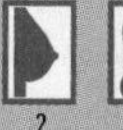
?
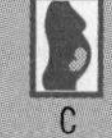
C

Tabs: 400, 600 mg
Oral suspension: 600 mg/5 mL

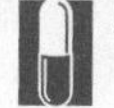

Lennox-Gastaut for child 2–14 yr (adjunctive therapy):
Start at 15 mg/kg/24 hr PO ÷ TID–QID; increase dosage by 15 mg/kg/24 hr increments at weekly intervals up to a **max. dose** of 45 mg/kg/24 hr or 3600 mg/24 hr (whichever is less). See remarks.
Child ≥14 yr–adult:
Adjunctive therapy: start at 1200 mg/24 hr PO ÷ TID–QID; increase dosage by 1200 mg/24 hr at weekly intervals up to a **max. dose** of 3600 mg/day. See remarks.
Monotherapy (as initial therapy): Start at 1200 mg/24 hr PO ÷ TID–QID. Increase dose under close clinical supervision at 600 mg increments Q 2 wk to 2400 mg/24 hr. **Max. dose:** 3600 mg/24 hr.
Conversion to monotherapy: Start at 1200 mg/24 hr ÷ PO TID–QID for 2 wk; then increase to 2400 mg/24 hr for 1 wk. At wk 3, increase to 3600 mg/24 hr. See remarks for dose reduction instructions of other antiepileptic drugs.

Continued

For explanation of icons, see p. 663.

FELBAMATE *continued*

Drug should be prescribed under strict supervision by a specialist. **Contraindicated** in blood dyscrasias or hepatic dysfunction (prior or current); and hypersensitivity to meprobamate. Aplastic anemia and hepatic failure leading to death have been associated with drug. May cause headache, fatigue, anxiety, GI disturbances, gingival hyperplasia, increased liver enzymes, and bone marrow suppression. Suicidal behavior or ideation have been reported. **Obtain serum levels of concurrent anticonvulsants.** Monitor liver enzymes, bilirubin, CBC with differential, platelets at baseline and every 1–2 wk. **Doses should be decreased by 50% in renally impaired patients.**

When initiating adjunctive therapy (all ages), doses of other antiepileptic drugs (AEDs) are reduced by 20% to control plasma levels of concurrent phenytoin, valproic acid, phenobarbital, and carbamazepine. Further reductions of concomitant AED dosage may be necessary to minimize side effects caused by drug interactions.

When converting to monotherapy, reduce other AEDs by one third at start of felbamate therapy. Then after 2 wk and at the start of increasing the felbamate dosage, reduce other AEDs by an additional one third. At wk 3, continue to reduce other AEDs as clinically indicated.

Carbamazepine levels may be decreased; whereas phenytoin and valproic acid levels may be increased. Phenytoin and carbamazepine may increase felbamate clearance; valproic acid may decrease its clearance.

Doses can be administered with or without food.

FENTANYL

Sublimaze, Duragesic, Fentora, Actiq, and many generics
Narcotic; analgesic, sedative

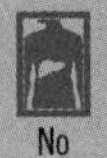
No
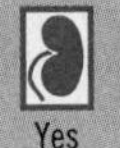
Yes
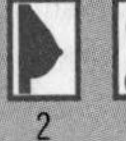
2
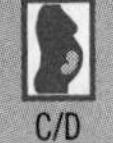
C/D

Injection: 50 mcg/mL
SR patch (Duragesic and others): 12.5, 25, 50, 75, 100 mcg/hr (5s)
Tabs for buccal administration:
Fentora: 100, 200, 300, 400, 600, 800 mcg (28s)
Lozenge on a stick:
Actiq and others: 200, 400, 600, 800, 1200, 1600 mcg (30s)

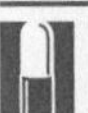

Titrate dose to effect.
Neonate and younger infant:
Sedation/analgesia: 1–4 mcg/kg/dose IV Q2–4 hr PRN.
Continuous IV infusion: 1–5 mcg/kg/hr; tolerance may develop.
Older infant and child:
Sedation/analgesia: 1–2 mcg/kg/dose IV/IM Q30–60 min PRN.
Continuous IV infusion: 1 mcg/kg/hr; titrate to effect; usual infusion range 1–3 mcg/kg/hr.
To prepare infusion, use the following formula:

$$50 \times \frac{\text{Desired dose (mcg/kg/hr)}}{\text{Desired infusion rate (mL/hr)}} \times \text{Wt (kg)} = \frac{\text{mcg Fentanyl}}{\text{50 mL fluid}}$$

Oral, breakthrough cancer pain for opioid-intolerant patients (see remarks):
Buccal tabs (≥18 yr): Start with 100 mcg by placing tablet in the buccal cavity (above a rear molar, between the upper cheek and gum) and letting the tablet dissolve for 15–25 min. A second 100 mcg dose, if needed, may be administered 30 min after the start of the first dose. If needed, increase dose initially in multiples of 100 mcg tablet when patients require >1 dose per breakthrough pain episode for several consecutive episodes. If titration requires >400 mcg/dose, use 200 mcg tabs.

Continued

FENTANYL *continued*

Lozenges (≥16 yr): Start with 200 mcg by placing lozenge in the mouth between the cheek and lower gum. If needed, may repeat dose 15 min after the completion of the first dose (30 min after start of prior dose). If therapy requires >1 lozenge per episode, consider increasing the dose to the next higher strength. Do not give more than 2 doses for each episode of breakthrough pain and re-evaluate long-acting opioid therapy if patient requires >4 doses/24 hr.

Transdermal (see remarks): Safety has not been established in children <2 yr and should be administered in children ≥2 yr who are opioid tolerant. Use is **contraindicated** in acute or post-operative pain in opiate-naïve patients.

Opioid-tolerant child receiving at least 60 mg morphine equivalents/24 hr: Use 25 mcg/hr patch Q 72 hr. Patch titration should not occur before 3 days of adiministration of the initial dose or more frequently than every 6 days thereafter.

See Chapter 6 for equianalgesic dosing and PCA dosing.

Intranasal route for acute and pre-procedure analgesia (see remarks):

≥1 yr–adolescent: 1–2 mcg/kg/dose intranasally (**max. dose:** 50 mcg) Q1 hr PRN

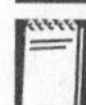

Use with caution in bradycardia, respiratory depression, and increased intracranial pressure. **Adjust dose in renal failure (see Chapter 31).** Fatalities and life-threatening respiratory depression have been reported with inappropriate use (overdoses, use in opioid-naïve patients, changing the patch too frequently, and exposing the patch to a heat source) of the transdermal route.

Highly lipophilic and may deposit into fat tissue. IV onset of action 1–2 min with peak effects in 10 min IV duration of action 30–60 min. Give IV dose over 3–5 min. Rapid infusion may cause respiratory depression and chest wall rigidity. Respiratory depression may persist beyond the period of analgesia. Transdermal onset of action 6–8 hr with a 72-hr duration of action. See Chapter 6 for pharmacodynamic information with transmucosal and transdermal routes.

Buccal tabs and oral lozenges are indicated only for the management of breakthrough cancer pain in patients who are already receiving and who are tolerant to opioid therapy. Buccal tabs (Fentora) and lozenge dosage forms are **NOT** bioequivalent; see package insert for conversion.

Intranasal route of administration for analgesia has an onset of action at 10–30 min. Pediatric studies has demonstrated that the intranasal fentanyl is equivalent to and better than morphine (PO/IV/IM) and equivalent to intravenous fentanyl for providing analgesia.

Fentanyl is a substrate for the CYP 450 3A4 enzyme. Be aware of medications that inhibit or induce this enzyme, for it may increase or decrease the effects of fentanyl, respectively.

Pregnancy category changes to "D" if drug is used for prolonged periods or in high doses at term.

FERRIC GLUCONATE

See *Iron—Injectable Preparations*

FERROUS SULFATE

See *Iron—Oral Preparations*

For explanation of icons, see p. 663.

FEXOFENADINE ± PSEUDOEPHEDRINE
Allegra, Allegra ODT, Allegra-D 12 Hour, Allegra-D 24 Hour, and other generics
Antihistamine, less-sedating ±decongestant

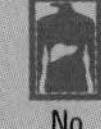
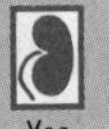
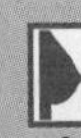
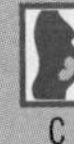

No Yes 2 C

Tabs: 30, 60, 180 mg
Tabs, orally disintegrating (Allegra ODT): 30 mg; contains phenylalanine
Oral suspension: 6 mg/mL (30, 300 mL)
Extended-release tab in combination with pseudoephedrine (PE):
Allegra-D 12 Hour: 60 mg fexofenadine + 120 mg pseudoephedrine
Allegra-D 24 Hour: 180 mg fexofenadine + 240 mg pseudoephedrine

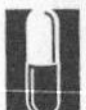

Fexofenadine:
6 mo–<2 yr: 15 mg PO BID
2–11 yr: 30 mg PO BID
≥12 yr–adult: 60 mg PO BID; 180 mg PO once daily may be used in seasonal rhinitis

Extended-release tabs of fexofenadine and pseudoephedrine:
≥12 yr–adult:
Allegra-D 12 Hour: 1 tablet PO BID
Allegra-D 24 Hour: 1 tablet PO once daily

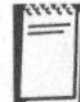

May cause drowsiness, fatigue, headache, dyspepsia, nausea, and dysmenorrhea. Has not been implicated in causing cardiac arrhythmias when used with other drugs that are metabolized by hepatic microsomal enzymes (e.g., ketoconazole, erythromycin). **Reduce dose to 30 mg PO once daily for child 6–11 yr old and 60 mg PO once daily for ≥12 yr old if CrCl <40 mL/min.** For use of Allegra-D 12 Hour and decreased renal function, an initial dose of 1 tablet PO once daily is recommended. Avoid use of Allegra-D 24 Hour in renal impairment. *See Pseudoephedrine* for additional remarks if using the combination product.

Medication as the single agent may be administered with or without food. **Do not** administer antacids with or within 2 hr of fexofenadine dose. The extended release combination product should be swallowed whole without food.

FILGRASTIM
Neupogen, G-CSF
Colony stimulating factor

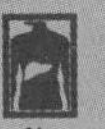
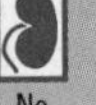
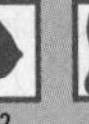
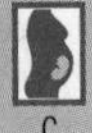

No No ? C

Injection: 300 mcg/mL (1, 1.6 mL)
Injection, prefilled syringes with 27-gauge 1/2-inch needles: 600 mcg/mL (0.5, 0.8 mL)
All dosage forms are preservative free.

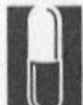

Individual protocols may direct dosing.
IV/SC: 5–10 mcg/kg/dose once daily × 14 days or until ANC >10,000/mm^3. Dosage may be increased by 5 mcg/kg/24 hr if desired effect is not achieved within 7 days. Discontinue therapy when ANC >10,000/mm^3.

May cause bone pain, fever, and rash. Monitor CBC, uric acid, and LFTs. **Use with caution** in patients with malignancies with myeloid characteristics. **Contraindicated** for patients sensitive to *E. coli*-derived proteins. **Do not** administer 24 hr before or after administration of chemotherapy.

SC routes of administration are preferred because of prolonged serum levels over IV route. If used via IV route and G-CSF final concentration <15 mcg/mL, add 2 mg albumin/1 mL of IV fluid to prevent drug adsorption to the IV administration set.

FLECAINIDE ACETATE
Tambocor and others
Antiarrhythmic, class Ic

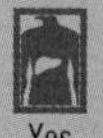 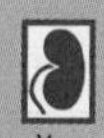  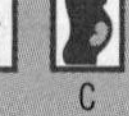
Yes Yes 2 C

Tabs: 50, 100, 150 mg
Oral suspension: 5, 20 mg/mL

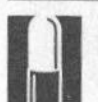

Child: Initial: 1–3 mg/kg/24 hr ÷ Q8 hr PO; usual range: 3–6 mg/kg/24 hr ÷ Q8 hr PO, monitor serum levels to adjust dose if needed.

Adult:

Sustained V tach: 100 mg PO Q12 hr; may increase by 50 mg Q12 hr (100 mg/24 hr) every 4 days to **max. dose** of 600 mg/24 hr.

Paroxysmal SVT/paroxysmal AF: 50 mg PO Q12 hr; may increase dose by 50 mg Q12 hr every 4 days to **max. dose** of 300 mg/24 hr.

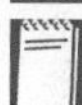

May aggravate LV failure, sinus bradycardia, pre-existing ventricular arrhythmias. May cause AV block, dizziness, blurred vision, dyspnea, nausea, headache, and increased PR or QRS intervals. **Reserve for life-threatening cases.** Use with caution in renal and/or hepatic impairment.

Flecainide is a substrate for the CYP P-450 2D6 enzyme. Be aware of medications that inhibit (e.g., certain SSRIs) or induce this enzyme for it may increase or decrease the effects of flecainide, respectively.

Therapeutic trough level: 0.2–1 mg/L. Recommended serum sampling time at steady-state: Obtain trough level within 30 min prior to the next scheduled dose after 2–3 days of continuous dosing for children; after 3–5 days for adults. **Adjust dose in renal failure (see Chapter 31).**

FLUCONAZOLE
Diflucan and others
Antifungal agent

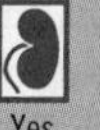 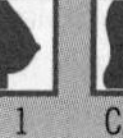 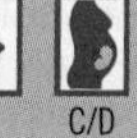
Yes Yes 1 C/D

Tabs: 50, 100, 150, 200 mg
Injection: 2 mg/mL (50, 100, 200 mL); contains 9 mEq Na/2 mg drug
Oral suspension: 10 mg/mL (35 mL), 40 mg/mL (35 mL)

Neonate (IV/PO):

Loading dose: 12 mg/kg

Maintenance dose: 6 mg/kg with the following dosing intervals (see following table)

Post-Conceptional Age (wk)	Postnatal Age (days)	Dosing Interval (hr) and Time (hr) to Start 1st Maint. Dose after Load
≤29	0–14	72
	>14	48
30–36	0–14	48
	>14	24
37–44	0–7	48
	>7	24
≥45	>0	24

Continued

For explanation of icons, see p. 663.

FLUCONAZOLE *continued*

Child (IV/PO):

Indication	Loading Dose	Maintenance Dose (Q24 hr) to Begin 24 hr after Loading Dose
Oropharyngeal candidiasis	6 mg/kg	3 mg/kg
Esophageal candidiasis	12 mg/kg	6 mg/kg
Invasive systemic candidiasis and cryptococcal meningitis	12 mg/kg	6–12 mg/kg
Suppressive therapy for HIV infected with cryptococcal meningitis	6 mg/kg	6 mg/kg

Max. dose: 12 mg/kg/24 hr

Adult:

Oropharyngeal and esophageal candidiasis: Loading dose of 200 mg PO/IV followed by 100 mg once daily 24 hr after; doses up to **max. dose** of 400 mg/24 hr should be used for esophageal candidiasis

Systemic candidiasis and cryptococcal meningitis: Loading dose of 400 mg PO/IV, followed by 200–800 mg once daily 24 hr later

Bone marrow transplant prophylaxis: 400 mg PO/IV Q24hr

Suppressive therapy in for HIV infected with cryptococcal meningitis: 200 mg PO/IV Q24 hr

Vaginal candidiasis: 150 mg PO × 1

Cardiac arrhythmias may occur when used with cisapride; concomitant use is **contraindicated.** May cause nausea, headache, rash, vomiting, abdominal pain, hepatitis, cholestasis, and diarrhea. Neutropenia, agranulocytosis, and thrombocytopenia have been reported. **Use with caution** in hepatic or renal dysfunction and in patients with proarrhythmic conditions.

Inhibits CYP 450 2C9/10 and CYP 450 3A3/4 (weak inhibitor). May increase effects, toxicity, or levels of cyclosporine, midazolam, phenytoin, rifabutin, tacrolimus, theophylline, warfarin, oral hypoglycemics, and AZT. Rifampin increases fluconazole metabolism.

Pediatric to adult dose equivalency: every 3 mg/kg pediatric dosage is equal to 100 mg adult dosage. Consider using higher doses in morbidly obese patients. **Adjust dose in renal failure (see Chapter 31).**

Pregnancy category is "C" for single 150 mg use for vaginal candidiasis; and category "D" for all other indications (high-dose use during first trimester of pregnancy may result in birth defects).

FLUCYTOSINE

Ancobon, 5-FC, 5-Fluorocytosine

Antifungal agent

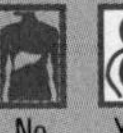
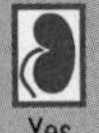
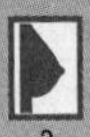
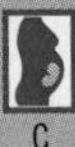

No Yes 3 C

Caps: 250, 500 mg

Oral liquid: 10, 50 mg/mL

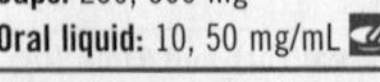

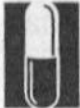

Neonate: 80–160 mg/kg/24 hr ÷Q6 hr PO

Child and adult: 50–150 mg/kg/24 hr ÷Q6 hr PO

Monitor CBC, BUN, serum creatinine, alkaline phosphatase, AST, and ALT. Common side effects: nausea, vomiting, diarrhea, rash, CNS disturbance, anemia, leukopenia, and thrombocytopenia. Use is **contraindicated** in the first trimester of pregnancy.

Therapeutic levels: 25–100 mg/L. Recommended serum sampling time at steady-state: Obtain peak level 2–4 hr after oral dose following 4 days of continuous dosing. Peak levels of 40–60 mg/L have been recommended for systemic candidiasis. Maintain trough levels above 25 mg/L. Prolonged levels above 100 mg/L can increase risk for bone marrow suppression. Bone marrow suppression in immunosuppressed patients can be irreversible and fatal.

Flucytosine interferes with creatinine assay tests using the dry-slide enzymatic method (Kodak Ektachem analyzer). **Adjust dose in renal failure (see Chaper 31).**

FLUDROCORTISONE ACETATE

Florinef acetate, 9-Fluorohydrocortisone, Fluohydrisone, and various generics

Corticosteroid

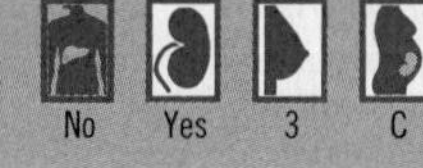

Tabs: 0.1 mg

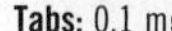

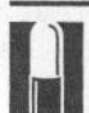

Infant and child: 0.05–0.1 mg/24 hr once daily PO

Congenital adrenal hyperplasia: 0.05–0.3 mg/24 hr once daily PO

Adult: 0.05–0.2 mg/24 hr once daily PO

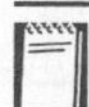

Contraindicated in CHF and systemic fungal infections. Has primarily mineralocorticoid activity. **Use with caution** in hypertension, edema, or renal dysfuction. May cause hypertension, hypokalemia, acne, rash, bruising, headaches, GI ulcers, and growth suppression.

Monitor BP and serum electrolytes. See Chapter 30 for steroid potency comparison.

Drug interactions: Drug's hypokalemic effects may induce digoxin toxicity; phenytoin and rifampin may increase fludrocortisone metabolism.

Doses 0.2–2 mg/24 hr has been used in the management of severe orthostatic hypotension in adults. Use a gradual dosage taper when discontinuing therapy.

FLUMAZENIL

Romazicon and other generics

Benzodiazepine antidote

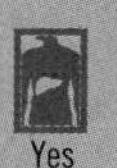
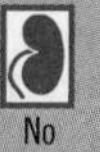
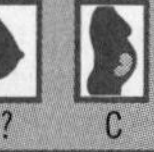

Injection: 0.1 mg/mL (5, 10 mL); contains parabens

Benzodiazepine overdose (IV, see remarks):

Child (limited data): 0.01 mg/kg (**max. dose:** 0.2 mg) Q 1 min PRN to **a max. total cumulative dose** of 1 mg. As an alternative for repeat bolus doses, a continuous infusion of 0.005–0.01 mg/kg/hr have been used.

Adult: Initial dose: 0.2 mg over 30 sec, if needed, give 0.3 mg 30 sec. later over 30 sec. Additional doses of 0.5 mg given over 30 sec Q 1 min PRN up to a cumulative dose of 3 mg (**usual cumulative dose:** 1–3 mg). Patients with only partial response to 3 mg may require additional slow titration to a total of 5 mg.

Reversal of benzodiazepine sedation (IV):

Child: Initial dose: 0.01 mg/kg (**max dose:** 0.2 mg) given over 15 sec, if needed after 45 sec, 0.01 mg/kg (**max. dose:** 0.2 mg) Q 1 min to a **max. total cumulative dose** of 0.05 mg/kg or 1 mg, whichever is lower. Usual total dose: 0.08–1 mg (average 0.65 mg).

Adult: Initial dose: 0.2 mg over 15 sec, if needed after 45 sec, give 0.2 mg Q 1 min to a **max. total cumulative dose** of 1 mg. Doses may be repeated at 20 min interval (**max. dose** of 1 mg per 20 min interval) up to a **max. dose** of 3 mg in 1 hr.

Does not reverse narcotics. Onset of benzodiazepine reversal occurs in 1–3 min. Reversal effects of flumazenil ($T_{1/2}$ approximately 1 hr) may wear off sooner than benzodiazepine effects. If patient does not respond after cummulative 1–3 mg dose, suspect agent other than benzodiazepines.

May precipitate seizures, especially in patients taking benzodiazepines for seizure control or in patients with tricyclic antidepressant overdose. Fear, panic attacks in patients with history of panic disorders have been reported.

Use with caution in liver dysfunction; flumazenil's clearance is significantly reduced. Use normal dose for initial dose and decrease the dosage and frequency for subsequent doses.

See Chapter 2 for complete management of suspected ingestions.

For explanation of icons, see p. 663.

FLUNISOLIDE
Nasarel, Aerospan, Aerobid, Aerobid-M
Corticosteroid

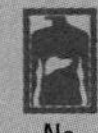
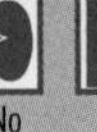
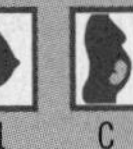

No No 1 C

Nasal solution:

Nasarel and others: 25 mcg/spray (200 sprays/bottle) (25 mL)

Oral aerosol inhaler:

Aerospan: 80 mcg/dose (60 doses/5.1 g, 120 doses/8.9 g); CFC-free (HFA)

Aerobid, Aerobid-M: 250 mcg/dose (100 doses/inhaler) (7 g); contains CFCs (to be discontinued June 30, 2011)

Aerobid-M: Contains menthol flavoring.

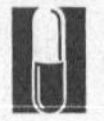

For all dosage forms, after symptoms are controlled, reduce to lowest effective maintenance dose (1 spray each nostril once daily) to control symptoms.

Nasal solution:

Child (6–14 yr):

Initial: 1 spray per nostril TID or 2 sprays per nostril BID; **max. dose:** 4 sprays per nostril/24 hr.

Adult:

Initial: 2 sprays per nostril BID; if needed in 4–7 days, increase to 2 sprays per nostril TID. **Max. dose:** 8 sprays per nostril/24 hr.

Inhaler (see remarks):

Aerobid or Aerobid-M:

Child (6–15 yr): 2 puffs BID; **max. dose:** 4 puffs/24 hr.

≥16 yr and adult: 2 puffs BID; **max. dose:** 8 puffs/24 hr.

Aerospan:

Child (6–11 yr): 1 puff BID; **max. dose:** 4 puffs/24 hr.

Adult: 2 puffs BID; **max. dose:** 8 puffs/24 hr.

May cause a reduction in growth velocity. Shake inhaler or nasal solution well before use. Patients using nasal solution should clear nasal passages before use.

Aerobid and Aerospan are not interchangeable on a mcg per mcg basis. Spacer devices may enhance drug delivery of Aerobid/Aerobid-M. **Do not use** a spacer with Aerospan because the product has a self-contained spacer. Rinse mouth after administering drug by inhaler to prevent thrush.

FLUORIDE
Luride, Fluoritab, Pediaflor, and others
Mineral

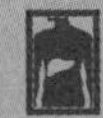
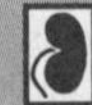
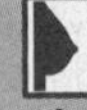
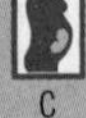

No No ? C

Concentrations and strengths based on fluoride ion:

Drops: 0.25 mg/drop, 0.5 mg/mL

Oral solution: 0.2 mg/mL

Chewable tabs: 0.25, 0.5, 1 mg

Tabs: 1 mg

Lozenges: 1 mg

See Chapter 21 for fluoride-containing multivitamins.

All doses/24 hr (see table below):

Recommendations from American Academy of Pediatrics and American Dental Association.

Continued

FLUORIDE *continued*

Age	Concentration of Fluoride in Drinking Water (ppm)		
	<0.3	0.3–0.6	>0.6
Birth–6 mo	0	0	0
6 mo–3 yr	0.25 mg	0	0
3–6 yr	0.5 mg	0.25 mg	0
6–16 yr	1 mg	0.5 mg	0

Contraindicated in areas where drinking water fluoridation is >0.7 ppm. **Acute overdose:** GI distress, salivation, CNS irritability, tetany, seizures, hypocalcemia, hypoglycemia, cardiorespiratory failure. Chronic excess use may result in mottled teeth or bone changes.

Take with food, but **not** milk, to minimize GI upset. The doses have been decreased owing to concerns over dental fluorosis.

FLUOXETINE HYDROCHLORIDE
Prozac, Sarafem, Prozac Weekly, and various generics
Antidepressant, selective serotonin reuptake inhibitor

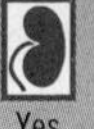
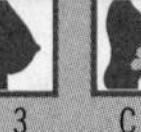
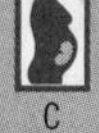

Yes Yes 3 C

Oral solution: 20 mg/5 mL; may contain alcohol
Caps: 10, 20, 40 mg
Delayed-released caps (Prozac Weekly): 90 mg
Tabs: 10, 20 mg

Depression:

Child, 8–18 yr: Start at 10–20 mg once daily PO. If started on 10 mg/24 hr, may increase dose to 20 mg/24 hr after 1 wk. Use lower 10 mg/24 hr initial dose for lower weight children; if needed, increase to 20 mg/24 hr after several weeks.

Adult: Start at 20 mg once daily PO. May increase after several wk by 20 mg/24 hr increments to **max. dose** of 80 mg/24 hr. Doses >20 mg/24 hr should be divided BID.

Obsessive-compulsive disorder:

Child, 7–18 yr:

Lower weight child: Start at 10 mg once daily PO. May increase after several wk. Usual dose range: 20–30 mg/24 hr. There is very minimal experience with doses >20 mg/24 hr and no experience with doses >60 mg/24 hr.

Higher weight child and adolescent: Start at 10 mg once daily PO and increase dose to 20 mg/24 hr after 2 wk. May further increase dose after several wk. Usual dose range: 20–60 mg/24 hr.

Bulimia:

Adult: 60 mg QAM PO; it is recommended to titrate up to this dose over several days.

Premenstrual dysphoric disorder:

Adult: Start at 20 mg once daily PO using the Sarafem product. **Max. dose:** 80 mg/24 hr. Systematic evaluation has shown that efficacy is maintained for periods of 6 mo at a dose of 20 mg/day. Reassess patients periodically to determine the need for continued treatment.

Continued

For explanation of icons, see p. 663.

FLUOXETINE HYDROCHLORIDE *continued*

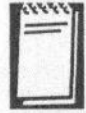

Contraindicated in patients taking MAO inhibitors due to possibility of seizures, hyperpyrexia, and coma. **Use with caution** in patients receiving diuretics, or with liver (reduce dose with cirrosis) or renal impairment. May increase the effects of tricyclic antidepressants. May cause headache, insomnia, nervousness, drowsiness, GI disturbance, and weight loss. Increased bleeding diathesis with unaltered prothrombin time may occur with warfarin. Hyponatremia has been reported. Monitor for clinical worsening of depression and suicidal ideation/behavior following the initiation of therapy or after dose changes.

May displace other highly protein-bound drugs. Inhibits CYP 450 2C19, 2D6, and 3A3/4 drug metabolism isoenzymes, which may increase the effects or toxicity of drugs metabolized by these enzymes.

Delayed-release capsule is currently indicated for depression and is dosed at 90 mg Q7 days. It is unknown if weekly dosing provides the same protection from relapse as does daily dosing.

FLUTICASONE PROPIONATE
Flonase HFA, Cutivate, Flovent Diskus, Veramyst, and others
Corticosteroid

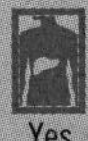
Yes
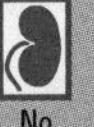
No
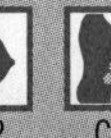
2
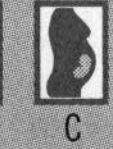
C

Nasal spray:
Flonase and other generics (as fluticasone propionate): 50 mcg/actuation (16 g = 120 doses)
Veramyst (as fluticasone furoate): 27.5 mcg/actuation (10 g = 120 doses)
Topical cream (Cutivate and others): 0.05% (15, 30, 60 g)
Topical ointment (Cutivate and others): 0.005% (15, 30, 60 g)
Topical lotion (Cutivate): 0.05% (120 mL)
Aerosol inhaler (MDI) (Flovent HFA): 44 mcg/actuation, 110 mcg/actuation, 220 mcg/actuation (7.9 g = 60 doses/inhaler, 13 g = 120 doses/inhaler)
Dry-powder inhalation (DPI) (Flovent Diskus): 50 mcg/dose, 100 mcg/dose, 250 mcg/dose; all strengths come in a package of 15 Rotadisks; each Rotadisk provides 4 doses for a total of 60 doses per package.

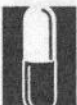

Intranasal (allergic rhinitis):
Fluticasone propionate (Flonase and others):

≥4 yr and adolescent: 1 spray (50 mcg) per nostril once daily. Dose may be increased to 2 sprays (100 mcg) per nostril once daily if inadequate response or severe symptoms. Reduce to 1 spray per nostril once daily when symptoms are controlled.

Adult: Initial 200 mcg/24 hr [2 sprays (100 mcg) per nostril once daily; OR 1 spray (50 mcg) per nostril BID]. Reduce to 1 spray per nostril once daily when symptoms are controlled.

Max dose (4 yr–adult): 2 sprays (100 mcg) per nostril/24 hr.

Fluticasone furoate (Veramyst):

2–11 yr: 1 spray (27.5 mcg) per nostril once daily. If needed, dose may be increased to 2 sprays each nostril once daily. Reduce to 1 spray per nostril once daily when symptoms are controlled.

≥11 and adult: 2 sprays (55 mcg) each nostril once daily. Reduce to 1 spray per nostril once daily when symptoms are controlled.

Max. dose (2 yr–adult): 2 sprays (55 mcg) per nostril/24 hr.

Oral inhalation (asthma): **Divide all 24 hr doses BID.** If desired response is not seen after 2 wk of starting therapy, increase dosage. Then reduce to the lowest effective dose when asthma symptoms are controlled. Administration of MDI with aerochamber enhances drug delivery.

Continued

FLUTICASONE PROPIONATE *continued*

Recommended dosages for asthma (see following table).

RECOMMENDED DOSAGES FOR ASTHMA

Age	Previous Use of Bronchodilators Only (max. dose)	Previous Use of Inhaled Corticosteroid (max. dose)	Previous Use of Oral Corticosteroid (max. dose)
Child (4–11 yr)	MDI: 88 mcg/24 hr (176 mcg/24 hr) DPI: 100 mcg/24 hr (200 mcg/24 hr)	MDI: 88 mcg/24 hr (176 mcg/24 hr) DPI: 100 mcg/24 hr (200 mcg/24 hr)	Dose not available
≥12 yr and adult	MDI: 176 mcg/24hr (880 mcg/24hr) DPI: 200 mcg/24 hr (1000 mcg/24 hr)	MDI: 176–440 mcg/24hr (880 mcg/24hr) DPI: 200–500 mcg/24 hr (1000 mcg/24 hr)	MDI: 880 mcg/24 hr (1760 mcg/24hr) DPI: 1000–2000 mcg/24 hr (2000 mcg/24 hr)

MDI = metered dose inhaler; DPI = dry powder inhaler.

Topical (reassess diagnosis if no improvement in 2 wk):

Cream (see Chaper 30 for topical steroid comparisons):

≥3 mo and adult: Apply thin film to affected areas once daily–BID; then reduce to a less potent topical agent when symptoms are controlled.

Lotion:

≥1 yr and adult: Apply thin film to affected areas once daily. Safety of use has not been evaluated longer than 4 wk.

Ointment:

Adult: Apply thin film to affected areas BID.

Concurrent administration with ritonavir and other CYP 450 3A4 inhibitors may increase fluticasone levels resulting in Cushing syndrome and adrenal suppression. **Use with caution** and monitor closely in hepatic impairment.

Intranasal: Clear nasal passages prior to use. May cause epistaxis and nasal irritation, which are usually transient. Taste and smell alterations, rare hypersensitivity reactions (angioedema, pruritis, urticaria, wheezing, dyspnea), and nasal septal perforation have been reported in post-marketing studies.

Oral inhalation: Rinse mouth after each use. May cause dysphonia, oral thrush, and dermatitis. Compared to beclomethasone, has been shown to have less of an effect on suppressing linear growth in asthmatic children. Eosinophilic conditions may occur with the withdrawal or decrease of oral corticosteroids after the initiation of inhaled fluticasone.

Topical use: **Avoid** application/contact to face, eyes, and open skin. Occlusive dressings are **not recommended** because they may increase local side effects (irritation, folliculits, acneiform eruptions, hypopigmentation, perioral dermatitis, contact dermatitis, secondary infection, skin atrophy, striae, hypertichosis and miliaria). **Do not use** lotion dosage form with formaldehyde hypersensitivity.

For explanation of icons, see p. 663.

FLUTICASONE PROPIONATE AND SALMETEROL
Advair Diskus, Advair HFA
Corticosteroid and long acting beta-2 adrenergic agonist

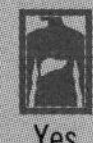 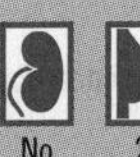 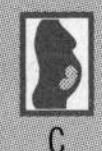
Yes No 2 C

Dry powder inhalation (DPI) (Advair Diskus):
100 mcg fluticasone propionate + 50 mcg salmeterol per inhalation (28, 60 inhalations)
250 mcg fluticasone propionate + 50 mcg salmeterol per inhalation (28, 60 inhalations)
500 mcg fluticasone propionate + 50 mcg salmeterol per inhalation (28, 60 inhalations)
Aerosol inhaler (MDI) (Advair HFA):
45 mcg fluticasone propionate + 21 mcg salmeterol per inhalation (12 g delivers 120 doses)
115 mcg fluticasone propionate + 21 mcg salmeterol per inhalation (12 g delivers 120 doses)
230 mcg fluticasone propionate + 21 mcg salmeterol per inhalation (12 g delivers 120 doses)

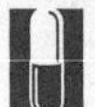

Asthma:
Without prior inhaled steroid use:
Dry powder inhalation (DPI):
4 yr–adult: Start with one inhalation BID of 100 mcg fluticasone propionate + 50 mcg salmeterol.
Aerosol inhaler (MDI):
≥12 yr and adult: 2 inhalations BID of 45 mcg fluticasone + 21 mcg salmeterol, OR 115 mcg fluticasone + 21 mcg salmeterol; max. dose: 2 inhalations BID of 230 mcg fluticasone + 21 mcg salmeterol.
With prior inhaled steroid use (conversion from other inhaled steroids; see following table):

Inhaled Corticosteroid	Current Daily Dose	Recommended Strength of Fluticasone Propionate + Salmeterol Diskus (DPI) (Advair Diskus) Administered at One Inhalation BID	Recommended Strength of Fluticasone Propionate + Salmeterol Aerosol Inhaler (MDI) (Advair HFA) Administered at Two Inhalations BID
Beclomethasone dipropionate (Qvar; CFC-free, HFA)	160 mcg	100 mcg + 50 mcg	45 mcg + 21 mcg
	320 mcg	250 mcg + 50 mcg	115 mcg + 21 mcg
	640 mcg	500 mcg + 50 mcg	230 mcg + 21 mcg
Budesonide	≤400 mcg	100 mcg + 50 mcg	45 mcg + 21 mcg
	800–1200 mcg	250 mcg + 50 mcg	115 mcg + 21 mcg
	1600 mcg	500 mcg + 50 mcg	230 mcg + 21 mcg
Flunisolide (Aerobid, Aerobid-M; containing CFCs)	≤1000 mcg	100 mcg + 50 mcg	45 mcg + 21 mcg
	1250–2000 mcg	250 mcg + 50 mcg	115 mcg + 21 mcg
Flunisolide (Aerospan; CFC-free, HFA)	≤320 mcg	100 mcg + 50 mcg	45 mcg + 21 mcg
	640 mcg	250 mcg + 50 mcg	115 mcg + 21 mcg
Fluticasone propionate aerosol (HFA)	≤176 mcg	100 mcg + 50 mcg	45 mcg + 21 mcg
	440 mcg	250 mcg + 50 mcg	115 mcg + 21 mcg
	660–880 mcg	500 mcg + 50 mcg	230 mcg + 21 mcg

Continued

FLUTICASONE PROPIONATE AND SALMETEROL *continued*

Inhaled Corticosteroid	Current Daily Dose	Recommended Strength of Fluticasone Propionate + Salmeterol Diskus (DPI) (Advair Diskus) Administered at One Inhalation BID	Recommended Strength of Fluticasone Propionate + Salmeterol Aerosol Inhaler (MDI) (Advair HFA) Administered at Two Inhalations BID
Fluticasone propionate dry powder (DPI)	≤200 mcg	100 mcg + 50 mcg	45 mcg + 21 mcg
	500 mcg	250 mcg + 50 mcg	115 mcg + 21 mcg
	1000 mcg	500 mcg + 50 mcg	230 mcg + 21 mcg
Mometasone furoate	220 mcg	100 mcg + 50 mcg	45 mcg + 21 mcg
	440 mcg	250 mcg + 50 mcg	115 mcg + 21 mcg
	880 mcg	500 mcg + 50 mcg	230 mcg + 21 mcg
Triamcinolone	≤1000 mcg	100 mcg + 50 mcg	45 mcg + 21 mcg
	1100–1600 mcg	250 mcg + 50 mcg	115 mcg + 21 mcg

Max. dose:

Dry powder inhalation (DPI): one inhalation BID of 500 mcg fluticasone propionate + 50 mcg salmeterol.

Aerosol inhaler (MDI): two inhalations BID of 230 mcg fluticasone propionate + 21 mcg salmeterol.

See *Fluticasone Propionate* and *Salmeterol* for remarks. Titrate to the lowest effective strength after asthma is adequately controlled. Proper patient education including dosage administration technique is essential; see patient package insert for detailed instructions. Rinse mouth after each use.

FLUVOXAMINE

Many generics; previously available as Luvox

Antidepressant, selective serotonin reuptake inhibitor

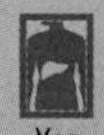
Yes
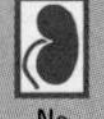
No
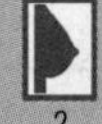
2
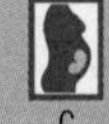
C

Tabs: 25, 50, 100 mg

Extended release capsules: 100, 150 mg

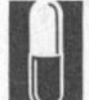

Obsessive compulsive disorder (use immediate release tablets unless noted otherwise):

8–17 yr: Start at 25 mg PO QHS. Dose may be increased by 25 mg/24 hr Q4–7 days. Total daily doses >50 mg/24 hr should be divided BID. Female patients may require lower dosages compared to males.

Max. dose: Child: 8–11 yr: 200 mg/24 hr; and child ≥12–17 yr: 300 mg/24 hr.

Adult: Start at 50 mg PO QHS. Dose may be increased by 50 mg/24 hr Q4–7 days up to a **max. dose** of 300 mg/24 hr. Total daily doses >100 mg/24 hr should be divided BID.

Extended release capsule (adults): Start at 100 mg PO QHS. Dose may be increased by 50 mg/24 hr Q7 days up to a **max. dose** of 300 mg/24 hr.

Continued

For explanation of icons, see p. 663.

FLUVOXAMINE *continued*

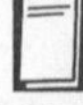

Contraindicated with coadministration of cisapride, pimozide, thioridazine, tizanidine, or MAO inhibitors. **Use with caution** in hepatic disease (dosage reduction may be necessary); drug is extensively metabolized by the liver. Monitor for clinical worsening of depression and suicidal ideation/behavior following the initiation of therapy or after dose changes.

Inhibits CYP 450 1A2, 2C19, 2D6, and 3A3/4 which may increase the effects or toxicity of drugs metabolized by these enzymes. Dose-related use of thioridazine with fluvoxamine may cause prolongation of QT interval and serious arrhythmias. May increase warfarin plasma levels by 98% and prolong PT. May increase toxicity and/or levels of theophylline, caffeine, and tricyclic antidepressants. Side effects include: headache, insomnia, somnolence, nausea, diarrhea, dyspepsia, and dry mouth.

Titrate to lowest effective dose.

FOLIC ACID

Folvite and many others

Water-soluble vitamin

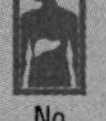 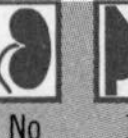 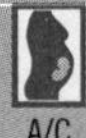

No No 1 A/C

Tabs (OTC): 0.4, 0.8, 1 mg
Oral solution: 50 mcg/mL
Injection: 5 mg/mL; contains 1.5% benzyl alcohol

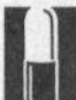

For U.S. RDA, see Chapter 21.
Folic acid deficiency PO, IM, IV, SC (see following table)

Infant	Child 1–10 yr	Child ≥11 yr and adult
INITIAL DOSE		
15 mcg/kg/ dose; **max. dose** 50 mcg/24 hr	1 mg/dose	1 mg/dose
MAINTENANCE		
30–45 mcg/ 24 hr once daily	0.1–0.4 mg/24 hr once daily	0.4 mg/24 hr once daily; Pregnant/lactating women: 0.8 mg/24 hr once daily

Normal levels: see Chapter 21. May mask hematologic effects of vitamin B_{12} deficiency, but will not prevent progression of neurologic abnormalities. High dose folic acid may decrease the absorption of phenytoin.

Women of child-bearing age considering pregnancy should take at least 0.4 mg once daily before and during pregnancy to reduce risk of neural tube defects in the fetus. Pregnancy category changes to "C" if used in doses above the RDA.

FOMEPIZOLE

Antizol and others

Antidote for ethylene glycol or methanol toxicity

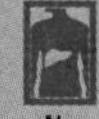 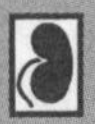  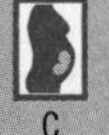

No Yes ? C

Injection: 1 g/mL (1.5 mL)

Child and adult not requiring hemodialysis (IV, all doses administered over 30 min):
Load: 15 mg/kg/dose × 1

Continued

FOMEPIZOLE *continued*

Maintenance: 10 mg/kg/dose Q12 hr × 4 doses, then 15 mg/kg/dose Q12 hr until ethylene glycol or methanol level decreases to <20 mg/dL and the patient is asymptomatic with normal pH.

Child and adult requiring hemodialysis (IV following the recommended doses at the intervals indicated here. Fomepizole is removed by dialysis. All doses administered over 30 min):

Dosing at the beginning of hemodialysis:

If <6 hr since last fomepizole dose: **DO NOT** administer dose.

If ≥6 hr since last fomepizole dose: Administer next scheduled dose.

Dosing during hemodialysis: Administer Q4 hr or as continuous infusion of 1–1.5 mg/kg/hr.

Dosing at the time hemodialysis is completed (based on the time between last dose and end of hemodialysis):

<1 hr: **DO NOT** administer dose at end of hemodialysis.

1–3 hr: Administer 1/2 of next scheduled dose.

>3 hr: Administer next scheduled dose.

Maintenance dose off hemodialysis: give next scheduled dose 12 hr from last dose administered.

Works by competitively inhibiting alcohol dehydrogenase. Safety and efficacy in pediatrics have not been established. **Contraindicated** in hypersensitivity to any components or other pyrazole compounds. Most frequent side effects include headache, nausea, and dizziness. Fomepizole is extensively eliminated by the kidneys (**use with caution in renal failure**) and removed by hemodialysis.

Drug product may solidify at temperatures <25° C (77° F); vial can be liquefied by running it under warm water (efficacy, safety, and stability are not affected). All doses must be diluted with at least 100 mL of D5W or NS to prevent vein irritation.

FORMOTEROL
Foradil Aerolizer, Perforomist
Beta-2-adrenergic agonist (long acting)

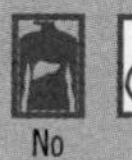
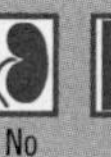
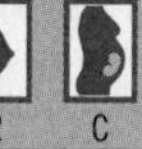

No No 2 C

Inhalation powder in capsules (Foradil Aerolizer): 12 mcg (12s and 60s); contains lactose. Use with Aerolizer inhaler.
Inhalation solution (Perforomist): 20 mcg/2 mL (60s)

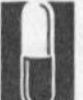

≥5 yr and adult:

Asthma/Bronchodilation (should be used with an inhaled corticosteroid):

Foradil Aerolizer: 12 mcg Q12 hr; **max. dose:** 24 mcg/24 hr (12 mcg spaced 12 hr apart)

Prevention of exercise-induced asthma for patients NOT receiving maintenance long-acting beta-2 agonists (e.g., formoterol or salmeterol):

Foradil Aerolizer: 12 mcg 15 min prior to exercise. If needed, an additional dose may be given AFTER 12 hr. **Max. dose:** 24 mcg/24 hr (12 mcg spaced 12 hr apart). Consider alternative therapy if maximum dosage is not effective.

Fast onset of action (1–3 min) with peak effects in 0.5–1 hr and long duration (up to 12 hr). Although long-acting beta-2 adrenergic agonists may decrease the frequency of asthma episodes, they may make asthma episodes more severe when they occur. Abdominal pain, dyspepsia, nausea, and tremor may occur.

Continued

For explanation of icons, see p. 663.

FORMOTEROL *continued*

Inhalation solution product (Perforomist) is indicated for COPD in adults [20 mcg Q12 hr; **max. dose:** 40 mcg/24 hr (20 mcg spaced 12 hr apart)].

WARNING: Long-acting beta-2-agonists may increase the risk of asthma-related death. Only use formoterol as additional therapy for patients not adequately controlled on other asthma-controller medications (e.g., low- to medium-dose inhaled corticosteroids) or whose disease severity clearly requires initiation of treatment with 2 maintenance therapies. Should **not** be used in conjunction with an inhaled, long-acting beta-2 agonist and is **not** a substitute for inhaled or systemic corticosteroids. See Chapter 24 for recommendations for asthma controller therapy.

FOSCARNET

Foscavir

Antiviral agent

No Yes 3 C

Injection: 24 mg/mL (250, 500 mL)

Adolescent and adult, IV:

CMV retinitis:

Induction: 180 mg/kg/24 hr ÷ Q8 hr × 14–21 days

Maintenance: 90–120 mg/kg/24 hr once daily

Acyclovir-resistant herpes simplex: 40 mg/kg/dose Q8 hr or 40–60 mg/kg/dose Q12 hr for up to 3 wk or until lesions heal

Use with caution in patients with renal insufficiency. Discontinue use in adults if serum Cr ≥2.9 mg/dL. **Adjust dose in renal failure (see Chapter 31).**

May cause peripheral neuropathy, seizures, hallucinations, GI disturbance, increased LFTs, hypertension, chest pain, ECG abnormalities, coughing, dyspnea, bronchospasm, and renal failure (adequate hydration and avoiding nephrotoxic medications may reduce risk). Hypocalcemia (increased risk if given with pentamidine), hypokalemia, and hypomagnesemia may also occur. Use with ciprofloxacin may increase risk for seizures.

FOSPHENYTOIN

Cerebyx and others

Anticonvulsant

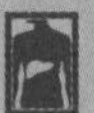 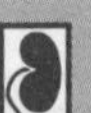  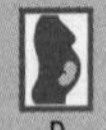

Yes Yes 2 D

Injection: 50 mg phenytoin equivalent (75 mg fosphenytoin)/1 mL (2, 10 mL)

1 mg phenytoin equivalent provides 0.0037 mmol phosphate.

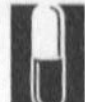

All doses are expressed as phenytoin sodium equivalents (PE) (see remarks for dose administration information):

Child: See Phenytoin and use the conversion of 1 mg phenytoin = 1 mg PE

Adult:

Loading dose:

Status epilepticus: 15–20 mg PE/kg IV

Nonemergent loading: 10–20 mg PE/kg IV/IM

Initial maintenance dose: 4–6 mg PE/kg/24 hr IV/IM ÷ once daily or BID

Continued

FOSPHENYTOIN *continued*

All doses should be prescribed and dispensed in terms of mg phenytoin sodium equivalents (PE) to avoid medication errors. Safety in pediatrics has not been fully established.

Use with caution in patients with renal or hepatic impairment and porphyria (consider amount of phosphate delivered by fosphenytoin in patients with phosphate restrictions). Drug is also metabolized to liberate small amounts of formaldehyde, which is considered clinically insignificant with short-term use (e.g., 1 wk). Side effects: hypokalemia (with rapid IV administration), slurred speech, dizziness, ataxia, rash, exfoliative dermatitis, nystagmus, diplopia, and tinnitus. Increased unbound phenytoin concentrations may occur in patients with renal disease or hypoalbuminemia; measure "free" or "unbound" phenytoin levels in these patients.

Abrupt withdrawal may cause status epilepticus. BP and ECG monitoring should be present during IV loading dose administration. **Max. IV infusion rate:** 3 mg PE/kg/min up to a **max.** of 150 mg PE/min. Administer IM via 1 or 2 injection sites and IM route is **not recommended** in status epilepticus.

Therapeutic levels: 10–20 mg/L (free and bound phenytoin) **OR** 1–2 mg/L (free only). Recommended peak serum sampling times: 4 hr following an IM dose or 2 hr following an IV dose.

See *Phenytoin* remarks for drug interactions. Drug is more safely administered via pheripheral IV than phenytoin.

FUROSEMIDE
Lasix and many other generics
Loop diuretic

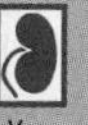
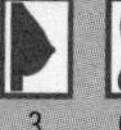
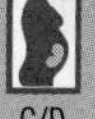

Yes Yes 3 C/D

Tabs: 20, 40, 80 mg
Injection: 10 mg/mL (2, 4, 10 mL)
Oral solution: 10 mg/mL (60, 120 mL), 40 mg/5 mL (5, 500 mL)

IM, IV:

Neonate: 0.5–1 mg/kg/dose Q8–24 hr; **max. dose:** 2 mg/kg/dose.
Infant and child: 1–2 mg/kg/dose Q6–12 hr.
Adult: 20–40 mg/24 hr ÷ Q6–12 hr; **max. dose:** 600 mg/24 hr or 80 mg/dose.

PO:

Neonate: Bioavailability by this route is poor; doses of 1–4 mg/kg/dose once daily to BID have been used.
Infant and child: Start at 2 mg/kg/dose; may increase by 1–2 mg/kg/dose no sooner than 6–8 hr following the previous dose. **Max. dose:** 6 mg/kg/dose. Dosages have ranged from 1–6 mg/kg/dose Q12–24 hr.
Adult: 20–80 mg/dose Q6–12 hr; max. dose: 600 mg/24 hr.

Continuous IV infusion:

Infant and child: 0.05 mg/kg/hr, titrate to effect.
Adult: 0.1 mg/kg/hr; titrate to effect; **max. dose:** 0.4 mg/kg/hr.

Contraindicated in anuria and hepatic coma. **Use with caution** in hepatic disease (hepatic encephalopathy has been reported); cirrhotic patients may require higher than usual doses. Ototoxicity may occur in presence of renal disease (especially when used with aminoglycosides), with rapid IV injection (do not infuse >4 mg/min in adults), or with hypoproteinemia. May cause hypokalemia, alkalosis, dehydration, hyperuricemia, and

Continued

For explanation of icons, see p. 663.

FUROSEMIDE *continued*

increased calcium excretion. Prolonged use in premature infants and in children <4 yr may result in nephrocalcinosis. May increase risk for PDA in premature infants during the first week of life.

Furosemide-resistant edema in pediatric patients may benefit with the addition of metolazone. Some of these patients may have an exaggerated response leading to hypovolemia, tachycardia, and orthostatic hypotension requiring fluid replacement. Severe hypokalemia has been reported with a tendency for diuresis persisting for up to 24 hr after discontinuing metolazone.

Max. rate of intermittent IV dose: 0.5 mg/kg/min.

Pregnancy category changes to "D" if used in pregnancy-induced hypertension.

GABAPENTIN

Neurontin, Gabarone

Anticonvulsant

No Yes ? C

Caps: 100, 300, 400 mg
Tabs: 100, 300, 400, 600, 800 mg
Oral solution: 250 mg/5 mL (480 mL)

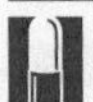

Seizures (maximum time between doses should not exceed 12 hr):

3–12 yr (PO, see remarks):

Day 1: 10-15 mg/kg/24 hr ÷ TID, then gradually titrate dose upward to the following dosages over a 3-day period:

3–4 yr: 40 mg/kg/24 hr ÷ TID

≥5–12 yr: 25–35 mg/kg/24 hr ÷ TID

Dosages up to 50 mg/kg/24 hr have been well tolerated.

>12 yr and adult (PO, see remarks): Start with 300 mg TID; if needed, increase dose up to 1800 mg/24 hr ÷ TID. Usual effective doses: 900–1800 mg/24 hr ÷ TID. Doses as high as 3.6 g/24 hr have been tolerated.

Neuopathic pain:

Child (PO; limited data):

Day 1: 5 mg/kg/dose at bedtime

Day 2: 5 mg/kg/dose BID

Day 3: 5 mg/kg/dose TID; then titrate dose to effect. Usual dosage range: 8–35 mg/kg/24 hr. **Maximum daily dose has not been evaluated.**

Adult (PO):

Day 1: 300 mg at bedtime

Day 2: 300 mg BID

Day 3: 300 mg TID; then titrate dose to effect. Usual dosage range: 1800–2400 mg/24 hr; **max. dose:** 3600 mg/24 hr. For post-herpetic neuralgia, dose may be titrated up PRN for pain relief to a daily dose of 1800 mg/24 hr ÷ TID (efficacy has been shown from 1800–3600 mg/24 hr; however, no additional benefit has been shown for doses >1800 mg/24 hr).

Generally used as adjunctive therapy for partial and secondary generalized seizures, and neuropathic pain.

Somnolence, dizziness, ataxia, fatigue, and nystagmus were common in use for seizures (≥12 yr). Viral infections, fever, nausea and/or vomiting, somnolence, and hostility have been reported in patients 3–12 yr receiving other antiepiletics. Dizziness, somnolence, and peripheral

Continued

G
FORMULARY

GABAPENTIN *continued*

edema are common side effects in adult with post-herpetic neuralgia. Suicidal behavior or ideation, and multi-organ hypersensitivity (DRESS) have been reported.

Do not withdraw medication abruptly (gradually over a minimum of 1 wk). Drug is not metabolized by the liver and is primarily excreted in the urine unchanged.

May be taken with or without food. In TID dosing schedule, **interval between doses should not exceed 12 hr. Adjust dose in renal impairment (see Chapter 31).**

GANCICLOVIR

Cytovene

Antiviral agent

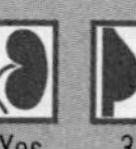
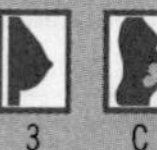

No Yes 3 C

Injection: 500 mg; contains 4 mEq Na per 1 g drug

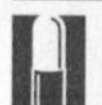

Cytomegalovirus (CMV) infections:

Neonate (Congenital CMV): 12 mg/kg/24 hr ÷ Q12 hr IV × 6 wk

Child >3 mo and adult:

Induction therapy (duration 14–21 days): 10 mg/kg/24 hr ÷ Q12 hr IV

IV maintenance therapy: 5 mg/kg/dose once daily IV for 7 days/wk or 6 mg/kg/dose once daily IV for 5 days/wk

Prevention of CMV in transplant recipients:

Child and adult:

Induction therapy (duration 7–14 days): 10 mg/kg/24 hr ÷ Q12 hr IV

IV maintenance therapy: 5 mg/kg/dose once daily IV for 7 days/wk or 6 mg/kg/dose once daily IV for 5 days/wk for 100–120 days post-transplant

Prevention of CMV in HIV-infected individuals (see www.aidsinfo.nih.gov for latest recommendations and guidelines for CMV treatment as well):

Recurrence prophylaxis:

Infant, child, adolescent, and adult: 5 mg/kg/dose IV once daily. Consider valganciclovir as an oral alternative.

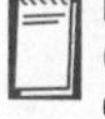

Limited experience with use in children <12 yr old. **Contraindicated** in severe neutropenia (ANC <500/microliter) or severe thrombocytopenia (platelets <25,000/microliter). **Use with extreme caution. Reduce dose in renal failure (see Chapter 31).** For oral route of administration, see valganciclovir.

Common side effects: neutropenia, thrombocytopenia, retinal detachment, confusion. Drug reactions alleviated with dose reduction or temporary interruption. Ganciclovir may increase didanosine and zidovudine levels, whereas, didanosine and zidovudine may decrease ganciclovir levels. Immunosuppressive agents may increase hematologic toxicities. Amphotericin B and cyclosporine and tacrolimus increases risk for nephrotoxicity. Imipenem/cilastatin may increase risk for seizures.

Minimum dilution is 10 mg/ml and should be infused IV over ≥1 hr. IM and SC administration are **contraindicated** because of high pH (pH = 11).

GCSF

See *Filgrastim*

For explanation of icons, see p. 663.

GENTAMICIN
Garamycin and many others
Antibiotic, aminoglycoside

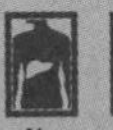 No 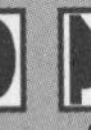 Yes 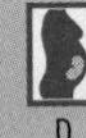 2 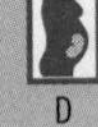 D

Injection: 10 mg/mL (2 mL), 40 mg/mL (2, 20 mL); some products may contain sodium metabisulfite
Pre-mixed injection in NS: 40 mg (50 mL), 60 mg (50 mL), 70 mg (50 mL), 80 mg (50, 100 mL), 90 mg (100 mL), 100 mg (50, 100 mL), 120 mg (50, 100 mL)
Ophthalmic ointment: 0.3% (3.5 g)
Ophthalmic drops: 0.3% (5, 15 mL)
Topical ointment: 0.1% (15, 30 g)
Topical cream: 0.1% (15, 30 g)

Initial empiric dosage; patient specific dosage defined by therapeutic drug monitoring (see remarks).

Parenteral (IM or IV):

Neonate/Infant (see table below):

Post-Conceptional Age (wk)	Postnatal Age (days)	Dose (mg/kg/dose)	Interval (hr)
≤29*	0–7	5	48
	8–28	4	36
	>28	4	24
30–33	0–7	4.5	36
	>7	4	24
34–37	0–7	4	24
	>7	4	18–24
≥38	0–7	4	24
	>7	4	12–18

*Or significant asphyxia, PDA, indomethacin use, poor cardiac output, reduced renal function.

Child: 7.5 mg/kg/24 hr ÷ Q8 hr
Adult: 3–6 mg/kg/24 hr ÷ Q8 hr
Cystic Fibrosis: 7.5–10.5 mg/kg/24 hr ÷ Q8 hr

Intrathecal/intraventricular (use preservative-free product only):
Newborn: 1 mg once daily
>3 mo: 1–2 mg once daily
Adult: 4–8 mg once daily

Ophthalmic ointment: apply Q8–12 hr
Ophthalmic drops: 1–2 drops Q2–4 hr

Use with caution in patients receiving anesthetics or neuromuscular blocking agents, and in patients with neuromuscular disorders. May cause nephrotoxicity and ototoxicity. Ototoxicity may be potentiated with the use of loop diuretics. Eliminated more quickly in patients with Cystic Fibrosis, neutropenia, and burns. **Adjust dose in renal failure (see Chapter 31).** Monitor peak and trough levels.

Therapeutic peak levels:
6–10 mg/L general
8–10 mg/L in pulmonary infections, Cystic Fibrosis, neutropenia, osteomyelitis, and severe sepsis

Continued

GENTAMICIN *continued*

To maximize bacterialcidal effects, an individualized peak concentration to target a peak/MIC ratio of 8–10 : 1 may be applied.

Therapeutic trough levels: <2 mg/L. Recommended serum sampling time at steady-state: trough within 30 min prior to the 3rd consecutive dose and peak 30–60 min after the administration of the 3rd consecutive dose.

For initial dosing in obese patients, use an adjusted body weight (ABW). ABW = Ideal Body Weight + 0.4 (Total Body Weight − Ideal Body Weight).

GLUCAGON HCl
GlucaGen, Glucagon Emergency Kit
Antihypoglycemic agent

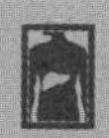 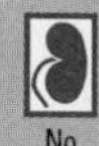 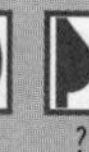 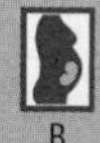
No No ? B

Injection: 1 mg vial (requires reconstitution)
1 unit = 1 mg

Hypoglycemia (IM, IV, SC):
Neonate, infant, and child <20 kg: 0.5 mg/dose (or 0.02–0.03 mg/kg/dose) Q20 min PRN
Child ≥20 kg and adult: 1 mg/dose Q20 min PRN

Beta-blocker and calcium channel blocker overdose: Load with 0.05–0.15 mg/kg (usually about 10 mg in adults) IV over 1 min followed by an IV infusion of 0.05–0.1 mg/kg/hr.
Alternatively, 5 mg IV bolus Q5–10 min PRN up to 4 doses. If patient is responsive at a particular bolus dose, initiate an hourly IV infusion at that same responsive dose. For example, if the patent responded at 10 mg, then start an infusion of 10 mg/hr.

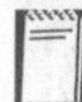

Use with caution in insulinoma and/or pheochromocytoma. Drug product is genetically engineered and identical to human glucagon. High doses have cardiac stimulatory effect and have had some success in beta-blocker and calcium channel blocker overdose. May cause nausea, vomiting, urticaria, and respiratory distress. **Do not delay** glucose infusion; dose for hypoglycemia is 2–4 mL/kg of dextrose 25%.

Onset of action: IM: 8–10 min; IV: 1 min. Duration of action: IM: 12–27 min; IV: 9–17 min.

GLYCERIN
Fleet Babylax, Sani-Supp, and others
Osmotic Laxative

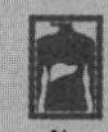 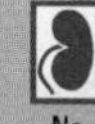 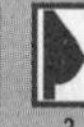 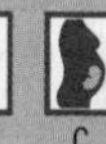
No No ? C

Rectal solution (OTC): 4 mL per application (6 doses), 7.5 mL per application (4 doses)
Suppository (OTC):
Infant/pediatric (10s, 12s, 25s)
Adult (10s, 12s, 24s, 25s, 50s)

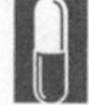

Constipation:
Neonate: 0.5 mL/kg/dose rectal solution PR as an enema once daily–BID PRN or half of infant suppository PR once daily PRN
Child <6 yr: 2–5 mL rectal solution PR as an enema or 1 infant suppository PR once daily–BID PRN
>6 yr–adult: 5–15 mL rectal solution PR as an enema or 1 adult suppository PR once daily–BID PRN

Onset of action: 15–30 min. May cause rectal irritation, abdominal pain, bloating, and dizziness. Insert suppository high into rectum and retain for 15 min.

For explanation of icons, see p. 663.

GLYCOPYRROLATE
Robinul and generics
Anticholinergic agent

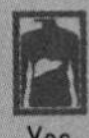 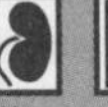 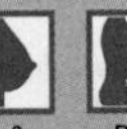 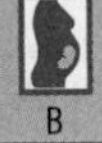
Yes Yes ? B

Tabs: 1, 2 mg
Injection: 0.2 mg/mL (1, 2, 5, 20 mL); some multidose vials contain 0.9% benzyl alcohol

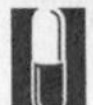

Respiratory antisecretory:
IM/IV:
Child: 0.004–0.01 mg/kg/dose Q4–8 hr
Adult: 0.1–0.2 mg/dose Q4–8 hr
Max. dose: 0.2 mg/dose or 0.8 mg/24 hr
Oral:
Child: 0.04–0.1 mg/kg/dose Q4–8 hr
Adult: 1–2 mg/dose BID–TID
Reverse neuromuscular blockade:
Child and adult: 0.2 mg IV for every 1 mg neostigmine or 5 mg pyridostigmine

Use with caution in hepatic and renal disease, ulcerative colitis, asthma, glaucoma, ileus, or urinary retention. Atropine-like side effects: tachycardia, nausea, constipation, confusion, blurred vision, and dry mouth. These may be potentiated if given with other drugs with anticholinergic properties. IV dosage form may be used orally.

Onset of action: PO: within 1 hr; IM/SC: 15–30 min; IV: 1 min. Duration of antisialogogue effect: PO: 8–12 hr; IM/SC/IV: 7 hr.

GRANISETRON
Kytril and others
Antiemetic agent, 5-HT$_3$ antagonist

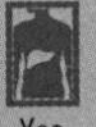 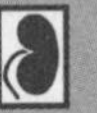  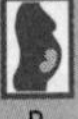
Yes No ? B

Injection: 1 mg/mL (1, 4 mL); 4 mL vials contain benzyl alcohol
Tabs: 1 mg
Oral liquid: 0.2 mg/mL (30 mL); contains sodium benzoate

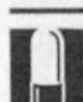

Chemotherapy-induced nausea and vomiting:
IV:
Child ≥2 yr and adult: 10–20 mcg/kg/dose 15–60 min before chemotherapy; the same dose may be repeated 2–3 times at ≥ 10-min intervals following chemotherapy (within 24 hr after chemotherapy) as a treatment regimen. **Max. dose:** 3 mg/dose or 9 mg/24 hr. Alternatively, a single 40 mcg/kg/dose 15–60 min before chemotherapy has been used.
PO:
Adult: 2 mg/24 hr ÷ once daily–BID; initiate first dose 1 hr prior to chemotherapy.
Post-operative nausea and vomiting prevention (dosed prior to anesthesia or immediately before anesthesia reversal) and treatment (IV):
≥4 yr: 20–40 mcg/kg/dose (**max. dose:** 1 mg) × 1
Adult: 1 mg × 1
Radiation-induced nausea and vomiting prevention:
Adult: 2 mg once daily PO administered 1 hr before radiation.

Use with caution in liver disease and pre-existing cardiac conduction disorders and arrhythmias. May cause hypertension, hypotension, arrhythmias, agitation, and insomnia. Inducers or inhibitors of the CYP 450 3A3/4 drug metabolizing enzymes may increase or decrease, respectively, the drug's clearance. QT prolongation has been reported.

Onset of action: IV: 4–10 min. Duration of action: IV: ≤24 hr.

GRISEOFULVIN
Grifulvin V, Grisactin, Fulvicin U/F, Fulvicin P/G, Gris-PEG, and others
Antifungal agent

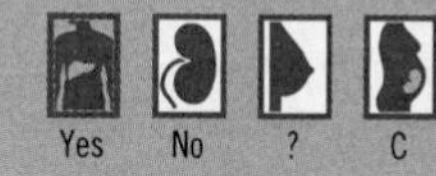

Microsize:
Tabs (Grifulvin V): 500 mg
Oral suspension (Grifulvin V, Griseofulvin Microsize): 125 mg/5 mL (120 mL); contains 0.2% alcohol, parabens and propylene glycol
Ultramicrosize (250 mg ultramicrosize is approximately 500 mg microsize):
Tabs (Gris-PEG): 125, 250 mg

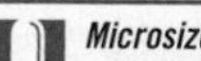

Microsize:
Child >2 yr: 10–20 mg/kg/24 hr PO ÷ once daily–BID; give with milk, eggs, fatty foods. Some have recommended a higher dose of 20–25 mg/kg/24 hr PO for tinea capitis to improve efficacy due to relative resistance of the organism.
Adult: 500–1000 mg/24 hr PO ÷ once daily–BID
Max. dose (all ages): 1 g/24 hr

Ultramicrosize:
Child >2 yr: 10–15 mg/kg/24 hr PO ÷ once daily–BID
Adult: 330–750 mg/24 hr PO ÷ once daily–BID
Max. dose (all ages): 750 mg/24 hr

Contraindicated in porphyria, pregnancy, and hepatic disease. Monitor hematologic, renal, and hepatic function. May cause leukopenia, rash, headache, paresthesias, and GI symptoms. Severe skin reactions (e.g., Stevens-Johnson, TEN), erythema multiforme, LFT elevations (AST, ALT, bilirubin), and jaundice have been reported. Possible cross-reactivity in penicillin-allergic patients. Usual treatment period is 8 wk for tinea capitis and 4–6 mo for tinea unguium. Photosensitivity reactions may occur. May reduce effectiveness or decrease level of oral contraceptives, warfarin, and cyclosporine. Induces CYP 450 1A2 isoenzyme. Phenobarbital may enhance clearance of griseofulvin. Coadministration with fatty meals will increase the drug's absorption.

HALOPERIDOL
Haldol, Haldol Decanoate 50, Haldol Decanoate 100, and other generics
Antipsychotic agent

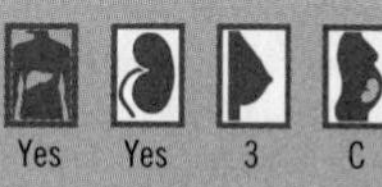

Injection (IM use only):
Lactate: 5 mg/mL (1, 10 mL); may contain parabens
Decanoate (long acting): 50, 100 mg/mL (1, 5 mL); in sesame oil with 1.2% benzyl alcohol
Tabs: 0.5, 1, 2, 5, 10, 20 mg
Oral solution: 2 mg/mL (15, 120 mL)

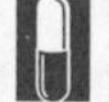

Child 3–12 yr:
PO: Initial dose at 0.025–0.05 mg/kg/24 hr ÷ BID–TID. If necessary, increase daily dosage by 0.25–0.5 mg/24 hr Q5–7 days PRN up to a **max. dose** of 0.15 mg/kg/24 hr. Usual maintenance doses for specific indications include the following:
Agitation: 0.01–0.03 mg/kg/24 hr once daily PO
Psychosis: 0.05–0.15 mg/kg/24 hr ÷ BID–TID PO

Continued

For explanation of icons, see p. 663.

HALOPERIDOL *continued*

Child 3–12 yr (cont'd):

Tourette's syndrome: 0.05–0.075 mg/kg/24 hr ÷ BID–TID PO; may increase daily dose by 0.5 mg Q5–7 days

IM, as lactate, for 6–12 yr: 1–3 mg/dose Q4–8 hr; **max. dose:** 0.15 mg/kg/24 hr

>12 yr:

Acute agitation: 2–5 mg/dose IM as lactate or 1–15 mg/dose PO; repeat in 1 hr PRN

Psychosis: 2–5 mg/dose Q4–8 hr IM PRN or 1–15 mg/24 hr ÷ BID–TID PO

Tourette's: 0.5–2 mg/dose BID–TID PO; 3–5 mg/dose BID–TID PO may be used for severe symptoms

Use with caution in patients with cardiac disease (risk of hypotension), renal or hepatic dysfunction, thyrotoxicosis, and in patients with epilepsy since the drug lowers the seizure threshold. Extrapyramidal symptoms, drowsiness, headache, tachycardia, ECG changes, nausea, and vomiting can occur. Higher than recommended doses are associated with a higher risk of QT prolongation and torsades de pointes. Leukopenia/neutropenia, including agranulcytosis has been reported.

Drug is metabolized by CYP P-450 1A2, 2D6, and 3A3/4 isoenzymes. May also inhibit CYP 450 2D6 and 3A3/4 isoenzymes. Serotonin specific reuptake inhibitors (e.g., fluoxetine) may increase levels and effects of haloperidol. Carbamazepine and phenobarbital may decrease levels and effects of haloperidol. Monitor for encephalopathic syndrome when used in combination with lithium.

Acutely aggravated patients may require doses as often as Q60 min. **Decanoate salt is given every 3–4 wk in doses that are 10–15 times the individual patient's stabilized oral dose.**

HEPARIN SODIUM

Various trade names

Anticoagulant

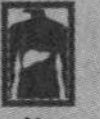
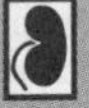
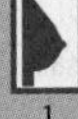
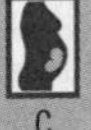

No No 1 C

Injection:

Porcine intestinal mucosa: 1000, 2000, 5000, 10,000, 20,000, 40,000 U/mL (some products may be preservative-free; multi-dosed vials contain benzyl alcohol)

Lock flush solution (porcine based): 1, 10, 100 U/mL (some products may be preservative-free or contain benzyl alcohol)

Injection for IV infusion (porcine based):

D_5W: 40 U/mL (500 mL), 50 U/mL (500 mL), 100 U/mL (100, 250 mL); contains bisulfite

NS (0.9% NaCl): 2 U/mL (500, 1000 mL)

0.45% NaCl: 50 U/mL (250, 500 mL), 100 U/mL (250 mL); contains EDTA

120 U = approximately 1 mg

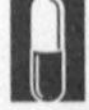

Anticoagulation empiric dosage (see Chapter 14, Table 14-8 for dosage adjustments):

Continuous IV infusion (initial doses for goal *unfractionated* heparin anti-Xa level of 0.3–0.7 units/mL):

Age	Loading Dose (IV)*	Initial IV infusion Rate (units/kg/hr)
Neonate and infant <1 yr	75 U/kg IV	28
Child ≥1–16 yr	75 U/kg IV (**max. dose:** 7700 U)	20 (max. initial rate: 1650 U/hr)
>16 yr	70 U/kg IV (**max. dose:** 7700 U)	15 (max. initial rate: 1650 U/hr)

***Do not give loading dose for stroke patients.**

Continued

HEPARIN SODIUM *continued*

DVT prophylaxis:

Adult: 5000 U/dose SC Q8–12 hr until ambulatory

Heparin flush (doses should be less than heparinizing dose):

Younger child: lower doses should be used to **avoid** systemic heparinization.

Older child and adult:

Peripheral IV: 1–2 mL of 10 U/mL solution Q4 hr

Central lines: 2–3 mL of 100 U/mL solution Q24 hr

TPN (central line) and arterial line: add heparin to make final concentration of 0.5–1 U/mL

Contraindicated in active major bleeding, known or suspected HIT and concurrent epidural therapy. Use with caution if platelets <50,000/mm^3. Avoid IM injections and other medications affecting platelet function (e.g., NSAIDS and ASA). Toxicities include bleeding, allergy, alopecia, and thrombocytopenia.

Adjust dose with one of the following laboratory goals:

Unfractionated heparin anti-Xa level: 0.3–0.7 units/mL

aPTT level (reagent specific to reflect anti-Xa level of 0.3–0.7 units/mL): 60–85 seconds.

These laboratory measurements are best measured 4–6 hr after initiation or changes in infusion rate. Do not collect blood levels from the heparinized line or same extremity as site of heparin infusion. If *unfractionated* heparin anti-Xa or aPTT levels are not available, a ratio of aPPT 1.5–2.5 times control value has been used in the past. Unfractionated heparin anti-Xa level is NOT THE SAME as *low molecular weight* heparin anti-Xa (used for monitoring *low molecular weight* heparin products such as enoxaparin).

Use preservative-free heparin in neonates. **NOTE:** heparin flush doses may alter aPTT in small patients; consider using more dilute heparin in these cases.

Use actual body weight when dosing obese patients. Due to recent regulatory changes to the manufacturing process, heparin products may exhibit decreased potency.

Antidote: Protamine sulfate (1 mg per 100 U heparin in previous 4 hr). For low molecular weight heparin, see *Enoxaparin.*

HYALURONIDASE

Amphadase, Hydase, Hylenex, Vitrase

Antidote, extravasation

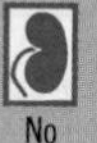
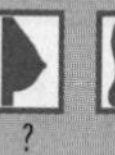

No No ? C

Injection:

Amphadase, Hydase: 150 U/mL (1 mL); bovine source and may contain thimerosal

Hylenex: 150 U/mL (1 mL); recombinant human source

Vitrase: 200 U/mL (2 mL); ovine source, preservative-free

Powder for injection (Vitrase): 6200 U; ovine source

Pharmacy can make a 15 U/mL dilution.

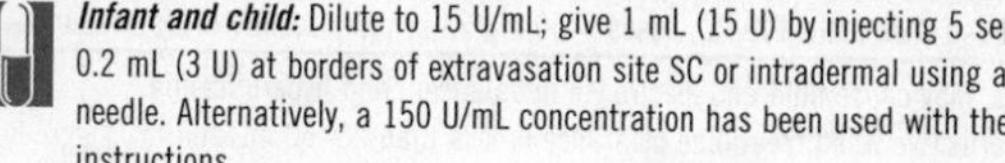

Infant and child: Dilute to 15 U/mL; give 1 mL (15 U) by injecting 5 separate injections of 0.2 mL (3 U) at borders of extravasation site SC or intradermal using a 25- or 26-gauge needle. Alternatively, a 150 U/mL concentration has been used with the same dosing instructions.

Contraindicated in dopamine and alpha-agonist extravasation and hypersensitivity to the respective product sources (bovine or ovine). May cause urticaria. Patients receiving large amounts of salicylates, cortisone, ACTH, estrogens, or antihistamines may decrease the effects of hyaluronidase (larger doses may be necessary). Administer as early as possible (minutes to 1 hour) after IV extravasation.

For explanation of icons, see p. 663.

HYDRALAZINE HYDROCHLORIDE
Apresoline and others
Antihypertensive, vasodilator

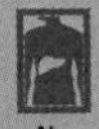 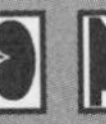 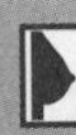 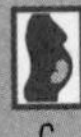
No Yes 1 C

Tabs: 10, 25, 50, 100 mg
Injection: 20 mg/mL (1 mL)
Oral liquid: 1.25, 4 mg/mL 
Some dosage forms may contain tartrazines or sulfites.

Hypertensive crisis (may result in severe and prolonged hypotension, see Chapter 4, Table 4-7 for alternatives):
Child: 0.1–0.2 mg/kg/dose IM or IV Q4–6 hr PRN; **max. dose:** 20 mg/dose. Usual IV/IM dosage range is 1.7–3.5 mg/kg/24 hr
Adult: 10–40 mg IM or IV Q4–6 hr PRN

Chronic hypertension:
Infant and child: Start at 0.75–1 mg/kg/24 hr PO ÷ Q6–12 hr (**max. dose:** 25 mg/dose). If necessary, increase dose over 3–4 wk up to a **max. dose** of 5 mg/kg/24 hr for infants and 7.5 mg/kg/24 hr for children; or 200 mg/24 hr
Adult: 10–50 mg/dose PO QID; **max. dose:** 300 mg/24 hr

Use with caution in severe renal and cardiac disease. Slow acetylators, patients receiving high-dose chronic therapy, and those with renal insufficiency are at highest risk of lupus-like syndrome (generally reversible). May cause reflex tachycardia, palpitations, dizziness, headaches, and GI discomfort. MAO inhibitors and beta-blockers may increase hypotensive effects. Indomethacin may decrease hypotensive effects.

Drug undergoes first pass metabolism. Onset of action: PO: 20–30 min; IV: 5–20 min. Duration of action: PO: 2–4 hr; IV: 2–6 hr. **Adjust dose in renal failure (see Chapter 31).**

HYDROCHLOROTHIAZIDE
Hydrodiuril and many generics
Diuretic, thiazide

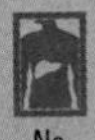 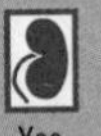  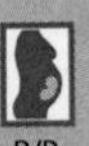
No Yes 2 B/D

Tabs: 12.5, 25, 50 mg
Caps: 12.5 mg

Edema:
Neonate and infant <6 mo: 2–4 mg/kg/24 hr ÷ BID PO; **max. dose:** 37.5 mg/24 hr
≥6 mo and child: 2 mg/kg/24 hr ÷ BID PO; **max. dose:** 100 mg/24 hr
Adult: 25–100 mg/24 hr ÷ once daily–BID PO; **max. dose:** 200 mg/24 hr

Hypertension:
Infant and child: Start at 0.5–1 mg/kg/24 hr once daily PO; dose may be increased to a **max. dose** of 3 mg/kg/24 hr up to 50 mg/24 hr.
Adult: 12.5–25 mg/dose once daily–BID PO; doses > 50 mg/24 hr often results in hypokalemia.

See *Chlorothiazide.* May cause fluid and electrolyte imbalances, and hyperuricemia. Drug may not be effective when creatinine clearance is less than 25–50 mL/min. Use with carbamazepine may result in symptomatic hyponatremia.

Hydrochlorothiazide is also available in combination with potassium-sparing diuretics (e.g., spironolactone), ACE inhibitors, angiotensin II receptor antagonists, hydralazine, methyldopa, reserpine, and beta-blockers.

Pregnancy category is "D" if used in pregnancy-induced hypertension.

HYDROCORTISONE
Solu-Cortef, Cortef, Cortifoam, Colocort, Cortenema, and many others
Corticosteroid

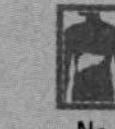
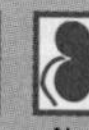
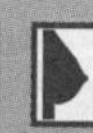
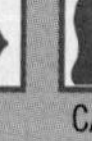
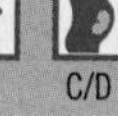

No No 3 C/D

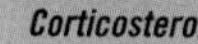

Hydrocortisone base:
Tabs: 5, 10, 20 mg
Oral suspension: 1, 2, 2.5 mg/mL
Rectal cream: 1% (30 g)
Rectal suspension (Colocort, Cortenema): 100 mg/60 mL (7s)
Topical ointment: 0.5% (OTC), 1% (OTC), 2.5%
Topical cream: 0.5% (OTC), 1% (OTC), 2.5%
Topical lotion: 1% (OTC), 2.5%

Na Succinate (Solu-Cortef):
Injection: 100, 250, 500, 1000 mg/vial; contains benzyl alcohol

Acetate:
Topical ointment (OTC): 0.5%, 1%
Topical cream (OTC): 0.5%, 1%
Rectal cream: 1%
Suppository: 25, 30 mg
Rectal foam aerosol (Cortifoam): 10% (90 mg/dose) (15 g)

Status asthmaticus:
Child:
Load (optional): 4–8 mg/kg/dose IV; **max. dose:** 250 mg
Maintenance: 8 mg/kg/24 hr ÷ Q6 hr IV
Adult: 100–500 mg/dose Q6 hr IV

Physiologic replacement: see Chapter 30 for dosing

Anti-inflammatory/immunosuppressive:
Child:
PO: 2.5–10 mg/kg/24 hr ÷ Q6–8 hr
IM/IV: 1–5 mg/kg/24 hr ÷ Q12–24 hr
Adolescent and adult:
PO/IM/IV: 15–240 mg/dose Q12 hr

Acute adrenal insufficiency: see Chapters 10 and 30 for dosing.

Topical use:
Child and adult: Apply to affected areas BID–QID, depending on severity

Rectal use:
Adolescent and adult: Insert 1 application once daily–BID × 2–3 weeks.

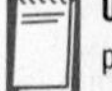

Use with caution in immunocompromised patients as they should avoid exposure to chicken pox or measles.

For doses based on body surface area and topical preparations (with comparisons), see Chapter 30. Pregnancy category changes to "D" if used in first trimester.

For explanation of icons, see p. 663.

HYDROMORPHONE HCL
Dilaudid, Dilaudid-HP, and other generics
Narcotic, analgesic

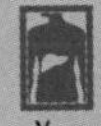 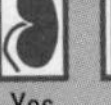 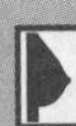 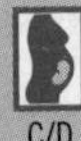

Yes Yes 3 C/D

Tabs: 2, 4, 8 mg
Injection: 1, 2, 4, 10 mg/mL (may contain methyl- and propylparabens)
Powder for injection (Dilaudid-HP): 250 mg
Suppository: 3 mg
Oral solution: 1 mg/mL

Analgesia, titrate to effect:
Child:
IV: 0.015 mg/kg/dose Q4–6 hr PRN
PO: 0.03–0.08 mg/kg/dose Q4–6 hr PRN; **max. dose:** 5 mg/dose
Adolescent and adult:
IM, IV, SC: 1–2 mg/dose Q4–6 hr PRN
PO: 1–4 mg/dose Q4–6 hr PRN

Refer to Chapter 6 for equianalgesic doses and for patient-controlled analgesia dosing. Less pruritus than morphine. Similar profile of side effects to other narcotics. **Use with caution** in infants and young children, and **do not use** in neonates due to potential CNS effects. Dose reduction recommended in renal insufficiency or severe hepatic impairment. Pregnancy category changes to "D" if used for prolonged periods or in high doses at term.

HYDROXYCHLOROQUINE
Plaquenil, Quineprox
Antimalarial, antirheumatic agent

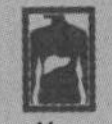 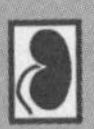 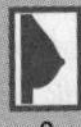 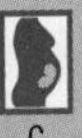

Yes Yes 2 C

Tabs: 200 mg (155 mg base)
Oral suspension: 25 mg/mL (19.375 mg/mL base)

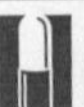

All doses expressed in mg of hydroxychloroquine base.
Malaria prophylaxis (start 1–2 wk prior to exposure and continue for 4 wk after leaving endemic area):
Child: 5 mg/kg/dose PO once weekly; **max. dose:** 310 mg.
Adult: 310 mg PO once weekly
Malaria treatment (acute uncomplicated cases):
For treatment of malaria, consult with ID specialist or see the latest edition of the AAP *Red Book.*
Child: 10 mg/kg/dose (**max. dose:** 620 mg) PO × 1 followed by 5 mg/kg/dose (**max. dose:** 310 mg) 6 hr later. Then 5 mg/kg/dose (**max. dose:** 310 mg) Q24 hr × 2 doses starting 24 hr after the first dose.
Adult: 620 mg PO × 1 followed by 310 mg 6 hr later. Then 310 mg Q24 hr × 2 doses starting 24 hr after the first dose.
Juvenile rheumatoid arthritis or systemic lupis erythematosus:
Child: 2.325–3.875 mg/kg/24 hr (base) PO ÷ once daily–BID; **max. dose:** 310 mg/24 hr **not to exceed** 5.425 mg/kg/24 hr.

Contraindicated in psoriasis, porphyria, retinal or visual field changes, and 4-aminoquinoline hypersensitivity. **Use with caution** in liver disease, G6PD deficiency, concomitant hepatic toxic drugs, renal impairment, metabolic acidosis, or hematologic disorders.

Continued

HYDROXYCHLOROQUINE *continued*

Long-term use in children is **not recommended.** May cause headaches, myopathy, GI disturbances, skin and mucosal pigmentation, agranulocytosis, visual disturbances, and increased digoxin serum levels.

For SLE and JRA, lower doses can be utilized when used in combination with other immunosuppressive agents.

HYDROXYZINE
Vistaril and various generics
Antihistamine, anxiolytic, antiemetic

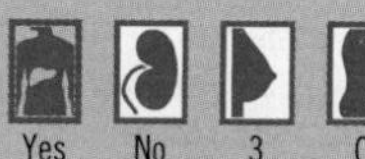

Tabs (HCl salt): 10, 25, 50 mg
Caps (pamoate salt): 25, 50, 100 mg
Syrup (HCl salt): 10 mg/5 mL (120, 473 mL); may contain alcohol
Oral suspension (pamoate salt): 25 mg/5 mL (473 mL)
Injection (HCl salt): 25, 50 mg/mL; may contain benzyl alcohol
NOTE: pamoate and HCL salts are equivalent in regards to mg of hydroxyzine.

Pruritus and anxiety:
Oral:
Child: 2 mg/kg/24 hr ÷ Q6–8 hr PRN, OR alternative dosing by age:
<6 yr: 50 mg/24 hr ÷ Q6–8 hr PRN
≥6 yr: 50–100 mg/24 hr ÷ Q6–8 hr PRN
Adult: 25 mg/dose TID–QID PRN; **max. dose:** 600 mg/24 hr
IM:
Child: 0.5–1 mg/kg/dose Q4–6 hr PRN
Adult: 25–100 mg/dose Q4–6 hr PRN; **max. dose:** 600 mg/24 hr

May potentiate barbiturates, meperidine, and other CNS depressants. May cause dry mouth, drowsiness, tremor, convulsions, blurred vision, and hypotension. May cause pain at injection site.

Increase dosage interval to Q24 hr or less in the presence of liver disease (e.g., primary biliary cirrhosis).

Onset of action within 15–30 min. Duration of action: 4–6 hr. **IV administration is not recommended.**

IBUPROFEN
PO: Motrin, Advil, Children's Advil, Children's Motrin, and others
IV: NeoProfen, Caldolor
Nonsteroidal anti-inflammatory agent

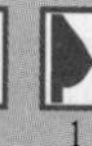
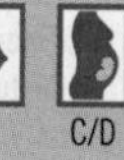

Oral suspension [OTC]: 100 mg/5 mL (60, 120, 480 mL)
Oral drops [OTC]: 40 mg/mL (15, 30 mL)
Chewable tabs [OTC]: 50, 100 mg
Caplets [OTC]: 100, 200 mg
Tabs: 100 [OTC], 200 [OTC], 400, 600, 800 mg
Capsules [OTC]: 200 mg

Continued

FORMULARY
For explanation of icons, see p. 663.

IBUPROFEN *continued*

Injection:

NeoProfen (lysine salt): 10 mg ibuprofen base/1 mL (2 mL)
Caldolor: 100 mg/mL (4, 8 mL); contains 78 mg/mL arginine

PO:

Child (≥6 mo):

Analgesic/antipyretic: 5–10 mg/kg/dose Q6–8 hr PO; **max. dose:** 40 mg/kg/24 hr.
JRA: 30–50 mg/kg/24 hr ÷ Q6 hr PO; **max. dose:** 2400 mg/24 hr.

Adult:

Inflammatory disease: 400–800 mg/dose Q6–8 hr PO; **max. dose:** 800 mg/dose or 3.2 g/24 hr.
Pain/fever/dysmenorrhea: 200–400 mg/dose Q4–6 hr PRN PO; **max. dose:** 1.2 g/24 hr.

IV:

Analgesic (≥17 yr and adult; see remarks): 400–800 mg/dose Q6 hr PRN; **max. dose:** 3200 mg/24 hr.
Antipyretic (≥17 yr and adult; see remarks): 400 mg/dose Q4–6 hr or 100–200 mg/dose Q4 hr PRN; **max. dose:** 3200 mg/24 hr.
Closure of ductus arteriosus:

<32 wk pf gestation and 0.5–1.5 kg (use birth weight to calculate all doses and infuse all doses over 15 min; see remarks): 10 mg/kg/dose IV ×1 followed by two doses of 5 mg/kg/dose each, after 24 and 48 hr. Hold second or third dose if urinary output is <0.6 mL/kg/hr; dosing should resume when laboratory studies indicate the return of normal renal function. If the ductus arteriosus fails to close or reopens, a second course of ibuprofen, the use of IV indomethacin, or surgery may be necessary.

Contraindicated with active GI bleeding and ulcer disease. **Use caution** with aspirin hypersensitivity, or hepatic/renal insufficiency, heart disease (risk for MI and stroke with prolonged use), dehydration, and in patients receiving anticoagulants. GI distress (lessened with milk), rashes, ocular problems, hypertension, granulocytopenia, and anemia may occur. Inhibits platelet aggregation. Consumption of more than three alcoholic beverages per day, use with corticosteroids or anticoagulants may increase risk for GI bleeding.

May increase serum levels and effects of digoxin, methotrexate, and lithium. May decrease the effects of antihypertensives, aspirin (anti-platelet effects) furosemide, and thiazide diuretics. Pregnancy category changes to "D" if used in 3rd trimester or near delivery.

IV USE for analgesia/antipyretic: Hydrate patient well before use. Doses must be diluted to a concentration ≤4 mg/mL with NS, D5W or LR and infused over ≥30 min. Most common reported side effects in clinical trials include nausea, flatulence, vomiting, and headache.

IV USE for PDA: Contraindicated in untreated infections, congenital heart diseases requiring a patent ductus arteriosus to facilitate satisfactory pulmonary and systemic blood flow, active intracranial or gastrointestinal bleeds, thrombocytopenia, coagulation defects, suspected/active NEC, and significant renal impairment. **Use with caution** in hyperbilirubinemia. Not indicated for IVH prophylaxis. When compared to IV indomethacin, renal side effects are generally less frequent and severe.

IMIPENEM AND CILASTATIN
Primaxin IV
Antibiotic, carbapenem

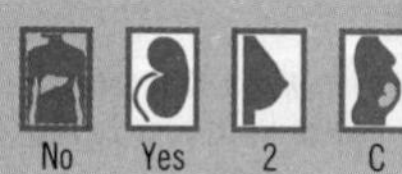

Injection: 250, 500 mg; contains 3.2 mEq Na/g drug
Each 1 mg drug contains 1 mg imipenem and 1 mg cilastatin

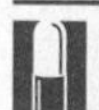

Neonate:
0–4 wk old and <1.2 kg: 50 mg/kg/24 hr ÷ Q12 hr IV
<1 wk old and ≥1.2 kg: 50 mg/kg/24 hr ÷ Q12 hr IV
≥1 wk old and ≥1.2 kg: 75 mg/kg/24 hr ÷ Q8 hr IV
Child (4 wk–3 mo): 100 mg/kg/24 hr ÷ Q6 hr IV
Child (>3 mo): 60–100 mg/kg/24 hr ÷ Q6 hr IV; **max. dose:** 4 g/24 hr
Cystic Fibrosis: 90 mg/kg/24 hr ÷ Q6 hr IV; **max. dose:** 4 g/24 hr
Adult:
IV: 1–4 g/24 hr ÷ Q6–8 hr; **max. dose:** 4 g/24 hr or 50 mg/kg/24 hr, whichever is less.
IM: 500–750 mg/dose Q12 hr

For IV use, give slowly over 30–60 min. Adverse effects: pruritus, urticaria, GI symptoms, seizures, dizziness, hypotension, elevated LFTs, blood dyscrasias, and penicillin allergy. CSF penetration is variable but best with inflamed meninges.

Do not administer with probenecid (increases imipenem/cilastatin levels) and ganciclovir (increased risk for seizures). May significantly reduce valproic acid levels.

Adjust dose in renal insufficiency (see Chapter 31).

IMIPRAMINE
Tofranil, Tofranil-PM, and many generics
Antidepressant, tricyclic

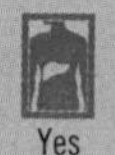
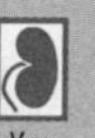
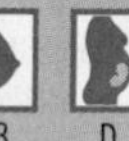
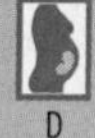

Tabs (HCl): 10, 25, 50 mg
Caps (Tofranil-PM, pamoate): 75, 100, 125, 150 mg; strengths are expressed as imipramine HCl equivalent

Antidepressant:
Child:
Initial: 1.5 mg/kg/24 hr ÷ TID PO; increase 1–1.5 mg/kg/24 hr Q3–4 days to a **max. dose** of 5 mg/kg/24 hr
Adolescent:
Initial: 25–50 mg/24 hr ÷ once daily–TID PO; **max. dose:** 200 mg/24 hr. Dosages exceeding 100 mg/24 hr are generally not necessary.
Adult:
Initial: 75–100 mg/24 hr ÷ TID PO
Maintenance: 50–300 mg/24 hr QHS PO; **max. dose:** 300 mg/24 hr
Enuresis (≥6 yr):
Initial: 10–25 mg QHS PO
Increment: 10–25 mg/dose at 1- to 2-wk intervals until **max. dose** (see below) for age or desired effect achieved. Continue × 2–3 mo, then taper slowly
Max. dose:
6–12 yr: 50 mg/24 hr
12–14 yr: 75 mg/24 hr

Continued

FORMULARY

For explanation of icons, see p. 663.

IMIPRAMINE *continued*

Augment analgesia for chronic pain:

Initial: 0.2–0.4 mg/kg/dose QHS PO; increase 50% every 2–3 days to a **max. dose** of 1–3 mg/kg/dose QHS PO

Contraindicated in narrow-angle glaucoma and patients who used MAO inhibitors within 14 days. See Chapter 2 for management of toxic ingestion. Monitor for clinical worsening of depression and suicidal ideation/behavior following the initiation of therapy or after dose changes. **Use with caution** in renal or hepatic impairment. Side effects include sedation, urinary retention, constipation, dry mouth, dizziness, drowsiness, and arrhythmia. QHS dosing during first weeks of therapy will reduce sedation. Monitor ECG, BP, CBC at start of therapy and with dose changes. Tricyclics may cause mania.

Therapeutic reference range (sum of imipramine and desipramine) = 150–250 ng/mL. Levels >1000 ng/mL are toxic, however, toxicity may occur at >300 ng/mL.

Recommended serum sampling times at steady-state: Obtain trough level within 30 min prior to the next scheduled dose after 5–7 days of continuous therapy. Carbamazepine may reduce imipramine levels; and cimetidine, fluoxetine, fluvoxamine, labetolol, quinidine may increase imipramine levels.

Onset of antidepressant effects: 1–3 wk. **Do not discontinue abruptly** in patients receiving long-term high dose therapy.

IMMUNE GLOBULIN
Immune globulins

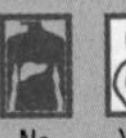
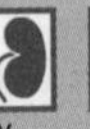
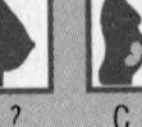
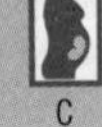

No Yes ? C

IM preparations:

GamaSTAN S/D: 150–180 mg/mL (2, 10 mL); contains 0.21–0.32 M glycine

IV preparations in solution:

Flebogamma 5% (50 mg/mL); contains 50 mg/mL sorbitol and ≤ 6 mg/mL polyethylene glycol
Gamunex: 10% (100 mg/mL); contains 0.16–0.24 M glycine
Gammagard liquid: 10% (100 mg/mL)
Octagam: 5% (50 mg/mL); contains 100 mg/mL maltose

IV preparations in powder for reconstitution:

Carimune NF: 1, 3, 6, 12 g (contains 1.67 g sucrose and <20 mg NaCl per 1 g Ig); dilute to 3, 6, 9, or 12%
Polygam S/D: 2.5, 5, 10 g (contains 3 mg/mL albumin, 22.5 mg/mL glycine, 20 mg/mL glucose, 2 mg/mL polyethylene glycol, 1 mcg/mL tri-n-butyl phosphate, 1 mcg/mL octoxynol 9, and 100 mcg/mL polysorbate 80); dilute to 5% or 10%

Subcutaneous (SC) preparations:

Hizentra: 200 mg/mL (5, 10, 20 mL); contains L-proline, polysorbate 80
Vivaglobin: 160 mg/mL (3, 10, 20 mL)

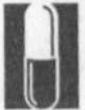

See indications and doses in Chapter 15.
General guidelines for administration (see package insert of specific products):
IV: Begin infusion at 0.01 mL/kg/min, double rate every 15–30 min, up to **max.** of 0.08 mL/kg/min. If adverse reactions occur, stop infusion until side effects subside and may restart at rate that was previously tolerated.
SC: Injection sites include the abdomen, thigh, upper arm and/or lateral hip. Doses may be administered into multiple sites (spaced ≥2 inches apart) simultaneously. See following table for product-specific guidelines.

Continued

IMMUNE GLOBULIN *continued*

SC Product	Max. Simultaneous Injection Sites	Max. Infusion Rate	Max. Infusion Volume
Hizentra	4	First infusion: 15 mL/hr per infusion site Subsequent infusions: 25 mL/hr per infusion site (**max.** 50 mL/hr for all simultaneous sites combined)	First 4 infusions: 15 mL per infusion site Subsequent infusions: 20–25 mL per infusion site
Vivaglobin	Child <45 kg: 3 Adult ≤65 yr: 6	20 mL/hr per infusion site (**max.** 1.13 mL/kg/hr for all simultaneous sites combined)	15 mL per infusion site

May cause flushing, chills, fever, headache, and hypotension. Hypersensitivity reaction may occur when IV form is administered rapidly. Gamimune-N contains maltose and may cause an osmotic diuresis. May cause **anaphylaxis** in IgA-deficient patients due to varied amounts of IgA. Some products are IgA depleted; consult a pharmacist.

Intravenous preparations containing sucrose **should not be infused** at a rate such that the amount of sucrose exceeds 3 mg/kg/min to decrease risk of renal dysfunction, including acute renal failure.

Subcutaneous route provides higher serum trough levels, lower rate of adverse reactions, and shorter administration time when compared with the IV route. Use an adjusted body weight [ABW = Ideal Body Weight + 0.5 (Actual Body Weight − Ideal Body Weight] dosing has been recommended for dosing in obese patients.

Delay immunizations after immune globulin administration (see latest AAP *Red Book* for details).

INDOMETHACIN
Indocin, Indocin SR, Indocin I.V., and various generics
Nonsteroidal antiinflammatory agent

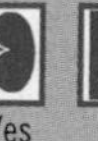
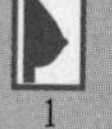
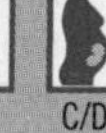
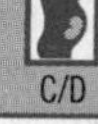

Yes Yes 1 C/D

Caps: 25, 50 mg
Sustained-release caps (Indocin SR and others): 75 mg
Oral suspension: 25 mg/5 mL (237 mL); contains 1% alcohol
Suppositories: 50 mg (30s)
Injection (Indocin I.V.): 1 mg

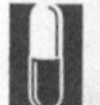

Anti-inflammatory/rheumatoid arthritis:
≥2 yr old: Start at 1–2 mg/kg/24 hr ÷ BID–QID PO; **max. dose:** the lesser of 4 mg/kg/24 hr or 200 mg/24 hr
Adult: 50–150 mg/24 hr ÷ BID–QID PO; **max. dose:** 200 mg/24 hr
Closure of ductus arteriosus:
Infuse intravenously over 20–30 min:

Postnatal Age	Dose (mg/kg/dose Q12–24 hr)* #1	#2	#3
<48 hr	0.2	0.1	0.1
2–7 days	0.2	0.2	0.2
>7 days	0.2	0.25	0.25

*Do not administer if urine output is <0.6 mL/kg/hr or anuric.

In infants <1500 g, 0.1–0.2 mg/kg/dose IV Q24 hr may be given for an additional 3–5 days.
Intraventricular hemorrhage prophylaxis: 0.1 mg/kg/dose IV Q24 hr × 3 doses, initiated at 6–12 hr of age (give in consultation with a neonatologist).

Continued

FORMULARY
For explanation of icons, see p. 663.

INDOMETHACIN *continued*

Contraindicated in active bleeding, coagulation defects, necrotizing enterocolitis, and renal insufficiency (urine output <0.6 mL/kg/hr). **Use with caution** in cardiac dysfunction, hypertension, heart disease (risk for MI and stroke with prolonged use), and renal or hepatic impairment. May cause (especially in neonates) decreased urine output, platelet dysfunction (thrombocytopenia), decreased GI blood flow, and reduce the antihypertensive effects of beta-blockers, hydralazine, and ACE inhibitors. **Fatal hepatitis reported in treatment of JRA.** Monitor renal and hepatic function before and during use.

Reduction in cerebral blood flow associated with rapid IV infusion; infuse all IV doses over 20–30 min.

Sustained-release capsules are dosed once daily–BID. Pregnancy category changes to "D" if used for >48 hr or after 34 wk gestation or close to delivery.

INSULIN PREPARATIONS

Pancreatic hormone

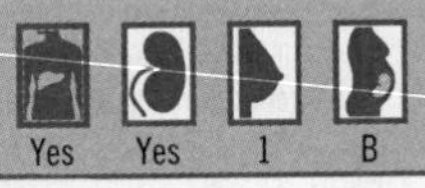

Many preparations, at concentrations of 40, 100, 500 U/mL. See Chapter 30, Table 30-4.

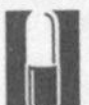 Diluted concentrations of 1 U/mL or 10 U/mL may be necessary for smaller doses in neonates and infants.

Hyperkalemia: See Chapter 11, Figure 11-2.
DKA: See Chapter 10, Figure 10-1.

When using insulin drip with new IV tubing, fill the tubing with the insulin infusion solution and wait for 30 min (before connecting tubing to the patient). Then flush the line and connect the IV line to the patient to start the infusion. This will ensure proper drug delivery. **Adjust dose in renal failure (see Chapter 31). Use with caution** and monitor closely in hepatic impairment.

IODIDE

See *Potassium Iodide*

IOHEXOL

Omnipaque 140, Omnipaque 240, Omnipaque 300, and Omnipaque 350

Radiopaque agent, contrast media

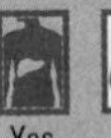

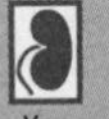

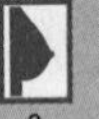

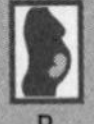

Injection:

Omnipaque 140: 302 mg iohexol equivalent to 140 mg iodine/mL (50 mL)
Omnipaque 240: 518 mg iohexol equivalent to 240 mg iodine/mL (10, 20, 50, 100, 150, 200 mL)
Omnipaque 300: 647 mg iohexol equivalent to 300 mg iodine/mL (10, 30, 50, 75, 100, 125, 150 mL)
Omnipaque 350: 755 mg iohexol equivalent to 350 mg iodine/mL (50, 75, 100, 125, 150, 200, 250 mL)

Continued

IOHEXOL *continued*

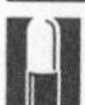

Contrast enhanced CT scan of the abdomen:

Oral (administered prior to IV dose):

Child: Mix 20 mL of Omnipaque 350 with 500 mL of noncarbonated beverage of patient's choice (apple juice works well for youger patients). Administer diluted contrast media PO 30–60 min prior to the IV dose and image acquisition using the following dosage:

- ***<6 mo:*** 40–60 mL
- ***6–18 mo:*** 120–160 mL
- ***18 mo–3 yr:*** 165–240 mL
- ***3 yr–12 yr:*** 250–360 mL
- ***>12 yr:*** 480–520 mL

Adult: Mix 50 mL of Omnipaque 350 with 1/2 gallon of noncarbonated beverage of patient's choice. Give 2–4 cups containing 480 mL (16 oz) of the diluted contrast media PO 20–40 min prior to the IV dose and image acquisition.

IV (administered after PO dose):

Child: 1–2 mL/kg IV of Omnipaque 240 or Omipaque 300 given 30–60 min after the oral dose. **Max. dose:** 3 mL/kg.

Adult: 100–150 mL IV of Omnipaque 300 given 20–40 min after the oral dose.

Use with caution in dehydration, previous allergic reaction to a contrast medium, iodine sensitivity, asthma, hay fever, food allergy, congestive heart failure, severe liver or renal impairment, diabetic nephropathy, multiple myeloma, pheochromocytoma, hyperthyroidism, and sickle cell disease. Allergic reactions, arrhythmias, and nephrotoxicity have been rarely reported. Children at higher risk for adverse events with contrast medium administration may include those having asthma, sensitivity to medication and/or allergens, congestive heart failure, serum creatinine >1.5 mg/dL, or <12 mo.

Use **NOT** recommended with drugs that lower seizure threshold (e.g., phenothiazines), amiodarone (increased risk of cardiotoxicity), and metformin (lactic acidosis and acute renal failure).

Many other uses exist, see package insert for additional information. Iohexol is particularly useful when barium sulfate is **contraindicated** in patients with suspected bowel perforation or those where aspiration of contrast medium is of concern. Oral dose is poorly absorbed from the normal GI tract (0.1%–0.5%); absorption increases with bowel perforation or bowel obstruction. Concentrations ≥518 mg iohexol/mL are hyperosmolar (1.8–3 times that of plasma).

IPRATROPIUM BROMIDE

Atrovent and other generics

Anticholinergic agent

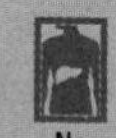

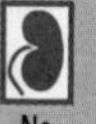

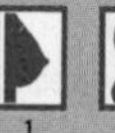

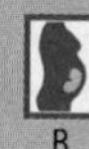

Aerosol (HFA): 17 mcg/dose (200 actuations per canister, 12.9 g)
Nebulized solution: 0.02% (500 mcg/2.5 mL, 25s, 30s, 60s)
Nasal spray: 0.03% (21 mcg per actuation, 30 mL); 0.06% (42 mcg per actuation, 15 mL)
In combination with albuterol:

Nebulized solution (DuoNeb): 0.5 mg ipratropium bromide and 2.5 mg albuterol in 3 mL (30s, 60s)

Aerosol (Combivent): 18 mcg ipratropium and 103 mcg albuterol per actuation (200 actuations per canister, 14.7 g)

Continued

For explanation of icons, see p. 663.

IPRATROPIUM BROMIDE *continued*

Acute use in the ED or ICU:

Nebulizer treatments:

<12 yr: 250 mcg/dose Q20 min × 3, then Q2–4 hr PRN

≥12 yr: 500 mcg/dose Q30 min × 3, then Q2–4 hr PRN

Inhaler:

Child and adult: 4–8 puffs PRN

Non-acute use:

Inhaler:

<12 yr: 1–2 puffs Q6 hr; **max. dose:** 12 puffs/24 hr

≥12 yr: 2–3 puffs Q6 hr; **max. dose:** 12 puffs/24 hr

Nebulized treatments: Infant: 125–250 mcg/dose Q8 hr

Child ≤12 yr: 250 mcg/dose Q6–8 hr

>12 yr and adult: 250–500 mcg/dose Q6–8 hr

Nasal spray:

Allergic and non-allergic rhinitis:

≥6 yr and adult: 2 sprays of 0.03% strength (42 mcg) per nostril BID–TID

Rhinitis associated with common cold (use up to a total of 4 days; safety and efficacy have not been evaluated >4 days):

5–11 yr: 2 sprays of 0.06% strength (84 mcg) per nostril TID

≥12 yr and adult: 2 sprays of 0.06% strength (84 mcg) per nostril TID–QID

Rhinitis associated with seasonal allergies (use up to a total of 3 weeks; safety and efficacy have not been evaluated >3 weeks):

≥5 yr and adult: 2 sprays of 0.06% strength (84 mcg) per nostril QID

Contraindicated in soy or peanut allergy (for aerosol inhaler) and atropine hypersensitivity. **Use with caution** in narrow-angle glaucoma or bladder neck obstruction, though ipratropium has fewer anticholinergic systemic effects than atropine. May cause anxiety, dizziness, headache, GI discomfort, and cough with inhaler or nebulized use. Epistaxis, nasal congestion, and dry mouth/throat have been reported with the nasal spray. Reversible anisocoria may occur with unintentional aerosolization of drug to the eyes; particularly with mask nebulizers. Proven efficacy of nebulized solution in pediatrics is currently limited to reactive airway disease management in the emergency room and intensive care unit areas.

Bronchodilation onset of action is 1–3 min with peak effects within 1.5–2 hr and duration of action of 4–6 hr.

Shake inhaler well prior to use with spacer. Nebulized solution may be mixed with albuterol (or use DuoNeb).

Breastfeeding safety **extrapolated** from safety of atropine.

IRON DEXTRAN

See *Iron—Injectable Preparations*

IRON SUCROSE

See *Iron—Injectable Preparations*

IRON—INJECTABLE PREPARATIONS
Ferric gluconate: Ferrlecit
Iron dextran: INFeD, DexFerrum
Iron sucrose: Venofer
Parenteral iron

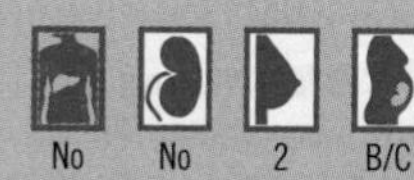

Injection:

Ferric gluconate (Ferrlecit): 62.5 mg/mL (12.5 mg elemental Fe/mL) (5 mL); contains 9 mg/mL benzyl alcohol and 20% sucrose
Iron dextran (INFeD, DexFerrum): 50 mg/mL (50 mg elemental Fe/mL) (1, 2 mL); products containing phenol 0.5% are only for IM administration; products containing sodium chloride 0.9% can be administered via the IM or IV route.
Iron sucrose (Venofer): 20 mg/mL (20 mg elemental Fe/mL) (5 mL); contains 300 mg/mL sucrose

FERRIC GLUCONATE (IV):
Iron deficiency anemia in patients undergoing chronic hemodialysis who are receiving supplemental erythropoietin therapy (most require 8 doses at 8 sequential dialysis treatments to achieve a favorable response):

Child ≥6 yr: 1.5 mg/kg elemental Fe (0.12 mL/kg) IV; **max. dose:** 125 mg elemental Fe/dose. Dilute dose in 25 mL NS and infuse over 1 hr.
Adult: 125 mg elemental Fe in 100 mL NS IV; infuse over 1 hr. Most require a minimum cumulative dose of 1 g elemental Fe administered over 8 sessions.

IRON DEXTRAN (IV or IM):
Iron deficiency anemia:

Test dose: 25 mg (12.5 mg for infants) IV (over 5 min) or IM. May initiate treatment dose 1 hr after test dose.
Total replacement dose of iron dextran (mL) = 0.0476 × lean body wt (kg) × (desired Hgb [g/dL] − measured Hgb [g/dL]) + 1 mL per 5 kg lean body weight (up to **max.** of 14 mL).

Acute blood loss: Total replacement dose of iron dextran (mL) = 0.02 × blood loss (mL) × hematocrit expressed as decimal fraction. Assumes 1 mL of RBC = 1 mg elemental iron. If no reaction to test dose, give remainder of replacement dose ÷ over 2–3 daily doses.

Max daily (IM) dose:

<5 kg: 0.5 mL (25 mg)
5–10 kg: 1 mL (50 mg)
>10 kg: 2 mL (100 mg)

IM administration: use "Z-track" technique.
IV administration: Dilute in NS at a max. concentration of 50 mg/mL and infuse over 1–6 hr at a **max.** rate of 50 mg/min.

IRON SUCROSE (IV):
Iron deficiency anemia in patients with chronic kidney disease:

Child (limited data from 14 children with ESRD on hemodialysis): 1 mg/kg/dialysis was adequate for correcting ferritin levels and 0.3 mg/kg/dialysis was successful in maintaining ferritin levels between 193–250 mcg/L. Doses were administered during the last hr of each dialysis and is recommended at a frequency of 3 times a week. A 10-mg test dose was administered.
Adult:

Hemodialysis-dependent: 100 mg elemental Fe 1–3 times a wk during dialysis up to a total cummulative dose of 1000 mg. May continue to administer at lowest dose to maintain target Hb, Hct, and iron levels.
Nonhemodialysis-dependent: 200 mg elemental Fe on 5 different days over a 2-wk period (total cummulative dose: 1000 mg).

Continued

For explanation of icons, see p. 663.

IRON—INJECTABLE PREPARATIONS *continued*

IRON SUCROSE (IV) (cont'd):

IV administration: May administer undiluted over 2–5 min. For an infusion, dilute each 100 mg with a **max.** of 100 mL NS and infuse over at least 15 min.

Oral therapy with iron salts is preferred, injectable routes are painful. Gluconate and sucrose salts may be better tolerated than iron dextran. Adverse effects include hypotension, GI disturbances, fever, rash, myalgia, arthralgias, cramps, and headaches. Hypersensitivity reactions (fatal anaphylaxis with iron dextran; use test dose prior to first therapeutic dose) have been reported.

IM administration is only possible with iron dextran salt. Follow infusion recommendations for specific product. Monitor vital signs during IV infusion. TIBC levels may not be meaningful within 3 wk after dosing.

Pregnancy category is "B" for ferric gluconate and iron sucrose and "C" for iron dextran.

IRON—ORAL PREPARATIONS

Fergon, Fer-In-Sol, Feosol, Niferex, Slow FE, and many others

Oral iron supplements

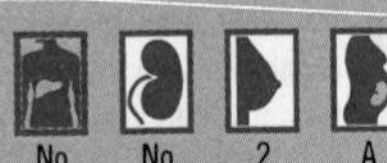

Ferrous sulfate (20% elemental Fe):

Drops (Fer-In-Sol, OTC): 75 mg (15 mg Fe)/0.6 mL (50 mL); contains 0.2% alcohol and sodium bisulfite
Elixir (OTC): 220 mg (44 mg Fe)/5 mL; contains 5% alcohol
Oral liquid (OTC): 300 mg (60 mg Fe)/5 mL
Tabs (OTC): 300 mg (60 mg Fe), 324 mg (65 mg Fe), 325 mg (65 mg Fe)

Ferrous gluconate (12% elemental Fe):

Tabs (OTC): 240 mg (27 mg Fe, as Fergon), 246 mg (28 mg Fe), 300 mg (34 mg Fe), 325 mg (36 mg Fe)

Ferrous sulfate, exsiccated/dried (30% elemental Fe):

Tabs (OTC): 200 mg (65 mg Fe)
Extended-release tabs (Slow FE, OTC): 160 mg (50 mg Fe)

Ferrous fumarate (33% elemental Fe):

Tabs (OTC): 90 mg (29.5 mg Fe), 200 mg (66 mg Fe), 324 mg (106 mg Fe), 325 mg (106 mg Fe), 350 mg (115 mg Fe)
Chewable tabs: 100 mg (33 mg Fe)
Timed-released tabs (OTC): 150 mg (50 mg Fe)

Polysaccharide-iron complex and ferrous bis-glycinate chelate (Niferex) (expressed in mg elemental Fe):

Caps (OTC): 60, 150 mg; 150 mg strength contains 50 mg vitamin C
Elixir (OTC): 100 mg/5 mL (237 mL); contains 10% alcohol

Iron deficiency anemia:

Premature infant: 2–4 mg elemental Fe/kg/24 hr ÷ once daily–BID PO; **max. dose:** 15 mg elemental Fe/24 hr
Child: 3–6 mg elemental Fe/kg/24 hr ÷ once daily–TID PO
Adult: 60–100 mg elemental Fe BID PO up to 60 mg elemental Fe QID

Prophylaxis:

Child: Give dose below PO ÷ once daily–TID
Premature: 2 mg elemental Fe/kg/24 hr; **max. dose:** 15 mg elemental Fe/24 hr
Full-term: 1–2 mg elemental Fe/kg/24 hr; **max. dose:** 15 mg elemental Fe/24 hr
Adult: 60–100 mg elemental Fe/24 hr PO ÷ once daily–BID

Continued

IRON—ORAL PREPARATIONS *continued*

Contraindicated in hemolytic anemia and hemochromatosis. **Avoid** use in GI tract inflammation.

Iron preparations are variably absorbed. Less GI irritation when given with or after meals. Vitamin C, 200 mg per 30 mg iron, may enhance absorption. Liquid iron preparations may stain teeth. Give with dropper or drink through straw. May produce constipation, dark stools (false positive guaiac is controversial), nausea, and epigastric pain. Iron and tetracycline inhibit each other's absorption. Antacids may decrease iron absorption.

ISONIAZID

INH, Nydrazid, Laniazid, and others
In combination with rifampin: Rifamate, IsonaRif
In combination with rifampin and pyrazinamide: Rifater
Antituberculous agent

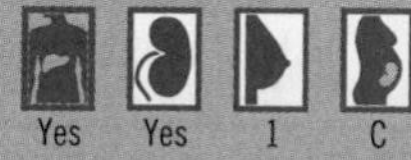

Tabs: 100, 300 mg
Syrup: 50 mg/5 mL (473 mL)
Injection: 100 mg/mL (10 mL); contains 0.25% chlorobutanol
In combination with rifampin:
Caps (Rifamate, IsonaRif): 150 mg isoniazid + 300 mg rifampin
In combination with rifampin and pyrazinamide:
Caps (Rifater): 50 mg isoniazid + 120 mg rifampin + 300 mg pyrazinamide

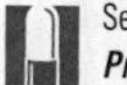

See most recent edition of the AAP *Red Book* for details and length of therapy.

Prophylaxis:

Infant and child: 10 mg/kg (**max. dose:** 300 mg) PO once daily. After 1 mo of daily therapy and in cases where daily compliance cannot be assured, may change to 20–40 mg/kg (**max. dose:** 900 mg) per dose PO, given twice weekly.

Adult: 300 mg PO once daily.

Treatment:

Infant and child:

10–15 mg/kg (**max. dose:** 300 mg) PO once daily or 20–30 mg/kg (**max. dose:** 900 mg) per dose twice weekly with rifampin for uncomplicated pulmonary tuberculosis in compliant patients. Additional drugs are necessary in complicated disease.

Adult:

5 mg/kg (**max. dose:** 300 mg) PO once daily or 15 mg/kg (**max. dose:** 900 mg) per dose twice weekly with rifampin. Additional drugs are necessary in complicated disease.

For INH-resistant TB: Discuss with Health Dept., or consult ID specialist.

Should not be used alone for treatment. Contraindicated in acute liver disease and previous isoniazid-associated hepatitis. Peripheral neuropathy, optic neuritis, seizures, encephalopathy, psychosis, hepatic side effects may occur with higher doses, especially in combination with rifampin. Severe liver injury has been reported in children and adults treated for latent TB. Follow LFTs monthly. Supplemental pyridoxine (1–2 mg/kg/24 hr) is recommended. May cause false-positive urine glucose test.

Inhibits CYP 450 1A2, 2C9, 2C19, and 3A3/4 microsomal enzymes; decrease dose of carbamazepine, diazepam, phenytoin, and prednisone. Prednisone may decrease isoniazid's effects. Also a substrate and inducer of CYP 450 2E1 and may potentiate acetaminophen hepatotoxicity.

May be given IM (same as oral doses) when oral therapy is not possible. Administer oral doses 1 hr prior to and 2 hr after meals. Aluminum salts may decrease absorption. **Adjust dose in renal failure (see Chapter 31).**

For explanation of icons, see p. 663.

ISOPROTERENOL
Isuprel and other generics
Adrenergic agonist

 No 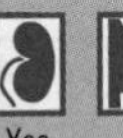 Yes 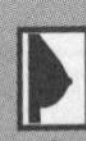 ? 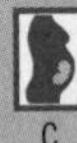 C

Isoproterenol HCl:
Injection, prefilled syringes: 0.02 mg/mL (10 mL); contains sulfites
Injection: 0.2 mg/mL (1, 5, 10 mL); contains sulfites

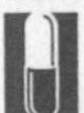

NOTE: The dosage units for adults are in mcg/min, compared to mcg/kg/min for children.
IV infusion:
Neonate–child: 0.05–2 mcg/kg/min; start at minimum dose and increase every 5–10 min by 0.1 mcg/kg/min until desired effect or onset of toxicity; **max. dose:** 2 mcg/kg/min.
Adult: 2–20 mcg/min.

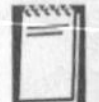

Use with caution in diabetes, hyperthyroidism, renal disease, CHF, ischemia, or aortic stenosis. May cause flushing, ventricular arrhythmias, profound hypotension, anxiety, and myocardial ischemia. Monitor heart rate, respiratory rate, and blood pressure. **Not** for treatment of asystole or for use in cardiac arrests, unless bradycardia is due to heart block.

Continuous infusion for bronchodilatation must be gradually tapered over a 24- to 48-hr period to prevent rebound bronchospasm. Tolerance may occur with prolonged use. Clinical deterioration, myocardial necrosis, congestive heart failure, and death have been reported with continuous infusion use in refractory asthmatic children.

ISOTRETINOIN
Accutane, Amnesteem, Claravis, Sotret
Retinoic acid, vitamin A derivative

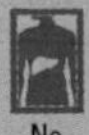 No 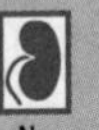 No 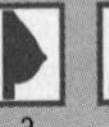 3 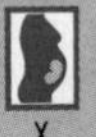 X

Caps: 10, 20, 30, 40 mg; may contain soybean oil, EDTA, and parabens

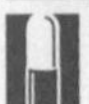

Cystic acne:
Child and adult: 0.5–2 mg/kg/24 hr ÷ BID PO × 15–20 wk or until the total cyst count decreases by 70%, whichever comes first.
Dosages as low as 0.05 mg/kg/24 hr have been reported to be beneficial.

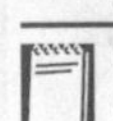

Contraindicated during pregnancy; known teratogen. Use with caution in females during childbearing years. May cause conjunctivitis, xerosis, pruritus, photosensitivity reactions (avoid exposure to sunlight and use sunscreen), epistaxis, anemia, hyperlipidemia, pseudotumor cerebri (especially in combination with tetracyclines; **avoid** this combination), cheilitis, bone pain, muscle aches, skeletal changes, lethargy, nausea, vomiting, elevated ESR, mental depression, aggressive/violent behavior, and psychosis.

To avoid additive toxic effects, **do not** take vitamin A concomitantly. Increases clearance of carbamazepine. Hormonal birth control (oral, injectable, and implantable) failures have been reported with concurrent use. Monitor CBC, ESR, triglycerides, and LFTs.

Prescribers, site pharmacists, patients, and wholesalers must register with the iPLEDGE system (a risk minimization program) at www.ipledgeprogram.com or 1-866-495-0654 before doses are dispensed. Prescriptions may not be written for more than a 1-mo supply.

ITRACONAZOLE
Sporanox
Antifungal agent

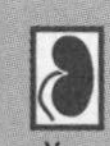

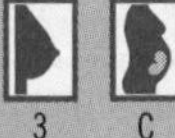
Yes Yes 3 C

Caps: 100 mg
Oral solution: 10 mg/mL (150 mL); contains sacharin and sorbitol

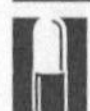

Child (limited data): 3–5 mg/kg/24 hr PO ÷ once daily–BID; dosages as high as 5–10 mg/kg/24 hr have been used for aspergillus prophylaxis in chronic granulomatous disease. Population pharmacokinetic data in pediatric Cystic Fibrosis and bone marrow transplant patients suggest an oral liquid dosage of 10 mg/kg/24 hr PO ÷ BID or oral capsule dosage of 20 mg/kg/24 hr PO ÷ BID to be more reliable for achieving trough plasma levels between 500 and 2000 ng/mL.

Prophylaxis for recurrence of opportunistic disease in HIV:

Cryptococcus neoformans: 2–5 mg/kg/dose PO Q12–24 hr

Histoplasma capsulatum or Coccidioides immitis: 2–5 mg/kg/dose PO Q12–48 hr

Adult:

Blastomycosis and nonmeningeal histoplasmosis:

PO: 200 mg once daily up to a max. dose of 400 mg/24 hr ÷ BID (**max. dose:** 200 mg/dose)

Aspergillosis and severe infections:

PO: 600 mg/24 hr ÷ TID × 3–4 days, followed by 200–400 mg/24 hr ÷ BID; **max. dose:** 600 mg/24 hr ÷ TID.

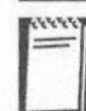

Oral solution and capsule dosage form should **NOT** be used interchangeably; oral solution is more bioavailable. Only the oral solution has been demonstrated effective for oral and/or esophageal candidiasis. Contraindicated in CHF and certain interacting drugs (see below). **Use with caution** in hepatic and/or renal impairment, cardiac dysrhythmias, and azole hypersensitivity. May cause GI symptoms, headaches, rash, liver enzyme elevation, hepatitis, and hypokalemia.

Like ketoconazole, it inhibits the activity of the CYP-450 3A4 drug metabolizing isoenzyme. Thus the coadministration of cisapride, dofetilide, pimozide, nisoldipine, levacetylmethadol, quinidine, triazolam, lovastatin, simvastatin, ergot derivatives, and oral midazolam is **contraindicated.** See remarks in *Ketoconazole* for additional drug interaction information.

Steady-state trough serum concentrations of >250 ng/mL itraconazole and >1000 ng/mL hydroxyitraconazole (metabolite) have been recommended. Recommended serum sampling time at steady-state: trough level after 2 wk after continuous dosing.

Administer oral solution on an empty stomach, but administer capsules with food. Achlorhydria reduces absorption of the drug.

KANAMYCIN
Kantrex and others
Antibiotic, aminoglycoside

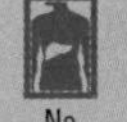
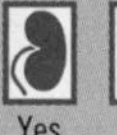
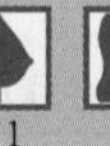
No Yes 1 D

Injection: 333 mg/mL (3 mL); may contain sulfites

Neonate IV/IM administration (see following table):

Birth Weight (kg)	<7 days	≥7 days
<2	15 mg/kg/ 24 hr ÷ Q12 hr	22.5 mg/kg/ 24 hr ÷ Q8 hr
≥2	20 mg/kg/ 24 hr ÷ Q12 hr	30 mg/kg/ 24 hr ÷ Q8 hr

Continued

For explanation of icons, see p. 663.

KANAMYCIN *continued*

Infant and child: IM/IV: 15–30 mg/kg/24 hr ÷ Q8–12 hr
Adult: IV/IM: 15 mg/kg/24 hr ÷ Q8–12 hr
PO administration for GI bacterial overgrowth: 150–250 mg/kg/24 hr ÷ Q6 hr; **max. dose:** 4 g/24 hr

Renal toxicity and ototoxicity may occur. Give over 30 min if IV route is used. **Use with caution** in neuromuscular disorders, anesthesia and muscle-relaxant medications, and hypermagnesemia. **Adjust dose in renal failure (see Chapter 31).** Poorly absorbed orally, PO used to treat GI bacterial overgrowth. Oral route is **contraindicated** in intestinal obstructions.

Therapeutic levels: peak: 15–30 mg/L; trough: <5–10 mg/L. Recommended serum sampling time at steady-state: trough within 30 min prior to the 3rd consecutive dose and peak 30–60 min after the administration of the 3rd consecutive dose.

KETAMINE

Ketalar and various generics
General anesthetic

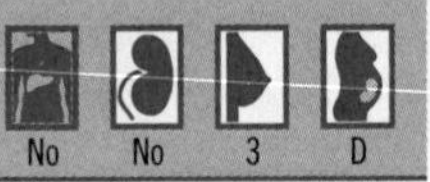

Injection: 10 mg/mL (20 mL), 50 mg/mL (10 mL), 100 mg/mL (5 mL); contains benzethonium chloride

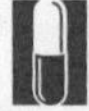

Child:
Sedation:
PO: 5 mg/kg × 1
IV (see remarks): 0.5–1 mg/kg
IM: 3–6 mg/kg × 1

Adult:
Analgesia with sedation:
IV (see remarks): 0.2–1 mg/kg
IM: 0.5–4 mg/kg

Contraindicated in elevated ICP, hypertension, aneurysms, thyrotoxicosis, CHF, angina, and psychotic disorders. May cause hypertension, hypotension, emergence reactions, tachycardia, laryngospasm, respiratory depression, and stimulation of salivary secretions. Intravenous use may induce general anesthesia. Benzodiazepine may be added to prevent emergence phenomenon. Anticholinergic agent may be added to decrease hypersalivation. Rate of IV infusion **should not exceed** 0.5 mg/kg/min and should **not be administered** in less than 60 sec. For additional information including onset and duration of action, see Chapter 6, Table 6-10.

KETOCONAZOLE

Nizoral, Nizoral A-D and others
Antifungal agent, imidazole

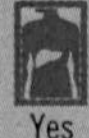

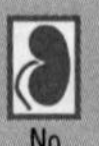

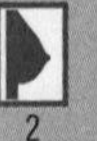

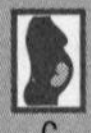

Tabs: 200 mg
Oral suspension: 100 mg/5 mL
Cream: 2% (15, 30, 60 g); contains sulfites
Shampoo: 1% [Nizoral A-D, OTC] (120, 210 mL), 2% (120 mL)
Gel: 2% [Xolegel] (15, 45 g)
Foam: 2% [Extina] (50, 100 g)

Continued

KETOCONAZOLE *continued*

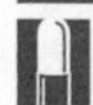

Oral:

Child ≥2 yr: 3.3–6.6 mg/kg/24 hr once daily

Adult: 200–400 mg/24 hr once daily

Max. dose: 800 mg/24 hr ÷ BID

Topical: 1–2 applications/24 hr

Shampoo (dandruff): Twice weekly with at least 3 days between applications for up to 8 weeks PRN. Thereafter, intermittently as needed to maintain control.

Suppressive therapy against mucocutaneous candidiasis in HIV:

Child: 5–10 mg/kg/24 hr ÷ once daily–BID PO; **max. dose:** 800 mg/24 hr ÷ BID

Adolescent and adult: 200 mg/dose once daily PO

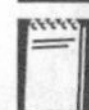

Monitor LFTs in long-term use. Drugs that decrease gastric acidity will decrease absorption. May cause nausea, vomiting, rash, headache, pruritus, and fever. Hepatotoxicity (including fatal cases) has been reported; use with caution in hepatic impairment. High doses may decrease adrenocortical function and serum testosterone levels.

Inhibits CYP 450 3A4. **Contraindicated** when used with cisapride, quinidine, terfinadine, and pimozide because of risk for cardiac arrhythmias. May increase levels/effects of phenytoin, digoxin, cyclosporine, corticosteroids, nevirapine, protease inhibitors, and warfarin. Achlorhydria, phenobarbital, rifampin, isoniazid, H_2 blockers, antacids, and omeprazole can decrease levels of ketoconazole.

Administering oral doses with food or acidic beverages and 2 hr prior to antacids will increase absorption.

To use shampoo, wet hair and scalp with water, apply sufficient amount to scalp and gently massage for about 1 min. Rinse hair thoroughly, reapply shampoo and leave on the scalp for an additional 3 min; then rinse.

KETOROLAC

Many generics (previously available as Toradol), Acular, Acular LS, Acular PF

Nonsteroidal anti-inflammatory agent

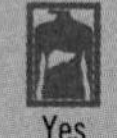
Yes

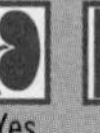
Yes

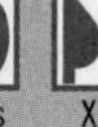
X

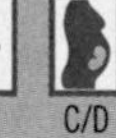
C/D

Injection: 15 mg/mL (1 mL), 30 mg/mL (1, 2 mL); contains 10% alcohol

Tabs: 10 mg

Ophthalmic:

Acular: 0.5% (3, 5, 10 mL); contains benzalkonium chloride

Acular PF: 0.5% (0.4 mL); preservative-free

Acular LS: 0.4% (5 mL); contains benzalkonium chloride

Systemic use is not to exceed 3–5 days; regardless of administration route (IM, IV, PO).

IM/IV:

Child: 0.5 mg/kg/dose IM/IV Q6–8 hr. **Max. dose:** 30 mg Q6 hr or 120 mg/24 hr. Alternatively, the manufacturer has recommended the following doses for children 2–16 yr with moderate/severe acute pain:

IV: 0.5 mg/kg ×1; **max. dose:** 15 mg

IM: 1 mg/kg ×1; **max. dose:** 30 mg

Adult: 30 mg IM/IV Q6 hr. **Max. dose:** 120 mg/24 hr

PO:

Child >50 kg and adult: 10 mg PRN Q6 hr; **max. dose:** 40 mg/24 hr

Ophthalmic (see remarks):

≥3 yr–adult: 1 drop in each affected eye QID

Continued

For explanation of icons, see p. 663.

KETOROLAC *continued*

May cause GI bleeding, nausea, dyspepsia, drowsiness, decreased platelet function, and interstitial nephritis. **Not recommended** in patients at increased risk of bleeding. **Do not use** in hepatic or renal failure. **Use with caution** in heart disease (risk for MI and stroke with prolonged use).

Use Acular PF for incisional refractive surgery and Acular LS for cornal refractive surgery. Duration of therapy for ophthalmic use: 14 days after cataract surgery; up to 4 days after cornal refractive surgery; and up to 3 days after incisional refractive surgery.

Pregnancy category changes to a "D" if used in the third trimester.

LABETALOL
Normodyne, Trandate, and various generics
Adrenergic antagonist (alpha and beta), antihypertensive

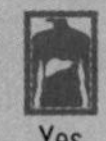 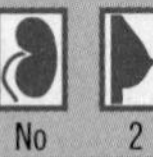 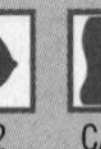 

Yes No 2 C/D

Tabs: 100, 200, 300 mg
Injection: 5 mg/mL (20, 40 mL); contains parabens
Oral suspension: 10, 40 mg/mL

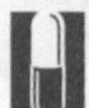

Child (see remarks):

PO: Initial: 4 mg/kg/24 hr ÷ BID. May increase up to 40 mg/kg/24 hr

IV: Hypertensive emergency (start at lowest dose and titrate to effect; see Chapter 4):

Intermittent dose: 0.2–1 mg/kg/dose Q10 min PRN; **max. dose:** 20 mg/dose

Infusion (hypertensive emergencies): 0.4–1 mg/kg/hr, to a **max. dose** of 3 mg/kg/hr; may initiate with a 0.2–1 mg/kg bolus; **max. bolus:** 20 mg.

Adult (see remarks):

PO: 100 mg BID, increase by 100 mg/dose Q2–3 days PRN to a **max. dose** of 2.4 g/24 hr. Usual range: 200–800 mg/24 hr ÷ BID

IV: Hypertensive emergency (start at lowest dose and titrate to effect with a **maximum** total dose of 300 mg for both methods of administration):

Intermittent dose: 20–80 mg/dose (begin with 20 mg) Q10 min PRN

Infusion: 2 mg/min, increase to titrate to response.

Contraindicated in asthma, pulmonary edema, cardiogenic shock, and heart block. May cause orthostatic hypotension, edema, CHF, bradycardia, AV conduction disturbances, bronchospasm, urinary retention, and skin tingling. **Use with caution** in hepatic disease (dose reduction may be necessary), diabetes, liver function test elevation, hepatic necrosis, hepatitis, and cholestatic jaundice have been reported. Use with digitalis glycosides may increase risk for bradycardia.

Patient should remain supine for up to 3 hr after IV administration. Pregnancy category changes to "D" if used in second or third trimesters.

Onset of action: PO: 1–4 hr; IV: 5–15 min.

LACTULOSE
Cephulac, Chronulac, Enuloase, and other generics
Ammonium detoxicant, hyperosmotic laxative

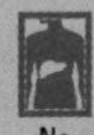 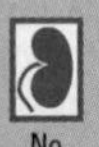  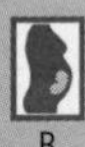

No No ? B

Syrup: 10 g/15 mL (15, 30, 237, 473, 960, 1893 mL); contains galactose, lactose, and other sugars
Crystals for reconstitution: 10 g (30s), 20 g (30s)

Continued

LACTULOSE *continued*

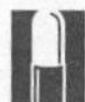

Chronic constipation:
- ***Child:*** 7.5 mL/24 hr PO after breakfast
- ***Adult:*** 15–30 mL/24 hr PO once daily to a **max. dose** of 60 mL/24 hr

Portal systemic encephalopathy (adjust dose to produce 2–3 soft stools/day):
- ***Infant:*** 2.5–10 mL/24 hr PO ÷ TID–QID
- ***Child:*** 40–90 mL/24 hr PO ÷ TID–QID
- ***Adult:*** 30–45 mL/dose PO TID–QID; acute episodes 30–45 mL Q1–2 hr until 2–3 soft stools/day
- ***Rectal (adult):*** 300 mL diluted in 700 mL water or NS in 30–60 min retention enema; may give Q4–6 hr

Contraindicated in galactosemia. **Use with caution** in diabetes mellitus. GI discomfort and diarrhea may occur. For portal systemic encephalopathy, monitor serum ammonia, serum potassium, and fluid status.

Adjust dose to achieve 2–3 soft stools per day. **Do not use** with antacids. Dissolve crystal dosage form with 4 ounces of water or juice. All doses may be adiministered with juice, milk, or water.

LAMIVUDINE

Epivir, Epivir-HBV, 3TC

Antiviral agent, nucleoside analogue reverse transcriptase inhibitor

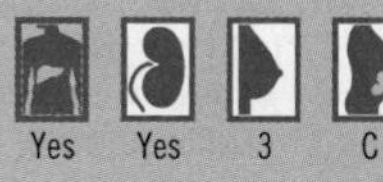

Yes Yes 3 C

Tabs: 100 mg (Epivir-HBV), 150, 300 mg
Oral solution: 5 mg/mL (Epivir-HBV), 10 mg/mL; contains parabens

HIV: See www.aidsinfo.nih.gov/guidelines.

Chronic hepatitis B (see remarks):
- ***2–17 yr:*** 3 mg/kg/dose PO once daily up to a **max. dose** of 100 mg/dose
- ***≥18 and adult:*** 100 mg/dose PO once daily

See aidsinfo.nih.gov/guidelines for remarks for use in HIV.

May cause headache, fatigue, GI disturbances, rash, and myalgia/arthralgia. Lactic acidosis, severe hepatomegaly with steatosis, post-treatment exacerbations of hepatitis B and ALT elevations, pancreatitis, and emergence of resistant viral strains have been reported. Concomitant use with cotrimoxazole (TMP/SMX) may result in increase lamivudine levels.

Use Epivir-HBV product for chronic hepatitis B indication. Safety and effectiveness beyond 1 yr have not been determined. Patients with both HIV and hepatitis B should use the higher HIV doses along with an appropriate combination regimen.

May be administered with food. **Adjust dose in renal impairment (see Chapter 31).**

LAMOTRIGINE

Lamictal, Lamictal ODT, Lamictal XR

Anticonvulsant

Yes Yes 2 C

Tabs: 25, 100, 150, 200 mg
Extended release tabs (Lamictal XR): 25, 50, 100, 200 mg
Chewable tabs: 2, 5, 25 mg
Orally disintegrated tabs (Lamictal ODT): 25, 50, 100, 200 mg
Oral suspension: 1 mg/mL

Continued

For explanation of icons, see p. 663.

LAMOTRIGINE *continued*

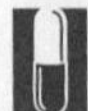

Child 2–12 yr adjunctive therapy (see remarks):
WITH anti-epileptic drugs (AEDs) other than carbamazepine, phenytoin, phenobarbital, primidone, or valproic acid (use immediate release dosage forms):

Wk 1 and 2: 0.3 mg/kg/24 hr PO ÷ once daily–BID; rounded down to the nearest whole tablet.
Wk 3 and 4: 0.6 mg/kg/24 hr PO ÷ BID; rounded down to the nearest whole tablet.
Usual maintenance dose: 4.5–7.5 mg/kg/24 hr PO ÷ BID titrate to effect; to achieve the usual maintenance dose, increase doses Q 1–2 wk by 0.6 mg/kg/24 hr (rounded down to the nearest whole tablet) as needed.
Max. dose: 300 mg/24 hr ÷ BID.

WITH enzyme inducing AEDs WITHOUT valproic acid (use immediate release dosage forms):

Wk 1 and 2: 0.6 mg/kg/24 hr PO ÷ BID; rounded down to the nearest whole tablet.
Wk 3 and 4: 1.2 mg/kg/24 hr PO ÷ BID; rounded down to the nearest whole tablet.
Usual maintenance dose: 5–15 mg/kg/24 hr PO ÷ BID titrate to effect; to achieve the usual maintenance dose, increase doses Q 1–2 wk by 1.2 mg/kg/24 hr (rounded down to the nearest whole tablet) as needed.
Max. dose: 400 mg/24 hr ÷ BID.

WITH AEDs WITH valproic acid (use immediate release dosage forms):

Wk 1 and 2: 0.15 mg/kg/24 hr PO ÷ once daily–BID; rounded down to the nearest whole tablet (see following table)
Wk 3 and 4: 0.3 mg/kg/24 hr PO ÷ once daily–BID; rounded down to the nearest whole tablet (see following table)

Weight (kg)	Weeks 1 & 2	Weeks 3 & 4
6.7–14	2 mg every other day	2 mg once daily
14.1–27	2 mg once daily	4 mg/24 hr ÷ once daily–BID
27.1–34	4 mg/24 hr ÷ once daily–BID	8 mg/24 hr ÷ once daily–BID
34.1–40	5 mg once daily	10 mg/24 hr ÷ once daily–BID

Usual maintenance dose: 1–5 mg/kg/24 hr PO ÷ once daily–BID titrate to effect; to achieve the usual maintenance dose, increase doses Q 1–2 wk by 0.3 mg/kg/24 hr (rounded down to the nearest whole tablet) as needed. If adding lamotrigine with valproic acid alone, usual maintenance dose is 1–3 mg/kg/24 hr.
Max. dose: 200 mg/24 hr.

>12 yr and adult adjunctive therapy:

WITH AEDs other than carbamazepine, phenytoin, phenobarbital, primidone, or valproic acid (use immediate release dosage forms):

Wk 1 and 2: 25 mg once daily PO
Wk 3 and 4: 50 mg once daily PO
Usual maintenance dose: 225–375 mg/24 hr ÷ BID PO titrate to effect; to achieve the usual maintenance dose, increase doses Q 1–2 wk by 50 mg/24 hr as needed.

WITH enzyme-inducing AEDs WITHOUT valproic acid (use immediate release dosage forms):

Wk 1 and 2: 50 mg once daily PO
Wk 3 and 4: 50 mg BID PO
Usual maintenance dose: 300–500 mg/24 hr ÷ BID PO titrate to effect; to achieve the usual maintenance dose, increase doses Q 1–2 wk by 100 mg/24 hr as needed. Doses as high as 700 mg/24 hr ÷ BID have been used.

WITH AEDs WITH valproic acid: (use immediate release dosage forms)

Wk 1 and 2: 25 mg every other day PO
Wk 3 and 4: 25 mg once daily PO

Continued

LAMOTRIGINE *continued*

Usual maintenance dose: 100–400 mg/24 hr ÷ once daily–BID PO titrate to effect; to achieve the usual maintenance dose, increase doses Q 1–2 wk by 25–50 mg/24 hr as needed. If adding lamotrigene to valproic acid alone, usual maintenance dose is 100–200 mg/kg/24 hr.

Extended-release dosage form (Lamictal XR):

≥13 yr and adult adjunctive therapy (maximum dose increases after week 8: 100 mg/24 hr at weekly intervals; see remarks):

	Weeks 1 & 2	Weeks 3 & 4	Week 5	Week 6	Week 7	Maintenance Dose
Patient NOT receiving enzyme-inducing drugs (e.g., carbamazepine) OR valproic acid	25 mg once daily	50 mg once daily	100 mg once daily	150 mg once daily	200 mg once daily	300–400 mg once daily
Patients receiving enzyme-inducing drugs (e.g., carbamazepine) WITHOUT valproic acid	50 mg once daily	100 mg once daily	200 mg once daily	300 mg once daily	400 mg once daily	400–600 mg once daily
Patients receiving valproic acid	25 mg every other day	25 mg once daily	50 mg once daily	100 mg once daily	150 mg once daily	200–250 mg once daily

Converting from a single enzyme-inducing AED to lamotrigine monotherapy for child ≥16 yr and adult (titrate lamotrigine to maintenance dose; then gradually withdraw enzyme-inducing AED by 20% decrements over a 4-wk period; use immediate release dosage forms):

Wk 1 and 2: 50 mg once daily PO

Wk 3 and 4: 50 mg BID PO

Usual maintenance dose: 500 mg/24 hr ÷ BID PO titrate to effect; to achieve the usual maintenance dose, increase doses Q 1–2 wk by 100 mg/24 hr as needed.

Bipolar disease (use immediate release dosage forms):

≥18 yr and adult (PO; see table below):

	Weeks 1 & 2	Weeks 3 & 4	Week 5	Weeks 6 and Thereafter
Patient NOT receiving enzyme-inducing drugs (e.g., carbamazepine) OR valproic acid	25 mg/24 hr	50 mg/24 hr	100 mg/24 hr	200 mg/24 hr (target dose)
Patents receiving enzyme-inducing drugs (e.g., carbamazepine) WITHOUT valproic acid	50 mg/24 hr	100 mg/24 hr ÷ once daily–BID	200 mg/24 hr ÷ once daily–BID	Week 6: 300 mg/24 hr ÷ once daily–BID Week 7 and thereafter: may increase to 400 mg/24 hr ÷ once daily–BID (target dose)*
Patients receiving valproic acid**	25 mg every other day	25 mg/24 hr	50 mg/24 hr	100 mg/24 hr (target dose)^

*If carbamazepine or other enzyme-inducing drug is discontinued, maintain current lamotrigine dose for 1 wk, then decrease daily lamotrigine dose in 100 mg increments at weekly intervals until 200 mg/24 hr.

^If valproic acid is discontinued, increase by 50 mg weekly intervals up to 200 mg/24 hr.

Continued

For explanation of icons, see p. 663.

LAMOTRIGINE *continued*

Enzyme-inducing antiepileptic drugs (AEDs) include carbamazepine, phenytoin, and phenobarbital. Stevens-Johnson syndrome, toxic epidermal necrolysis, and other potentially life-threatening rashes have been reported in children (0.8%) and adults (0.3%) for adjunctive therapy in seizures. Reported rates for adults treated for bipolar/mood disorders as monotherapy and adjunctive therapy are 0.08% and 0.13%, respectively. May cause fatigue, drowsiness, ataxia, rash (especially with valproic acid), headache, nausea, vomiting, and abdominal pain. Diplopia, nystagmus, aseptic meningitis, and alopecia have also been reported. Use during the first 3 mo of pregnancy may result in a higher chance for cleft lip or cleft palate in the newborn. Suicidal behavior or ideation have been reported.

If converting from immediate release to extended release dosage form, initial dose of extended release should match the total daily dose of the immediate release dosage and be administered once daily. Adjust dose as needed with the recommended dosage guidelines.

Reduce maintenance dose in renal failure. Reduce all doses (initial, escalation, and maintenance) in liver dysfunction defined by the Child-Pugh grading system as follows:

Grade B: moderate dysfunction, decrease dose by ~50%

Grade C: severe dysfunction, decrease dose by ~75%

Withdrawal symptoms may occur if discontinued suddenly. A stepwise dose reduction over ≥2 wk (~50% per week) is recommended unless safety concerns require a more rapid withdrawal.

Acetaminophen, carbamazepine, oral contraceptives (ethinylestradiol), phenobarbital, primidone, phenytoin, and rifampin may decrease levels of lamotrigine. Valproic acid may increase levels.

LANSOPRAZOLE
Prevacid
Gastric acid pump inhibitor

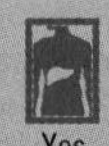
Yes
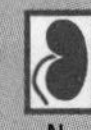
No
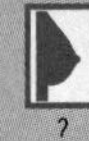
?
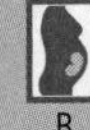
B

Caps, delayed-release: 15, 30 mg
Tabs, disintegrating delayed-release: 15, 30 mg; contains aspartame
Granules for delayed release oral suspension: 15, 30 mg packets (30s)
Oral suspension: 3 mg/mL; contains ~0.3 mEq sodium bicarbonate per 1 mg drug
Injection: 30 mg; contains 60 mg mannitol

1–11 yr (short-term treatment of GERD and erosive esophagitis, for up to 12 wk):

Initial dose:

- ***≤30 kg:*** 15 mg PO once daily
- ***>30 kg:*** 30 mg PO once daily–BID

Subsequent dosage increase (if needed): may be increased up to 30 mg PO BID after ≥2 wk of therapy without response at initial dose level.

12 yr–adult:

GERD: 15 mg PO once daily for up to 8 wk

Erosive esophagitis:

- ***PO:*** 30 mg once daily × 8–16 wk; maintenance dose: 15 mg PO once daily
- ***IV:*** 30 mg once daily for up to 7 days and convert to PO as soon as possible.

Duodenal ulcer: 15 mg PO once daily × 4 wk

Gastric ulcer and NSAID induced ulcer: 30 mg PO once daily for up to 8 wk

Hypersecretory conditions: 60 mg PO once daily; dosage may be increased up to 90 mg PO BID, where doses >120 mg/24 hr are divided BID.

Continued

LANSOPRAZOLE *continued*

Common side effects include GI discomfort, headache, fatigue, rash, and taste perversion. Microscopic colitis resulting in watery diarrhea has been reported and switching to an alternative proton-pump inhibitor may be beneficial in resolving diarrhea.

Drug is a substrate for CYP 450 2C19 and 3A3/4. May decrease absorption of itraconazole, ketoconazole, iron salts, and ampicillin esters; and increase the effects of warfarin. Theophylline clearance may be enhanced. Reduce dose in severe hepatic impairment. May be used in combination with clarithromycin and amoxicillin for *H. pylori* infections.

Administer all oral doses before meals and 30 min prior to sucralfate. **Do not** crush or chew the granules (all dosage forms). Capsule may be opened and intact granules may be administered in an acidic beverage (e.g., apple or cranberry juice) or apple sauce. **Do not** break or cut the orally disintegrating tablets. The extemporaneously compounded oral suspension may be less bioavailable owing to the loss of the enteric coating. For IV use, use a 1.2-micron in-line filter.

LEVALBUTEROL

Xopenex, Xopenex HFA

Beta-2 adrenergic agonist

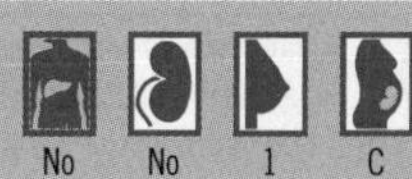

Prediluted nebulized solution: 0.31 mg in 3 mL, 0.63 mg in 3 mL, 1.25 mg in 3 mL (24s)
Concentrated nebulized solution: 1.25 mg/0.5 mL (0.5 mL)
Aerosol inhaler (MDI; Xopenex HFA): 45 mcg/actuation (15 g delivers 200 doses)

Nebulizer:

<4 yr: Start at 0.31 mg inhaled Q4–6 hr PRN; dose may be increased up to 1.25 mg Q4–6 hr PRN

5–11 yr: Start at 0.31 mg inhaled Q8 hr PRN; dose may be increased to 0.63 mg Q8 hr PRN

≥12 yr and adult: Start at 0.63 mg inhaled Q8 hr PRN; dose may be increased to 1.25 mg inhaled Q8 hr PRN

Aerosol inhaler (MDI):

≥4 yr and adult: 2 puffs Q4–6 hr PRN

For use in acute exacerbations, more aggressive dosing may be employed.

R-isomer of racemic albuterol. Side effects include tachycardia, palpitations, tremor, insomnia, nervousness, nausea, and headache.

Current clinical data in children indicate levalbuterol is as effective as albuterol with fewer cardiac side effects at equi-potent doses (0.31–0.63 mg levalbuterol ~2.5 mg albuterol).

More frequent dosing may be necessary in asthma exacerbation.

LEVETIRACETAM

Keppra, Keppra XR, and generics

Anticonvulsant

No | Yes | 2 | C

Tabs: 250, 500, 750, 1000 mg
Extended release tabs (Keppra XR): 500, 750 mg
Oral solution: 100 mg/mL (480 mL); dye free and contains parabens
Injection: 100 mg/mL (5 mL); contains 45 mg sodium chloride and 8.2 mg sodium acetate trihydrate per 100 mg drug

Continued

For explanation of icons, see p. 663.

LEVETIRACETAM *continued*

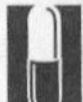

Partial seizures (adjunctive therapy; using immediate release dosage forms):

Child 4–15 yr: Start at 10 mg/kg/dose PO BID; may increase by 10 mg/kg/dose BID every 2 wk as tolerated up to a **max. dose** of 30 mg/kg/dose BID.

16 yr–adult: Start at 500 mg PO BID; may increase by 500 mg/dose BID every 2 wk as tolerated up to a **max. dose** of 1500 mg BID.

Myoclonic seizure (adjunctive therapy; using immediate release dosage forms):

≥12 yr and adult: Start at 500 mg PO BID; then increase dosage by 500 mg/dose BID every 2 wk to reach the target dosage of 1500 mg BID.

Tonic-clonic seizure (primary generalized, adjunctive therapy; use immediate release dosage forms):

Child 6–15 yr: Start at 10 mg/kg/dose PO BID; may increase by 10 mg/kg/dose BID every 2 wk to reach the target dosage of 30 mg/kg/dose BID.

16 yr–adult: Start at 500 mg PO BID; then increase dosage by 500 mg/dose BID every 2 wk to reach the target dosage of 1500 mg BID.

Refractory seizures (add-on therapy; data limited to): See remarks.

Do not abruptly withdrawal therapy to reduce risk for seizures. **Use with caution** in renal impairment **(reduce dose; see Chapter 31),** hemodialysis, and neuropsychiatric conditions.

May cause loss of appetite, vomiting, dizziness, headaches, somnolence, agitation, depression, and mood swings. Drowsiness, fatigue, nervousness, and aggressive behavor have been reported in children. Suicidal behavior or ideation, and hematologic abnormalities have been reported. Levetiracetam may decrease carbamazepine's effects. Ginkgo may decrease levetriacetam's effects.

Use in children 6 mo–4 yr have been reported in refractory seizures of various types and as an add-on therapy. The following dosage had been used: Start at 5–10 mg/kg/24 hr PO ÷ BID–TID, if needed and tolerated, increase dose by 10 mg/kg/24 hr at weekly intervals up to a **max. dose** of 60 mg/kg/24 hr.

Drug has excellent PO absorption. For IV use, use similar immediate release PO dosages only when the oral route of administration is not feasible. Extended release tablet is designed for once daily administration at similar daily dosage of the immediate release forms (e.g., 1000 mg once daily of the extended release tablet is equivalent to 500 mg BID of the immediate release tablet).

LEVOCARNITINE

See *Carnitine*

LEVOFLOXACIN

Levaquin, Quixin, Iquix, and generics

Antibiotic, quinolone

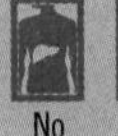
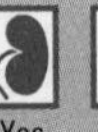
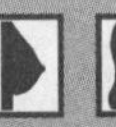
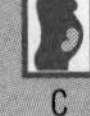

No Yes 3 C

Tabs: 250, 500, 750 mg

Oral solution: 25 mg/mL (480 mL)

Injection: 25 mg/mL (20, 30 mL)

Prediluted injection in D_5W: 250 mg/50 mL, 500 mg/100 mL, 750 mg/150 mL

Ophthalmic drops:

Quixin: 0.5% (5 mL)

Iquix: 1.5% (5 mL)

Continued

LEVOFLOXACIN *continued*

Child:

Recurrent or persistent acute otitis media (6 mo–<5 yr): 10 mg/kg/dose PO Q12 hr × 10 days; **max. dose:** 500 mg/24 hr

Community acquired pneumonia (see remarks) and data from a single-dose pharmacokinetic study to provide similar drug exposures associated with clinical efficacy and safety as seen in adults:

6 mo–<5 yr: 10 mg/kg/dose PO/IV Q12 hr

5–12 yr: 10 mg/kg/dose PO/IV Q24 hr; **max. dose:** 500 mg/24 hr

Adult:

Community acquired pneumonia: 500 mg PO/IV Q24 hr × 7–14 days; OR 750 mg PO/IV Q24 hr × 5 days

Complicated UTI/acute pyelonephritis: 250 PO/IV Q24 hr × 10 days; OR 750 mg PO/IV Q24 hr × 5 days

Uncomplicated UTI: 250 mg PO/IV Q24 hr × 3 days

Uncomplicated skin/skin structure infection: 500 mg PO/IV Q24 hr × 7–10 days

Acute bacterial sinusitis: 500 mg PO/IV Q24 hr × 10–14 days; OR 750 mg PO/IV Q24 hr × 5 days

Inhalational anthrax (post-exposure): Initiate immediately after exposure at 500 mg PO/IV Q24 hr × 60 days

Conjunctivitis:

≥1 yr and adult: Instill 1–2 drops of the 0.5% solution to affected eye(s) Q2 hr up to 8 times/24 hr while awake for the first 2 days, then Q4 hr up to 4 times/24 hr while awake for the next 5 days.

Corneal ulcer:

≥6 yr and adult: Instill 1–2 drops of the 1.5% solution to affected eye(s) Q30 min–2 hr while awake and 4 and 6 hr after retiring for the first 3 days, then Q1–4 hr while awake.

Contraindicated in hypersensitivity to other quinolones. **Avoid** in patients with history of QTc prolongation or taking QTc prolonging drugs, and excessive sunlight exposure. **Use with caution** in diabetes, seizures, children <18 yr, and renal impairment **(adjust dose, see Chapter 31).** May cause GI disturbances, headache, and blurred vision with the ophthalmic solution. Like other quinolones, tendon rupture can occur during or after therapy (risk increases with concurrent corticosteroids). Use with NSAIDs may increase risk of CNS stimulation and seizures.

Levofloxacin was well tolerated with equal efficacy in a comparative study to standard-of-care antibiotics in children 0.5 to 16 yr with community-acquired pneumonia. Long-term safety trials are underway in children treated for pneumonia and otitis media.

Infuse IV over 1–1.5 hr; **avoid** IV push or rapid infusion because of risk of hypotension. **Do not** administer antacids or other divalent salts with or within 2 hr of oral levofloxacin dose; otherwise may be administered with or without food.

LEVOTHYROXINE (T_4)
Synthroid, Levothroid, Levoxyl, and others
Thyroid product

No No 1 A

Tabs: 25, 50, 75, 88, 100, 112, 125, 137, 150, 175, 200, 300 mcg
Injection: 200, 500 mcg
Oral suspension: 25 mcg/mL

Continued

For explanation of icons, see p. 663.

LEVOTHYROXINE (T_4) *continued*

Child PO dosing:

- ***0–6 mo:*** 8–10 mcg/kg/dose once daily
- ***6–12 mo:*** 6–8 mcg/kg/dose once daily
- ***1–5 yr:*** 5–6 mcg/kg/dose once daily
- ***6–12 yr:*** 4–5 mcg/kg/dose once daily
- ***>12 yr:*** 2–3 mcg/kg/dose once daily

Child: IM/IV dose: 50%–75% of oral dose once daily

Adult:

PO: Start with 12.5–50 mcg/dose once daily. Increase by 25–50 mcg/24 hr at intervals of Q2–4 wk until euthyroid. Usual adult dose: 100–200 mcg/24 hr.

IM/IV dose: 50% of oral dose once daily

Myxedema coma or stupor: 200–500 mcg IV × 1, then 75–300 mcg IV once daily; convert to oral therapy once patient is stabilized.

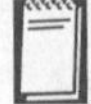

Contraindications include acute MI, thyrotoxicosis, and uncorrected adrenal insufficiency. May cause hyperthyroidism, rash, growth disturbances, hypertension, arrhythmias, diarrhea, and weight loss. Pseudotumor cerebri has been reported in children. Overtreatment may cause craniosynostosis in infants and premature closure of the epiphyses in children.

Total replacement dose may be used in children unless there is evidence of cardiac disease; in that case, begin with one-fourth of maintenance and increase weekly. Titrate dosage with clinical status and serum T_4 and TSH. Increases the effects of warfarin. Phenytoin, rifampin, carbamazepine, iron and calcium supplements, antacids, and orlistat may decrease levothyroxine levels. Tricyclic antidepressants and SSRIs may enhance toxic effects.

100 mcg levothyroxine = 65 mg thyroid USP. Administer oral doses on an empty stomach and tablets with a full glass of water. Iron and calcium supplements and antacids may decrease absorption; **do not** administer within 4 hr of these agents. Excreted in low levels in breast milk; preponderance of evidence suggests no clinically significant effect in infants.

LIDOCAINE

Xylocaine, L-M-X, Lidoderm, and various generics

Anti-arrhythmic class Ib, local anesthetic

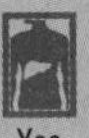
Yes

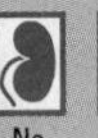
No

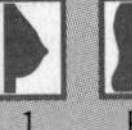
1

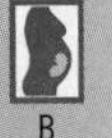
B

Injection: 0.5%, 1%, 1.5%, 2%, 4%, 10%, 20% (1% sol = 10 mg/mL)
IV infusion (in D_5W): 0.4% (4 mg/mL) (250, 500 mL); 0.8% (8 mg/mL) (250, 500 mL)
Injection with 1:50,000 epi: 2%
Injection with 1:100,000 epi: 1%, 2%
Injection with 1:200,000 epi: 0.5%, 1%, 1.5%, 2%
Ointment: 5% (50 g)
Cream, topical: 3% (30 g), 4% (L-M-X-4)[OTC] (5, 15, 30 g); may contain benzyl alcohol
Cream, rectal: 5% (L-M-X-5; 15, 30 g); contains benzyl alcohol
Jelly: 2% (5, 15, 30 mL); may contain benzalkonium chloride
Liquid (topical): 2.5% (7.5 mL)
Liquid (viscous): 2% (20, 100 mL)
Solution (topical): 2% (180 mL), 4% (50 mL)
Topical spray: 0.5% (60 mL), 9.6% (13 mL)
Topical 2.5% (with 2.5% prilocaine): See *Lidocaine* and *Prilocaine*
Transdermal patch (Lidoderm): 5% (30s)

Continued

LIDOCAINE *continued*

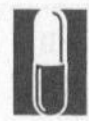

Anesthetic:
Injection:

Without epinephrine: **max. dose** of 4.5 mg/kg/dose (up to 300 mg); **do not** repeat within 2 hr.

With epinephrine: **max. dose** of 7 mg/kg/dose (up to 500 mg); **do not** repeat within 2 hr.

Topical:

Cream (child and adult): Apply to affected intact skin areas BID–QID

Gel or ointment (child and adult): Apply to affected intact skin areas once daily–QID; **max. dose:** 4.5 mg/kg up to 300 mg

Patch (adult): Apply to most painful area with up to 3 patches at a time. Patch(es) may be applied for up to 12 hr in any 24-hr period.

Antiarrhythmic:

Bolus: 1 mg/kg/dose (**max. dose:** 100 mg) slowly IV; may repeat in 10–15 min × 2; **max. total dose** 3–5 mg/kg within the first hr. ETT dose = 2–3 × IV dose.

Continuous infusion: 20–50 mcg/kg/min IV/IO (do not exceed 20 mcg/kg/min for patients with shock or CHF); see IV Infusions on page i for infusion preparation. Administer a 1 mg/kg bolus when infusion is initiated if bolus has not been given within previous 15 min.

Oral use (viscous liquid):

Child (≥3 yr): up to the lesser of 4.5 mg/kg/dose or 300 mg/dose swish and spit Q3 hr PRN up to a **max. dose** of 4 doses per 12-hr period

Adult: 15 mL swish and spit Q3 hr PRN up to a **max. dose** of 8 doses/24 hr

For cardiac arrest, amiodarone is the perferred agent over lidocaine; lidocaine may be used only when amiodarone is not available.

Contraindicated in Stokes-Adams attacks, SA, AV, or intraventricular heart block without a pacemaker. Side effects include hypotension, asystole, seizures, and respiratory arrest.

CYP 450 2D6 and 3A3/4 substrate. Decrease dose in hepatic failure or decreased cardiac output. **Do not use** topically for teething. Prolonged infusion may result in toxic accumulation of lidocaine, especially in infants. **Do not use** epinephrine-containing solutions for treatment of arrhythmias.

Therapeutic levels 1.5–5 mg/L. Toxicity occurs at >7 mg/L. Toxicity in neonates may occur at >5 mg/L. Elimination $T_{1/2}$: premature infant: 3.2 hr, adult: 1.5–2 hr.

When using the topical patch, avoid exposing the application site to external heat sources as they may increase the risk for toxicity.

LIDOCAINE AND PRILOCAINE
EMLA, Eutectic mixture of lidocaine and prilocaine
Topical analgesic

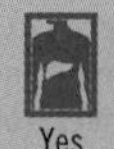
Yes
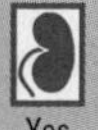
Yes

?
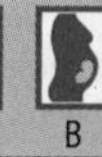
B

Cream: Lidocaine 2.5% + prilocaine 2.5%; 5 g kit (with dressings); 30 g tube

Topical anesthetic disc: Lidocaine 2.5% + prilocaine 2.5%; 1 g (contact surface ~10 cm^2) (box of 2s or 10s)

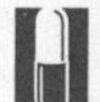

See Chapter 6, Table 6-5, for general use information.

Newborn ≥37 wk gestation, infant, child, and adult:

Minor procedures: 2.5 g/site for at least 60 min

Painful procedures: 2 g/10 cm^2 of skin for at least 2 hr

See following table for **max. dose** and application information.

Continued

For explanation of icons, see p. 663.

LIDOCAINE AND PRILOCAINE *continued*

Age and Weight	Maximum Total EMLA Dose (g)	Maximum Application Area (cm^2)	Maximum Application Time
Birth–3 mo or <5 kg	1	10	1 hr
3–12 mo and >5 kg*	2	20	4 hr
1–6 yr and >10 kg	10	100	4 hr
7–12 yr and >20 kg	20	200	4 hr

*If patient is >3 months and is not >5 kg, use the **maximum** total dose which corresponds to the patient's weight.

Should not be used in neonates <37 wk of gestation nor in infants <12 mo old receiving treatment with methoglobin-inducing agents (e.g., sulfa drugs, acetaminophen, nitrofurantoin, nitroglycerin, nitroprusside, phenobarbital, phenytoin). **Use with caution** in patients with G6PD deficiency, patients treated with class I or III anti-arrhythmic drugs (additive or toxic cardiac effects), and in patients with renal and hepatic impairment. Prilocaine has been associated with methemoglobinemia. Long duration of application, large treatment area, small patients, or impaired elimination may result in high blood levels.

Apply topically to intact skin and cover with occlusive dressing; **avoid** mucous membranes or the eyes. Wipe cream off before procedure.

LINDANE

Various brands, Gamma benzene hexachloride

Scabicidal agent, pediculocide

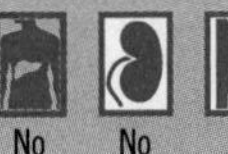
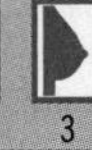
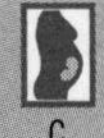

No No 3 C

Shampoo: 1% (60 mL)
Lotion: 1% (60 mL)

Scabies: Apply thin layer of lotion to skin. Bathe and rinse off medication in adults after 8–12 hr; children 6–8 hr. May repeat × 1 in 7 days PRN.

Pediculosis capitis: Apply 15–30 mL of shampoo, lather for 4–5 min, rinse hair and comb with fine comb to remove nits. May repeat × 1 in 7 days PRN.

Pediculosis pubis: May use lotion or shampoo (applied locally) as for scabies and pediculosis capitis.

Contraindicated in premature infants and seizure disorders. **Use with caution** with drugs that lower seizure threshold. Systemically absorbed. Risk of toxic effects is greater in young children; use other agents (permethrin) in infants, young children, and during pregnancy.

Lindane is considered second-line therapy owing to side-effect risk and reports of resistance. May cause a rash; rarely may cause seizures or aplastic anemia. For scabies, change clothing and bedsheets after starting treatment and treat family members. For pediculosis pubis, treat sexual contacts.

Avoid contact with face, urethral meatus, damaged skin, or mucous membranes. **Do not use** any covering (e.g., plastic lining or clothing) over the applied lindane.

LINEZOLID
Zyvox
Antibiotic, oxazolidinone

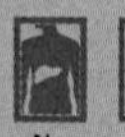 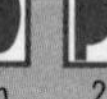 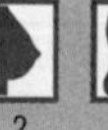 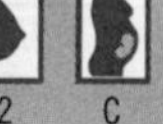
No No 2 C

Tabs: 400, 600 mg; contains ~0.45 mEq Na per 200 mg drug
Oral suspension: 100 mg/5 mL (240 mL); contains phenylalanine and sodium benzoate and 0.8 mEq Na per 200 mg drug
Injection, premixed: 200 mg in 100 mL, 400 mg in 200 mL, 600 mg in 300 mL; contains 1.7 mEq Na per 200 mg drug

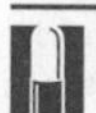

Neonate <7 days old: 10 mg/kg/dose IV/PO Q12 hr; if response is suboptimal, increase dose to 10 mg/kg/dose Q8 hr.
Neonate ≥7 days old–11 yr:
Pneumonia, bacteremia, complicated skin/skin structure infections, vancomycin-resistant E. faecium (VRE): 10 mg/kg/dose IV/PO Q8 hr. Duration of therapy: 10–14 days, except for VRE (14–28 days).
Uncomplicated skin/skin structure infections:
<5 yr: 10 mg/kg/dose PO Q8 hr × 10–14 days.
5–11 yr: 10 mg/kg/dose PO Q12 hr × 10–14 days.

≥12 yr and adult:
MRSA Infections: 600 mg Q12 hr IV/PO.
Vancomycin-resistant E. faecium: 600 mg Q12 hr IV/PO × 14–28 days.
Community-acquired and nosocomial pneumonia; and bacteremia: 600 mg Q12 hr IV/PO × 10–14 days.
Uncomplicated skin infections:
≥12 yr and adolescent: 600 mg Q12 hr PO × 10–14 days.
Adult: 400 mg Q12 hr PO ×10–14 days.

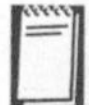

Most common side effects include diarrhea, headache, and nausea. Anemia, leukopenia, pancytopenia, thrombocytopenia may occur in patients who are at risk for myelosuppression and who receive regimens >2 wk. Complete blood count monitoring is recommended in these individuals. Pseudomembranous colitis and neuropathy (peripheral and optic) have also been reported.

Do not use with SSRIs (e.g., fluoxetine, paroxetine), tricyclic antidepressants, venlafaxine, and trazodone; may cause serotonin syndrome. **Avoid** use with monoamine oxidase inhibitors (e.g., phenelzine); and in patients with uncontrolled hypertension, pheochromocytoma, thyrotoxicosis, and taking sympathomimetics or vasopressive agents (may elevate blood pressure). **Use caution** when consuming large amounts of foods and beverages containing tyramine; may increase blood pressure. Dosing information in severe hepatic failure and renal impairment with multi-doses have not been completed.

Protect all dosage forms from light and moisture. Oral suspension product must be gently mixed by inverting the bottle 3–5 times prior to each use (**do not shake**). All oral doses may be administered with or without food.

LISDEXAMFETAMINE
Vyvanse
CNS stimulant

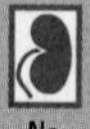 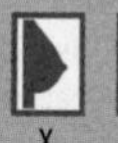 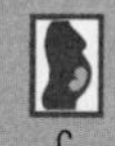
No No X C

Capsules: 20, 30, 40, 50, 60, 70 mg

Continued

For explanation of icons, see p. 663.

LISDEXAMFETAMINE *continued*

Attention deficit hyperactivity disorder:

Child ≥6 yr and adult: Start with 30 mg PO QAM. May increase dose by 10–20 mg/24 hr at weekly intervals if needed, up to a **maximum dose** of 70 mg/24 hr.

Lisdexamfetamine is a pro-drug of dextroamphetamine, which requires activation by intestinal/hepatic metabolism.

Contraindicated in amphetamine or sympathomimetic hypersensitivity, symptomatic cardiovascular disease, moderate/severe hypertension, hyperthyroidism, glaucoma, agitated states, drug/alcohol abuse history, and MAO inhibitors (concurrent or use within 14 days). As with other CNS simulant medications, serious cardiovascular events, including **death,** have been reported in patients with pre-existing structural cardiac abnormalities or other serious heart problems. **Use with caution** in patients with hypertension, psychiatric conditions, and epilepsy. May cause insomnia, irritability, rash, appetite suppression/weight loss, dizziness, xerostomia, and GI disturbances. Stevens-Johnson syndrome and TEN have been reported.

Urinary acidifying agents may reduce levels of amphetamines and urinary alkalinizing agent may increase levels. May increase the effects of TCAs; increase or decrease the effects of phenytoin, and phenobarbital; and decrease the effects of adrenergic blockers, antihistamines, and antihypertensives. Norepinephrine may increase the effects of amphetamines.

See *Dextroamphetamine ± Amphetamine* for additional remarks.

LISINOPRIL

Prinivil, Zestril, and others

Angiotensin converting enzyme inhibitor, antihypertensive

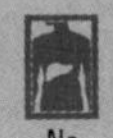
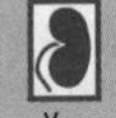
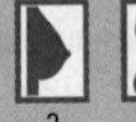
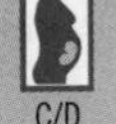

No Yes 3 C/D

Tabs: 2.5, 5, 10, 20, 30, 40 mg

Oral suspension: 1, 2 mg/mL

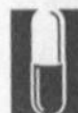

Hypertension (see remarks):

6–16 yr: Start with 0.07 mg/kg/dose PO once daily; **max. initial dose:** 5 mg/dose. If needed, titrate dose upward to doses up to 0.61 mg/kg/24 hr or 40 mg/24 hr (higher doses have not been evaluated).

Adult: Start with 10 mg PO once daily. If needed, increase dose by 5–10 mg/24 hr at 1–2 week intervals. Usual dosage range: 10–40 mg/24 hr. **Max. dose:** 80 mg/24 hr.

Use lower initial dose (50% of recommended dose) if using with a diuretic or with the presence of hyponatremia, hypovolemia, and severe CHF.

Contraindicated in hypersensitivity and history of angioedemia with other ACE inhibitors. **Avoid** use with dialysis with high-flux membranes because of anaphylactoid reactions have been reported. **Use with caution** in aortic or bilateral renal artery stenosis. Side effects include cough, dizziness, headache, hyperkalemia, hypotension (especially with concurrent diuretic or antihypertensive agent use), rash, and GI disturbances. Mood alterations, including depressive symptoms, has been reported. Use with diabetic patients treated with oral antidiabetic agents should be monitored for hypoglycemia, especially during the first month of use. NSAIDs (e.g., indomethacin) may decrease linsinopril's effects. **Adjust dose in renal impairment (see Chapter 31).**

Onset of action: 1 hr with maximal effect in 6–8 hr. Pregnancy category is a "C" during the first trimester but changes to a "D" for the second and third trimesters. Despite the pregnancy category, an increased risk for major congenital malformations has been reported with use of ACE inhibitors during the first trimester. Lisinopril should be discontinued as soon as possible when pregnancy is detected.

LITHIUM
Lithobid and many other generics (previously available as Eskalith)
Antimanic agent

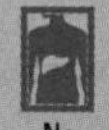
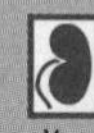

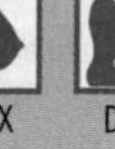
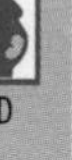

No Yes X D

Carbonate:
300 mg carbonate = 8.12 mEq lithium
Caps: 150, 300, 600 mg
Tabs: 300 mg
Extended-release tabs: 300 mg (Lithobid), 450 mg
Citrate:
Syrup: 8 mEq/5 mL (5, 480 mL); 5 mL is equivalent to 300 mg lithium carbonate

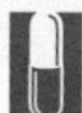

Child:
Initial (immediate release dosage forms): 15–60 mg/kg/24 hr ÷ TID–QID PO. Adjust as needed (weekly) to achieve therapeutic levels.
Adolescent: 600–1800 mg/24 hr ÷ TID–QID PO (divided BID using controlled/slow release tablets).
Adult:
Initial: 300 mg TID PO. Adjust as needed to achieve therapeutic levels. Usual dose is about 300 mg TID–QID with immediate release dosage form. For controlled/slow release tablets, 900–1800 mg/24 hr PO ÷ BID.
Max. dose: 2400 mg/24 hr.

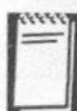

Contraindicated in severe cardiovascular or renal disease. Decreased sodium intake or increased sodium wasting will increase lithium levels. May cause goiter, nephrogenic diabetes insipidus, hypothyroidism, arrhythmias, or sedation at therapeutic doses.

Co-administration with thiazide diuretics, metronidazole, ACE inhibitors, or nonsteroidal anti-inflammatory drugs may increase risk for lithium toxicity. Iodine may increase risk for hypothyroidism. If used in combination with haloperidol, closely monitor neurologic toxicities because an encephalopathic syndrome followed by irreversible brain damage has been reported.

Therapeutic levels: 0.6–1.5 mEq/L. In either acute or chronic toxicity, confusion, and somnolence may be seen at levels of 2–2.5 mEq/L. **Seizures or death** may occur at levels >2.5 mEq/L. Recommended serum sampling: trough level within 30 min prior to the next scheduled dose. Steady-state is achieved within 4–6 days of continuous dosing. **Adjust dose in renal failure (see Chapter 31).**

LOPERAMIDE
Imodium, Imodium AD, and others
Antidiarrheal

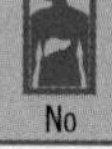
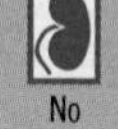
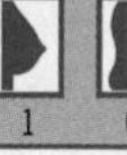

No No 1 C

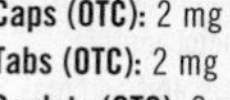

Caps (OTC): 2 mg
Tabs (OTC): 2 mg
Caplets (OTC): 2 mg
Liquid (OTC): 1 mg/5 mL, 1 mg/7.5 mL; may contain alcohol (60, 120 mL)

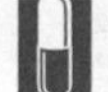

Active diarrhea:
Child (initial doses within the first 24 hr):
2–5 yr (13–20 kg): 1 mg PO TID
6–8 yr (20–30 kg): 2 mg PO BID
9–12 yr (>30 kg): 2 mg PO TID
Max. single dose: 2 mg

Continued

For explanation of icons, see p. 663.

LOPERAMIDE *continued*

Child (initial doses within the first 24 hr) (cont'd):

Follow initial day's dose with 0.1 mg/kg/dose after each loose stool (**not to exceed** the aforementioned initial doses).

≥12 yr and adult: 4 mg/dose × 1, followed by 2 mg/dose after each stool up to **max. dose** of 16 mg/24 hr.

Chronic diarrhea:

Child: 0.08–0.24 mg/kg/24 hr ÷ BID–TID; **max. dose:** 2 mg/dose

Contraindicated in acute dysentery; acute ulcerative colitis; bacterial enterocolitis caused by *Salmonella, Shigella, Campylobacter,* and *C. difficile*; and abdominal pain in the absence of diarrhea. **Avoid** use in children <2 yr due to reports of paralytic ileus associated with abdominal distention. Rare hypersensitivity reactions including anaphylactic shock have been reported. May cause nausea, rash, vomiting, constipation, cramps, dry mouth, and CNS depression. **Discontinue use if no clinical improvement is observed within 48 hr.** Naloxone may be administered for CNS depression.

LORATADINE ± PSEUDOEPHEDRINE
Claritin, Claritin Children's Allergy, Claritin RediTabs, Claritin-D 12 Hour, Claritin-D 24 Hour, and others
Antihistamine, less sedating ± decongestant

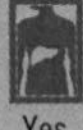
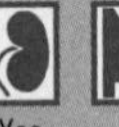
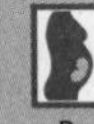
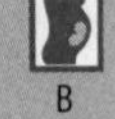

Yes Yes 2 B

Tabs (OTC): 10 mg
Chewable tabs (Claritin Children's Allergy) (OTC): 5 mg; contains aspartame
Disintegrating tabs (RediTabs) (OTC): 5, 10 mg; contains aspartame
Syrup (OTC): 1 mg/mL (480 mL)
Time-release tabs in combination with pseudoephedrine (PE):
Claritin-D 12 Hour (OTC): 5 mg loratadine + 120 mg PE
Claritin-D 24 Hour (OTC): 10 mg loratadine + 240 mg PE

Loratadine:

2–5 yr: 5 mg PO once daily

≥6 yr and adult: 10 mg PO once daily

Time-release tabs of loratidine and pseudoephedrine:

≥12 yr and adult:

Claritin-D 12 Hour: 1 tablet PO BID

Claritin-D 24 Hour: 1 tablet PO once daily

May cause drowsiness, fatigue, dry mouth, headache, bronchospasams, palpitations, dermatitis, and dizziness. Has **not** been implicated in causing cardiac arrhythmias when used with other drugs that are metabolized by hepatic microsomal enzymes (e.g., ketoconazole, erythromycin). May be administered safely in patients who have allergic rhinitis and asthma.

In hepatic and renal function impairment (GFR <30 mL/min), prolong loratadine (single agent) dosage interval to every other day. **Adjust dose in renal failure (see Chapter 31).**

For time-release tablets of the combination product (loratadine and pseudoephedrine), prolong dosage interval in renal impairment (GFR <30 mL/min) as follows: Claritin-D 12 Hour: 1 tablet PO once daily; Claritin-D 24 Hour: 1 tablet PO every other day. **Do not use** the combination product in hepatic impairment because drugs cannot be individually titrated.

Administer doses on an empty stomach. For use of RediTabs, place tablet on tongue and allow it to disintegrate in the mouth with or without water. For Claritin-D, also see remarks in *Pseudoephedrine.*

LORAZEPAM
Ativan and many generics
Benzodiazepine anticonvulsant

Yes Yes 2 D

Tabs: 0.5, 1, 2 mg
Injection: 2, 4 mg/mL (each contains 2% benzyl alcohol and propylene glycol)
Oral solution: 2 mg/mL (10, 30 mL); alcohol and dye free

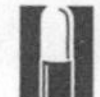

Status epilepticus:

Neonate, infant, child, and adolescent: 0.05–0.1 mg/kg/dose IV over 2–5 min. May repeat 0.05 mg/kg × 1 in 10–15 min.

Max. dose: 2 mg/dose.

Adult: 4 mg/dose given slowly over 2–5 min. May repeat in 10–15 min. **Usual total max. dose** in 12-hr period is 8 mg.

Antiemetic adjunct therapy:

Child: 0.02–0.05 mg/kg/dose IV Q6 hr PRN; **max. single dose:** 2 mg.

Anxiolytic/sedation:

Infant and child: 0.05 mg/kg/dose Q4–8 hr PO/IV; **max. dose:** 2 mg/dose.
May also give IM for preprocedure sedation.

Adult: 1–10 mg/24 hr PO ÷ BID–TID

Contraindicated in narrow-angle glaucoma and severe hypotension. **Use with caution** in renal insufficiency (glucoronide metabolite clearance is reduced), hepatic insufficiency (may worsen hepatic encephalopahy), compromised pulmonary function, and use of CNS depressant medications. May cause respiratory depression, especially in combination with other sedatives. May also cause sedation, dizziness, mild ataxia, mood changes, rash, and GI symptoms. Paradoxical excitation has been reported in chlidren (10%–30% of patients <8 year old).

Significant respiratory depression and/or hypotension has been reported when used in combination with loxapine. Probenecid and valproic acid may increase the effects/toxicity of lorazepam and oral contraceptive steroids may decrease lorazepam's effects.

Injectable product may be given rectally. Benzyl alcohol and propylene glycol may be toxic to newborns at high doses.

Onset of action for sedation: PO, 20–30 min; IM, 30–60 min; IV, 1–5 min. Duration of action: 6–8 hr. **Flumazenil is the antidote.**

LOSARTAN
Cozaar
Angiotensin II receptor antagonist

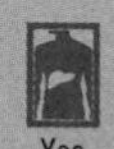 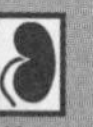 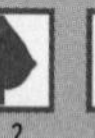 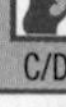

Yes Yes ? C/D

Tabs: 25, 50, 100 mg
Oral suspension: 2.5 mg/mL
Contains 2.12 mg potassium per 25 mg drug

Hypertension (see remarks):

6–16 yr: Start with 0.75 mg/kg/dose PO once daily up to 50 mg/24 hr. Adjust dose to desired blood pressure response. **Max. dose:** 1.4 mg/kg/24 hr or 100 mg/24 hr.

Adult: Start with 50 mg PO once daily. Usual maintenance dose is 25–100 mg/24 hr PO ÷ once daily–BID

Continued

For explanation of icons, see p. 663.

LOSARTAN *continued*

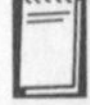

Use with caution in angioedema (current or past), excessive hypotension (volume depletion), hepatic (use lower starting dose) or renal (contains potassium) impairment, hyperkalemia, renal artery stenosis and severe CHF. **Not recommended** in patients <6 yr or in children with GFR <30 mL/min/1.73 m^2 due to the lack of data.

Discontinue use as soon as possible when pregnancy is detected because injury and death to developing fetus may occur. Pregnancy category is "C" during the first trimester but changes to "D" for the second and third trimesters.

Diarrhea, asthenia, dizziness, fatigue, and hypotension are common. Thrombocytopenia, rhabdomyolysis, and angioedema have been rarely reported. Losartan is a substrate for CYP 450 2C9 (major) and 3A4. Fluconazole and cimetidine may increase losartan effects/toxicity. Rifampin, phenobarbital, and indomethacin may decrease its effects. Losartan may increase the risk of lithium toxicity.

LOW MOLECULAR WEIGHT HEPARIN

See *Enoxaparin*

MAGNESIUM CITRATE

Various
16.17% Elemental Magnesium
Laxative/cathartic

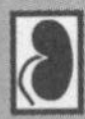
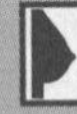
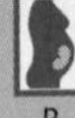

No Yes 1 B

Oral solution (OTC): 1.75 g/30 mL (300 mL); 5 mL = 3.9–4.7 mEq Mg

Cathartic:
- ***<6 yr:*** 2–4 mL/kg/24 hr PO ÷ once daily–BID
- ***6–12 yr:*** 100–150 mL/24 hr PO ÷ once daily–BID
- ***>12 yr and adult:*** 150–300 mL/24 hr PO ÷ once daily–BID

Use with caution in renal insufficiency and patients receiving digoxin. May cause hypermagnesemia, diarrhea, muscle weakness, hypotension, and respiratory depression. Up to about 30% of dose is absorbed. May decrease absorption of H_2 antagonists, phenytoin, iron salts, tetracycline, steroids, benzodiazepines, and quinolone antibiotics.

MAGNESIUM HYDROXIDE

Milk of Magnesia and various generics
41.69% Elemental Magnesium
Antacid, laxative

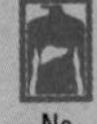
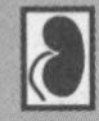

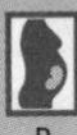

No Yes 1 B

Oral liquid (OTC): 400 mg/5 mL (Milk of Magnesia and others)
Concentrated oral liquid (OTC): 800 mg/5 mL (Milk of Magnesia concentrate)
Chewable tabs (OTC): 311 mg
400 mg magnesium hydroxide is equivalent to 166.76 mg elemental magnesium
Combination product with aluminum hydroxide: See *Aluminum Hydroxide.*

Continued

MAGNESIUM HYDROXIDE *continued*

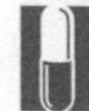

Laxative (all liquid mL doses based on 400 mg/5 mL magnesium hydroxide, unless noted otherwise):

Dose/24 hr ÷ once daily–QID PO

- ***<2 yr:*** 0.5 mL/kg
- ***2–5 yr:*** 5–15 mL OR 311–622 mg (1–2 chewable tabs)
- ***6–11 yr:*** 15–30 mL OR 933–1244 mg (3–4 chewable tabs)
- ***≥12 yr and adult:*** 30–60 mL OR 1866–2488 mg (6–8 chewable tabs)

Antacid:

Child:

- ***Liquid:*** 2.5–5 mL/dose once daily–QID PO
- ***Tabs:*** 311 mg once daily–QID PO

Adult:

- ***Liquid:*** 5–15 mL/dose once daily–QID PO
- ***Concentrated liquid (800 mg/5 mL):*** 2.5–7.5 mL/dose once daily–QID PO
- ***Tabs:*** 622–1244 mg/dose once daily–QID PO

See *Magnesium Citrate.*

MAGNESIUM OXIDE

Mag-200, Mag-Ox 400, Uro-Mag, and others
60.32% Elemental Magnesium
Oral magnesium salt

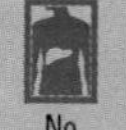 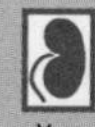 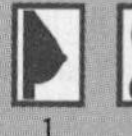 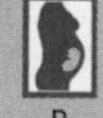

No Yes 1 B

Tabs (OTC): 200, 400, 420, 500 mg
Caps (Uro-Mag and others; OTC): 140 mg
400 mg Magnesium oxide is equivalent to 241.3 mg elemental Mg or 20 mEq Mg

Doses expressed in magnesium oxide salt.

Magnesium suplementation:

- ***Child:*** 5–10 mg/kg/24 hr ÷ TID–QID PO
- ***Adult:*** 400–800 mg/24 hr ÷ BID–QID PO

Hypomagnesemia:

- ***Child:*** 65–130 mg/kg/24 hr ÷ QID PO
- ***Adult:*** 2000 mg/24 hr ÷ QID PO

See *Magnesium Citrate.* For dietary recommended intake (U.S. RDA) for magnesium, see Chapter 21.

MAGNESIUM SULFATE

Epsom salts and others
9.9% Elemental Magnesium
Magnesium salt

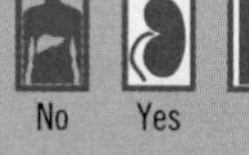 

No Yes 1 A

Injection: 100 mg/mL (0.8 mEq/mL), 125 mg/mL (1 mEq/mL), 500 mg/mL (4 mEq/mL)
Injection, pre-diluted in sterile water for injection; ready to use: 40 mg/mL (0.325 mEq/mL) (100, 500, 1000 mL); 80 mg/mL (0.65 mEq/mL) (50 mL)
Injection, pre-diluted in D_5W; ready to use: 10 mg/mL (0.081 mEq/mL) (100 mL); 20 mg/mL (0.163 mEq/mL) (500, 1000 mL)

Continued

For explanation of icons, see p. 663.

MAGNESIUM SULFATE *continued*

Granules: Approx. 40 mEq Mg per 5 g (120, 454, 1810 g)
500 mg magnesium sulfate is equivalent to 49.3 mg elemental Mg or 4.1 mEq Mg

All doses expressed in magnesium sulfate salt.

Cathartic:

Child: 0.25 g/kg/dose PO Q4–6 hr
Adult: 10–30 g/dose PO Q4–6 hr

Hypomagnesemia or hypocalcemia:

IV/IM: 25–50 mg/kg/dose Q4–6 hr × 3–4 doses; repeat PRN. **Max. single dose:** 2 g
PO: 100–200 mg/kg/dose QID PO

Daily maintenance:

30–60 mg/kg/24 hr or 0.25–0.5 mEq/kg/24 hr IV
Max. dose: 1 g/24 hr

Adjunctive therapy for moderate to severe reactive airway disease exacerbation (bronchodilation):

Child: 25–75 mg/kg/dose (max. dose: 2 g) × 1 IV over 20 min
Adult: 2 g/dose × 1 IV over 20 min

When given IV **beware** of hypotension, respiratory depression, complete heart block, and/or hypermagnesemia. Calcium gluconate (IV) should be available as **antidote. Use with caution** in patients with renal insufficiency and with patients on digoxin. **Serum level dependent toxicity** includes the following: >3 mg/dL: CNS depression; >5 mg/dL: decreased deep tendon reflexes, flushing, somnolence; and >12 mg/dL: respiratory paralysis, heart block.

Max. IV intermittent infusion rate: 1 mEq/kg/hr or 125 mg $MgSO_4$ salt/kg/hr.

MANNITOL
Osmitrol, Resectisol, and various generics
Osmotic diuretic

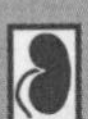
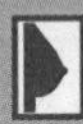
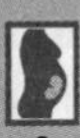
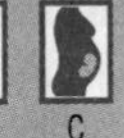

No Yes ? C

Injection: 50, 100, 150, 200, 250 mg/mL (5%, 10%, 15%, 20%, 25%)

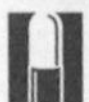

Anuria/oliguria (Child and adult):

Test dose to assess renal function: 0.2 g/kg/dose IV; **max. dose:** 12.5 g over 3–5 min. If there is no diuresis within 2 hr, discontinue mannitol.
Initial: 0.5–1 g/kg/dose
Maintenance: 0.25–0.5 g/kg/dose Q4–6 hr IV

Contraindicated in severe renal disease, active intracranial bleed, dehydration, and pulmonary edema. May cause circulatory overload and electrolyte disturbances. For hyperosmolar therapy, keep serum osmolality at 310–320 mOsm/kg.

Caution: may crystallize at low temperatures with concentrations ≥15%; redissolve crystals by warming solution up to 70° C with agitation. Use an in-line filter. May cause hypovolemia, headache, and polydipsia. Reduction in ICP occurs in 15 min and lasts 3–6 hr.

MEBENDAZOLE
Vermox and others
Anthelmintic

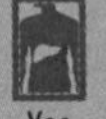
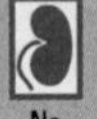
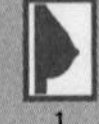
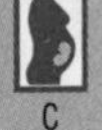

Yes No 1 C

Chewable tabs: 100 mg (may be swallowed whole or chewed) (boxes of 12s, 60s)

Child (>2 yr) and adult:

Pinworms (Entererobius): 100 mg PO × 1, repeat in 2 wk if not cured.

Continued

MEBENDAZOLE *continued*

Child (>2 yr) and adult (cont'd):

Hookworms, roundworms (Ascaris), and whipworm (Trichuris): 100 mg PO BID × 3 days. Repeat in 3–4 wk if not cured. Alternatively, may administer 500 mg PO ×1.

Capillariasis: 200 mg PO BID × 20 days

Visceral larva migrans (Toxocariasis): 100–200 mg PO BID × 5 days.

Trichinellosis (Trichinella spiralis): 200-400 mg PO TID × 3 days, then 400–500 mg PO TID × 10 days; use with steroids for severe symptoms.

Ancylostoma caninum (Eosinophilic enterocolitis): 100 mg PO BID × 3 days.

See latest edition of the AAP *Red Book* for additional information.

Experience in children <2 yr is limited. May cause rash, headache, diarrhea, and abdominal cramping in cases of massive infection. Liver function test elevations and hepatitis have been reported with prolonged courses; monitor hepatic function with prolonged therapy. Family may need to be treated as a group. Therapeutic effect may be decreased if administered to patients receiving carbamazepine or phenytoin. Administer with food.

MEDROXYPROGESTERONE

Depo-Provera, Provera, and various generics; Depo-Sub Q Provera 104.

Contraceptive, progestin

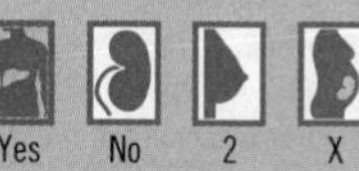

Tabs (Provera and others): 2.5, 5, 10 mg

Injection, suspension as acetate:

Depo-Provera and others, for IM use only: 150 mg/mL (1 mL), 400 mg/mL (2.5 mL); may contain parabens

Injection, pre-filled syringe:

Depo-Sub Q Provera 104, for SC use only: 104 mg (0.65 mL of 160 mg/mL); contains parabens.

Adolescent and adult:

Contraception: Initiate therapy during the first 5 days after onset of a normal menstrual period, within 5 days postpartum if not breastfeeding, or if breastfeeding, at 6-wk postpartum. When converting contraceptive method to Depo-Sub Q Provera, dose should be administered within 7 days after the last day of using the previous method (pill, ring, patch).

IM (Depo-Provera): 150 mg Q3 mo

SC (Depo-Sub Q Provera 104): 104 mg Q3 mo (every 12–14 wk)

Amenorrhea: 5–10 mg PO once daily × 5–10 days

Abnormal uterine bleeding: 5–10 mg PO once daily × 5–10 days initiated on the 16th or 21st day of the menstrual cycle.

Endometriosis-associated pain (Depo-Sub Q Provera 104): 104 mg SC Q 3 mo. **Do not use** longer than 2 yr due to impact on bone mineral density.

Consider patient's risk for osteoporosis because of the potential for decrease in bone mineral density with long-term use. **Contraindicated** in pregnancy, breast or genital cancer, liver disease, missed abortion, thrombophlebitis, thromboembolic disorders, cerebral vascular disease and undiagnosed vaginal bleeding. **Use with caution** in patients with family history of breast cancer, drepression, diabetes and fluid retention. May cause dizziness, headache, insomnia, fatigue, nausea, weight increase, appetite changes, amenorrhea, and breakthrough bleeding. Cholestatic jaundice and increased intracranial pressure have been reported.

Aminoglutethimide may decrease medroxyprogesterone levels. May alter thyroid and liver function tests, prothrombin time, factors VII, VIII, IX, and X, and metyrapone test.

Do not inject IM or SC product intravenously. Shake IM injection vial well before use and administer in the upper arm or buttock. Administer SC injection product into the anterior thigh or abdomen. Administer oral doses with food.

For explanation of icons, see p. 663.

MEFLOQUINE HCL
Lariam and others
Antimalarial

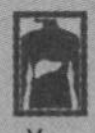 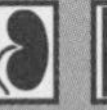  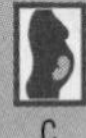
Yes No ? C

Tabs: 250 mg (228 mg base)

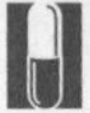

Doses expressed in mg mefloquine HCl salt
Malaria prophylaxis (start 1–2 wk prior to exposure and continue for 4 wk after leaving edemic area):
Child (PO, administered Q weekly):
<10 kg: 5 mg/kg
10–19 kg: 62.5 mg (¼ tablet)
20–30 kg: 125 mg (½ tablet)
31–45 kg: 187.5 mg (¾ tablet)
>45 kg: 250 mg (1 tablet)
Adult: 250 mg PO Q weekly
Malaria treatment:
<45 kg: 15 mg/kg × 1 PO followed by 10 mg/kg × 1 PO 12 hr later
Adult: 750 mg × 1 PO followed by 500 mg × 1 PO 12 hr later
See latest edition of the *Red Book* for additional information.

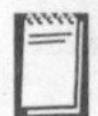

Contraindicated in active or recent history of depression, anxiety disorders, psychosis or schizophrenia, seizures, or hypersensitivity to quinine or quinidine. **Use with caution** in cardiac dysrhythmias and neurologic disease. May cause dizziness, headache, syncope, seizures, ocular abnormalities, GI symptoms, leukopenia, and thrombocytopenia (most adverse events occur within 3 doses with prophylaxis use). Monitor liver enzymes and ocular exams for therapies greater than 1 yr. Mefloquine may reduce valproic acid levels. ECG abnormalities may occur when used in combination with quinine, quinidine, chloroquine, halofantrine, and beta blockers. If any of the aforementioned antimalarial drugs is used in the initial treatment of severe malaria, initiate mefloquine at least 12 hours after the last dose of any of these drugs.

Do not take on an empty stomach. Administer with at least 240 mL (8 oz) water. Treatment failures in children may be related to vomiting of administered dose. If vomiting occurs less than 30 min after the dose, administer a second full dose. If vomiting occurs 30–60 min after the dose, administer an additional half-dose. If vomiting continues, monitor patient closely and consider alternative therapy.

MEROPENEM
Merrem
Carbapenem antibiotic

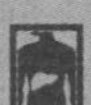 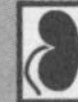  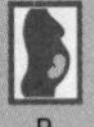
No Yes 2 B

Injection: 0.5, 1 g
Contains 3.92 mEq Na/g drug

Neonate: 20 mg/kg/dose IV using the following dosage intervals:
<7 days old: Q12 hr
≥7 days old:
1.2–2 kg: Q 12 hr
>2 kg: Q8 hr
Infant >3 mo and child:
Skin and subcutaneous tissue infections: 30 mg/kg/24 IV ÷ Q8 hr; **max. dose:** 1.5 g/24 hr
Intra-abdominal and mild/moderate infections: 60 mg/kg/24 hr IV ÷ Q8 hr; **max. dose:** 3 g/24 hr
Meningitis, Cystic Fibrosis, and severe infections: 120 mg/kg/24 hr IV ÷ Q8 hr; **max. dose:** 6 g/24 hr

Continued

MEROPENEM *continued*

Adult:

Skin and subcutaneous tissue infections: 1.5 g/24 hr IV ÷ Q8 hr
Intra-abdominal and mild/moderate infections: 3 g/24 hr IV ÷ Q8 hr
Meningitis and severe infections: 6 g/24 hr IV ÷ Q8 hr

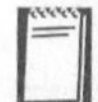

Contraindicated in patients sensitive to carbapenems, or with a history of anaphylaxis to beta-lactam antibiotics. **Use with caution** in meningitis and CNS disorders (may cause seizures) and renal impairment (**adjust dose; see Chapter 31**). Drug penetrates well into the CSF.

May cause diarrhea, rash, nausea, vomiting, oral moniliasis, glossitis, pain and irritation at the IV injection site, and headache. Hepatic enzyme and bilirubin elevation, leukopenia, thrombocytopenia (in renal dysfunction), and neutropenia have been reported. Probenecid may increase serum meropenem levels. May reduce valproic acid levels.

MESALAMINE

Asacol, Asacol HD, Canasa, Lialda, Pentasa, Rowasa, FIV-ASA, and others; 5-aminosalicylic acid, 5-ASA
Salicylate, GI anti-inflammatory agent

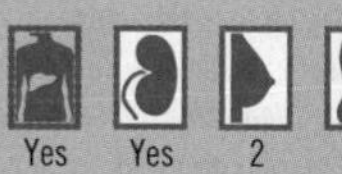

Caps, controlled release (Pentasa): 250, 500 mg
Tabs, delayed release: 400 mg (Asacol), 800 mg (Asacol HD), 1200 mg (Lialda)
Suppository (Canasa, FIV-ASA): 1000 mg (30s)
Rectal suspension (Rowasa and others): 4 g/60 mL (7s, 28s); contains sulfites and sodium benzoate

Child:

Caps, controlled release: 50 mg/kg/24 hr ÷ Q6–12 hr PO
Tabs, delayed release: 50 mg/kg/24 hr ÷ Q8–12 hr PO

Adult:

Caps, controlled release: 1 g QID PO up to 8 wk
Tabs, delayed release:

Asacol: 800 mg TID PO for 6 wk; for ulcerative colitis remission, use 1.6 g/24 hr ÷ BID–QID. PO up to 6 mo.
Asacol HD: 1.6 g TID PO up to 6 wk.
Lialda: 2.4–4.8 g once daily PO up to 8 wk.

Suppository: 500 mg BID PR × 3–6 wk; may increase dose to TID if inadequate response for 2 wk. Alternately, 1000 mg QHS PR may be used. Retain each dose in the rectum for 1–3 hr or longer.
Rectal suspension: 60 mL (4 g) QHS × 3–6 wk, retaining each dose for about 8 hr; lie on left side during administration to improve delivery to the sigmoid colon.

Generally **not recommended** in children <16 yr with chicken pox or flu-like symptoms (risk of Reye's syndrome). **Contraindicated** in active peptic ulcer disease, severe renal failure, and salicylate hypersensitivity. Rectal suspension **should not** be used in patients with history of sulfite allergy. **Use with caution** in sulfasalazine hypersensitivity, impaired hepatic or renal function, pyloric stenosis, and concurrent thrombolytics. May cause headache, GI discomfort, pancreatitis, pericarditis, rash, and Stevens-Johnson syndrome.

Do not administer with lactulose or other medications that can lower intestinal pH. Oral capsules are designed to release medication throughout the GI tract and oral tablets release medication at the terminal ileus and beyond. 400 mg PO mesalamine is equivalent to 1 g sulfasalazine PO. Tablets should be swallowed whole.

For explanation of icons, see p. 663.

METFORMIN
Glucophage, Glucophage XR, Fortamet, Riomet, and others
Antidiabetic, biguanide

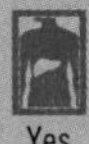 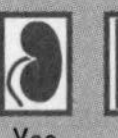 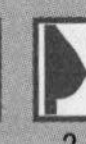 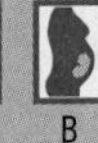

Yes Yes 2 B

Tabs: 500, 850, 1000 mg
Tabs, extended release (Glucophage XR, Fortamet, and others): 500, 750 mg
Oral suspension (Riomet): 100 mg/mL (120, 480 mL); contains saccharin

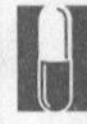

Administer all doses with meals (e.g., BID: morning and evening meals).
Child (10–16 yr) (see remarks): Start with 500 mg BID; may increase dose weekly by 500 mg/24 hr in 2 divided doses up to a **max. dose** of 2000 mg/24 hr.
Child ≥17 yr and adult (see remarks):
500 mg tabs: Start with 500 mg PO BID; may increase dose weekly by 500 mg/24 hr in 2 divided doses up to a **max. dose** of 2500 mg/24 hr. Administer 2500 mg/24 hr doses by dividing daily dose TID with meals.
850 mg tabs: Start with 850 mg PO once daily with morning meal; may increase by 850 mg every 2 wk up to a **max. dose** of 2550 mg/24 hr (first dosage increment: 850 mg PO BID; second dosage increment: 850 mg PO TID).
Extended released tabs: Start with 500 mg PO once daily with evening meal; may increase by 500 mg every wk up to a **max. dose** of 2000 mg/24 hr (if glycemic control is not achieved at max. dose, divide dose to 1000 mg PO BID). If a dose >2000 mg is needed, switch to non-extended released tablets in divided doses and increase dose to a **max. dose** of 2550 mg/24 hr.

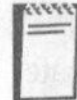

Contraindicated in renal impairment, CHF, metabolic acidosis, and during radiology studies using iodinated contrast media. **Use with caution** when transferring patients from chlorpropamide therapy (potential hypoglycemia risk), excessive alcohol intake, hypoxemia, dehydration, surgical procedures, hepatic disease, anemia, and thyroid disease.

Fatal lactic acidosis (diarrhea; severe muscle pain, cramping; shallow and fast breathing; unusual weakness and sleepiness) and decrease in vitamin B_{12} levels have been reported. May cause GI discomfort (~50% incidence), anorexia, and vomiting. Transient abdominal discomfort or diarrhea have been reported in 40% of pediatric patients. Cimetidine, furosemide, and nifedipine may increase the effects/toxicity of metformin. In addition to monitoring serum glucose and glycosylated hemoglobin, monitor renal function and hematologic parameters (baseline and annual).

Adult patients initiated on 500 mg PO BID may also have their dose increased to 850 mg PO BID after 2 wk.

COMBINATION THERAPY WITH SULFONYLUREAS: If patient has not responded to 4 wk of maximum doses of metformin monotherapy, consider gradual addition of an oral sulfonylurea with continued maximum metformin dosing (even if failure with sulfonylurea has occurred). Attempt to identify the minimum effective dosage for each drug (metformin and sulfonylurea), since the combination can increase risk for sulfonylurea-induced hypoglycemia. If patient does not respond to 1–3 mo of combination therapy with maximum metformin doses, consider discontinuing combination therapy and initiating insulin therapy.

Administer all doses with food.

METHADONE HCL
Dolophine, Methadose, and others
Narcotic, analgesic

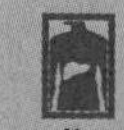
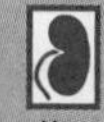

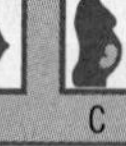
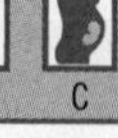

No Yes 2 C

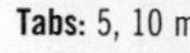

Tabs: 5, 10 mg
Tabs (dispersible): 40 mg
Oral solution: 5 mg/5 mL, 10 mg/5 mL; contains 8% alcohol
Concentrated solution: 10 mg/mL
Injection: 10 mg/mL (20 mL), contains 0.5% chlorobutanol

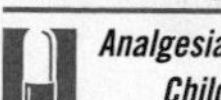

Analgesia:
Child: 0.7 mg/kg/24 hr ÷ Q4–6 hr PRN pain PO, SC, IM, or IV. **Max. dose:** 10 mg/dose.
Adult: 2.5–10 mg/dose Q3–4 hr PRN pain PO, SC, IM, or IV.
Detoxification or maintenance: See package insert.

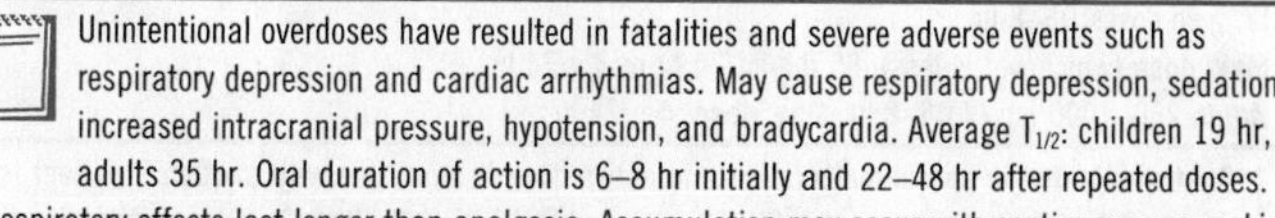

Unintentional overdoses have resulted in fatalities and severe adverse events such as respiratory depression and cardiac arrhythmias. May cause respiratory depression, sedation, increased intracranial pressure, hypotension, and bradycardia. Average $T_{1/2}$: children 19 hr, adults 35 hr. Oral duration of action is 6–8 hr initially and 22–48 hr after repeated doses. Respiratory effects last longer than analgesia. Accumulation may occur with continuous use making it necessary to adjust dose. Nevirapine may decrease serum levels of methadone. Methadone is a substrate for CYP 450 3A3/4, 2D6, 1A2; and inhibitor of 2D6.

See Chapter 6 for equianalgesic dosing and onset of action. **Adjust dose in renal failure (see Chapter 31).**

METHIMAZOLE
Tapazole and others
Antithyroid agent

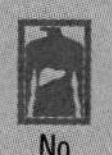
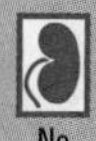
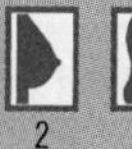
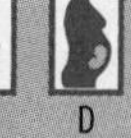

No No 2 D

Tabs: 5, 10 mg

Hyperthyroidism:
Child:
Initial: 0.4–0.7 mg/kg/24 hr or 15–20 mg/m^2/24 hr PO ÷ Q8 hr
Maintenance: ⅓ – ⅔ of initial dose PO ÷ Q8 hr
Max. dose: 30 mg/24 hr
Adult:
Initial: 15–60 mg/24 hr PO ÷ TID
Maintenance: 5–15 mg/24 hr PO ÷ TID

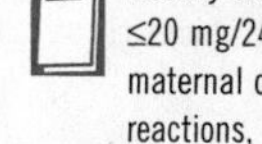

Readily crosses placental membranes and distributes into breast milk (maternal doses ≤20 mg/24 hr is considered safe but there are insufficient data to support safe use with maternal doses >20 mg/24 hr). Blood dyscrasias, dermatitis, hepatitis, arthralgia, CNS reactions, pruritis, nephritis, hypoprothrombinemia, agranulocytosis, headache, fever, and hypothyroidism may occur.

May increase the effects of oral anticoagulants. When correcting hyperthyroidism, existing beta-blocker, digoxin, and theophylline doses may need to be reduced to avoid potential toxicities.

Switch to maintenance dose when patient is euthyroid. Administer all doses with food.

For explanation of icons, see p. 663.

METHYLDOPA
Various brand names
Central alpha-adrenergic blocker, antihypertensive

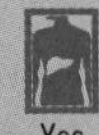 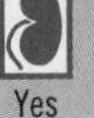 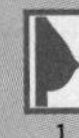 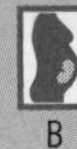
Yes Yes 1 B

Tabs: 250, 500 mg
Injection: 50 mg/mL; may contain sulfites
Oral suspension: 50 mg/mL

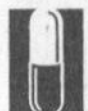

Hypertension:
Child: 10 mg/kg/24 hr ÷ Q6–12 hr PO; increase PRN Q2 days. **Max. dose:** 65 mg/kg/24 hr or 3 g/24 hr, whichever is less.
Adult: 250 mg/dose BID–TID PO. Increase PRN Q2 days to **max. dose** of 3 g/24 hr.

Hypertensive crisis:
Child: 2–4 mg/kg/dose IV, if no response within 4–6 hr, may increase dose to 5–10 mg/kg/dose IV; give doses Q6–8 hr.
Max. dose (whichever is less): 65 mg/kg/24 hr or 3 g/24 hr.
Adult: 250–1000 mg IV Q6–8 hr. **Max. dose:** 4 g/24 hr.

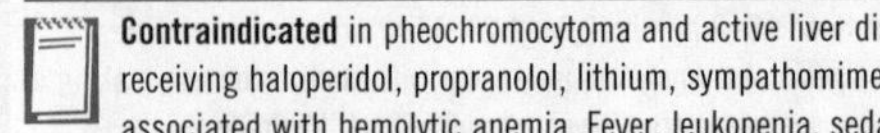

Contraindicated in pheochromocytoma and active liver disease. **Use with caution** if patient is receiving haloperidol, propranolol, lithium, sympathomimetics. Positive Coombs' test rarely associated with hemolytic anemia. Fever, leukopenia, sedation, memory impairment, hepatitis, GI disturbances, orthostatic hypotension, black tongue, and gynecomastia may occur. May interfere with lab tests for creatinine, urinary catecholamines, uric acid, and AST.

Do not co-administer oral doses with iron; decreases methyldopa absorption. **Adjust dose in renal failure (see Chaper 31).**

METHYLENE BLUE
Urolene Blue and many generics
Antidote, drug-induced methemoglobinemia, and cyanide toxicity

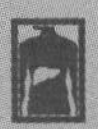 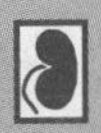  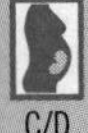 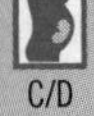
No Yes ? C/D

Tabs (Urolene Blue): 65 mg
Injection: 10 mg/mL (1%) (1, 10 ml)

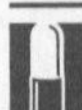

Methemoglobinemia:
Child and adult: 1–2 mg/kg/dose or 25–50 mg/m²/dose IV over 5 min. May repeat in 1 hr if needed.

At high doses, may cause methemoglobinemia. **Avoid** subcutaneous or intrathecal routes of administration. **Use with caution** in G6PD deficiency or renal insufficiency. May cause nausea, vomiting, dizziness, headache, diaphoresis, stained skin, and abdominal pain. Causes blue-green discoloration of urine and feces. Pregnancy category changes to "D" if injected intra-amniotically.

METHYLPHENIDATE HCL
Ritalin, Methylin, Metadate ER, Methylin ER, Concerta, Ritalin SR, Metadate CD, Ritalin LA, Daytrana, and others
CNS stimulant

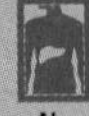 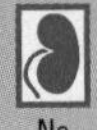  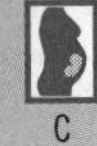
No No ? C

Tabs: 5, 10, 20 mg
Chewable tabs: 2.5, 5, 10 mg; contains phenylalanine

Continued

METHYLPHENIDATE HCL *continued*

Oral solution (Methylin): 1 mg/mL, 2 mg/mL
Extended-release tabs:
8-hr duration (Metadate ER, Methylin ER): 10, 20 mg
24-hr duration (Concerta): 18, 27, 36, 54 mg
Sustained-release tabs:
8-hr duration (Ritalin SR): 20 mg
Extended-release caps:
24-hr duration (Metadate CD, Ritalin LA): 10, 20, 30, 40, 50, 60 mg
Transdermal patch (Daytrana): 10 mg/9 hr (each 12.5 cm^2 patch contains 27.5 mg), 15 mg/9 hr (each 18.75 cm^2 patch contains 41.3 mg), 20 mg/9 hr (each 25 cm^2 patch contains 55 mg), 30 mg/9 hr (each 37.5 cm^2 patch contains 82.5 mg) (10s and 30s)

Attention deficit hyperactivity disorder:
Immediate release oral dosage forms (Methylin, Ritalin; ≥6 yr):
Initial: 0.3 mg/kg/dose (or 2.5–5 mg/dose) given before breakfast and lunch. May increase by 0.1 mg/kg/dose PO (or 5–10 mg/24 hr) weekly until maintenance dose achieved. May give extra afternoon dose if needed.
Maintenance dose range: 0.3–1 mg/kg/24 hr
Max. dose: 2 mg/kg/24 hr or 60 mg/24 hr
Extended release once daily oral dosage form (Concerta; ≥6 yr):
Methylphenidate naiive patients: Start with 18 mg PO QAM for children and adolescents and 18–36 mg PO QAM for adults, dosage may be increased at weekly intervals at 18 mg increments up to the following **max. dose:**
6–12 yr: 54 mg/24 hr
13–17 yr: 72 mg/24 hr not to exceed 2 mg/kg/24 hr
Patients currently receiving methylphenidate: See following table.

Recommended Dose Conversion from Methylphenidate Regimens to Concerta

Previous Methylphenidate Daily Dose	Recommended Concerta Dose
5 mg PO BID–TID or 20 mg SR PO once daily	18 mg PO QAM
10 mg PO BID–TID or 40 mg SR PO once daily	36 mg PO QAM
15 mg PO BID–TID or 60 mg SR PO once daily	54 mg PO QAM
20 mg PO BID–TID	72 mg PO QAM

After a week of receiving the above-recommended Concerta dose, dose may be increased in 18 mg increments at weekly intervals up to a **maximum** of 54 mg/24 hr for 6–12 yr and 72 mg/24 hr (not to exceed 2 mg/kg/24 hr) for 13–17 yr.

Other extended release oral dosage forms:
Metadate CD (≥6 yr): Start with 20 mg PO once daily, dosage may be increased at weekly intervals at 20-mg increments up to a **max. dose** of 60 mg/24 hr.
Ritalin LA (≥6 yr): Start with 20 mg PO once daily, dosage may be increased at weekly intervals at 10 mg increments up to a **max. dose** of 60 mg/24 hr.
Transdermal patch (Daytrana): Apply to the hip 2 hr before the effect is needed and remove 9 hr later. Patch may be removed before 9 hr if shorter duration of effect is desired or if late day adverse effects appear.
6–17 yr: Start with 10 mg/9 hr patch once daily. Increase dose PRN Q7 days by increasing to the next dosage strength.

Continued

For explanation of icons, see p. 663.

METHYLPHENIDATE HCL *continued*

Contraindicated in glaucoma, anxiety disorders, motor tics, and Tourette's syndrome. Medication should generally **not** be used in children <5 yr old as diagnosis of ADHD in this age group is extremely difficult and should be only done in consultation with a specialist. **Sudden death** (children, adolescents, and adults), stroke (adults), and MI (adults) have been reported in patients with pre-existing structural cardiac abnormalities or other serious heart problems. **Use with caution** in patients with hypertension, psychiatric conditions, and epilepsy. Insomnia, weight loss, anorexia, rash, nausea, emesis, abdominal pain, hyper- or hypotension, tachycardia, arrhythmias, palpitations, restlessness, headaches, fever, tremor, visual disturbances, and thrombocytopenia may occur. Abnormal liver function, cerebral arteritis and/or occlusion, leukopenia and/or anemia, transient depressed mood, paranoia, mania, auditory hallucination, and scalp hair loss have been reported. Skin irritation may occur and contact dermatitis has been reported with transdermal route. High doses may slow growth by appetite suppression. GI obstruction has been reported with Concerta.

May increase serum concentrations/effects of tricyclic antidepressants, dopamine agonists (e.g., haloperidol), phenytoin, phenobarbital, and warfarin. May decrease the effects of antihypertensive drugs. Effect of methylphenidate may be potentiated by MAO inhibitors; hypertensive crisis may also occur if used within 14 days of discontinuance of the MAO inhibitor.

Extended/sustained-release dosage forms have either an 8- or 24-hour dosage interval (as stipulated previously). Concerta dosage form delivers 22.2% of its dose as an immediate-release product with the remaining amounts as an extended-release product (e.g., 18 mg strength: 4 mg as immediate release and 14 mg as extended release). **Do not expose transdermal application site to external heat sources** (e.g., electric blankets, heating pads); this may increase drug release.

METHYLPREDNISOLONE

Medrol, Medrol Dosepack, Solu-Medrol, Depo-Medrol, and others
Corticosteroid

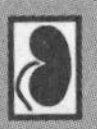 No  No 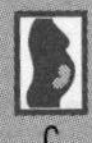 2 C

Tabs: 2, 4, 8, 16, 24, 32 mg
Tabs, dose pack (Medrol Dosepack and others): 4 mg (21s)
Injection, Na succinate (Solu-Medrol and others): 40, 125, 500, 1000, 2000 mg (IV or IM use); may contain benzyl alcohol
Injection, Acetate (Depo-Medrol and others): 20, 40, 80 mg/mL (IM repository)

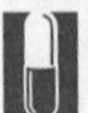

Anti-inflammatory/immunosuppressive:
PO/IM/IV: 0.5–1.7 mg/kg/24 hr ÷ Q6–12 hr.

Asthma exacerbations (2007 National Heart, Lung, and Blood Institute Guideline Recommendations; dose until peak expiratory flow reaches 70% of predicted or personal best):

Child ≤12 yr (IM/IV/PO): 1 mg/kg/24 hr ÷ Q12 hr (**max. dose:** 60 mg/24 hr). Higher alternative regimen of 1 mg/kg/dose Q6 hr × 48 hr followed by 1–2 mg/kg/24 hr (**max. dose:** 60 mg/24 hr) ÷ Q12 hr has been suggested.

>12 yr and adult (IV/IM/PO): 40–80 mg/24 hr ÷ Q12–24 hr. Higher alternative regimen of 120–180 mg/24 hr ÷ Q6–8 hr × 48 hr followed by 60–80 mg/24 hr ÷ Q12 hr has been suggested.

Continued

METHYLPREDNISOLONE *continued*

Outpatient asthma exacerbation burst therapy (longer durations may be necessary):

PO:

Child ≤12 yr: 1–2 mg/kg/24 hr ÷ Q12–24 hr (**max. dose:** 60 mg/24 hr) × 3–10 days.

Child >12 yr and adult: 40–60 mg/24 hr ÷ Q12–24 hr × 3–10 days.

IM (use methylprednisolone acetate product) for patients vomiting or with adherence issues:

Child ≤12 yr: 7.5 mg/kg (**max. dose:** 240 mg) IM × 1.

Child >12 yr and adult: 240 mg IM × 1.

Acute spinal cord injury:

30 mg/kg IV over 15 min followed in 45 min by a continuous infusion of 5.4 mg/kg/hr × 23 hr.

See Chapter 30 for relative, steroid potencies and doses based on body surface area. Acetate form may also be used for intra-articular and intralesional injection and has longer times to max. effect and duration of action; it should **NOT** be given IV. Like all steroids, may cause hypertension, pseudotumor cerebri, acne, Cushing syndrome, adrenal axis suppression, GI bleeding, hyperglycemia, and osteoporosis.

Barbiturates, phenytoin, and rifampin may enhance methylprednisolone clearance. Erythromycin, itraconazole, and ketoconazole may increase methylprednisone levels. Methylprednisolone may increase cyclosporine and tacrolimus levels.

METOCLOPRAMIDE
Reglan, Maxolon, Metozolv, and many other generics
Antiemetic, prokinetic agent

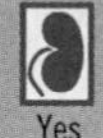
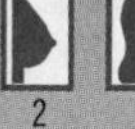
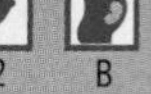

No Yes 2 B

Tabs: 5, 10 mg
Tabs, orally disintegrating (ODT) (Metozolv): 5, 10 mg
Injection: 5 mg/mL (2, 10, 30 mL)
Syrup: 5 mg/5 mL

Gastroesophageal reflux (GER) or GI dysmotility:

Infant and child: 0.1–0.2 mg/kg/dose up to QID IV/IM/PO; **max. dose:** 0.8 mg/kg/24 hr

Adult: 10–15 mg/dose QAC and QHS IV/IM/PO

Antiemetic (all ages): Premedicate with diphenydramine to reduce EPS.

1–2 mg/kg/dose Q2–6 hr IV/IM/PO.

Postoperative nausea and vomiting:

Child: 0.1–0.2 mg/kg/dose Q6–8 hr PRN IV

>14 yr and adult: 10 mg Q6–8 hr PRN IV

Contraindicated in GI obstruction, seizure disorder, pheochromocytoma, or in patients receiving drugs likely to cause extrapyramidal symptoms (EPS). May cause EPS, especially at higher doses. Sedation, headache, anxiety, depression, leukopenia, and diarrhea may occur. Neuroleptic malignant syndrome and tardive dyskinesia have been reported.

For GER, give 30 min before meals and at bedtime. **Reduce dose in renal impairment (see Chapter 31).**

METOLAZONE
Zaroxolyn and many other generics
Diuretic, thiazide-like

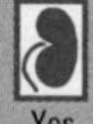
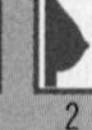
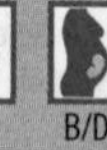

Yes Yes 2 B/D

Tabs: 2.5, 5, 10 mg
Oral suspension: 0.25, 1 mg/mL 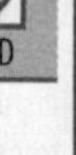

Continued

For explanation of icons, see p. 663.

METOLAZONE *continued*

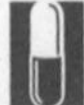

Dosage based on Zaroxolyn (for oral suspension, see remarks):
Child: 0.2–0.4 mg/kg/24 hr ÷ once daily–BID PO
Adult:
Hypertension: 2.5–5 mg once daily PO
Edema: 2.5–20 mg once daily PO

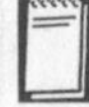

Contraindicated in patients with anuria, hepatic coma, or hypersensitivity to sulfonamides or thiazides. **Use with caution** in severe renal disease, impaired hepatic function, gout, lupus erythematosus, diabetes mellitus, and elevated cholesterol and triglycerides. Electrolyte imbalance, GI disturbance, hyperglycemia, marrow suppression, chills, hyperuricemia, chest pain, hepatitis, and rash may occur.

Oral suspension have increased bioavailability; therefore, lower doses may be necessary when using these dosage forms. More effective than thiazide diuretics in impaired renal function; may be effective in GFRs as low as 20 mL/min. Furosemide-resistant edema in pediatric patients may benefit with the addition of metolazone.

Pregnancy category changes to "D" if used for pregnancy-induced hypertension.

METOPROLOL
Lopressor, Toprol-XL, and others
Adrenergic blocking agent (beta-1 selective), class II antiarrhythmic

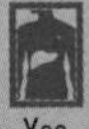
Yes
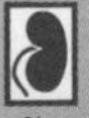
No
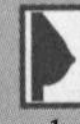
1
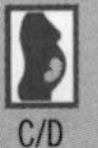
C/D

Tabs: 25, 50, 100 mg
Extended-released tabs (Toprol-XL and others): 25, 50, 100, 200 mg
Oral liquid: 10 mg/mL
Injection: 1 mg/mL (5 mL)

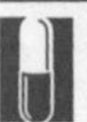

Hypertension:
Child ≥1 yr and adolescent (non-extended released oral dosage forms): Start at 1–2 mg/kg/24 hr PO ÷ BID; **max. dose:** 6 mg/kg/24 hr **up to** 200 mg/24 hr.
Adult:
Nonextended released tabs: Start at 50–100 mg/24 hr PO ÷ once daily–BID; if needed, increase dosage at weekly intervals to desired blood pressure. Usual effective dosage range is 100–450 mg/24 hr. Doses >450 mg/24 hr have not been studied. Patients with bronchospastic diseases should receive the lowest possible daily dose divided TID.
Extended released tabs: Start at 25–100 mg/24 hr PO once daily; if needed, increase dosage at weekly intervals to desired blood pressure. Usual dosage range is 50–100 mg/24 hr. Doses >400 mg/24 hr have not been studied.

Contraindicated in sinus bradycardia, heart block >1st degree, sick sinus syndrome (except with functioning pacemaker), cardiogenic shock, and uncompensated CHF. **Use with caution** in hepatic dysfunction, peripheral vascular disease, history of severe anaphylactic hypersensitivity drug reactions, pheochromocytoma, and concurrent use with verapamil, diltiazem, or anesthetic agents that may decrease myocardial function. Should not be used with bronchospastic diseases. Reserpine and other drugs that deplete catecholamines (e.g., MAO inhibitors) may increase the effects of metoprolol. Metoprolol is a CYP 450 2D6 substrate.

Avoid abrupt cessation of therapy in ischemic heart disease; angina and MI have occurred. Common side effects include bradyarrhythmia, heart block, heart failure, pruritus, rash, GI disturbances, dizziness, fatigue, and depression. Bronchospasm, dyspnea and elevations in transaminase, alkaline phosphatase, and LDH have all been reported.

Pregnancy category changes to "D" if used in second or third trimesters.

METRONIDAZOLE
Flagyl, Flagyl ER, Protostat, MetroGel, MetroLotion, MetroCream, Noritate, MetroGel-Vaginal, and others
Antibiotic, antiprotozoal

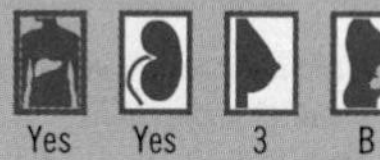

Tabs: 250, 500 mg
Tabs, extended release (Flagyl ER): 750 mg
Caps: 375 mg
Oral suspension: 10, 50 mg/mL
Oral syrup: 5 mg/mL
Injection: 500 mg; contains 830 mg mannitol/g drug
Ready-to-use injection: 5 mg/mL (100 mL); contains 28 mEq Na/g drug
Gel, topical (MetroGel): 0.75% (28, 60 g)
Lotion (MetroLotion): 0.75% (60 mL); contains benzyl alcohol
Cream, topical:
MetroCream: 0.75% (45 g); contains benzyl alcohol
Noritate: 1% (60 g)
Gel, vaginal (MetroGel-Vaginal): 0.75% (70 g with 5 applicators)

Amebiasis:
Child: 35–50 mg/kg/24 hr PO ÷ TID × 10 days
Adult: 500–750 mg/dose PO TID × 10 days

Anaerobic infection:
Neonate: PO/IV:
<7 days:
<1.2 kg: 7.5 mg/kg/dose Q48 hr
1.2–2 kg: 7.5 mg/kg/dose Q24 hr
≥2 kg: 15 mg/kg/24 hr ÷ Q12 hr
≥7 days:
<1.2 kg: 7.5 mg/kg Q24 hr
1.2–2 kg: 15 mg/kg/24 hr ÷ Q12 hr
≥2 kg: 30 mg/kg/24 hr ÷ Q12 hr
Infant/child/adult:
IV/PO: 30 mg/kg/24 hr ÷ Q6 hr
Max. dose: 4 g/24 hr

Other parasitic infections:
Infant/child: 15–30 mg/kg/24 hr PO ÷ Q8 hr
Adult: 250 mg PO Q8 hr or 2 g PO × 1

Bacterial vaginosis:
Adolescent and adult:
PO:
Immediate release tabs: 500 mg BID × 7 days
Extended release tabs: 750 mg once daily × 7 days
Vaginal: 5 g (1 applicator full) BID × 5 days

Giardiasis:
Child: 15 mg/kg/24 hr PO ÷ TID × 5 days; **max. dose:** 750 mg/24 hr
Adult: 250 mg PO TID × 5 days

Trichomoniasis: Treat sexual contacts.
Child: 15 mg/kg/24 hr PO ÷ TID × 7 days
Adolescent/adult: 2 g PO × 1 or 250 mg PO TID or 375 mg PO BID × 7 days

Continued

For explanation of icons, see p. 663.

METRONIDAZOLE *continued*

C. difficile infection (IV may be less efficacious):

Child: 30 mg/kg/24 hr ÷ Q6 hr PO/IV × 10 days

Adult: 250–500 mg TID–QID PO × 10–14 days, or 500 mg Q8 hr IV × 10–14 days

H. pylori infection (use in combination with amoxicillin and bismuth subsalicylate):

Child: 15–20 mg/kg/24 hr ÷ BID PO × 4 wk

Adult: 250–500 mg TID PO × 14 days

Inflammatory bowel disease (as alternative to sulfasalazine):

Adult: 400 mg BID PO

Topical use: apply and rub a thin film to affected areas at the following frequencies specific to product concentration.

0.75% cream: BID

1% cream: once daily

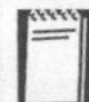

Avoid use in first-trimester pregnancy. **Use with caution** in patients with CNS disease, blood dyscrasias, severe liver or **renal disease (GFR <10 mL/min), see Chapter 31.** Nausea, diarrhea, urticaria, dry mouth, leukopenia, vertigo, metallic taste, and peripheral neuropathy may occur. Candidiasis may worsen. May discolor urine. Patients **should not** ingest alcohol for 24–48 hr after dose (disulfuram-type reaction).

Single dose oral regimen no longer recommended in bacterial vaginosis due to poor efficacy. May increase levels or toxicity of phenytoin, lithium, and warfarin. Phenobarbital and rifampin may increase metronidazole metabolism.

IV infusion must be given slowly over 1 hr. For intravenous use in all ages, some references recommend a 15 mg/kg loading dose.

MICAFUNGIN SODIUM

Mycamine

Antifungal, echinocandin

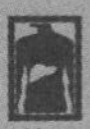 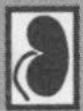  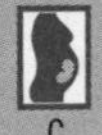

Yes Yes ? C

Injection: 50, 100 mg; contains lactose

Invasive candidiasis (see remarks):

Neonate and infant (based on a multi-dose pharmacokinetic and safety trial in 13 neonates/infants >48 hr and <120 days old with suspected or invasive candidiasis; minimum of 4–5 days of therapy):

<1 kg: 10 mg/kg/dose IV once daily; additional data from another multi-dose trial in 12 pre-term neonates (median birth weight: 775 g, 27 wk gestation) suggest 15 mg/kg/dose IV once daily will provide similar AUC drug exposure of approximately 5 mg/kg/dose in adults.

≥1 kg: 7 mg/kg/dose IV once daily.

Child, adolescent: 3–4 mg/kg/dose IV once daily; **max. dose:** 200 mg/dose.

Adult: 100–150 mg IV once daily.

Esophageal candidiasis (see remarks):

Child–adult:

<50 kg: 3–4 mg/kg/dose IV once daily; **max. dose:** 200 mg/dose.

≥50 kg: 150 mg IV once daily; mean duration for successful therapy was 15 days (range: 10–30 days).

Candida prophylaxis in hematopoietic stem cell transplant:

Child–adult:

<50 kg: 1 mg/kg/dose IV once daily; **max. dose:** 50 mg/dose.

≥50 kg: 50 mg IV once daily; mean duration 19 days (range: 6–51 days).

Continued

MICAFUNGIN SODIUM *continued*

Invasive aspergilosis (see remarks; doses under investigation):

Child–adult:

<50 kg: 3–4 mg/kg/dose IV once daily; dosages as high as 7.5 mg/kg/24 hr have been tolerated.

≥50 kg: 150 mg IV once daily.

Prior hypersensitivity to other echinocandins (anidulafungin, casopofungin) increases risk; anaphylaxis with shock has been reported. **Use with caution** in hepatic and renal impairment.

No dosing adjustments are required based on race or gender, or in patients with severe renal dysfunction or mild to moderate hepatic function impairment. Effect of severe hepatic function impairment on micafungin pharmacokinetics has not been evaluated. Higher dosage requirements in premature and young infants may be attributed to the faster drug clearance due to lower protein binding. Higher treatment doses in infants and children have been reported at 8.6–12 mg/kg/dose IV once daily.

May cause GI disturbances, phlebitis, rash, hyperbilirubinemia, liver function test elevation, headache, fever, and rigor. Anemia, leukopenia, neutropenia, thrombocytopenia, and hemolysis have been reported. Micafungin is CYP450 3A isoenzyme substrate and weak inhibitor. May increase the effects/toxicity of nifedipine and sirolimus.

MICONAZOLE

Topical products: Micatin, Lotrimin AF, and others

Vaginal products: Monistat, Vagistat-3, and others

Antifungal agent

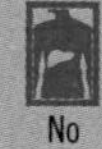
No

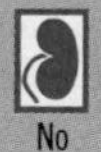
No

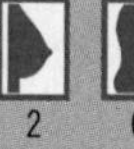
2 C

Cream (OTC): 2% (15, 30, 90 g)
Lotion (OTC): 2% (30, 60 mL)
Ointment (OTC): 2% (28.4 g)
Solution (OTC): 2% with alcohol (30.3 mL)
Gel (OTC): 2% with alcohol (24 g)
Topical solution (OTC): 2% with alcohol (30.3 mL)
Powder (OTC): 2% (70, 90 g)
Spray, liquid (OTC): 2% (105 mL); contains alcohol
Spray, powder (OTC): 2% (90, 120 g); contains alcohol
Vaginal cream (OTC): 2% (15, 25, 45 g), 4% (15, 25 g)
Vaginal suppository (OTC): 100 mg (7s), 200 mg (3s)
Vaginal combination packs:

Monistat 1 Combination Pack (OTC): 1200 mg suppository (1) and 2% cream (9 g)
Monistat 3, Vagistat-3 (OTC): 200 mg suppository (3s) and 2% cream (9 g)
Monistat 7 (OTC): 100 mg suppository (7s) and 2% cream (9 g)

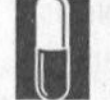

Topical: Apply BID × 2–4 wk

Vaginal:

7 day regimen: 1 applicator full of 2% cream or 100 mg suppository QHS × 7 days

3 day regimen: 1 applicator full of 4% cream or 200 mg suppository QHS × 3 days

Monistat 1: 1200 mg suppository × 1 at bedtime or during the day

Use with caution in hypersensitivity to other imidazole antifungal agents (e.g., clotrimazole, ketoconazole). Side effects include pruritis, rash, burning, phlebitits, headaches, and pelvic cramps.

Drug is a substrate and inhibitor of the CYP 450 3A3/4 isoenzymes. Vaginal use with concomitant warfarin use has also been reported to increase warfarin's effect. Vegetable oil base in vaginal suppositories may interact with latex products (e.g., condoms and diaphragms); consider switching to the vaginal cream.

For explanation of icons, see p. 663.

MIDAZOLAM
Various generics; previously available as Versed
Benzodiazepine

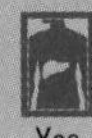
Yes
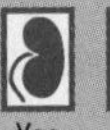
Yes
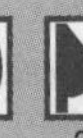
2
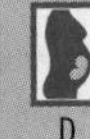
D

Injection: 1, 5 mg/mL; some preparations may contain 1% benzyl alcohol
Oral syrup: 2 mg/mL; contains sodium benzoate

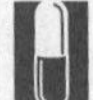

Titrate to effect under controlled conditions.
See Chapter 6 for additional routes of administration.

Sedation for procedures:

Child:

IV:

6 mo–5 yr: 0.05–0.1 mg/kg/dose over 2–3 min. May repeat dose PRN in 2–3 min intervals up to a **max. total dose** of 6 mg. A total dose up to 0.6 mg/kg may be necessary for desired effect.

6–12 yr: 0.025–0.05 mg/kg/dose over 2–3 min. May repeat dose PRN in 2–3 min intervals up to a **max. total dose** of 10 mg. A total dose up to 0.4 mg/kg may be necessary for desired effect.

>12–16 yr: Use adult dose; up to **max. total dose** of 10 mg.

PO:

≥6 mo: 0.25–0.5 mg/kg/dose × 1; **max. dose:** 20 mg. Younger patients (6 mo–5 yr) may require higher doses of 1 mg/kg/dose, whereas older patients (6–15 yr) may require only 0.25 mg/kg/dose. Use 0.25 mg/kg/dose for patients with cardiac or respiratory compromise, concurrent CNS depressive drug, or high-risk surgery.

Adult:

IV: 0.5–2 mg/dose over 2 min. May repeat PRN in 2–3 min intervals until desired effect. Usual total dose: 2.5–5 mg. **Max. total dose:** 10 mg.

Sedation with mechanical ventilation:

Intermittent:

Infant and child: 0.05–0.15 mg/kg/dose IV Q1–2 hr PRN.

Continuous IV infusion (initial doses, titrate to effect):

Neonate:

<32 wk gestation: 0.5 mcg/kg/min.

≥32 wk gestation: 1 mcg/kg/min.

Infant and child: 1–2 mcg/kg/min.

Refractory status epilepticus:

≥2 mo and child: Load with 0.15 mg/kg IV × 1 followed by a continuous infusion of 1 mcg/kg/min and titrate dose upward Q5 min to effect (mean dose of 2.3 mcg/kg/min with a range of 1–18 mcg/kg/min has been reported).

Contraindicated in patients with narrow angle glaucoma and shock. **Use with caution** in CHF, **renal impairment (adjust dose; see Chapter 31),** pulmonary disease, hepatic dysfunction, and in neonates. Causes respiratory depression, hypotension, and bradycardia. Cardiovascular monitoring is recommended. Use lower doses or reduce dose when given in combination with narcotics or in patients with respiratory compromise.

Drug is a substrate for CYP 450 3A4. Serum concentrations may be increased by cimetidine, clarithromycin, diltiazem, erythromycin, itraconazole, ketoconazole, and protease inhibitors (use contraindicated). Sedative effects may be antagonized by theophylline. **Effects can be reversed by flumazenil.** For pharmacodynamic information, see Chapter 6.

MILRINONE
Primacor
Inotrope

No Yes ? C

Injection: 1 mg/mL (10, 20, 50 mL)
Pre-mixed injection in D_5W: 200 mcg/mL (100, 200 mL)

Child (limited data): 50 mcg/kg IV bolus over 15 min, followed by a continuous infusion of 0.25–0.75 mcg/kg/min and titrate to effect.
Adult: 50 mcg/kg IV bolus over 10 min, followed by a continuous infusion of 0.375–0.75 mcg/kg/min and titrate to effect. **Max. dose:** 1.13 mg/kg/24 hr.

Contraindicated in severe aortic stenosis, severe pulmonic stenosis, and acute MI. May cause headache, dysrhythmias, hypotension, hypokalemia, nausea, vomiting, anorexia, abdominal pain, hepatotoxicity, and thrombocytopenia. Pediatric patients may require higher mcg/kg/min doses because of a faster elimination $T_{1/2}$ and larger volume of distribution, when compared to adults. Hemodynamic effects can last up to 3–5 hr after discontinuation of infusion in children. **Reduce dose in renal impairment.**

MINERAL OIL
Kondremul, Fleet Mineral Oil, and others
Laxative, lubricant

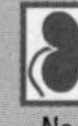

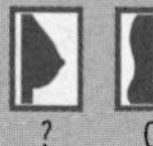

No No ? C

Liquid, oral (OTC): 480 mL
Emulsion, oral (Kondremul; OTC): 480 mL
Rectal liquid (Fleet Mineral Oil, OTC): 133 mL

Child 5–11 yr (see remarks):
Oral liquid: 5–15 mL/24 hr ÷ once daily–TID PO
Oral emulsion (Kondremul): 10–25 mL/24 hr ÷ once daily–TID PO
Rectal: 30–60 mL as single dose
Child ≥12 yr and adult (see remarks):
Oral liquid: 15–45 mL/24 hr ÷ once daily–TID PO
Oral emulsion (Kondremul): 30–75 mL/24 hr ÷ once daily–TID PO
Rectal: 60–150 mL as single dose

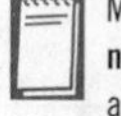

May cause diarrhea, cramps, and lipid pneumonitis via aspiration. Use as a laxative **should not exceed** >1 wk. Onset of action is approximately 6–8 hr. Higher doses may be necessary to achieve desired effect. Do **not** give QHS dose and **use with caution** in children <5 yr to minimize risk of aspiration. May impair the absorption of fat-soluble vitamins, calcium, phosphorus, oral contraceptives, and warfarin. Emulsified preparations are more palatable and are dosed differently than the oral liquid preparation.

For disimpaction, doses up to 1 ounce (30 mL) per yr of age (**max. dose** of 240 mL) BID can be given.

For explanation of icons, see p. 663.

MINOCYCLINE
Minocin, Dynacin, Arestin, Solodyn, and others
Antibiotic, tetracycline derivative

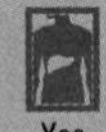 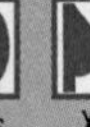 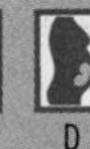 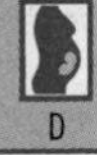
Yes Yes X D

Tabs: 50, 75, 100 mg
Caps: 50, 75, 100 mg
Extended-release tabs (Solodyn): 45, 65, 90, 115, 135 mg
Caps (pellet filled): 50, 100 mg
Sustained-release microspheres (Arestin): 1 mg (12s)
Oral suspension: 50 mg/5 mL (60 mL); contains 5% alcohol

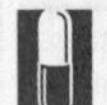

General infections:
Child (8–12 yr): 4 mg/kg/dose × 1 PO, then 2 mg/kg/dose Q12 hr PO; **max. dose:** 200 mg/24 hr
Adolescent and adult: 200 mg/dose × 1 PO, then 100 mg Q12 hr PO
Chlamydia trachomatis/Ureaplasma urealyticum:
Adolescent and adult: 100 mg PO Q12 hr × 7 days
Acne (≥12 yr–adult):
Immediate release dosage forms: 50–100 mg PO once daily–BID
Extended-release tabs:
45–54 kg: 45 mg PO once daily
55–77 kg: 65 mg PO once daily
78–102 kg: 90 mg PO once daily
103–125 kg: 115 mg PO once daily
126–136 kg: 135 mg PO once daily

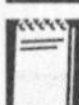

Not recommended for children <8 yr and during the last half of pregnancy due to risk of permanent tooth discoloration. **Use with caution** in renal failure, lower dosage may be necessary. High incidence of vestibular dysfunction (30%–90%). Nausea, vomiting, allergy, increased intracranial pressure, photophobia, and injury to developing teeth may occur. Hepatitis, including autoimmune hepatitis, liver failure, hypersensitivity reactions (e.g., anaphylaxis, Stevens Johnson syndrome, erythema multiforme), and lupus-like syndrome have been reported.

May increase effects/toxicity of warfarin and decrease the efficacy of live attenuated oral typhoid vaccine. May be administered with food but **NOT** with milk or dairy products. See *Tetracycline* for additional drug/food interactions and comments.

MINOXIDIL
Various generics (previously available as Loniten), Rogaine, Men's Rogaine Extra Strength
Antihypertensive agent, hair growth stimulant

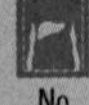 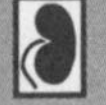 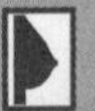 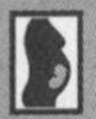
No Yes 2 C

Tabs: 2.5, 10 mg
Topical solution:
Rogaine (OTC): 2% (60 mL)
Men's Rogaine Extra Strength (OTC): 5% (60 mL); contains 30% alcohol
Topical aerosol foam:
Men's Rogaine Extra Strength (OTC): 5% (60 g); contains alcohol

Continued

MINOXIDIL *continued*

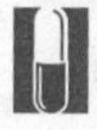

Child <12 yr:
Start with 0.1–0.2 mg/kg/24 hr PO once daily; **max. dose:** 5 mg/24 hr. Dose may be increased in increments of 0.1–0.2 mg/kg/24 hr at 3-day intervals. Usual effective range: 0.25–1 mg/kg/24 hr PO ÷ once daily–BID; **max. dose:** 50 mg/24 hr.

≥12 yr and adult:
Oral: Start with 5 mg once daily. Dose may be gradually increased at 3-day intervals. Usual effective range: 10–40 mg/24 hr ÷ once daily–BID; **max. dose:** 100 mg/24 hr.

Topical (alopecia):
Adult: Apply 1 mL to the total affected areas of the scalp BID (QAM and QHS). **Max. dose:** 2 mL/24 hr.

Contraindicated in acute MI, dissecting aortic aneurysm, and pheochromocytoma. Concurrent use with a beta-blocker and diuretic is recommended to prevent reflex tachycardia and reduce water retention, respectively. May cause drowsiness, dizziness, CHF, pulmonary edema, pericardial effusion, pericarditis, thrombocytopenia, leukopenia, Stevens-Johnson syndrome, and hypertrichosis (reversible) with systemic use. Concurrent use of guanethidine may cause profound orthostatic hypotension; use with other antihypertensive agents may cause additive hypotension. Patients with renal failure or receiving dialysis may require a dosage reduction. Antihypertensive onset of action within 30 min and peak effects within 2–8 hr.

TOPICAL USE: Local irritation, contact dermatitis may occur. **Do not use** in conjunction with other topical agents including topical corticosteroids, retinoids or petrolatum, or agents that are known to enhance cutaneous drug absorption. Onset of hair growth (topical use) is 4 mo. The 5% solution is flammable.

MOMETASONE FUROATE ± FORMOTEROL FUMARATE
Asmanex Twisthaler, Nasonex, Elocon, and other generic topical products
In combination with fomoterol: Dulera
Corticosteroid

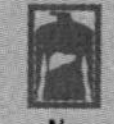 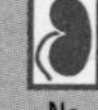 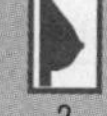 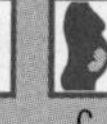 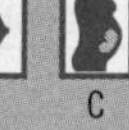

No No 2 C

Nasal spray (Nasonex): 0.05%, 50 mcg per actuation (17 g = 120 doses)
Powder for inhalation (Asmanex Twisthaler, see remarks): 110 mcg per actuation (30 units), 220 mcg per actuation (14, 30, 60, 120 units); contains lactose
Topical cream and ointment (Elocon and others): 0.1% (15, 45 g)
Topical lotion and solution (Elocon and others): 0.1% (30, 60 mL); contains isopropyl alcohol
In combination with fomoterol:
Aerosol inhaler (Dulera):
100 mcg mometasone furoate + 5 mcg formoterol fumarate dihydrate per inhalation (13 g delivers 120 inhalations)
200 mcg mometasone furoate + 5 mcg formoterol fumarate dihydrate per inhalation (13 g delivers 120 inhalations)

MOMETASONE FUROATE:
Intranasal (allergic rhinitis): Patients with known seasonal allergic rhinitis should initiate therapy 2–4 wk prior to anticipated pollen season.
2–11 yr: 50 mcg (1 spray) each nostril once daily
≥12 yr: 100 mcg (2 sprays) each nostril once daily

Oral inhalation:
4–11 yr: Start with 110 mcg (1 inhalation) QHS of the 110 mcg inhaler regardless of prior therapy. **Max. dose:** 110 mcg/24 hr.

Continued

For explanation of icons, see p. 663.

MOMETASONE FUROATE ± FORMOTEROL FUMARATE *continued*

Oral inhalation (cont'd):

≥12 yr: Max. effects may not be achieved until 1–2 wk or longer. Titrate doses to the lowest effective dose once asthma stabilized.

Previously treated with bronchodilators alone or with inhaled corticosteroids: Start with 220 mcg (1 inhalation) QHS. Dose may be increased up to a **max. dose** of 440 mcg/24 hr ÷ QHS or BID.

Previously treated with oral corticosteroids: Start with 440 mcg BID; **max. dose:** 880 mcg/24 hr.

Topical:

Cream and ointment:

≥2 yr: Apply a thin film to affected area once daily. Safety and efficacy for >3 wk has not been established for pediatric patients.

Lotion:

≥12 yr: Apply a few drops to affected area and massage lightly into skin until it disappears once daily.

MOMETASONE FUROATE + FORMOTEROL FUMARATE (Dulera):

≥12 yr and adult: Two inhalations BID of either 100 mcg mometasone + 5 mcg formoterol or 200 mcg mometasone + 5 mcg formoterol based on prior asthma therapy (see Table below).
Maximum dose: Two inhalations BID of 200 mcg mometasone + 5 mcg formoterol.

Previous Therapy	Recommended Starting Dose	Recommended Maximum Daily Dose
Medium dose inhaled corticosteroids	100 mcg mometasone + 5 mcg formoterol: 2 inhalations BID	400 mcg mometasone + 20 mcg formoterol
High dose inhaled corticosteroids	200 mcg mometasone + 5 mcg formoterol: 2 inhalations BID	800 mcg mometasone + 20 mcg formoterol

Concurrent administration with ketoconazole and other CYP 450 3A4 inhibitors may increase mometasone levels, resulting in Cushing syndrome and adrenal suppression.

INTRANASAL: Clear nasal passages and shake nasal spray well before each use. Onset of action for nasal symptoms of allergic rhinitis has been shown to occur within 11 hr after the first dose. Nasal burning and irritation may occur. Nasal septal perforation, taste and smell disturbances have been rarely reported.

ORAL INHALATION (all forms): Rinse mouth after each use. Fever, allergic rhinitis, URI, UTI, GI discomfort, and sore throat have been reported in children. Musculoskeletal pain, oral candidiasis, arthralgia, and fatigue may occur. Do not use Asmanex Twisthaler if allergic to milk proteins.

MOMETASONE + FOMOTEROL (Dulera): Breastfeeding information is currently unknown. Common side effects include nasopharyngitis, sinusitis, and headache. See *Formoterol* for additional remarks.

TOPICAL USE: Avoid application/contact to face, eyes, underarms, groin, and open skin. Occlusive dressings and use in diaper dermatitis are **not recommended.**

MONTELUKAST
Singulair
Anti-asthmatic, anti-allergy, leukotriene receptor antagonist

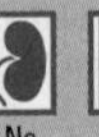
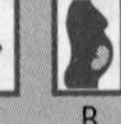

No No ? B

Chewable tabs: 4, 5 mg; contains phenylalanine
Tabs: 10 mg
Oral granules: 4 mg per packet (30s)

Continued

MONTELUKAST *continued*

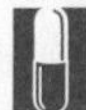

Asthma and seasonal allergic rhinitis:

Child (6 mo–5 yr): 4 mg (oral granules or chewable tablet) PO QHS

Child (6–14 yr): 5 mg (chewable tablet) PO QHS

>14 yr and adult: 10 mg PO QHS

Prevention of exercise-induced bronchospasm:

≥15 yr and adult: 10 mg PO at least 2 hr prior to exercise; additional doses should not be administered within 24 hr.

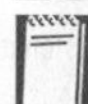

Chewable tablet dosage form is **contraindicated** in phenylketonuric patients. Side effects include: headache, abdominal pain, dyspepsia, fatigue, dizziness, cough, and elevated liver enzymes. Diarrhea, eosinophilia, hypersensitivity reactions, pharyngitis, nausea, otitis, sinusitis, and viral infections have been reported in children. Neuropsychiatric events, including aggression, anxiety, dream abnormalities, hallucinations, depression, suicidal behavior, and insomnia, have been reported.

Drug is a substrate for CYP 450 3A4 and 2C9. Phenobarbital and rifampin may induce hepatic metabolism to increase the clearance of montelukast.

Doses may administered with or without food.

MORPHINE SULFATE

Roxanol, MS Contin, Oramorph SR, and many others

Narcotic, analgesic

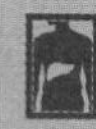 No 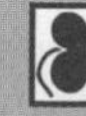 Yes 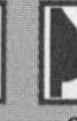 2 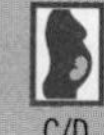 C/D

Oral solution: 10 mg/5 mL, 20 mg/5 mL

Concentrated oral solution: 100 mg/5 mL

Caps/tabs: 15, 30 mg

Controlled release tabs (MS Contin, Oramorph SR): 15, 30, 60, 100*, 200* mg

Extended-release tabs: 15, 30, 60, 100*, 200* mg

Soluble tabs: 10, 15, 30 mg

Extended-release caps: 30, 60*, 90*, 120* mg

Sustained-release pellets in caps: 10, 20, 30, 50, 60, 100*, 200* mg

Rectal suppository: 5, 20 mg

Injection: 0.5, 1, 2, 4, 5, 8, 10, 15, 25, 50 mg/mL

*Use only for opioid-tolerant patients

Titrate to effect.

Analgesia/tetralogy (cyanotic) spells:

Neonate: 0.05–0.2 mg/kg/dose IM, slow IV, SC Q4 hr

Neonatal opiate withdrawal: 0.08–0.2 mg/dose Q3–4 hr PRN

Infant and child:

PO: 0.2–0.5 mg/kg/dose Q4–6 hr PRN (immediate release) or 0.3–0.6 mg/kg/dose Q12 hr PRN (controlled release)

IM/IV/SC: 0.1–0.2 mg/kg/dose Q2–4 hr PRN; **max. dose:** 15 mg/dose

Adult:

PO: 10–30 mg Q4 hr PRN (immediate release) or 15–30 mg Q8–12 hr PRN (controlled release)

IM/IV/SC: 2–15 mg/dose Q2–6 hr PRN

Continuous IV infusion: (dosing ranges, titrate to effect)

Neonate: 0.01–0.02 mg/kg/hr

Infant and child:

Postoperative pain: 0.01–0.04 mg/kg/hr

Sickle cell and cancer: 0.04–0.07 mg/kg/hr

Adult: 0.8–10 mg/hr

Continued

For explanation of icons, see p. 663.

MORPHINE SULFATE *continued*

Continuous IV infusion: (dosing ranges, titrate to effect) ***(cont'd):***

To prepare infusion for neonates, infants, and children, use the following formula:

$$50 \times \frac{\text{Desired dose (mg/kg/hr)}}{\text{Desired infusion rate (mL/hr)}} \times \text{Wt (kg)} = \frac{\text{mg morphine}}{\text{50 mL fluid}}$$

Dependence, CNS and respiratory depression, nausea, vomiting, urinary retention, constipation, hypotension, bradycardia, increased ICP, miosis, biliary spasm, and allergy may occur. **Naloxone may be used to reverse effects, especially respiratory depression.** Causes histamine release resulting in itching and possible bronchospasm. Low-dose naloxone infusion may be used for itching. Inflammatory masses (e.g., granulomas) have been reported with continuous infusions via indwelling intrathecal catheters.

See Chapter 6 for equianalgesic dosing. Pregnancy category changes to "D" if used for prolonged peroids or in higher doses at term. Rectal dosing is same as oral dosing but is **not recommended** due to poor absorption.

Controlled/sustained-released oral tablets must be administered whole. Controlled-released oral capsules may be opened and the entire contents sprinkled on applesauce immediately prior to ingestion. Be aware of the various oral solution concentrations; the concentrated oral solution (100 mg/5 mL) has been associated with accidental overdoses. **Adjust dose in renal failure (see Chapter 31).**

MUPIROCIN

Bactroban, Bactroban Nasal, and others

Topical antibiotic

No No 2 B

Ointment: 2% (22, 30 g); contains polyethylene glycol
Cream: 2% (15, 30 g); contains benzyl alcohol
Nasal ointment: 2% (1 g), as calcium salt

Topical:

≥3 mo–adult: Apply small amount TID to affected area × 5–10 days. Topical ointment may be used in infants ≥2 mo.

Intranasal: Apply small amount intranasally 2–4 times/24 hr for 5–14 days.

Avoid contact with the eyes. Topical cream is **not** intended for use in lesions >10 cm in length or 100 cm^2 in surface area. **Do not use** topical ointment preparation on open wounds because of concerns about systemic absorption of polyethylene glycol. May cause minor local irritation and dry skin. Intranasal route may cause nasal stinging, taste disorder, headache, rhinitis, and pharyngitis.

If clinical response is not apparent in 3–5 days with topical use, reevaluate infection. Intranasal administration may be used to eliminate carriage of *S. aureus,* including MRSA.

MYCOPHENOLATE

Mycophenolate mofetil: CellCept
Mycophenolate sodium: Myfortic
Immunosuppressant agent

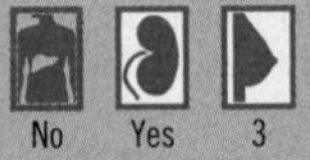

Mycophenolate mofetil:

Caps: 250 mg
Tabs: 500 mg
Oral suspension: 200 mg/mL (225 mL); contains phenylalanine (0.56 mg/mL) and methylparabens
Injection: 500 mg

Continued

MYCOPHENOLATE *continued*

Mycophenolate sodium:

Delayed released tabs (Myfortic): 180, 360 mg

Child (see remarks):

Renal transplant:

Caps, tabs, or suspension: 600 mg/m^2/dose PO BID up to a **max. dose** of 2000 mg/24 hr; alternatively, patients with body surface areas (BSAs) ≥1.25 m^2 may be dosed as follows:

1.25–1.5 m^2: 750 mg PO BID

>1.5 m^2: 1000 mg PO BID

Delayed-release tabs (Myfortic): 400–450 mg/m^2/dose PO BID; **max. dose:** 720 mg BID; this dosage form not recommended in patients with BSAs <1.19 m^2. Alternatively, patients with body surface areas ≥1.19 m^2 may be dosed as follows:

1.19–1.58 m^2: 540 mg PO BID

>1.58 m^2: 720 mg PO BID

Nephrotic syndrome:

Frequently relapsing: 12.5–18 mg/kg/dose PO BID up to a **max. dose** of 2000 mg/24 hr for 1–2 years and taper prednisone regimen.

Steroid dependent: 12–18 mg/kg/dose or 600 mg/m^2/dose PO BID up to a **max. dose** of 2000 mg/24 hr.

Adult (in combination with corticosteroids and cyclosporine; check specific transplantation protocol for specific dosage):

IV: 2000–3000 mg/24 hr ÷ BID

Oral:

Caps, tabs, or suspension: 2000–3000 mg/24 hr PO ÷ BID

Delayed-release tabs (Myfortic): 720 mg PO BID

Check specific transplantation protocol for specific dosage. Mycophenolate mofetil is a pro-drug for mycophenolic acid. Due to differences in absorption, the delayed-release tablets **should not** be interchanged with the other oral dosage forms on an equivalent mg-to-mg basis. Increases risk of first trimester pregnancy loss and increased risk of congenital malformations (especially external ear and facial abnormalities including cleft lip and palate, and anomalies of the distal limbs, heart, and esophagus).

Common side effects may include headache, hypertension, diarrhea, vomiting, bone marrow suppression, anemia, fever, opportunistic infections, and sepsis. May also increase the risk for lymphomas or other malignancies. GI bleeds and increased risk for rejection in heart transplant patients switched from calcineurin inhibitors (e.g., cyclosporine and tacrolimus) and CellCept to sirolimus and CellCept have been reported. Cases of progressive multifocal leukoencephalopathy (PML) and pure red cell aplasia (PRCA) have also been reported.

Use with caution in patients with active GI disease or renal impairment (GFR <25 mL/min/1.73 m^2) outside of the immediate post-transplant period. In adults with renal impairment, **avoid** doses >2 g/24 hr and observe carefully. No dose adjustment is needed for patients experiencing delayed graft function postoperatively.

Drug interactions: (1) Displacement of phenytoin or theophylline from protein binding sites will decrease total serum levels and increase free serum levels of these drugs. Salicylates displace mycophenolate to increase free levels of mycophenolate. (2) Competition for renal tubular secretion results in increased serum levels of acyclovir, ganciclovir, probenecid, and mycophenolate (when any of these are used together). (3) **Avoid** live and live attenuated vaccines (including influenza); decreases vaccine effectiveness.

Administer oral doses on an empty stomach. Cholestyramine and antacid use may decrease mycophenolic acid levels. Infuse intravenous doses over 2 hr. Oral suspension may be administered via NG tube with a minimum size of 8 French.

For explanation of icons, see p. 663.

NAFCILLIN
Unipen, Nallpen, and others
Antibiotic, penicillin (penicillinase resistant)

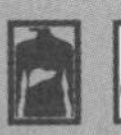 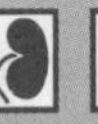  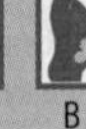 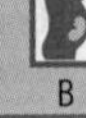
Yes Yes 2 B

Injection: 1, 2, 10 g; contains 2.9 mEq Na/g drug
Injection, premixed in iso-osmotic dextrose: 1 g in 50 mL, 2 g in 100 mL

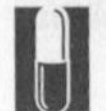

Neonate (IM/IV):
≤7 days:
<2 kg: 50 mg/kg/24 hr ÷ Q12 hr
≥2 kg: 75 mg/kg/24 hr ÷ Q8 hr
>7 days:
<1.2 kg: 50 mg/kg/24 hr ÷ Q12 hr
1.2–2 kg: 75 mg/kg/24 hr ÷ Q8 hr
≥2 kg: 100 mg/kg/24 hr ÷ Q6 hr

Infant and child (IM/IV):
Mild to moderate infections: 50–100 mg/kg/24 hr ÷ Q6 hr
Severe infections: 100–200 mg/kg/24 hr ÷ Q4–6 hr; give 200 mg/kg/24 hr ÷ Q4–6 hr; for staphylococcal endocarditis.
Max. dose: 12 g/24 hr

Adult:
IV: 500–2000 mg Q4–6 hr
IM: 500 mg Q4–6 hr
Max. dose: 12 g/24 hr

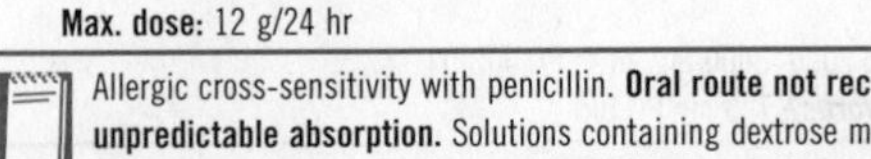

Allergic cross-sensitivity with penicillin. **Oral route not recommended because of unpredictable absorption.** Solutions containing dextrose may be **contraindicated** in patients with known allergy to corn or corn products. High incidence of phlebitis with IV dosing. CSF penetration is poor unless meninges are inflammed. **Use with caution** in patients with combined renal and hepatic impairment (reduce dose by 33%–50%). Nafcillin may increase elimination of cyclosporine and warfarin. Acute interstitial nephritis is rare. May cause rash and bone marrow suppression.

NALOXONE
Narcan and many generics
Narcotic antagonist

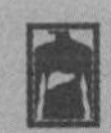 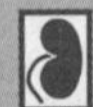 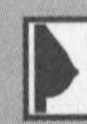 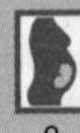
No No ? C

Injection: 0.4 mg/mL (1, 10 mL); some preparations may contain parabens
Injection, in syringe: 1 mg/mL (2 mL)

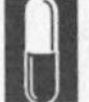

Opiate intoxication (IM/IV/SC, use 2–10 times IV dose for ETT route; see remarks):
Neonate, infant, child ≤20 kg or ≤5 yr: 0.1 mg/kg/dose. May repeat PRN Q2–3 min.
Child >20 kg or >5 yr: 2 mg/dose. May repeat PRN Q2–3 min.
Continuous infusion (child and adult): 0.005 mg/kg loading dose followed by infusion of 0.0025 mg/kg/hr has been recommended. A range of 0.0025–0.16 mg/kg/hr has been reported. Taper gradually to avoid relapse.
Adult: 0.4–2 mg/dose. May repeat PRN Q2–3 min. Use 0.1- to 0.2-mg increments in opiate-dependent patients.

Short duration of action may necessitate multiple doses. For severe intoxication, doses of 0.2 mg/kg may be required. If no response is achieved after a cumulative dose of 10 mg,

Continued

NALOXONE *continued*

reevaluate diagnosis. **In the nonarrest situation, use the lowest dose effective (may start at 0.001 mg/kg/dose). See Chapter 6 for additional information.**

Will produce narcotic withdrawal syndrome in patients with chronic dependence. **Use with caution** in patients with chronic cardiac disease. Abrupt reversal of narcotic depression may result in nausea, vomiting, diaphoresis, tachycardia, hypertension, and tremulousness.

May be used simultaneously with opiates at lower dosages (~0.25–2 mcg/kg/hr) to abate opiate-related pruritus.

IV administration is preferred. Onset of action may be delayed with other routes of adminstration.

NAPROXEN/NAPROXEN SODIUM
Naprosyn, Anaprox, EC-Naprosyn, Naprelan, Aleve [OTC], and many others
Nonsteroidal antinflammatory agent

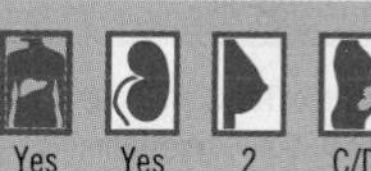

Naproxen:
Tabs: 250, 375, 500 mg
Delayed release tabs (EC-Naprosyn): 375, 500 mg
Oral suspension: 125 mg/5 mL; contains 0.34 mEq Na/1 mL and parabens

Naproxen Sodium:
Tabs:
Aleve and others (OTC): 220 mg (200 mg base); contains 0.87 mEq Na
Anaprox: 275 mg (250 mg base), 550 mg (500 mg base); contains 1 mEq, 2 mEq Na, respectively
Controlled-release tabs (Naprelan): 412.5 mg (375 mg base), 550 mg (500 mg base)

All doses based on naproxen base.
Child >2 yr:
Analgesia: 5–7 mg/kg/dose Q8–12 hr PO
JRA: 10–20 mg/kg/24 hr ÷ Q12 hr PO
Usual max. dose: 1000 mg/24 hr

Adult:
Analgesia (includes adolescents):
Over the counter dosage forms: 200 mg Q8–12 hr PRN PO; if needed, 400 mg initial dose may be needed. **Max. dose:** 600 mg/24 hr.
Prescription strength dosage forms: 250 mg Q8–12 hr PRN (500 mg initial dose may be needed) or 500 mg Q12 hr PRN PO. **Max. dose:** 1250 mg/24 hr for first day then 1000 mg/24 hr.

Rheumatoid arthritis, ankylosing spondylitis:
Immediate release forms: 250–500 mg BID PO
Delayed release tabs (EC-Naprosyn): 375–500 mg BID PO
Controlled-release tabs (Naprelan): 750–1000 mg once daily PO. For patients converting from immediate and delayed release forms, calculate daily dose and administer Naprelan as a single daily dose.
Max. dose (all dosage forms): 1500 mg/24 hr.

Dysmenorrhea:
500 mg × 1, then 250 mg Q6–8 hr PRN PO or 500 mg Q12 hr PRN PO; **max. dose:** 1250 mg/24 hr for first day then 1000 mg/24 hr.

Contraindicated in treating perioperative pain for coronary artery bypass graft surgery. May cause GI bleeding, thrombocytopenia, heartburn, headache, drowsiness, vertigo, and tinnitus.

Continued

For explanation of icons, see p. 663.

NAPROXEN/NAPROXEN SODIUM *continued*

Use with caution in patients with GI disease, cardiac disease (risk for thrombotic events, MI, stroke), renal or hepatic impairment, and those receiving anticoagulants. See *Ibuprofen* for other side effects.

Pregnancy category changes to "D" if used in the third trimester or near delivery. Administer doses with food or milk to reduce GI discomfort.

NEOMYCIN SULFATE
Mycifradin, Neo-fradin, Neo-Tabs, and others
Antibiotic, aminoglycoside; ammonium detoxicant

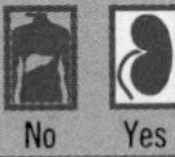 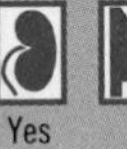 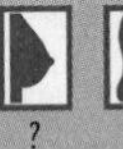 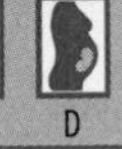
No Yes ? D

Tabs (Neo-Tabs): 500 mg
Oral solution (Mycifradin, Neo-Fradin): 125 mg/5 mL; contains parabens

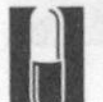

Diarrhea:
Preterm and newborn: 50 mg/kg/24 hr ÷ Q6 hr PO
Hepatic encephalopathy:
Infant and child: 50–100 mg/kg/24 hr ÷ Q6–8 hr PO × 5–6 days. **Max. dose:** 12 g/24 hr
Adult: 4–12 g/24 hr ÷ Q4–6 hr PO × 5–6 days
Bowel prep:
Child: 90 mg/kg/24 hr PO ÷ Q4 hr × 2–3 days
Adult: 1 g Q1 hr PO × 4 doses, then 1 g Q4 hr PO × 5 doses. (Many other regimens exist.)

Contraindicated in ulcerative bowel disease, intestinal obstruction, or aminoglycoside hypersensitivity. Monitor for nephrotoxicity and ototoxicity. Oral absorption is limited, but levels may accumulate. Consider dosage reduction in the presence of renal failure. May cause itching, redness, edema, colitis, candidiasis, or poor wound healing if applied topically. Prevalence of neomycin hypersensitivity has increased. May decrease absorption of penicillin V, vitamin B_{12}, digoxin, and methotrexate. May potentiate oral anticoagulants and the adverse effects of other neurotoxic, ototoxic, or nephrotoxic drugs.

NEOMYCIN/POLYMYXIN B/± BACITRACIN
Neosporin GU Irrigant, Neosporin, Neosporin Ophthalmic, and others
Topical antibiotic

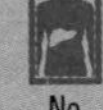 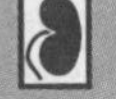 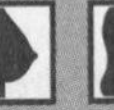 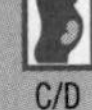
No No ? C/D

Solution, genitourinary irrigant: 40 mg neomycin sulfate, 200,000 U polymyxin B/mL (1, 20 mL); multidose vial contains methylparabens
In combination with bacitracin:
Ointment, topical (Neosporin) (OTC): 3.5 mg neomycin sulfate, 400 U bacitracin, 5000 U polymyxin B/g (0.9, 14, 28 g)
Ointment, ophthalmic (Neosporin Ophthalmic): 3.5 mg neomycin sulfate, 400 U bacitracin, 10,000 U polymyxin B/g (3.5 g)

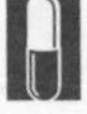

Topical: Apply to minor wounds and burns once daily–TID
Ophthalmic: Apply small amount to conjunctiva Q3–4 hr × 7–10 days, depending on the severity of infection.
Bladder irrigation:
Child–adult: Mix 1 ml in 1000 ml NS and administer via a 3-way catheter at a rate adjusted to the patient's urine output. **Do not exceed** 10 days of continuous use.

Continued

NEOMYCIN/POLYMYXIN B/± BACITRACIN *continued*

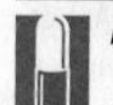

Do not use for extended periods. May cause superinfection, delayed healing. See *Neomycin* for additional remarks. Ophthalmic preparation may cause stinging and sensitivity to bright light. **Avoid** use of bladder irrigant in patients with defects in the bladder mucosa or wall.

Pregnancy category is a "C" for neomycin/polymixin B/bacitracin and a "D" for neomycin/polymixin B.

NEOSTIGMINE

Prostigmin and others

Anticholinesterase (cholinergic) agent

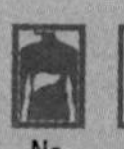
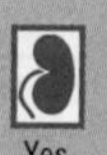
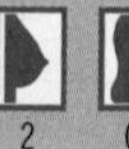
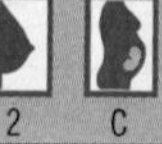

No Yes 2 C

Tabs: 15 mg (bromide)

Injection: 0.25, 0.5, 1 mg/mL (methylsulfate); may contain parabens or phenol

Myasthenia gravis diagnosis: Use with atropine (see remarks).

Child: 0.025–0.04 mg/kg IM × 1

Adult: 0.02 mg/kg IM × 1

Treatment:

Child:

IM/IV/SC: 0.01–0.04 mg/kg/dose Q2–4 hr PRN

PO: 2 mg/kg/24 hr ÷ Q3–4 hr; **max. dose:** 375 mg/24 hr.

Adult: IM/IV/SC: 0.5–2.5 mg/dose Q1–3 hr PRN up to **max. dose** of 10 mg/24 hr.

PO: Start with 15 mg/dose TID. May increase every 1–2 days. Dosage requirements may vary from 15–375 mg/24 hr with an average of 150 mg/24 hr. Some patients may require as much as 30–40 mg Q2–4 hr.

Reversal of nondepolarizing neuromuscular blocking agents: Administer with atropine or glycopyrrolate.

Infant: 0.025–0.1 mg/kg/dose IV

Child: 0.025–0.08 mg/kg/dose IV

Adult: 0.5–2.5 mg/dose IV

Max. dose: 5 mg/dose

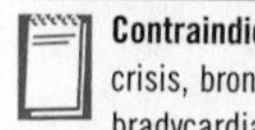

Contraindicated in GI and urinary obstruction. **Caution** in asthmatics. May cause cholinergic crisis, bronchospasm, salivation, nausea, vomiting, diarrhea, miosis, diaphoresis, lacrimation, bradycardia, hypotension, fatigue, confusion, respiratory depression, and seizures. Titrate for each patient, but **avoid** excessive cholinergic effects.

For diagnosis of myasthenia gravis (MG), administer atropine 0.011 mg/kg/dose IV immediately before or IM (0.011 mg/kg/dose) 30 min before neostigmine. For treatment of MG, patients may need higher doses of neostigmine at times of greatest fatigue.

Antidote: Atropine 0.01–0.04 mg/kg/dose. Atropine and epinephrine should be available in the event of a hypersensitivity reaction.

Adjust dose in renal failure (see Chapter 31).

NEVIRAPINE

Viramune, NVP

Antiviral, non-nucleoside reverse transcriptase inhibitor

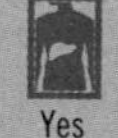
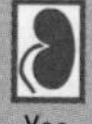

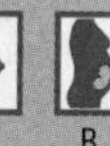

Yes Yes 3 B

Tabs: 200 mg

Oral suspension: 10 mg/mL (240 mL); contains parabens

Continued

For explanation of icons, see p. 663.

NEVIRAPINE *continued*

HIV: See www.aidsinfo.nih.gov/guidelines

Prevention of vertical transmission (see Chapter 17 for additional information):

Mother, at onset of labor (use in combination with IV zidovudine infusion during labor and consider adding zidovudine/lamivudine during labor or immediately postpartum to reduce development of nevirapine resistance): 200 mg PO × 1.

Neonate (<14 days old; consider adding lamivudine to reduce development of nevirapine resistance): 2 mg/kg/dose PO × 1 within 72 hr after birth; give dose as soon as possible if maternal dose given ≤2 hr prior to delivery or if not given at all.

See www.aidsinfo.nih.gov/guidelines for additional remarks.

Use with caution in patients with hepatic or renal dysfunction. Most frequent side effects include: skin rash (may be life-threatening, including Stevens-Johnson Syndrome; **permanently discontinue and never restart**), fever, abnormal liver function tests, headache, and nausea. **Discontinue therapy** if any of the following occurs: severe rash; rash with fever, blistering, oral lesions, conjunctivitis, or muscle aches with or without organ dysfunction; rash with increased ALT or AST; or symptoms of hepatitis**. Life-threatening** hepatotoxicity has been reported primarily during the first 12 wk of therapy. Patients with increased serum transaminase or a history of hepatitis B or C infection prior to nevirapine are at greater risk for hepatotoxicity. Women, including pregnant women, with CD_4 counts >250 cells/mm^3 or men with CD_4 counts >400 cells/mm^3 are at risk for hepatotoxicity. Monitor liver function tests and CBCs.

Nevirapine induces the CYP 450 3A4 drug metabolizing isoenzyme to cause an autoinduction of its own metabolism within the first 2–4 wk of therapy and has the potential to interact with many drugs. **Carefully review the patient's drug profile for other drug interactions each time nevirapine is initiated or when a new drug is added to a regimen containing nevirapine.**

Doses can be administered with food and concurrently with didanosine.

NIACIN/VITAMIN B_3

Niacor, Niaspan, Slo-Niacin, Nicotinic acid, Vitamin B_3, and many other generics

Vitamin, water soluble

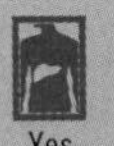 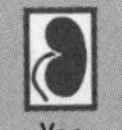 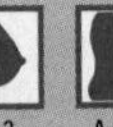 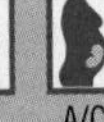

Yes Yes ? A/C

Tabs (OTC): 50, 100, 250, 500 mg

Timed or extended-release tabs (all OTC except 1000 mg): 250, 500, 750, 1000 mg

Timed or extended-release caps (OTC): 125, 250, 400, 500 mg

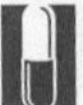

US RDA: **See Chapter 21.**

Pellagra (PO):

Child: 50–100 mg/dose TID

Adult: 50–100 mg/dose TID–QID

Max. dose: 500 mg/24 hr

Contraindicated in hepatic dysfunction, active peptic ulcer, and severe hypotension. **Use with caution** in unstable angina, acute MI (especially if receiving vasoactive drugs), renal dysfunction, and in patients with history of jaundice, hepatobiliary disease, or peptic ulcer.

Adverse reactions of flushing, pruritis, or GI distress may occur with PO administration. May cause hyperglycemia, hyperuricemia, blurred vision, abnormal liver function tests, dizziness, and headaches. Burning sensation of the skin, skin discoloration, hepatitis, and elevated creatine kinase have been reported. May cause false-positive urine catecholamines (fluorometric methods) and urine glucose (Benedict's reagent).

Pregnancy category changes to "C" if used in doses above the RDA or for typical doses used for lipid disorders. See Chapter 21 for multivitamin preparations.

NICARDIPINE
Cardene, Cardene SR, and others
Calcium channel blocker, antihypertensive

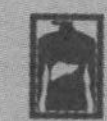 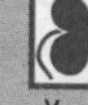 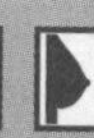 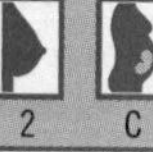
Yes Yes 2 C

Caps (immediate release): 20, 30 mg
Sustained-release caps: 30, 45, 60 mg
Injection: 2.5 mg/mL (10 mL)

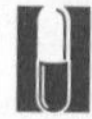
Child (see remarks):
Hypertension:
Continuous IV infusion: Start at 0.5–1 mcg/kg/min, dose may be increased as needed every 15–30 min up to a maximum of 4–5 mcg/kg/min.

Adult:
Hypertension:
Oral:
Immediate release: 20 mg PO TID, dose may be increased after 3 days to 40 mg PO TID if needed.
Sustained release: 30 mg PO BID, dose may be increased after 3 days to 60 mg PO BID if needed.
Continuous IV infusion: Start at 5 mg/hr, increase dose as needed by 2.5 mg/hr Q5–15 min up to a **max. dose** of 15 mg/hr. Following attainment of desired BP, decrease infusion to 3 mg/hr and adjust rate as needed to maintain desired response.

Reported use in children has been limited to a small number of preterm infants, infants, and children. **Contraindicated** in advanced aortic stenosis. **Avoid** systemic hypotension in patients following an acute cerebral infarct or hemorrhage. **Use with caution** in hepatic or renal dysfunction by carefully titrating dose. The drug undergoes significant first pass metabolism through the liver and is excreted in the urine (60%).

May cause headache, dizziness, asthenia, peripheral edema, and GI symptoms. Cimetidine increases the effects/toxicity of nicardipine. **See *Nifedipine* for additional drug and food interactions.**

Onset of action for PO administration is 20 min with peak effects in 0.5–2 hr. IV onset of action is 1 min. Duration of action following a single IV or PO dose is 3 hr. To reduce the risk for venous thrombosis, phlebitis, and vascular impairment with IV administration, do not use small veins (e.g., dorsum of hand or wrist). Avoid intra-arterial administration or extravasation. For additional information, see Chapter 4.

NIFEDIPINE
Adalat CC, Nifediac CC, Procardia, Procardia XL, and many others
Calcium channel blocker, antihypertensive

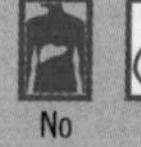 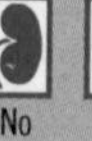 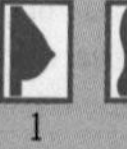
No No 1 C

Caps: (Procardia and others): 10 mg (0.34 mL), 20 mg (0.45 mL)
Sustained-release tabs: (Adalat CC, Nifediac CC, Procardia XL and others): 30, 60, 90 mg
Oral solution: 10 mg/mL
Oral suspension: 1 mg/mL

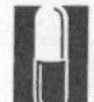
Child (see remarks for precautions):
Hypertensive urgency: 0.25–0.5 mg/kg/dose Q4–6 hr PRN PO/SL. **Max. dose:** 10 mg/dose or 1–2 mg/kg/24 hr.

Continued

For explanation of icons, see p. 663.

NIFEDIPINE *continued*

Child (see remarks for precautions) (cont'd):

Hypertension:

Sustained release: Start with 0.25–0.5 mg/kg/24 hr ÷ Q12–24 hr. May increase to **max. dose:** 3 mg/kg/24 hr up to 120 mg/24 hr.

Hypertrophic cardiomyopathy: 0.6–0.9 mg/kg/24 hr ÷ Q6–8 hr PO/SL.

Adult:

Hypertension:

Caps: Start with 10 mg/dose PO TID. May increase to 30 mg/dose PO TID–QID. **Max. dose:** 180 mg/24 hr.

Sustained release: Start with 30 mg PO once daily; usual range: 30–60 mg once daily. May increase to **max. dose:** 120 mg/24 hr.

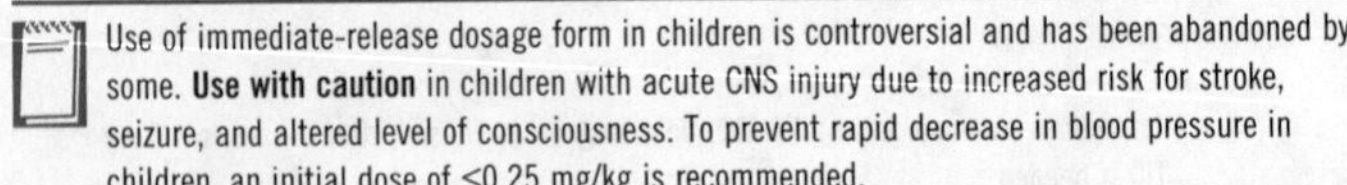

Use of immediate-release dosage form in children is controversial and has been abandoned by some. **Use with caution** in children with acute CNS injury due to increased risk for stroke, seizure, and altered level of consciousness. To prevent rapid decrease in blood pressure in children, an initial dose of ≤0.25 mg/kg is recommended.

Use with caution in patients with CHF, aortic stenosis, GI obstruction/narrowing (bezoar formation), and cirrhosis (reduced drug clearance). May cause severe hypotension, peripheral edema, flushing, tachycardia, headaches, dizziness, nausea, palpitations, and syncope. Although overall use in adults has been abandoned, the immediate-release dosage form is **contraindicated** in adults with severe obstructive coronary artery disease or recent MI, and hypertensive emergencies.

Nifedipine is a substrate for CYP 450 3A3/4, and 3A5-7. **Do not administer** with grapefruit juice; may increase bioavailability and effects. Itraconazole and ketoconazole may increase nifedipine levels/effects. CYP 3A inducers (e.g., rifampin, rifabutin, penobarbital, phenytoin, carbamazepine) may reduce nifedipine's effects. Nifedipine may increase phenytoin, cyclosporine, and digoxin levels. For hypertensive emergencies, see Chapter 4.

For sublingual administration, capsule must be punctured and liquid expressed into mouth. A small amount is absorbed via the SL route. Most effects are due to swallowing and oral absorption. **Do not** crush or chew sustained-release tablet dosage form.

NITROFURANTOIN

Furadantin, Macrodantin, Macrobid, and others

Antibiotic

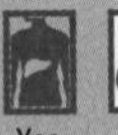
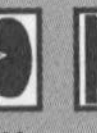
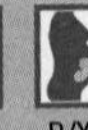
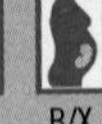

Yes Yes 2 B/X

Caps (macrocrystals; Macrodantin): 50, 100 mg
Caps (dual release; Macrobid): 100 mg (25 mg macrocrystal/75 mg monohydrate)
Oral suspension (Furadantin): 25 mg/5 mL (230 mL); contains parabens and saccharin

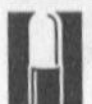

Child (>1 mo):

Treatment: 5–7 mg/kg/24 hr ÷ Q6 hr PO; **max. dose:** 400 mg/24 hr

UTI prophylaxis: 1–2 mg/kg/dose QHS PO; **max. dose:** 100 mg/24 hr

≥12 yr and adult:

Macrocrystals: 50–100 mg/dose Q6 hr PO

Dual-release (Macrobid): 100 mg/dose Q12 hr PO

UTI prophylaxis (macrocrystals): 50–100 mg/dose PO QHS

Contraindicated in severe renal disease, infants <1 mo of age, GFR <60 mL/min (reduced drug distribution in the urine), active/previous choletatic jaunice/hepatic dysfunction, and pregnant women at term. **Use with caution** in G6PD deficiency, anemia, lung disease, and

Continued

NITROFURANTOIN *continued*

peripheral neuropathy. May cause nausea, hypersensitivity reactions, vomiting, cholestatic jaundice, headache, hepatotoxicity, polyneuropathy, and hemolytic anemia.

Anticholinergic drugs and high-dose probenecid may increase nitrofurantoin toxicity. Magnesium salts may decrease nitrofurantoin absorption. Causes false-positive urine glucose with Clinitest. Administer doses with food or milk.

Pregnancy category changes to "X" at term (38–42 wk gestation). Breastfeeding in mothers receiving nitrofurantoin is not recommended for infants <1 mo and those with G6PD deficiency; use in infants ≥1 mo and without G6PD deficiency is compatible.

NITROGLYCERIN
Nitro-Bid, Nitrostat, Nitro-Time, Nitro-Dur, NitroMist, and many others
Vasodilator, antihypertensive

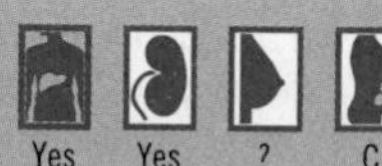

Injection: 5 mg/mL (5, 10 mL); may contain alcohol or propylene glycol
Prediluted injection in D_5W: 100 mcg/mL, 200 mcg/mL, 400 mcg/mL (250, 500 mL)
Sublingual tabs (Nitrostat and others): 0.3, 0.4, 0.6 mg
Sustained-release caps (Nitro-Time and others): 2.5, 6.5, 9 mg
Ointment, topical (Nitro-Bid and others): 2% (30, 60 g)
Patch (Nitro-Dur and others): 2.5 mg/24 hr (0.1 mg/hr), 5 mg/24 hr (0.2 mg/hr), 7.5 mg/24 hr (0.3 mg/hr), 10 mg/24 hr (0.4 mg/hr), 15 mg/24 hr (0.6 mg/hr), 20 mg/24 hr (0.8 mg/hr)
Spray, translingual: 0.4 mg per metered spray (4.9, 12 g; delivers 60 and 200 doses, respectively); may contain 20% alcohol
NitroMist: 0.4 mg per metered spray (8.5 g; delivers 230 doses)

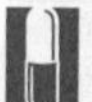

NOTE: The IV dosage units for children are in mcg/kg/min, compared to mcg/min for adults.

Child:

Continuous IV infusion: Begin with 0.25–0.5 mcg/kg/min; may increase by 0.5–1 mcg/kg/min Q3–5 min PRN. Usual dose: 1–5 mcg/kg/min. **Max. dose:** 20 mcg/kg/min.

Adult:

Continuous IV infusion: 5 mcg/min IV, then increase Q3–5 min PRN by 5 mcg/min up to 20 mcg/min. If no response, increase by 10 mcg/min Q3–5 min PRN up to a **max.** of 200 mcg/min.
Sublingual: 0.2–0.6 mg Q5 min. **Max.** of three doses in 15 min.
Oral: 2.5–9 mg BID–TID; up to 26 mg QID
Ointment: Apply 1–2 inches Q8 hr, up to 4–5 inches Q4 hr
Patch: 0.2–0.4 mg/hr initially, then titrate to 0.4–0.8 mg/hr; apply new patch daily (tolerance is minimized by removing patch for 10–12 hr/24 hr)

Contraindicated in glaucoma and severe anemia. In small doses (1–2 mcg/kg/min) acts mainly on systemic veins and decreases preload. At 3–5 mcg/kg/min acts on systemic arterioles to decrease resistance. May cause headache, flushing, GI upset, blurred vision, and methemoglobinemia. **Use with caution** in severe renal impairment, increased ICP, and hepatic failure. IV nitroglycerin may antagonize anticoagulant effect of heparin.

Decrease dose gradually in patients receiving drug for prolonged periods to **avoid** withdrawal reaction. Must use polypropylene infusion sets to **avoid** adsorption of drug to plastic tubing. Use in heparized patients may result in a decrease of PTT with subsequent rebound effect upon discontinuation of nitroglycerin.

Onset (duration) of action: IV: 1–2 min (3–5 min); sublingual: 1–3 min (30–60 min); PO sustained release: 40 min (4–8 hr); topical ointment: 20–60 min (2–12 hr); and transdermal patch: 40–60 min (18–24 hr).

For explanation of icons, see p. 663.

NITROPRUSSIDE

Nitropress and others (previously available as Nipride)
Vasodilator, antihypertensive

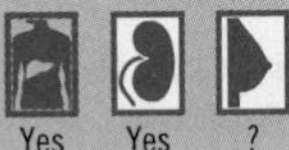
Yes Yes ? C

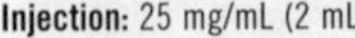

Injection: 25 mg/mL (2 mL)

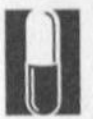

Child and adult: IV, continuous infusion
Dose: Start at 0.3–0.5 mcg/kg/min, titrate to effect. Usual dose is 3–4 mcg/kg/min. **Max. dose:** 8–10 mcg/kg/min.

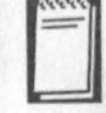

Contraindicated in patients with decreased cerebral perfusion and in situations of compensatory hypertension (increased ICP). Monitor for hypotension and acidosis. Dilute with D_5W and protect from light.

Nitroprusside is nonenzymatically converted to cyanide, which is converted to thiocyanate. Cyanide may produce metabolic acidosis and methemoglobinemia; thiocyanate may produce psychosis and seizures. Monitor thiocyanate levels if used for >48 hr or if dose ≥4 mcg/kg/min. **Thiocyanate levels should be <50 mg/L.** Monitor **cyanide levels (toxic levels >2 mcg/mL)** in patients with hepatic dysfunction and thiocyanate levels in patients with renal dysfunction.

Onset of action is 2 min with a 1- to 10-min duration of effect.

NOREPINEPHRINE BITARTRATE

Levophed and others
Adrenergic agonist

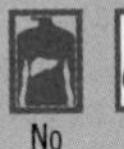 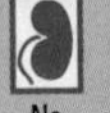  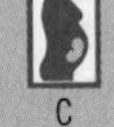
No No ? C

Injection: 1 mg/mL as norepinephrine base (4 mL); contains sulfites

NOTE: The dosage units for children are in mcg/kg/min; compared to mcg/min for adults.
Child: Continuous IV infusion **doses as norepinephrine base.** Start at 0.05–0.1 mcg/kg/min. Titrate to effect. **Max. dose:** 2 mcg/kg/min.
Adult: Continuous IV infusion **doses as norepinephrine base.** Start at 4 mcg/min and titrate to effect. Usual dosage range: 8–12 mcg/min.

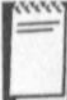

May cause cardiac arrhythmias, hypertension, hypersensitivity, headaches, vomiting, uterine contractions, and organ ischemia. May cause decreased renal blood flow and urine output. **Avoid** extravasation into tissues; may cause severe tissue necrosis. If this occurs, treat locally with phentolamine.

NORFLOXACIN

Noroxin, Chibroxin
Antibiotic, quinolone

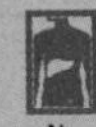 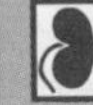 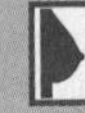 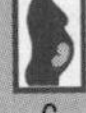
No Yes 2 C

Tabs: 400 mg
Oral suspension: 20 mg/mL
Ophthalmic drops (Chibroxin): 3 mg/mL (5 mL)

Child:
UTI (limited data in children 5 mo–19 yr; see remarks): 9–14 mg/kg/24 hr PO ÷ Q12 hr; **max. dose:** 800 mg/24 hr. For UTI prophylaxis, give 2–6 mg/kg/24 hr.

Continued

NORFLOXACIN *continued*

Adult:

UTI: 400 mg PO Q12 hr (× 7–10 days for uncomplicated cases and × 10–21 days for complicated cases)

Prostatitis: 400 mg PO Q12 hr × 28 days

Ophthalmic:

≥1 yr–adult: 1–2 drops QID × ≤7 days. May give up to Q2 hr for severe infections during the first day of therapy.

Like other quinolones, there is concern regarding development of arthropathy. Norfloxacin does **not** adequately treat chlamydia co-infections. UTI dosing can be used for BK virus nephropathy in immunocompromised patients. Fluoroquinolones are no longer recommended for gonorrhea by the CDC due to resistance. **Use with caution** in children <18 yr, seizures, proarrhythmic conditions, diabetes, patients receiving Class Ia or Class III antiarrhythmics, and impaired renal function **(adjust dose in renal failure; see Chapter 31).**

Inhibits CYP 450 1A2. May increase serum theophylline levels and decrease mycophenolate levels. May prolong PT in patients on warfarin. See *Ciprofoxacin* for common side effects and drug interactions. QTc prolongation, peripheral neuropathy, and tendon rupture (with all ages; especially with corticosteroid use) have been reported.

Ophthalmic dosage form may cause local burning or discomfort, photophobia, and bitter taste. Administer oral doses on an empty stomach.

NORTRIPTYLINE HYDROCHLORIDE

Pamelor, Aventyl, and various generics

Antidepressant, tricyclic

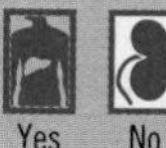
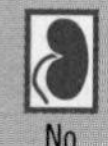
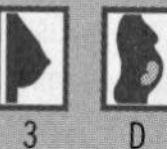

Yes No 3 D

Caps: 10, 25, 50, 75 mg; may contain benzyl alcohol, EDTA

Oral solution: 10 mg/5 mL; contains up to 4% alcohol

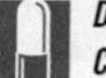

Depression:

Child 6–12 yr: 1–3 mg/kg/24 hr ÷ TID–QID PO or 10–20 mg/24 hr ÷ TID–QID PO

Adolescent: 1–3 mg/kg/24 hr ÷ TID–QID PO or 30–50 mg/24 hr ÷ TID–QID PO

Adult: 75–100 mg/24 hr ÷ TID–QID PO

Max. dose (all ages): 150 mg/24 hr

Nocturnal enuresis:

6–7 yr (20–25 kg): 10 mg PO QHS

8–11 yr (26–35 kg): 10–20 mg PO QHS

>11 yr (36–54 kg): 25–35 mg PO QHS

See *Imipramine* for **contraindications** and common side effects. Fewer CNS and anticholinergic side effects than amitriptyline. Lower doses and slower dose titration is recommended in hepatic impairment. Therapeutic antidepressant effects occur in 7–21 days. Monitor for clinical worsening of depression and suicidal ideation/behavior following the initiation of therapy or after dose changes. **Do not** discontinue abruptly. Nortriptyline is a substrate for the CYP 450 1A2 and 2D6 drug metabolizing enzymes. Rifampin may increase the metabolism of nortriptyline.

Therapeutic nortriptyline levels for depression: 50–150 ng/mL. Recommended serum sampling time: obtain a single level 8 or more hr after an oral dose (following 4 days of continuous dosing for children and after 9–10 days for adults).

Administer with food to decrease GI upset.

For explanation of icons, see p. 663.

NYSTATIN
Mycostatin, Nilstat, and others
Antifungal agent

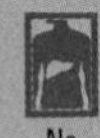
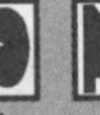
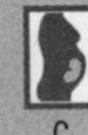

No No 1 C

Tabs: 500,000 U
Troches/pastilles: 200,000 U
Oral suspension: 100,000 U/mL (5, 60, 480 mL)
Cream/ointment: 100,000 U/g (15, 30 g)
Topical powder: 100,000 U/g (15, 30 g)
Vaginal tabs: 100,000 U (15 s)

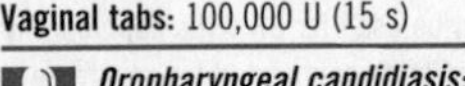

Oropharyngeal candidiasis:
Preterm infant: 0.5 mL (50,000 U) to each side of mouth QID
Term infant: 1 mL (100,000 U) to each side of mouth QID
Child/adult:
Suspension: 4–6 mL (400,000–600,000 U) swish and swallow QID
Troche: 200,000–400,000 U 4–5 ×/24 hr

Vaginal:
Adolescent and adult: 1 tab QHS × 14 days
Topical: Apply to affected areas BID–QID

May produce diarrhea and GI side effects. Local irritation, contact dermatitis and Stevens-Johnson syndrome have been reported. Treat until 48–72 hr after resolution of symptoms. Drug is poorly absorbed through the GI tract. **Do not** swallow troches whole (allow to dissolve slowly). Oral suspension should be swished about the mouth and retained in the mouth as long as possible before swallowing.

OCTREOTIDE ACETATE
Sandostatin, Sandostatin LAR Depot
Somatostatin analog, antisecretory agent

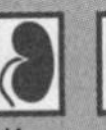
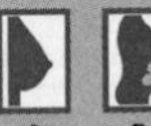
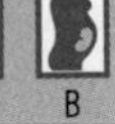

No Yes ? B

Injection (amps): 0.05, 0.1, 0.5 mg/mL (1 mL)
Injection (multi-dose vials): 0.2, 1 mg/mL (5 mL)
Injection, microspheres for suspension (Sandostatin LAR Depot): 10, 20, 30 mg (in kits with 2 mL diluent and 1.5 inch 20-gauge needles)

Infant and child (limited data):
Intractable diarrhea:
IV/SC: 1–10 mcg/kg/24 hr ÷ Q12–24 hr. Dose may be increased within the recommended range by 0.3 mcg/kg/dose every 3 days as needed. **Max. dose:** 1500 mcg/24 hr.
IV continuous infusion: 1 mcg/kg/dose bolus followed by 1 mcg/kg/hr has been used in diarrhea associated with graft versus host disease.

Cholelithiasis, hyperglycemia, hypoglycemia, hypothyroidism, nausea, diarrhea, abdominal discomfort, headache, dizziness, and pain at injection site may occur. Growth hormone suppression may occur with long-term use. Bradycardia and increased risk for pregnancy in patients with acromegaly and pancreatitis have been reported. Cyclosporine levels may be reduced in patients receiving this drug. May increase the effects/toxicity of bromocriptine.

Patients with severe renal failure requiring dialysis may require dosage adjustments due to an increase in half-life. The effects of hepatic dysfunction on octreotide have not been evaluated.

Sandostatin LAR Depot is administered once every 4 wk **only** by the IM route and is currently indicated for use in adults who have been stabilized on IV/SC therapy. See package insert for details.

OFLOXACIN
Floxin, Floxin Otic, Ocuflox, and others
Antibiotic, quinolone

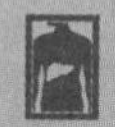
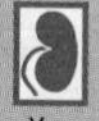
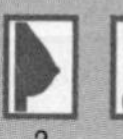
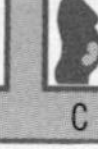

Yes Yes 2 C

Otic solution (Floxin Otic): 0.3% (5, 10 mL)
Ophthalmic solution (Ocuflox): 0.3% (5, 10 mL)
Tabs: 200, 300, 400 mg
Prediluted inj in D_5W: 200 mg/50 mL, 400 mg/100 mL

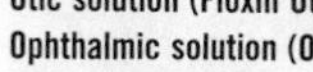

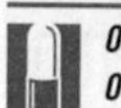

Otitic use:
Otitis externa:
6 mo–12 yr: 5 drops to affected ear(s) BID × 7 days
≥13 yr–adult: 10 drops to affected ear(s) BID × 7 days
Chronic suppurative otitis media:
≥12 yr–adult: 10 drops to affected ear(s) BID × 10–14 days
Acute otitis media with tympanostomy tubes:
1–12 yr: 5 drops to affected ear(s) BID × 10 days
Ophthalmic use:
>1 yr: 1–2 drops to affected eye(s) Q2–4 hr × 2 days, then QID for an additional 5 days

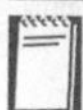

Pruritus, local irritation, taste perversion, dizziness, earache have been reported with otic use. Ocular burning/discomfort is frequent with ophthalmic use. Consult with ophthalmology in corneal ulcers.

When using otic solution, warm solution by holding the bottle in the hand for 1–2 min. Cold solutions may result in dizziness. For otitis externa, patient should lie with affected ear upward before instillation and remain in the same position after dose administration for 5 min to enhance drug delivery. For acute otitis media with tympanostomy tubes, patient should lie in the same position prior to instillation and the tragus should be pumped 4 times after the dose to assist in drug delivery to the middle ear.

Adjust dose in severe renal or hepatic impairment (max. dose: 400 mg/24 hr) with systemic use. Systemic use of ofloxacin is typically replaced by its S-isomer, levofloxacin, which has a more favorable side effect profile than ofloxacin. See *Levofloxacin.*

OLOPATADINE
Patanol, Pataday, Patanase
Antihistamine

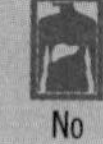
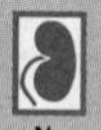
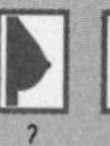
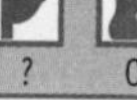

No No ? C

Ophthalmic solution:
Patanol: 0.1% (5 mL); contains benzalkonium chloride
Pataday: 0.2% (2.5 mL); contains benzalkonium chloride
Nasal spray (Patanase): 0.6% (30.5 g provides 240 metered spray doses); contains benzalkonium chloride

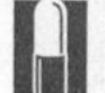

Allergic conjunctivitis:
≥3 yr and adult:
0.1% solution (Patanol): 1 drop in affected eye(s) BID (spaced 6–8 hr apart).
0.2% solution (Pataday): 1 drop in affected eye(s) once daily.
Allergic rhinitis:
≥12 yr and adult: Inhale 2 sprays into each nostril BID.

Continued

For explanation of icons, see p. 663.

OLOPATADINE *continued*

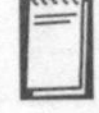

Ocular use: **DO NOT** use while wearing contact lenses; wait at least 10 min after instilling drops before inserting lenses. Ocular side effects include burning or stinging, dry eye, foreign body sensation, hyperemia, keratitis, lid edema, and pruritis. May also cause headaches, asthenia, pharyngitis, rhinitis, and taste perversion.

Nasal use: common side effects include bitter taste and headaches. Nasal ulceration, epistaxis, throat pain, and post-nasal drip have been reported.

OLSALAZINE
Dipentum, Di-mesalazine, Di-5-ASA
Salicylate, GI anti-inflammatory agent

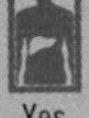 Yes 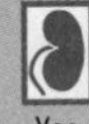 Yes 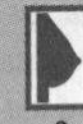 2 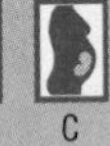 C

Caps: 250 mg

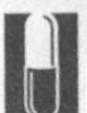

Ulcerative colitis:
Child: see remarks
Adult: 500 mg PO BID

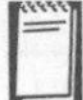

Drug is converted to 5-aminosalicylic acid (mesalamine) by colonic bacteria. 1 g olsalazine generally delivers 0.9 g of mesalamine to the colon. Only 1%–3% of olsalazine is systemically absorbed.

Contraindicated in salicylate hypersensitivity. **Use with caution** in severe liver disease, renal dysfunction, sulfasalazine hypersensitivity, and bronchial asthma. Diarrhea is the most common dose-related side effect. May also cause GI discomfort, headaches, rash, dizziness, and increase risk of bleeding with low molecular weight heparins or heparinoids and warfarin. Use with 6-mercaptopurine or thioguanine may increase risk of myelosuppression. Pancreatitis in children and hepatotoxicity have been reported. Monitor urinalysis and renal function.

Administer all doses with food to enhance efficacy.

Use in children (2–18 yr) has been limited to a trial where olsalazine 30 mg/kg/24 hr (**max. dose:** 2 g/24 hr) was found to be less efficacious than sulfasalazine 60 mg/kg/24 hr (**max. dose:** 4 g/24 hr) in treating mild/moderate ulcerative colitis. This may suggest inadequate dosing in this trial; additional studies are needed.

OMEPRAZOLE
Prilosec, Prilosec OTC, and others
In combination with sodium bicarbonate: Zegerid
Gastric acid pump inhibitor

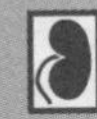 Yes 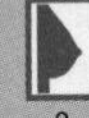 No 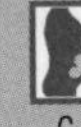 2 C

Caps, sustained-release: 10, 20, 40 mg
Tabs, delayed-release (OTC): 20 mg
Oral suspension: 2 mg/mL; contains ~0.5 mEq sodium bicarbonate per 1 mg drug
In combination with sodium bicarbonate:
Powder for oral suspension (Zegerid): 20, 40 mg packets (30s); each packet (regardless of strength) contains 1680 mg (20 mEq) sodium bicarbonate
Caps, immediate-release (Zegerid): 20, 40 mg; each capsule (regardless of strength) contains 1100 mg (13.1 mEq) sodium bicarbonate

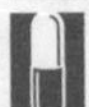

Child:
Esophagitis, GERD, or ulcers: 1 mg/kg/24 hr PO ÷ once daily–BID. Reported effective range: 0.2–3.5 mg/kg/24 hr. Children 1–6 yr may require higher doses due to enchanced drug clearance. Alternative dosing for patients ≥2 yr:

Continued

OMEPRAZOLE *continued*

Child: Esophagitis, GERD, or ulcers: Alternative dosing for patients ≥2 yr ***(cont'd):***
- ***5–<10 kg:*** 5 mg PO once daily
- ***10–<20 kg:*** 10 mg PO once daily
- ***≥20 kg:*** 20 mg PO once daily

Adult:

Duodenal ulcer or GERD: 20 mg/dose PO once daily × 4–8 wk; may give up to 12 wk for erosive esophagitis

Gastric ulcer: 40 mg/24 hr PO ÷ once daily–BID × 4–8 wk

Pathological hypersecretory conditions: Start with 60 mg/24 hr PO once daily. If needed, dose may be increased up to 120 mg/24 hr PO ÷ TID. Daily doses >80 mg should be administered in divided doses.

Common side effects: headache, diarrhea, nausea, and vomiting. Allergic reactions including anaphylaxis have been reported. Drug induces CYP 450 1A2 (decreases theophylline levels) and is also a substrate and inhibitor of CYP 2C19. Increases $T_{1/2}$ of citalopram, diazepam, phenytoin, and warfarin. May decrease the effects of itraconazole, ketoconazole, clopiogrel, iron salts, and ampicillin esters. May be used in combination with clarithromycin and amoxicillin for *H. pylori* infections.

Bioavailability may be increased with hepatic dysfunction or in patients of Asian decent.

Administer all doses before meals. Administer 30 min prior to sulcralfate. Capsules contain enteric-coated granules to ensure bioavailability. **Do not** chew or crush capsule. For doses unable to be divided by 10 mg, capsule may be opened and intact pellets may be administered in an acidic beverage (e.g., apple juice, cranberry juice) or apple sauce. The extemporaneously compounded oral suspension product may be less bioavailable due to the loss of the enteric-coating.

OMNIPAQUE

See *Iohexol*

ONDANSETRON

Zofran and generics

Antiemetic agent, 5-HT$_3$ antagonist

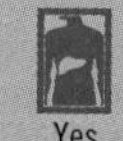
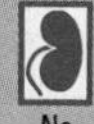
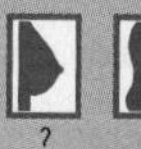

Yes No ? B

Injection: 2 mg/mL (2, 20 mL); may contain parabens
Premix injection in D$_5$W: 32 mg/50 mL
Tabs: 4, 8 mg
Tabs, orally disintegrating (ODT): 4, 8 mg; contains aspartame
Oral solution: 4 mg/5 mL (50 mL); contains sodium benzoate

Preventing nausea and vomiting associated with chemotherapy:
Oral (give initial dose 30 min before chemotherapy):
Child, dose based on body surface area:
- ***<0.3 m²:*** 1 mg TID PRN nausea
- ***0.3–0.6 m²:*** 2 mg TID PRN nausea
- ***0.6–1 m²:*** 3 mg TID PRN nausea
- ***>1 m²:*** 4–8 mg TID PRN nausea

Dose based on age:
- ***<4 yr:*** Use dose based on body surface area from preceding dosages.
- ***4–11 yr:*** 4 mg TID PRN nausea
- ***>11 yr and adult:*** 8 mg TID or 24 mg once daily PRN nausea

Continued

For explanation of icons, see p. 663.

ONDANSETRON *continued*

Preventing nausea and vomiting associated with chemotherapy (cont'd):

IV (child and adult):

Moderately emetogenic drugs: 0.15 mg/kg/dose at 30 min before, 4 and 8 hr after emetogenic drugs. Then same dose Q4 hr PRN.

Highly emetogenic drugs: 0.45 mg/kg/dose (**max. dose:** 32 mg/dose) 30 min before emetogenic drugs. Then 0.15 mg/kg/dose Q4 hr PRN.

Preventing nausea and vomiting associated with surgery (additional doses for controlling nausea and vomiting may not provide any benefits):

IV/IM (administered prior to anesthesia over 2–5 min):

Child (2–12 yr):

≤40 kg: 0.1 mg/kg/dose × 1

>40 kg: 4 mg × 1

Adult: 4 mg × 1

PO:

Adult: 16 mg × 1, 1 hr prior to induction of anesthesia

Preventing nausea and vomiting associated with radiation therapy:

Child: use above dosage for preventing nausea and vomiting assocated with chemotherapy and give initial dose 1–2 hr prior to radiation.

Adult:

Total body irradiation: 8 mg PO 1–2 hr prior to radiation once daily

Single high-dose fraction radiation to abdomen: 8 mg PO 1–2 hr prior to radiation with subsequent doses Q8 hr after first dose × 1–2 days after completion of radiation.

Daily fractionated radiation to abdomen: 8 mg PO 1–2 hr prior to radiation with subsequent doses Q8 hr after first dose for each day radiation is given.

Vomiting in acute gastroenteritis (PO route is preferred, use IV when PO is not possible):

PO (use oral disintegrating tablet):

8–15 kg: 2 mg × 1

>15 and ≤30 kg: 4 mg × 1

>30 kg: 8 mg × 1

IV: 0.1–0.5 mg/kg/dose × 1; **max. dose:** 4 mg/dose

Avoid use in congenital long QTc syndrome. Bronchospasm, tachycardia, hypokalemia, seizures, headaches, lightheadedness, constipation, diarrhea and transient increases in AST, ALT, and bilirubin may occur. Transient blindness (resolution within a few min up to 48 hr), arthralgia, hepatic dysfunction, and rare/transient ECG changes (including QT interval prolongation) have been reported with IV route of administration. Data limited for use in children <3 yr.

ECG monitoring is recommended in patients with electrolyte abnormalities, CHF, or bradyarrhythmias.

Ondansetron is a substrate for CYP 450 1A2, 2D6, 2E1, and 3A3/4 drug metabolizing enzymes. It is likely that the inhibition/loss of one of the previously listed enzymes will be compensated by others and may result in insignificant changes to ondansetron's elimination. Ondansetron's elimination may be affected by CYP 450 enzyme inducers. Follow theophylline, phenytoin, or warfarin levels closely, if used in combination. Use with apomorphine may result in profound hypotension and loss of consciousness, and is contraindicated.

OPIUM TINCTURE

Deodorized tincture of opium

Narcotic, analgesic

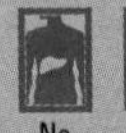
No

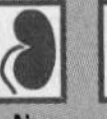
No

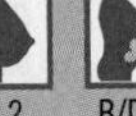
2

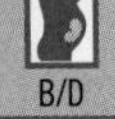
B/D

Oral liquid: 10% opium. Contains 17%–21% alcohol (1 mL equivalent to 10 mg morphine)

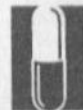

Dilute 25-fold with water to make a final concentration of 0.4 mg/mL morphine equivalent.

Neonatal opiate withdrawal (doses based on mg morphine equivalent):

Continued

0
FORMULARY

OPIUM TINCTURE *continued*

Start with 0.04 mg/kg/dose Q3–4 hr, if needed, increase dose by 0.04 mg/kg/dose Q3–4 hr until symptoms abate. Usual doses range from 0.08–0.12 mg (or 0.2–0.3 mL)/dose Q3–4 hr and it is rare that doses exceed 0.28 mg (or 0.7 mL)/dose.

Use 25-fold dilution to treat neonatal abstinence syndrome (NAS). Follow neonatal abstinence scores. **Doses for the dilution are equivalent to paregoric doses.** Morphine is considered a safer agent for NAS because tincture of opium contains alcohol and requires a dilution (potential calculation error). May cause respiratory depression, hypotension, bradycardia, and CNS depression. Pregnancy category changes to "D" if used for prolonged periods or in high doses at term.

OSELTAMIVIR PHOSPHATE

Tamiflu

Antiviral

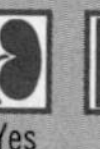
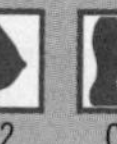
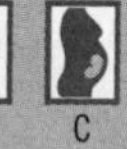

No Yes 2 C

Caps: 30, 45, 75 mg

Oral suspension: 6 mg/mL (60 mL, \Rx); may contain saccharin and sodium benzoate

NOTE: Previous oral suspension concentration of 12 mg/mL has been replaced with a 6 mg/mL concentration so that both commerically available and compounded products are similar in concentration to prevent dosing errors.

Treatment of influenza (initiate therapy within 2 days of onset of symptoms):

Pre-term neonate (24–37 weeks gestation; based on pharmacokinetic data from 20 neonates): 1 mg/kg/dose PO BID

Child <1 yr: see following table.

Age (Months)	Dosage for 5 Days	Volume of Oral Suspension (6 mg/mL)
<3	12 mg PO BID	2 mL
3–5	20 mg PO BID	3.33 mL
6–11	25 mg PO BID	4.2 mL

Child ≥1 yr: see following table.

Weight (kg)	Dosage for 5 Days	Volume of Oral Suspension (6 mg/mL)
≤15	30 mg PO BID	5 mL
>15–23	45 mg PO BID	7.5 mL
>23–40	60 mg PO BID	10 mL
>40	75 mg PO BID	12.5 mL

≥12 yr and adults: 75 mg PO BID × 5 days.

Prophylaxis of influenza (initiate therapy within 2 days of exposure; see remarks):

Child 3 mo–<1 yr: 3 mg/kg/dose PO once daily; alternative dosage based on age:

3–5 mo: 20 mg PO once daily

6–11 mo: 25 mg PO once daily

Child 1–12 yr:

≤15 kg: 30 mg PO once daily

16–23 kg: 45 mg PO once daily

24–40 kg: 60 mg PO once daily

>40 kg: 75 mg PO once daily

≥13 yr and adult: 75 mg PO once daily for a minimum of 7 days and up to 6 wk; initiate therapy within 2 days of exposure.

Continued

For explanation of icons, see p. 663.

OSELTAMIVIR PHOSPHATE *continued*

Currently indicated for the treatment of influenza A and B strains. **Do not** use in children <1 yr due to concerns of fatalities related to excessive CNS penetration in 7-day-old rats. Nausea and vomiting generally occurring within the first 2 days and are the most common adverse effects. Insomnia, vertigo, seizures, hypothermia, neuropsychiatric events (may result in fatal outcomes), arrhythmias, rash, and toxic epidermal necrolysis have also been reported. Reduce dosage treatment dose if GFR is 10–30 mL/min to 75 mg PO once daily × 5 days. **(See Chapter 31.)**

PROPHYLAXIS USE: Oseltamivir is not a substitute for annual flu vaccination. Safety and efficacy have been demonstrated for ≤6 wk; duration of protection lasts for as long as dosing is continued. Adjust prophylaxis dose if GFR is 10–30 mL/min by extending the dosage interval to once every other day.

Probenecid increases oseltamivir levels. Oseltamivir decreases the efficacy of the nasal influenza vaccine (FluMist; discontinue oseltamivir 48 hr before and **do not** restart for at least 1–2 wk after fluMist administration.

Dosage adjustments in hepatic impairment, severe renal disease, and dialysis have not been established for either treatment or prophylaxis use. The safety and efficacy of repeated treatment or prophylaxis courses have not been evaluated. Doses may be administered with or without food.

OXACILLIN

Various generic brands
Antibiotic, penicillin (penicillinase resistant)

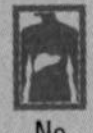
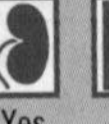
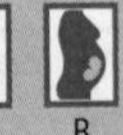

No Yes 2 B

Oral solution: 250 mg/5 mL (100 mL); contains 0.8 mEq Na per 250 mg drug and may contain saccharin
Injection: 1, 2, 10 g
Injection, premixed in iso-osmotic dextrose: 1 g/50 mL, 2 g/50 mL
Injectable products contain 2.8–3.1 mEq Na per 1 g drug

Neonate: IM/IV
<7 days:
- ***<1.2 kg:*** 50 mg/kg/24 hr ÷ Q12 hr
- ***<1.2–2 kg:*** 50–100 mg/kg/24 hr ÷ Q12 hr
- ***≥2 kg:*** 75–150 mg/kg/24 hr ÷ Q8 hr

≥7 days:
- ***<1.2 kg:*** 50 mg/kg/24 hr ÷ Q12 hr
- ***1.2–2 kg:*** 75–150 mg/kg/24 hr ÷ Q8 hr
- ***≥2 kg:*** 100–200 mg/kg/24 hr ÷ Q6 hr

Infant and child:
- ***Oral:*** 50–100 mg/kg/24 hr ÷ Q6 hr
- ***IM/IV:*** 100–200 mg/kg/24 hr ÷ Q4–6 hr
- **Max. dose:** 12 g/24 hr

Adult:
- ***Oral:*** 500–1000 mg/dose Q4–6 hr
- ***IM/IV:*** 250–2000 mg/dose Q4–6 hr

Rash and GI disturbances are common. Leukopenia, reversible hepatotoxicity, and acute interstitial nephritis has been reported. Hematuria and azotemia have occurred in neonates and infants with high doses. May cause false-positive urinary and serum proteins.

CSF penetration is poor unless meninges are inflamed. Use the lower end of the usual dosage range for patients with creatinine clearances <10 mL/min. Oral form should be administered on an empty stomach. **Adjust dose in renal failure (see Chapter 31).**

OXCARBAZEPINE
Trileptal
Anticonvulsant

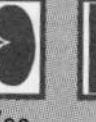 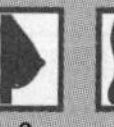 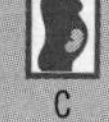 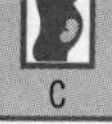

No Yes 2 C

Tabs: 150, 300, 600 mg
Oral suspension: 300 mg/5 mL (250 mL); contains saccharin and ethanol

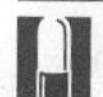

Child (2–<4 yr):
Adjunctive therapy: Start with 8–10 mg/kg/24 hr PO ÷ BID up to a **max. dose** of 600 mg/24 hr. For children <20 kg, may consider using a starting dose of 16–20 mg/kg/24 hr PO ÷ BID; gradually increase the dose over a 2- to 4-week period and do not exceed 60 mg/kg/24 hr ÷ BID.

Child (4–16 yr, see remarks):
Adjunctive therapy: Start with 8–10 mg/kg/24 hr PO ÷ BID up to a **max. dose** of 600 mg/24 hr. Then gradually increase the dose over a 2-wk period to the following maintenance doses:
20–29 kg: 900 mg/24 hr PO ÷ BID
29.1–39 kg: 1200 mg/24 hr PO ÷ BID
>39 kg: 1800 mg/24 hr PO ÷ BID
Conversion to monotherapy: Start with 8–10 mg/kg/24 hr PO ÷ BID and simultaneously initiate dosage reduction of concomitant AEDs and withdrawal completely over 3–6 wk. Dose may be increased at weekly intervals, as clinically indicated, by a **maximum** of 10 mg/kg/24 hr to achieve the recommended monotherapy maintenance dose as described in the following table.
Initiation of monotherapy: Start with 8–10 mg/kg/24 hr PO ÷ BID. Then increase by 5 mg/kg/24 hr every 3 days up to the recommended monotherapy maintenance dose as described in the following table:

Recommended Monotherapy Maintenance Doses for Children by Weight

Weight (kg)	Daily Oral Maintenance Dose (mg/24 hr) Divided BID
20	600–900
25–30	900–1200
35–40	900–1500
45	1200–1500
50–55	1200–1800
60–65	1200–2100
70	1500–2100

Adult:
Adjunctive therapy: Start with 600 mg/24 hr PO ÷ BID. Dose may be increased at weekly intervals, as clinically indicated, by a **maximum** of 600 mg/24 hr. Usual maintenance dose is 1200 mg/24 hr PO ÷ BID. Doses ≥2400 mg/24 hr are generally not well tolerated due to CNS side effects.
Conversion to monotherapy: Start with 600 mg/24 hr PO ÷ BID and simultaneously initiate dosage reduction of concomitant AEDs. Dose may be increased at weekly intervals, as clinically indicated, by a **maximum** of 600 mg/24 hr to achieve a dose of 2400 mg/24 hr PO ÷ BID. Concomitant AEDs should be terminated gradually over approximately 3–6 wk.
Initiation of monotherapy: Start with 600 mg/24 hr PO ÷ BID. Then increase by 300 mg/24 hr every 3 days up to 1200 mg/24 hr PO ÷ BID.

Continued

For explanation of icons, see p. 663.

OXCARBAZEPINE *continued*

Clinically significant hyponatremia may occur; generally seen within the first 3 mo of therapy. May also cause headache, dizziness, drowsiness, ataxia, fatigue, nystagmus, urticaria, diplopia, abnormal gait, and GI discomfort. About 25% to 30% of patients with cabamazepine hypersensitivity will experience a cross reaction with oxcarbazepine. Serious dermatological reactions (Stevens-Johnson and TEN), multi-organ hypersensitivity reactions, rare cases of anaphylaxis and angioedema, and suicidal behavior or ideation have been reported.

Inhibits CYP 450 2C19 and induces CYP 450 3A4/5 drug metabolizing enzymes. Carbamazepine, phenobarbital, phenytoin, valproic acid, and verapamil may decrease oxcarbazepine levels. Oxcarbazepine may increase phenobarbital and phenytoin levels. Oxcarbazepine can decrease the effects of oral contraceptives, felodipine, and lamotrigine.

A median pediatric maintenance dose of 31 mg/kg/24 hr (range: 6–51 mg/kg/24 hr) was achieved in a clinical trial. Adjust dosage if GFR <30 mL/min by administering 50% of the normal starting dose (**max. dose:** 300 mg/24 hr) followed by a slower than normal increase in dose if necessary **(see Chapter 31.)** No dosage adjustment is required in mild/moderate hepatic impairment.

Doses may be administered with or without food.

OXYBUTYNIN CHLORIDE
Ditropan, Ditropan XL, Oxytrol, and others
Anticholinergic agent, antispasmodic

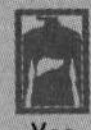
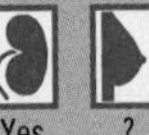
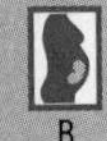
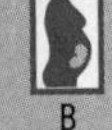

Yes Yes ? B

Tabs: 5 mg
Tabs, extended-release (Ditropan XL and others): 5, 10, 15 mg
Syrup: 1 mg/mL (473 mL); contains parabens
Transdermal system (Oxytrol): delivers 3.9 mg/24 hr (8s); contains 36 mg per system

Child ≤5 yr:
Immediate release: 0.2 mg/kg/dose BID–QID PO; **max. dose:** 15 mg/24 hr
Child >5 yr:
Immediate release: 5 mg/dose BID–TID PO; **max. dose:** 15 mg/24 hr
Extended release (≥6 yr): Start with 5 mg/dose once daily PO; if needed, increase as tolerated by 5 mg increments up to a **maximum** of 20 mg/24 hr
Adult:
Immediate release: 5 mg/dose BID–QID PO
Extended release (Ditropan XL): 5–10 mg/dose once daily PO up to a **max. dose** of 30 mg/dose once daily PO
Transdermal system: 1 patch (3.9 mg/24 hr) every 3–4 days (twice weekly)

Use with caution in hepatic or renal disease, hypterthyroidism, IBD, or cardiovascular disease. Anticholinergic side effects may occur, including drowsiness and hallucinations. **Contraindicated** in glaucoma, GI obstruction, megacolon, myasthenia gravis, severe colitis, hypovolemia, and GU obstruction. Memory impairment and QT interval prolongation have been reported. Oxybutynin is a CYP 450 3A4 substrate; inhibitors and inducers of CYP 450 3A4 may increase and decrease the effects of oxybutynin, respectively.

Dosage adjustments for the extended-release dosage form are at weekly intervals. **Do not** crush, chew, or divide the extended-release tablets. Apply transdermal system on dry intact skin on the abdomen, hip, or buttock by rotating the site and avoiding same site application within 7 days.

OXYCODONE

Roxicodone, OxyContin, and many others
Narcotic, analgesic

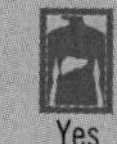 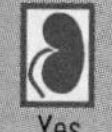  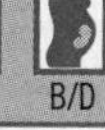 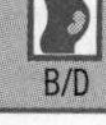

Yes Yes 2 B/D

Solution: 1 mg/mL (5, 500 mL); contains alcohol
Concentrated solution: 20 mg/mL (30 mL); may contain saccharin
Tabs: 5, 15, 30 mg
Controlled-release tabs (OxyContin and others): 10, 15, 20, 30, 40, 80 mg (80 mg strength for opioid-tolerant patients only)
Caps: 5 mg

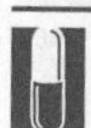

Opioid naïve doses based upon oxycodone salt:
Child: 0.05–0.15 mg/kg/dose Q4–6 hr PRN up to 5 mg/dose PO
Adult: 5–10 mg Q4–6 hr PRN PO; see remarks for use of controlled-release tablets.

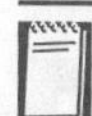

Abuse potential, CNS and respiratory depression, increased ICP, histamine release, constipation, and GI distress may occur. **Use with caution** in severe renal impairment (increases $T_{1/2}$) and mild/moderate hepatic dysfunction (use ⅓ to ½ of usual dose has been recommended). **Naloxone is the antidote.** See Chapter 6 for equianalgesic dosing. Check dosages of acetaminophen or aspirin when using combination products (e.g., Tylox, Percodan). Aspirin is **not recommended** in children due to concerns of Reye's syndrome. Oxycodone is metabolized by the CYP 450 2D6 isoenzyme.

When using controlled-released tablets (Oxycontin), determine patient's total 24-hr requirements and divide by 2 to administer on a Q12 hr dosing interval. Oxycontin 80 mg tablet is **USED ONLY** for opioid tolerant patients; this strength can cause fatal respiratory depression in opioid naïve patients. Controlled-release dosage form **should not be used** as a PRN analgesic and must be swallowed whole.

Pregnancy category changes to "D" if used for prolonged periods or in high doses at term.

OXYCODONE AND ACETAMINOPHEN

Tylox, Roxilox, Percocet, Endocet, Roxicet, and many others
Combination analgesic with a narcotic

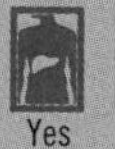 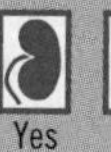 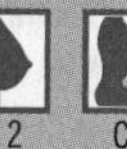

Yes Yes 2 C

Capsule (Tylox, Roxilox)/caplet: Oxycodone HCl 5 mg + acetaminophen 500 mg
Tabs (Percocet, Endocet, and others):
  Most common strength: oxycodone HCl 5 mg + acetaminophen 325 mg
  Other strengths:
    Oxycodone HCl 2.5 mg + acetaminophen 325 mg
    Oxycodone HCl 7.5 mg + acetaminophen 325 mg or 500 mg
    Oxycodone HCl 10 mg + acetaminophen 325 mg or 650 mg
Oral solution (Roxicet): Oxycondone HCl 5 mg + acetaminophen 325 mg/5 mL (5, 500 mL); contains 0.4% alcohol and saccharin

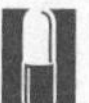

Dose based on amount of oxycodone and acetaminophen.

See *Oxycodone* and *Acetaminophen*. Check dosages of acetaminophen when using these combination products.

For explanation of icons, see p. 663.

OXYCODONE AND ASPIRIN
Percodan, Roxiprin, and many others
Combination analgesic (narcotic and salicylate)

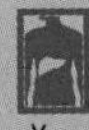 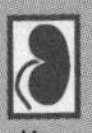  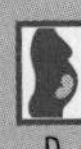
Yes Yes 2 D

Tabs:
Percodan, Roxiprin, and others: Oxycodone HCl 4.5 mg, oxycodone tereph 0.38 mg, and aspirin 325 mg

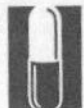
Dose based on amount of oxycodone (combined salts) and aspirin.

See *Oxycodone* and *Aspirin.* **Do not use** in children <16 yr because of risk for Reye's syndrome. Check dosages of aspirin when using these combination products.

OXYMETAZOLINE
Nasal: Afrin, Duramist 12-Hr Nasal, Neo-Synephrine 12-Hour Nasal, Nostrilla, and many others
Ophthalmic: Visine LR
Nasal decongestant, vasoconstrictor

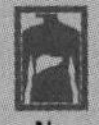 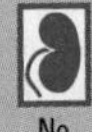 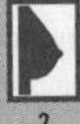 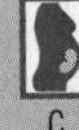 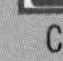
No No ? C

Nasal spray [OTC]: 0.05% (15, 30 mL)
Ophthalmic drops [OTC]: 0.025% (15, 30 mL); contains benzalkonium chloride and EDTA

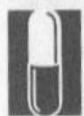
Nasal decongestant (not to exceed 3 days in duration):
≥6 yr–adult: 2–3 sprays or 2–3 drops or 1–2 metered sprays (Nostrilla) in each nostril BID. Do not exceed 2 doses/24 hr period.

Ophthalmic:
≥6 yr–adult: Instill 1–2 drops in the affected eye(s) Q6 hr.

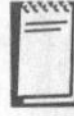
Contraindicated in patients on MAO inhibitor therapy. Rebound nasal congestion may occur with excessive use (>3 days) via the nasal route. Systemic absorption may occur with either route of administration. Headache, dizziness, hypertension, transient burning, stinging, dryness, nasal mucosa ulceration, sneezing, blurred vision, and mydriasis have occurred.

Do not use ophthalmic solution if it changes color or becomes cloudy.

PALIVIZUMAB
Synagis
Monoclonal antibody

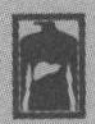 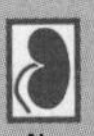 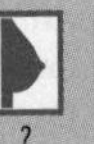 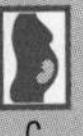
No No ? C

Injection, solution: 100 mg/mL (0.5, 1 mL; single use); contains glycine and histidine.

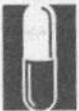
RSV prophylaxis (see latest edition of *Red Book* for most recent indications):
Chronic lung disease ≤2 yr requiring medical therapy within 6 mo of age prior to RSV season, premature infant (≤28 wk of gestation) <12 mo of age, premature infant (29–32 wk of gestation) <6 mo of age, hemodynamically significant cyanotic and acyanotic congenital heart disease ≤2 yr, or congenital airway abnormality or neuromuscular disorder <12 mo of age: 15 mg/kg/dose IM Q monthly just prior to and during the RSV season.

Continued

PALIVIZUMAB *continued*

RSV season typically November through April in the northern hemisphere but may begin earlier or persist later in certain communities. **Use with caution** in patients with thrombocytopenia or any coagulation disorder because of IM route of administration. IM is currently the only route of administration. The following adverse effects have been reported at slightly higher incidences when compared to placebo: rhinitis, rash, pain, increased liver enzymes, pharyngitis, cough, wheeze, diarrhea, vomiting, conjunctivitis, and anemia. Rare acute hypersensitivity reactions have been reported (first or subsequent doses).

Does not interfere with the response to routine childhood vaccines. Palivizumab is currently indicated for RSV prophylaxis in high-risk infants only. Efficacy and safety have not been demonstrated for treatment of RSV.

Each dose should be administered IM in the anterolateral aspect of the thigh. It is recommended to divide doses with total injection volumes >1 mL. **Avoid** injection in the gluteal muscle because of risk for damage to the sciatic nerve.

PANCREATIC ENZYMES

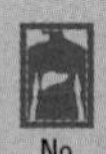
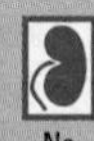

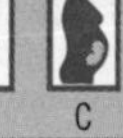

No No 2 C

See Chapter 30 for description and contents of lipase, protease, and amylase.

Initial doses (actual requirements are patient specific):
Enteric-coated microspheres and microtabs:

- ***Infant:*** 2000–4000 U lipase per 120 mL formula or per breast-feeding.
- ***Child <4 yr:*** 1000 U lipase/kg/meal
- ***Child ≥4 yr and adult:*** 500 U lipase/kg/meal
- **Max. dose:** 2500 U lipase/kg/meal

The total daily dose should include approximately three meals and two to three snacks per day. Snack doses are approximately half of meal doses.

May cause occult GI bleeding, allergic reactions to porcine proteins, hyperuricemia, and hyperuricosuria with high doses. Dose should be titrated to eliminate diarrhea and to minimize steatorrhea. **Do not** chew microspheres or microtabs. Concurrent administration with H_2 antagonists or gastric acid pump inhibitors may enhance enzyme efficacy. Doses higher than 6000 U lipase/kg/meal have been associated with colonic strictures in children <12 yr. Powder dosage form is **not** preferred due to potential GI mucosal ulceration.

Avoid use of generic pancreatic enzyme products, since they been associated with treatment failures. Unapproved products by the FDA are no longer allowed to be distributed in the United States.

PANCURONIUM BROMIDE

Various generic brands
Nondepolarizing neuromuscular blocking agent

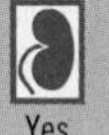
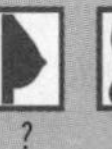
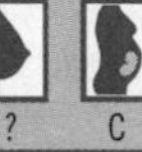

Yes Yes ? C

Injection: 1 mg/mL (10 mL), 2 mg/mL (2, 5 mL); contains benzyl alcohol

Intermitent dosing (see remarks):
Neonate:
- ***Initial:*** 0.02 mg/kg/dose IV
- ***Maintenance:*** 0.05–0.1 mg/kg/dose IV Q0.5–4 hr PRN

Continued

For explanation of icons, see p. 663.

PANCURONIUM BROMIDE *continued*

1 mo–adult:

Initial: 0.04–0.1 mg/kg/dose IV

Maintenance: 0.015–0.1 mg/kg/dose IV Q30–60 min

Continuous IV infusion (see remarks):

Neonate: 0.02–0.04 mg/kg/hr

Child: 0.03–1 mg/kg/hr

Adolescent and adult: 0.02–0.04 mg/kg/hr

Onset of action is 1–2 min. May cause tachycardia, salivation, and wheezing. Severe anaphylactic reactions have been reported; crossreactivity between neuromuscular blocking agents has been reported.

Drug effects may be accentuated by hypothermia, acidosis, neonatal age, decreased renal function, halothane, succinylcholine, hypokalemia, hyponatremia, hypocalcemia, clindamycin, tetracycline, and aminoglycoside antibiotics. Drug effects may be antagonized by alkalosis, hypercalcemia, peripheral neuropathies, diabetes mellitus, demyelinating lesions, carbamazepine, phenytoin, theophylline, anticholinesterases (e.g., neostigmine, pyridostigmine), and azathioprine. For obese patients, use of lean body weight for dose calculation has been recommended to prevent intense block of long duration and possible overdose.

Antidote is neostigmine (with atropine or glycopyrrolate). **Avoid** use in severe renal impairment (<10 mL/min). Patients with cirrhosis may require a high initial dose to achieve adequate relaxation, but muscle paralysis will be prolonged.

PANTOPRAZOLE

Protonix and others

Gastric acid pump inhibitor

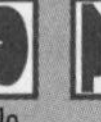

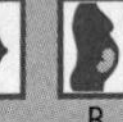

No No 2 B

Tab, enteric coated: 20, 40 mg

Injection: 40 mg; contains edetate sodium

Oral suspension: 2 mg/mL; contains 0.25 mEq sodium bicarbonate per 1 mg drug

Powder for delayed-release oral suspension: 40 mg (30s)

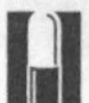

Child:

GERD with erosive esophagitis (limited data): 0.5–1 mg/kg/dose PO once daily × 28 days; dosed as 20 mg PO once daily × 28 days in 15 children 6–13 yr weighing 20–40 kg.

IV (data limited to pharmacokinetic trials): Some doses ranging from 0.32–1.88 mg/kg/dose have been reported from three separate trials (total N = 31; 0.01–16.4 yr). Patients with systemic inflammatory response syndrome (SIRS) cleared the drug more slowly, resulting in higher $T_{1/2}$ and AUC, than patients without. Despite limited data, 1–2 mg/kg/24 hr ÷ Q12–24 hr have been used. Additional studies are needed.

Adult:

GERD: 40 mg PO once daily × 8–16 wk or 40 mg IV once daily × 7–10 days.

Peptic ulcer: 40–80 mg PO once daily × 4–8 wk

Hypersecretory conditions:

PO: 40 mg BID; dose may be increased as needed up to a **max. dose** of 240 mg/24 hr.

IV: 80 mg Q12 hr; dose may be increased as needed to Q8 hr (**max. dose:** 240 mg/24 hr). Therapy >6 days at 240 mg/24 hr has not been evaluated.

Convert from IV to PO therapy as soon as patient is able to tolerate PO. Common side effects include diarrhea and headache. May cause transient elevation in LFTs. Drug is a substrate for CYP 450 2C19 and 3A3/4 isoenzymes. May decrease the absorption of itraconazole, ketoconazole, iron salts, and ampicillin esters.

Continued

PANTOPRAZOLE *continued*

All oral doses may be taken with or without food. **Do not** crush or chew tablets. The extemporaneously compounded oral suspension may be less bioavailable owing to the loss of the enteric coating. Powder for delayed-release oral suspension product may be mixed with 5 mL apple juice (administer immediately followed by rinsing container with more apple juice), or sprinkled on 1 teaspoonful of apple sauce (administer within 10 min); see package insert for NG administration.

For IV infusion, doses may be administer over 15 min at a concentration of 0.4–0.8 mg/mL or over 2 min at a concentration of 4 mg/mL. Midazolam and zinc are **not compatible** with the IV dosage form. Parenteral routes other than IV **are not recommended.**

PAREGORIC

Camphorated opium tincture
Narcotic, analgesic

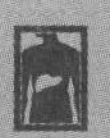 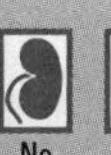 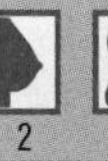 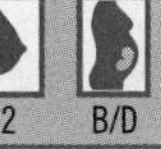

No No 2 B/D

Camphorated tincture: 2 mg (morphine equivalent)/5 mL (contains 45% alcohol and may contain benzoic acid or camphor) (473 mL)

Neonatal opiate withdrawal:
Start with 0.08–0.12 mg (or 0.2–0.3 mL)/dose Q3–4 hr, increase dose by 0.02 mg (or 0.05 mL)/dose Q3–4 hr until symptoms abate; **max. dose:** 0.28 mg (or 0.7 mL)/dose. Maintain withdrawal symptoms for 3–5 days and then gradually taper dosage by maintaining same dosage amount and widen dosing interval over a 2- to 4-week period.

Analgesia:
Child: 0.1–0.2 mg/kg (or 0.25–0.5 mL/kg)/dose PO once daily–QID
Adult: 2–4 mg (or 5–10 mL)/dose PO once daily–QID

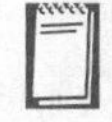

Morphine is preferred over paregoric because of excipients (alcohol, camphor, benzoic acid) found in paregoric. Each 5 mL paregoric contains 2 mg morphine equivalent, 0.02 mL anise oil, 20 mg benzoic acid, 20 mg camphor, 0.2 mL glycerin and alcohol. The final concentration of morphine equivalent is 0.4 mg/mL. This is 25-fold less potent than undiluted deodorized tincture of opium (DTO: 10 mg morphine equivalent/mL). **If using DTO to treat neonatal abstinence, must dilute 25-fold prior to use.** Similar side effects to morphine. After symptoms are controlled for several days, dose for opiate withdrawal should be decreased gradually over a 2- to 4-wk period (e.g., by 10% Q2–3 days). Monitor neonatal abstinence scores for NAS. Pregnancy category changes to "D" if used for prolonged periods or in high doses.

PAROMOMYCIN SULFATE

Humatin
Amebicide, antibiotic (aminoglycoside)

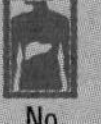 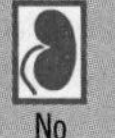 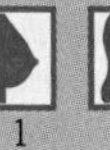

No No 1 C

Caps: 250 mg

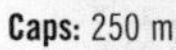

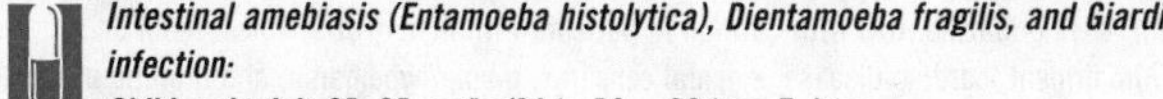

Intestinal amebiasis (Entamoeba histolytica), Dientamoeba fragilis, and Giardia lamblia infection:
Child and adult: 25–35 mg/kg/24 hr PO ÷ Q8 hr × 7 days

Tapeworm (T. saginata, T. solium, D. latum, and D. caninum):
Child: 11 mg/kg/dose PO Q15 min × 4 doses
Adult: 1 g PO Q15 min × 4 doses

Tapeworm (Hymenolepis nana):
Child and adult: 45 mg/kg/dose PO once daily × 5–7 days

Continued

For explanation of icons, see p. 663.

PAROMOMYCIN SULFATE *continued*

Cryptosporidial diarrhea:

Adult: 1.5–2.25 g/24 hr PO ÷ 3–6 × daily. Duration varies from 10–14 days to 4–8 wk. Maintenance therapy has also been used. Alternatively, 1 g PO BID × 12 wk in conjunction with azithromycin 600 mg PO once daily × 4 wk has been used in patients with AIDS.

Contraindicated in intestinal obstruction. **Use with caution** in ulcerative bowel lesions to avoid renal toxicity via systemic absorption. Drug is generally poorly absorbed and therefore **not** indicated for sole treatment of extraintestinal amebiasis. Side effects include GI disturbance, hematuria, rash, ototoxicity, and hypocholesterolemia. May decrease the effects of digoxin.

PAROXETINE

Paxil, Pexeva, Paxil CR, and others

Antidepressant, selective serotonin reuptake inhibitor

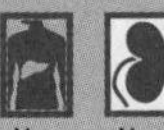
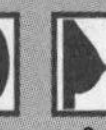
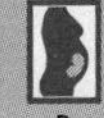

Yes Yes 2 D

Tabs: 10, 20, 30, 40 mg
Controlled-release tabs (Paxil CR): 12.5, 25, 37.5 mg
Oral suspension: 10 mg/5 mL (250 mL); contains saccharin and parabens

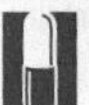

Child:

Depression: Well-controlled clinical trials have failed to demonstrate efficacy in children. The FDA recommends paroxetine not to be used for this indication.

Obsessive compulsive disorder (limited data, based on a 10-wk randomized controlled trial in 207 children 7–17 yr; mean age 11.1 ± 3.03 yr): Start with 10 mg PO once daily. If needed, adjust upwards by increasing dose no more than 10 mg/24 hr no more frequently than Q7 days up to a **max. dose** of 50 mg/24 hr. A mean doses of 20.3 mg/24 hr (children) and 26.8 mg/24 hr (adolescents) were used.

Social anxiety disorder (8–17 yr): Start with 10 mg PO once daily. If needed, increase dose by 10 mg/24 hr no more frequently than Q7 days up to a **max. dose** of 50 mg/24 hr.

Adult:

Depression: Start with 20 mg PO QAM × 4 wk. If no clinical improvement, increase dose by 10 mg/24 hr Q7 days PRN up to a **max. dose** of 50 mg/24 hr.

Paxil CR: Start with 25 mg PO QAM × 4 wk. If no improvement, increase dose by 12.5 mg/24 hr Q7 days PRN up to a **max. dose** of 62.5 mg/24 hr.

Obsessive compulsive disorder: Start with 20 mg PO once daily; increase dose by 10 mg/24 hr Q7 days PRN up to a **max. dose** of 60 mg/24 hr. Usual dose is 40 mg PO once daily.

Panic disorder: Start with 10 mg PO QAM; increase dose by 10 mg/24 hr Q7 days PRN up to a **max. dose** of 60 mg/24 hr.

Paxil CR: Start with 12.5 mg PO QAM; increase dose by 12.5 mg/24 hr Q7 days PRN up to a **max. dose** of 75 mg/24 hr.

Contraindicated in patients taking MAO inhibitors (within 14 days of discontinuing MAO inhibitors), or thioridazine. **Use with caution** in patients with history of seizures, renal or hepatic impairment, cardiac disease, suicidal concerns, mania/hypomania, and diuretic use.

Patients with severe renal or hepatic impairment should initiate therapy at 10 mg/24 hr and increase dose as needed up to a **maximum** of 40 mg/24 hr.

Common side effects include anxiety, nausea, anorexia, and decreased appetite. Monitor for clinical worsening of depression and suicidal ideation/behavior following the initiation of therapy or after dose changes.

Continued

PAROXETINE *continued*

Paroxetine is an inhibitor and substrate for CYP 450 2D6. May increase the effects/toxicity of tricyclic antidepressants, theophylline, and warfarin. Cimetidine, ritonavir, MAO inhibitors (fatal serotonin syndrome), dextromethorphan, phenothiazines, and type 1C antiarrhythmics may increase the effect/toxicity of paroxetine. Weakness, hyperreflexia, and poor coordination have been reported when taken with sumatriptan.

Do not discontinue therapy abruptly, may cause sweating, dizziness, confusion, and tremor. May be taken with or without food.

PENICILLAMINE
Cuprimine, Depen
Heavy metal chelator

No Yes 3 D

Tabs: 250 mg
Caps: 250 mg
Oral suspension: 50 mg/mL

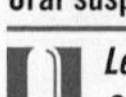

Lead chelation therapy (third-line therapy):
Child: 30–40 mg/kg/24 hr or 600–750 mg/m^2/24 hr PO ÷ TID–QID; **max. dose:** 1.5 g/24 hr. Administer doses 2 hr before or 3 hr after meals.
Adult: 1–1.5 g/24 hr PO ÷ BID–TID.
Durations of treatment vary from 1 to 6 mo.

Wilson's disease (see remarks for titration information):
Infant and child: 20 mg/kg/24 hr PO ÷ BID–QID; **max. dose:** 1 g/24 hr.
Adult: 250 mg/dose PO QID; **max. dose:** 2 g/24 hr.

Arsenic poisoning:
Child: 100 mg/kg/24 hr PO ÷ Q6 hr × 5 days; **max. dose:** 1 g/24 hr.

Cystinuria (see remarks for titration information):
Infant and young child: 30 mg/kg/24 hr ÷ QID PO; **max. dose:** 4 g/24 hr.
Older child and adult: 1–4 g/24 hr ÷ QID PO.

Primary biliary cirrhosis (adult):
Initial: 250 mg/24 hr PO; increase by 250 mg Q2 wk to a total of 1 g/24 hr (given as 250 mg QID).

Juvenile rheumatoid arthritis:
5 mg/kg/24 hr ÷ once daily–BID PO × 2 mo, then 10 mg/kg/24 hr ÷ once daily–BID PO × 4 mo.

Dose should be given 1 hr before or 2 hr after meals. **AAP relegates this drug as a third-line agent for lead chelation indicated only after unacceptable reaction with oral succimer and calcium EDTA.** If used, must be in lead-free environment, since it can increase absorption of lead if present in GI tract. **Avoid use** if patient's creatinine clearance is <50 mL/min. Follow CBC, LFTs, and urinalysis; and monitor the patient's skin, lymph nodes, and body temperature. Can cause optic neuritis, fever, rash, GI disturbances, altered taste, vomiting, lupus-like syndrome, nephrotic syndrome, peripheral neuropathy, leukopenia, eosinophilia, and thrombocytopenia. May reduce serum digoxin levels. **Avoid** concomitant administration with iron, antacids, and food.

Patients treated for Wilson's disease, rheumatoid arthritis, or cystinuria should be treated with pyridoxine 25–50 mg/24 hr. Titrate urinary copper excretion to >1 mg/24 hr for patients with Wilson's disease. Patients with cystinuria should have doses titrated to maintain urinary cystine excretion at <100–200 mg/24 hr.

For explanation of icons, see p. 663.

PENICILLIN G PREPARATIONS—AQUEOUS POTASSIUM AND SODIUM
Pfizerpen and others
Antibiotic, aqueous penicillin

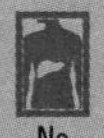
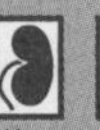
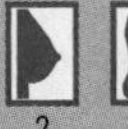
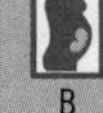

No Yes 2 B

Injection (K^+): 5, 20 million units (contains 1.7 mEq K and 0.3 mEq Na/1 million units penicillin G)
Premixed frozen injection (K^+): 1 million units in 50 mL dextrose 4%; 2 million units in 50 mL dextrose 2.3%; 3 million units in 50 mL dextrose 0.7% (contains 1.7 mEq K and 0.3 mEq Na/1 million units penicillin G)
Injection (Na^+): 5 million units (contains 2 mEq Na/1 million units penicillin G)
Conversion: 250 mg = 400,000 U

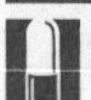

Neonate (IM/IV; use higher end of dosage range for meningitis and severe infections):
≤7 days:
≤2 kg: 50,000–100,000 U/kg/24 hr ÷ Q12 hr
>2 kg: 75,000–150,000 U/kg/24 hr ÷ Q8 hr
>7 days:
<1.2 kg: 50,000–100,000 U/kg/24 hr ÷ Q12 hr
1.2–2 kg: 75,000–150,000 U/kg/24 hr ÷ Q8 hr
≥2 kg: 100,000–200,000 U/kg/24 hr ÷ Q6 hr
Group B streptococcal meningitis:
≤7 days: 250,000–450,000 U/kg/24 hr ÷ Q8 hr
>7 days: 450,000–500,000 U/kg/24 hr ÷ Q4–6 hr
Congenital syphilis (total of 10 days of therapy; if >1 day of therapy is missed, restart the entire course):
≤7 days: 100,000 U/kg/24 hr ÷ Q12 hr IV; increase to dosage below at day 8 of life
>7 days: 150,000 U/kg/24 hr ÷ Q8 hr IV
Infant and child:
IM/IV (use higher end of dosage range and Q4 hr interval for meningitis and severe infections): 100,000–400,000 U/kg/24 hr ÷ Q4–6 hr; **max. dose:** 24 million U/24 hr
Neurosyphilis: 200,000–300,000 U/kg/24 hr ÷ Q4–6 hr IV × 10–14 days; **max. dose:** not to exceed the adult dose
Adult:
IM/IV: 4–24 million U/24 hr ÷ Q4–6 hr
Neurosyphilis: 18–24 million U/24 hr ÷ Q4–6 hr IV × 10–14 days

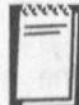

Use penicillin V potassium for oral use. Side effects: anaphylaxis, urticaria, hemolytic anemia, interstitial nephritis, Jarisch-Herxheimer reaction (syphilis). $T_{1/2}$ = 30 min; may be prolonged by concurrent use of probenecid. For meningitis, use higher daily dose at shorter dosing intervals. For the treatment of anthrax (*Bacillus anthracis*), see www.bt.cdc.gov for additional information. **Adjust dose in renal impairment (see Chapter 31).**

Tetracyclines, chloramphenicol, and erythromycin may antagonize penicillin's activity. Probenecid increases penicillin levels. May cause false-positive or negative urinary glucose (Clinitest method), false-positive direct Coombs' test, and false-positive urinary and/or serum proteins.

P

FORMULARY

PENICILLIN G PREPARATIONS—BENZATHINE
Bicillin L-A
Antibiotic, penicillin (very long-acting IM)

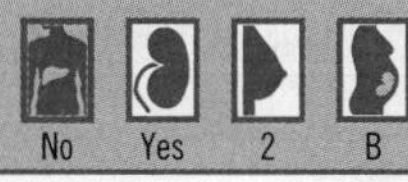

Injection: 600,000 U/mL (1, 2, 4 mL); contains parabens and povidone
Injection should be IM only.

Group A streptococci:

Infant and child: 25,000–50,000 U/kg/dose IM × 1. **Max. dose:** 1.2 million U/dose **OR**
>1 mo and <27 kg: 600,000 U/dose IM × 1
≥27 kg and adult: 1.2 million U/dose IM × 1

Rheumatic fever prophylaxis (Q3 week administration is recommended for high-risk situations):

Infant and child (>1 mo and <27 kg): 600,000 U/dose IM Q3–4 wk
Adult: 1.2 million U/dose IM Q3–4 wk

Syphilis (if >1 day of therapy is missed, restart the entire course; divided total dose into two injection sites):

Infant and child:

Early acquired: 50,000 U/kg/dose (**max. dose:** 2.4 million/dose) × 1
>1 yr duration: 50,000 U/kg/dose (**max. dose:** 2.4 million/dose) Q7 days × 3 doses

Provides sustained levels for 2–4 wk. **Use with caution** in renal failure, asthma, and cephalosporin hypersensitivity. Side effects and drug interactions same as for penicillin G preparations—aqueous potassium and sodium. Injection site reactions are common. **Do not administer intravenously (cardiac arrest and death may occur)** and **do not inject** into or near an artery or nerve (may result in permanent neurological damage).

PENICILLIN G PREPARATIONS—PENICILLIN G BENZATHINE AND PENICILLIN G PROCAINE
Bicillin C-R, Bicillin C-R 900/300
Antibiotic, penicillin (very long-acting IM)

No Yes 2 B

Bicillin CR: 300,000 U penicillin G procaine + 300,000 U penicillin G benzathine/mL to provide 600,000 U penicillin per 1 mL (1, 2 mL tubex, 4 mL syringe)
Bicillin CR (900/300): 150,000 U penicillin G procaine + 450,000 U penicillin G benzathine/mL (2 mL tubex)
All preparations contain parabens and povidone.
Injection should be for IM use only.

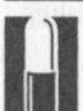

Dosage based on total amount of penicillin.
Group A streptococci:

Child <14 kg: 600,000 U/dose IM × 1
Child 14–27 kg: 900,000–1,200,000 U/dose IM × 1
Child >27 kg and adult: 2,400,000 U/dose IM × 1

This preparation provides early peak levels in addition to prolonged levels of penicillin in the blood. **Do not use this product to treat syphilis because of treatment failure. Use with caution** in renal failure, asthma, significant allergies, and cephalosporin hypersensitivity. The addition of procaine penicillin has not been shown to be more efficacious than benzathine alone. However, it may reduce injection discomfort.

Do not administer intravenously (cardiac arrest and death may occur) and **do not inject** into or near an artery or nerve (may result in permanent neurological damage).

Side effects and drug interactions same as for penicillin G preparations—aqueous potassium and sodium. Immune hypersensitivity reaction has been reported.

For explanation of icons, see p. 663.

PENICILLIN G PREPARATIONS—PROCAINE
Wycillin and others
Antibiotic, penicillin (long-acting IM)

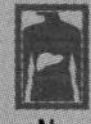 No 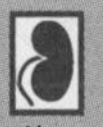 Yes 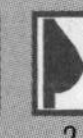 2 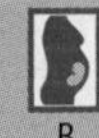 B

Injection: 600,000 U/ml (1, 2 mL); may contain parabens, phenol, povidone, and formaldehyde
Contains 120 mg procaine per 300,000 U penicillin.
Injection should be for IM use only.

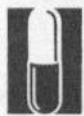

Newborn (see remarks): 50,000 U/kg/24 hr IM once daily
Infant and child: 25,000–50,000 U/kg/24 hr ÷ Q12–24 hr IM. **Max. dose:** 4.8 million U/24 hr
Adult: 0.6–4.8 million U/24 hr ÷ Q12–24 hr IM
Congenital syphilis, syphilis (if >1 day of therapy is missed, restart the entire course):
Neonate, infant, child: 50,000 U/kg/dose once daily IM × 10 days
Neurosyphilis:
Adult: 2.4 million U/dose once daily IM × 10 days with Probenecid 500 mg Q6 hr PO

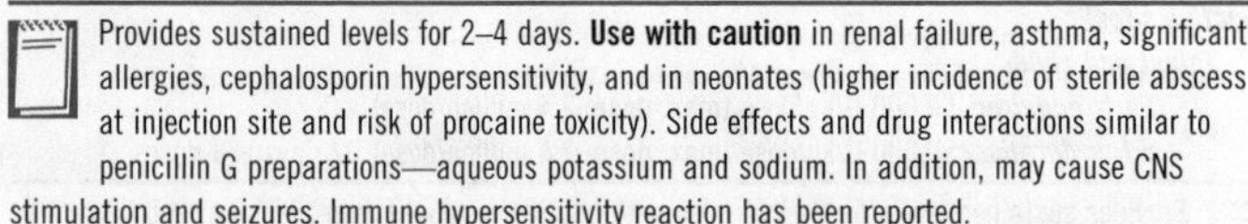

Provides sustained levels for 2–4 days. **Use with caution** in renal failure, asthma, significant allergies, cephalosporin hypersensitivity, and in neonates (higher incidence of sterile abscess at injection site and risk of procaine toxicity). Side effects and drug interactions similar to penicillin G preparations—aqueous potassium and sodium. In addition, may cause CNS stimulation and seizures. Immune hypersensitivity reaction has been reported.

Do not administer intravenously (cardiac arrest and death may occur) and **do not inject** into or near an artery or nerve (may result in permanent neurological damage). Large doses may be administered in two injection sites. No longer recommended for empiric treatment of gonorrhea due to resistant strains.

PENICILLIN V POTASSIUM
Veetids and others
Antibiotic, penicillin

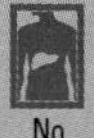 No 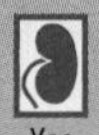 Yes  2 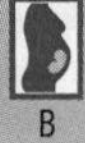 B

Tabs: 250, 500 mg
Oral solution: 125 mg/5 mL, 250 mg/5 mL (100, 200 mL); may contain saccharin
Contains 0.7 mEq potassium/250 mg drug
250 mg = 400,000 U

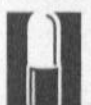

Child: 25–50 mg/kg/24 hr ÷ Q6–8 hr PO. **Max. dose:** 3 g/24 hr
Adolescent and adult: 125–500 mg/dose PO Q6–8 hr
Acute group A streptococcal pharyngitis (use BID dosing regimen ONLY if good compliance is expected):
Child <27 kg: 250 mg PO BID–TID × 10 days
≥27 kg, adolescent and adult: 500 mg PO BID–TID × 10 days
Rheumatic fever prophylaxis, and pneumococcal prophylaxis for sickle cell disease and functional or anatomical asplenia (regardless of immunization status):
2 mo–<3 yr: 125 mg PO BID
3–5 yr: 250 mg PO BID; for sickle cell and asplenia, use may be discontinued after 5 yr of age if child received recommended pneumococcal immunizations and did not experience invasive pneumococcal infection.
Recurrent rheumatic fever prophylaxis:
Child and adult: 250 mg PO BID

Continued

PENICILLIN V POTASSIUM *continued*

See *Penicillin G Preparations—Aqueous Potassium and Sodium* for side effects and drug interactions. GI absorption is better than penicillin G. **NOTE:** Must be taken 1 hr before or 2 hr after meals. Penicillin will prevent rheumatic fever if started within 9 days of the acute illness. **Adjust dose in renal failure (see Chapter 31).**

PENTAMIDINE ISETHIONATE
Pentam 300, NebuPent
Antibiotic, antiprotozoal

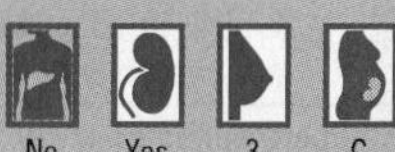

Injection (Pentam 300 and others): 300 mg
Inhalation (NebuPent): 300 mg

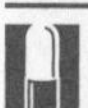

Treatment:
Pneumocystis jiroveci (formerly carinii): 4 mg/kg/24 hr IM/IV once daily × 14–21 days (IV is the preferred route)
Trypanosomiasis (T. gambiense, T. rhodesiense): 4 mg/kg/24 hr IM once daily × 7 days
Visceral leishmaniasis (L. donovani, L. infantum, L. chagasi): 4 mg/kg/dose IM once daily, or once every other day × 15–30 doses
Cutaneous leishmaniasis (L. [V.] panamensis): 2–3 mg/kg/dose IM once daily, or once every other day × 4–7 doses
Prophylaxis:
Pneumocystis jiroveci (formerly carinii):
IM/IV: 4 mg/kg/dose Q2–4 wk
Inhalation:
≥5 yr: 300 mg in 6 ml H_2O via inhalation Q month. Use with a Respigard II nebulizer.
Max. single dose: 300 mg

Use with caution in ventricular tachycardia, Stevens-Johnson syndrome, and daily doses >21 days. May cause hypoglycemia, hyperglycemia, hypotension (both IV and IM administration), nausea, vomiting, fever, mild hepatotoxicity, pancreatitis, megaloblastic anemia, nephrotoxicity, hypocalcemia, and granulocytopenia. Additive nephrotoxicity with aminoglycosides, amphotericin B, cisplatin, and vancomycin may occur. Aerosol administration may also cause bronchospasm, cough, oxygen desaturation, dyspnea, and loss of appetite. Infuse IV over 1–2 hr to reduce the risk of hypotension. Sterile abscess may occur at IM injection site.

Adjust dose in renal impairment (see Chapter 31) with systemic use.

PENTOBARBITAL
Nembutal and others
Barbiturate

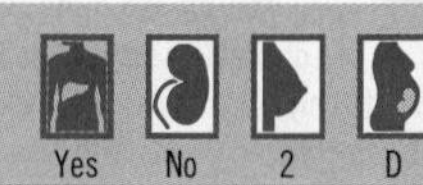

Injection: 50 mg/mL (2 mL); contains prophylene glycol and 10% alcohol

Hypnotic:
Child:
IM: 2–6 mg/kg/dose. **Max. dose:** 100 mg
Adult:
IM: 150–200 mg

Continued

For explanation of icons, see p. 663.

PENTOBARBITAL *continued*

Pre-procedure sedation:

Child:

IM: 2–6 mg/kg/dose. **Max. dose:** 150 mg

IV: 1–3 mg/kg/dose. **Max. dose:** 150 mg

Barbiturate coma:

Child and adult:

IV: Load: 10–15 mg/kg given slowly over 1–2 hr

Maintenance: Begin at 1 mg/kg/hr. Dose range: 1–3 mg/kg/hr as needed.

Contraindicated in liver failure and history of porphyria. **Use with caution** in hypovolemic shock, CHF, hypotension, and hepatic impairment. No advantage over phenobarbital for control of seizures. Adjunct in treatment of ICP. May cause drug-related isoelectric EEG. **Do not administer** for >2 wk in treatment of insomnia. May cause hypotension, arrhythmias, hypothermia, respiratory depression, and dependence.

Onset of action: IM: 10–15 min; IV: 1 min. Duration of action: IV: 15 min.

Administer IV at a rate of <50 mg/min.

Therapeutic serum levels: Sedation: 1–5 mg/L; Hypnosis: 5–15 mg/L; Coma: 20–40 mg/L (steady state is achieved after 4–5 days of continuous IV dosing).

PERMETHRIN
Elimite, Acticin, Nix, and others
Scabicidal agent

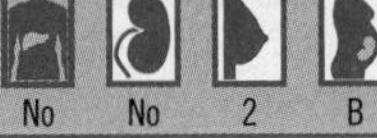

Cream (Elimite, Acticin): 5% (60 g); contains 0.1% formaldehyde
Liquid cream rinse (Nix-OTC): 1% (60 mL with comb); contains 20% isopropyl alcohol
Lotion (OTC): 1% (60 mL with comb)

Pediculus capitis, Phthirus pubis (>2 mo):

Head lice: Saturate hair and scalp with 1% cream rinse after shampooing, rinsing, and towel drying hair. Leave on for 10 min, then rinse. May repeat in 9–10 days. May be used for lice in other areas of the body (e.g., pubic lice) in same fashion. If the 1% cream rinse is resistant, the 5% cream may be used after shampooing, rinsing, and towel drying hair. Leave on for 8–14 hr overnight under a shower cap; then rinse off. May repeat in 9–10 days.

Scabies (see remarks): Apply 5% cream from neck to toe (head to toe for infants and toddlers) wash off with water in 8–14 hr. May repeat in 7 days. Use in infants <1 mo is safe and effective when applied for a 6-hr period.

Ovicidal activity generally makes single-dose regimen adequate. However, resistance to permethrin has been reported. **Avoid** contact with eyes during application. Shake well before using. May cause pruritus, hypersensitivity, burning, stinging, erythema, and rash. For either lice or scabies, instruct patient to launder bedding and clothing. For lice, treat symptomatic contacts only. For scabies, treat all contacts even if asymptomatic. The 5% cream has been used safely in children <1 mo with neonatal scabies (a 6-hr application time was utilized). Topical cream dosage form contains formaldehyde. Dispense 60 g per adult or 2 small children.

PHENAZOPYRIDINE HCL
Pyridium, Azo-Standard [OTC], and others
Urinary analgesic

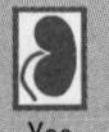
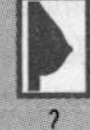
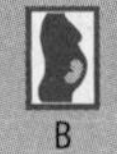

Tabs: 95 mg [OTC], 97.2 mg, 100 mg [OTC and Rx], 150 mg 200 mg
Oral suspension: 10 mg/mL

Continued

PHENAZOPYRIDINE HCL *continued*

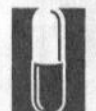

UTI (use with an appropriate antibacterial agent):

Child 6–12 yr: 12 mg/kg/24 hr ÷ TID PO until symptoms of lower urinary tract irritation are controlled or 2 days.

Adult: 95–200 mg TID PO until symptoms are controlled or 2 days.

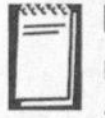

May cause hepatitis, GI distress, vertigo, and headache. Anaphylactoid-like reaction, methemoglobinemia, hemolytic anemia, renal and hepatic toxicity have been reported, usually at overdosage levels. Colors urine orange; stains clothing. May also stain contact lenses and interfere with urinalysis tests based on spectrometry or color reactions. Give doses after meals.

Avoid use in moderate/severe renal impairment; adjust dose in mild renal impairment (see Chapter 31).

PHENOBARBITAL
Luminal and many others
Barbiturate

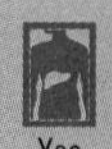
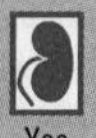
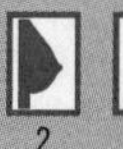
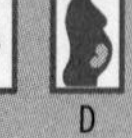

Yes Yes 2 D

Tabs: 15, 16, 30, 60, 90, 100 mg
Elixir: 20 mg/5 mL; contains alcohol
Injection: 60, 65, 130 mg/mL; may contain 10% alcohol and propylene glycol

Status epilepticus:

Loading dose, IV:

Neonate, infant, and child: 15–20 mg/kg/dose in a single or divided dose. May give additional 5 mg/kg doses Q15–30 min to a **max. total** of 40 mg/kg.

Maintenance dose, PO/IV: Monitor levels.

Neonate: 3–5 mg/kg/24 hr ÷ once daily–BID
Infant: 5–6 mg/kg/24 hr ÷ once daily–BID
Child 1–5 yr: 6–8 mg/kg/24 hr ÷ once daily–BID
Child 6–12 yr: 4–6 mg/kg/24 hr ÷ once daily–BID
>12 yr: 1–3 mg/kg/24 hr ÷ once daily–BID

Hyperbilirubinemia (<12 yr): 3–8 mg/kg/24 hr PO ÷ BID–TID. Doses up to 12 mg/kg/24 hr have been used.

Preoperative sedation (child): 1–3 mg/kg/dose IM/IV/PO × 1. Give 60–90 min prior to procedure.

Contraindicated in porphyria, severe respiratory disease with dyspnea or obstruction. **Use with caution** in hepatic or renal disease (reduce dose). IV administration may cause respiratory arrest or hypotension. Side effects include drowsiness, cognitive impairment, ataxia, hypotension, hepatitis, skin rash, respiratory depression, apnea, megaloblastic anemia, and anticonvulsant hypersensitivity syndrome. Paradoxical reaction in children (not dose related) may cause hyperactivity, irritability, insomnia. Induces several liver enzymes (CYP 450 1A2, 2B6, 2C8, 3A3/4, 3A5-7), thus decreases blood levels of many drugs (e.g., anticonvulsants). IV push **not to exceed** 1 mg/kg/min.

$T_{1/2}$ is variable with age: neonates, 45–100 hr; infants, 20–133 hr; children, 37–73 hr. Due to long half-life, consider other agents for sedation for procedures.

Therapeutic levels: 15–40 mg/L. Recommended serum sampling time at steady-state: trough level obtained within 30 minutes prior to the next scheduled dose after 10–14 days of continuous dosing.

Adjust dose in renal failure (see Chapter 31).

For explanation of icons, see p. 663.

PHENTOLAMINE MESYLATE
Regitine and others
Adrenergic blocking agent (alpha); antidote, extravasation

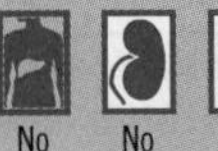 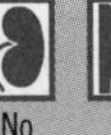 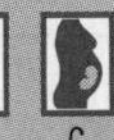 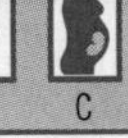

No No ? C

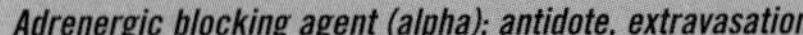

Injection: 5 mg vial; may contain mannitol

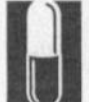

Treatment of alpha adrenergic drug extravasation (most effective within 12 hr of extravasation)

Neonate: Make a solution of 0.25–0.5 mg/mL with preservative-free normal saline. Inject 1 mL (in 5 divided doses of 0.2 mL) SC around site of extravasation within 12 hr of extravasation; **max. total dose:** 0.1 mg/kg or 2.5 mg total.

Infant, child, and adult: Make a solution of 0.5–1 mg/mL with preservative-free normal saline. Inject 1–5 mL (in 5 divided doses) SC around site of extravasation within 12 hr of extravasation; **max. total dose:** 0.1–0.2 mg/kg or 5 mg total.

Diagnosis of pheochromocytoma, IM/IV:

Child: 0.05–0.1 mg/kg/dose up to a **max. dose** of 5 mg.

Adult: 5 mg/dose

Hypertension, prior to surgery for pheochromocytoma, IM/IV:

Child: 0.05–0.1 mg/kg/dose up to a **max. dose** of 5 mg 1–2 hr prior to surgery, repeat Q2–4 hr PRN.

Adult: 5 mg/dose 1–2 hr prior to surgery, repeat Q2–4 hrs PRN.

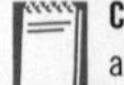

Contraindicated in MI, coronary insufficiency and angina. **Use with caution** in hypotension, arrhythmias, and cerebral vascular spasm/occlusion.

For diagnosis of pheochromocytoma, patient should be resting in a supine position. A blood pressure reduction of more than 35 mmHg systolic and 24 mmHg diastolic is considered a positive test for pheochromocytoma. For treatment of extravasation, use 27- to 30-gauge needle with multiple small injections and monitor site closely as repeat doses may be necessary.

PHENYLEPHRINE HCL
Neo-Synephrine and many others
Adrenergic agonist

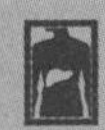 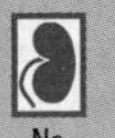 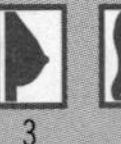 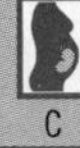 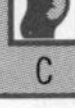

No No 3 C

Nasal drops [OTC]: 0.125, 0.25, 0.5, 1% (15, 30 mL)
Nasal spray [OTC]: 0.25, 0.5, 1% (15, 30 mL)
NOTE: For Neo-Synephrine 12-hr Nasal, see Oxymetazoline
Ophthalmic drops: 0.12% [OTC] (15 mL), 2.5% (2, 3, 5, 15 mL), 10% (2, 5 mL)
Injection: 10 mg/mL (1%)
Tabs (Sudafed PE) [OTC]: 10 mg
Chewable tabs (AH-chew): 10 mg
Orally disintegrating tabs (Nasop): 10 mg; contains phenylalanine
Oral liquid: 7.5 mg/5 mL (472 mL); contains phenylalanine
Oral solution [OTC]: 2.5 mg/5 mL
Oral drops [OTC]: 2.5 mg/1 mL
Orally disintegrating filmstrip [OTC]: 1.25, 2.5, 10 mg
Oral suspension (Phenylephrine Tannate)
AH-chewD: 10 mg/5 mL (118 mL)
NaSop: 7.5 mg/5 mL (120 mL)

Continued

PHENYLEPHRINE HCL *continued*

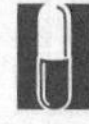

Hypotension:

NOTE: The IV drip dosage units for children are in mcg/kg/min, compared to mcg/min for adults. To prepare infusion: See IV Infusions on page i.

Child:

IV bolus: 5–20 mcg/kg/dose Q10–15 min PRN

IV drip: 0.1–0.5 mcg/kg/min; titrate to effect

IM/SC: 0.1 mg/kg/dose Q1–2 hr PRN; **max. dose:** 5 mg

Adult:

IV bolus: 0.1–0.5 mg/dose Q10–15 min PRN

IV drip: Initial rate at 100–180 mcg/min; titrate to effect. Usual maintenance dose: 40–60 mcg/min

IM/SC: 2–5 mg/dose Q1–2 hr PRN; **max. dose:** 5 mg

Pupillary dilation (<1 yr): 2.5% solution; 1 drop in each eye 15–30 min before exam

Nasal decongestant (in each nostril; give up to 3 days):

Infant (>6 mo): 1–2 drops of 0.16% solution (see remarks) Q3 hr PRN

Child 1–6 yr: 2–3 drops of 0.125% solution Q4 hr PRN

Child 6–12 yr: 2–3 drops or 1–2 sprays of 0.25% solution Q4 hr PRN

>12 yr–adult: 2–3 drops or 1–2 sprays of 0.25% or 0.5% solution Q4 hr PRN

Oral decongestant (see remarks):

2–<6 yr:

Oral drops (2.5 mg/mL): 1 mL (2.5 mg) PO Q4 hr; not to exceed 6 doses in 24 hr

Oral liquid (7.5 mg/5 mL): 2.5 mL (3.75 mg) PO Q6 hr up to 10 mL (15 mg) per 24 hr

Oral solution (2.5 mg/5 mL): 5 mL (2.5 mg) PO Q4 hr, up to 30 mL (15 mg) per 24 hr

Oral suspension (Phenylephrine Tannate):

NaSop (7.5 mg/5 mL): 1.25–2.5 mL (1.88–3.75 mg) PO Q12 hr

≥ 6–<12 yr:

Oral liquid (7.5 mg/5 mL): 5 mL (7.5 mg) PO Q6 hr up to 20 mL (30 mg) per 24 hr

Oral solution (2.5 mg/5 mL): 10 mL (5 mg) PO Q4 hr up to 60 mL (30 mg) per 24 hr

Oral suspension (Phenylephrine Tannate):

AH-chewD (10 mg/5 mL): 2.5–5 mL (5–10 mg) PO Q12 hr

NaSop (7.5 mg/5 mL): 2.5–5 mL (3.75–7.5 mg) PO Q12 hr

Tabs or chewable tabs: 10 mg PO Q4 hr

≥12 yr and adult:

Tabs or Chewable tabs: 10–20 mg PO Q4 hr

Oral liquid (7.5 mg/5 mL): 10 mL (15 mg) PO Q6 hr up to 40 mL (60 mg) per 24 hr.

Oral suspension (Phenylephrine Tannate):

AH-chewD (10 mg/5 mL): 5–10 mL (10–20 mg) PO Q12 hr

NaSop (7.5 mg/5 mL): 5–10 mL (7.5–15 mg) PO Q12 hr

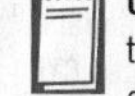

Use with caution in presence of arrhythmias, hyperthyroidism, or hyperglycemia. May cause tremor, insomnia, palpitations. Metabolized by MAO. **Contraindicated** in pheochromocytoma and severe hypertension. Injectable product may contain sulfites.

Nasal decongestants may cause rebound congestion with excessive use (>3 days). The 0.16% nasal drops are no longer available; may use the 0.125% solution or dilute the 0.25% or 0.5% concentrations with normal saline. The 1% nasal spray can be used in adults with extreme congestion.

Oral phenylephrine is found in a variety of combination cough and cold products and has replaced pseudoephedrine and phenylpropanolamine. Over the counter (OTC or nonprescription) use of this product is **not recommended** for children <6 years old due to reports of serious adverse effects (cardiac and respiratory distress, convulsions, and hallucinations) and fatalities (from unintentional overdosages, including combined use of other OTC products containing the same active ingredients).

For explanation of icons, see p. 663.

PHENYTOIN

Dilantin, Dilantin Infatab, Phenytek, and others

Anticonvulsant, class Ib antiarrhythmic

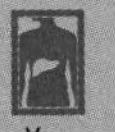
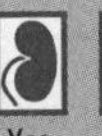
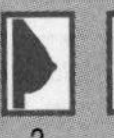
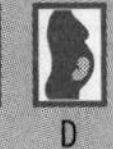

Yes Yes 2 D

Chewable tabs (Infatab): 50 mg
Prompt-release caps: 100 mg
Extended-release caps: 30, 100, 200, 300 mg
Oral suspension: 125 mg/5 mL (240 mL); contains ≤0.6% alcohol
Injection: 50 mg/mL; contains alcohol and propylene glycol

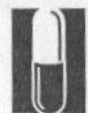

Status epilepticus: **See Chapter 1.**
Loading dose (all ages): 15–20 mg/kg IV
Max. dose: 1500 mg/24 hr
Maintenance for seizure disorders:
- ***Neonate:*** start with 5 mg/kg/24 hr PO/IV ÷ Q12 hr; usual range 5–8 mg/kg/24 hr PO/IV ÷ Q8–12 hr.
- ***Infant/child:*** start with 5 mg/kg/24 hr ÷ BID–TID PO/IV; usual dose range (doses divided BID–TID):
  - ***6 mo–3 yr:*** 8–10 mg/kg/24 hr
  - ***4–6 yr:*** 7.5–9 mg/kg/24 hr
  - ***7–9 yr:*** 7–8 mg/kg/24 hr
  - ***10–16 yr:*** 6–7 mg/kg/24 hr
- **NOTE:** Use once daily–BID dosing with extended release caps.
- ***Adult:*** Start with 100 mg/dose Q8 hr IV/PO and carefully titrate (if needed) by 100 mg increments Q2–4 wk to 300–600 mg/24 hr (or 6–7 mg/kg/24 hr) ÷ Q8–24 hr IV/PO.

Antiarrhythmic (secondary to digitalis intoxication):
Load (all ages): 1.25 mg/kg IV Q5 min up to a total of 15 mg/kg
Maintenance:
- ***Child (IV/PO):*** 5–10 mg/kg/24 hr ÷ Q8–12 hr
- ***Adult:*** 250 mg PO QID × 1 day, then 250 mg PO Q12 hr × 2 days, then 300–400 mg/24 hr ÷ Q6–24 hr

Contraindicated in patients with heart block or sinus bradycardia. IM administration is **not recommended** because of erratic absorption and pain at injection site; consider fosphenytoin. Side effects include gingival hyperplasia, hirsutism, dermatitis, blood dyscrasia, ataxia, lupus-like and Stevens-Johnson syndromes, lymphadenopathy, liver damage, and nystagmus. Suicidal behavior or ideation have been reported. The FDA is currently investigating the possible increased risk for serious skin reactions (e.g., TEN and Stevens-Johnson) in patients with the HLA-B*1502 allele.

Many drug interactions: levels may be increased by cimetidine, chloramphenicol, INH, sulfonamides, trimethoprim, etc. Levels may be decreased by some antineoplastic agents. Phenytoin induces hepatic microsomal enzymes (CYP 450 1A2, 2C8/9/19, and 3A3/4) leading to decreased effectiveness of oral contraceptives, quinidine, valproic acid, theophylline, and other substrates to the previously listed CYP 450 hepatic enzymes.

Suggested dosing intervals for specific oral dosage forms: extended release caps (once daily–BID); chewable and immediate release tablets, and oral suspension (TID). Oral absorption reduced in neonates. $T_{1/2}$ is variable (7–42 hr) and dose-dependent. Drug is highly protein-bound; free fraction of drug will be increased in patients with hypoalbuminemia.

For seizure disorders, therapeutic levels: 10–20 mg/L (free and bound phenytoin) **OR** 1–2 mg/L (free only). Monitor free phenytoin levels in hypoalbuminemia or renal insufficiency. Recommended serum sampling times: trough level (PO/IV) within 30 min prior to the next scheduled dose; peak or post-load

Continued

PHENYTOIN *continued*

level (IV) 1 hr after the end of IV infusion. Steady state is usually achieved after 5–10 days of continuous dosing. For routine monitoring, measure trough.

IV push/infusion rate: **Not to exceed** 0.5 mg/kg/min in neonates, or 1 mg/kg/min infants, children, and adults with **maximum** of 50 mg/min; may cause cardiovascular collapse. Consider fosphenytoin in situations of tenuous IV access and risk for extravasation.

PHOSPHORUS SUPPLEMENTS
K-PHOS Neutral, Uro-KP-Neutral, PHOS-NaK, Sodium Phosphate, Potassium Phosphate, and many generics for injections

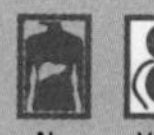
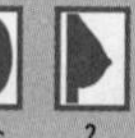
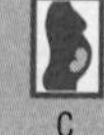

No Yes ? C

Oral: (reconstitute in 75 mL H_2O per capsule or packet)

Na and K phosphate:

PHOS-NaK; powder (OTC): 250 mg (8 mM) P, 6.96 mEq (160 mg) Na, 7.16 mEq (280 mg) K per packet of powder

K-PHOS Neutral; tabs: 250 mg P (8 mM), 13 mEq Na, 1.1 mEq K

Uro-KP-Neutral; tabs: 250 mg (8 mM) P, 10.9 mEq Na, 1.27 mEq K

Injection:

Na phosphate: 3 mM (94 mg) P, 4 mEq Na/mL

K phosphate: 3 mM (94 mg) P, 4.4 mEq K/mL

Conversion: 31 mg P = 1 mM P

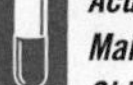

Acute hypophosphatemia: 0.16–0.32 mM/kg/dose (or 5–10 mg/kg/dose) IV over 6 hr

Maintenance/replacement:

Child:

IV: 0.5–1.5 mM/kg (or 15–45 mg/kg) over 24 hr

PO: 30–90 mg/kg/24 hr (or 1–3 mM/kg/24 hr) ÷ TID–QID

Adult:

IV: 50–65 mM (or 1.5–2 g) over 24 hr

PO: 3–4.5 g/24 hr (or 100–150 mM/24 hr) ÷ TID–QID

Recommended IV infusion rate: ≤0.1 mM/kg/hr (or 3.1 mg/kg/hr) of phosphate. When potassium salt is used, the rate will be limited by the **max.** potassium infusion rate. **Do not** co-infuse with calcium containing products.

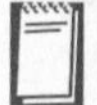

May cause tetany, hyperphosphatemia, hyperkalemia, hypocalcemia. **Use with caution** in patients with renal impairment. Be aware of sodium and/or potassium load when supplementing phosphate. IV administration may cause hypotension and renal failure, or arrhythmias, heart block, cardiac arrest with potassium salt. PO dosing may cause nausea, vomiting, abdominal pain, or diarrhea. See Chapter 21 for daily requirements and Chapter 11 for additional information on hypophosphatemia and hyperphosphatemia.

PHYSOSTIGMINE SALICYLATE
Antilirium
Cholinergic agent

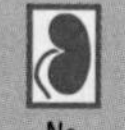
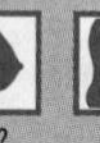
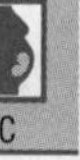

No No ? C

Injection: 1 mg/mL (2 mL); contains 2% benzyl alcohol and 0.1% sodium bisulfite

Reversal of toxic anticholinergic effects from antihistamine or anticholinergic agents:

Child: 0.01–0.03 mg/kg/dose IV administered over 3–5 min, dose may be repeated every 20 min if no response or return of anticholinergic symptoms up to a maximum total of 2 mg.

Adult: 0.5–2 mg IV (administered over 5 min)/IM/SQ, if needed repeat dose every 20 min until response is seen or when adverse effects occurs.

Continued

For explanation of icons, see p. 663.

PHYSOSTIGMINE SALICYLATE *continued*

Physostigmine antidote: Atropine always should be available. **Contraindicated** in asthma, gangrene, diabetes, cardiovascular disease, GI or GU tract obstruction, any vagotonic state, and patients receiving choline esters or depolarizing neuromuscular blocking agents (e.g., decamethonium, succinylcholine). May cause seizures, arrhythmias, bradycardia, GI symptoms, and other cholingeric effects. Rapid IV administration can cause bradycardia and hypersalivation leading to respiratory distress and seizures.

PHYTONADIONE/VITAMIN K_1
Mephyton and others

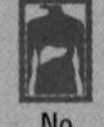
No
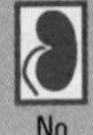
No
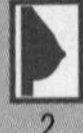
2
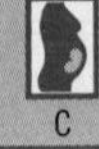
C

Tabs (Mephyton): 5 mg
Oral suspension: 1 mg/mL
Injection, emulsion: 2 mg/mL (0.5 mL), 10 mg/mL (1 mL); contains 0.9% benzyl alcohol

Neonatal hemorrhagic disease:
Prophylaxis: 0.5–1 mg IM × 1 within 1 hr after birth
Treatment: 1–2 mg/24 hr IM/SC/IV
Oral anticoagulant (warfarin) overdose:
INR ≥5 and no serious bleeding:
<40 kg: 30 mcg/kg PO/IV
≥40 kg: 1–2.5 mg PO/IV
Serious bleeding (any elevated INR): 2.5–5 mg PO/IV
Life threatening bleeding (any elevated INR): 5–10 mg PO/IV
Vitamin K deficiency:
Infant and child:
PO: 2.5–5 mg/24 hr
IM/SC/IV: 1–2 mg/dose × 1
Adolescent and adult:
PO: 2.5–25 mg/24 hr
IM/SC/IV: 10 mg/dose × 1

Monitor PT/PTT. Large doses (10–20 mg) in newborns may cause hyperbilirubinemia and severe hemolytic anemia. Blood coagulation factors increase within 6–12 hr after oral doses and within 1–2 hr following parenteral administration.

IV injection rate **not to exceed** 3 mg/m^2/min or 1 mg/min. IV or IM doses may cause flushing, dizziness, cardiac/respiratory arrest, hypotension, and anaphylaxis. IV or IM administration is indicated only when other routes of administration are not feasible (or in emergency situations).

Mineral oil may decrease GI absorption of vitamin K with concurrent oral administration. Protect product from light. See Chapter 21 for multivitamin preparations.

PILOCARPINE HCL
Akarpine, Isopto Carpine, Pilocar, Salagen, Pilopine HS, and others
Cholinergic agent

Yes
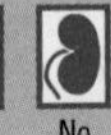
No
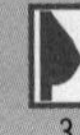
3
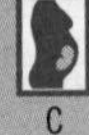
C

Ophthalmic solution: 0.5% (15 mL), 1% (2, 15, 30 mL), 2% (2, 15, 30 mL), 3% (15, 30 mL), 4% (1, 2, 15, 30 mL), 5% (15 mL), 6% (15, 30 mL), 8% (2, 15 mL), 10% (15 mL); may contain benzalkonium chloride
Ophthalmic gel (Pilopine HS): 4% (3.5 g); contains benzalkonium chloride
Tab (Salagen and others): 5, 7.5 mg

Continued

PILOCARPINE HCL *continued*

For elevated intraocular pressure:
Drops: 1–2 drops in each eye 4–6 times a day; adjust concentration and frequency as needed.
Gel: 0.5-inch ribbon applied to lower conjunctival sac QHS. Adjust dose as needed.

Xerostomia:
Adult: 5 mg/dose PO TID, dose may be titrated to 10 mg/dose PO TID in patients who do not respond to lower dose and who are able to tolerate the drug.

Contraindicated in acute iritis or anterior chamber inflammation and uncontrolled asthma. May cause stinging, burning, lacrimation, headache, and retinal detachment with ophthalmic use. **Use with caution** in patients with corneal abrasion or significant cardiovascular disease.

Use with topical NSAIDs (e.g., ketorolac) may decrease topical pilocarpine effects. Sweating, nausea, rhinitis, chills, flushing, urinary frequency, dizziness, asthenia, and headaches have also been reported with oral dosing. Reduce oral dosing in the presence of mild hepatic insufficiency (Child-Pugh score of 5–6); use in severe hepatic insufficiency is **not recommended.**

PIMECROLIMUS
Elidel
Topical immunosuppressant

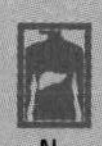
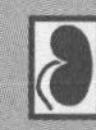

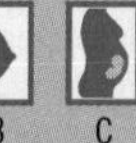

No No 3 C

Cream: 1% (30, 60, 100 g); contains benzyl alcohol and propylene glycol

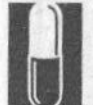

≥2 yr and adult (see remarks): Apply a thin layer to affected area BID and rub in gently and completely. Re-evaluate patient in 6 wk if lesions are not healed.

Do not use in children <2 yr (higher rate of upper respiratory infections), immunocompromised patients, or with occlusive dressings (promotes systemic absorption). Approved as a second-line therapy for atopic dermatitis for patients who fail to respond, or do not tolerate, other approved therapies. Use medication for short periods of time by using the minimum amounts to control symptoms; long-term safety is unknown. **Avoid** contact with eyes, nose, mouth, and cut, infected, or scraped skin. Minimize and **avoid** exposure to natural and artificial sunlight, respectively.

Most common side effects include burning at the application site, headache, viral infections, and pyrexia. Skin discoloration, skin flushing associated with alcohol use, anaphylactic reactions, ocular irritation after application to the eye lids or near the eyes, angioneurotic edema, and facial edema have been reported. Although the risk is uncertain, the FDA has issued an alert about the potential cancer risk with the use of this product. See www.fda.gov/medwatch for the latest information. Drug is a CYP 450 3A3/4 substrate.

PIPERACILLIN
Pipracil and others
Antibiotic, penicillin (extended spectrum)

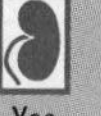
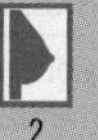
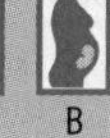

No Yes 2 B

Injection: 2, 3, 4, 40 g
Contains 1.85 mEq Na/g drug

Neonate, IV:
≤7 days:
≤36 wk of gestation: 150 mg/kg/24 hr ÷ Q12 hr
>36 wk of gestation: 225 mg/kg/24 hr ÷ Q8 hr

Continued

P
FORMULARY
For explanation of icons, see p. 663.

PIPERACILLIN *continued*

Neonate, IV (cont'd):

>7 days:

≤36 wk of gestation: 225 mg/kg/24 hr ÷ Q8 hr

>36 wk of gestation: 300 mg/kg/24 hr ÷ Q6 hr

Infant and child: 200–300 mg/kg/24 hr IM/IV ÷ Q4–6 hr; **max. dose:** 24 g/24 hr

Cystic Fibrosis: 350–600 mg/kg/24 hr IM/IV ÷ Q4–6 hr; **max. dose:** 24 g/24 hr

Adult: 2–4 g/dose IV Q4–6 hr or 1–2 g/dose IM Q6 hr; **max. dose:** 24 g/24 hr

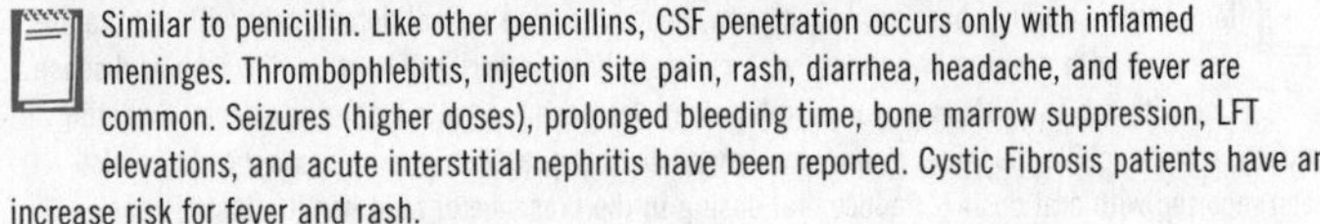

Similar to penicillin. Like other penicillins, CSF penetration occurs only with inflamed meninges. Thrombophlebitis, injection site pain, rash, diarrhea, headache, and fever are common. Seizures (higher doses), prolonged bleeding time, bone marrow suppression, LFT elevations, and acute interstitial nephritis have been reported. Cystic Fibrosis patients have an increase risk for fever and rash.

Coagulation parameters should be tested more frequently and monitored regularly with high doses of heparin, warfarin, or other drugs affecting blood coagulation or thrombocyte function. May falsely lower aminoglycoside serum levels if the drugs are infused close to one another; allow a minimum of 2 hr between infusions to prevent this interaction.

For IM use, drug may be diluted to 400 mg/mL with 0.5% or 1% lidocaine without epinephrine. **Adjust dose in renal impairment (see Chapter 31).**

PIPERACILLIN WITH TAZOBACTAM

Zosyn

Antibiotic, penicillin (extended spectrum with beta-lactamase inhibitor)

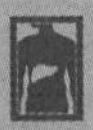
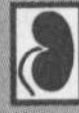
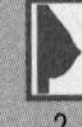
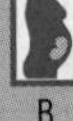

No Yes 2 B

8 : 1 ratio of piperacillin to tazobactam:

Injection, powder: 2 g piperacillin and 0.25 g tazobactam; 3 g piperacillin and 0.375 g tazobactam; 4 g piperacillin and 0.5 g tazobactam; 36 g piperacillin and 4.5 g tazobactam

Injection, premixed in iso-osmotic dextrose: 2 g piperacillin and 0.25 g tazobactam in 50 mL; 3 g piperacillin and 0.375 g tazobactam in 50 mL; 4 g piperacillin and 0.5 g tazobactam in 100 mL

Contains 2.35 mEq Na/g piperacillin

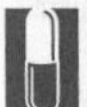

All doses based on piperacillin component.

Infant <6 mo: 150–300 mg/kg/24 hr IV ÷ Q6–8 hr

Infant >6 mo and child: 300–400 mg/kg/24 hr IV ÷ Q6–8 hr

Adult:

Intra-abdominal or soft tissue infections: 3 g IV Q6 hr

Nosocomial pneumonia: 4 g IV Q6 hr

Cystic Fibrosis: see *Piperacillin*

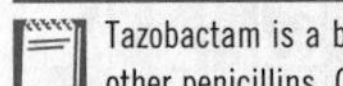

Tazobactam is a beta-lactamase inhibitor, thus extending the spectrum of piperacillin. Like other penicillins, CSF penetration occurs only with inflammed meninges. See *Piperacillin* and *Penicillin Preparations—Aqueous Potassium and Sodium* for additional comments.

Prolonging the dose administration time to 4 hr will maximize the pharmacokinetic/pharmacodyamic properties by prolonging the time of drug concentration above the MIC. **Adjust dose in renal impairment (see Chapter 31).**

POLYCITRA

See *Citrate Mixtures*

POLYETHYLENE GLYCOL—ELECTROLYTE SOLUTION
GoLYTELY, CoLyte, NuLYTELY, OCL, TriLyte, MiraLax, and others
Bowel evacuant, osmotic laxative

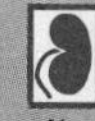
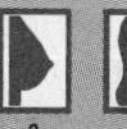
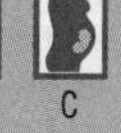

No No ? C

Powder for oral solution:

GoLYTELY: Polyethylene glycol 3350 236 g, Na sulfate 22.74 g, Na bicarbonate 6.74 g, NaCl 5.86 g, KCl 2.97 g. Contents vary somewhat. See package insert for specific contents of other products.

MiraLax [OTC] and others: Polyet

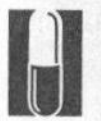

Bowel cleansing (use products containing supplemental electrolytes for bowel cleansing such as GoLYTELY, CoLyte, NuLYTELY, OCL, TriLyte; and patients should be NPO 3–4 hr prior to dosing):

Child:

Oral/nasogastric: 25–40 mL/kg/hr until rectal effluent is clear (usually in 4–10 hr)

Adult:

Oral: 240 ml PO Q10 min up to 4 L or until rectal effluent is clear

Nasogastric: 20–30 mL/min (1.2–1.8 L/hr) up to 4 L

Constipation (MiraLax; see remarks):

Child (limited data in 20 children with chronic constipation, 18 mo–11 yr; see remarks): a mean effective dose of 0.84 g/kg/24 hr PO ÷ BID for 8 wk (range: 0.25–1.42 g/kg/24 hr) was used to yield 2 soft stools per day. **Do not exceed** 17 g/24 hr. If patient >20 kg, use adult dose.

Adult: 17 g (one heaping tablespoonful) mixed in 240 mL of water, juice, soda, coffee, or tea PO once daily

Contraindicated in polyethylene glycol hypersensitivity. Monitor electrolytes, BUN, serum glucose, and urine osmolality with prolonged administration. Seizures resulting from electrolyte abnormalities have been reported.

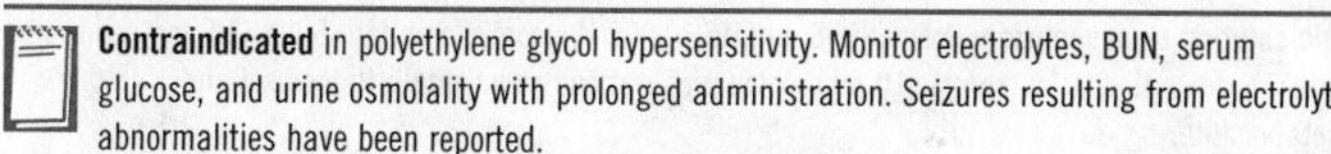

BOWEL CLEANSING: Contraindicated in toxic megacolon, gastric retention, colitis, and bowel perforation. **Use with caution** in patients prone to aspiration or with impaired gag reflex. Effect should occur within 1–2 hr. Solution generally more palatable if chilled. MiraLax at higher dosages of 1–1.5 g/kg/24 hr (**max. dose:** 100 g/24 hr) PO × 3 days has been shown to be safe and effective in treating childhood fecal impaction.

CONSTIPATION (MiraLax): Contraindicated in bowel obstruction.

Child: Dilute powder using the ratio of 17 g powder to 240 mL of water, juice, or milk. An onset of action within 1 wk in 12 of 20 patients, with the remaining 8 patients reporting improvement during the second wk of therapy. Side effects reported in this trial included diarrhea, flatulence, and mild abdominal pain. (See *J Pediatr* 2001;139[3]:428–432 for additional information.)

Adult: 2 to 4 days may be required to produce a bowel movement. Most common side effects include nausea, abdominal bloating, cramping and flatulence. Use beyond 2 wk has not been studied.

POLYMYXIN B SULFATE AND BACITRACIN

See *Bacitracin ± Polymyxin B*

For explanation of icons, see p. 663.

POLYMYXIN B SULFATE AND TRIMETHOPRIM SULFATE
Polytrim Ophthalmic Solution and various others
Topical antibiotic (ophthalmic preparations listed)

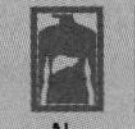 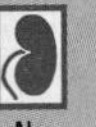 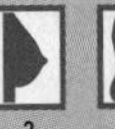 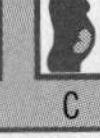
No No ? C

Ophthalmic solution: Polymyxin B sulfate 10,000 U, trimethoprim sulfate 1 mg/mL (10 mL); some preparations may contain 0.04 mg/mL benzalkonium chloride

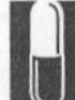

≥2 mo and adult: Instill 1 drop in the affected eye(s) Q3 hr (**max.** of 6 doses/24 hr) × 7–10 days.

Active against susceptible strains of *S. aureus, S. epidermidis, S. pneumoniae, S. viridans, H. influenzae,* and *P. aeruginosa.* **Not indicated** for the prophylaxis or treatment of ophthalmia neonatorum. Local irritation consisting of redness, burning, stinging, and/or itching is common. Hypersensitivity reactions consisting of lid edema, itching, increased redness, tearing, and/or circumocular rash has been reported.

Apply finger pressure to lacrimal sac during and for 1–2 min after dose application.

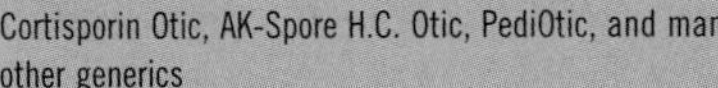

POLYMYXIN B SULFATE, NEOMYCIN SULFATE, HYDROCORTISONE
Cortisporin Otic, AK-Spore H.C. Otic, PediOtic, and many other generics
Topical antibiotic (otic and ophthalmic preparations listed)

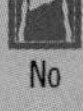 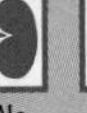 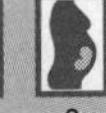
No No ? C

Otic solution or suspension: Polymyxin B sulfate 10,000 U, neomycin sulfate 5 mg (3.5 mg neomycin base), hydrocortisone 10 mg/mL (10 mL); some preparations may contain thimerosol and metabisulfite.
Ophthalmic suspension: Polymyxin B sulfate 10,000 U, neomycin sulfate 5 mg (3.5 mg neomycin base), hydrocortisone 10 mg/mL (7.5 mL); may contain thimerosol and propylene glycol

Otitis externa:
≥2 yr–adult: 3–4 drops TID–QID × 7–10 days. If preferred, a cotton wick may be saturated and inserted into ear canal. Moisten wick with antibiotic every 4 hr. Change wick Q24 hr.

Ophthalmic:
Child, adolescent and adult: Instill 1–2 drops into the affected eye(s) Q3–4 hr

Neomycin may cause sensitization. Prolonged treatment may result in overgrowth of nonsusceptible organisms and fungi. May cause cutaneous sensitization.

OTIC USE: Shake suspension well before use. **Contraindicated** in patients with active varicella and herpes simplex and in cases with perforated eardrum (possible ototoxicity). **Use with caution** in chronic otitis media and when the integrity of the tympanic membrane is in question. Metabisulfite containing products may cause allergic reactions to susceptible individuals. Hypersensitivity (itching, skin rash, redness, swelling, or other sign of irritation in or around the ear) may occur. Warm the medication to body temperature prior to use.

OPHTHALMIC USE: Use with caution in glaucoma. Blurred vision, burning, and stinging may occur. Increased intraocular pressure and mycosis may occur with prolonged use. Apply finger pressure to lacrimal sac during and for 1–2 min after dose application.

POLYTRIM OPHTHALMIC SOLUTION

See *Polymyxin B Sulfate and Trimethoprim Sulfate*

PORACTANT ALFA

See *Surfactant, pulmonary*

POTASSIUM IODIDE

Iosat, Pima, SSKI, ThyroShield, ThyroSafe, and others
Antithyroid agent

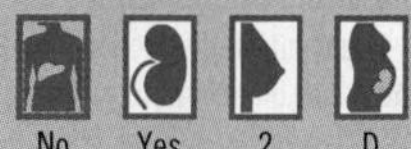

Tabs:

ThyroSafe (OTC): 65 mg (50 mg iodine)
Iosat: 130 mg

Syrup (Pima): 325 mg/5 mL (249 mg iodide/5 mL) (473 mL, 4000 mL)

Oral solution:

ThyroShield: 65 mg/mL (30 mL); contains parabens and saccharin
Saturated solution (SSKI): 1000 mg/mL (30, 240 mL); 10 drops = 500 mg potassium iodide
Lugol's (strong iodine) solution: Iodine 50 mg and potassium iodide 100 mg per mL (15, 473 mL)

Potassium content is 6 mEq (234 mg) K^+/gram potassium iodide

Neonatal Grave's disease: 1 drop strong iodine (Lugol's solution) PO Q8 hr

Thyrotoxicosis:

Child: 50–250 mg PO TID (about 1–5 drops of SSKI TID)
Adult: 50–500 mg PO TID (1–10 drops SSKI PO TID)

Cutaneous or lymphocutaneous sporotrichosis (see remarks):

Child and adult: Start with 250 mg PO TID. Doses may be gradually increased as tolerated to the following **max. doses:**

Child max.: 1250–2000 mg PO TID
Adult max.: 2000–2500 mg PO TID

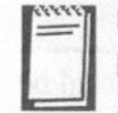

Contraindicated in pregnancy, hyperkalemia, iodine-induced goiter, and hypothyroidism. **Use with caution** in cardiac disease and renal failure. GI disturbance, metallic taste, rash, salivary gland inflammation, headache, lacrimation, and rhinitis are symptoms of iodism.

Give with milk or water after meals. Monitor thyroid function tests. Onset of antithyroid effects: 1–2 days.

Lithium carbonate and iodide-containing medications may have synergistic hypothyroid activity. Potassium-containing medications, potassium-sparing diuretics, and ACE inhibitors may increase serum potassium levels.

For sporotrichosis, continue treatment for 4–6 wk after lesions have completely healed. Increase dose until either **max. dose** is achieved or signs of intolerance appear.

For use as a thyroid blocking agent in radiation emergencies, see www.fda.gov/cder/guidance/4825fnl.pdf.

POTASSIUM SUPPLEMENTS

Many brand names
Electrolyte

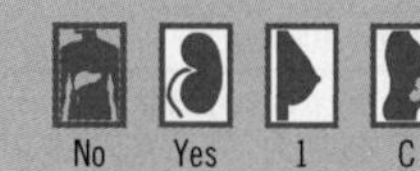

Potassium chloride (40 mEq K = 3 g KCl):

Sustained-release caps: 8, 10 mEq
Sustained-release tabs: 8, 10, 15, 20 mEq
Powder: 15, 20, 25 mEq/packet
Oral solution: 10% (6.7 mEq/5 mL), 20% (13.3 mEq/5 mL)
Concentrated injection: 2 mEq/mL

Continued

For explanation of icons, see p. 663.

POTASSIUM SUPPLEMENTS *continued*

Potassium gluconate (40 mEq K = 9.4 g K gluconate):

Tabs [OTC]: 500 mg (2.15 mEq), 595 mg (2.56 mEq)

Oral liquid: 20 mEq/15 mL; may contain alcohol

Potassium acetate (40 mEq K = 3.9 K acetate):

Concentrated injection: 2 mEq/mL

Potassium bicarbonate (10 mEq K = 1 g K bicarbonate):

Effervescent tab for oral solution: 10, 20 mEq

Potassium phosphate:

See Phosphorus Supplements

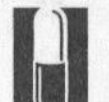

***Normal daily requirements:* See Chapter 21.**

Replacement: Determine based on maintenance requirements, deficit and ongoing losses. **See Chapter 11.**

Hypokalemia:

Oral:

Child: 1–4 mEq/kg/24 hr ÷ BID–QID. Monitor serum potassium.

Adult: 40–100 mEq/24 hr ÷ BID–QID

***IV:* MONITOR SERUM K CLOSELY.**

Child: 0.5–1 mEq/kg/dose given as an infusion of 0.5 mEq/kg/hr × 1–2 hr.

Max. IV infusion rate: 1 mEq/kg/hr. This may be used in critical situations (i.e., hypokalemia with arrhythmia).

Adult:

Serum K ≥2.5 mEq/L: Replete at rates up to 10 mEq/hr. **Total dosage not to exceed** 200 mEq/24 hr.

Serum K <2 mEq/L: Replete at rates up to 40 mEq/hr. **Total dosage not to exceed** 400 mEq/24 hr.

Max. peripheral IV solution concentration: 40 mEq/L

Max. concentration for central line administration: 150–200 mEq/L

PO administration may cause GI disturbance and ulceration. Oral liquid supplements should be diluted in water or fruit juice prior to administration. Sustained-release tablets must be swallowed whole, and **NOT** dissolved in the mouth or chewed.

Do not administer IV potassium undiluted. IV administration may cause irritation, pain, and phlebitis at the infusion site. **Rapid or central IV infusion may cause cardiac arrhythmias.** Patients receiving infusion >0.5 mEq/kg/hr (>20 mEq/hr for adults) should be placed on an ECG monitor.

PRALIDOXIME CHLORIDE

Protopam, 2-PAM

Antidote, organophosphate poisoning

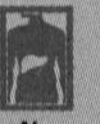

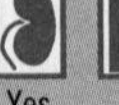

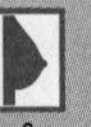

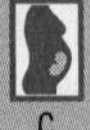

Injection: 1000 mg

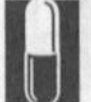

Organophosphate poisoning (use with atropine):

Child: 20–50 mg/kg/dose × 1 IM/IV/SC. May repeat in 1–2 hr if muscle weakness is not relieved, then at Q10–12 hr if cholinergic signs reappear.

Continuous infusion: loading dose of 20–50 mg/kg/dose (**max. dose:** 2000 mg) IV over 15–30 min followed by 10–20 mg/kg/hr.

Adult: 1–2 g/dose × 1 IM/IV/SC. May repeat in 1–2 hr if muscle weakness is not relieved, then at Q10–12 hr if cholinergic signs reappear.

Continued

PRALIDOXIME CHLORIDE *continued*

Contraindicated in poisonings due to phosphorus, inorganic phosphates, or organic phosphates without anticholinesterase activity. **Do not use** as an antidote for carbamate classes of pesticides. Removal of secretions and maintaining a patent airway is critical. May cause muscle rigidity, laryngospasm, and tachycardia after rapid IV infusion. Drug is generally ineffective if administered 36–48 hr after exposure. Additional doses may be necessary.

For IV administration, dilute to 50 mg/mL or less and infuse over 15–30 min (**not to exceed** 200 mg/min). Reduce dosage in renal impairment since 80%–90% of the drug is excreted unchanged in the urine 12 hr after administration.

PREDNISOLONE
Orapred, Orapred ODT, Prelone, Pediapred, and others
Corticosteroid

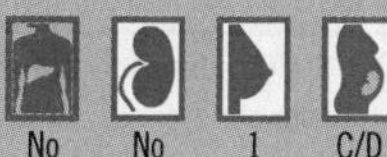

No No 1 C/D

Tabs: 5 mg
Syrup (Prelone and others): 5 mg/5 mL (120 mL), 15 mg/5 mL (240 mL); may contain alcohol and saccharin
Tablets, orally disintegrating (as Na phosphate) (Orapred ODT): 10, 15, 30 mg
Oral solution (as Na phosphate):
Pediapred: 5 mg/5 mL (120 mL); may contain alcohol and dye free
Orapred and others: 15 mg/5 mL (237 mL); may contain 2% alcohol and is dye free
Ophthalmic suspension (as acetate): 0.12% (5, 10 mL), 1% (5, 10, 15 mL); contains benzalkonium chloride and may contain bisulfites
Ophthalmic solution (as Na phosphate): 1% (5, 10, 15 mL); contains benzalkonium chloride

See *Prednisone* (equivalent dosing).
Ophthalmic (consult ophthalmologist before use):
Child and adult: Start with 1–2 drops Q1 hr during the day and Q2 hr during the night until favorable response, then reduce dose to 1 drop Q4 hr. Dose may be further reduced to 1 drop TID–QID.

See *Prednisone* for remarks. See Chapter 30 for relative steroid potencies. Pregnancy category changes to "D" if used in the first trimester. Orapred oral solution product should be stored in the refrigerator.

OPHTHALMIC USE: Contraindicated in viral (e.g., herpes simplex, vaccinia, and varicella), fungal, and mycobacterial infections of the cornea and conjunctiva. Increase in intraocular pressure, cataract formation, and delayed wound healing may occur.

PREDNISONE
Orasone, Deltasone, Liquid Pred, and others
Corticosteroid

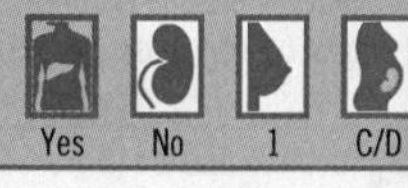

Yes No 1 C/D

Tabs: 1, 2.5, 5, 10, 20, 50 mg
Oral syrup/solution: 1 mg/mL (120, 500 mL); contains 5% alcohol and saccharin
Concentrated solution: 5 mg/mL (30 mL); contains 30% alcohol

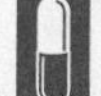

Anti-inflammatory/immunosuppressive:
Child: 0.5–2 mg/kg/24 hr PO ÷ once daily–BID
Acute asthma:
Child: 2 mg/kg/24 hr PO ÷ once daily–BID × 5–7 days; **max. dose:** 80 mg/24 hr. Patients may benefit from tapering if therapy exceeds 5–7 days.

Continued

For explanation of icons, see p. 663.

PREDNISONE *continued*

Asthma exacerbations (2007 National Heart, Lung, and Blood Institute Guideline Recommendations; dose until peak expiratory flow reaches 70% of predicted or personal best):

Child ≤12 yr: 1–2 mg/kg/24 hr PO ÷ Q12 hr (**max. dose:** 60 mg/24 hr).

>12 yr and adult: 40–80 mg/24 hr PO ÷ Q12–24 hr.

Outpatient asthma exacerbation burst therapy (longer durations may be necessary):

Child ≤12 yr: 1–2 mg/kg/24 hr PO ÷ Q12–24 hr (**max. dose:** 60 mg/24 hr) × 3–10 days.

Child >12 yr and adult: 40–60 mg/24 hr PO ÷ Q12–24 hr × 5–10 days.

Nephrotic syndrome:

Child: Starting dose of 2 mg/kg/24 hr PO (**max. dose:** 80 mg/24 hr) ÷ once daily–TID is recommended. Further treatment plans are individualized. Consult a nephrologist.

See Chapter 30 for physiologic replacement, relative steroid potencies, and doses based on body surface area. Methylprednisolone is preferable in hepatic disease because prednisone must be converted to methylprednisolone in the liver.

Side effects may include: mood changes, seizures, hyperglycemia, diarrhea, nausea, abdominal distension, GI bleeding, HPA axis suppression, osteopenia, cushingoid effects, and cataracts with prolonged use. Prednisone is a CYP 450 3A3/4 substrate and inducer. Barbiturates, carbamazepine, phenytoin, rifampin, isoniazid, may reduce the effects of prednisone, whereas estrogens may enhance the effects. Pregnancy category changes to "D" if used in the first trimester.

PRIMAQUINE PHOSPHATE

Various generic brands

Antimalarial

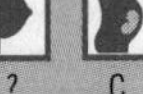

No No ? C

Tabs: 26.3 mg (15 mg base)

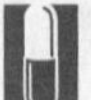

Doses expressed in mg of primaquine base:

Malaria:

Prevention of relapses for P. vivax or P. ovale only (initiate therapy during the last 2 wk of, or following a course of, suppression with chloroquine or comparible drug):

Child: 0.5 mg/kg/dose (**max. dose:** 30 mg/dose) PO once daily × 14 days

Adult: 30 mg PO once daily × 14 days

Prevention of chloroquine-resistant strains (initiate 1 day prior to departure and continued until 3–7 days after leaving endemic area):

Child: 0.5 mg/kg/dose PO once daily; **max. dose:** 30 mg/24 hr

Adult: 30 mg PO once daily

Pneumocystis jiroveci (formerly carinii) pneumonia (in combination with clindamycin):

Child: 0.3 mg/kg/dose (**max. dose:** 30 mg/dose) PO once daily × 21 days

Adult: 30 mg PO once daily × 21 days

Contraindicated in granulocytopenia (e.g., rheumatoid arthritis, lupus erythematosus) and bone marrow suppression. **Avoid use** with quinacrine and with other drugs that have a potential for causing hemolysis or bone marrow suppression. **Use with caution** in G6PD and NADH methemoglobin-reductase deficient patients due to increased risk for hemolytic anemia and leukopenia, respectively. Use in pregnancy is **not recommended** by the AAP *Red Book*. Cross sensitivity with iodoquinol.

May cause headache, visual disturbances, nausea, vomiting, and abdominal cramps. Hemolytic anemia, leukopenia, and methemoglobinemia have been reported. Administer all doses with food to mask bitter taste.

PRIMIDONE
Mysoline and others
Anticonvulsant, barbiturate

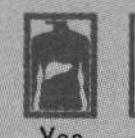 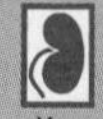  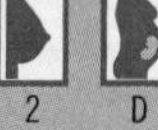 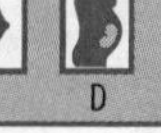
Yes Yes 2 D

Tabs: 50, 250 mg

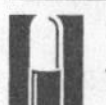
Neonate: 12–20 mg/kg/24 hr PO ÷ BID–QID; initiate therapy at the lower dosage range and titrate upwards.
Child, adolescent, and adult:

Day of Therapy	<8 yr	≥8 yr and adult
Days 1–3	50 mg PO QHS	100–125 mg PO QHS
Days 4–6	50 mg PO BID	100–125 mg PO BID
Days 7–9	100 mg PO BID	100–125 mg PO TID
Day 10 and thereafter	125–250 mg PO TID or 10–25 mg/kg/ 24 hr ÷ TID–QID	250 mg PO TID–QID; **max. dose:** 2 g/24 hr

Use with caution in renal or hepatic disease and pulmonary insufficiency. Primidone is metabolized to phenobarbital and has the same drug interactions and toxicities (see *Phenobarbital*). Additionally, primidone may cause vertigo, nausea, leukopenia, malignant lymphoma-like syndrome, diplopia, nystagmus, systemic lupus-like syndrome. Monitor for suicidal behavior or ideation. Acetazolamide may decrease primidone absorption. **Adjust dose in renal failure (see Chapter 31).**

Follow both primidone and phenobarbital levels. Therapeutic levels: 5–12 mg/L of primidone and 15–40 mg/L of phenobarbital. Recommended serum sampling time at steady-state: trough level obtained within 30 min prior to the next scheduled dose after 1–4 days of continuous dosing.

PROBENECID
Various generic brands
Penicillin therapy adjuvant, uric acid lowering agent

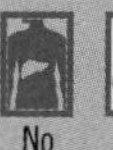 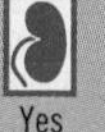 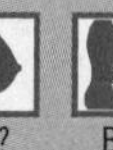 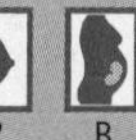
No Yes ? B

Tabs: 500 mg

To prolong penicillin levels.
Child (2–14 yr): 25 mg/kg PO × 1, then 40 mg/kg/24 hr ÷ QID; **max. single dose:** 500 mg/dose. Use adult dose if >50 kg.
Adult: 500 mg PO QID

Hyperuricemia:
Adult: 250 mg PO BID × 1 wk, then 500 mg PO BID; may increase by 500 mg increments Q4 wk PRN up to a **max. dose** of 2–3 g/24 hr ÷ BID.

Gonorrhea, antibiotic adjunct (just prior to antibiotic):
≤45 kg: 23 mg/kg/dose PO × 1 just prior to antibiotic
>45 kg: 1 g PO × 1

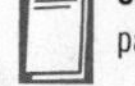
Use with caution in patients with peptic ulcer disease. **Contraindicated** in children <2 yr and patients with renal insuficiency. **Do not use** if GFR <30 mL/min.

Increases uric acid excretion. Inhibits renal tubular secretion of acyclovir, ganciclovir, ciprofloxacin, levofloxacin, nalidixic acid, moxifloxacin, organic acids, penicillins, cephalosporins, AZT, dapsone, methotrexate, nonsteroidal anti-inflammatory agents, and benzodiazepines. Salicylates may decrease probenecid's activity. Alkalinize urine in patients with gout. May cause headache, GI symptoms, rash, anemia, and hypersensitivity. False-positive glucosuria with Clinitest may occur.

For explanation of icons, see p. 663.

PROCAINAMIDE
Pronestyl, Procanbid, and various generic brands
Antiarrhythmic, class Ia

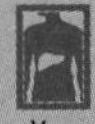 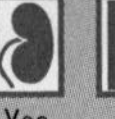  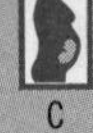
Yes Yes 2 C

Injection: 500 mg/mL; contains methylparabens and bisulfites

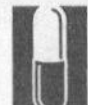

Child:

V. tach with poor perfusion: Consider 15 mg/kg/dose IV × 1 over 30–60 min if cardioversion ineffective; follow with continuous infusion if effective (see information that follows).

IM: 20–30 mg/kg/24 hr ÷ Q4–6 hr; **max. dose:** 4 g/24 hr (peak effect in 1 hr).

IV: Load: 3–6 mg/kg/dose over 5 min (**max. dose:** 100 mg/dose); repeat dose Q5–10 min PRN up to a total **max. dose** of 15 mg/kg. **Do not exceed** 500 mg in 30 min.

Maintenance: 20–80 mcg/kg/min by continuous infusion; **max. dose:** 2 g/24 hr.

Adult:

IM: 50 mg/kg/24 hr ÷ Q3–6 hr.

IV: Load: 50–100 mg/dose; repeat dose Q5 min PRN to a **max. dose** of 1000–1500 mg.

Maintenance: 1–6 mg/min by continuous infusion.

NOTE: The IV infusion dosage units for adults are in mg/min; compared to mcg/kg/min for children.

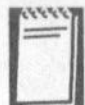

Contraindicated in myasthenia gravis, complete heart block, SLE, and torsade de pointes. **Use with caution** in asymptomatic premature ventricular contractions, digitalis intoxication, CHF, renal or hepatic dysfunction. **Adjust dose in renal failure (see Chapter 31).**

May cause lupus-like syndrome, positive Coombs' test, thrombocytopenia, arrhythmias, GI complaints, and confusion. Increased LFTs and liver failure have been reported. Monitor BP and ECG when using IV. QRS widening by >0.02 sec suggests toxicity.

Do not use with desipramine and other TCAs. Cimetidine, ranitidine, amiodarone, beta-blockers, and trimethoprim may increase procainamide levels. Procainamide may enhance the effects of skeletal muscle relaxants and anticholinergic agents. Therapeutic levels: 4–10 mg/L of procainamide or 10–30 mg/L of procainamide and NAPA levels combined.

Recommended serum sampling times:

IM intermittent dosing: Trough level within 30 minutes prior to the next scheduled dose after 2 days of continuous dosing (steady-state).

IV continuous infusion: 2 and 12 hr after start of infusion and at 24-hr intervals thereafter.

PROCHLORPERAZINE
Compazine and others
Antiemetic, phenothiazine derivative

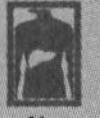 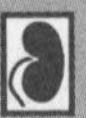 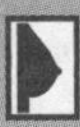 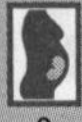
No No 2 C

Tabs (as maleate): 5, 10 mg
Slow-release caps (as maleate): 10, 15 mg
Suppository: 25 mg (12s)
Injection (as edisylate): 5 mg/mL (2, 10 mL); may contain bisulfites and benzyl alcohol

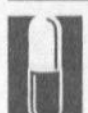

Antiemetic doses:

Child (>10 kg or >2 yr):

PO or PR: 0.4 mg/kg/24 hr ÷ TID–QID or alternative dosing by weight:

10–14 kg: 2.5 mg once daily–BID; **max. dose:** 7.5 mg/24 hr

15–18 kg: 2.5 mg BID–TID; **max. dose:** 10 mg/24 hr

19–39 kg: 2.5 mg TID or 5 mg BID; **max. dose:** 15 mg/24 hr

IM: 0.1–0.15 mg/kg/dose TID–QID; **max. dose:** 40 mg/24 hr

Continued

PROCHLORPERAZINE *continued*

Adult:

PO:

Immediate release: 5–10 mg/dose TID–QID

Extended release: 10 mg/dose BID or 15 mg/dose once daily

PR: 25 mg/dose BID

IM: 5–10 mg/dose Q3–4 hr

IV: 2.5–10 mg/dose; may repeat Q3–4 hr

Max. IM/IV dose: 40 mg/24 hr

Psychoses:

Child 2–12 yr:

PO or PR: Start with 2.5 mg BID–TID with a **max. first day dose** of 10 mg/24 hr. Dose may be increased as needed to 20 mg/24 hr for children 2–5 yr and 25 mg/24 hr for 6–12 yr.

IM: 0.13 mg/kg/dose × 1 and convert to PO immediately.

Adult:

PO: 5–10 mg TID–QID; may be increased as needed to a **max. dose** of 150 mg/24 hr.

IM: 10–20 mg Q2–4 hr PRN convert to PO immediately.

Toxicity as for other phenothiazines (see *Chlorpromazine*). Extrapyramidal reactions (reversed by diphenhydramine) or orthostatic hypotension may occur. May mask signs and symptoms of overdosage of other drugs and may obscure the diagnosis and treatment of conditions such as intestinal obstruction, brain tumor, and Reye's syndrome. May cause false-positive test for phenylketonuria, urinary amylase, uroporphyrins, and urobilinogen. **Do not use** IV route in children. Use only in management of prolonged vomiting of known etiology.

A 0.15 mg/kg/dose IV over 10 min was effective in migraine headaches presenting in the emergency departments for children 5–18 yr (see *Ann Emerg Med* 2004;43:256–262).

PROMETHAZINE

Phenergan and others

Antihistamine, antiemetic, phenothiazine derivative

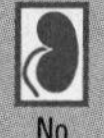

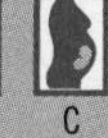

No No 3 C

Tabs: 12.5, 25, 50 mg

Syrup: 6.25 mg/5 mL (240, 473 mL); contains alcohol

Suppository: 12.5, 25, 50 mg (12s)

Injection: 25, 50 mg/mL (1 mL); may contain sulfites

Antihistaminic:

Child ≥2 yr: 0.1 mg/kg/dose (**max. dose:** 12.5 mg/dose) Q6 hr PO during the day hours and 0.5 mg/kg/dose (**max. dose:** 25 mg/dose) QHS PO PRN

Adult: 12.5 mg PO/PR TID and 25 mg QHS

Nausea and vomiting PO/IM/IV/PR (see remarks):

Child ≥2 yr: 0.25–1 mg/kg/dose Q4–6 hr PRN; **max. dose:** 25 mg/dose

Adult: 12.5–25 mg Q4–6 hr PRN

Motion sickness: (1st dose 0.5–1 hr before departure):

Child ≥2 yr: 0.5 mg/kg/dose Q12 hr PO/PR PRN; **max. dose:** 25 mg/dose

Adult: 25 mg PO Q8–12 hr PRN

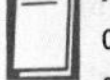

Avoid use in children <2 yr because of risk for fatal respiratory depression. Toxicity similar to other phenothiazines (see *Chlorpromazine*). **Do not** administer SQ or intra-arterially because of severe local reactions. IV route of administration is **not recommended** (IM preferred) due to

Continued

For explanation of icons, see p. 663.

PROMETHAZINE *continued*

severe tissue injury (tissue necrosis and gangrene). If using IV route, dilute 25 mg/mL strength product with 10–20 mL NS and administer over 10–15 min, consider lower initial doses, administer through a large-bore vein and check patency of line before administering, administer through an IV line at the port farthest from the patient's vein, and monitor for burning or pain during or after injection. Administer oral doses with meals to decrease GI irritation.

May cause profound sedation, blurred vision, respiratory depression (use lowest effective dose in children and **avoid** concomitant use of respiratory depressants), and dystonic reactions (reversed by diphenhydramine). Cholestatic jaundice and neuroleptic malignant syndrome has been reported. May intefere with pregnancy tests (immunological reactions between hCG and anti-hCG). For nausea and vomiting, use only in management of prolonged vomiting of known etiology.

PROPRANOLOL

Inderal and many other generics

Adrenergic blocking agent (beta), class II antiarrhythmic

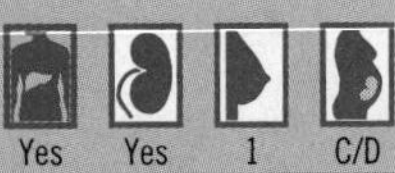

Tabs: 10, 20, 40, 60, 80 mg
Extended-release caps: 60, 80, 120, 160 mg
Oral solution: 20, 40 mg/5 mL; contains parabens and saccharin
Concentrated solution: 80 mg/mL; alcohol and dye free
Injection: 1 mg/mL (1 mL)

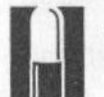

Arrhythmias:
Child:
IV: 0.01–0.1 mg/kg/dose IV push over 10 min, repeat Q6–8 hr PRN
Max. dose: 1 mg/dose for infant; 3 mg/dose for child
PO: Start at 0.5–1 mg/kg/24 hr ÷ Q6–8 hr; increase dosage Q3–5 days PRN. Usual dosage range: 2–4 mg/kg/24 hr ÷ Q6–8 hr. **Max. dose:** 60 mg/24 hr or 16 mg/kg/24 hr
Adult:
IV: 1 mg/dose Q5 min up to total 5 mg
PO: 10–20 mg/dose TID–QID; increase PRN. Usual range 40–320 mg/24 hr ÷ TID–QID.

Hypertension:
Child:
PO: Initial: 0.5–1 mg/kg/24 hr ÷ Q6–12 hr. May increase dose Q5–7 days PRN; **max. dose:** 8 mg/kg/24 hr
Adult:
PO: 40 mg/dose PO BID or 60–80 mg/dose (sustained-release capsule) PO once daily. May increase 10–20 mg/dose Q3–7 days; **max. dose:** 640 mg/24 hr.

Migraine prophylaxis:
Child:
<35 kg: 10–20 mg PO TID
≥35 kg: 20–40 mg PO TID
Adult: 80 mg/24 hr ÷ Q6–8 hr PO; increase dose by 20–40 mg/dose Q3–4 wk PRN. Usual effective dose range: 160–240 mg/24 hr.

Tetralogy spells:
IV: 0.15–0.25 mg/kg/dose slow IV push. May repeat in 15 min × 1. See also Chapter 7.
PO: Start at 2–4 mg/kg/24 hr ÷ Q6 hr PRN. Usual dose range: 4–8 mg/kg/24 hr ÷ Q6 hr PRN. Doses as high as 15 mg/kg/24 hr have been used with careful monitoring.

Continued

P
FORMULARY

PROPRANOLOL *continued*

Thyrotoxicosis:

Neonate: 2 mg/kg/24 hr PO ÷ Q6–12 hr

Adolescent and adult:

IV: 1–3 mg/dose over 10 min. May repeat in 4–6 hr.

PO: 10–40 mg/dose PO Q6 hr.

Infantile hemangioma (see remarks):

Start at 1 mg/kg/24 hr ÷ Q8 hr PO. If tolerated after one day, increase dose to 2 mg/kg/24 hr ÷ Q8 hr PO.

Contraindicated in asthma, Raynaud's syndrome, heart failure, and heart block. **Not indicated** for the treatment of hypertensive emergencies. **Use with caution** in presence of obstructive lung disease, diabetes mellitus, renal or hepatic disease. May cause hypoglycemia, hypotension, nausea, vomiting, depression, weakness, impotence, bronchospasm, and heart block. Cutaneous reactions, including Stevens-Johnson, TEN, exfoliative dermatitis, erythema multiforme, and utricaria have been reported. Acute hypertension has occurred after insulin-induced hypoglycemia in patients on propranolol.

Therapeutic levels: 30–100 ng/mL. Drug is metabolized by CYP 450 1A2, 2C18, 2C19, and 2D6 isoenzymes. Concurrent administration with barbiturates, indomethacin, or rifampin may cause decreased activity of propranolol. Concurrent administration with cimetidine, hydralazine, flecainide, quinidine, chlorpromazine, or verapamil may lead to increased activity of propranolol. **Avoid** IV use of propranolol with calcium channel blockers; may increase effect of calcium channel blocker. Use with amiodarone may increase negative chronotropic effects.

For infantile hemangioma, monitor BP, HR, and blood glucose. Infants <6 mo must be fed every 4 hr. Successful use in infantile hepatic hemangiomas has also been reported.

Pregnancy category changes to "D" if used in second or third trimesters.

PROPYLTHIOURACIL

PTU

Antithyroid agent

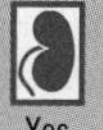

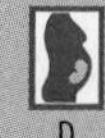

Yes Yes 2 D

Tabs: 50 mg

Oral suspension: 5 mg/mL

100 mg PTU = 10 mg methimazole

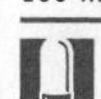

Dosages should be adjusted as required to achieve and maintain T_4, TSH levels in normal ranges.

Neonate: 5–10 mg/kg/24 hr ÷ Q8 hr PO

Child:

Initial: 5–7 mg/kg/24 hr ÷ Q8 hr PO, OR by age:

6–10 yr: 50–150 mg/24 hr ÷ Q8 hr PO

>10 yr: 150–300 mg/24 hr ÷ Q8 hr PO

Maintenance: Generally begins after 2 mo. Usually $\frac{1}{3}$ – $\frac{2}{3}$ the initial dose in divided doses (Q8–12 hr) when the patient is euthyroid.

Adult:

Initial: 300–450 mg/24 hr ÷ Q6–8 hr PO; some may require larger doses of 600–1200 mg/24 hr

Maintenance: 100–150 mg/24 hr ÷ Q8–12 hr PO

May cause blood dyscrasias, fever, liver disease, dermatitis, urticaria, malaise, CNS stimulation or depression, and arthralgias. Glomerulonephritis, severe liver injury/failure, agranulocytosis, interstitial pneumonitis, exfoliative dermatitis, and erythema nodosum have

Continued

For explanation of icons, see p. 663.

PROPYLTHIOURACIL *continued*

also been reported. May decrease the effectiveness of warfarin. Monitor thyroid function. A dose reduction of beta-blocker may be necessary when the hyperthyroid patient becomes euthyroid.

For neonates, crush tablets, weigh appropriate dose, and mix in formula/breast milk. **Adjust dose in renal failure (see Chapter 31).**

PROSTAGLANDIN E_1

See *Alprostadil*

PROTAMINE SULFATE

Various generic brands
Antidote, heparin

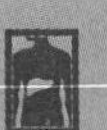
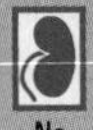
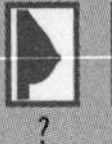
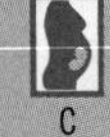

No No ? C

Injection: 10 mg/mL (5, 25 mL); preservative free

Heparin antidote, IV:
1 mg protamine will neutralize 115 U porcine intestinal heparin, 90 U beef lung heparin, or 100 U (1 mg) low molecular weight heparin.
Consider time since last heparin dose:

If <0.5 hr: give 100% of specified dose
If within 0.5–1 hr: give 50%–75% of aforementioned dose
If within 1–2 hr: give 37.5%–50% of aforementioned dose
If ≥2 hr: give 25%–37.5% of aforementioned dose
Max. dose: 50 mg IV
Max. infusion rate: 5 mg/min
Max. IV concentration: 10 mg/mL

If heparin was administered by deep SC injection, give 1–1.5 mg protamine per 100 U heparin as follows:

Load with 25–50 mg via slow IV infusion followed by the rest of the calculated dose via continuous infusion over 8–16 hr or the expected duration of heparin absorption.

Enoxaparin overdosage, IV (see remarks): Approximately 1 mg protamine will neutralize 1 mg enoxaparin.

Consider time since last enoxaparin dose:

If <8 hr: Give 100% of aforementioned dose.
If within 8–12 hr: Give 50% of aforementioned dose.
If >12 hr: Protamine not required but if serious bleeding is present, give 50% of aforementioned dose.
If aPTT remains prolonged 2–4 hr after the first protamine dose, a second infusion of 0.5 mg protamine per 1 mg enoxaparin may be given.
Max. dose: 50 mg. See *Heparin* antidote IV dosage for **max.** administration concentration and rate.

Risk factors for protamine hypersensitivity include known hypersensitivity to fish, and exposure to protamine-containing insulin or prior protamine therapy.

May cause hypotension, bradycardia, dyspnea, and anaphylaxis. Monitor aPTT or ACT. Heparin rebound with bleeding has been reported to occur 8–18 hr later.

Use in enoxaparin overdose may not be complete despite using multiple doses of protamine.

PSEUDOEPHEDRINE
Sudafed, Efidac/24-Pseudoephedrine, and others
Sympathomimetic, nasal decongestant

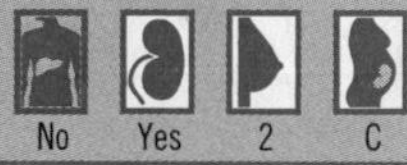

Tabs (OTC): 30, 60 mg
Extended-release tab (OTC): 120 mg, 240 mg (Efidac/24)
Caps (OTC): 30, 60 mg
Sustained-release caps (OTC): 120 mg
Liquid (OTC): 15, 30 mg/5 mL (120, 473 mL)
Syrup (OTC): 15 mg/5 mL (118 mL); contains parabens
Drops (OTC): 7.5 mg/0.8 mL (15, 30 mL)
Purchases of OTC products are limited to behind the pharmacy counter sales with monthly sale limits due to the methamphetamine epidemic

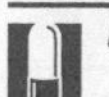

Child <12 yr: 4 mg/kg/24 hr ÷ Q6 hr PO or by age:
- ***<2 yr:*** 4 mg/kg/24 hr ÷ Q6 hr PO
- ***2–5 yr:*** 15 mg/dose Q6 hr PO; **max. dose:** 60 mg/24 hr
- ***6–12 yr:*** 30 mg/dose Q6 hr PO; **max. dose:** 120 mg/24 hr

Child ≥12 yr and adult:
- ***Immediate release:*** 30–60 mg/dose Q6 hr PO; **max. dose:** 240 mg/24 hr
- ***Sustained release:*** 120 mg PO Q12 hr
  - ***Efidac/24:*** 240 mg PO Q24 hr

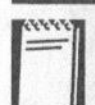

Contraindicated with MAO inhibitor drugs and in severe hypertension and severe coronary artery disease. **Use with caution** in mild/moderate hypertension, hyperglycemia, hyperthyroidism, and cardiac disease. May cause dizziness, nervousness, restlessness, insomnia, and arrhythmias. Pseudoephedrine is a common component of OTC cough and cold preparations and is combined with several antihistamines; these products are not recommended for children <6 yr. Since drug and active metabolite are primarily excreted renally, **doses should be adjusted in renal impairment.** May cause false-positive test for amphetamines (EMIT assay).

PSYLLIUM
Metamucil, Fiberall, Serutan, Konsyl, Perdiem Fiber Therapy, and many others
Bulk-forming laxative

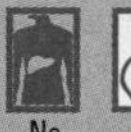
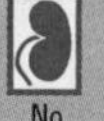
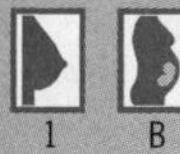

Granules [OTC]: Serutan: 2.5 g/rounded teaspoonful (170, 540 g), Perdiem: 4.03 g/rounded teaspoonful (100, 250 g)
Powder [OTC]: 50% psyllium, 50% dextrose (sugar-free version available) (Metamucil: 3.4 g/rounded teaspoon); 100% psyllium (Konsyl: 6 g/rounded teaspoon); for other products check the label for the amount of psyllium per unit of measurement
Wafers [OTC]: 3.4 g
Caps: 0.52 g

Child (granules or powder must be mixed with a full glass of water or juice):
- ***<6 yr:*** 1.25–2.5 g/dose PO once daily–TID; **max. dose:** 7.5 g/24 hr
- ***6–11 yr:*** 2.5–3.75 g/dose PO once daily–TID; **max. dose:** 15 g/24 hr
- **≥12 yr:** 2.5–7.5 g/dose PO once daily–TID; **max. dose:** 30 g/24 hr

Contraindicated in cases of fecal impaction or GI obstruction. **Use with caution** in patients with esophageal strictures and rectal bleeding. Phenylketonurics should be aware that certain preparations may contain aspartame. Should be taken with a full glass (240 mL) of liquid. Onset of action: 12–72 hr.

For explanation of icons, see p. 663.

PYRANTEL PAMOATE
Antiminth, Reese's Pinworm, Pamix, Pin-Rid, and Pin-X
Anthelmintic

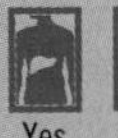 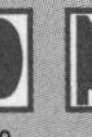 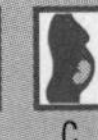 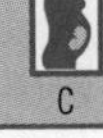
Yes No ? C

Oral suspension (OTC): 50 mg/mL pyrantel base (144 mg/mL pyrantel pamoate) (30, 60 mL)
Liquid (OTC): 50 mg/mL pyrantel base (144 mg/mL pyrantel pamoate) (30 mL); may contain parabens
Caps (OTC) and tabs (OTC): 62.5 mg pyrantel base (180 mg pyrantel pamoate)

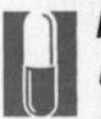

All doses expressed in terms of pyrantel base.
Child and adult:
Ascaris (roundworm) and Trichostrongylus: 11 mg/kg/dose PO × 1
Enterobius (pinworm): 11 mg/kg/dose PO × 1. Repeat same dose 2 wk later.
Hookworm or eosinophilic enterocolitis: 11 mg/kg/dose PO once daily × 3 days
Max. dose (all indications): 1 g/dose

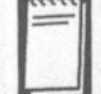

Use with caution in liver dysfunction. **Do not use** in combination with piperazine because of antagonism. May cause nausea, vomiting, anorexia, transient AST elevations, headaches, rash, and muscle weakness. Limited experience in children <2 yr. May increase theophylline levels. Drug may be mixed with milk or fruit juice and may be taken with food.

PYRAZINAMIDE
Pyrazinoic acid amide
Antituberculous agent

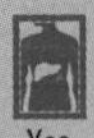 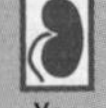 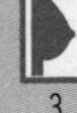 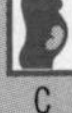 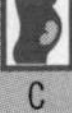
Yes Yes 3 C

Tab: 500 mg
Oral suspension: 10, 100 mg/mL
In combination with isoniazid and rifampin (Rifater):
Tab: 300 mg with 50 mg isoniazid and 120 mg rifampin; contains povidone and propylene glycol

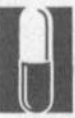

Tuberculosis: Use as part of a multidrug regimen for tuberculosis. See latest edition of the AAP *Red Book* for recommended treatment for tuberculosis.
Child:
Daily dose: 30–40 mg/kg/24 hr PO ÷ once daily–BID; **max. dose:** 2 g/24 hr
Twice-weekly dose: 50 mg/kg/dose PO 2 × per week; **max. dose:** 2 g/dose
Adult:
Daily dose: 15–30 mg/kg/24 hr PO ÷ once daily–QID; **max. dose:** 2 g/24 hr
Twice-weekly dose: 50–70 mg/kg/dose PO 2 × per week; **max. dose:** 4 g/dose
Mycobacterium tuberculosis in HIV, prophylaxis to prevent first episode:
Infant and child: not recommended because of increased risk of severe/fatal hepatotoxity.

See latest edition of the AAP *Red Book* for recommended treatment for tuberculosis. **Contraindicated** in severe hepatic damage and acute gout. The CDC and ATS **do not recommend** the combination of pyazinamide and rifampin for latent TB infections. **Use with caution** in patients with renal failure (dosage reduction has been recommended), gout, or diabetes mellitus. Monitor liver function tests (baseline and periodic) and serum uric acid.

Hepatoxicity is most common dose-related side effect; doses ≤30 mg/kg/24 hr minimize effect. Hyperuricemia, maculopapular rash, arthralgia, fever, acne, porphyria, dysuria, and photosensitivity may occur. Severe hepatic toxicity may occur with rifampin use. May decrease isoniazid levels.

PYRETHRINS
Tisit, A-200, Pyrinyl, Pronto, RID, and others
Pediculicide

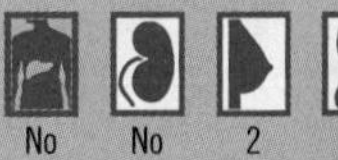

All products are available without a prescription.
Lotion (Tisit): 0.3% pyrethrins and 2% piperonyl butoxide (59, 118 mL); contains petroleum distillate and equivalent to 1.6% ether
Gel (Tisit): 0.3% pyrethrins and 3% piperonyl butoxide (30 mL)
Shampoo (Tisit, RID, Pronto, A-200): 0.33%pyrethrins and 4% piperonyl butoxide (60, 120, 240 mL); may contain alcohol
Mousse (RID): 0.33% pyrethrins and 4% piperonyl butoxide (165 mL); contains alcohol

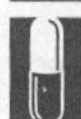

Pediculosis: Apply to hair or affected body area for 10 min, then wash thoroughly and comb with fine-tooth comb or nit-removing comb; repeat in 7–10 days.

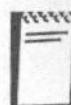

Contraindicated in ragweed hypersensitivity; drug is derived from the chrysanthemum flowers. For topical use only. **Avoid** use in and around the eyes, mouth, nose, or vagina. **Avoid** repeat applications in <24 hr. Low ovicidal activity requires repeat treatment. Dead nits require mechanical removal. Wash bedding and clothing to eradicate infestation.

Local irritation including erythema, pruritis, urticaria, edema, and eczema may occur.

PYRIDOSTIGMINE BROMIDE
Mestinon and others
Cholinergic agent

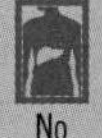
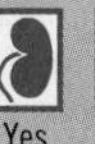
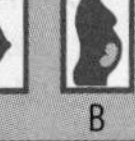

Syrup: 60 mg/5 mL (480 mL); contains 5% alcohol
Tabs: 60 mg
Sustained-release tab: 180 mg
Injection: 5 mg/mL; may contain 0.2% parabens

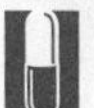

Myasthenia gravis:
Neonate:
- ***PO:*** 5 mg/dose Q4–6 hr
- ***IM/IV:*** 0.05–0.15 mg/kg/dose Q4–6 hr; **max. single IM/IV dose:** 10 mg

Child:
- ***PO:*** 7 mg/kg/24 hr in 5–6 divided doses
- ***IM/IV:*** 0.05–0.15 mg/kg/dose Q4–6 hr; **max. single IM/IV dose:** 10 mg

Adult:
- ***PO (immediate release):*** 60 mg TID; increase Q48 hr PRN. Usual effective dose: 60–1500 mg/24 hr
- ***PO (sustained release):*** 180–540 mg once daily–BID
- ***IM/IV:*** 2 mg/dose Q2–3 hr

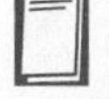

Contraindicated in mechanical intestinal or urinary obstruction. **Use with caution** in patients with epilepsy, asthma, bradycardia, hyperthyroidism, arrhythmias, or peptic ulcer. May cause nausea, vomiting, diarrhea, rash, headache, and muscle cramps. Pyridostigmine is mainly excreted unchanged by the kidney. Therefore, lower doses titrated to effect in renal disease may be necessary.

Changes in oral dosages may take several days to show results. **Atropine is the antidote.**

For explanation of icons, see p. 663.

PYRIDOXINE
Aminoxin, Vitamin B_6, and various
Vitamin, water soluble

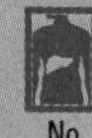
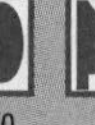
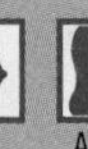
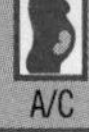

No No 1 A/C

Tabs (HCl) [OTC]: 25, 50, 100 mg
Tabs, enteric-coated (pyridoxal-5′-phosphate) (Aminoxin) [OTC]: 20 mg
Oral solution (HCl): 1 mg/mL
Injection (HCl): 100 mg/mL (1 mL); contains chorobutanol

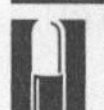

Deficiency, IM/IV/PO (PO preferred):
Child: 5–25 mg/24 hr × 3 wk, followed by 1.5–2.5 mg/24 hr as maintenance therapy (via multivitamin preparation)
Adolescent and adult: 10–20 mg/24 hr × 3 wk, followed by 2–5 mg/24 hr as maintenance therapy (via multivitamin preparation)

Drug-induced neuritis (PO):
Prophylaxis:
Child: 1–2 mg/kg/24 hr
Adolescent and adult: 25–100 mg/24 hr
Treatment:
Child: 10–50 mg/24 hr
Adolescent and adult: 100–300 mg/24 hr

Pyridoxine dependent seizures:
Neonate and infant:
Initial: 50–100 mg/dose IM or rapid IV × 1
Maintenance: 50–100 mg/24 hr PO

Recommended daily allowance: See Chapter 21.

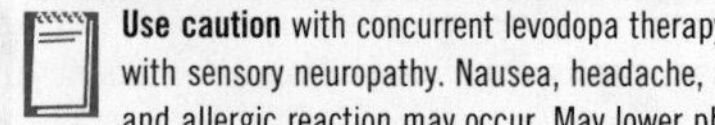

Use caution with concurrent levodopa therapy. Chronic administration has been associated with sensory neuropathy. Nausea, headache, increased AST, decreased serum folic acid level, and allergic reaction may occur. May lower phenobarbital and phenytoin levels. **See Chapter 20 for management of neonatal seizures.** Pregnancy category changes to "C" if dosage exceeds U.S. RDA recommendation.

PYRIMETHAMINE
Daraprim
Antiparasitic agent

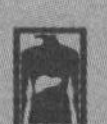
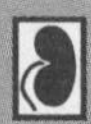
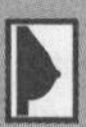
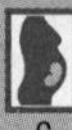

Yes Yes 2 C

Tabs: 25 mg
Oral suspension: 2 mg/mL

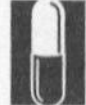

Congenital toxoplasmosis (administer with sulfadiazine and leucovorin; see remarks):
Load: 2 mg/kg/24 hr PO ÷ Q12 hr × 2 days
Maintenance: 1 mg/kg/24 hr PO once daily × 2–6 mo, then 1 mg/kg/24 hr 3 × per wk to complete total 12 mo of therapy

Toxoplasmosis (administer with sulfadiazine or trisulfapyrimidines, and leucovorin):
Child:
Load: 2 mg/kg/24 hr PO ÷ BID × 3 days; **max. dose:** 100 mg/24 hr
Maintenance: 1 mg/kg/24 hr PO ÷ once daily–BID × 4 wk; **max. dose:** 25 mg/24 hr
Adult: 50–75 mg/24 hr × 3–4 wk depending on response. After response, decrease dose by 50% and continue for an additional 4–5 wk.

Continued

PYRIMETHAMINE *continued*

Pyrimethamine is a folate antagonist. Supplementation with folinic acid leucovorin at 5–15 mg/24 hr is recommended. **Contraindicated** in megaloblastic anemia secondary to folate deficiency. **Use with caution** in G6PD deficiency, malabsorption syndromes, alcoholism, pregnancy, and renal or hepatic impairment. Pyrimethamine can cause glossitis, bone marrow suppression, seizures, rash, and photosensitivity. For congenital toxoplasmosis, see *Clin Infect Dis* 1994;18:38–72. Zidovudine and methotrexate may increase risk for bone marrow suppression. Aurothioglucose, trimethoprim, and sulfamethoxazole may increase risk for blood dyscrasias. Administer doses with meals. Most cases of acquired toxoplasmosis **do not** require specific antimicrobial therapy.

Pyrimethamine and sulfadoxine combination product (Fansidar) is no longer available in the United States.

QUINIDINE
Quinidex and various generic brands
Class Ia antiarrhythmic

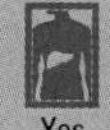 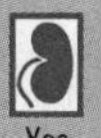 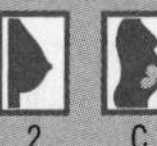
Yes Yes 2 C

As gluconate (62% quinidine):
- **Slow-release tabs:** 324 mg
- **Injection:** 80 mg/mL (50 mg/mL quinidine) (10 mL); contains phenol

As sulfate (83% quinidine):
- **Tabs:** 200, 300 mg
- **Slow-release tab (Quinidex):** 300 mg
- **Oral suspension:** 10 mg/mL

Equivalents: 200 mg sulfate = 267 mg gluconate

All doses expressed as salt forms.

Antiarrhythmic:

Child (Give PO as sulfate; give IM/IV as gluconate):

Test dose: 2 mg/kg ×1 IM/PO; **max. dose:** 200 mg.

Therapeutic dose:

IV (as gluconate): 2–10 mg/kg/dose Q3–6 hr PRN.

PO (as sulfate): 15–60 mg/kg/24 hr ÷ Q6 hr.

Adult (Give PO as sulfate; give IM as gluconate):

Test dose: 200 mg ×1 IM/PO.

Therapeutic dose:

As sulfate:

PO, immediate-release: 100–600 mg/dose Q4–6 hr. Begin at 200 mg/dose and titrate to desired effect.

PO, sustained release: 300–600 mg/dose Q 8–12 hr.

As gluconate:

IM: 400 mg/dose Q4–6 hr.

IV: 200–400 mg/dose, infused at a rate of ≤10 mg/min.

PO: 324–972 mg Q8–12 hr.

Malaria:

Child and adult (give IV as gluconate; see remarks):

Loading dose: 10 mg/kg/dose (**max. dose:** 600 mg) IV over 1–2 hr followed by maintenance dose. Omit or decrease load if patient has received quinine or mefloquine.

Maintenance dose: 0.02 mg/kg/min IV as continuous infusion until oral therapy can be initiated. If more than 48 hr of IV therapy is required, reduce dose by 30%–50%.

Continued

For explanation of icons, see p. 663.

QUINIDINE *continued*

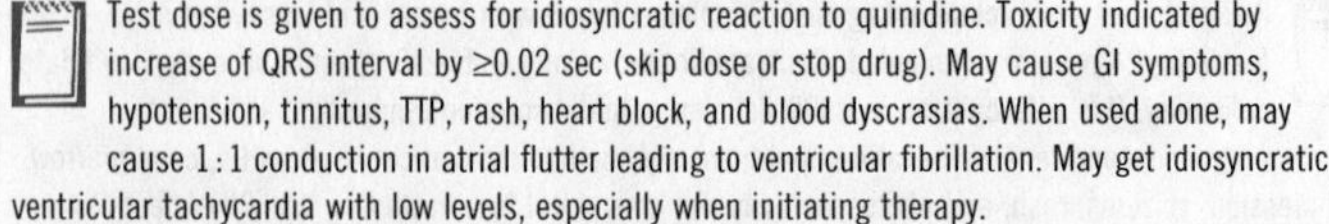

Test dose is given to assess for idiosyncratic reaction to quinidine. Toxicity indicated by increase of QRS interval by ≥0.02 sec (skip dose or stop drug). May cause GI symptoms, hypotension, tinnitus, TTP, rash, heart block, and blood dyscrasias. When used alone, may cause 1 : 1 conduction in atrial flutter leading to ventricular fibrillation. May get idiosyncratic ventricular tachycardia with low levels, especially when initiating therapy.

Quinidine is a substrate of CYP 450 3A3/4 and 3A5-7 enzymes, and an inhibitor of CYP 450 2D6 and 3A3/4 enzymes. Can cause increase in digoxin levels. Quinidine potentiates the effect of neuromuscular blocking agents, beta-blockers, anticholinergics, and warfarin. Amiodarone, antacids, delavirdine, diltiazem, grapefruit juice, saquinavir, ritonavir, verapamil, or cimetidine may enhance the drug's effect. Barbiturates, phenytoin, cholinergic drugs, nifedipine, sucralfate, or rifampin may reduce quinidine's effect. **Use with caution** in renal insufficiency (15%–25% of drug is eliminated unchanged in the urine), myocardial depression, sick sinus syndrome, G6PD deficiency, and hepatic dysfunction.

Therapeutic levels: 3–7 mg/L. Recommended serum sampling times at steady-state: trough level obtained within 30 min prior to the next scheduled dose after 1–2 days of continuous dosing (steady-state).

MALARIA USE: Continuous monitoring of ECG, blood pressure, and serum glucose are recommended, especially in pregnant women and young children.

QUINUPRISTIN AND DALFOPRISTIN

Synercid

Antibiotic, streptogramin

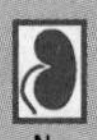

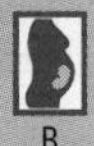

Yes No ? B

Injection: 500 mg (150 mg quinupristin and 350 mg dalfopristin)

Doses expressed in mg of combined quinupristin and dalfopristin.

Vancomycin-resistant Enterococcus faecium (VREF):

Child <16 yr (limited data), ≥16 yr and adult: 7.5 mg/kg/dose IV Q8 hr

Complicated skin infections:

Child <16 yr (limited data), ≥16 yr and adult: 7.5 mg/kg/dose IV Q12 hr for at least 7 days

VREF endocarditis:

Child and adult: 7.5 mg/kg/dose IV Q8 hr for at least 8 wk

Not active against *Enterococcus faecalis.* **Use with caution** in hepatic impairment; dosage reduction may be necessary. Most common side effects include pain, burning, inflammation and edema at the IV infusion site, thrombophlebitis, and thrombosis, GI distubances, rash, arthralgia, myalgia, increased liver enzymes, hyperbilirubinemia, and headache. Dose frequency reductions (Q8 hr to Q12 hr) or discontinuation can improve severe cases of arthralgia and myalgia. Use total body weight for obese patients when calculating dosages.

Drug is an inhibitor to the CYP 450 3A4 isoenzyme. **Avoid use** with CYP 450 3A4 substrates, which can prolong QTc interval (e.g., cisapride). May increase the effects/toxicity of cyclosporine, tacrolimus, sirolimus, delavirdine, nevirapine, indinavir, ritonavir, diazepam, midazolam, carbamazepine, methylprednisolone, vinca alkaloids, docetaxel, paclitaxel, quinidine, and some calcium channel blockers.

Pediatric pharmacokinetic studies have not been completed. Reduce dose for patients with hepatic cirrhosis (Child-Pugh A or B).

Drug is compatible with D5W and incompatible with saline and heparin. Infuse each dose over 1 hr using the following **max.** IV concentrations: peripheral line: 2 mg/mL, central line: 5 mg/mL. If injection site reaction occurs, dilute infusion to <1 mg/mL.

RANITIDINE HCL
Zantac, Zantac 75 [OTC], Zantac 150 Maximum Strength [OTC], and many generics
Histamine-2-antagonist

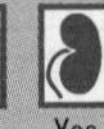  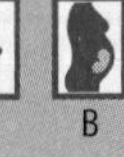
Yes Yes 1 B

Tabs: 75 [OTC], 150 [OTC and Rx], 300 mg
Effervescent tabs: 25, 150 mg
Syrup: 15 mg/mL (480 mL); contains 7.5% alcohol and parabens
Oral liquid: 15 mg/mL (473 mL); contains parabens and may contain alcohol
Carbohydrate-free oral solution: 5, 10 mg/mL [dissolve 150 mg effervescent granules with 30 mL (5 mg/mL) or 15 mL (10 mg/mL) water; solution good for 24 hr]
Injection: 25 mg/mL (2, 6, 40 mL); contains 0.5% phenol
Injection (pre-mixed): 1 mg/mL (preservative-free in 1/2 normal saline, 50 mL)

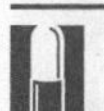

Neonate:
- ***PO:*** 2–4 mg/kg/24 hr ÷ Q8–12 hr
- ***IV:*** 2 mg/kg/24 hr ÷ Q6–8 hr

≥1 mo–16 yr:
- ***Duodenal/gastric ulcer (see remarks):***
  - ***PO:***
    - ***Treatment:*** 4–8 mg/kg/24 hr ÷ Q12 hr; **max. dose:** 300 mg/24 hr
    - ***Maintenance:*** 2–4 mg/kg/24 hr ÷ Q12 hr; **max. dose:** 150 mg/24 hr
  - ***IV/IM:*** 2–4 mg/kg/24 hr ÷ Q6–8 hr; **max. dose:** 200 mg/24 hr
- ***GERD/erosive esophagitis:***
  - ***PO:*** 5–10 mg/kg/24 hr ÷ Q8–12 hr; GERD **max. dose:** 300 mg/24 hr, erosive esophagitis **max. dose:** 600 mg/24 hr
  - ***IV/IM:*** 2–4 mg/kg/24 hr ÷ Q6–8 hr; **max. dose:** 200 mg/24 hr

Adult:
- ***PO:*** 150 mg/dose BID or 300 mg/dose QHS
- ***IM/IV:*** 50 mg/dose Q6–8 hr; **max. dose:** 400 mg/24 hr

Continuous infusion, all ages: Administer daily IV dosage over 24 hr (may be added to parenteral nutrition solutions).

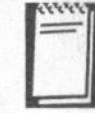

May cause headache and GI disturbance, malaise, insomnia, sedation, arthralgia, and hepatotoxicity. May increase levels of nifedipine and midazolam. May decrease levels of ketoconazole, itraconazole, and delavirdine. May cause false-positive urine protein test (Multistix).

Duodenal/gastric ulcer doses for ≥1 mo–16 yr are extrapolated from clinical adult trials and pharmacokinetic data in children. Extemporaneously compounded carbohydrate-free oral solution dosage form is useful for patients receiving the ketogenic diet. The syrup dosage form has a peppermint flavor and may not be tolerated. **Adjust dose in renal failure (see Chapter 31).**

RASBURICASE
Elitek
Antihyperuricemic agent

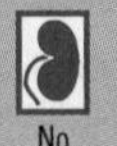 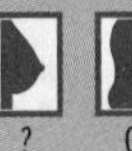 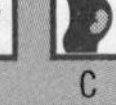
No No ? C

Injection: 1.5, 7.5 mg; contains mannitol

Hyperuricemia: 0.1–0.2 mg/kg/dose (rounded down to the nearest whole 1.5 mg multiple) IV over 30 min × 1. Patients generally respond to 1 dose but, if needed, dose may be repeated Q24 hr for up to 4 additional doses.

Continued

For explanation of icons, see p. 663.

RASBURICASE *continued*

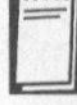

Contraindicated in G6PD deficiency or history of hypersensitivity, hemolytic reactions, or methemoglobinemia with rasburicase. **Use with caution** in asthma, allergies, hypersensitivity with other medications, and children <2 yr (decreased efficacy and increased risk for rash, vomiting, diarrhea, and fever).

Common side effects include nausea, vomiting, abdominal pain, discomfort, diarrhea, constipation, mucositis, fever, and rash.

During therapy, uric acid blood samples must be sent to the laboratory immediately. Blood should be collected in prechilled tubes containing heparin, and placed in an ice-water bath to avoid potential falsely low uric acid levels (degradation of plasma uric acid occurs in the presence of rasburicase at room temperature). Centrifugation in a precooled centrifuge (4°C) is indicated. Plasma samples must be assayed within 4 hr of sample collection.

RH_0(D) IMMUNE GLOBULIN INTRAVENOUS (HUMAN)
WinRho-SDF
Immune Globulin

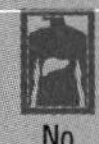 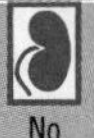  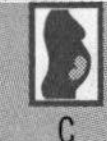 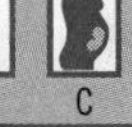

No No 1 C

Injection: 1500, 2500, 5000, 15,000 IU
Conversion: 1 mcg = 5 IU

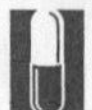

All doses based on international units (IU).
Immune thrombocytopenic purpura (nonsplenectomized Rh_0(D)-positive patients):
Initial dose (may be given in two divided doses on separate days or as a single dose):
- ***Hemoglobin ≥10 mg/dL:*** 250 IU/kg/dose IV × 1
- ***Hemoglobin <10 mg/dL:*** 125–200 IU/kg/dose IV × 1. See remarks for hemoglobin <8 mg/dL.

Additional doses: 125–300 IU/kg/dose IV; actual dose and frequency of adminstration is determined by the patient's response and subsequent hemoglobin level.

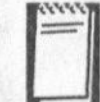

WinRho SDF is currently the only Rh_0(D) immune globulin product indicated for ITP. **Contraindicated** in IgA deficiency. **Use with extreme caution** in patients with a hemoglobin <8 mg/dL and thrombocytopenia or bleeding disorders. Adverse events associated with ITP include headache, chills, fever, and reduction in hemoglobin (due to the destruction of Rh_0(D) antigen-positive red cells). Intravascular hemolysis resulting in anemia and renal insufficiency has been reported. May interfere with immune response to live virus vaccines (e.g., MMR, varicella). Rh_0(D)-positive patients should be monitored for signs and symptoms of intravascular hemolysis, anemia, and renal insufficiency. Administer IV doses over 3–5 min.

RIBAVIRIN
Oral: Rebetol, Copegus, Ribaspheres, and others
Inhalation: Virazole
Antiviral agent

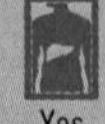 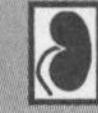 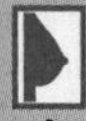 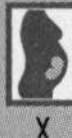

Yes Yes ? X

Oral solution (Rebetol): 200 mg/5 mL (120 mL); contains sodium benzoate
Oral caps (Rebetol, Ribaspheres): 200 mg
Tabs (Copegus, Ribaspheres): 200 mg
Aerosol (Virazole): 6 g

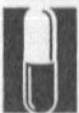

Hepatitis C (PO, see remarks):
***Child ≥3 yr** (in combination with interferon alfa-2b at 3 million units 3 × per wk SC; use oral solution or capsule):*

Continued

RIBAVIRIN *continued*

Child ≥3 yr (cont'd):

25–36 kg: 200 mg BID
37–49 kg: 200 mg QAM and 400 mg QPM
50–61 kg: 400 mg BID
>61–75 kg: 400 mg QAM and 600 mg QPM
>75 kg: 600 mg BID
Dosage modification for toxicity: See remarks.

Adult:

Oral capsules in combination with interferon alfa-2b at 3 million units 3 × per week SC:
≤75 kg: 400 mg QAM and 600 mg QPM
>75 kg: 600 mg BID
Oral capsules in combination with Peginterferon alfa-2b: 400 mg BID
Oral tablets in combination with Peginterferon alfa-2a for hepatitis C genotype 1, 4:
≤75 kg: 500 mg BID × 48 wk
>75 kg: 600 mg BID × 48 wk
Oral tablets in combination with Peginterferon alfa-2a for genotype 2, 3: 400 mg BID × 24 wk
Oral tablets in combination with Peginterferon alfa-2a for HIV coinfected patient (regardless of genotype): 400 mg BID × 48 wk
Dosage modification for toxicity: See remarks.

Inhalation:

Continuous: Administer 6 g by aerosol over 12–18 hr once daily for 3–7 days. The 6 g ribavirin vial is diluted in 300 mL preservative-free sterile water to a final concentration of 20 mg/mL. **Must be administered** with Viratek Small Particle Aerosol Generator (SPAG-2).

Intermittent (for non-ventilated patients): Administer 2 g by aerosol over 2 hr TID for 3–7 days. The 6 g ribavirin vial is diluted in 100 mL preservative-free sterile water to a final concentration of 60 mg/mL. The intermittent use is **not recommended** in patients with endotracheal tubes.

ORAL RIBAVIRIN: Contraindicated in pregnancy, significant or unstable cardiac disease, autoimmune hepatitis, hepatic decompensation (Child-Pugh score >6; class B or C), hemoglobinpathies, and creatinine clearance <50 mL/min. **Use with caution** in pre-exisiting cardiac disease, pulmonary disease, and sarcoidosis. Anemia (most common), insomnia, depression, irritability, and suicidal behavior (higher in adolescent and pediatric patients) have been reported with the oral route.

Tinnitus, hearing loss, vertigo, and severe hypertriglyceridemia have been reported in combination with interferon. Pancytopenia has been reported in combination with interferon and azathoprine. Increased risk for hepatic decompensation with cirrotic chronic hepatitis C patients treated with alpha interferons or with HIV co-infection receiving HAART and interferon alfa-2a.

May decrease the effects of zidovudine, stavudine; and increase risk for lactic acidosis with nucleoside analogues. **Reduce or discontinue dosage for toxicity as follows:**

Patient with no cardiac disease:

Hgb <10 g/dL and ≥8.5 g/dL:

Child: 12 mg/kg/dose PO once daily; may further reduce to 8 mg/kg/dose PO once daily.
Adult: 600 mg PO once daily (capsules or solution) or 200 mg PO QAM and 400 mg PO QPM (tablets).

Hgb <8.5 g/dL: Discontinue therapy permanently.

Patient with cardiac disease:

≥2 mg/dL decrease in Hgb during any 4-wk period during therapy:

Child: 12 mg/kg/dose PO once daily; may further reduce to 8 mg/kg/dose PO once daily (monitor weekly).

Continued

For explanation of icons, see p. 663.

RIBAVIRIN *continued*

Patient with cardiac disease (cont'd):

Adult: 600 mg PO once daily (capsules or solution) or 200 mg PO QAM and 400 mg PO QPM (tablets).

Hgb <12 g/dL after 4 wk of reduced dose: Discontinue therapy permanently.

INHALED RIBAVIRIN: Use of ribavirin for RSV is controversial and **not** routinely indicated. Aerosol therapy may be considered for selected infants and young children at high risk for serious RSV disease (see most recent edition of the AAP *Redbook*). Most effective if begun early in course of RSV infection; generally in the first 3 days. May cause worsening respiratory distress, rash, conjunctivitis, mild bronchospasm, hypotension, anemia, and cardiac arrest. **Avoid** unnecessary occupational exposure to ribavirin due to its teratogenic effects. Drug can precipitate in the respiratory equipment.

RIBOFLAVIN
Vitamin B_2 and various brands
Water-soluble vitamin

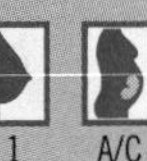

No No 1 A/C

Tabs [OTC]: 50, 100 mg

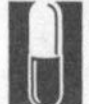

Riboflavin deficiency:

Child: 2.5–10 mg/24 hr ÷ once daily–BID PO

Adult: 5–30 mg/24 hr ÷ once daily–BID PO

U.S. RDA requirements: see Chapter 21.

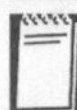

Hypersensitivity may occur. Administer with food. Causes yellow to orange discoloration of urine. For multivitamin information, see Chapter 21.

Pregnancy category changes to "C" if used in doses above the RDA.

RIFABUTIN
Mycobutin
Antituberculous agent

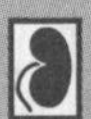
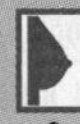
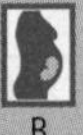

Yes Yes 3 B

Caps: 150 mg
Oral suspension: 20 mg/mL

MAC prophylaxis for first episode and recurrence of opportunistic disease in HIV (may be in combination with a macrolide antibiotic; see remarks for interactions and www.aidsinfo.nih.gov/guideline):

<6 yr: 5 mg/kg/24 hr PO once daily; **max. dose:** 300 mg/24 hr.

≥6 yr and adult: 300 mg PO once daily; doses may be administered as 150 mg PO BID if GI upset occurs.

MAC prophylaxis for recurrence of opportunistic disease in HIV (in combination with ethambutol and a macrolide antibiotic; see remarks for interactions):

Infant and child: 5 mg/kg/24 hr PO once daily; **max. dose:** 300 mg/24 hr.

Adolescent and adult: 300 mg PO once daily.

MAC treatment:

Child: 10–20 mg/kg/24 hr PO once daily or intermittently BID–TID; **max. dose:** 300 mg/24 hr as part of a multi-drug regimen.

Adult: 300 mg PO once daily; may be used in combination with azithromycin and ethambutol.

In combination with non-nucleoside reverse transcriptase inhibitors:

With efavirenz: 450 mg PO once daily or 600 mg PO 3× per wk.

With nevirapine: 300 mg PO 3× per wk.

Continued

RIFABUTIN *continued*

MAC treatment: Adult (cont'd):

In combination with protease inhibitors:

With amprenavir, indinavir, or nelfinavir: 150 mg PO once daily or 300 mg PO 3× per wk.

With ritonavir boosted regimens (e.g., saquinavir/ritonavir, or lopinavir/ritonavir): 150 mg PO once every other day or 150 mg PO 3× per wk.

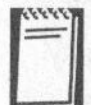

Should not be used for MAC prophylaxis with active TB. May cause GI distress, discoloration of skin and body fluids (brown-orange color), and marrow suppression. **Use with caution** in renal and liver impairment. **Adjust dose in renal impairment (see Chapter 31).** May permanently stain contact lenses. Uveitis can occur when using high doses (>300 mg/24 hr in adults) in combination with macrolide antibiotics.

Rifabutin is an inducer of CYP 450 3A enzyme and is structurally similar to rifampin (similar drug interactions, see *Rifampin*). Clarithromycin, fluconazole, itraconazole, nevirapine, and protease inhibitors increase rifabutin levels. Efavirenz may decrease rifabutin levels. May decrease effectiveness of dapsone, delavirdine, nevirapine, amprenavir, indinavir, nelfinavir, saquinavir, itraconazole, warfarin, oral contraceptives, digoxin, cyclosporine, ketoconazole, and narcotics.

Doses may be administered with food if patient experiences GI intolerance.

RIFAMPIN
Rimactane, Rifadin, and others
Antibiotic, antituberculous agent, rifamycin

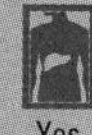

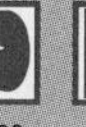

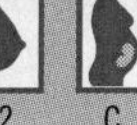

Yes Yes 2 C

Caps: 150, 300 mg
Oral suspension: 10, 15, 25 mg/mL
Injection: 600 mg

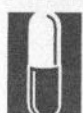

Staphylococcus aureus infections (as part of synergistic therapy with other antistaphylococcal agents):

0–1 mo:

IV: 10–20 mg/kg/24 hr ÷ Q12 hr

PO: 10–20 mg/kg/dose Q24 hr

>1 mo: 10–20 mg/kg/24 hr ÷ Q12 hr IV/PO; ***max. dose:*** 600 mg/24 hr

Adult: 300–600 mg Q12 hr IV/PO

Prosthetic valve endocarditis: 300 mg Q8 hr IV/PO in combination with antistaphylococcal penicillin with or without gentamicin for a minimum of 6 wk.

Tuberculosis (see latest edition of the AAP Red Book, for duration of therapy and combination therapy): Twice weekly therapy may be used after 1–2 mo of daily therapy

Infant, child, and adolescent:

Daily therapy: 10–20 mg/kg/24 hr ÷ Q12–24 hr IV/PO

Twice weekly therapy: 10–20 mg/kg/24 hr PO twice weekly

Max. daily dose: 600 mg/24 hr

Adult:

Daily therapy: 10 mg/kg/24 hr once daily PO

Twice weekly therapy: 10 mg/kg/24 hr once daily twice weekly

Max. daily dose: 600 mg/24 hr

Prophylaxis for N. meningitidis (see latest edition of the AAP Red Book for additional information):

0–<1 mo: 10 mg/kg/24 hr ÷ Q12 hr PO × 2 days

≥1 mo: 20 mg/kg/24 hr ÷ Q12 hr PO × 2 days

Adult: 600 mg PO Q12 hr × 2 days

Max. dose (all ages): 1200 mg/24 hr

Continued

For explanation of icons, see p. 663.

RIFAMPIN *continued*

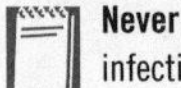

Never use as monotherapy except when used for prophylaxis. Patients with latent tuberculosis infection should not be treated with rifampin and pyrazinamide because of the risk of severe liver injury. Use is **not recommended** in porphyria. **Use with caution** in diabetes.

May cause GI irritation, allergy, headache, fatigue, ataxia, muscle weakness, confusion, fever, hepatitis, transient LFT abnormalities, blood dyscrasias, interstitial nephritis, and elevated BUN and uric acid. Causes red discoloration of body secretions such as urine, saliva, and tears (which can permanently stain contact lenses). Induces hepatic enzymes (CYP 450 2C9, 2C19, and 3A4) which may decrease plasma concentration of digoxin, corticosteroids, buspirone, benzodiazepines, fentanyl, calcium channel blockers, beta-blockers, cyclosporine, tacrolimus, itraconazole, ketoconazole, oral anticoagulants, barbiturates, and theophylline. May reduce the effectiveness of oral contraceptives and anti-retroviral agents (protease inhibitors and non-nucleoside reverse transcriptase inhibitors). Hepatotoxicity is a concern when used in combination with pyrazinamide and ritonavir-boosted saquinavir **(use is contraindicated).**

Adjust dose in renal failure (see Chapter 31). Reduce dose in hepatic impairment. Give 1 hr before or 2 hr after meals.

For *H. influenza* prophylaxis, see latest edition of the *Red Book.*

RIMANTADINE
Flumadine
Antiviral agent

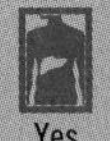
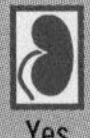
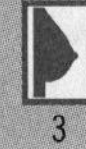
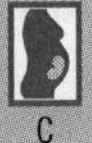

Yes Yes 3 C

Syrup: 50 mg/5 mL (240 mL); contains saccharin and parabens
Tabs: 100 mg

Influenza A prophylaxis (for at least 10 days after known exposure; usually for 6–8 wk during influenza A season or local outbreak):

Child:

- ***1–9 yr:*** 5 mg/kg/24 hr PO once daily; **max. dose:** 150 mg/24 hr
- ***≥10 yr:***
  - ***<40 kg:*** 5 mg/kg/24 hr PO ÷ BID; **max. dose:** 150 mg/24 hr
  - ***≥40 kg:*** 100 mg/dose PO BID

Adult: 100 mg PO BID

Influenza A treatment (within 48 hr of illness onset):

Use the aforementioned prophylaxis dosage × 5–7 days.

Resistance to influenza A and recommendations against the use for treatment and prophylaxis have been reported by the CDC. Check with local microbiology laboratories and the CDC for seasonal susceptibility/resistance.

Preferred over amantadine for influenza due to lower incidence of adverse events. Individuals immunized with live attenuated influenza vaccine (e.g., FluMist) should **not** receive rimantadine prophylaxis for 14 days after the vaccine. Chemoprophylaxis does not interfere with immune response to inactivated influenza vaccine.

May cause GI disturbance, xerostoma, dizziness, headache, and urinary retention. CNS disturbances are less than with amantadine. **Contraindicated** in amantadine hypersensitivity. **Use with caution** in renal or hepatic insufficiency; dosage reduction may be necessary. A dosage reduction of 50% has been recommended in severe hepatic or renal impairment. Subjects with severe renal impairment have been reported to have an 81% increase in systemic exposure.

RISPERIDONE
Risperdal, Risperdal M-Tab, and Risperdal Consta
Atypical antipsychotic, serotonin (5-HT_2) and dopamine (D_2) antagonist

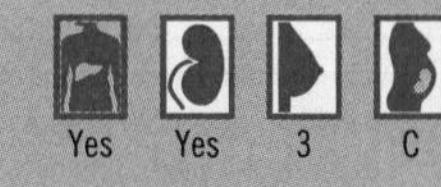

Tabs: 0.25, 0.5, 1, 2, 3, 4 mg
Oral solution: 1 mg/mL (30 mL)
Orally disintegrating tabs (Risperdal M-Tab): 0.5, 1, 2, 3, 4 mg; contains phenylalanine
Injection (Risperdal Consta): 25, 37.5, 50 mg (pre-filled syringe with 2 mL diluent); for IM administration only

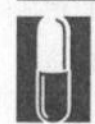

Irritability associated with autistic disorder:
5–16 yr (PO daily doses may be administer once daily–BID; patients experiencing somnolence may benefit from QHS or BID dosing or dose reduction):
Initial dose:
<20 kg: 0.25 mg/24 hr PO for a minimum of 4 days; use with caution if <15 kg as dosing recommendation is not established.
≥20 kg: 0.5 mg/24 hr PO for a minimum of 4 days.
Dose increment (if needed) after 4 days of initial dose:
<20 kg: 0.5 mg/24 hr PO for a minimum of 14 days, if additional increments needed, increase dose by 0.25 mg/24 hr at intervals of at least 14 days.
≥20 kg: 1 mg/24 hr PO for a minimum of 14 days, if additional increments needed, increase dose by 0.5 mg/24 hr at intervals of at least 14 days.
Max. daily dose for plateau of therapeutic effect (from one pivotal clinical trial):
<20 kg: 1 mg/24 hr
≥20–45 kg: 2.5 mg/24 hr
>45 kg: 3 mg/24 hr

Bipolar mania: Oral doses may be administer once daily–BID and patients experiencing somnolence may benefit from QHS or BID dosing or dose reduction. Long-term use beyond 3 wk and doses (all ages) >6 mg/24 hr have not been evaluated.
Child (10–17 yr): Start with 0.5 mg/24 hr PO once daily (QAM or QHS). If needed, increase dose at intervals not <24 hr in increments of 0.5 or 1 mg/24 hr, as tolerated, up to a recommended dose of 2.5 mg/24 hr. Although efficacy has been demonstrated between 0.5–6 mg/24 hr, no additional benefit was seen above 2.5 mg/24 hr. Higher doses were associated with more adverse effects.
Adult: Start with 2–3 mg PO once. Dosage increases or decreases of 1 mg/24 hr can be made at 24-hr intervals. Dosage range: 1–6 mg/24 hr.

Schizophrenia: Oral doses may be administered once daily–BID and patients experiencing somnolence may benefit from BID dosing (see remarks).
Adolescent (13–17 yr): No data are available to support long-term use of >8 wk.
PO: Start with 0.5 mg once daily (QAM or QHS). If needed, increase dose at intervals not <24 hr in increments of 0.5 to 1 mg/24 hr, as tolerated, to a recommended dose of 3 mg/24 hr. Although efficacy has been demonstrated between 1–6 mg/24 hr, no additional benefit was seen above 3 mg/24 hr. Doses >6 mg/24 hr have not been studied.
Adult:
PO: Start with 1 mg BID on day 1, if tolerated, increase to 2 mg BID on day 2 and to 3 mg BID thereafter. Dosage increases or decreases of 1–2 mg can be made on a weekly basis if needed. Usual effective dose: 2–8 mg/24 hr. Doses above 16 mg/24 hr have not been evaluated.
IM: Start with 25 mg Q2 wk; if no response, dose may be increased to 37.5 mg or 50 mg at 4-wk intervals. **Max. IM dose:** 50 mg Q2 wk.

Continued

For explanation of icons, see p. 663.

RISPERIDONE *continued*

Use with caution in cardiovascular disorders, diabetes, renal or hepatic impairment (dose reduction necessary), hypothermia or hyperthermia, seizures, breast cancer or other prolactin dependent tumors, and dysphagia. Common side effects include abdominal pain and other GI disturbances, arthralgia, anxiety, dizziness, headache, insomnia, somnolence (use QHS dosing), EPS, cough, fever, pharyngitis, rash, rhinitis, sexual dysfunction, tachycardia, and weight gain. Weight gain, somnolence, and fatigue were common side effects reported in the autism studies. Priapism, sleep apnea syndrome, urinary retention, diabetes mellitus, and hypoglycemia have been reported in post marketing reports.

In the presence of severe renal or hepatic impairment or risk for hypotension, the following adult dosing has been recommended: Start with 0.5 mg PO BID. Increase dose, if needed and tolerated, in increments no more than 0.5 mg BID. Increases to doses >1.5 mg BID should occur at intervals of at least 1 wk; slower titration may be required in some patients.

Limited studies in pediatric related Tourette's syndrome, schizophrenia, and aggressive behavior in psychiatric disorders are reported. Autistic disorder safety and efficacy in children <5 yr have not been established. If therapy has been discontinued for a period of time, therapy should be reinitiated with the same initial titration regimen.

Drug is a CYP 450 2D6 and 3A4 isoenzyme substrate. Concurrent use of isoenzyme inhibitors (e.g., fluoxetine, paroxetine, sertraline, cimetidine) and inducers (e.g., carbamazepine, rifampin, phenobarbital, phenytoin) may increase and decrease the effects of risperidone, respectively. Alcohol, CNS depressants, and St. John's wort may potentiate the drug's side effect. Risperidone may enhance the hypotensive effects of levodopa and dopamine agonists.

Oral dosage forms may be administered with or without food. Oral solution can be mixed in water, coffee, orange juice, or low-fat milk but is incompatible with cola or tea. **Do not** split or chew the orally disintegrating tablet. Use IM suspension preparation within 6 hr after reconstitution.

ROCURONIUM

Zemuron

Nondepolarizing neuromuscular blocking agent

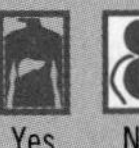 Yes 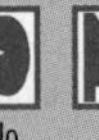 No 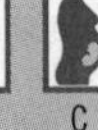 ? 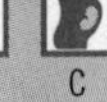 C

Injection: 10 mg/mL (5, 10 mL)

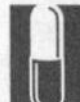

Use of a peripheral nerve stimulator to monitor drug effect is recommended.

Infant:

IV: 0.5 mg/kg/dose; may repeat Q20–30 min PRN.

Child:

IV: 0.6 mg/kg/dose × 1; if needed, give maintenance doses of 0.075–0.125 mg/kg/dose Q 20–30 min.

Adolescent and adult:

IV: Start with 0.6–1.2 mg/kg/dose × 1; if needed, maintenance doses at 0.1–0.2 mg/kg/dose Q20–30 min.

Continuous IV infusion:

Child and adult: Start at 7–10 mcg/kg/min and titrate to effect. Maintenance infusion rates have ranged from 4–16 mcg/kg/min in adults.

Use with caution in hepatic impairment and history of anaphylaxis with other neuromuscular blocking agents. Hypertension, hypotension, arrhythmia, tachycardia, nausea, vomiting, bronchospasm, wheezing, hiccups, rash, and edema at the injection site may occur. Myopathy after long-term use in an ICU, and QT interval prolongation in pediatric patients receiving general anestetic agents have been reported. Increased neuromuscular blockade may occur with

Continued

ROCURONIUM *continued*

concomitant use of aminoglycosides, clindamycin, tetracycline, magnesium sulfate, quinine, quinidine, succinylcholine, and inhalation anesthetics (for continuous infusion, reduce infusion by 30%–50% at 45–60 min after intubating dose).

Caffeine, calcium, carbamazepine, phenytoin, phenylephrine, azathioprine, and theophylline may reduce neuromuscular blocking effects.

Use must be accompanied by adequate anesthesia or sedation. Peak effects occur in 0.5–1 min for children and in 1–3.7 min for adults. Duration of action: 30–40 min in children and 20–94 min in adults (longer in geriatrics). Recovery time in children 3 mo to 1 yr is simular to adults. To prevent residual paralysis, extubate patient only after the patient has sufficiently recovered from neuromuscular blockade. In obese patients, use actual body weight for dosage calculation.

SALMETEROL
Serevent Diskus
Beta-2-adrenergic agonist (long acting)

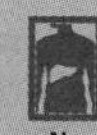
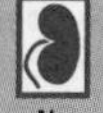
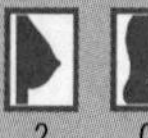

No No 2 C

Dry powder inhalation (DPI; Diskus): 50 mcg/inhalation (28, 60 inhalations)
In combination with fluticasone: see *Fluticasone Propionate* and *Salmeterol*

Persistent asthma (see remarks):
≥4 yr and adult: 1 inhalation (50 mcg) Q12 hr
Prevention of exercise-induced bronchospasm:
≥4 yr and adult: 1 inhalation 30–60 min before exercise. Additional doses should not be used for another 12 hr. Patients who are already using Q12 hr dosing for persistent asthma, should not use additional salmeterol doses for this indication and use alternative therapy (e.g., cromolyn) prior to exercise.

For long-term asthma control, should be used in combination with inhaled corticosteroids. **Should not be used to relieve symptoms of acute asthma.** It is long acting and has its onset of action in 10–20 min with a peak effect at 3 hr. May be used QHS (1 inhalation of the DPI) for nocturnal symptoms. Salmeterol is a chronic medication and is not used in similar fashion to short-acting beta agonists (e.g., albuterol). Patients already receiving salmeterol Q12 hr should not use additional doses for prevention of exercise-induced bronchospasm; consider alternative therapy. Asthma exacerbations or hospitalizations were reported to be lower when used with an inhaled corticosteroid.

WARNING: Long-acting beta-2-agonists may increase the risk of asthma-related death. A subgroup analysis suggested higher risk in African-American patients compared to Caucasians. Use salmeterol only as additional therapy for patients not adequately controlled on other asthma-controller medications (e.g., low- to medium-dose inhaled corticosteroids) or whose disease severity clearly requires initiation of treatment with 2 maintenance therapies.

Should not be used in conjunction with an inhaled, long-acting beta-2 agonist and is **not** a substitute for inhaled or systemic corticosteroid. Use with strong CYP 3A4 inhibitors (e.g., ketoconazole, HIV protease inhibitors, clarithromycin, itraconazole, nefazodone, and telithromycin) are not recommended due to risk for cardiovascular adverse events (e.g., QTc prolongation, tachycardia). Salmeterol is a P450 3A4 substrate.

Proper patient education is essential. Side effects are similar to albuterol. Hypertension and arrhythmias have been reported. See Chapter 24 for recommendations for asthma controller therapy.

For explanation of icons, see p. 663.

SCOPOLAMINE HYDROBROMIDE
Transderm Scop, Isopto Hyoscine, Scopace, and others
Anticholinergic agent

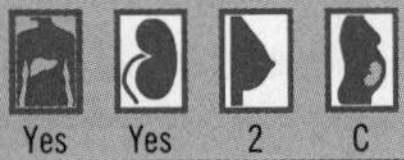

Injection: 0.4 mg/mL (1 mL); may contain alcohol
Transdermal: 1.5 mg/patch (10s and 24s); delivers ~1 mg over 3 days
Ophthalmic solution (Isopto Hyoscine): 0.25% (5 mL); contains benzalkonium chloride
Tabs, soluble (Scopace): 0.4 mg

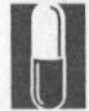

Antiemetic (SC/IM/IV):
Child: 6 mcg/kg/dose Q6–8 hr PRN; **max. dose:** 300 mcg/dose
Adult: 0.32–0.65 mg/dose Q6–8 hr PRN

Transdermal (≥12 yr) (see remarks):
Motion sickness: Apply patch behind the ear at least 4 hr prior to exposure to motion; remove after 72 hr.
Antiemetic prior to surgery: Apply patch behind the ear the evening before surgery.
Antiemetic prior to cesarean section: Apply patch behind the ear 1 hr prior to surgery to minimize infant exposure.

Ophthalmic:
Child refraction: 1 drop BID for 2 days before procedure.
Child iridocyclitis: 1 drop up to TID.

Toxicities similar to atropine. **Contraindicated** in urinary or GI obstruction and glaucoma. **Use with caution** in hepatic or renal dysfunction, cardiac disease, seizures, or psychoses. May cause dry mouth, drowsiness, and blurred vision.

Transdermal route should **NOT** be used in children <12 yr. Drug withdrawal symptoms (nausea, vomiting, headache, and vertigo) have been reported following removal of transdermal patch in patients using the patch for >3 days. For perioperative use, the patch should be kept in place for 24 hr following surgery. Systemic effects have been reported with both transdermal and ophthalmic preparations. Compress nasolacrimal ducts to minimize systemic effects when using ophthalmic preparations.

SELENIUM SULFIDE
Selsun and others
Topical antiseborrheic agent

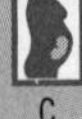

No No 2 C

Lotion/Shampoo: 1% [OTC] (210, 325, 400 mL)
Lotion: 2.5% (120 mL)

Seborrhea/Dandruff (≥2 yr): Massage 5–10 mL of 1% or 2.5% into wet scalp and leave on scalp × 2–3 min. Rinse thoroughly and repeat. Shampoo twice weekly × 2 wk. Maintenance applications once every 1–4 wk.
Tinea versicolor (≥2 yr): Apply 2.5% lotion to affected areas of skin. Allow to remain on skin × 30 min for children and 10 min adults. Rinse thoroughly. Repeat once daily × 7 days. Follow with monthly applications for 3 mo to prevent recurrences.

Rinse hands and body well after treatment. May cause local irritation, hair loss, and hair discoloration. **Avoid** eyes, genital areas, and skin folds. Shampoo may be used for tinea capitis to reduce risk of transmission to others (does **not** eradicate tinea infection).

For tinea versicolor, 15%–25% sodium hyposulfite or thiosulfate (Tinver lotion) applied to affected areas BID × 2–4 wk is an alternative. Topical antifungals (e.g., clotrimazole, miconazole) may be used for small, focal infections. **Do not use** for tinea versicolor during pregnancy.

SENNA/SENNOSIDES
Senokot, Senna-Gen, Lax-Pills, Fletcher's Castoria, and many others
Laxative, stimulant

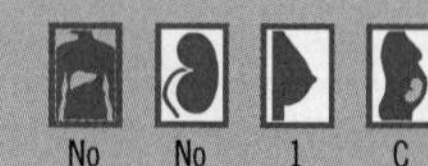

Based on mg of senna (all products are OTC):

Granules: 326 mg/tsp
Syrup: 176 mg/5 mL, 218 mg/5 mL (60 mL, 240 mL)
Tabs: 187, 217, 374 mg
Liquid concentrate (Fletcher's Castoria): 33.3 mg/mL (75 mL); contains sodium benzoate
187 mg senna extract is approximately 8.6 mg sennosides.

Based on mg of sennosides (all products are OTC):

Granules: 15 mg/tsp, 20 mg/tsp
Syrup: 8.8 mg/5 mL (60 mL, 240 mL)
Tabs: 6, 8.6, 15, 17, 25 mg
Chewable tabs: 10, 15 mg
8.6 mg sennosides is approximately 187 mg senna extract.

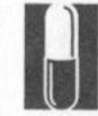

Constipation:
Dosing based on mg senna:
Child:

Oral: 10–20 mg/kg/dose PO QHS (**max. dose:** as shown below) or dosage by age:
- ***1 mo–1 yr:*** 55–109 mg PO QHS to **max. dose:** 218 mg/24 hr
- ***1–5 yr:*** 109–218 mg PO QHS to **max. dose:** 436 mg/24 hr
- ***5–15 yr:*** 218–436 mg PO QHS to **max. dose:** 872 mg/24 hr

Adult:

Granules: 326 mg (1 tsp) PO at bedtime; **max. dose:** 652 mg (2 tsp) BID
Syrup: 436–654 mg PO at bedtime; **max. dose:** 654 mg (15 mL) BID
Tabs: 374 mg PO at bedtime; **max. dose:** 748 mg BID

Dosing based on mg sennosides:
Child:

Syrup:
- ***1 mo–2 yr:*** 2.2–4.4 mg (1.25–2.5 mL) PO QHS to **max. dose:** 8.8 mg/24 hr
- ***2–5 yr:*** 4.4–6.6 mg (2.5–3.75 mL) PO QHS to **max. dose:** 6.6 mg BID
- ***6–12 yr:*** 8.8–13.2 mg (5–7.5 mL) PO QHS to **max. dose:** 13.2 mg BID

Tabs:
- ***2–5 yr:*** 4.3 mg PO QHS to **max. dose:** 8.6 mg BID
- ***6–12 yr:*** 8.6 mg PO QHS to **max. dose:** 17.2 mg BID

>12 yr and adult:

Granules: 15 mg PO QHS to **max. dose:** 30 mg BID
Syrup: 17.6–26.4 mg (10–15 mL) PO QHS to **max. dose:** 26.4 mg BID
Tabs: 17.2 mg PO QHS to **max. dose:** 34.4 mg BID

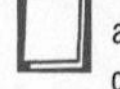

Effects occur within 6–24 hr after oral administration. Prolonged use (>1 wk) should be avoided as it may lead to dependency. May cause nausea, vomiting, diarrhea, abdominal cramps. Active metabolite stimulates Auerbach's plexus. Syrup may be adminstered with juice, milk, or mixed with ice cream. Granules may be sprinkled onto food or mixed with drinks.

For explanation of icons, see p. 663.

SERTRALINE HCL
Zoloft and generics
Antidepressant (selective serotonin reuptake inhibitor)

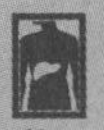 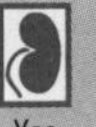 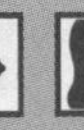 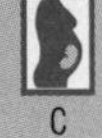
Yes Yes 2 C

Tabs: 25, 50, 100 mg
Oral concentrate solution: 20 mg/mL (60 mL); contains alcohol and menthol

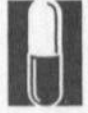

Depression:

Child ≥6–12 yr (data limited in this age group): Start at 12.5–25 mg PO once daily. May increase dosage by 25 mg at 1-wk intervals up to a **max. dose** of 200 mg/24 hr.

Child ≥13 yr and adult: Start at 25–50 mg PO once daily. May increase dosage by 50 mg at 1-wk intervals up to a **max. dose** of 200 mg/24 hr.

Obesessive compulsive disorder:

Child ≥6–12 yr: Start at 25 mg PO once daily. May increase dosage by 25 mg at 3–4 day intervals or by 50 mg at 7-day intervals up to a **max. dose** of 200 mg/24 hr.

Child ≥13 yr and adult: Start at 50 mg PO once dialy. May increase dosage by 50 mg at 1-wk intervals up to **max. dose** of 200 mg/24 hr.

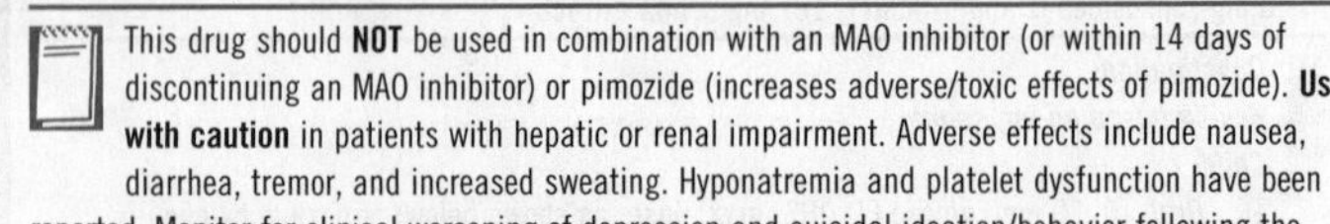

This drug should **NOT** be used in combination with an MAO inhibitor (or within 14 days of discontinuing an MAO inhibitor) or pimozide (increases adverse/toxic effects of pimozide). **Use with caution** in patients with hepatic or renal impairment. Adverse effects include nausea, diarrhea, tremor, and increased sweating. Hyponatremia and platelet dysfunction have been reported. Monitor for clinical worsening of depression and suicidal ideation/behavior following the initiation of therapy or after dose changes.

Use with drugs that interfere with hemostasis (e.g., NSAIDs, aspirin, and warfarin) may increase risk for GI bleeds. Use with warfarin may increase PT. Inhibits the CYP 450 2D6 drug metabolizing enzyme. Serotonin syndrome may occur when taken with selective serotonin reuptake inhibitors (e.g., amitriptyline, amphetamines, buspirone, dihydroergotamine, sumatriptan, sympathomimetics).

Mix oral concentrate solution with 4 oz. of water, ginger ale, lemon/lime soda, lemonade, or orange juice. After mixing, a slight haze may appear; this is normal. This dosage form should be **used cautiously** in patients with latex allergy because the dropper contains dry natural rubber.

SILDENAFIL
Revatio, Viagra
Phosphodiesterase type-5 (PDE5) inhibitor

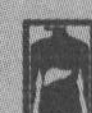 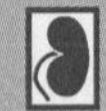  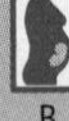
Yes Yes ? B

Tabs:

Revatio: 20 mg

Viagra: 25, 50, 100 mg

Oral suspension: 2.5 mg/mL

Injection:

Revatio: 4 mg/mL (2.5 mL)

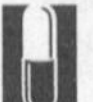

Pulmonary hypertension:

Neonate (limited data from case reports and small clinical trials):

PO: Several dosages have been reported and have ranged from 0.5–3 mg/kg/dose Q6–12 hr PO. A single ~0.3 mg/kg/dose PO has been used in select patients to facilitate weaning from inhaled nitric oxide.

IV (case report from 4 neonates >34 wk gestation and <72 hr old): Start with 0.4 mg/kg/dose IV over 3 hr followed by a continuous infusion of 1.6 mg/kg/24 hr (0.067 mg/kg/hr) for up to 7 days.

Continued

Infant and child:

Child 1–17 yr (results from a 16 week dose-ranging study in 235 treatment naïve children > 8 kg with pulmonary arterial hypertension, see remarks):

PO:

>8–20 kg: 10–20 mg TID
> 20–45 kg: 20–40 mg TID
> 45 kg: 40–80 mg TID

PO: Several dosages have been reported. Start at 0.25–0.5 mg/kg/dose Q4–8 hr PO; if needed and tolerated, increase to 1 mg/kg/dose Q4–8 hr PO. Doses as high as 2 mg/kg/dose Q4 hr PO have been given in case reports. A single ~0.4 mg/kg/dose PO has been used in select patients to facilitate weaning from inhaled nitric oxide.

Contraindicated with concurrent use of nitrates (e.g., nitroglycerin) and other nitric oxide donors; potentiates hypotensive effects. **Use with caution** in sepsis (high levels of cGMP may potentiate hypotension), and with concurrent CYP 450 3A4 inhibiting medications (see discussion that follows) and anti-hypertensive medications. Hepatic insufficiency or severe renal impairment (GFR <30 mL/min) significantly reduces sildenafil clearance.

Findings from the dose-ranging study in 1–17 year old with pulmonary arterial hypertension: Headache, pyrexia, URTIs, vomiting and diarrhea were the most frequently reported side effect. Optimal dosing based on age and body weight still needs to be determined.

In adults, a transient impairment of color discrimination may occur; this effect could increase risk of severe retinopathy of prematurity in neonates. Common side effects reported in adults have included flushing, rash, diarrhea, indigestion, headache, abnormal vision, and nasal congestion. Hearing loss has been reported.

Sildenafil is substrate for CYP 450 3A4 (major) and 2C8/9 (minor). Azole antifungals, cimetidine, ciprofloxacin, clarithromycin, erythromycin, nicardipine, propofol, protease inhibitors, quinidine, verapamil, and grapefruit juice may increase the effects/toxicity of sildenafil. Bosentin, efavirenz, carbamazepine, phenobarbital, phenytoin, rifampin, St. John's wort, and high-fat meals decreases sildenafil effects.

SILVER SULFADIAZINE

Silvadene, Thermazene, SSD Cream, SSD AF Cream
Topical antibiotic

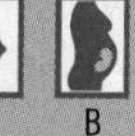

Cream: 1% (20, 25, 50, 85, 400, 1000 g); contains methylparabens

Child and adult: Cover affected areas completely once daily–BID. Apply cream to a thickness of ⅟₁₆ inch using sterile technique.

Contraindicated in premature infants and infant ≤ to 2 mo of age due to concerns of kernicterus; and pregnancy (approaching term). **Use with caution** in G6PD and renal and hepatic impairment. Discard product if cream has darkened. Significant systemic absorption may occur in severe burns. Adverse effects include pruritus, rash, bone marrow suppression, hemolytic anemia, and interstitial nephritis. **NOT** for ophthalmic use. See Chapter 4 for more information.

SIMETHICONE

Mylicon, Phazyme, Mylanta Gas, Gas-X, and others
Antiflatulent

No No 1 C

All dosage forms available OTC
Oral drops: 40 mg/0.6 mL (30 mL)
Caps: 125, 180 mg
Tabs: 60, 95 mg
Chewable tabs: 80, 125 mg
Strip, orally disintegrating: 62.5 mg (18s)

For explanation of icons, see p. 663.

SIMETHICONE *continued*

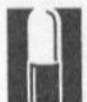

Infant and child <2 yr: 20 mg PO QID PRN; **max. dose:** 240 mg/24 hr
2–12 yr: 40 mg PO QID PRN
>12 yr and adult: 40–250 mg PO QPC and QHS PRN; **max. dose:** 500 mg/24 hr

Efficacy has not been demonstrated for treating infant colic. **Avoid** carbonated beverages and gas-forming foods. Oral liquid may be mixed with water, infant formula, or other suitable liquids for ease of oral administration.

SIROLIMUS
Rapamune
Immunosuppressant agent

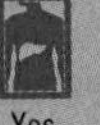 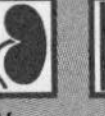 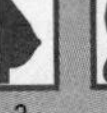 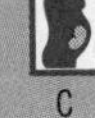

Yes Yes 3 C

Tabs: 1, 2 mg
Oral solution: 1 mg/mL (60 mL); contains 1.5-2.5% ethanol

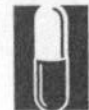

Child ≥13 yr and <40 kg: 3 mg/m²/dose PO × 1 immediately after transplantation, followed by 1 mg/m²/24 hr PO ÷ Q12–24 hr on the next day. Adjust dose to achieve desired trough blood levels.

Adult:

Patients at low/moderate immunologic risk:

In combination with cyclosporine (adjust dose to achieve desired trough blood levels):

<40 kg: 3 mg/m²/dose PO × 1 immediately after transplantation, followed by 1 mg/m²/dose PO once daily on the next day

≥40 kg: 6 mg PO × 1 immediately after transplantation, followed by 2 mg PO once daily on the next day.

Patients at high immunologic risk:

In combination with cyclosporine (withdrawal of cyclosporine is not recommended): 15 mg PO × 1 immediately after transplantation, followed by 5 mg PO once daily on the next day. Adjust dose to achieve desired trough blood levels.

Increased susceptibility to infection and development of lymphoma may result from immunosupression. **Fatal** bronchial anastomotic dehiscence has been reported in lung transplantation. Excess mortality, graft loss, and hepatic artery thrombosis have been reported in liver transplantation when used with tacrolimus. Patients with the greatest amount of urinary protein excretion prior to sirolimus conversion were those whose protein excretion increased the most after conversion. Increase risk of BK virus associated nephropathies have been reported. Increased mortality in stable liver transplant patients has been reported after conversion from a calcineurin inhibitor-based regimen to sirolimus.

Monitor whole blood trough levels (just prior to a dose at steady-state); especially with pediatric patients; hepatic impairment; concurrent use of CYP 450 3A4 and/or P-gp inducers and inhibitors; and/or if cyclosporine dosage is markedly changed or discontinued. Steady-state is generally achieved after 5–7 days of continuous dosing. Interpretation will vary based on specific treatment protocol and assay methodology (HPLC vs. immunoassay vs. LC/MS/MS). Younger children may exhibit faster siolimus clearance compared to adolescents.

Sirolimus is a substrate for CYP 450 3A4 and P-gp. Cyclosporine, diltiazem, protease inhibitors, erythromycin, grapefruit juice, and other inhibitors of CYP 3A4 may increase the toxicity of sirolimus. Phenobarbital, carbamazepine, phenytoin, and St John's wort may decrease the effects of sirolimus. Strong inhibitors (e.g., azole antifungals and clarithromycin) and strong inducers (e.g., rifamycins) are **not recommended.**

Continued

SIROLIMUS *continued*

Hypertension, peripheral edema, increase serum creatinine, dyspnea, epistaxis, headache, anemia, thrombocytopenia, hyperlipidemia, hypercholesterolemia, and arthralgia may occur. Urinary tract infections have been reported in pediatric renal transplant patients with high immunologic risk.

2 mg of the oral solution has been demonstrated to be clinically equivalent to the 2 mg tablets. However, it is not known whether they are still therapeutically equivalent at higher doses. Reduce maintenance dosage by ⅓ in the presence of hepatic function impairment. Administer doses consistently with or without food. When administered with cyclosporine, give dose 4 hr after cyclosporine. **Do not** crush or split tablets. Measure the oral liquid dosage form with an amber oral syringe and dilute in a cup with 60 mL of water or orange juice only. Take dose immediately after mixing, add/mix additional 120 mL diluent into the cup, and drink immediately after mixing.

SODIUM BICARBONATE
Neut and many other generics
Alkalinizing agent, electrolyte

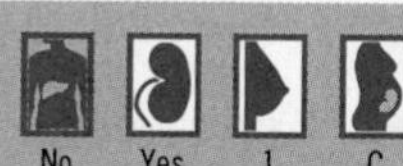

Injection: 4% (Neut) (0.48 mEq/mL) (5 mL), 4.2% (0.5 mEq/mL) (10 mL), 7.5% (0.89 mEq/mL) (50 mL), 8.4% (1 mEq/mL) (10, 50 mL)
Injection, pre-mixed: 5% (0.6 mEq/mL) (500 mL)
Tabs: 325 mg (3.8 mEq), 650 mg (7.6 mEq)
Powder: 120, 480 g; contains 30 mEq Na^+ per ½ teaspoon
Each 1 mEq bicarbonate provides 1 mEq Na^+.

Cardiac arrest: See Resuscitation Medications on page ii.
Correction of metabolic acidosis: Calculate patient's dose with the following formulas.

Neonate, infant, and child:

HCO_3^- (mEq) = 0.3 × weight (kg) × base deficit (mEq/L), **OR**
HCO_3^- (mEq) = 0.5 × weight (kg) × [24 – serum HCO_3^- (mEq/L)]

Adult:

HCO_3^- (mEq) = 0.2 × weight (kg) × base deficit (mEq/L), **OR**
HCO_3^- (mEq) = 0.5 × weight (kg) × [24 – serum HCO_3^- (mEq/L)]

Urinary alkalinization (titrate dose accordingly to urine pH):

Child: 84–840 mg (1–10 mEq)/kg/24 hr PO ÷ QID
Adult: 4 g (48 mEq) × 1 followed by 1–2 g (12–24 mEq) PO Q4 hr. Doses up to 16 g (192 mEq)/24 hr have been used.

Contraindicated in respiratory alkalosis, hypochloremia, and inadequate ventilation during cardiac arrest. **Use with caution** in CHF, renal impairment, cirrhosis, hypocalcemia, hypertension, and concurrent corticosteroids. Maintain high urine output. Monitor acid-base balance and serum electrolytes. May cause hypernatremia (contains sodium), hypokalemia, hypomagnesemia, hypocalcemia, hyperreflexia, edema, and tissue necrosis (extravasation). Oral route of administration may cause GI discomfort and gastric rupture from gas production.

For direct IV administration (cardiac arrest) in neonates and infants, use the 0.5 mEq/mL (4.2%) concentration or dilute the 1 mEq/mL (8.4%) concentration 1 : 1 with sterile water for injection and infuse at a rate **no greater than** 10 mEq/min. The 1 mEq/mL (8.4%) concentration may be used in children and adults for direct IV administration.

For IV infusions (for all ages), dilute to a **max. concentration** of 0.5 mEq/mL in dextrose or sterile water for injection and infuse over 2 hr using a **max. rate** of 1 mEq/kg/hr.

Sodium bicarbonate should **not** be mixed with or be in contact with calcium, norepinephrine, or dobutamine.

For explanation of icons, see p. 663.

SODIUM CHLORIDE—INHALED PREPARATIONS
Hypersal, Simply Saline, Ocean, Ayr Saline, Rhinaris, and many other brands
Electrolyte, inhalation

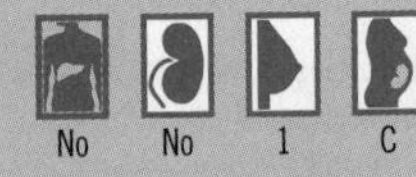

Nebulized solution: 0.9% (5 mL), 3% (15 mL)
Hypersal (preservative-free): 3.5% (4 mL), 7% (4 mL)
Nasal solution spray/drops/mist (OTC): 0.2% (30 mL), 0.4% (15, 50 mL), 0.65% (15, 30, 45 mL), 0.75% (20, 50 mL), 0.9% (45, 90 mL), 3% (44 mL)
Nasal gel: 0.2% (28.4 g), 0.65% (30 g), 3% (20 g)

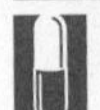

Intranasal as moisturizer:
Child and adult:
Spray/Mist: 2–6 sprays into each nostril Q2 hr PRN.
Drops: 2–6 drops into each nostril Q2 hr PRN.
Nasal gel: Use PRN to relieve nasal discomfort. Use at bedtime helps in preventing drying and crusting.

Cystic Fibrosis (Pre-treatment with albuterol is recommended to prevent bronchospasms; see remarks):
≥6 yr and adult: Nebulize 4 mL of 7% solution once daily–BID. If unable to tolerate the 7% strength, lower strengths of 3%, 3.5% or 5% may be used.

Acute viral bronchiolitis (for hospitalized patients only; pre-treatment with albuterol is recommended to prevent bronchospasms; see remarks):
Infant (>34 wk gestation up to 18 mo old): Nebulize 4 mL of 3% solution Q2 hr × 3 doses followed by Q4 hr × 5 doses, followed by Q6 hr until discharge.

INTRANASAL USE: May be used as a nasal wash for sinuses, restore moisture, thin nasal secretions, or relieve dry, crusted, and inflamed nasal membranes from colds, low humidity, allergies, nasal decongestant overuse, minor nose bleeds, and other irritations. Nasal adminstration instructions:
Nasal drops: Tilt head back and hold bottle upside down.
Nasal spray: Hold head in upright position and give short, firm squeezes into each nostril. Sniff deeply.
Nasal gel: Apply around nostrils, under nose, or in nostrils as needed to help relieve discomfort.

NEBULIZATION: Hypertonic solutions lowers sputum viscosity and enhances mucociliary clearance.

Cystic Fibrosis: Improves FEV_1 and reduces pulmonary exacerbation frequency. May cause bronchospasm, cough, pharyngitis, hempotysis, and acute decline in pulmonary function (administer first dose in a medical facility). It is recommended to withhold therapy in the presence of massive hemoptysis.

Acute viral bronchiolitis: Reduces length of hospitalization when compared to normal saline. May cause acute bronchospasm and local irritation.

SODIUM PHOSPHATE
Fleet, Fleet Phospho-Soda, Visicol, OsmoPrep, and others
Laxative, enema/oral

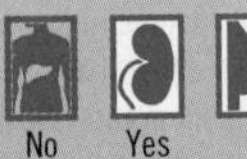
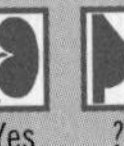
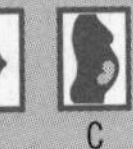
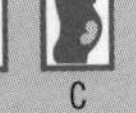

Enema (Fleet) [OTC]: 7 g dibasic sodium phosphate and 19 g monobasic sodium phosphate/118 mL; contains 4.4 g sodium per 118 mL
Pediatric size: 66 mL
Adult size: 133 mL

Continued

SODIUM PHOSPHATE *continued*

Oral solution (Fleet Phospho-Soda) [OTC]: 2.4 g monobasic sodium phosphate and 0.9 g dibasic sodium phosphate/5 mL (45, 90, 240 mL); contains 96.4 mEq Na per 20 mL and 62.25 mEq phospate/5 mL
Oral tablets (Visicol, OsmoPrep): 1.5 g

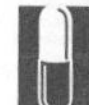

Not to be used for phosphorus supplementation. See *Phosphorus Supplements.*
Enema (see remarks):
2–12 yr: 66 mL enema × 1. May repeat × 1.
>12 yr and adult: 133 mL enema × 1. May repeat × 1.
Oral laxative (Fleet Phospho-Soda); mix with equal volume of water:
5–9 yr: 5 mL PO × 1
10–12 yr: 10 mL PO × 1
≥12 yr and adult: 20–30 mL PO × 1

Contraindicated in patients with severe renal failure, megacolon, bowel obstruction, and congestive heart failure. May cause hyperphosphatemia, hypernatremia, hypocalcemia, hypotension, dehydration, and acidosis. **Avoid** retention of enema solution and **do not exceed** recommended doses, as this may lead to severe electrolyte disturbances due to enhanced systemic absorption. Rare but serious form of kidney failure (acute phosphate nephropathy) has been reported with the use of bowel cleansing preparations such as Fleet Phospho-Soda and Visicol.

Onset of action: PO, 3–6 hr; PR, 2–5 min.

SODIUM POLYSTYRENE SULFONATE
Kayexalate, SPS, Kionex, and others
Potassium-removing resin

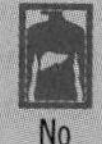
No
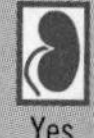
Yes

2
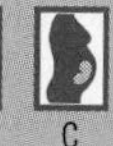
C

Powder: 454, 480 g
Suspension: 15 g/60 mL (60, 500 mL); contains 21.5 mL sorbitol per 60 mL and 0.1%–0.3% alcohol
Contains 4.1 mEq Na^+/g drug.

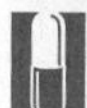

Infant and child:
Usual dose: 1 g/kg/dose Q6 hr PO or Q2–6 hr PR
Adult:
PO: 15 g once daily–QID
PR: 30–50 g Q6 hr

NOTE: Suspension may be given PO or PR. Practical exchange ratio is 1 mEq K per 1 g resin. May calculate dose according to desired exchange.

Contraindicated in obstructive bowel disease, neonates with reduced gut motility, and oral administration in neonates. **Use cautiously** in presence of renal failure, CHF, hypertension, or severe edema. May cause hypokalemia, hypernatremia, hypomagnesemia, and hypocalcemia. Cases of colonic necrosis, GI bleeding, ischemic colitis, and perforation have been reported with the concomitant use of sorbitol in patients with GI risk factors (prematurity, history of intestinal disease or surgery hypovolemia, and renal insufficieny/failure).

1 mEq Na delivered for each mEq K removed. **Do not administer** with antacids or laxatives containing Mg^{2+} or Al^{3+}. Systemic alkalosis may result. Retain enema in colon for at least 30–60 min.

For explanation of icons, see p. 663.

SPIRONOLACTONE
Aldactone and others
Diuretic, potassium sparing

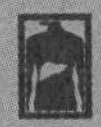 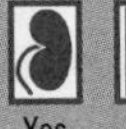 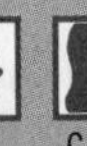 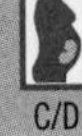
Yes Yes 1 C/D

Tabs: 25, 50, 100 mg
Oral suspension: 1, 2, 2.5, 5, 10, 25 mg/mL 

Diuretic:
Neonate: 1–3 mg/kg/24 hr ÷ once daily–BID PO
Child: 1–3.3 mg/kg/24 hr ÷ once daily–QID PO
Adult: 25–200 mg/24 hr ÷ once daily–QID PO (see remarks)
Max. dose: 200 mg/24 hr

Diagnosis of primary aldosteronism:
Child: 125–375 mg/m²/24 hr ÷ BID–QID PO
Adult: 400 mg once daily PO × 4 days (short test) or 3–4 wk (long test), then 100–400 mg once daily maintenance.

Hirsutism in women:
Adult: 50–200 mg/24 hr ÷ once daily–BID PO

Contraindicated in severe renal failure (see Chapter 31). Use with caution in dehydration, hyponatremia, and renal or hepatic dysfunction. May cause hyperkalemia (especially with severe heart failure), GI distress, rash, and gynecomastia. May potentiate ganglionic blocking agents and other antihypertensives. Monitor potassium levels and be aware of other K^+ sources, K^+ sparing diuretics, and angiotensin-converting enzyme inhibitors (all can increase K^+). May cause false elevation in serum digoxin levels measured by radioimmuneassay.

Although TID–QID regimens have been recommended, data suggests once daily–BID dosing to be adequate. Pregnancy category changes to "D" if used in pregnancy induced hypertension.

STREPTOMYCIN SULFATE
Various
Antibiotic, aminoglycoside; antituberculous agent

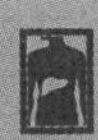 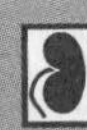 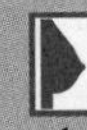 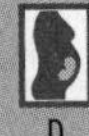
No Yes 1 D

Powder for injection: 1 g

Tuberculosis: Use as part of multidrug regimen; see latest edition of AAP *Red Book*
Infant, child, and adolescent:
Daily therapy: 20–40 mg/kg/24 hr IM once daily
Max. daily dose: 1 g/24 hr
Twice weekly therapy: 20–40 mg/kg/dose IM twice weekly under direct observation
Max. daily dose: 1.5 g/24 hr

Adult:
Daily therapy: 15 mg/kg/24 hr IM once daily
Max. daily dose: 1 g/24 hr
Twice weekly therapy: 25–30 mg/kg/dose IM twice weekly under direct observation
Max. daily dose: 1.5 g/24 hr

Brucellosis, tularemia, plague, and rat bite fever: See latest edition of the *Red Book.*

Contraindicated with aminoglycoside and sulfite hypersensitivity. **Use with caution** in pre-existing vertigo, tinnitus, hearing loss, and neuromuscular disorders. Drug is administered via deep IM injection only. Follow auditory status. May cause CNS depression, other neurologic

Continued

STREPTOMYCIN SULFATE *continued*

problems, myocarditis, serum sickness, nephrotoxicity, and ototoxicity. Concomitant neurotoxic, ototoxic, or nephrotoxic drugs and dehydration may increase risk for toxicity.

Therapeutic levels: peak 15–40 mg/L; trough: <5 mg/L. Recommended serum sampling time at steady-state: trough within 30 min prior to the third consecutive dose and peak 30–60 min after the administration of the third consecutive dose. Therapeutic levels are **not** achieved in CSF.

Adjust dose in renal failure (see Chapter 31).

SUCCIMER
Chemet, DMSA [dimercaptosuccinic acid]
Chelating agent

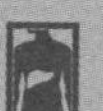 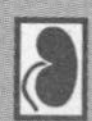 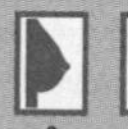 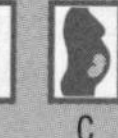

Yes Yes ? C

Cap: 100 mg

Lead chelation, child:

10 mg/kg/dose (or 350 mg/m²/dose) PO Q8 hr × 5 days, then 10 mg/kg/dose (or 350 mg/m²/dose) PO Q12 hr × 14 days.

Manufacturer recommendation (see following table):

Weight (kg)	Dose (mg) Q8 hr × 5 Days Followed by Same Dose Q12 hr × 14 Days
8–15	100
16–23	200
24–34	300
35–44	400
≥45	500

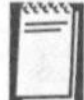

Use caution in patients with compromised renal or hepatic function. Repeated courses may be necessary. Follow serum lead levels. Allow minimum of 2 wk between courses, unless blood levels require more aggressive management. Side effects: GI symptoms, increased LFTs (10%), rash, headaches, and dizziness. **Coadministration with other chelating agents is not recommended.** Treatment of iron deficiency is recommended as well as environmental remediation. Contents of capsule may be sprinkled on food for those who are unable to swallow capsule.

SUCCINYLCHOLINE
Anectine and Quelicin
Neuromuscular blocking agent

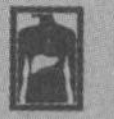 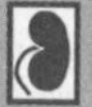 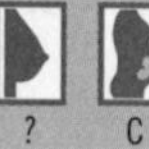

Yes No ? C

Injection: 20 mg/mL (10 mL), 100 mg/mL (10 mL); may contain parabens and/or benzyl alcohol

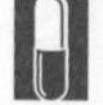

Paralysis for intubation (see remarks):
Infant and child:
Initial:
IV: 1–2 mg/kg/dose × 1
IM: 2.5–4 mg/kg/dose × 1
Max. dose: 150 mg/dose
Maintenance: 0.3–0.6 mg/kg/dose IV Q5–10 min PRN. **Continuous infusion not recommended** due to risk of malignant hyperthermia.

Continued

For explanation of icons, see p. 663.

SUCCINYLCHOLINE *continued*

Paralysis for intubation (see remarks) (cont'd):

Adult:

Initial:

IV: 0.3–1.1 mg/kg/dose × 1

IM: 2.5–4 mg/kg/dose × 1

Max. dose: 150 mg/dose

Maintenance: 0.04–0.07 mg/kg/dose IV Q5–10 min PRN

Continuous infusion not recommended.

Pretreatment with atropine is recommended to reduce incidence of bradycardia. For rapid sequence intubation, see Chapter 1.

Contraindicated after the acute phase of an injury following major burns, multiple trauma, extensive denervation of skeletal muscle, or upper motor neuron injury because severe hyperkalemia and subsequent **cardiac arrest** may occur.

Cardiac arrest has been reported in children and adolescents primarily with skeletal muscle myopathies (e.g., Duchenne's muscular dystrophy). Identify developmental delays suggestive of a myopathy prior to use. Pre-dose creatine kinase may be useful for identifying patients at risk. Monitoring of ECG for peaked T-waves may be useful in detecting early signs of this adverse effect.

May cause malignant hyperthermia (use dantrolene to treat), bradycardia, hypotension, arrhythmia, and hyperkalemia. Severe anaphylactic reactions have been reported; use caution if previous anaphylactic reaction to other neuromuscular blocking agents. **Use with caution** in patients with severe burns, paraplegia, or crush injuries and in patients with preexisting hyperkalemia. Beware of prolonged depression in patients with liver disease, malnutrition, pseudocholinesterase deficiency, hypothermia, and those receiving aminoglycosides, phenothiazines, quinidine, beta-blockers, amphotericin B, cyclophosphamide, diuretics, lithium, acetylcholine, and anticholinesterases. Diazepam may decrease neuromuscular blocking effects. Prior use of succinylcholine may enhance the neuromuscular blocking effect of vecuronium and its duration of action.

Duration of action 4–6 min IV, 10–30 min IM. Must be prepared to intubate within 1 min.

SUCRALFATE

Carafate and many other generics

Oral anti-ulcer agent

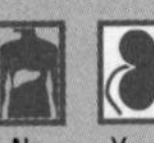
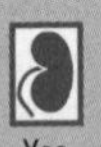

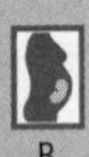

No Yes 1 B

Tabs: 1 g

Suspension: 100 mg/mL (420 mL); contains sorbitol and parabens

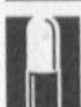

Child:

Duodenal or gastric ulcer: 40–80 mg/kg/24 hr ÷ Q6 hr PO.

Stomatitis: 5–10 mL (500–1000 mg of suspension) swish and spit or swish and swallow QID.

Adult:

Duodenal ulcer:

Treatment: 1 g PO QID (1 hr before meals and QHS) or 2 g PO BID × 4–8 wk.

Maintenance/prophylaxis: 1 g PO BID.

Stress ulcer:

Treatment: 1 g PO Q4 hr.

Prophylaxis: 1 g PO QID.

Stomatitis: 10 mL (1000 mg of suspension) swish and spit or swish and swallow QID.

Proctitis (use oral suspension as rectal enema): 20 mL (2 g) PR once daily–BID.

Continued

SUCRALFATE *continued*

May cause vertigo, constipation, and dry mouth. Hyperglycemia has been reported in diabetic patients. Aluminum may accumulate in patients with renal failure. This may be augmented by the use of aluminum-containing antacids. Decreases absorption of phenytoin, digoxin, theophylline, cimetidine, fat-soluble vitamins, ketoconazole, omeprazole, quinolones, and oral anticoagulants. Administer these drugs at least 2 hr before or after sucralfate doses.

Drug requires an acidic environment to form a protective polymer coating for damaged GI tract mucosa. Administer oral doses on an empty stomach (1 hr before meals and QHS).

SULFACETAMIDE SODIUM OPHTHALMIC

AK-Sulf, Bleph 10, Ocusulf-10, and various generic products

Ophthalmic antibiotic, sulfonamide derivative

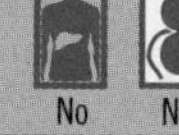 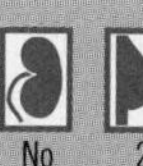 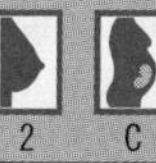

No No 2 C

Ophthalmic solution: 10% (5, 15 mL); may contain methylparaben and propylparben.
Ophthalmic ointment: 10% (3.5 g); may contain phenylmercuric acetate

Ophthalmic (usual duration of therapy for ophthalmic use is 7–10 days):
>2 mo and adult:
Ointment: Apply ribbon once daily–QID and QHS (5 ×/24 hr)
Drops: 1–2 drops Q2–3 hr to affected eye(s)

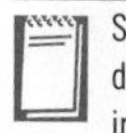

See *Sulfisoxazole.* 10% solution is used most frequently. Hypersensitivity reactions between different sulfonamides can occur regardless of route of administration. May cause local irritation, stinging, burning, conjunctival hyperemia, excessive tear production, and eye pain. Rare toxic epidermal necrolysis and Stevens-Johnson syndrome have been reported. Sulfacetamide preparations are incompatible with silver preparations.

To reduce risk of systemic absorption with ophthalmic solution, apply finger pressure to lacrimal sac during and 1–2 min after instillation.

SULFADIAZINE

Various trade names

Antibiotic, sulfonamide derivative

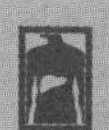 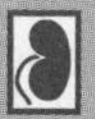  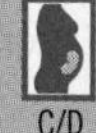

Yes Yes 3 C/D

Tabs: 500 mg
Oral suspension: 100 mg/mL

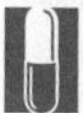

Congenital toxoplasmosis (administer with pyrimethamine and folinic acid; see *Pyrimethamine* for dosage information):
Infant: 100 mg/kg/24 hr PO ÷ BID × 12 mo

Toxoplasmosis (administer with pyrimethamine and folinic acid): See *Pyrimethamine* for dosage information.
Child: 100–200 mg/kg/24 hr ÷ Q6 hr PO × 3–4 wk
Adult: 4–6 g/24 hr PO ÷ Q6 hr × 3–4 wk

Rheumatic fever prophylaxis:
≤27 kg: 500 mg PO once daily
>27 kg: 1000 mg PO once daily

Most cases of acquired toxoplasmosis do not require specific antimicrobial therapy. **Contraindicated** in porphyria and hypersensitivity to sulfonamides. **Use with caution** in premature infants and infants <2 mo because of risk of hyperbilirubinemia, and in hepatic or

Continued

For explanation of icons, see p. 663.

SULFADIAZINE *continued*

renal dysfunction (30%–44% eliminated in urine). Maintain hydration. May cause fever, rash, hepatitis, SLE-like syndrome, vasculitis, bone marrow suppression and hemolysis in patients with G6PD deficiency, and Stevens-Johnson syndrome.

May cause increased effects of warfarin, methotrexate, thiazide diuretics, uricosuric agents, and sulfonylureas due to drug displacement from protein binding sites. Large quantities of vitamin C or acidifying agents (e.g., cranberry juice) may cause crystalluria. Pregnancy category changes from "C" to "D" if administered near term. Administer on an empty stomach with plenty of water.

SULFAMETHOXAZOLE AND TRIMETHOPRIM
Trimethoprim-sulfamethoxazole, Co-Trimoxazole, TMP-SMX;
Bactrim, Septra, Sulfatrim, and others
Antibiotic, sulfonamide derivative

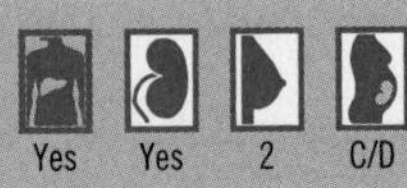

Tabs (reg strength): 80 mg TMP/400 mg SMX
Tabs (double strength): 160 mg TMP/800 mg SMX
Suspension: 40 mg TMP/200 mg SMX per 5 mL (100, 480 mL)
Injection: 16 mg TMP/mL and 80 mg SMX/mL (5, 10, 30 mL); some preparations may contain propylene glycol and benzyl alcohol

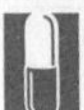

Doses based on TMP component.
Minor/moderate infections (PO or IV):
Child: 8–12 mg/kg/24 hr ÷ BID
Adult (>40 kg): 160 mg/dose BID
Severe infections (PO or IV):
Child and adult: 20 mg/kg/24 hr ÷ Q6–8 hr
UTI prophylaxis:
Child: 2–4 mg/kg/24 hr PO once daily
Pneumocystic (formerly jiroveci) carinii pneumonia (PCP):
Treatment (PO/IV): 20 mg/kg/24 hr ÷ Q6–8 hr
Prophylaxis (PO or IV):
≥1 mo and child: 5–10 mg/kg/24 hr ÷ BID or 150 mg/m^2/24 hr ÷ BID for 3 consecutive days/wk; **max. dose:** 320 mg/24 hr
Adult: 80–160 mg once daily or 160 mg 3 days/wk

Not recommended for use with infants <2 mo (excluding PCP prophylaxis). **Contraindicated** in patients with sulfonamide or trimethoprim hypersensitivity, and megaloblastic anemia due to folate deficiency. May cause kernicterus in newborns; may cause blood dyscrasias, crystalluria, glossitis, renal or hepatic injury, GI irritation, rash, Stevens-Johnson syndrome, hemolysis in patients with G6PD deficiency. Hyperkalemia may appear in HIV/AIDS patients. **Do not use drug at term during pregnancy.** Pregnancy risk factor changes to "D" if administered near term. **Use with caution** in renal and hepatic impairment, and G6PD deficiency.

Sulfamethoxazole is a CYP 450 2C9 substrate and inhibitor. Trimethoprim is a CYP 450 2C9, 3A4 substrate and 2C8/9 inhibitor. **Reduce dose in renal impairment (see Chapter 31).** See Chapter 17 for PCP prophylaxis guidelines.

SULFASALAZINE
Salicylazosulfapyridine, SAS, Azulfidine, Azulfidine EN-tabs and others
Anti-inflammatory agent

Yes Yes 2 B/D

Tabs: 500 mg
Enteric-coated tabs (Azulfidine EN-tabs): 500 mg
Oral suspension: 100 mg/mL

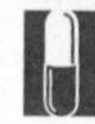

Ulcerative colitis:
Child ≥2 yr:
Initial dosing:
Mild: 40–50 mg/kg/24 hr ÷ Q6 hr PO
Moderate/severe: 50–75 mg/kg/24 hr ÷ Q4–6 hr PO; **max. dose:** 4 g/24 hr
Maintenance: 30–50 mg/kg/24 hr ÷ Q4–8 hr PO; **max. dose:** 2 g/24 hr
Adult:
Initial: 3–4 g/24 hr ÷ Q4–8 hr PO
Maintenance: 2 g/24 hr ÷ Q6 hr PO
Max. dose: 6 g/24 hr
Juvenile rheumatoid arthritis:
Child >6 yr: Start with 10 mg/kg/24 hr ÷ BID PO and increase by 10 mg/kg/24 hr Q7 days until planned maintenance dose is achieved. Usual maintenance dose is 30–50 mg/kg/24 hr ÷ BID PO up to a **max.** of 2 g/24 hr.

Contraindicated in sulfa or salicylate hypersensitivity, porphyria, and GI or GU obstruction. **Use with caution** in renal impairment, blood dyscrasias, or asthma. Maintain hydration. May cause orange-yellow discoloration of urine and skin. May permanently stain contact lenses. May cause photosensitivity, hypersensitivity, blood dyscrasias, CNS changes, nausea, vomiting, anorexia, diarrhea, and renal damage. Hepatotoxicity/hepatic failure, drug rash with eosinophilia and systemic symptoms (DRESS), interstitial lung disease have been reported. May cause hemolysis in patients with G6PD deficiency. Decreases folic acid absorption; and reduces serum digoxin and cyclosporine levels. Slow acetylators may require lower dosage due to accumulation of active sulfapyridine metabolite. Pregnancy category changes to "D" if administered near term.

SUMATRIPTAN SUCCINATE
Imitrex
Antimigraine agent, selective serotonin agonist

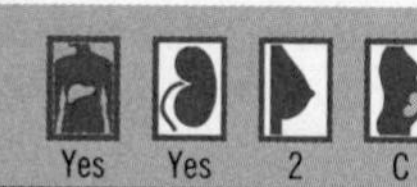

Injection: 8, 12 mg/mL (0.5 mL)
Tabs: 25, 50, 100 mg
Oral suspension: 5 mg/mL
Nasal spray (as a unit-dose spray device): 5 mg dose in 100 microliters (6 units per pack); 20 mg dose in 100 microliters (6 units per pack)

Adolescent and adult (see remarks):
PO: 25 mg as soon as possible after onset of headache. If no relief in 2 hr, give 25–100 mg Q 2 hr up to a **daily max.** of 200 mg.
Max. single dose: 100 mg/dose.
Max. daily dose: 200 mg/24 hr (with exclusive PO dosing or with an initial SC dose and subsequent PO dosing).

Continued

For explanation of icons, see p. 663.

SUMATRIPTAN SUCCINATE *continued*

Adolescent and adult (cont'd):

SC: 6 mg × 1 as soon as possible after onset of headache. If no response, may give an additional dose 1 hr later.

Max. daily dose: 12 mg/24 hr.

Nasal: 5–20 mg/dose into one nostril or divided into each nostril after onset of headache. Dose may be repeated in 2 hr up to a **max.** of 40 mg/24 hr.

Contraindicated with concomitant administration of ergotamine derivatives, MAO inhibitors (and use within the past 2 wk) or other vasoconstrictive drugs. **Not** for migraine prophylaxis. **Use with caution** in renal or hepatic impairment. A **max. single dose** of 50 mg has been recommended in adults with hepatic dysfunction. Acts as selective agonist for serotonin receptor. Induration and swelling at the injection site, flushing, dizziness, chest, jaw and neck tightness may occur with SC administration. Weakness, hyper-reflexia, incoordination, and serotonin syndrome have been reported with use in combination with selective serotonin reuptake inhibitors (e.g., fluoxetine, fluvoxamine, paroxetine, sertraline).

May cause coronary vasospasm if administered IV. **Use injectable form SC only!** Onset of action is 10–120 min SC, and 60–90 min PO. For nasal use, the safety of treating more than 4 headaches in a 30-day period has not been established.

Oral and nasal efficacy were not established in placebo-controlled trial in adolescents. Some **do not recommend** use in patients <18 yr due to poor efficacy and reports of serious adverse events (e.g., stroke, visual loss, and death) in both children and adults.

SURFACTANT, PULMONARY/BERACTANT

Survanta

Bovine lung surfactant

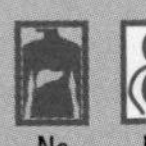
No

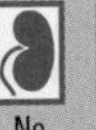
No

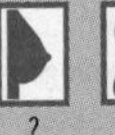
?

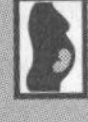

Suspension for inhalation: 25 mg/mL (4, 8 mL); contains 0.5–1.75 mg triglycerides, 1.4–3.5 mg free fatty acids and <1 mg protein/1 mL drug

Prophylatic therapy: 4 mL/kg/dose intratracheally as soon as possible; up to 4 doses may be given at intervals no shorter than Q6 hr during the first 48 hr of life.

Rescue therapy: 4 mL/kg/dose intratracheally, immediately following the diagnosis of respiratory distress syndrome (RDS). May repeat dose as needed Q6 hr to **max.** of 4 doses total.

Method of administration for previously listed therapies (see remarks): Suction infant prior to administration. Each dose is divided into four 1 mL/kg aliquots; administer 1 mL/kg in each of four different positions (slight downward inclination with head turned to the right, head turned to the left; slight upward inclination with the head turned to the right, head turned to the left).

Transient bradycardia, O_2 desaturation, pallor, vasoconstriction, hypotension, endotracheal tube blockage, hypercarbia, hypercapnea, apnea, and hypertension may occur during the administration process. Other side effects may include pulmonary interstitial emphysema, pulmonary air leak, and post-treatment nosocomial sepsis. Monitor heart rate and transcutaneous O_2 saturation during dose administration; and arterial blood gases for post-dose hyperoxia and hypocarbia after administration.

All doses are administered intratracheally via a 5 french feeding catheter. If the suspension settles during storage, gently swirl the contents—**do not shake.** Drug is stored in the refrigerator, protected from light, and needs to be warmed by standing at room temperature for at least 20 min or warm in the hand for at least 8 min. Artificial warming methods should **NOT** be used.

S

FORMULARY

SURFACTANT, PULMONARY/CALFACTANT

Infasurf

Bovine lung surfactant

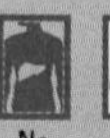
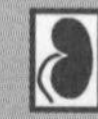
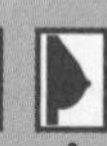
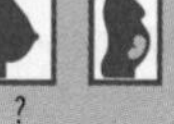

No No ?

Intratracheal suspension: 35 mg/mL (3, 6 mL); contains 26 mg phosphatidylcholine and 0.26 mg surfactant protein B per 1 mL

Prophylactic therapy: 3 mL/kg/dose intratracheally as soon as possible; up to a total of 3 doses may be given Q12 hr.

Rescue therapy (see remarks): 3 mL/kg/dose intratracheally immediately after the diagnosis of respiratory distress syndrome (RDS). May repeat dose as needed Q12 hr to **max.** of 3 doses total.

Method of administration for previously listed therapies (see remarks): Suction infant prior to administration. Manufacturer recommends administration through a side-port adapter into the endotracheal tube with two attendants (one to instill drug and another to monitor and position patient). Each dose is divided into two 1.5-mL/kg aliquots; administer 1.5 mL/kg in each of two different positions (infant positioned to the right or left-side dependent). Drug in administered while ventilation is continued over 20–30 breaths for each aliquot, with small bursts timed only during the inspiratory cycles. A pause followed by evaluation of respiratory status and repositioning should separate the two aliquots. The drug has also been administered by divided dose into four equal aliquots and administered with repositioning in the prone, supine, right and left lateral positions.

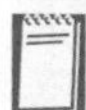

Common adverse effects include cyanosis, airway obstruction, bradycardia, reflux of surfactant into the ET tube, requirement for manual ventilation, and reintubation. Monitor O_2 saturation and lung compliance after each dose such that oxygen therapy and ventilator pressure are adjusted as necessary.

All doses administered intratracheally via a 5 french feeding catheter. If suspension settles during storage, gently swirl the contents—**do not shake.** Drug is stored in the refrigerator, protected from light, and does not need to be warmed before administration. Unopened vials that have been warmed to room temperature (once only) may be refrigerated within 24 hours and stored for future use.

For rescue therapy, repeat doses may be administered as early as 6 hr after the previous dose for a total of up to 4 doses if the infant is still intubated and requires at least 30% inspired oxygen to maintain a PaO_2 ≥80 torr.

SURFACTANT, PULMONARY/PORACTANT ALFA

Curosurf

Porcine lung surfactant

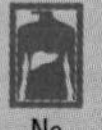
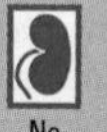
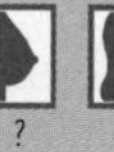
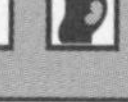

No No ?

Intratracheal suspension: 80 mg/mL (1.5, 3 mL): contains 0.3 mg surfactant protein B per 1 mL drug

Prophylaxis therapy: 2.5 mL/kg/dose × 1 intratracheally as soon as possible; up to 2 subsequent 1.25 mL/kg/doses may be given at 12-hr intervals for a **max. total dose** of 5 mL/kg.

Rescue therapy: 2.5 mL/kg/dose × 1 intratracheally, immediately following the diagnosis of respiratory distress syndrome (RDS). May administer 1.25 mL/kg/dose Q12 hr × 2 doses as needed up to a **max. total dose** of 5 mL/kg.

Continued

For explanation of icons, see p. 663.

SURFACTANT, PULMONARY/PORACTANT ALFA *continued*

Method of administration for previously listed therapies (see remarks): Suction infant prior to administration. Each dose is divided into two aliquots, with each aliquot administered into one of the two main bronchi by positioning the infant with either the right or left side dependent. After the first aliquot is administered, remove the catheter from the ET tube and manually ventilate the infant with 100% oxygen at a rate of 40–60 breaths/min for 1 min. When the infant is stable, reposition the infant and administer the second dose. Then remove the catheter without flushing.

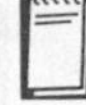

Transient episodes of bradycardia, decreased oxygen saturation, reflux of surfactant into the ET tube, and airway obstruction have occurred during dose administration. Monitor O_2 saturation and lung compliance after each dose, and adjust oxygen therapy and ventilator pressure as necessary. Pulmonary hemorrhage has been reported.

All doses administered intratracheally via a 5 french feeding catheter. Suction infant prior to administration and 1 hr after surfactant instillation (unless signs of significant airway obstruction).

Drug is stored in the refrigerator and protected from light. Each vial of drug should be slowly warmed to room temperature and gently turned upside-down for uniform suspension **(do not shake)** before administration. Unopened vials that have been warmed to room temperature (once only) may be refrigerated within 24 hr and stored for future use.

TACROLIMUS

Prograf, FK506, Protopic

Immunosuppressant

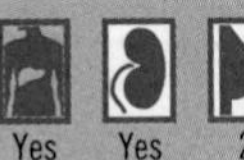

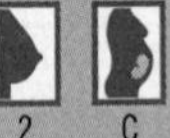

Yes Yes 2 C

Caps: 0.5, 1, 5 mg

Oral suspension: 0.5, 1 mg/mL

Injection: 5 mg/mL (1 mL); contains alcohol and polyoxyl 60 hydrogenaed castor oil

Topical ointment (Protopic): 0.03%, 0.1% (30, 60, 100 g)

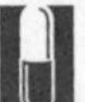

Child:

Liver transplantation without pre-existing renal or hepatic dysfunction (initial doses; titrate to therapeutic levels):

IV: 0.03–0.15 mg/kg/24 hr by continuous infusion.

PO: 0.15–0.2 mg/kg/24 hr ÷ Q12 hr.

Adult (initial doses; titrate to therapeutic levels):

IV: 0.03–0.1 mg/kg/24 hr by continuous infusion.

PO: 0.15–0.3 mg/kg/24 hr ÷ Q12 hr.

Liver transplantation: 0.1–0.15 mg/kg/24 hr ÷ Q12 hr.

Kidney transplantation: 0.2 mg/kg/24 hr ÷ Q12 hr.

Cardiac transplantation: 0.075 mg/kg/24 hr ÷ Q12 hr.

Atopic dermatitis (continue treatment for 1 wk after clearing of signs and symptoms; see remarks):

Child ≥2 yr old: Apply a thin layer of the 0.03% ointment to the affected skin areas BID and rub in gently and completely.

Adult: Apply a thin layer of the 0.03% or 0.1% ointment to the affected skin areas BID and rub in gently and completely.

IV dosage form **contraindicated** in patients allergic to polyoxyl 60 hydrogenated castor oil. Experience in pediatric kidney transplantation is limited. Pediatric patients have required higher mg/kg doses than adults. For BMT use (beginning 1 day before BMT), dose and therapeutic levels similar to those in liver transplantation have been used.

Continued

TACROLIMUS *continued*

Major adverse events include tremor, headache, insomnia, diarrhea, constipation, hypertension, nausea, and renal dysfunction. Hypokalemia, hypomagnesemia, hyperglycemia, confusion, depression, infections, lymphoma, liver enzyme elevation, and coagulation disorders may also occur. Tacrolimus is a substrate of the CYP 450 3A4 drug metabolizing enzyme. Calcium channel blockers, imidazole antifungals (ketoconazole, itraconazole, fluconazole, clotrimazole, posaconazole), macrolide antibiotics (erythromycin, clarithromycin, troleandomycin), cisapride, cimetidine, cyclosporine, danazol, methylprednisolone, and grapefruit juice can increase tacrolimus serum levels. In contrast, carbamazepine, caspofungin, phenobarbital, phenytoin, rifampin, rifabutin, and sirolimus may decrease levels. Use with sirolimus may increase risk for hepatic artery thrombosis. Reduce dose in renal or hepatic insufficiency.

Monitor trough levels (just prior to a dose at steady-state). Steady-state is generally achieved after 2–5 days of continuous dosing. Interpretation will vary based on treatment protocol and assay methodology (whole blood ELISA vs. MEIA vs. HPLC). Whole blood trough concentrations of 5–20 ng/mL have been recommended in liver transplantation at 1–12 mo. Trough levels of 7–20 ng/mL (whole blood) for the first 3 mo and 5–15 ng/mL after 3 mo have been recommended in renal transplantation.

Tacrolimus therapy generally should be initiated 6 hr or more after transplantation. PO is the preferred route of administration and should be administered on an empty stomach. IV infusions should be administered at concentrations between 0.004 and 0.02 mg/mL diluted NS or D_5W.

TOPICAL USE: Do not use in children <2 yr, immunocompromised patients, or with occlusive dressings (promotes systemic absorption). Approved as a second-line therapy for short-term and intermittent treatment of atopic dermatitis for patients who fail to respond, or do not tolerate, other approved therapies. Long-term safety is unknown. Skin burn sensation, pruritus, flu-like symptoms, allergic reaction, skin erythema, headache, and skin infection are the most common side effects. Although the risk is uncertain, the FDA has issued an alert about the potential cancer risk with the use of this product. See www.fda.gov/medwatch for the latest information.

TERBUTALINE
Brethine and others
Beta-2-adrenergic agonist

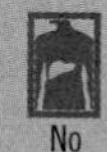
No
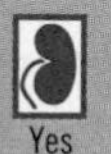
Yes
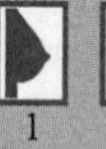
1
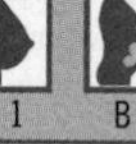
B

Tabs: 2.5, 5 mg
Oral suspension: 1 mg/mL
Injection: 1 mg/mL (1 mL)

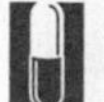

Oral:

≤12 yr: Initial: 0.05 mg/kg/dose Q8 hr, increase as required. **Max. dose:** 0.15 mg/kg/dose Q8 hr or total of 5 mg/24 hr.

>12 yr and adult: 2.5–5 mg/dose PO Q6–8 hr.

Max. dose:

12–15 yr: 7.5 mg/24 hr.

>15 yr: 15 mg/24 hr.

Nebulization:

<2 yr: 0.5 mg in 2.5 ml NS Q4–6 hr PRN.

2–9 yr: 1 mg in 2.5 ml NS Q4–6 hr PRN.

>9 yr: 1.5–2.5 mg in 2.5 ml NS Q4–6 hr PRN.

SC injection:

≤12 yr: 0.005–0.01 mg/kg/dose (**max. dose:** 0.4 mg/dose) Q15–20 min × 3; if needed, Q2–6 hr PRN.

>12 yr and adult: 0.25 mg/dose Q15–30 min PRN × 3; **max. total dose:** 0.75 mg.

Continued

For explanation of icons, see p. 663.

TERBUTALINE *continued*

Continuous infusion, IV: 2–10 mcg/kg loading dose followed by infusion of 0.1–0.4 mcg/kg/min. May titrate in increments of 0.1–0.2 mcg/kg/min Q30 min depending on clinical response. Doses as high as 10 mcg/kg/min have been used.
To prepare infusion: See IV Infusions on page i.

Nervousness, tremor, headache, nausea, tachycardia, arrhythmias, and palpitations may occur. Paradoxical bronchoconstriction may occur with excessive use; if it occurs, discontinue drug immediately. Injectable product may be used for nebulization. For acute asthma, nebulizations may be given more frequently than Q4–6 hr. Use spacer device with inhaler to optimize drug delivery.

Monitor heart rate, blood pressure, respiratory rate, and serum potassium when using the continuous IV infusion route of administration. **Adjust dose in renal failure (see Chapter 31).**

TETRACYCLINE HCL

Sumycin and various generics
Antibiotic

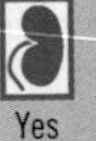
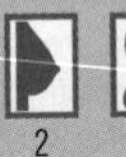
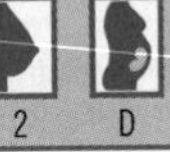

Yes Yes 2 D

Caps: 250, 500 mg
Oral suspension: 25 mg/mL

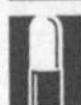

Do not use in children <8 yr.
Child ≥8 yr: 25–50 mg/kg/24 hr PO ÷ Q6 hr; **max. dose:** 3 g/24 hr
Adult: 1–2 g/24 hr PO ÷ Q6–12 hr

Not recommended in patients <8 yr due to tooth staining and decreased bone growth. Also **not recommended** for use in pregnancy because these side effects may occur in the fetus. The risk for these adverse effects are highest with long-term use. May cause nausea, GI upset, hepatotoxicity, stomatitis, rash, fever, and superinfection. Photosensitivity reaction may occur. **Avoid** prolonged exposure to sunlight.

Never use outdated tetracyclines because they may cause Fanconi-like syndrome. **Do not** give with dairy products or with any divalent cations (i.e., Fe^{2+}, Ca^{2+}, Mg^{2+}). Give 1 hr before or 2 hr after meals.

May decrease the effectiveness of oral contraceptives, increase serum digoxin levels, and increase effects of warfarin. Use with methoxyflurane increases risk for nephrotoxicity and use with isotretinoin is associated with pseudotumor cerebri. **Adjust dose in renal failure (see Chapter 31).**

THEOPHYLLINE

Theo-24, Theochron, Uniphyl, TheoCap, Elixophyllin, and many others
Bronchodilator, methylxanthine

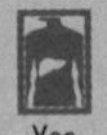
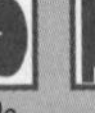

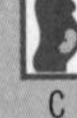

Yes No 2 C

Other dosage forms may exist.
Immediate release:
Elixir (Elixophyllin): 80 mg/15 mL. Contains up to 20% alcohol.
Sustained/extended release (see remarks):
Tabs: 100, 200, 300, 400, 600 mg
Caps: 100, 125, 200, 300, 400 mg
Sustained-release forms should not be chewed or crushed. Capsules may be opened and contents may be sprinkled on food.

Continued

THEOPHYLLINE *continued*

Dosing intervals are for immediate-release preparations.
For sustained-release preparations, divide daily dose >Q8–24 hr based on product.

Neonatal apnea:

Load: 5 mg/kg/dose PO × 1

Maintenance: 3–6 mg/kg/24 hr PO ÷ Q6–8 hr

Bronchospasm; PO:

Loading dose: 1 mg/kg/dose for each 2 mg/L desired increase in serum theophylline level.

Maintenance, infant (<1 yr):

Preterm:

<24 days old (postnatal): 1 mg/kg/dose PO Q12 hr

≥24 days old (postnatal): 1.5 mg/kg/dose PO Q12 hr

Full-term up to 1 yr old: Total daily dose (mg) = [(0.2 × age in weeks) + 5] × (kg body weight)

≤6 mo: Divide daily dose Q8 hr

>6 mo: Divide daily dose Q6 hr

Maintenance, child >1 yr and adult without risk factors for altered clearance (see remarks):

<45 kg: Begin therapy at 12–14 mg/kg/24 hr ÷ Q4–6 hr up to **max. dose** of 300 mg/24 hr. If needed based on serum levels, gradually increase to 16–20 mg/kg/24 hr ÷ Q4–6 hr. **Max. dose:** 600 mg/24 hr.

≥45 kg: Begin therapy with 300 mg/24 hr ÷ Q6–8 hr. If needed based on serum levels, gradually increase to 400–600 mg/24 hr ÷ Q6–8 hr.

Drug metabolism varies widely with age, drug formulation, and route of administration. Most common side effects and toxicities are nausea, vomiting, anorexia, abdominal pain, gastroesophageal reflux, nervousness, tachycardia, seizures, and arrhythmias.

Serum levels should be monitored. Therapeutic levels: bronchospasm: 10–20 mg/L; apnea: 7–13 mg/L. Half-life is age-dependent: 30 hr (newborns); 6.9 hr (infants); 3.4 hr (children); 8.1 hr (adults). See *Aminophylline* for guidelines for serum level determinations. Liver impairment, cardiac failure and sustained high fever may increase theophylline levels. Theophylline is a substrate for CYP 450 1A2. Levels are increased with allopurinol, alcohol, ciprofloxacin, cimetidine, clarithromycin, disulfiram, erythromycin, estrogen, isoniazid, propranolol, thiabendazole, and verapamil. Levels are decreased with carbamazepine, isoproterenol, phenobarbital, phenytoin, and rifampin. May cause increased skeletal muscle activity, agitation, and hyperactivity when used with doxapram.

Use ideal body weight in obese patients when calculating dosage because of poor distribution into body fat. Risk factors for increased clearance include: smoking, Cystic Fibrosis, hyperthyroidism, and high-protein carbohydrate diet. Factors for decreased clearance include CHF, correction of hyperthyroidism, fever, viral illness, and sepsis.

Suggested dosage intervals for sustained-released products (see following table):

Theophylline Sustained Release Products

Trade Name	Available Strengths	Dosage Interval
CAPSULES:		
Theo-24	100, 200, 300, 400 mg	Q24 hr
TheoCap	125, 200, 300 mg	Q12–24 hr
TABLETS:		
Theocron	100, 200, 300, 450 mg	Q12–24 hr
Uniphyl	400, 600 mg	Q24 hr

For explanation of icons, see p. 663.

THIABENDAZOLE
Mintezol
Anthelmintic

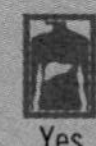 Yes 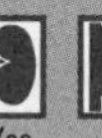 Yes 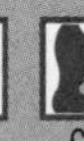 ? 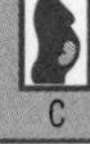 C

Oral suspension: 500 mg/5 mL
Chew tabs: 500 mg; contains saccharin
Topical suspension: 10%–15% 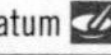
Topical ointment: 10% in white petrolatum

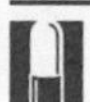

Child and adult: 50 mg/kg/24 hr PO ÷ BID; **max. dose:** 3 g/24 hr
Duration of therapy (consecutive days):
Strongyloides: × 2 days (5 days for disseminated disease)
Cutaneous larva migrans: × 2–5 days
Visceral larva migrans: × 5–7 days
Trichinosis: × 2–4 days
Angiostrongylosis: 75 mg/kg/24 hr PO ÷ BID-TID × 3 days; **max. dose:** 3 g/24 hr
Dracunculosis: 50–75 mg/kg/24 hr PO ÷ BID × 3 days; **max. dose:** 3 g/24 hr

Topical therapy for cutaneous larva migrans: Apply sparingly to all lesions 4–6 ×/24 hr until lesions are inactivated. See *Arch Dermatol* 1993;129:588 for additional information.

Contraindicated in prophylatic treatment for pinworm infestation. **Not** suitable for prophylactic use and for treatment of mixed infections with ascaris. **Use with caution** in renal or hepatic impairment. Nausea, vomiting, and vertigo are frequent side effects. May cause abnormal sensation in eyes, xanthopsia, blurred vision, dry mucous membranes, rash, hypersensitivity, erythema multiforme, leukopenia, and hallucinations. Stevens-Johnson syndrome and liver damage have been reported. May increase serum levels of theophylline or caffeine. Clinical experience in children weighing <13.6 kg (30 lbs) is limited.

THIAMINE
Vitamin B_1, Thiamilate, and others
Water-soluble vitamin

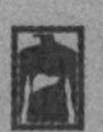 No 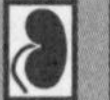 No 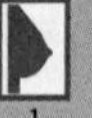 1 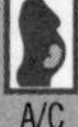 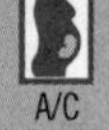 A/C

Tabs (OTC): 50, 100 mg
Enteric-coated tabs (OTC; Thiamilate): 20 mg
Injection: 100 mg/mL (1, 2 mL); contains benzyl alcohol

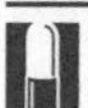

For US RDA, see Chapter 21.
Beriberi (thiamine deficiency):
Child: 10–25 mg/dose IM/IV once daily (if critically ill) or 10–50 mg/dose PO once daily × 2 wk, followed by 5–10 mg/dose once daily × 1 mo.
Adult: 5–30 mg/dose IM/IV TID (if critically ill) × 2 wk, followed by 5–30 mg/24 hr PO ÷ once daily or TID × 1 mo.

Wernicke's encephalopathy syndrome (adult): 100 mg IV × 1, then 50–100 mg IM/IV once daily until patient resumes a normal diet. (Administer thiamine before starting glucose infusion.)

Multivitamin preparations contain amounts meeting RDA requirements. Allergic reactions and anaphylaxis may occur, primarily with IV administration. Therapeutic range: 1.6–4 mg/dL. High carbohydrate diets or IV dextrose solutions may increase thiamine requirements. Large doses may interfere with serum theophylline assay. Pregnancy category changes to "C" if used in doses above the RDA.

THIORIDAZINE
Various generics, previously avaiable as Mellaril
Antipsychotic, phenothiazine derivative

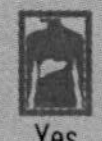
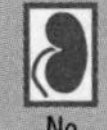
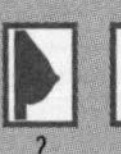
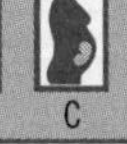
Yes No ? C

Tabs: 10, 25, 50, 100 mg

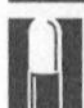

Child 2–12 yr: Start with 0.5 mg/kg/24 hr PO ÷ BID–TID; dosage range: 0.5–3 mg/kg/24 hr PO ÷ BID–TID. **Max. dose:** 3 mg/kg/24 hr.

>12 yr and adult: Start with 75–300 mg/24 hr PO ÷ TID. Then gradually increase PRN to **max. dose** 800 mg/24 hr ÷ BID–QID.

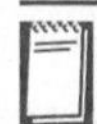

Indicated for schizophrenia unresponsive to standard therapy. **Contraindicated** in severe CNS depression, brain damage, narrow-angle glaucoma, blood dyscrasias, and severe liver or cardiovascular disease. **DO NOT** co-administer with drugs which may inhibit the CYP 450 2D6 isoenzymes (e.g., SSRIs such as fluoxetine, fluvoxamine, paroxetine; and beta-blockers such as propranolol and pindolol); drugs which may widen the QTc interval (e.g., disopyramide, procainamide, quinidine); and in patients with known reduced activity of CYP 450 2D6.

May cause drowsiness, extrapyramidal reactions, autonomic symptoms, ECG changes (QTc prolongation in a dose-dependent manner), arrhythmias, paradoxical reactions, and endocrine disturbances. Long-term use may cause tardive dyskinesia. Pigmentary retinopathy may occur with higher doses; a periodic eye exam is recommended. More autonomic symptoms and less extrapyramidal effects than chlorpromazine. Concurrent use with epinephrine can cause hypotension. Increased cardiac arrhythmias may occur with tricyclic antidepressants.

In an overdose situation, monitor ECG and avoid drugs that can widen QTc interval.

TIAGABINE
Gabitril
Anticonvulsant

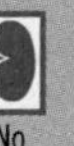
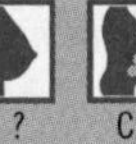
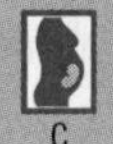
Yes No ? C

Tabs: 2, 4, 12, 16 mg
Oral suspension: 1 mg/mL

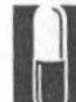

Adjunctive therapy for refractory seizures (see remarks):

Child ≥2 yr (limited data from a safety and tolerability study in 52 children 2–17 yr, mean 9.3 ± 4.1): Initial dose of 0.25 mg/kg/24 hr PO ÷ TID × 4 wk. Dosage was increased at 4-wk intervals to 0.5, 1, and 1.5 mg/kg/24 hr until an effective and well-tolerated dose was established. Criteria for dose increase required tolerance of the current dosage level and <50% reduction in seizures. Patients receiving enzyme-inducing antiepileptic drugs (AEDs) received a **max. daily dose** of 0.73 ± 0.44 mg/kg/24 hr and patients receiving non-enzyme inducing AEDs received a **max.** of 0.61 ± 0.32 mg/kg/24 hr.

Adjunctive therapy for partial seizures (dosage based on use with enzyme-inducing AEDs; see remarks). **NOTE:** Patients receiving non-enzyme-inducing AEDs results in tiagabine blood levels about two times higher than patients receiving enzyme-inducing AEDs.

≥12 yr and adult: Start at 4 mg PO once daily × 7 days. If needed, increase dose to 8 mg/24 hr PO ÷ BID. Dosage may be increased further by 4–8 mg/24 hr at weekly intervals (daily doses may be divided BID–QID) until a clinical response is achieved or up to specified **max. dose.**

Max. dose:

12–18 yr: 32 mg/24 hr

Adult: 56 mg/24 hr

Continued

For explanation of icons, see p. 663.

TIAGABINE *continued*

Use with caution in hepatic insufficiency (may need to reduce dose and/or increase dosing interval). Most common side effects include dizziness, somnolence, depression, confusion, and asthenia. Nervousness, tremor, nausea, abdominal pain, confusion, and difficulty in concentrating may also occur. Cognitive/neuropsychiatric symptoms resulting in nonconvulsive status epilepticus requiring subsequent dose reduction or drug discontinuation have been reported. Suicidal behavior or ideation has been reported. **Off-label use in patients WITHOUT epilepsy is discouraged** due to reports of seizures in these patients.

Tiagabine's clearance is increased by concurrent hepatic enzyme-inducing antiepileptic drugs (e.g., phenytoin, carbamazepine, and barbiturates). Lower doses or a slower titration for clinical response may be necessary for patients receiving non-enzyme-inducing drugs (e.g., valproate, gabapentin, and lamotrigine). **Avoid** abrupt discontinuation of drug.

TID dosing schedule may be preferred since BID schedule may not be well tolerated. Doses should be administered with food.

TICARCILLIN AND CLAVULANATE

Timentin

Antibiotic, penicillin (extended spectrum with beta-lactamase inhibitor)

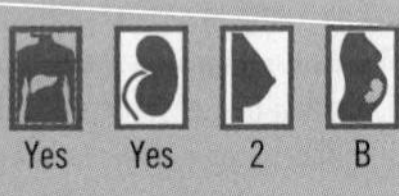

Injection: 3.1 g (3 g ticarcillin and 0.1 g clavulanate); contains 4.51 mEq Na^+ and 0.15 mEq K^+ per 1 g drug

Premixed injection: 3.1 g (3 g ticarcillin and 0.1 g clavulanate) in 100 mL; contains 18.7 mEq Na^+ and 0.5 mEq K^+ per 100 mL

All doses based on tiarcillin component.

Neonate (IV):

≤7 days:

<2 kg: 150 mg/kg/24 hr ÷ Q12 hr

≥2 kg: 225 mg/kg/24 hr ÷ Q8 hr

>7 days:

<1.2 kg: 150 mg/kg/24 hr ÷ Q12 hr

1.2–2 kg: 225 mg/kg/24 hr ÷ Q8 hr

>2 kg: 300 mg/kg/24 hr ÷ Q8 hr

Term neonate and infant <3 mo: 200–300 mg/kg/24 hr IV ÷ Q 4–6 hr

Infant ≥3 mo and child <60 kg:

Mild/moderate infections: 200 mg/kg/24 hr IV ÷ Q6 hr

Severe infections: 300 mg/kg/24 hr IV ÷ Q4–6 hr

Max. dose: 18–24 mg/24 hr

Cystic Fibrosis: 300–600 mg/kg/24 hr IV ÷ Q4-6 hr IV; **max. dose:** 24 g/24 hr

Adult: 3 g/dose IV Q4–6 hr IV

UTI: 3 g/dose IV Q6–8 hr

Max. dose: 18–24 g/24 hr

Beta-lactamase inhibitor broadens spectrum to include *S. aureus* and *H. influenzae.*

Thrombophlebitis, rash, and immune hypersensitivity are common side effects. May also cause decreased platelet aggregation, bleeding diathesis, hypernatremia, hematuria, hypokalemia, hypocalcemia, allergy, and increased AST. Hemorrhagic cystitis has been reported. Use with caution with cephalosporin hypersensitivity and CHF (high sodium content). Like other penicillins, CSF penetration occurs only with inflamed meninges. May cause false-positive tests for urine protein and serum Coombs' test.

Do not mix with aminoglycoside in same solution. Ticarcillin elimination is prolonged with impaired hepatic and/or renal function **(adjust dosage in renal impairment; see Chapter 31).**

TOBRAMYCIN
Nebcin, Tobrex, AKTob, TOBI and others
Antibiotic, aminoglycoside

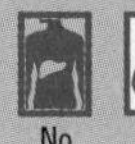
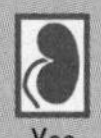

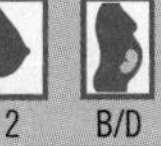
No Yes 2 B/D

Injection: 10, 40 mg/mL; may contain phenol and bisulfites
Powder for injection: 1.2 g; preservative free
Ophthalmic ointment (Tobrex, AKTob): 0.3% (3.5 g)
  In combination with dexamethasone (TobraDex): 0.3% tobramycin with 0.1% dexamethasone (3.5 g); contains 0.5% chlorbutanol
Ophthalmic solution (Tobrex): 0.3% (5 mL)
  In combination with dexamethasone: 0.3% tobramycin with 0.1% dexamethasone (2.5, 5, 10 mL); contains 0.01% benzalkonium chloride and EDTA
Nebulizer solution: 300 mg/5 mL (TOBI, preservative free) (56s), 170 mg/3.4 mL (mixed in 0.45% NS, preservative free, use with eFlow/Trio nebulizer)

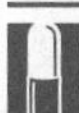
Initial empiric dosage; patient specific dosage defined by therapeutic drug monitoring (see remarks).
Neonate, IM/IV (see following table):

Post-conceptional Age (wk)	Postnatal Age (days)	Dose (mg/kg/dose)	Interval (hr)
≤29*	0–7	5	48
	8–28	4	36
	>28	4	24
30–33	0–7	4.5	36
	>7	4	24
34–37	0–7	4	24
	>7	4	18–24
≥38	0–7	4	24
	>7	4	12–18

*Or significant asphyxia, PDA, indomethacin use, poor cardiac output, reduced renal function.

Child: 7.5 mg/kg/24 hr ÷ Q8 hr IV/IM
Cystic Fibrosis (if available, use patient's previous therapeutic mg/kg dosage):
  Conventional Q8 hr dosing: 7.5–10.5 mg/kg/24 hr ÷ Q8 hr IV
  High dose extended interval (once daily) dosing: 10–12 mg/kg/dose Q24 hr IV
Adult: 3–6 mg/kg/24 hr ÷ Q8 hr IV/IM
Ophthalmic:
  Tobramycin:
    Child and adult:
      Ophthalmic ointment: Apply ½ inch ribbon into conjunctival sac(s) BID–TID; for severe infections, apply Q3–4 hr
      Ophthalmic drop: Instill 1–2 drops of solution to affected eye(s) Q4 hr; for severe infections, instill 2 drops Q30–60 min initially, then reduce dosing frequency.
  Tobramycin with dexamethasone:
    ≥2 yr and adult:
      Ophthalmic ointment: Apply ½ inch ribbon of ointment into conjunctival sac(s) TID–QID
      Ophthalmic drop: Instill 1–2 drops of solution to affected eye(s) Q2 hr × 24–48 hr, then 1–2 drops Q4–6 hr.

Continued

For explanation of icons, see p. 663.

TOBRAMYCIN *continued*

Inhalation:

Cystic Fibrosis prophylaxis therapy:

≥6 yr and adult:

TOBI: 300 mg Q12 hr administered in repeated cycles of 28 days on drug followed by 28 days off drug.

Use with eFlow/Trio nebulizer: 170 mg Q12 hr administered in repeated cycles of 28 days on drug followed by 28 days off drug.

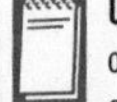

Use with caution in combination with neurotoxic, ototoxic, or nephrotoxic drugs; anesthetics or neuromuscular blocking agents; pre-existing renal, vestibular or auditory impairment; and in patients with neuromuscular disorders. May cause ototoxicity, nephrotoxicity, and neuromuscular blockade. Serious allergic reactions including anaphylaxis and dermatologic reactions including exfoliative dermatitis, toxic epidermal necrolysis, erythema multiforme, and Stevens-Johnson syndrome have been reported rarely. **Ototoxic effects synergistic with furosemide.**

Higher doses are recommended in patients with Cystic Fibrosis, neutropenia, or burns. **Adjust dose in renal failure (see Chapter 31).** Monitor peak and trough levels.

Therapeutic peak levels:

6–10 mg/L in general

8–10 mg/L in pulmonary infections, neutropenia, osteomyelitis, and severe sepsis

Therapeutic trough levels: <2 mg/L. Recommended serum sampling time at steady-state: trough within 30 min prior to the third consecutive dose and peak 30–60 min after the administration of the third consecutive dose.

To maximize bacterialcidal effects, an individualized peak concentration to target a peak/MIC ratio of 8–10 : 1 may be applied.

For initial dosing in obese patients, use an adjusted body weight (ABW). ABW = Ideal Body Weight + 0.4 (Total Body Weight – Ideal Body Weight).

INHALATIONAL USE: Transient voice alteration, bronchospasm, dyspnea, pharyngitis, and increased cough may occur. Transient tinnitus has been reported. Use with other medications in Cystic Fibrosis, use the following order of administration: bronchodilator first, chest physiotherapy, other inhaled medications (if indicated), and tobramycin last.

Pregnancy category is a "D" for injection and inhalation routes of administration and a "B" for the ophthalmic route.

TOLNAFTATE

Tinactin, Aftate, and many others

Antifungal agent

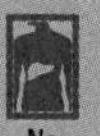
No

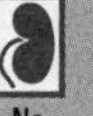
No

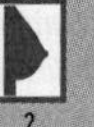
?

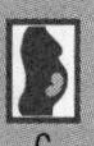
C

Topical aerosol liquid [OTC]: 1% (60, 120 mL); may contain 36% alcohol
Aerosol powder [OTC]: 1% (100, 105, 150 g); contains 14% alcohol and talc
Cream [OTC]: 1% (15, 21, 30 g)
Gel [OTC]: 1% (15 g)
Topical powder [OTC]: 1% (45, 90 g)
Topical solution [OTC]: 1% (10 mL)

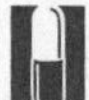

Child (≥2 yr) and adult:

Topical: apply 1–3 drops of solution or small amount of gel, liquid, cream, or powder to affected areas BID–TID for 2–4 wk.

May cause mild irritation and sensitivity. Contact dermatitis has been reported. **Avoid** eye contact. **Do not use** for nail or scalp infections. Discontinue use if sensitization develops.

TOPIRAMATE
Topamax
Anticonvulsant

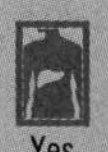 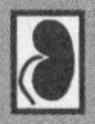  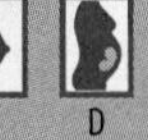
Yes Yes 2 D

Caps, sprinkle: 15, 25 mg
Tabs: 25, 50, 100, 200 mg
Oral suspension: 6 mg/mL 

Adjunctive therapy for partial onset seizures or Lennox-Gastaut syndrome:

Child 2–16 yr: Start with 1–3 mg/kg/dose (**max. dose:** 25 mg/dose) PO QHS × 7 days, then increase by 1–3 mg/kg/24-hr increments at 1- to 2-wk intervals (divided daily dose BID) to response. Usual maintenance dose is 5–9 mg/kg/24 hr PO ÷ BID

≥17 yr and adult: Start with 25–50 mg PO QHS × 7 days, then increase by 25–50 mg/24 hr increments at 1-wk intervals until adequate response. Doses >50 mg should be divided BID. Usual maintenance dose: 100–200 mg/24 hr. Doses above 1600 mg/24 hr have not been studied.

Adjunctive therapy for primary generalized tonic clonic seizures:

Child 2–16 yr: Use above initial dose and slower titration rate by reaching 6 mg/kg/24 hr by the end of 8 wk.

≥17 yr and adult: Use above initial dose and slower titration rate by reaching 200 mg BID by the end of 8 wk.

Monotherapy for partial onset seizures or primary generalized tonic clonic seizures:

Child ≥10 yr and adult: Start with 25 mg PO BID × 7 days, then increase by 50 mg/24 hr increments at 1-wk intervals up to a max. dose of 100 mg PO BID at wk 4. If needed, dose may be further increased at weekly intervals by 100 mg/24 hr up to a recommended max. dose of 200 mg PO BID.

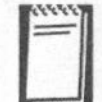

Use with caution in renal and hepatic dysfunction (decreased clearance) and sulfa hypersensitivity. **Reduce dose by 50% when creatinine clearance is <70 mL/min.** Common side effects (incidence lower in children) include ataxia, cognitive dysfunction, dizziness, nystagmus, paresthesia, sedation, visual disturbances, nausea, dyspepsia, and kidney stones. Secondary angle closure glaucoma characterized by ocular pain, acute myopia, and increased intraocular pressure has been reported and may lead to blindness if left untreated. Patients should be instructed to seek immediate medical attention if they experience blurred vision or periorbital pain. Oligohidrosis and hyperthermia has been reported primarily in children and should be monitored especially during hot weather and with use of drugs that predispose patients to heat-related disorders (e.g., carbonic anyhdrase inhibitors and anticholinergics). Hyperchloremic, non-anion gap metabolic acidosis has also been reported. Suicidal behavior or ideation have been reported.

Drug is metabolized by and inhibits the CYP 450 2C19 isoenzyme. Phenytoin, valproic acid, and carbamazepine may decrease topiramate levels. Topiramate may decrease valproic acid, digoxin, and ethinyl estradiol (to decrease oral contraceptive efficacy), but may increase phenytoin levels. Alcohol and CNS depressants may increase CNS side effects. Carbonic anhydrase inhibitors (e.g., acetazolamide) may increase risk of metabolic acidosis, nephrolithiasis, or paresthesia.

Doses may be administered with or without food. Capsule may be opened and sprinkled on small amount of food (e.g., 1 teaspoonful of applesauce) and swallowed whole **(do not chew).** Maintain adequate hydration to prevent kidney stone formation.

For explanation of icons, see p. 663.

TRAZODONE
Many generics, previously available as Desyrel
Antidepressant, triazolopyridine-derivative

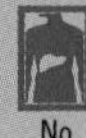 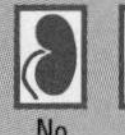 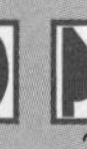 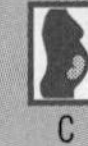

No No 2 C

Tabs: 50, 100, 150, 300 mg

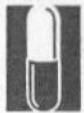
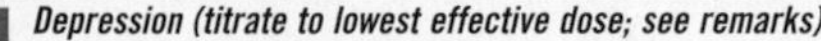

Depression (titrate to lowest effective dose; see remarks):
Child (6–18 yr): Start at 1.5–2 mg/kg/24 hr PO ÷ BID–TID; if needed, gradually increase dose Q3–4 days up to a **maximum** of 6 mg/kg/24 hr ÷ TID
Adult: Start at 150 mg/24 hr PO ÷ TID; if needed, increase by 50 mg/24 hr Q 3–4 days up a **max.** of 600 mg/24 hr for hospitalized patients (400 mg/24 hr for ambulatory patients).

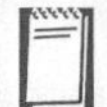

Use with caution in pre-existing cardiac disease, initial recovery phase of MI, in patients receiving antihypertensive medications, and electroconvulsive therapy. Common side effects include dizziness, drowsiness, dry mouth, and diarrhea. Seizures, tardive dyskinesia, EPS, arrhythmias, priapism, blurred vision, neuromuscular weakness, anemia, orthostatic hypotension, and rash have been reported. Monitor for clinical worsening of depression and suicidal ideation/behavior following the initiation of therapy or after dose changes.

Trazodone is CYP 450 3A4 isoenzyme substrate (may interact with inhibitors and inducers) and may increase digoxin levels and increase CNS effects of alcohol, barbiturates, and other CNS depressants. **Max.** antidepressant effect is seen at 2–6 wk.

TRETINOIN
Retin-A, Retin-A Micro, Avita, Renova, and many others
Retinoic acid derivative, topical acne product

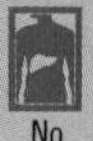 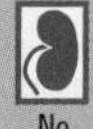 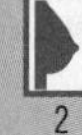 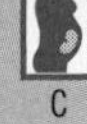

No No 2 C

Cream: 0.02% (40 g), 0.025% (20, 45 g), 0.05% (20, 40, 45, 60 g), 0.1% (20, 45 g)
Topical gel: 0.01% (15, 45 g), 0.025% (15, 20, 45 g), 0.04% (20, 40 g); may contain 90% alcohol and may contain propylene glycol
Topical gel (Retin-A Micro): 0.04% (20, 45 g), 0.1% (20, 45 g); contains glycerin, propylene glycol, benzyl alcohol

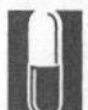

Topical:
Child >12 yr and adult: Gently wash face with a mild soap, pat the skin dry, and wait 20 to 30 min before use. Initiate therapy with either 0.025% cream or 0.01% gel and apply a small pea-sized amount to the affected areas of the face QHS or on alternate days. See remarks.

Contraindicated in sunburns. **Avoid** excessive sun exposure. If stinging or irritation occurs, decrease frequency of administration to every other day. **Avoid** contact with eyes, ears, nostrils, mouth, or open wounds. Local adverse effects include irritation, erythema, excessive dryness, blistering, crusting, hyperpigmentation or hypopigmentation, and acne flare-ups. Concomitant use of other topical acne products may lead to significant skin irritation. Onset of therapeutic benefits may be experienced within 2–3 wk with optimal effects in 6 wk. The gel dosage form is flammable and should not be exposed to heat or temperatures >120°F.

TRIAMCINOLONE
Azmacort, Nasacort HFA, Nasacort AQ, Kenalog, Aristospan and others
Corticosteroid

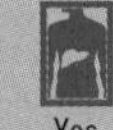 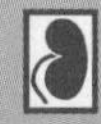  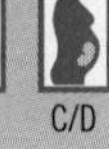 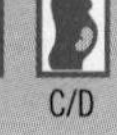
Yes Yes 2 C/D

Nasal spray:
Nasacort AQ: 55 mcg/actuation (30 actuations per 6.5 g, 120 actuations per 16.5 g); contains benzalkonium chloride and EDTA
Cream (Kenalog and others): 0.025%, 0.1% (15, 80, 454 g), 0.5% (15 g)
Ointment (Kenalog and others): 0.025%, 0.1% (15, 80, 454 g), 0.5% (15 g)
Lotion (Kenalog and others): 0.025%, 0.1% (60 mL)
Topical aerosol (Kenalog): 0.2 mg/2 second spray (23, 63 g); contains 10.3% alcohol
Dental paste (Kenalog in Orabase and others): 0.1% (5 g)
See Chapter 30 for potency rankings and sizes of topical preparations.
Injection as acetonide: 10 mg/mL (Kenalog-10) (5 mL), 40 mg/mL (Kenalog-40) (1, 5, 10 mL); contains benzyl alcohol
Injection as hexacetonide: 5 mg/mL (Aristospan Intralesional) (5 mL), 20 mg/mL (Aristospan Intra-articular) (1, 5 mL); contains benzyl alcohol

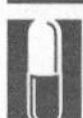

Intranasal (titrate to lowest effective dose after symptoms are controlled; discontinue use if no relief of symptoms occur after 3 wk of use):
Nasacort AQ:
Child 2–5 yr: 1 spray in each nostril once daily (110 mcg/24 hr; starting and **max. dose**).
Child 6–11 yr: Start with 1 spray in each nostril once daily (110 mcg/24 hr). If no benefit in 1 wk, dose may be increased to 2 sprays in each nostril once daily (220 mcg/24 hr). Decrease dose back to 1 spray each nostril when symptoms are controlled.
≥12 yr and adult: 2 sprays in each nostril once daily (220 mcg/24 hr; starting and **max. dose**). Decrease dose to 1 spray each nostril when symptoms are controlled.

Topical:
Child and adult: Apply a thin film to affected areas BID–TID.

Intralesional:
≥12 yr and adult:
Acetonide salt (Kenalog-10; 10 mg/mL): Up to 1 mg/site at intervals of 1 wk or more. May give separate doses in sites >1 cm apart, **not to exceed** 30 mg.
Hexacetonide salt (Aristospan Intralesional; 5 mg/mL): Up to 0.5 mg/square inch of affected skin; additional injections should be administered according to patient response.

Rinse mouth thoroughly with water after each use of the oral inhalation dosage form. Rare reports of bone mineral density loss and osteoporosis has been reported with prolonged use of inhaled dosage form. Nasal preparations may cause epistaxis, cough, fever, nausea, throat irritation, dyspepsia, and fungal infections (rarely). Topical preparations may cause dermal atrophy, telangiectasias and hypopigmentation. Topical steroids should be **used with caution** on the face and in intertriginous areas. See Chapter 8.

Dosage adjustment for hepatic failure with systemic use may be necessary. **Use with caution** in thyroid dysfunction, respiratory TB, ocular herpes simplex, peptic ulcer disease, osteoporosis, hypertension, CHF, myasthenia gravis, ulcerative colitis, and renal dysfunction. With systemic use, pregnancy category changes to "D" if used in the first trimester. Pregnancy category is "D" with the ophthalmic route.

Shake intranasal dosage forms before each use. **Avoid** SQ and IV administration with injectable dosage forms. Injectable forms contain benzyl alcohol.

For explanation of icons, see p. 663.

TRIAMTERENE
Dyrenium
Diuretic, potassium sparing

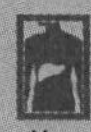 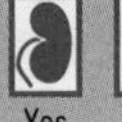 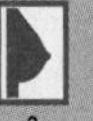 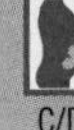
Yes Yes ? C/D

Caps: 50, 100 mg; contains benzyl alcohol and povidone

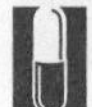

Child: 1–2 mg/kg/24 hr ÷ BID PO. May increase up to a **max.** of 3–4 mg/kg/24 hr up to 300 mg/24 hr.

Adult: 50–100 mg/24 hr ÷ once daily–BID PO; **max. dose:** 300 mg/24 hr.

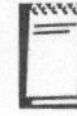

Do not use if GFR <10 mL/hr. **Adjust dose in renal impairment (see Chapter 31)** and cirrhosis. Monitor serum electrolytes. May cause hyperkalemia, hyponatremia, hypomagnesemia, and metabolic acidosis. Interstitial nephritis, thrombocytopenia, and anaphylaxis have been reported.

Concurrent use of ACE inhibitors may increase serum potassium. **Use with caution** when administering medications with high potassium load (e.g., some penicillins), and in patients with hepatic impairment or on high potassium diets. Cimetidine may increase effects. This drug is also available as a combination product with hydrochlorothiazide; erythema multiforme and toxic epidermal necrolysis have been reported with this combination product. Administer doses with food to minimize GI upset. Pregnancy category changes to "D" if used in pregnancy induced hypertension.

TRILISATE

See *Choline Magnesium Trisalicylate*

TRIMETHOBENZAMIDE HCL
Tigan and others
Antiemetic

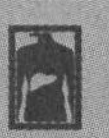 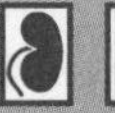 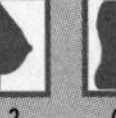 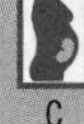
Yes Yes ? C

Caps: 300 mg
Injection: 100 mg/mL (2, 20 mL); may contain phenol or parabens

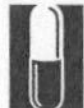

Child (PO): 15–20 mg/kg/24 hr ÷ TID–QID

Alternative dosing:

- ***<13.6 kg:*** 100 mg TID–QID
- ***13.6–40 kg:*** 100–200 mg/dose TID–QID
- ***>40 kg:*** 300 mg/dose TID–QID

Adult:

- ***PO:*** 300 mg/dose TID–QID
- ***IM:*** 200 mg/dose TID–QID

Do not use in premature or newborn infants. **Avoid** use in patients with hepatotoxicity, acute vomiting, or allergic reaction. CNS disturbances are common in children (extrapyramidal symptoms, drowsiness, confusion, dizziness). Hypotension, especially with IM use, may occur.

IM not recommended in children. Consider reducing dosage in the presence of renal impairment since a significant amount of drug is excreted and eliminated by the kidney.

TRIMETHOPRIM AND SULFAMETHOXAZOLE

See *Sulfamethoxazole and Trimethoprim*

URSODIOL

Actigall, Urso 250, Urso Forte, and others
Gallstone solubilizing agent, cholelitholytic agent

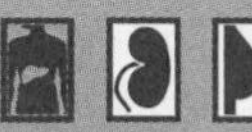
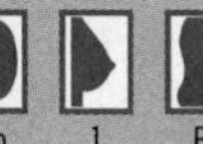
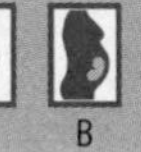

Yes No 1 B

Oral suspension: 20, 25, 50, 60 mg/mL
Caps (Actigall and others): 300 mg
Tabs:
Urso 250: 250 mg
Urso Forte: 500 mg

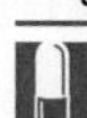

Biliary atresia:
Infant (limited data): 10–15 mg/kg/24 hr once daily PO
TPN-induced cholestasis:
Infant and child (limited data, Gastroenterology. 1996;111[3]:716–719): 30 mg/kg/24 hr ÷ TID PO
Gallstone disolution:
Adult: 8–10 mg/kg/24 hr ÷ BID–TID PO
Cystic Fibrosis (to improve fatty acid metabolism in liver disease):
Child: 15–30 mg/kg/24 hr ÷ once daily–TID PO

Contraindicated in calcified cholesterol stones, radiopaque stones, bile pigment stones, or stones >20 mm in diameter. **Use with caution** in patients with nonvisualizing gallbladder and chronic liver disease. May cause GI disturbance, rash, arthralgias, anxiety, headache, and elevated liver enzymes. Thrombocytopenia has been reported in clinical trials. Aluminum-containing antacids, cholestyramine, and oral contraceptives decrease ursodiol effectiveness. Dissolution of stones may take several mo. Stone recurrence occurs in 30%–50% of patients within 5 yr.

VALACYCLOVIR

Valtrex
Antiviral agent

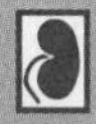

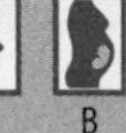

Yes Yes 1 B

Tabs/Caplets: 500, 1000 mg
Oral suspension: 25, 50 mg/mL

Herpes labialis (cold sores; initiated at earliest symptoms):
≥12 yr and adult: 2 g/dose PO Q12 hr × 1 day.
Chickenpox (immunocompetent patient):
2–<18 yr: 20 mg/kg/dose PO TID × 5 days; **max. dose:** 1 g/dose TID.
Child: Recommended dosages based on steady-state pharmacokinetic data in immunocompromised children. Efficacy data is incomplete.
To mimic an IV acyclovir regimen of 250 mg/m²/dose or 10 mg/kg/dose TID:
30 mg/kg/dose PO TID OR alternatively by weight:
4–12 kg: 250 mg PO TID.
13–21 kg: 500 mg PO TID.
22–29 kg: 750 mg PO TID.
≥30 kg: 1000 mg PO TID.

Continued

For explanation of icons, see p. 663.

VALACYCLOVIR *continued*

To mimic a PO acyclovir regimen of 20 mg/kg/dose 4 or 5 times a day:

20 mg/kg/dose PO TID OR alternatively by weight:

6–19 kg: 250 mg PO TID.

20–31 kg: 500 mg PO TID.

≥32 kg: 750 mg PO TID.

Herpes zoster (see remarks):

Adult (immunocompetent): 1 g/dose PO TID × 7 days within 48–72 hours of onset of rash.

Genital herpes:

Adolescent and adult:

Initial episodes: 1 g/dose PO BID × 10 days.

Recurrent episodes: 500 mg/dose PO BID × 3 days.

Suppressive therapy:

Immunocompetent patient: 500–1000 mg/dose PO once daily × 1 yr, then reassess for recurrences. Patients with <9 recurrances per yr may be dosed at 500 mg/dose PO once daily × 1 yr.

HIV patient with CD4 ≥100 cells/mm³: 500 mg PO BID.

This pro-drug is metabolized to acyclovir and L-valine with better oral absorption than acyclovir. **Use with caution in hepatic or renal insufficiency (adjust dose; see Chapter 31).** Thrombotic thrombocytopenic purpura/hemolytic uremic syndrome (TTP/HUS) has been reported in patients with advanced HIV infection and in bone marrow and renal transplant recipients. Probenecid or cimetidine can reduce the rate of conversion to acyclovir. Headache, nausea, and abdominal pain are common adverse events in adults. Headache is common in children. See *Acyclovir* for additional drug interactions and adverse effects.

For initial episodes of genital herpes, therapy is most effective when initiated within 48 hr of symptom onset. Therapy should be initiated immediately after the onset of symptoms in recurrent episodes (no efficacy data when initiating therapy >24 hr after onset of symptoms). Data are not available for use as suppressive therapy for periods >1 yr.

Valacyclovir **CANNOT** be substituted for acyclovir on a one-to-one basis. Doses may be administered with or without food.

VALGANCICLOVIR

Valcyte

Antiviral agent

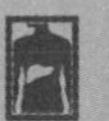
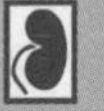
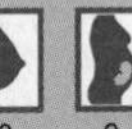
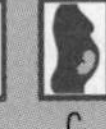

No Yes 3 C

Tabs: 450 mg

Oral solution: 50 mg/mL (100 mL)

Oral suspension: 60 mg/mL

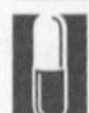

Neonate and infant:

Symptomatic congenital CMV (from pharmacokinetic [PK] data in 8 infants 4–90 days old, mean: 20 days; and 24 neonates 8–34 days old): 15–16 mg/kg/dose PO BID. Additional PK, safety, and efficacy studies are required.

Child:

CMV prophylaxis in kidney or heart transplantation: Once daily PO dosage is calculated with the following equation.

Daily mg dose (**max. dose:** 900 mg) = 7 × BSA × CrCl. BSA is determined by the Mosteller equation and CrCL is determined by a modified Schwartz equation (Max. value: 150 mL/min/1.73 m²).

Continued

VALGANCICLOVIR *continued*

Mosteller BSA (m^2) equation: square root of [(height (cm) × weight (kg)) ÷ 3600]

Modified Schwartz (mL/min/1.73 m^2) equation (max. value = 150 mL/min/1.73 m^2): k × height (cm) ÷ serum creatinine (mg/dL); where k = 0.45 if patient is 4 mo to <2 years old or; k = 0.55 for boys 2–<13 yr and girls aged 2 to 16 yr or; k = 0.7 if boys 13–16 yr old.

CMV prophylaxis in liver transplantation (limited data based on a retrospective review in 10 patients, mean age 4.9 ± 5.6 yr): 15–18 mg/kg/dose PO once daily × 100 days following transplantation resulted in 1 case of asymptomatic CMV infection detected by CMV antigenemia at day 7 of therapy. This patient then received a higher dose of 15 mg/kg/dose BID until 3 consecutive negative CMV antigenemia were achieved. The dose was switched back to a prophylactic regimen at day 46 posttransplant.

Adolescent and adult:

CMV retinitis:

Induction therapy: 900 mg PO BID × 21 days with food.

Maintenance therapy: 900 mg PO once daily with food.

CMV prophylaxis in heart, kidney, and kidney-pancreas transplantation: 900 mg PO once daily starting within 10 days of transplantation until 100 days post heart or kidney-pancreas transplantation; or until 200 days post kidney transplantation.

This pro-drug is metabolized to ganciclovir with better oral absorption than ganciclovir. **Contraindicated** with hypersensitivity to valganciclovir/ganciclovir; ANC <500 mm^3; platelets <25,000 mm^3; hemoglobin <8 g/dL; and patients on hemodialysis. **Use with caution in renal insufficiency (adjust dose; see Chapter 31)**, bone marrow suppression, or receiving myelosuppressive drugs or irradiation. May cause headache, insomnia, peripheral neuropathy, diarrhea, vomiting, neutropenia, anemia, and thrombocytopenia. Use effective contraception during and for at least 90 days after therapy. See *Ganciclovir* for drug interactions and additional adverse effects.

Valganciclovir **CANNOT** be substituted for ganciclovir on a one-to-one basis. All doses are administered with food. **Avoid** direct contact with broken or crushed tablets with the skin or mucous membranes.

VALPROIC ACID

Depakene, Depacon, and various generics

[Depakote: See *Divalproex Sodium*]

Anticonvulsant

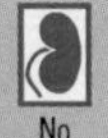
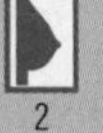
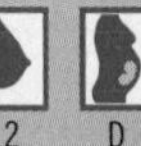

Yes No 2 D

Caps: 250 mg

Syrup: 250 mg/5 mL (473 mLl); may contain parabens

Injection (Depacon): 100 mg/mL (5 mL)

Oral:

Initial: 10–15 mg/kg/24 hr ÷ once daily–TID

Increment: 5–10 mg/kg/24 hr at weekly intervals to max. dose of 60 mg/kg/24 hr.

Maintenance: 30–60 mg/kg/24 hr ÷ BID–TID. Due to drug interactions, higher doses may be required in children on other anticonvulsants. If using divalproex sodium, administer BID.

Intravenous (use only when PO is not possible):

Use same PO daily dose ÷ Q6 hr. Convert back to PO as soon as possible.

Rectal (use syrup, diluted 1 : 1 with water, given PR as a retention enema):

Load: 20 mg/kg/dose.

Maintenance: 10–15 mg/kg/dose Q8 hr.

Continued

For explanation of icons, see p. 663.

VALPROIC ACID *continued*

Migrane prophylaxis:

Child (limited data): 15–30 mg/kg/24 hr PO ÷ BID.

Adult: Start with 500 mg/24 hr ÷ PO BID. Dose may be increased to a **max.** of 1000 mg/24 hr ÷ PO BID. If using divalproex sodium extended-release tablets, administer daily dose once daily.

Contraindicated in hepatic disease. May cause GI, liver, blood, and CNS toxicity; weight gain; transient alopecia; pancreatitis (potentially life-threatening); nausea; sedation; vomiting; headache; thrombocytopenia; platelet dysfunction; rash (especially with lamotrigine); and hyperammonemia. Hepatic failure has occurred especially in children <2 yr (especially those receiving multiple anticonvulsants, with congenital metabolic disorders, with severe seizure disorders with mental retardation, and with organic brain disease). Idiosyncratic life-threatening pancreatitis has been reported in children and adults. Hyperammonemic encephalopathy has been reported in patients with urea cycle disorders. Suicidal behavior or ideation have been reported.

Valproic acid is a substrate for CYP 450 2C19 isoenzyme and an inhibitor of CYP 450 2C9, 2D6 and 3A3/4 (weak). It increases amitriptyline/nortriptyline, phenytoin, diazepam, and phenobarbital levels. Concomitant phenytoin, phenobarbital, topiramate, meropenem, and carbamazepine may decrease valproic acid levels. Amitriptyline or nortriptyline may increase valproic acid levels. May interfere with urine ketone and thyroid tests.

Do not give syrup with carbonated beverages. Use of IV route has not been evaluated for >14 days of continuous use. Infuse IV over 1 hr up to a **max. rate** of 20 mg/min. Depakote and Depakote ER are **NOT** bioequivalent; see package insert for dose conversion.

Therapeutic levels: 50–100 mg/L. Recommendations for serum sampling at steady-state: Obtain trough level within 30 min prior to the next scheduled dose after 2–3 days of continuous dosing. Levels of 50–60 mg/L and as high as 85 mg/L have been recommended for bipolar disorders. Monitor CBC and LFTs prior to and during therapy.

Increased risk of neural tube defects, craniofacial defects, and cardiovascular malformations have been reported in babies exposed to valproic acid and divalproex sodium.

VANCOMYCIN

Vancocin and others

Antibiotic

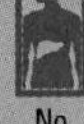 No 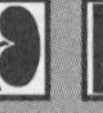 Yes 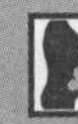 2 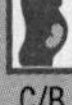 C/B

Injection: 0.5, 0.75, 1, 5, 10 g

Premixed injection: 500 mg/100 mL in dextrose; 1000 mg/200 mL in dextrose (iso-osmotic solutions)

Caps: 125, 250 mg

Oral solution: 1 g (reconstitute to 250 mg/5 mL), 10 g (reconstitute to 500 mg/6 mL)

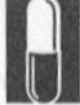

Initial empiric dosage; patient specific dosage defined by therapeutic drug monitoring (see remarks).

Neonate, IV (see following table for dosage interval):

Bacteremia: 10 mg/kg/dose

Meningitis, pneumonia: 15 mg/kg/dose

Continued

VANCOMYCIN *continued*

Neonate, IV (cont'd):

Post-menstrual Age (wk)*	Post-natal Age (days)	Dosage Interval (hr)
≤29	0–14	18
	>14	12
30–36	0–14	12
	>14	8
37–44	0–7	12
	>7	8
≥45	All	6

*Post-menstrual age = gestational age + post-natal age.

Infant, child, adolescent, and adult, IV:

Age	General Dosage	CNS Infections, Endocarditis, Osteomyelitis, Pneumonia, and MRSA Bacteremia
1 mo–12 yr	15 mg/kg Q6 hr	20 mg/kg Q6 hr
Adolescent	15 mg/kg Q6–8 hr	20 mg/kg Q6–8 hr
Adult	15 mg/kg Q8–12 hr	20 mg/kg Q8–12 hr

C. difficile colitis:

Child: 40–50 mg/kg/24 hr ÷ Q6 hr PO × 7–10 days

Max dose: 500 mg/24 hr; higher **max.** of 2 g/24 hr have also been used.

Adult: 125 mg/dose PO Q6 hr × 7–10 days; dosages as high as 2 g/24 hr ÷ Q6–8 hr have also been used.

Endocarditis prophylaxis for GU or GI (excluding esophageal) procedures (complete all antibiotic dose infusion(s) within 30 min of starting procedure):

Moderate-risk patients allergic to ampicillin or amoxicillin:

Child: 20 mg/kg/dose IV over 1–2 hr × 1

Adult: 1 g/dose IV over 1–2 hr × 1

High-risk patients allergic to ampicillin or amoxicillin:

Child and adult: Same dose as moderate-risk patients plus gentamicin 1.5 mg/kg/dose (**max. dose:** 120 mg/dose) IV/IM ×1

Ototoxicity and nephrotoxicity may occur and may be exacerbated with concurrent aminoglycoside use. Greater nephrotoxicity risk has been associated with higher therapeutic serum trough concentrations (≥15 mg/mL), and receiving furosemide in the intensive care unit. **Adjust dose in renal failure (see Chapter 31).** Use total body weight for obese patients when calculating dosages. Low concentrations of the drug may appear in CSF with inflamed meninges. Nausea, vomiting, and drug-induced erythroderma are common. "Red man syndrome" associated with rapid IV infusion may occur. Infuse over 60 min (may infuse over 120 min if 60 min infusion is not tolerated). **NOTE:** Diphenhydramine is used to reverse red man syndrome. Allergic reactions, including drug rash with eosinophilia and systemic symptoms (DRESS), have been reported.

Current recommendations extrapolated from adult guidelines suggest measuring only trough levels. However, an additional post-distributional level may be useful in characterizing enhanced/altered drug clearance for quicker dosage modification to attain target levels; consult a pharmacist. The following therapeutic trough level recommendations are based on the assumption that the pathogen's vancomycin MIC is ≤1 mg/L.

Continued

For explanation of icons, see p. 663.

VANCOMYCIN *continued*

Indication	Goal Trough Level
Uncomplicated skin and soft tissue infection, non-MRSA bacteremia, febrile neutropenia	10–15 mg/L
CNS infections, endocarditis, pneumonia, osteomyelitis, MRSA bacteremia	15–20 mg/L

Peak level measurement (20–50 mg/L) has also been recommended for patients with burns, clinically nonresponsive in 72 hr of therapy, persistent positive cultures, and CNS infections (≥30 mg/L).

Recommended serum sampling time at steady-state: Trough within 30 min prior to the fourth consecutive dose and peak 60 min after the administration of the fourth consecutive dose. Infants with faster elimination (shorter $T_{1/2}$) may be sampled around the third consecutive dose.

Metronidazole (PO) is the drug of choice for *C. difficile* colitis; vancomycin should be **avoided** due to the emergence of vancomycin-resistant enterococcus. Pregnancy category "B" is assigned with the oral route of administration.

VARICELLA-ZOSTER IMMUNE GLOBULIN (HUMAN)

VariZig, VZIG

Hyperimmune globulin, varicella-zoster

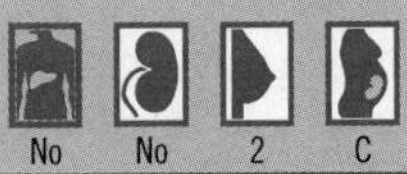

Injection: 125 U; contains 60–200 mg human immunoglobulin G, 0.1 M glycine, 0.04 M sodium chloride, and 0.01% polysorbate 80.

Product is available via an FDA-approved Expanded Access Protocol; see www.fffenterprises.com or call FFF Enterprises at 1-800-843-7477 for additional information.

Dose should be given within 48 hr of varicella exposure and no later than 96 hr post exposure.

IM (preferred route) or IV (see remarks):

≤10 kg: 125 U
10.1–20 kg: 250 U
20.1–30 kg: 375 U
30.1–40 kg: 500 U
>40 kg: 625 U
Max. dose: 625 U/dose

If patient is high risk and re-exposed to varicella >3 weeks after a prior dose, another full dose may be given.

Contraindicated in severe thrombocytopenia due to IM injection, immunoglobulin A-deficiency (anaphylactic reactions may occur), and known immunity to varicella zoster virus. See Chapter 16 for indications. Local discomfort, redness and swelling at the injection site, and headache may occur.

Hyperviscosity of the blood may increase risk for thrombotic events. IM route is preferred over IV in patients with pre-existing respiratory conditions. Interferes with immune response to live virus vaccines such as measles, mumps and rubella; defer administration of live vaccines 5 mo or longer after VZIG dose. See latest AAP *Red Book* for additional information.

IM route is the preferred route by diluting each vial with 1.25 mL of diluent for a 100 U/mL concentration. **Avoid** IM injection into the gluteal region due to risk for sciatic nerve damage and **do not exceed** age specific **single max. IM injection** volume. For IV administration, dilute each vial with 2.5 mL of diluent for a 50 U/mL concentration. IV doses are administered over 3–5 min.

VASOPRESSIN
Pitressin and various generics, 8-Arginine Vasopressin
Antidiuretic hormone analog

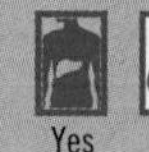
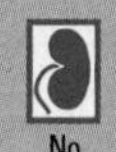

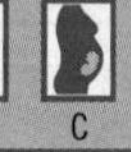
Yes No 2 C

Injection: 20 U/mL (aqueous) (0.5, 1, 10 mL); contains 0.5% chlorobutanol

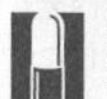

Diabetes insipidus: Titrate dose to effect.
SC/IM:
Child: 2.5–10 U BID–QID
Adult: 5–10 U BID–QID
Continuous infusion (adult and child): Start at 0.5 milliunit/kg/hr (0.0005 U/kg/hr). Double dosage every 30 min PRN up to **max. dose** of 10 milliunit/kg/hr (0.01 U/kg/hr).
Growth hormone and corticotropin provocative tests:
Child: 0.3 U/kg IM; **max. dose:** 10 U
Adult: 10 U IM
GI hemorrhage (IV):
Child: Start at 0.002–0.005 U/kg/min. Increase dose as needed to **max. dose** of 0.01 U/kg/min.
Adult: Start at 0.2–0.4 U/min. Increase dose as needed to **max. dose** of 0.9 U/min.
Cardiac arrest, ventricular fibrillation, and pulseless ventricular tachycardia:
Child (use following 2 doses of epinephrine; limited data): 0.4 U/kg IV × 1
Adult: 40 U IV or IO × 1

Use with caution in seizures, migrane, asthma, and renal, cardiac, or vascular diseases. Side effects include tremor, sweating, vertigo, abdominal discomfort, nausea, vomiting, urticaria, anaphylaxis, hypertension, and bradycardia. May cause vasoconstriction, water intoxication, and bronchoconstriction. Drug interactions: lithium, demeclocycline, heparin, and alcohol reduce activity; carbamazepine, tricyclic antidepressants, fludrocortisone, and chlorpropamide increase activity.

Do not abruptly discontinue IV infusion (taper dose). Patients with variceal hemorrhage and hepatic insufficiency may respond to lower dosages. Monitor fluid intake and output, urine specific gravity, urine and serum osmolality and sodium.

VECURONIUM BROMIDE
Norcuron and various generics
Nondepolarizing neuromuscular blocking agent

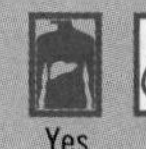
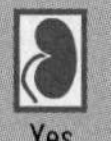
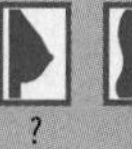
Yes Yes ? C

Injection: 10, 20 mg; diluent for reconstitution may contain benzyl alcohol

Neonate:
Initial: 0.1 mg/kg/dose IV.
Maintenance: 0.03–0.15 mg/kg/dose IV Q1–2 hr PRN.
Infants (>7 wk–1 yr) (see remarks):
Initial: 0.08–0.1 mg/kg/dose IV.
Maintenance: 0.05–0.1 mg/kg/dose IV Q1 hr PRN; may administer via continuous infusion at 0.06–0.09 mg/kg/hr IV.
>1 yr–adult (see remarks):
Initial: 0.08–0.1 mg/kg/dose IV.
Maintenance: 0.05–0.1 mg/kg/dose IV Q1 hr PRN; may administer via continuous infusion at 0.09–0.15 mg/kg/hr IV.

Continued

For explanation of icons, see p. 663.

VECURONIUM BROMIDE *continued*

Use with caution in patients with renal or hepatic impairment, and neuromuscular disease. Dose reduction may be necessary in hepatic insufficiency. Infants (7 wk to 1 yr) are more sensitive to the drug and may have a longer recovery time. Children (1–10 yr) may require higher doses and more frequent supplementation than adults. Enflurane, isoflurane, aminoglycosides, beta blockers, calcium channel blockers, clindamycin, furosemide, magnesium salts, quinidine, procainamide, and cyclosporine may increase the potency and duration of neuromuscular blockade. Calcium, caffeine, carbamazepine, phenytoin, steroids (chronic use), acetylcholinesterases, and azthioprine may decrease effects. May cause arrhythmias, rash, and bronchospasm. Severe anaphylactic reactions have been reported.

Neostigmine, pyridostigmine or edrophonium are antidotes. Onset of action within 1–3 min. Duration is 30–40 min. **See Chapter 1 for rapid sequence intubation.**

VERAPAMIL
Isoptin, Isoptin SR, Calan, Calan SR, Verelan, Verelan PM, Covera-HS, and others
Calcium channel blocker

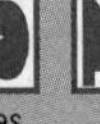
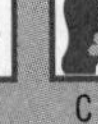

Yes Yes 1 C

Tabs: 40, 80, 120 mg
Extended/sustained-release tabs: 120, 180, 240 mg
Extended/sustained-release caps: 120, 180, 200, 240, 300, 360 mg
Injection: 2.5 mg/mL (2, 4 mL)
Oral suspension: 50 mg/mL

IV for dysrhthmias: Give over 2–3 min. May repeat once after 30 min.

1–16 yr, for PSVT: 0.1–0.3 mg/kg/dose × 1 may repeat dose in 30 min; **max. dose:** 5 mg first dose, 10 mg second dose.

Adult, for SVT: 5–10 mg (0.075–0.15 mg/kg) × 1 may administer second dose of 10 mg (0.15 mg/kg) 15–30 min later.

PO for hypertension:

Child: 4–8 mg/kg/24 hr ÷ TID or by age:

1–5 yr: 40–80 mg Q8 hr

>5 yr: 80 mg Q6–8 hr

Adult: 240–480 mg/24 hr ÷ TID–QID or divide once daily–BID for sustained-release preparations.

Contraindications include hypersensitivity, cardiogenic shock, severe CHF, sick sinus syndrome, or AV block. **Use with caution** in hepatic and renal **(reduce dose in renal insufficiency; see Chapter 31)** impairment. **Due to negative inotropic effects, verapamil should not be used to treat SVT in an emergency setting in infants. Avoid IV use** in neonates and young infants due to apnea, bradycardia, and hypotension. Monitor ECG. **Have calcium and isoproterenol available to reverse myocardial depression.** May decrease neuromuscular transmission in patients with Duchenne's muscular dystrophy, and worsen myasthenia gravis.

Drug is a substrate of CYP 450 1A2, and 3A3/4; and an inhibitor of CYP 3A4 and P-gp transporter. Barbiturates, sulfinpyrazone, phenytoin, vitamin D, and rifampin may decrease serum levels/effects of verapamil; quinidine and grapefruit juice may increase serum levels/effects. Verpamil may increase effects/toxicity of beta-blockers (severe myocardial depression), carbamazepine, cyclosporine, digoxin, ethanol, fentanyl, lithium, nondepolarizing muscle relaxants, prazosin, and tizanidine. Use with telithromycin has resulted in hypotension, bradyarrhythmias, and lactic acidosis. Bradycardia has been reported with concurrent use of clonidine.

VIGABATRIN
Sabril
Anticonvulsant

Yes Yes ? C

Tabs: 500 mg
Powder for oral solution: 500 mg per packet to be dissolved in 10 mL water (50s)

Infantile spasms (1 mo–2 yr; see remarks for discontinuation of therapy): Start at 50 mg/kg/24 hr ÷ BID PO, if needed and tolerated, may titrate dosage upwards by 25–50 mg/kg/24 hr increments Q3 days up to a **maximum** of 150 mg/kg/24 hr.

Adjunctive therapy for refractory complex partial seizures (see remarks for discontinuation of therapy):

Child (≥10 kg): Start at 40 mg/kg/24 hr ÷ BID PO, if needed and tolerated, adjust dose to the following maintenance dose:

10–15 kg: 500–1000 mg/24 hr ÷ BID
16–30 kg: 1000–1500 mg/24 hr ÷ BID
31–50 kg: 1500–3000 mg/24 hr ÷ BID
>50 kg: 2000–3000 mg/24 hr ÷ BID

Adolescent (≥16 yr) and adult (see remarks for discontinuation of therapy): Start at 500 mg BID PO, if needed and tolerated, increase daily dose by 500 mg increments at 7-day intervals. Usual dose: 1500 mg BID; **max. dose:** 6000 mg/24 hr. Doses >3 g/24 hr has not shown to provide additional benefit and is associated with more side effects.

Use with caution in renal impairment **(reduce dose; see Chapter 31)** and other CNS depressants (enhanced effects). Can cause progressive and permanent vision loss (risk increases with dose and duration); periodic vision testing is required. Common side effects include rash, weight gain, GI disturbances, arthralgia, visual disturbances, vertigo, sedation, headache, confusion, and URIs. Liver failure, anemia, psychotic disorder, and suicidal ideation have been reported. Dose-dependent abnormal MRIs have been reported in infants treated for infantile spasms.

Ketorolac, naproxen, and mefloquine may decrease the effect of vigabitrin. Vigabitrin may decrease the effects/levels of phenytoin but increase the levels/toxicity of carbamazepine.

DO NOT rapidly withdrawal therapy. Dosage needs to be tapered when discontinuing therapy to minimize increased seizure frequency. The following tapering guidelines have been recommended:

Infants and children: decrease by 25–50 mg/kg every 3–4 days
Adult: decrease by 1 g/24 hr every 7 days.

Doses may be administered with or without food. Access to this medication is restricted to prescribers and pharmacies registered under a special restricted distribution program (SHARE) in the United States. Call 888-45-SHARE for more information.

VITAMIN A
Aquasol A, Palmitate-A 5000, and many generics
Vitamin, fat soluble

No No 1 A/X

Caps: 10,000 IU [OTC], 15,000 IU [OTC], 25,000 IU
Tabs (Palmitate-A 5000): 5000 IU [OTC]
Injection (Aquasol A): 50,000 IU/mL (2 mL); contains polysorbate 80

Continued

For explanation of icons, see p. 663.

VITAMIN A *continued*

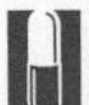

US RDA: See Chapter 21.

Supplementation in measles (6 mo to 2 yr; see remarks):

6 mo–1 yr: 100,000 IU/dose once daily PO × 2 days. Repeat 1 dose at 4 wk.

1–2 yr: 200,000 IU/dose once daily PO × 2 days. Repeat 1 dose at 4 wk.

Malabsorption syndrome prophylaxis:

Child >8 yr and adult: 10,000–50,000 IU/dose once daily PO of water miscible product.

High doses above the U.S. RDA are teratogenic (category X). The use of vitamin A in measles is recommended in children 6 mo to 2 yr of age who are either hospitalized or who have any of the following risk factors: immunodeficiency, ophthalmologic evidence of vitamin A deficiency, impaired GI absorption, moderate to severe malnutrition, and recent immigration from areas with high measles mortality. May cause GI disturbance, rash, headache, increased ICP (pseudotumor cerebri), papilledema, and irritability. Large doses may increase the effects of warfarin. Mineral oil, cholestyramine, and neomycin will reduce vitamin A absorption. See Chapter 21 for multivitamin preparations.

VITAMIN B_1

See *Thiamine*

VITAMIN B_2

See *Riboflavin*

VITAMIN B_3

See *Niacin*

VITAMIN B_6

See *Pyridoxine*

VITAMIN B_{12}

See *Cyanocobalamin*

VITAMIN C

See *Ascorbic Acid*

VITAMIN D_2

See *Ergocalciferol*

VITAMIN D_3

See *Cholecalciferol*

VITAMIN E/ALPHA-TOCOPHEROL
Aquasol E, Aquavit-E, Nutr-E-sol, and others
Vitamin, fat soluble

No No 1 A/C

Tabs [OTC]: 100, 200, 400, 500, 800 IU
Caps [OTC]: 100, 200, 400, 1000 IU
Drops (Aquasol E, Aquavit-E) [OTC]: 50 IU/mL (12, 30 mL)
Liquid (Nutr-E-sol) [OTC]: 400 IU/15 mL (473 mL)

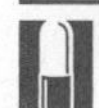

US RDA: See Chapter 21.
Vitamin E deficiency, PO: Follow levels.
Use water miscible form with malabsorption.
Neonate: 25–50 IU/24 hr
Child: 1 IU/kg/24 hr
Adult: 60–75 IU/24 hr
Cystic Fibrosis (use water miscible form): 5–10 IU/kg/24 hr PO once daily; **max. dose:** 400 IU/24 hr.

Adverse reactions include GI distress, rash, headache, gonadal dysfunction, decreased serum thyroxine and triiodothyronine, and blurred vision. Necrotizing enterocolitis has been associated with large doses (>200 units/24 hr). May increase hypoprothrombinemic response of oral anticoagulants (e.g., warfarin), especially in doses >400 IU/24 hr.

One unit of vitamin E = 1 mg of DL-alpha-tocopherol acetate. In malabsorption, water miscible preparations are better absorbed. Therapeutic levels: 6–14 mg/L.

Pregnancy category changes to "C" if used in doses above the RDA. See Chapter 21 for multivitamin preparations.

VITAMIN K

See *Phytonadione*

VORICONAZOLE
VFEND
Antifungal, triazole

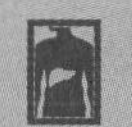 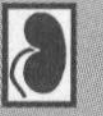  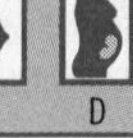

Yes Yes ? D

Tabs: 50, 200 mg; contains povidone
Oral suspension: 40 mg/mL (75 mL); contains sodium benzoate
Injection: 200 mg; contains 3200 mg sulfobutyl ether beta-cyclodextrin (SBECD)

IV:
2–11 yr (Pediatric dosing not well established; see remarks):
Loading dose: 6 mg/kg/dose Q12 hr × 2 doses.
Maintenance dose: 4 mg/kg/dose Q12 hr; a pharmacokinetic/pharmacodynamic evaluation in 46 children suggests 7 mg/kg/dose Q12 hr is required to achieve therapeutic trough levels >1 mg/L. Between-patient and inter-occasion pharmacokinetic variability was high; thus requiring serum level monitoring (see remarks).
Invasive aspergillosis: 5–7 mg/kg/dose Q12 hr.

Continued

For explanation of icons, see p. 663.

VORICONAZOLE *continued*

IV: 2–11 yr (cont'd):

>12 yr and adult:

Loading dose: 6 mg/kg/dose Q12 hr × 2 doses.

Maintenance dose:

Candidemia: 3–4 mg/kg/dose Q12 hr

Invasive aspergilosis or other serious fungal infection: 4 mg/kg/dose Q12 hr; if patient unable to tolerate, reduce dose to 3 mg/kg/dose Q12 hr.

PO:

2–11 yr: The following oral dosages are currently being investigated in Phase III clinical trials (see www.clinicaltrials.gov):

Invasive aspergillosis, serious candida infections, esophageal candidiasis, and other rare molds: 9 mg/kg/dose Q12 hr PO; maximum initial dose: 350 mg Q12 hr.

Prophylaxis in pediatric acute leukemia (up to 15 yrs old): 6 mg/kg/dose Q12 hr PO × 2 doses, followed by 4 mg/kg/dose Q12 hr PO.

≥12 yr (see remarks):

Invasive aspergillosis/Fusarium/Scedosporium/and other serious infections:

<40 kg: 100 mg PO Q12 hr; if response is inadequate, increase to 150 mg PO Q12 hr (if unable to tolerate, reduce dose by 50-mg increments to a minimum of 100 mg Q12 hr).

≥40 kg: 200 mg PO Q12 hr; if response is inadequate, increase to 300 mg PO Q12 hr (if unable to tolerate, reduce dose by 50-mg increments to a minimum of 200 mg Q12 hr).

Esophageal candidiasis (treat for a minimum 14 days and until 7 days after resolution of symptoms):

<40 kg: 100 mg PO Q12 hr; if response is inadequate, dose may be increased to 150 mg PO Q12 hr (if unable to tolerate, reduce dose by 50-mg increments to a minimum of 100 mg Q12 hr).

≥40 kg: 200 mg PO Q12 hr; if response is inadequate, dose may be increased to 300 mg PO Q12 hr (if unable to tolerate, reduce dose by 50 mg increments to a minimum of 200 mg Q12 hr).

Contraindicated with concomitant administration with CYP 450 3A4 substrates that can lead to prolonged QTc interval (e.g., cisapride, pimozide, and quinidine); concomitant administration with rifampin, carbamazepine, barbiturates, ritonavir, efavirenz, rifabutin, and St. John's wort (decreases voriconazole levels); concomitant administration with sirolimus, efavirenz, rifabutin, and ergot alkaloids (voriconazole increases levels of these drugs). Drug is a substrate and inhibitor for CYP 450 2C9, 2C19 (major substrate), and 3A4 isoenzymes. **Use with caution** in severe hepatic disease and galactose intolerance.

Currently approved for use in invasive aspergillosis, candidal esophagitis, and *Fusarium* and *Scedosporium apiospermum* infections. Common side effects include GI disturbances, fever, headache, hepatic abnormalities, photosensitivity (avoid direct sunlight), rash (6%), and visual disturbances (30%). Serious but rare side effects include anaphylaxis, liver or renal failure, and Stevens-Johnsons syndrome. Pancreatitis has been reported in children.

Adjust dose in hepatic impairment by decreasing only the maintenance dose by 50% for patients with a Child-Pugh Class A or B. **Do not use** IV dosage form for patients with GFR <50 mL/min because of accumulation of the cyclodextrin excipient; switch to oral therapy if possible. Patients receiving concurrent phenytoin should increase their voriconazole maintenance doses (IV: 5 mg/kg/dose Q 12 hr; PO: double the usual dose).

Therapeutic levels: trough: 1–5.5 mg/L. Levels <1 mg/L have resulted in treatment failures and levels >5.5 mg/L have resulted in neurotoxicity such as encephalopathy. Recommended serum sampling time: obtain trough within 30 min prior to a dose. Steady-state is typically achieved after 5–7 days of initiating therapy.

Administer IV over 1–2 hr with a **max. rate** of 3 mg/kg/hr at a concentration ≤5 mg/mL. Administer oral doses 1 hr before and after meals.

WARFARIN
Coumadin and others
Anticoagulant

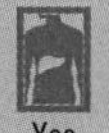 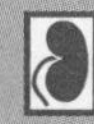 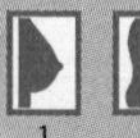 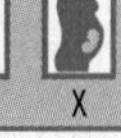
Yes Yes 1 X

Tabs: 1, 2, 2.5, 3, 4, 5, 6, 7.5, 10 mg
Injection: 5 mg

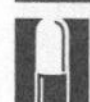

Infant and child (see remarks): To achieve an INR between 2 and 3.
Loading dose on day 1:
Baseline INR 1–1.3: 0.2 mg/kg/dose PO; **max. dose:** 7.5 mg/dose
Liver dysfunction, baseline INR >1.3, undergone Fontan procedure, NPO status/poor nutrition, receiving broad spectrum antibiotics, receiving medications that significantly inhibit CYP 450 2C9, or slow metabolizers of warfarin (see remarks): 0.1 mg/kg/dose PO; **max. dose:** 5 mg/dose
Loading dose on days 2–4:
If INR 1.1–1.3: Repeat day 1 loading dose
If INR 1.4–1.9: 50% of day 1 loading dose
If INR 2–3: 50% of day 1 loading dose
If INR 3.1–3.5: 25% of day 1 loading dose
If INR >3.5: Hold doses until INR <3.5 and restart at 50% of previous dose.
Maintenance dose (therapy day ≥5):
If INR 1.1–1.4: Increase previous dose by 20%
If INR 1.5–1.9: Increase previous dose by 10%
If INR 2–3: No change
If INR 3.1–3.5: Decrease previous dose by 10%
If INR >3.5: Hold doses until INR <3.5 and restart at 20% less than the last dose.
Usual maintenance dose: ~0.1 mg/kg/24 hr PO once daily; range: 0.05–0.34 mg/kg/24 hr. See remarks.

Adult (see remarks): 5–10 mg PO once daily × 2–5 days. Adjust dose to achieve the desired INR or PT. Maintenance dose range: 2–10 mg/24 hr PO once daily.

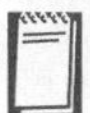

Contraindicated in severe liver or kidney disease, uncontrolled bleeding, GI ulcers, and malignant hypertension. Acts on vitamin K-dependent coagulation factors II, VII, IX, and X. Side effects include: fever, skin lesions, skin necrosis (especially in protein C deficiency), anorexia, nausea, vomiting, diarrhea, hemorrhage, and hemoptysis.

Warfarin is a substrate for CYP 450 1A2, 2C8, 2C9, 2C18, 2C19, and 3A3/4. Chloramphenicol, chloral hydrate, cimetidine, delavirdine, fluconazole, fluoxetine, metronidazole, indomethacin, large doses of vitamins A or E, nonsteroidal anti-inflammatory agents, omeprazole, oxandrolone, quinidine, salicylates, SSRIs (e.g., fluoxetine, paroxetine, sertraline), sulfonamides, and zafirlukast may increase warfarin's effect. Ascorbic acid, barbituates, carbamazepine, cholestyramine, dicloxacillin, griseofulvin, oral contraceptives, rifampin, spironolactone, sucralfate, and vitamin K (including foods with high content) may decrease warfarin's effect.

Younger children generally require higher doses to achieve desired effect. A cohort study of 319 children found that infants <1 yr required an average daily dose of 0.33 mg/kg and teenagers 11–18 yr required 0.09 mg/kg to maintain a target INR of 2–3. Children receiving Fontan cardiac surgery may require smaller doses than children with either congenital heart disease (without Fontan) or no congenital heart disease. (See *Chest* 2004;126:645–687S and *Blood* 1999;94[9]:3007–3014 for additional information.)

Continued

For explanation of icons, see p. 663.

WARFARIN *continued*

Lower initial doses should be considered for patients with pharmacogenetic variations in CYP 2C9 (e.g., *2 and *3 alleles) and VKORC1 (e.g., 1639G>A allele) enzymes, elderly and/or debilitated patients, and patients with a potential to exhibit greater than expected PT/INR response to warfarin.

The INR (international ratio) is the recommended test to monitor warfarin anticoagulant effect. Monitor INR after 5–7 days of new dosage. The particular INR desired is based upon the indication and have been extrapolated from adults. An INR of 2–3 has been recommended for prophylaxis and treatment of DVT, pulmonary emboli, and bioprosthetic heart valves. An INR of 2.5–3.5 has been recommended for mechanical prosthetic heart valves and the prevention of recurrent systemic emboli. If PT is monitored, it should be 1.5–2 times the control. Patients at high risk for bleeding may benefit from more frequent INR monitoring.

Onset of action occurs within 36–72 hr and peak effects occur within 5–7 days. IV dosing is equivalent to PO doses and is used in situations where oral dosing is not possible. **The antidote is vitamin K and fresh frozen plasma.**

ZAFIRLUKAST

Accolate

Anti-asthmatic, leukotriene receptor antagonist

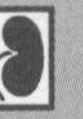
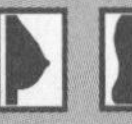
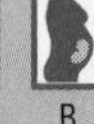

Yes No 3 B

Tabs: 10, 20 mg

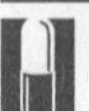

Asthma:

Child 5–11 yr: 10 mg PO BID

Child ≥12 yr and adult: 20 mg PO BID

Use with caution in hepatic insufficiency; 50%–60% reduction in clearance occurs in alcoholic cirrhosis. Contraindicated in hepatic impairment including hepatic cirrhosis. May cause headache, dizziness, nausea, diarrhea, abdominal pain, vomiting, generalized pain, asthenia, myalgia, fever, LFT elevation and dyspepsia. Eosinophilia, vasculitic rash, worsening pulmonary symptoms, cardiac complications, and/or neuropathy have been reported primarily in patients with oral steroid dose reduction. Hepatitis, hyperbilirubinemia, hepatic failure, hypersensitivity reactions (e.g., urticaria, angioedema and rashes), and neuropsychiatric events (e.g., aggression, anxiety, dream abnormalities, hallucinations, depression, suicidal behavior, and insomnia) have also been reported.

Drug is a substrate for CYP 450 2C9 and inhibits CYP 450 2C9 and 3A4 isoenzymes. Erythromycin, terfenadine, and theophylline decrease zafirlukast levels; aspirin increases levels. Zafirlukast may increase the effects of warfarin. Administer doses on an empty stomach, at least 1 hr prior or 2 hr after eating.

ZIDOVUDINE

Retrovir, AZT

Antiviral agent, nucleoside analogue reverse transcriptase inhibitor

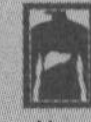
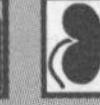
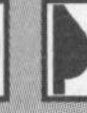
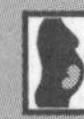

Yes Yes 3 C

Caps: 100 mg
Tabs: 300 mg
Liquid: 50 mg/5 mL (240 mL); contains 0.2% sodium benzoate
Injection: 10 mg/mL (20 mL)
In combination with lamivudine (3TC) as Combivir:
Tabs: 300 mg zidovudine + 150 mg lamivudine

Continued

ZIDOVUDINE *continued*

In combination with abacavir and lamivudine (3TC) as Trizivir:
Tabs: 300 mg zidovudine + 300 mg abacavir + 150 mg lamivudine

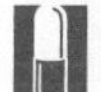

HIV: See www.aidsinfo.nih.gov/guidelines.

Prevention of vertical transmission:

14–34 wk of pregnancy:

Until labor: 600 mg/24 hr PO ÷ BID–TID.

During labor: 2 mg/kg/dose IV over 1 hour followed by 1 mg/kg/hr IV infusion until umbilical cord clamped.

Neonate and infant <6 wk: 2 mg/kg/dose Q6 hr PO or 1.5 mg/kg/dose Q6 hr IV over 60 min. Begin within 12 hr of birth and continue until 6 wk of age.

Premature infant:

<30 wk of gestation: 2 mg/kg/dose PO Q12 hr or 1.5 mg/kg/dose IV Q12 hr for first 4 wk of life, then increase dosing interval to Q8 hr thereafter.

≥30 wk of gestation: 2 mg/kg/dose PO Q12 hr or 1.5 mg/kg/dose IV Q12 hr for first 2 wk of life, then increase dosing interval to Q8 hr thereafter. Dosage interval may be further reduced to Q6 hr when the child reaches full term (40 wk postconceptional age [PCA]).

HIV post exposure prophylaxis (all therapies to begin within 2 hr of exposure if possible):

≥12 yr and adult: 200 mg/dose PO TID or 300 mg/dose PO BID × 28 days. Use in combination with lamivudine or emtricitabine, and with or without lopinavir/ritonavir × 28 days. Many other regimens exist, see above website for the most updated information.

See www.aidsinfo.nih.gov/guidelines for additional remarks.

Use with caution in patients with impaired renal or hepatic function. Dosage reduction is recommended in severe renal impairment and may be necessary in hepatic dysfunction. Drug penetrates well into the CNS. Most common side effects include: anemia, granulocytopenia, nausea, and headache (dosage reduction, erythropoietin, filgrastim/GCSF, or discontinuance may be required depending on event). Seizures, confusion, rash, myositis, myopathy (use >1 yr), hepatitis, and elevated liver enzymes have been reported. Macrocytosis is noted after 4 wk of therapy and can be used as an indicator of compliance. Lactic acidosis and severe hepatomegaly with steatosis, including fatal cases have been reported.

Do not use in combination with stavudine because of poor antiretroviral effect. Effects of interacting drugs include: increased toxicity (acyclovir, trimethoprim-sulfamethoxazole); increased hematological toxicity (ganciclovir, interferon-alpha, marrow suppressive drugs); and granulocytopenia (drugs which affect glucuronidation). Methadone, atovaquone, cimetidine, valproic acid, probenecid, and fluconazole may increase levels of zidovudine. Whereas, rifampin, rifabutin, and clarithromycin may decrease levels.

Do not administer IM. IV form is incompatible with blood product infusions and should be infused over 1 hr (intermittent IV dosing). Despite manufacturer recommendations of administering oral doses 30 min prior to or 1 hr after meals, doses may be administered with food.

ZINC SALTS, SYSTEMIC

Galzin, Orazinc, Zincate, and others
Trace mineral

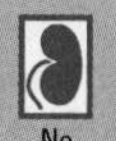
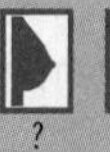
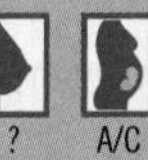

No No ? A/C

Tabs as sulfate (Orazinc and others) [OTC], 23% elemental: 66, 110, 200 mg
Caps as sulfate (Orazinc, Zincate, and others) [OTC], 23% elemental: 220 mg
Tabs as gluconate, 14.3% elemental [OTC]: 10, 15, 50 mg
Caps as acetate (Galzin), 25, 50 mg elemental per capsule

Continued

For explanation of icons, see p. 663.

ZINC SALTS, SYSTEMIC *continued*

Liquid as acetate: 5 mg elemental Zn/mL
Liquid as sulfate: 10 mg elemental Zn/mL
Injection as sulfate: 1 mg, 5 mg elemental Zn/mL; may contain benzyl alcohol
Injection as chloride: 1 mg elemental Zn/mL (10, 50 mL)

Zinc deficiency (see remarks):
Infant and child: 0.5–1 mg elemental Zn/kg/24 hr PO ÷ once daily–TID
Adult: 25–50 mg elemental Zn/dose (100–220 mg Zn sulfate/dose) PO TID
Wilson's disease:
Child (≥10 yr): 75 mg/24 hr elemental Zn PO ÷ TID; if needed, may increase to 150 mg/24 hr elemental Zn PO ÷ TID
U.S. RDA: See Chapter 21.
For supplementation in parenteral nutrition, see Chapter 21.

Nausea, vomiting, GI disturbances, leukopenia, and diaphoresis may occur. Gastric ulcers, hypotension, and tachycardia may occur at high doses. Patients with excessive losses (burns) or impaired absorption require higher doses. Therapeutic levels: 70–130 mcg/dL.

May decrease the absorption of penicillamine, tetracycline, and fluoroquinolones (e.g., ciprofloxacin). Drugs that increase gastric pH (e.g., H_2 antagonists and proton pump inhibitors) can reduce the absorption of zinc. Excessive zinc administration can cause copper deficiency.

Approximately 20%–30% of oral dose is absorbed. Oral doses may be administered with food if GI upset occurs. Pregnancy category is "A" for zinc acetate.

ZONISAMIDE
Zonegran and generics
Anticonvulsant

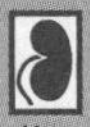 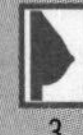 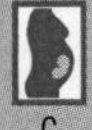 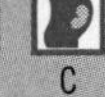
Yes Yes 3 C

Caps: 25, 50, 100 mg
Oral syrup: 10 mg/mL

Infant and child (data are incomplete):
Suggested dosing from a review of Japanese open-label studies for partial and generalized seizures: Start with 1–2 mg/kg/24 hr ÷ BID PO. Increase dosage by 0.5–1 mg/kg/24 hr Q2 wk to the usual dosage range of 5–8 mg/kg/24 hr ÷ BID PO.
Recommended higher alternative dosing: Start with 2–4 mg/kg/24 hr PO ÷ BID–TID. Gradually increase dosage at 1- to 2-wk intervals to 4–8 mg/kg/24 hr; **max. dose:** 12 mg/kg/24 hr.
Infantile spasms (regimen that was effective in a small study from Japan; additional studies are needed): Start with 2–4 mg/kg/24 hr PO ÷ BID. Then increase by 2–5 mg/kg/24 hr every 2–4 days until seizures disappear, up to a **maximum** of 20 mg/kg/24 hr.
>16 yr–adult:
Adjunctive therapy for partial seizures: 100 mg PO once daily × 2 wk. Dose may be increased to 200 mg PO once daily × 2 wk. Additional dosage increments of 100 mg/24 hr can be made at 2-wk intervals to allow attainment of steady-state levels. Effective doses have ranged from 100–600 mg/24 hr ÷ once daily–BID (BID dosing may provide better efficacy). No additional benefit has been shown for doses >400 mg/24 hr.

Because zonisamide is a sulfonamide, it is **contraindicated** in patients allergic to sulfonamides (may result in Stevens-Johnson syndrome or TEN). Common side effects of drowsiness, ataxia, anorexia, gastrointestinal discomfort, headache, rash, and pruritis usually

Continued

ZONISAMIDE *continued*

occur early in therapy and can be minimized with slow dose titration. Urolithiasis and metabolic acidosis (more frequent and severe in younger patients) have been reported. Children are at increased risk for hyperthermia and oligohydrosis, especially in warm or hot weather. Suicidal behavior or ideation have been reported.

Although not fully delineated, therapeutic serum levels of 20–30 mg/L have been suggested as higher rates of adverse reactions have been seen at levels >30 mg/L.

Zonisamide is a CYP P450 3A4 substrate. Phenytoin, carbamazepine, and phenobarbital can decrease levels of zonisamide.

Use with caution in renal or hepatic impairment; slower dose titration and more frequent monitoring is recommended. **Do not use** if GFR is <50 ml/min. **Avoid** abrupt discontinuation or radical dose reductions. Swallow capsules whole and **do not** crush or chew.

BIBLIOGRAPHY

1. Package inserts of medications.
2. Drugs and Lactation Database (LactMed). United States National Library of Medicine, Toxicology Data Network. http://toxnet.nlm.nih.gov/cgi-bin/sis/htmlgen?LACT.
3. Briggs GG, Freeman RK, Yaffe SJ. *A Reference Guide to Fetal and Neonatal Risk: Drugs in Pregnancy and Lactation.* 8th ed. Baltimore, MD: Lippincott Williams & Wilkins, 2008.
4. Pickering LK, ed. *Red Book: 2009 Report of the Committee on Infectious Diseases.* 28th ed. Elk Grove Village, IL: American Academy of Pediatrics; 2009.
5. AIDSinfo: Information on HIV/AIDS Treatment, Prevention, and Research. U.S. Department of Health and Human Services. www.aidsinfo.nih.gov.
6. Young TE, Mangum OB. *Pediatrics and Neofax electronic version.* New York, NY: Thomson Healthcare, USA; http://neofax.thomsonhc.com/neofax/neofax.php.
7. Field JM, Hazinski MF, Gilmore D, eds. *Handbook of Emergency Cardiovascular Care for Healthcare Providers: Guidelines CPR ECC 2005.* American Heart Association; 2005.
8. McEvoy GK, Snow EK, eds. *AHFS Drug Information. Stat!Ref electronic version.* Bethesda, MD: American Society of Health-System Pharmacists. www.ahfsdruginformation.com.
9. Facts and Comparisons: Online 4.0, electronic drug information service 21, Facts and Comparisons. Philadelphia, PA: Wolters Luwer Health and Pharma Solutions Division. www.online.factsandcomparisons.com.
10. Micromedex(r) Healthcare Series 2.0. Electronic database. New York, NY: Thomson Healthcare USA. Updated periodically. www.thomsonhc.com/micromedex2/librarian.
11. Takemoto CK, Hodding JH, Kraus DM. *Pediatric Dosage Handbook, electronic intranet database.* Hudson, OH: Lexi-Comp, Inc. Updated periodically. www.crlonline.com/crlsql/servlet/crlonline.
12. National Institutes of Health: National Heart, Lung and Blood Institute–Expert Panel. Clinical Practice Guidelines: Guidelines for the Diagnosis and Management of Asthma. http://www.nhlbi.nih.gov/guidelines/asthma/asthsumm.htm.
13. National High Blood Pressure Education Program Working Group on High Blood Pressure in Children and Adolescents. The Fourth Report on the Diagnosis, Evaluation, and Treatment of High Blood Pressure in Children and Adolescents. *Pediatrics* 2004;114:555–576.

For explanation of icons, see p. 663.

14. Flynn JT, Daniels SR. Pharmacologic Treatment of Hypertension in Children and Adolescents. *Journal of Pediatrics* 2006;149:746–754.
15. Lande MB, Flynn JT. Treatment of Hypertension in Children and Adolescents. *Pediatric Nephrology* 2009;(24):1939–1949.
16. Monagle P, Chalmers E, Chan A, deVeber G, Kirkham F, Massicotte, P, Michelson AD. Antithrombotic Therapy in Neonates and Children: American College of Chest Physicians Evidence-Based Clinical Practice Guidelines, 8th edition. *Chest* 2008;133:887–968.
17. Yin T, Miyata T. Warfarin dose and the pharmacogenomics of CYP2C9 and VKORC1–Rationale and Perspectives. *Thrombosis Research* 2007;(120):1–10.
18. American Thoracic Society. Targeted Tuberculin Testing and Treatment of Latent Tuberculosis Infection. American Journal of Respiratory *Critical Care Medicine* 2000;161:1376–1395.
19. Food and Drug Administration Drug Safety Labeling Changes. www.fda.gov/Safety/MedWatch/SafetyInformation/Safety-RelatedDrugLabelingChanges/default.htm.
20. Wagner CL, Greer FR, and the Section on Breastfeeding and Committee on Nutrition. Prevention of Rickets and Vitamin D Deficiency in Infants, Children, and Adolescents. *Pediatrics* 2008;122:1142–1152.
21. Committee to Review Reference Intakes for Vitamin D and Calcium. Ross AC (Chair). Institute of Medicine of the National Academies. Brief Report: Dietary Reference Intakes for Calcium and Vitamin D. November 2010. www.iom.edu/vitamind.
22. Jew RK, Soo-Hoo W, Erush SC. *Extemporaneous Formulations for Pediatrics, Geriatric, and Special Needs Patients*. 2nd ed. Bethesda, MD: American Society of Health-System Pharmacists; 2010.

Chapter 30

Formulary Adjunct

Kristin M. Arcara, MD

Special thanks go to the following people who provided guidance in preparing the elements of Chapter 30: Sande Okelo, MD; Allison Kirk, MD; Bernard Cohen, MD; Katherine Puttgen, MD; Amy Schwartz, RD; Michael Repka, MD; Elizabeth Shumann, MD; Alix Dabb, Pharm D.

I. WEBSITES

Physician's Desk Reference: http://www.pdr.net/Default.aspx
Lexi-Comp Drug Reference: http://online.lexi.com
G6PD Deficiency: http://g6pddeficiency.org/index.php?cmd=contraindicated

II. SYSTEMIC CORTICOSTEROIDS

A. Endocrine[1]

1. **Glucocorticoid deficiency:**

a. **Etiology:** Central adrenocorticotropic hormone (ACTH) deficiency or hypopituitarism, adrenal suppression (e.g., treatment for >2 weeks with exogenous glucocorticoid), adrenalectomy, congenital adrenal hyperplasia (CAH), Addison's disease

b. **Chronic physiologic replacement:**
   (1) Hydrocortisone: By mouth (PO) 12–18 mg/m^2/24 hr ÷ q8hr
   (2) Prednisone/prednisolone: PO 2.5–3.5 mg/m^2/24 hr ÷ q12hr

NOTE: See the body surface area nomogram (Fig. 30-1)
   (3) Doses may need to be titrated based on variability in metabolism among patients. Consultation with an endocrinologist is strongly encouraged

c. **Acute stress dosing:**
   (1) Minor ambulatory illnesses: Three times physiologic replacement dose
   (2) Severe stress/illness/surgery/adrenal crisis: Hydrocortisone sodium succinate (Solu-Cortef): Intravenous (IV): 50 mg/m^2 IV bolus, then 25–100 mg/m^2/24 hr (give as continuous infusion). If IV access not available, administer 25 mg/m^2/dose IM q6hr

2. **Mineralocorticoid deficiency:**

a. **Etiology:** Salt-losing CAH, Addison's disease, adrenalectomy
Mineralocorticoid therapy is not necessary with adrenal suppression or central ACTH deficiency

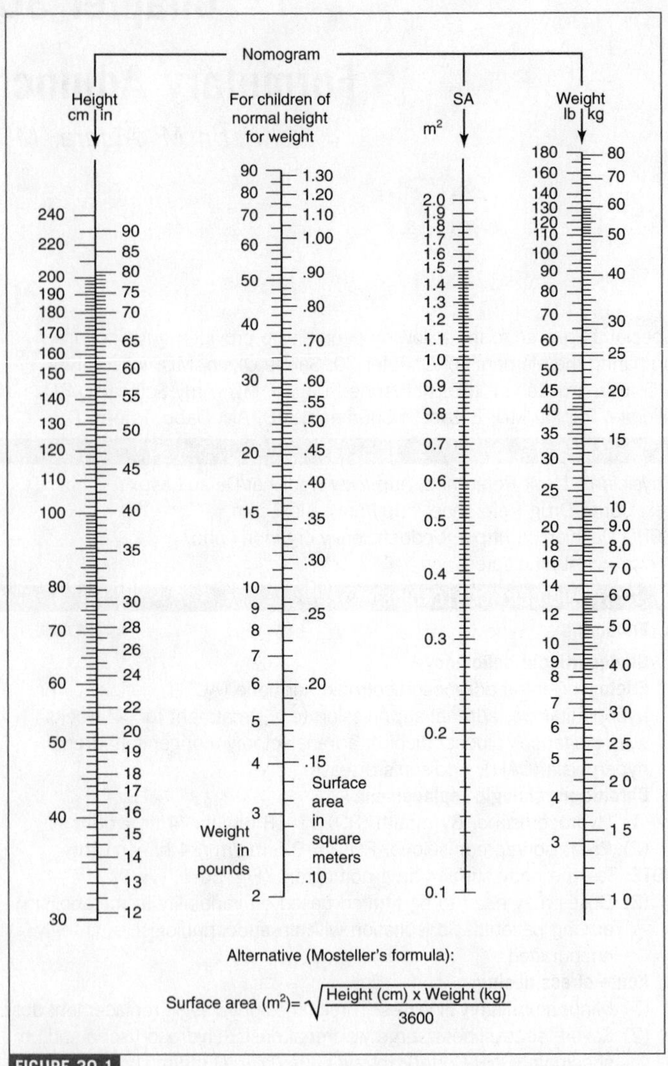

$$\text{Surface area (m}^2) = \sqrt{\frac{\text{Height (cm)} \times \text{Weight (kg)}}{3600}}$$

FIGURE 30-1

Body surface area nomogram and equation. *(From Briars GL, Bailey BJ: Surface area estimation: pocket calculator V nomogram. Arch Dis Child 1994;70:246–247.)*

b. **Chronic physiologic replacement:** Fludrocortisone acetate (Florinef): PO: Usually 0.1 mg/m^2/24 hr, with a range of 0.05–0.15 mg/24 hr. Dose adjusted for blood pressure and plasma renin activity[1,2]
c. No change in dose in the face of stress

B. Pulmonary

1. **Airway edema:**
a. Peri-extubation: Dexamethasone: PO/IV/intramuscular (IM): 0.5–2 mg/kg/24 hr ÷ q6hr. Begin 24 hr before extubation, and continue for 4–6 doses after extubation
b. Croup: Dexamethasone, 0.6 mg/kg/dose PO/IM/IV, regardless of severity.[3] Recent studies have suggested comparable efficacy of prednisolone 1mg/kg, dexamethasone 0.6mg/kg and dexamethasone 0.15 mg/kg PO doses.[4] Inhaled budesonide, 2 mg q12hr (maximum: 4 doses)[5]
2. **Acute asthma[6]:**
a. Prednisone/prednisolone:
   (1) PO: 1–2 mg/kg/day divided 1–2 times daily for 3–10 days (maximum 60 mg/day in children <12 years and 80 mg/day in children ≥12 years)
   (2) Treatment should be continued until symptoms resolve or peak expiratory flow is 70% of predicted or 80%–100% of personal best
b. Methylprednisolone:
   (1) IV/PO: 1–2 mg/kg/day divided 1–2 times daily for 3–10 days (maximum 60 mg/day in children <12 years and 80 mg/day in children ≥12 years)
   (2) Treatment should be continued until symptoms resolve or peak expiratory flow is 70% of predicted or 80%–100% of personal best
   (3) IM: (if compliance or vomiting are a concern) 7.5 mg/kg × one for children ≤4 years or 240 mg × one dose in children 5–11 years of age

C. Miscellaneous

1. **Antiemetic (chemotherapy induced): Dexamethasone[7]**
a. IV: Initial: 10 mg/m^2/dose (maximum dose: 20 mg)
b. Subsequent: 5 mg/m^2/dose q6hr
2. **Cerebral edema (due to trauma): Dexamethasone[7]**
a. PO/IM/IV: Loading dose: 1–2 mg/kg/dose × 1 dose
b. Maintenance: 1–1.5 mg/kg/24 hr ÷ q4–6hr (maximum dose: 16 mg/24 hr)
3. **Spinal cord injury: Methylprednisolone[8]**
a. 30 mg/kg bolus dose over 15 min, followed 45 min later by a continuous infusion of 5.4 mg/kg/hr
   (1) Continue infusion for 23 hour if therapy initiated within 3 hours of injury

30

TABLE 30-1

POTENCY OF VARIOUS THERAPEUTIC STEROIDS (Set Relative to the Potency of Cortisol)

Steroid	Glucocorticoid Effect* (in mg of cortisol per mg of steroid)	Mineralocorticoid Effect† (in mg of cortisol per mg of steroid)
Cortisol (hydrocortisone)	1.0	1.0
Cortisone acetate (oral)	0.8	0.8
Cortisone acetate (IM)	0.8	0.8
Prednisone	4	0.25
Prednisolone	4	0.25
Methyl prednisolone	5	0.4
Betamethasone	25	0
Triamcinolone	5	0
Dexamethasone	30	0
9α–fluorocortisone (fludrocortisone)	15	200
DOC acetate	0	20
Aldosterone	0.3	200–1,000

*To determine cortisol equivalent of a given steroid dose, multiply dose of steroid by the corresponding number in the column for glucocorticoid or mineralocorticoid effect. To determine dose of a given steroid based on desired cortisol dose, divide desired hydrocortisone dose by corresponding number in the column.

†Total physiologic replacement for salt retention is usually 0.1 mg Florinef, regardless of patient size.

Modified from Sperling MA: Pediatric endocrinology, 3rd ed. Philadelphia, Saunders, 2008, p. 476.

(2) Continue infusion for 48 hours if initiated between 3–8 hours after injury. Should be administered within 8 hours of injury for efficacy

b. Methylprednisolone does not appear to be of benefit in acute head injury

4. **Bacterial meningitis[9]:**

a. Indications:

(1) Dexamethasone may be beneficial for children >6 weeks with *Haemophilus influenzae* type b meningitis

(2) Dexamethasone could be considered for children >6 weeks with pneumococcal meningitis; still controversial

b. Dose: Dexamethasone: 0.6 mg/kg/day IV divided q6hr for the first 4 days of antibiotic therapy. Start at the time of the first parenteral antibiotic dose. Initiation >4 hours after parenteral antibiotics unlikely to be effective. Do not delay antibiotic therapy because of steroid administration

5. **Idiopathic thrombocytic purpura[10]:**

a. Indications: Clinical bleeding

b. Dose: Prednisone 1–2 mg/kg/day for up to 14 days. Alternatively, 4 mg/kg/day for 3–4 days

D. Dose Equivalence of Commonly Used Steroids (Table 30-1)

III. INHALED CORTICOSTEROIDS FOR AIRWAY INFLAMMATION (TABLE 30-2)

TABLE 30-2

ESTIMATED COMPARATIVE DAILY DOSAGES FOR INHALED CORTICOSTEROIDS

Inhaled Corticosteroids (ICS)		<12 years old			>12 years old		
		Low Dose	Medium Dose	High Dose	Low Dose	Medium Dose	High Dose
Beclomethasone/QVar MDI	40 mcg	2–4 puffs/day	5–8 puffs/day	>8 puffs/day	2–6 puffs/day	7–12 puffs/day	>12 puffs/day
	80 mcg	1–2 puffs/day	3–4 puffs/day	>4 puffs/day	1–3 puffs/day	3–6 puffs/day	>6 puffs/day
Budesonide/Pulmicort DPI Flexhaler	90 mcg	2–4 puffs/day	4–8 puffs/day	>8 puffs/day	2–6 puffs/day	7–12 puffs/day	>12 puffs/day
	180 mcg	1–2 puffs/day	2–4 puffs/day	>4 puffs/day	1–3 puffs/day	4–6 puffs/day	>6 puffs/day
Budesonide/Pulmicort Respule	0.25 mg neb	2 nebs/day	4 nebs/day	8 nebs/day	N/A	N/A	N/A
	0.5 mg neb	1 neb/day	2 nebs/day	4 nebs/day	N/A	N/A	N/A
Flunisolide/Aerospan MDI	80 mcg	2 puffs/day	4 puffs/day	>8 puffs/day	4 puffs/day	5–8 puffs/day	>8 puffs/day
	250 mcg	2–3 puffs/day	4–5 puffs/day	>5 puffs/day	2–4 puffs/day	5–8 puffs/day	>8 puffs/day
Fluticasone/Flovent MDI	44 mcg	2–4 puffs/day	5–8 puffs/day	>8 puffs/day	2–6 puffs/day	7–10 puffs/day	>10 puffs/day
	110 mcg	1 puff/day	2–3 puffs/day	>3 puffs/day	1–2 puffs/day	3–4 puffs/day	>4 puffs/day
	220 mcg	N/A	1 puff/day	>1 puff/day	1 puff/day	2 puffs/day	>2 puffs/day
Fluticasone/Flovent Diskus DPI	50 mcg	2–4 puffs/day	5–8 puffs/day	>8 puffs/day	2–6 puffs/day	7–10 puffs/day	>10 puffs/day
	100 mcg	1–2 puffs/day	2–4 puffs/day	>4 puffs/day	1–3 puffs/day	4–5 puffs/day	>5 puffs/day
	250 mcg	N/A	1 puff/day	>1 puff/day	1 puff/day	2 puffs/day	>2 puffs/day
Mometasone/Asmanex Twisthaler	220 mcg	N/A	N/A	N/A	1 puff	2 puffs	>2 puffs

Continued

TABLE 30-2

ESTIMATED COMPARATIVE DAILY DOSAGES FOR INHALED CORTICOSTEROIDS (Continued)

Inhaled Corticosteroids (ICS)		<12 years old			>12 years old		
		Low Dose	Medium Dose	High Dose	Low Dose	Medium Dose	High Dose
Combination Drugs–ICS + LABA**							
Fluticasone/Salmeterol MDI	45/21 mcg	2 puffs/day	2–3 puffs/day	4 puffs/day	2 puffs/day	3–4 puffs/day	
	115/21 mcg		2 puffs/day	2–4 puffs/day	2 puffs/day	2 puffs/day	3–4 puffs/day
	230/21 mcg			2–4 puffs/day			3–4 puffs/day
Fluticasone/Salmeterol Diskus DPI	100/50 mcg	1 puff/day	2 puffs/day	2 puffs/day		2 puffs/day	
	250/50 mcg			2 puffs/day		1 puff/day	2 puffs/day
	500/50 mcg			2 puffs/day			2 puffs/day
Budesonide/Formoterol	80/4.5 mcg MDI	1–2 puffs/day	2–4 puffs/day		1–3 puffs/day	4 puffs/day	
	160/4.5 mcg MDI		1–2 puffs/day	2–4 puffs/day		2 puffs/day	4 puffs/day

**For ICS+LABA combination drugs, patient should not take more than 2 puffs per dose of the MDI, 1 puff per dose of the DPI, or 2 doses per day.

DPI, Dry powder inhaler; ICS, inhaled corticosteroid; LABA, long acting β-agonist; LTRA, leukotriene receptor antagonist; MDI, metered dose inhaler.

Modified from Expert Panel Report III. Guidelines for the diagnosis and management of asthma—full report 2007; National Institutes of Health Pub. No. 08-4051. Bethesda, MD, National Asthma Education and Prevention Program, 2007.

IV. TOPICAL CORTICOSTEROIDS

A. Potency

Table 30-3 provides a listing of topical steroids from the most potent (class 1) to the least potent (class 7). Use intermediate- and low-potency steroids (class 4–7) for pediatric patients. Topical steroid use is contraindicated in the treatment of varicella.

TABLE 30-3

TOPICAL STEROID POTENCY RANKING

Brand Name	Generic Name
CLASS 1—SUPERPOTENT	
Clobex Lt/Spray/Shampoo, 0.05%	Clobetasol propionate
Cormax Cr/Sol, 0.05%	Clobetasol propionate
Diprolene Ot, 0.05%	Betamethasone dipropionate
Olux E Foam, 0.05%	Clobetasol propionate
Olux Foam, 0.05%	Clobetasol propionate
Temovate Cr/Ot/Sol, 0.05%	Clobetasol propionate
Ultravate Cr/Ot, 0.05%	Halobetasol propionate
Vanos Cr, 0.1%	Fluocinonide
Psorcon Ot, 0.05%	Diflorasone diacetate
Psorcon E Ot, 0.05%	Diflorasone diacetate
CLASS 2—POTENT	
Diprolene Cr AF, 0.05%	Betamethasone dipropionate
Elocon Ot, 0.1%	Mometasone furoate
Florone Ot, 0.05%	Diflorasone diacetate
Halog Ot/Cr, 0.1%	Halcinonide
Lidex Cr/Gel/Ot, 0.05%	Fluocinonide
Psorcon Cr, 0.05%	Diflorasone diacetate
Topicort Cr/Ot, 0.25%	Desoximetasone
Topicort Gel, 0.05%	Desoximetasone
CLASS 3—UPPER MID-STRENGTH	
Cutivate Ot, 0.005%	Fluticasone propionate
Lidex-E Cr, 0.05%	Fluocinonide
Luxiq Foam, 0.12%	Betamethasone valerate
Topicort LP Cr, 0.05%	Desoximetasone
CLASS 4—MID-STRENGTH	
Cordran Ot, 0.05%	Flurandrenolide
Elocon Cr, 0.1%	Mometasone furoate
Kenalog Cr/Spray, 0.1%	Triamcinolone acetonide
Synalar Ot, 0.03%	Fluocinolone acetonide
Westcort Ot, 0.2%	Hydrocortisone valerate
CLASS 5—LOWER MID-STRENGTH	
Capex Shampoo, 0.01%	Fluocinolone acetonide
Cordran Cr/Lt/Tape, 0.05%	Flurandrenolide

Continued

TABLE 30-3

TOPICAL STEROID POTENCY RANKING (Continued)

Brand Name	Generic Name
CLASS 5—LOWER MID-STRENGTH	
Cutivate Cr/Lt, 0.05%	Fluticasone propionate
DermAtop Cr, 0.1%	Prednicarbate
DesOwen Lt, 0.05%	Desonide
Locoid Cr/Lt/Ot/Sol, 0.1%	Hydrocortisone
Pandel Cr, 0.1%	Hydrocortisone
Synalar Cr, 0.03%/0.01%	Fluocinolone acetonide
Westcort Cr, 0.2%	Hydrocortisone valerate
CLASS 6—MILD	
Aclovate Cr/Ot, 0.05%	Alclometasone dipropionate
Derma-Smoothe/FS Oil, 0.01%	Fluocinolone acetonide
Desonate Gel, 0.05%	Desonide
Synalar Cr/Sol, 0.01%	Fluocinolone acetonide
Verdeso Foam, 0.05%	Desonide
CLASS 7—LEAST POTENT	
Cetacort Lt, 0.5%/1%	Hydrocortisone
Cortaid Cr/Spray/Ot	Hydrocortisone
Hytone Cr/Lt, 1%/2.5%	Hydrocortisone
Micort-HC Cr, 2%/2.5%	Hydrocortisone
Nutracort Lt, 1%/2.5%	Hydrocortisone
Synacort Cr, 1%/2.5%	Hydrocortisone

National Psoriasis Foundation: http://www.psoriasis.org/netcommunity/sublearn03_mild_potency. Accessed August 16, 2010.

B. Cautions

1. Occlusive dressings (including waterproof diapers) increase systemic absorption of topical steroids; should not be used with high-potency preparations
2. Topical steroids should be used with caution in intertriginous areas and on the face

C. Application

Apply once or twice daily. Penetration of the skin is greatest with ointments, with decreasing effectiveness in gels, creams, and lotions. Prolonged use may result in cutaneous and systemic side effects.

D. Coverage

A gram of topical cream or ointment should cover a 10 × 10-cm area. A 30- to 60-g tube will cover the entire body of an adult once.

V. INSULIN (TABLE 30-4)

For the management of diabetic ketoacidosis, see Chapter 10.

VI. PANCREATIC ENZYME SUPPLEMENTS (TABLE 30-5)

TABLE 30-4

CURRENTLY AVAILABLE INSULIN PRODUCTS

Insulin*	Onset	Peak	Effective Duration
Rapid acting	5–15 min	30–90 min	5 hr
Lispro (Humalog)			
Aspart (NovoLog)			
Glulisine (Apidra)			
Short acting	30–60 min	2–3 hr	5–8 hr
Regular U100			
Regular U500 (concentrated)			
Intermediate acting	2–4 hr	4–10 hr	10–16 hr
Isophane insulin (NPH, Humulin N/Novolin N)			
Long acting			
Glargine (Lantus)	2–4 hr[†]	No peak	20–24 hr
Detemir (Levemir)	Slow	6–8 hr	6–24 hr (dose-related)
Premixed			
70% NPH/30% regular (Humulin 70/30)	30–60 min	Dual	10–16 hr
75% NPL/25% lispro (Humalog Mix 75/25)	5–15 min	Dual	10–16 hr
50% NPL/50% lispro (Humalog Mix 50/50)	5–15 min	Dual	10–16 hr
70% NPA/30% aspart (NovoLog Mix 70/30)	5–15 min	Dual	10–16 hr

*Assuming 0.1–0.2 U/kg per injection. Onset and duration vary significantly by injection site.

[†]Time to steady state.

L, Lente; NPA, insulin aspart protamine (neutral protamine aspart); NPH, neutral protamine Hagedom; NPL, insulin lispro protamine (neutral protamine lispro).

Adapted from American Diabetes Association: Practical insulin: a handbook for prescribing providers, 2nd ed. American Diabetes Association, 2007;

http://www.novonordisk-us.com/documents/promotion_page/document/diabetes_care.asp

http://www.lilly.com/products/

TABLE 30-5

PANCRELIPASE*

Product	Lipase (USP) Units	Amylase (USP) Units	Protease (USP) Units
Creon			
6	6,000	30,000	19,000
12	12,000	60,000	38,000
24	24,000	120,000	76,000
Pancreaze MT			
4	4,200	17,500	10,000
10	10,500	43,750	25,000
16	16,800	70,000	40,000
20	21,000	61,000	37,000
Zenpep			
5	5,000	27,000	17,000
10	10,000	55,000	34,000
15	15,000	82,000	51,000
20	20,000	109,000	68,000

*See Formulary for side effects associated with administration. As of April 12, 2010, these are the only 3 products approved by the Food and Drug Administration (FDA) as many were recently removed from the market. Products are all supplied as delayed release capsules.

Data from http://www.creon-us.com/Healthcare-Professional/default.htm

http://www.zenpep.com/site/cfpatient.aspx

http://newdrugreview.com/index.php/gastrointestinal-drugs/pancreaze-3-dosage-forms-and-strengths

U.S. Food and Drug Administration: Updated questions and answers for healthcare professionals and the public: use an approved pancreatic enzyme product (PEP). Accessed August 11, 2010.

http://www.fda.gov/Drugs/DrugSafety/PostmarketDrugSafetyInformationforPatientsandProviders/ucm204745.htm

VII. COMMON INDUCES AND INHIBITORS OF THE CYTOCHROME P450 SYSTEM (TABLE 30-6)

Table 30-6 is meant to give some common pediatric examples of inducers/inhibitors. Other resources have more complete listings.[7]

TABLE 30-6

EXAMPLES OF INDUCERS AND INHIBITORS OF THE CYTOCHROME P450 SYSTEM

Isoenzyme	Substrates (Drugs Metabolized by Isoenzyme)	Inhibitors*	Inducers
CYP1A2	Caffeine, theophylline, estradiol, propranolol	Cimetidine, quinolones, fluvoxamine, ketoconazole, lidocaine	Carbamazepine, smoking, phenobarbital, rifampin
CYP2B6	Cyclophosphamide, efavirenz, propofol	Paroxetine, sertraline	Carbamazepine, (fos)phenytoin, phenobarbital, rifampin
CYP2 C9/10	Warfarin, phenytoin, tolbutamide, fluoxetine, sulfamethoxazole, fosphenytoin	Amiodarone, fluconazole, ibuprofen, indomethacin, nicardipine	Carbamazepine, (fos)phenytoin, rifampin, phenobarbital
CYP2 C19	Diazepam, PPIs, phenytoin, desogestrel, ifosfamide, phenobarbital, sertraline	Cimetidine fluvoxamine, fluconazole, isoniazid, PPIs, sertraline	Carbamazepine, (fos)phenytoin, rifampin
CYP2D6	Captopril, codeine, haloperidol, dextromethorphan, tricyclic antidepressants, hydrocodone, oxycodone, phenothiazines, metoprolol, propranolol, paroxetine, venlafaxine, risperidone, flecainide, sertraline, ariprazole, fluoxetine, lidocaine, fosphenytoin, ritonavir	Chlorpromazine, cinacalcet, dexmedetomidine, cocaine, cimetidine, quinidine, ritonavir, fluoxetine, sertraline, amiodarone	None known

CYP2E1	Acetaminophen, alcohol, isoniazid, theophylline, Isoflurane	Disulfiram	Alcohol
CYP3A4	Amlodipine, ariprazole, budesonide, cocaine, clonazepam, diltiazem, efavirenz, erythromycin, estradiol, fentanyl, fluticasone, nifedipine, verapamil, cyclosporine, carbamazepine, cisapride, tacrolimus, midazolam, alfentanil, diazepam, ifosfamide, imatinib, itraconazole, ketoconazole, cyclophosphamide, PPIs, haloperidol, lidocaine, medroxyprogesterone, methadone, methylprednisolone, salmeterol, theophylline, quetiapine, ritonavir, indinavir, sildenafil	Erythromycin, cimetidine, clarithromycin, isoniazid, ketoconazole, itraconazole, metronidazole, sertraline, ritonavir, indinavir, imatinib, nicardipine, propofol, quinidine	Rifampin, (fos)phenytoin, phenobarbital, carbamazepine, dexamethasone

*Only strong and some moderate inhibitors are listed here. Weak inhibitors also exist.

NOTE: The cytochrome P450 enzyme system is composed of different isoenzymes. Each isoenzyme metabolizes a unique group of drugs or substrates. When an ***inhibitor*** of a particular isoenzyme is introduced, the serum concentration of any drug or ***substrate*** metabolized by that particular isoenzyme will ***increase.*** When an ***inducer*** of a particular isoenzyme is introduced, the serum concentration of drugs or ***substrates*** metabolized by that particular isoenzyme will ***decrease.***

CYP, Cytochrome P450; PPI, proton pump inhibitor.

Data from Taketomo CK, Hodding JH, Kraus DM: American Pharmaceutical Association pediatric dosage handbook, 16th ed. Hudson, OH, Lexi-Comp, 2009; Zevin S, Benowitz NL. Drug interactions with tobacco smoking. An update. Clin Phamacokinet 1999;36(6):425–438; Cupp MJ, Tracy TS: Cytochrome P450: new nomenclature and clinical implications. Am Fam Physician 1998;57(1):107–116.

VIII. OPHTHALMIC DRUGS (TABLE 30-7)

TABLE 30-7

OPHTHALMIC DRUGS

Brand Name	Ingredient	Indication	Dose
Alocril (≥3 yr) Sol: 5 mL	Nedocromil sodium 2% (mast cell stabilizer), benzalkonium chloride	Allergic conjunctivitis	1–2 gtt several times a day; remove contact lenses during therapy
Alomide (>2 yr) Sol: 10 mL	Lodoxamide tromethamine 0.1% (mast cell stabilizer)	Vernal conjunctivitis and keratitis, keratoconjunctivitis	1–2 gtt qid up to 3 mo
Azasite (≥1 yr) Sol: 2.5 mL	Azithromycin 1% (contains benzalkonium chloride)	Conjunctivitis	1 gtt bid × 2 days, then q day × 5 days
Bleph-10 (>2 mo) Sol: 2.5 mL, 5 mL, 15 mL Oint: 3.5 g	Sulfacetamide sodium 10% Sol: benzalkonium chloride Oint: phenylmercuric acetate	Conjunctivitis Ophthalmic solution used as adjunct in trachoma	1–2 gtt q2–3hr or small amount of oint q3–4hr for 7–10 days Trachoma: 2 gtt q2hr w/systemic therapy
Cortisporin Oph susp: 7.5 mL Oph oint: 3.5 g	Susp (per mL): polymyxin B sulfate (10,000 U), neomycin sulfate (0.35%), hydrocortisone (1%) Oint (per g): polymyxin B sulfate (10,000 U), neomycin sulfate (0.35%), bacitracin zinc (400 U), hydrocortisone (1%)	Ocular inflammation associated with infection **Contraindicated in fungal, viral, or mycobacterial infection** Use with caution in glaucoma, or in corneal or scleral thinning	1–2 gtt or small amount of oint tid–qid
Erythromycin Oint: 1, 3.5 g	Erythromycin (5 mg/g)	Conjunctivitis Prophylaxis of ophthalmia neonatorum	Small amount up to 6 times daily 0.5–1 cm to each conjunctival sac
Neosporin Oint: 3.75 g Sol: 10 mL	Oint (per g): polymyxin B sulfate (10,000 U), bacitracin zinc (400 U), neomycin sulfate (3.5 mg) Sol (per mL): polymyxin B sulfate (10,000 U), neomycin sulfate (1.75 mg), gramicidin (0.025 mg), 0.5% alcohol	Conjunctivitis	1–2 gtt or small amount of oint q 4 hr for 7–10 days For acute infections, 1–2 gtt 2–4 × q1hr initially

Ocuflox (>1 yr) Sol: 5 mL, 10 mL	Ofloxacin 0.3%, benzalkonium chloride	Conjunctivitis Corneal ulcer	1–2 gtt q2–4hr × 2 days, then qid × 5 days 1–2 gtt q30min while awake; at 4 hr and 6 hr during sleep × 2 days; then 1–2 gtt q1hr while awake × 5–7 days, then qid until treatment completion
Patanol/Pataday (≥3 yr) Sol: 5 mL	Olopatadine 0.1% (H_1-antagonist and mast cell stabilizer)	Allergic conjunctivitis	1 gtt bid
Poly-Pred Susp: 5 mL, 10 mL	Susp (per mL): prednisolone acetate (0.5%), neomycin sulfate (0.35%), polymyxin B sulfate (10,000 U)	Ocular inflammation associated with infection **Contraindicated in fungal, viral, or mycobacterial infections** Use with caution in glaucoma, or in corneal or scleral thinning	1–2 gtt q3–4hr
Polysporin Oint: 3.5 g	Oint (per g): polymyxin B sulfate (10,000 U), bacitracin zinc (500 U)	Conjunctivitis	1–2 gtt q3–4hr; do not use >7 days
Polytrim (>2 mo) Sol: 10 mL	Trimethoprim sulfate (1 mg), polymyxin B sulfate (10,000 U/mL), benzalkonium chloride	Conjunctivitis	1 gtt q3hr × 7–10 days
Pred-Forte Sol: 1, 5, 10, 15 mL Pred-Mild Sol: 5, 10 mL	Prednisolone acetate 1% Prednisolone acetate 0.12%	Ocular/conjunctival inflammation. **Contraindicated in fungal, viral or mycobacterial infections.** Prolonged use may cause glaucoma, corneal/scleral thinning	1–2 gtt 2–4 × per day Safety and efficacy not established in children

Continued

TABLE 30-7

OPHTHALMIC DRUGS (Continued)

Brand Name	Ingredient	Indication	Dose
Tobrex Sol: 5 mL Oint: 3.5 g	Sol: tobramycin 0.3%, benzalkonium chloride Oint: tobramycin 0.3%, chlorobutanol	Conjunctivitis	Severe infections: 2 gtt q1hr or ½ inch of ointment q3–4hr Mild-moderate infections: 1–2 gtt q4hr or ½ inch of ointment bid–tid
Vigamox (≥1 yr) Sol: 3 mL	Moxifloxacin hydrochloride 0.5% (fluoroquinolone)	Bacterial conjunctivitis	1 gtt tid × 7 days
Viroptic (>6 yr) Sol: 7.5 mL	Trifluridine 1%, contains thimerosal	Primary keratoconjunctivitis, recurrent epithelial keratitis caused by HSV 1 and 2	1 gtt q2hr while awake (maximum 9 gtt/day) 1 gtt q4hr × 7 days after re-epithelialization (maximum 21 days)
Zaditor (≥3 yr) Sol: 5 mL	Ketotifen fumarate 0.025% (H_1-antagonist and mast cell stabilizer)	Allergic conjunctivitis	1 gtt q 8–12 hr
Zymar (≥1 yr) Sol: 5 mL	Gatifloxacin 0.3% (fluoroquinolone)	Bacterial conjunctivitis	1 gtt q2h while awake, up to 8 times/day × 2 days; then 1 gtt up to qid × 5 days

Adapted from Physician's Desk Reference, 64th ed. Montvale, NJ, Medical Economics, 2010.

IX. PSYCHIATRIC DRUG FORMULARY (TABLE 30-8)

NOTE: See Formulary for stimulants (methylphenidate and amphetamine preparations), non-psychostimulants (clonidine), mood stabilizers (lithium, divalproex sodium, and carbamazepine), and tricyclic antidepressants (nortriptyline and imipramine).

TABLE 30-8

PSYCHIATRIC DRUG FORMULARY

Agent	Suggested Dose	Side Effects/Comments
ANTIPSYCHOTICS		
Aripiprazole (Abilify)	For depression (as adjunctive therapy) or mood stabilization: 2–5 mg/day (all ages) For true psychosis: Starting dose: 2 mg/day × 2 days, increase to 5 mg/day × 2 days, then up to target 10 mg/day Titrate upward by 5 mg/day as needed Max dose: 30 mg/day	Side effects include orthostatic hypotension, sedation, weight gain, hyperlipidemia, hyperglycemia, dystonic reactions, tardive dyskinesia, akathisia, neuroleptic malignant syndrome, nausea Monitoring: Fasting lipid profile, fasting blood glucose/Hgb A1c (prior to treatment, at 3 months, then annually or as symptoms warrant), measurement of weight/BMI/blood pressure/heart rate at least q3 months
Clozapine (Clozaril)	Starting dose: 12.5 mg/day Titrate upward by 25 mg/day q 3–5 days Max dose (in adults): 900 mg/day	See comments for ariprazole Very rarely used in pediatrics Obtain baseline ECG Monitor CBC. Because of potentially lethal hematologic changes, use is reserved for patients resistant to treatment
Haloperidol (Haldol)	See Formulary	See comments for ariprazole Additional side effects: QT prolongation, hyperprolactinemia, amenorrhea, galactorrhea, hyponatremia, hypomagnesemia, leukopenia/leukocytosis, anemia, agranulocytosis (rare), hepatotoxicity (rare) Additional monitoring: ECG (with non-FDA approved IV administration); CBC with differential; LFTs (with long term use)
Olanzapine (Zyprexa)	≥13 years: 2.5–5 mg q day Increase by 2.5–5 mg/day q week to maximum 20 mg/day	See comments for ariprazole
Risperidone (Risperdal)	Children <20 kg: 0.25 mg q day Child 6 yr–Adolescent: 0.5–0.75 mg/day or greater divided q day to BID Adult: 1 mg bid Increase by 0.25–1 mg/day Max dose: 3 mg/day	Renal/hepatic dosing See comments for ariprazole Additional side effects: hyperprolactinemia, galactorrhea, amenorrhea Interval between dose increases depends on indication (≥24 hr up to ≥14 days)

Continued

30

TABLE 30-8

PSYCHIATRIC DRUG FORMULARY (Continued)

Agent	Suggested Dose	Side Effects/Comments
ANTIPSYCHOTICS		
Quetiapine (Seroquel)	Prepubescent: 12.5–75 mg/day Children 10–17 years: 50 mg/day on day 1, 100 mg/day on day 2, then increase of 100 mg/day q day up to maximum of 800 mg	See comments for ariprazole Other side effect: hyperprolactinemia
Ziprasidone (Geodon)	Adult dose: 20–40 mg bid titrating up to max of 80 mg bid	See comments for ariprazole; low incidence of extrapyramidal side effects Other side effects: dyspepsia, constipation, abdominal pain, prolonged QTc
ANTIDEPRESSANTS/ANXIOLYTICS		
Selective Serotonin Reuptake Inhibitors (SSRIs)*†		
Fluoxetine (Prozac)	Starting dose ≤11 yr: 5–10 mg/day Maintenance: 10–30 mg/day Starting dose ≥12 yr: 10 mg/day Maintenance: 20–40 mg/day Max dose: 60 mg/day	Do not use if MAOIs have been used in previous 14 days Side effects: GI upset/emesis, CNS side effects (headaches, anxiety, sedation), behavioral activation (restlessness, hyperkinesis, hyperactivity, agitation) Monitoring: LFTs, weight, serum glucose Dose may be titrated up after 1 wk of therapy if no activating symptoms occur
Fluvoxamine (Luvox)	Starting dose 8–17 yr: 25 mg qhs Increase by 25 mg/day q 7–14 days Maximum dose: (8–11 yr) 200 mg/day; (adolescents) 300 mg/day	Contraindications: MAOIs, alosetron, pimozide, sibutramine, thioridazine, tizanidine Smoking increases levels See comments for fluoxetine
Sertraline (Zoloft)	Starting dose ≤12 yr (not FDA approved): 12.5–25 mg/day. Increase by 25–50 mg/day q ≥1 week Starting dose >12 yr: 25–50 mg/day Maximum: 200 mg/day	See comments for fluoxetine Other side effects: SIADH
Citalopram (Celexa)	Initial dose <12 yr: 10 mg/day Increase by 5 mg/day q 2 wk Initial dose ≥12 yr: 20 mg/day Increase by 10 mg/day q 2 wk Max dose: 60 mg	Not FDA approved for use in children Side effects: GI upset/emesis, anxiety, sedation, behavioral activation (restlessness, hyperkinesis, hyperactivity, agitation)
Escitalopram (Lexapro)	Initial dose ≥12 yr: 10 mg/day; may increase to 20 mg/day after 3 weeks Initial dose 6–17 yr (autism): 2.5 mg/day, increase by 5 mg q week up to 20 mg/day	Not FDA approved for children <12 yr or for indications other than depression although some limited data exists regarding efficacy in autism and social anxiety disorder See comments for sertraline

TABLE 30-8

PSYCHIATRIC DRUG FORMULARY (Continued)

Agent	Suggested Dose	Side Effects/Comments
Other Antidepressants/Anxiolytics*		
Venlafaxine (Effexor) *Serotonin norepinephrine reuptake inhibitor*	Not FDA approved in children—doses are not well studied Starting dose age 7–17 yr: 37.5 mg/day, increased to 75 mg/day after 1 week Maximum adult dose: 375 mg/day divided tid (severe depression)	Hypertension, orthostatic hypotension, weight loss, hypercholesterolemia, SIADH, nausea, somnolence, constipation, xerostomia Renal/hepatic dosing Monitoring: BP, serum lipids, weight, serum sodium Discontinuation withdrawal—must be tapered very slowly to prevent flu-like symptoms and orthostatic hypotension
Bupropion (Wellbutrin)	<15 yr: 50 mg bid. Titrate dose up as needed Max dose: 300–450 mg/day ≥15 yr: 150 mg q day; increase to 300–400 mg divided bid as needed SR and XL formulations: SR doses greater than 150 mg/day should be divided BID due to risk of seizure. XL doses are given once daily.	Tachycardia, hypertension/hypotension, headache, anxiety, somnolence, tics, fever, CNS stimulation, weight loss, dry mouth, nausea, insomnia Contraindications: Seizures, eating disorders, MAOIs Safe and effective pediatric doses have not been established
Mirtazapine (Remeron)	≥18 yr: Initially 15 mg qhs; increase q1–2wk to maximum of 45 mg/day Not approved for use in children	Side effects: Increased appetite, weight gain, dizziness, nausea, dry mouth, constipation, CNS effects (somnolence), hypotension/hypertension, elevated triglycerides/cholesterol
Buspirone (BuSpar) *Anxiolytic*	Prepubescent: 2.5–5 mg/day; increase by 2.5 mg/day q3–4 days Max dose: 20 mg/day Adolescent: 5–10 mg/day; increase by 5 mg/day q3–4 days Max dose: 60 mg/day	Nausea, headache, insomnia, restlessness, confusion, dizziness, anxiety, fatigue, akathisia
Trazodone	Initial adolescent dose: 25 mg/day, increase every 3–4 days to 100–150 mg/day in divided doses	Orthostatic hypotension, sedation, extrapyramidal reactions, headache, priapism, hepatitis, blurred vision Monitoring: LFTs, BP

*In clinical trials, antidepressants increased the risk of suicidal thinking and behavior in children, adolescents, and young adults with major depressive disorder and other psychiatric disorders.

†Multiple drug interactions exist.

BP, Blood pressure; CBC, complete blood count; CNS, central nervous system; ECG, electrocardiogram; GI, gastrointestinal; HR, heart rate; LFT, liver function test; MAOIs, monoamine oxidase inhibitors; SIADH, syndrome of inappropriate antidiuretic hormone; SR, sustained release; XL, extended release.

Adapted from Physician's Desk Reference, 64th ed. Montvale, NJ, Medical Economics, 2010; Taketomo CK, Hodding JH, Kraus DM: American Pharmaceutical Association pediatric dosage handbook, 16th ed. Hudson, OH, Lexi-Comp, 2009.

X. CHEMOTHERAPEUTIC AGENTS (TABLE 30-9)

TABLE 30-9

CHARACTERISTICS OF CHEMOTHERAPEUTIC AGENTS

Drug Name *(Drug Class)*	Toxicity*
Asparaginase (L-Asp, PEG-Asp, Elspar, Erwinia) *(Enzyme)*	DLT: Pancreatitis, seizures, hypersensitivity reactions (both acute and delayed; less with PEG-modified), encephalopathy Other: Nausea, pancreatitis, hyperglycemia, azotemia, fever, coagulopathy, sagittal sinus thrombosis and other venous thromboses, hyperammonemia Long-term: Stroke
Bevacizumab (Avastin) *(VEGF inhibitor)*	DLT: wound healing, hemorrhage, thromboembolic events, CHF Other: abdominal pain, constipation, mucositis, dizziness, headache, dyspnea, epistaxis
Bleomycin (Blenoxane) *(DNA strand breaker)*	DLT: Anaphylaxis, pneumonitis Other: Pain, fever, chills, mucositis, skin reactions Long-term: Pulmonary fibrosis
Busulfan (Myleran) *(Alkylator)*	DLT: Myelosuppression, mucositis, seizures, veno-occlusive disease Other: Hyperpigmentation, hypotension Long-term: Infertility, endocardial fibrosis, secondary malignancy
Carboplatin (CBDCA, Paraplatin) *(DNA cross-linker)*	DLT: Thrombocytopenia, nephrotoxicity Other: Severe emesis, ototoxicity, peripheral neuropathy, optic neuritis (rare) Long-term: Renal insufficiency, hearing loss
Carmustine (bis-chloronitrosourea, BCNU, BiCNU) *(Alkylator)*	DLT: Myelosuppression (prolonged cumulative) Other: Vesicant; brownish discoloration of skin, hepatic and renal toxicity, severe emesis Long-term: Pulmonary fibrosis, infertility, secondary malignancy
Cisplatin (*cis*-platinum, CDDP, Platinol) *(DNA cross-linker)*	DLT: Tubular and glomerular nephrotoxicity (related to cumulative dose), peripheral neuropathy, severe emesis Other: myelosuppression, ototoxicity, SIADH (rare), papilledema and retrobulbar neuritis (rare) Long-term: Renal insufficiency, hearing loss, peripheral neuropathy
Cladribine (2-CdA, Leustatin) *(Nucleotide analogue)*	Myelosuppression, nausea and vomiting, headache, fever, chills, fatigue
Clofarabine (Clolar) *(Purine analog)*	Capillary leak syndrome, veno-occlusive disease, increased creatinine, hyperbilirubinemia
Cyclophosphamide (CTX, Cytoxan) *(Alkylator prodrug)*	DLT: Leukopenia, cardiomyopathy Other: Hemorrhagic cystitis (improved by mesna), emesis, direct ADH effect, SIADH Long-term: Infertility, cardiomyopathy, secondary malignancy, leukoencephalopathy
Cytarabine (Ara-C) *(Nucleotide analog)*	DLT: Myelosuppression, cerebellar toxicity Other: Rash, fever, conjunctivitis, nausea and vomiting, anorexia, diarrhea, metallic taste, severe GI ulceration, lethargy, ataxia, nystagmus, slurred speech, respiratory distress rapidly progressing to pulmonary edema, influenza-like syndrome

TABLE 30-9

CHARACTERISTICS OF CHEMOTHERAPEUTIC AGENTS (Continued)

Drug Name *(Drug Class)*	**Toxicity***
Dacarbazine (DIC, DTIC, imidazole carboxamide, DTIC-Dome) *(Alkylator)*	DLT: Myelosuppression Other: Severe emesis, transaminitis, facial paresthesias (rare), rash Long-term: Infertility
Dactinomycin (actinomycin D) *(Antibiotic)*	DLT: Myelosuppression, severe diarrhea Other: Vesicant; nausea, acne, erythema, radiation recall, veno-occlusive disease Long-term: Secondary malignancy
Daunorubicin (daunomycin) *(Anthracycline)*	DLT: Leukopenia, arrhythmia, congestive heart failure (related to cumulative dose) Other: Stomatitis, emesis, vesicant, red urine, radiation recall Long-term: Cardiomyopathy
Doxorubicin (Adriamycin) *(Anthracycline)*	Refer to daunorubicin
Etoposide (VP-16, VePesid) *(Topoisomerase inhibitor)*	DLT: Leukopenia, anaphylaxis (rare), transient cortical blindness Other: Hyperbilirubinemia, transaminitis, peripheral neuropathy (rare), hypotension Long-term: Secondary malignancy (AML)
Fludarabine (Fludara) *(Nucleotide analogue)*	Myelosuppression, anorexia, increased AST, somnolence, fatigue Long-term: Peripheral neuropathy, immune suppression
Fluorouracil (5-FU, Adrucil) *(Nucleotide analogue)*	DLT: Myelosuppression, mucositis, severe diarrhea Other: Hand-foot syndrome, tear duct stenosis, hyperpigmentation, loss of nails, cerebellar syndrome (rare), anaphylaxis
Gemcitabine *(Pyrimidine analog)*	Peripheral edema, rash, nausea, vomiting, constipation, transaminase elevation, myalgias, neuropathy, HUS, pulmonary edema
Hydroxyurea (Hydrea) *(Ribonucleotide reductase inhibitor)*	DLT: Leukopenia, pulmonary edema (rare) Other: Megaloblastic erythropoiesis, hyperpigmentation, azotemia, transaminitis, radiation recall
Idarubicin (idamycin) *(Anthracycline)*	DLT: Arrhythmia, cardiomyopathy (cumulative) Other: Vesicant; diarrhea, mucositis, enterocolitis Long-term: Cardiomyopathy
Ifosfamide (isophosphamide, Ifex) *(Alkylator prodrug)*	DLT: Myelosuppression, mental status changes, dizziness, encephalopathy (rarely progressing to death), renal tubular damage Other: Emesis, hemorrhagic cystitis (improved with Mesna), direct ADH effect, SIADH, Fanconi syndrome Long-term: Secondary malignancy, infertility
Irinotecan (Camptosar, IRN) *(Topoisomerase I inhibitor)*	DLT: diarrhea Other: nausea and vomiting, asthenia, hyperbilirubinemia, dizziness, cough, dyspnea
Imatinib (Gleevec) *(Tyrosine kinase inhibitor)*	CHF, edema, pleural effusion, rash, night sweats, weight gain, myalgias, fever

Continued

TABLE 30-9

CHARACTERISTICS OF CHEMOTHERAPEUTIC AGENTS (Continued)

Drug Name *(Drug Class)*	Toxicity*
Lomustine (CCNU) *(Alkylating agent)*	Myelosuppression, nausea and vomiting, disorientation, fatigue Long-term: Secondary malignancy (leukemia)
Mechlorethamine (nitrogen mustard, HN_2 [mustine], Mustargen) *(Alkylator)*	DLT: Leukopenia, thrombocytopenia Other: Severe emesis; vesicant; peptic ulcer (rare) Long-term: Secondary malignancy, infertility
Melphalan (L-PAM, Alkeran) *(Alkylator)*	DLT: Prolonged leukopenia, mucositis, diarrhea Other: Pruritus, emesis Long-term: Pulmonary fibrosis, secondary malignancy, infertility, cataracts
Mercaptopurine (6-MP) *(Nucleotide analogue)*	DLT: Hepatic necrosis and encephalopathy Other: Headache, diarrhea, nausea Long-term: Cirrhosis
Methotrexate (MTX, amethopterin, Folex, Mexate) *(Folate antagonist)*	DLT: Mucositis, diarrhea, renal dysfunction, encephalopathy, cortical blindness, ventriculitis (intrathecal) Other: Photosensitivity, erythema, excessive lacrimation, transaminitis, pleuritis Long-term: Leukoencephalopathy, cirrhosis, pulmonary fibrosis, aseptic necrosis of bone, osteoporosis
Mitoxantrone (dihydroxyanthracenedione dihydrochloride, Novantrone) *(DNA intercalator)*	DLT: Myelosuppression, cardiomyopathy Other: Mucositis, blue-green urine Long-term: Cardiomyopathy
Paclitaxel (Taxol) *(Tubulin inhibitor)*	DLT: Neutropenia, anaphylaxis, ventricular tachycardia and myocardial infarction (rare) Other: Mucositis, peripheral neuropathy, bradycardia, hypertriglyceridemia
Procarbazine (Matulane) *(Alkylating agent)*	DLT: Encephalopathy; pancytopenia, especially thrombocytopenia Other: Emesis, paresthesias, dizziness, ataxia, hypotension; adverse effects with tyramine-rich foods, ethanol, MAOIs, meperidine, and many other drugs Long-term: Secondary malignancy, infertility
Temozolomide (Temodar) *(Alkylating agent)*	DLT: Myelosuppression Other: Constipation, headache, nausea, seizures
Teniposide (VM-26) *(Topoisomerase inhibitor)*	DLT: Leukopenia, anaphylaxis (rare) Other: Hyperbilirubinemia, transaminitis Long-term: Secondary malignancy (AML)
Thioguanine (6-TG, 6-thioguanine) *(Nucleotide analogue)*	DLT: Myelosuppression, mucositis, diarrhea Other: Hyperbilirubinemia, transaminitis, decreased vibratory sensation, ataxia, dermatitis

TABLE 30-9

CHARACTERISTICS OF CHEMOTHERAPEUTIC AGENTS (Continued)

Drug Name *(Drug Class)*	Toxicity*
Thiotepa *(Alkylating agent)*	DLT: Cognitive impairment, leukopenia Other: Increased AST, headache, dizziness, rash, desquamation Long-term: Secondary malignancy (leukemia), impaired fertility, lower extremity weakness
Topotecan (Hycamptin) *(Topoisomerase inhibitor)*	DLT: Leukopenia, peripheral neuropathy (rare), Horner syndrome Other: Nausea, diarrhea, transaminitis, headache
Vinblastine (VBL, vincaleukoblastine, Velban) *(Microtubule inhibitor)*	DLT: Leukopenia Other: Vesicant; constipation, bone pain (especially in the jaw), peripheral and autonomic neuropathy, SIADH (rare)
Vincristine (VCR, Oncovin) *(Microtubule inhibitor)*	DLT: Peripheral and autonomic neuropathy, constipation, jaw pain, encephalopathy, foot drop, ptosis Other: Vesicant; bone pain, hoarseness, SIADH (rare), hyperbilirubinemia
Vinorelbine (Navelbine) *(Microtubule inhibitor)*	Peripheral neuropathy, asthenia, hyperbilirubinemia, constipation, diarrhea, nausea, emesis
CHEMOTHERAPY ADJUNCTS	
Amifostine	Indication: Reduces the toxicity of radiation Side effects: Hypotension (62%), nausea and vomiting, flushing, chills, dizziness, somnolence, hiccups, sneezing, hypocalcemia in susceptible patients (<1%), rigors (<1%), mild skin rash
Dexrazoxane	Indication: Protective agent for anthracycline-induced cardiotoxicity Side effects: Myelosuppression
Leucovorin	Indication: Reduces methotrexate toxicity Side effects: Allergic sensitization (rare)
Mesna	Indication: Reduces risk of hemorrhagic cystitis Side effects: Headache, limb pain, abdominal pain, diarrhea, rash

*The dose-limiting toxicity (DLT) is the toxicity most likely to require adjustment or withholding of drug.

ADH, antidiuretic hormone; AML, acute myeloid leukemia; AST, aspartate transaminase; CHF, congestive heart failure; HUS, hemolytic uremic syndrome; MAOI, monoamine oxidase inhibitors; SIADH, syndrome of inappropriate antidiuretic hormone; VEGF, vascular endothelial growth factor.

Adapted from Physician's Desk Reference, 64th ed. Montvale, NJ, Medical Economics, 2010; Taketomo CK, Hodding JH, Kraus DM: American Pharmaceutical Association pediatric dosage handbook, 16th ed. Hudson, OH, Lexi-Comp, 2009; Micromedex 2.0: http://www.thomsonhc.com/micromedex2/librarian

XI. OXIDIZING AGENTS AND GLUCOSE-6-PHOSPHATE DEHYDROGENASE (G6PD) DEFICIENCY

See the following website for a comprehensive listing of drugs: http://g6pddeficiency.org/index.php?cmd=contraindicated

XII. DOSING OF COMMONLY USED ANTIBIOTICS IN THE NEONATAL INTENSIVE CARE UNIT (TABLE 30-10)

TABLE 30-10

DOSING OF COMMONLY USED ANTIBIOTICS IN THE NEONATAL INTENSIVE CARE UNIT BASED ON POST-MATERNAL AND POSTNATAL AGE

AMPICILLIN (GBS bacteremia = 150–200 mg/kg/day; GBS meningitis = 300–400 mg/kg/day)
CEFOTAXIME 50 mg/kg/dose (gonococcal infections = 25 mg/kg/dose) (GC ophthalmia PPX if maternal GC infection is present = 100 mg/kg × 1 dose)
OXACILLIN 25–50 mg/kg/dose

Dosing Interval Chart

PMA (weeks)	Postnatal (days)	Interval (hours)
≤29	0–28	12
	>28	8
30–36	0–14	12
	>14	8
37–44	0–7	12
	>7	8
≥45	All	6

VANCOMYCIN (bacteremia = 10 mg/kg/dose; meningitis = 15 mg/mg/dose)

Dosing Interval Chart

PMA(weeks)	Postnatal (days)	Interval (hours)
≤29	0–14	18
	>14	12
30–36	0–14	12
	>14	8
37–44	0–7	12
	>7	8
≥45	All	6

METRONIDAZOLE[†] (loading = 15 mg/kg/dose; maintenance = 7.5 mg/kg/dose)

Dosing Interval Chart

PMA (weeks)	Postnatal (days)	Interval (hours)
≤29	0–28	48
	>28	24
30–36	0–14	24
	>14	12
37–44	0–7	24
	>7	12
≥45	All	8

GENTAMICIN

Dosing Chart

PMA (weeks)	Postnatal (days)	Dose (mg/kg)	Interval (hours)
≤29*	0–7	5	48
	8–28	4	36
	≥29	4	24
30–34	0–7	4.5	36
	≥8	4	24
≥35	All	4	24

FLUCONAZOLE[†] (Invasive candidiasis: loading = 12–25 mg/kg/dose; maintenance = 6–12 mg/kg/dose)

Dosing Interval Chart

Gest. Age (weeks)	Postnatal (days)	Interval (hours)
≤29	0–14	48
	>14	24
30 and older	0–7	48
	>7	24

[†]Thrush = 6 mg/kg/dose on day 1, then 3 mg/kg/dose PO q24hr regardless of gestational or postnatal age.

*Or significant asphyxia, PDA, or treatment with indomethacin.

GC, Gonococcus; GBS, group B streptococcus; PDA, patent ductus arteriosus; PMA, post-maternal age; Ppx, prophylaxis.

Online Neofax: http://neofax.thomsonhc.com/neofax/index.php. 2010. Thomson Reuters Inc. • Application Version: 3.0.0.4 • User Manual Version: 200901.

REFERENCES

1. Kappy MS, Blizzard RM, Migeon CJ, et al, eds. *Diagnosis and treatment of endocrine disorders in childhood and adolescence*, 4th ed. Springfield, IL: Charles C Thomas; 1994.
2. Migeon CJ, Wisniewski AB. Congenital adrenal hyperplasia owing to 21-hydroxylase deficiency: Growth, development, and therapeutic considerations. *Endocrinol Metab Clin North Am*. 2001;30(1):193–206.
3. Bjornson CL, Klassen TP, Williamson J, et al. A randomized trial of a single dose of oral dexamethasone for mild croup. *N Engl J Med*. 2004;351(13): 1306–1313.
4. Fifoot AA, Ting JYS. Comparison between single dose oral prednisolone and oral dexamethasone in the treatment of croup: a randomised double-blinded clinical trial. *Emerg Med Australas*. 2007;19:51–58.
5. Roberts GW. Repeated dose inhaled budesonide versus placebo in the treatment of croup. *J Pediatr Child Health*. 1999;35(2):170–174.
6. Expert Panel Report III. *Guidelines for the diagnosis and management of asthma—full report 2007. National Institutes of Health Pub. No. 08-4051*. Bethesda, MD: National Asthma Education and Prevention Program; 2007.
7. Taketomo CK, Hodding JH, Kraus DM. *American Pharmaceutical Association pediatric dosage handbook*, 16th ed. Hudson, OH: Lexi-Comp; 2009.
8. Bracken MB, Shepard MJ, Holford TR, et al. Administration of methylprednisolone for 24 or 48 hours or tirilazad mesylate for 48 hours in the treatment of acute spinal cord injury. Results of the Third National Acute Spinal Cord Injury Randomized Controlled Trial. National Acute Spinal Cord Injury Study. *JAMA*. 1997;277(20):1597–1604.
9. Pickering LK, ed. *2009 Red book: report of the committee on infectious diseases*, 28th ed. Elk Grove Village, IL: American Academy of Pediatrics; 2009.
10. Provan D, Stasi R, Newland AC, et al. International consensus report on the investigation and management of primary immune thrombocytopenia. *Blood*. 2010;115(2):168.

Chapter 31

Drugs in Renal Failure

Megan M. Tschudy, MD

I. DOSE ADJUSTMENT METHODS

A. Maintenance Dose

In patients with renal insufficiency, the dose may be adjusted using the following methods:

1. **Interval extension (I):** Lengthen the intervals between individual doses, keeping the dose size normal. For this method, the suggested interval is shown
2. **Dose reduction (D):** Reduce the amount of individual doses, keeping the interval between the doses normal. This method is particularly recommended for drugs in which a relatively constant blood level is desired. For this method, the percentage of the usual dose is shown
3. **Interval extension and dose reduction (DI):** Lengthen the interval and reduce the dose
4. **Interval extension or dose reduction (D, I):** In some instances, either the dose or the interval can be changed

NOTE: These dose adjustments are for beyond the neonatal period. For neonatal renal dosing please consult a neonatal dosage reference. These dose modifications are only approximations. **Each patient must be monitored closely for signs of drug toxicity, and serum levels must be measured when available.** Drug dose and interval should be adjusted accordingly. When in doubt please consult a nephrologist or pharmacist with a specialty in renal dosing.

B. Dialysis

Quantitative effects of hemodialysis (He) and peritoneal dialysis (P) on drug removal are shown. *Y* indicates the need for a supplemental dose with dialysis. The supplemental dose may not be a full dose, but instead a lower than standard dose. *N* indicates no need for adjustment. The designation *No* does not preclude the use of dialysis or hemoperfusion for drug overdose. *?* indicates insufficient data available. **Please consult with a nephrologist or pharmacist who is very familiar with renal dosing in dialysis.**

Text continued on page 1027

II. ANTIMICROBIALS REQUIRING ADJUSTMENT IN RENAL FAILURE (TABLE 31-1)

TABLE 31-1

ANTIMICROBIALS REQUIRING ADJUSTMENT IN RENAL FAILURE[1–4]

	Pharmacokinetics			Adjustments in Renal Failure				
Drug	Route of Excretion*	Normal $t_{1/2}$ (hr)	Normal Dose Interval	Method	CrCl (mL/min)	Dose	Interval	Supplemental Dose for Dialysis
Acyclovir (IV)	Renal	2–4	q8hr	D,I	25–50	Nl	q12hr	Y (He)
					10–25	Nl	q24hr	N (P)
					<10	50% ↓	q24hr	
Amantadine[†]	Renal	10–28	q12–24hr	D,I	30–50	50% ↓	q24hr	N (He)[α]
					15–29	50% ↓	q48	N (P)
					<15	Nl daily dose	q7 days	
Amikacin	Renal	1.5–3	q8–12hr	I	Loading dose 5–7.5 mg/kg; subsequent doses are best determined by serum levels and assessment of renal insufficiency.[1]			Y (He) Y (P)
Amoxicillin[‡]	Renal	0.7–2	q8–12hr	I	10–30	Nl	q12hr	Y (He)
					<10	Nl	q24hr	? (P)
Amoxicillin/ clavulanate[‡]	Renal	1	q8–12hr	I	10–30	Nl	q12hr	Y (He)
					<10	Nl	q24hr	? (P)

*Route in parentheses indicates secondary route of excretion.

[†]In adults; guidelines not established in children.

[α]On day one normal dose should be given then decreased for subsequent doses based on renal insufficiency.

[‡]Should not use 875-mg tablet or extended release tablets in patients with CrCl <30 mL/min.

Continued

TABLE 31-1

ANTIMICROBIALS REQUIRING ADJUSTMENT IN RENAL FAILURE (Continued)

	Pharmacokinetics			Adjustments in Renal Failure				
Drug	**Route of Excretion***	**Normal $t_{1/2}$ (hr)**	**Normal Dose Interval**	**Method**	**CrCl (mL/min)**	**Dose**	**Interval**	**Supplemental Dose for Dialysis**
Amphotericin B	Renal (40% over 7 days)	Initial 15–48 hr Terminal 15 days	q24hr	D,I	Dosage adjustments are unnecessary with preexisting renal impairment; "if decreased renal function is due to amphotericin B, daily dose can be decreased by 50% or dose given every other day. Therapy may be held until serum creatinine begins to decline. Can give 1–4 mg/L of peritoneal dialysis fluid ± low-dose IV therapy."[1]			N (He) ? (P)
Amphotericin B lipid complex (Abelcet)	Renal (1%)	173	q24hr	I	Renal toxicity is dose dependent. No firm guidelines for dose adjustments.			N (He) ? (P)
Amphotericin B, liposomal (AmBisome)	Renal (≤10%)	100–153	q24hr	I	No guidelines established.			N (He) ? (P)
Ampicillin[†]	Renal	1–1.8	q6–12hr	I	10–30 <10	NI NI	q6–12hr q12hr	Y (He) ? (P)
Ampicillin/ sulbactam	Renal	1–1.8	q4–8hr	I	15–29 <15	NI NI	q12hr q24hr	Y (He) ? (P)
Aztreonam	Renal (hepatic)	1.3–2.2	q6–12hr	D	10–30 <10	50% ↓ 75% ↓	NI NI	Y (He) Y (P)
Cefaclor	Renal	0.5–1	q8–12hr	D	<10	50% ↓	NI	Y (He) ? (P)
Cefadroxil	Renal	1–2	q12–24hr	I	10–25 <10	NI NI	q24hr q36hr	? (He) ? (P)

Cefazolin	Renal	1.5–2.5	q6–8hr	D,I	40–70 20–40 <20	40%↓[Σ] 75%↓[Σ] 90%↓[Σ]	q12hr q12hr q12hr	Y (He) ? (P)
Cefdinir	Renal	1.1–2.3	q12–24hr	D,I	<30	7 mg/kg/dose (children; max 300 mg) 300 mg (adults)	q24hr q24hr	Y (He)[Ω] ? (P)
Cefepime[†]	Renal	1.8–2	q8–12hr	I	10–50 <10	NI NI	q24hr q48hr	Y (He) ? (P)
Cefixime	Renal (hepatic)	3–4	q12–24hr	D	21–60 <20	25% ↓ 50% ↓	NI NI	Y (He) ? (P)
Cefotaxime	Renal	1–1.5	q6–12hr	D	<20	50% ↓	NI	Y (He) ? (P)
Cefotetan	Renal (hepatic)	3.5	q12hr	I	10–30 <10	NI NI	q24hr q48hr	Y (He) ? (P)
Cefoxitin	Renal	0.75–1.5	q4–8hr	I	30–50 10–30 <10	NI NI NI	q8–12hr q12–24hr q24–48hr	Y (He) ? (P)
Cefpodoxime	Renal	2.2	q12hr	I	<30	NI	q24hr	Y (He)[§] ? (P)

*Route in parentheses indicates secondary route of excretion.

[†]In adults; guidelines not established in children.

[Σ]After initial loading dose is administered then decrease dose based on renal insufficiency.

[Ω]Patients on hemodialysis should have a dose of 300 mg or 7 mg/kg/dose at the conclusion of each hemodialysis session with subsequent doses q48hr.

[§]For patients on hemodialysis, administer 3 times per week.

Continued

TABLE 31-1

ANTIMICROBIALS REQUIRING ADJUSTMENT IN RENAL FAILURE (Continued)

	Pharmacokinetics			Adjustments in Renal Failure				
Drug	Route of Excretion*	Normal $t_{1/2}$ (hr)	Normal Dose Interval	Method	CrCl (mL/min)	Dose	Interval	Supplemental Dose for Dialysis
Cefprozil	Renal	1.3	q12–24hr	D	<30	50% ↓	NI	Y (He)
								? (P)
Ceftazidime	Renal	1–2	q8–12hr	I	30–50	NI	q12hr	Y (He)
					10–30	NI	q24hr	? (P)
					<10	NI	q24–48hr	
Ceftibuten	Renal	1.9–3	q24hr	D	30–49	50% ↓	NI	Y (He)[αα]
					5–29	75% ↓	NI	? (P)
Ceftizoxime	Renal	1.6	q6–12hr	I	50–80	NI	q8–12hr	Y (He)
					10–50	NI	q36–48hr	? (P)
					<10	NI	q48–72hr	
Cefuroxime (IV)	Renal	1–2	q8–12hr	I	10–20	NI	q12hr	Y (He)
					<10	NI	q24hr	? (P)
Cephalexin	Renal	0.5–2.5	q6–8hr	I	10–40	NI	q8–12hr	Y (He)
					<10	NI	q12–24hr	? (P)
Cephradine	Renal	0.7–2	q6–12hr	D,I	10–50	50% ↓	NI	? (He)
					<10	75% ↓	NI	? (P)
					OR			
					25–50	NI	q12hr	
					10–25	NI	q24hr	
					<10	NI	q36hr	
Ciprofloxacin[†]	Renal (hepatic)	3–5	q8–12hr	D,I	<30 (IV)	200–400 mg[†]	q18–24hr	Y (He)
					30–50 (PO)	250–500 mg[†]	q12hr	? (P)
					<30 (PO)	250–500 mg[†]	q18hr	

Clarithromycin	Renal/hepatic	3–9	q12hr	D,I	<30	50% ↓	q12–24hr	? (He) ? (P)
Ertapenem†	Renal	2.5–4	q12–24hr	D	≤30	50% ↓	NI	Y (He) ? (P)
Erythromycin	Hepatic (renal)	1.5–2	q6–12hr	D	<10	25%–50%	↓NI	N (He) N (P)
Ethambutol	Renal (hepatic)	2.5–3.6	q24hr	I	10–50 <10	NI NI or reduced	q24–36hr q48hr	Y (He) ? (P)
Famciclovir†	Renal (hepatic)	2–3	q8hr	D,I	**Herpes Zoster Treatment†,*****			Y (He) ? (P)
					40–59	500 mg	q12hr	
					20–39	500 mg	q24hr	
					<20	250 mg	q24hr	
					Recurrent Genital Herpes Treatment†,***			
					40–59	500 mg	q12hr × 1 day	
					20–39	500 mg	Single dose	
					<20	250 mg	Single dose	
					Recurrent Genital Herpes Suppression†,ΣΣ			
					>40	250 mg	q12hr	
					20–39	125 mg	q12hr	
					<20	125 mg	q24hr	

*Route in parentheses indicates secondary route of excretion.
†In adults; guidelines not established in children.
ααWith hemodialysis administer 9 mg/kg (max dose 400 mg) after hemodialysis.
***Patients on hemodialysis administer 250 mg after each dialysis session.
ΣΣPatients on hemodialysis administer 125 mg after each dialysis session.

Continued

TABLE 31-1

ANTIMICROBIALS REQUIRING ADJUSTMENT IN RENAL FAILURE (Continued)

	Pharmacokinetics			Adjustments in Renal Failure				
Drug	**Route of Excretion***	**Normal $t_{1/2}$ (hr)**	**Normal Dose Interval**	**Method**	**CrCl (mL/min)**	**Dose**	**Interval**	**Supplemental Dose for Dialysis**
Famciclovir—cont'd					**Recurrent Herpes Labialis—Single Dose Regimen[†,***]**			
					>60	1,500 mg as single dose		
					40–59	750 mg as single dose		
					20–39	500 mg as single dose		
					<20	250 mg as single dose		
					Recurrent Orolabial or Genital Herpes in HIV-Infected Patients[†,*]**			
					40–59	500 mg	q12hr	
					20–39	500 mg	q12hr	
					<20	250 mg	q24hr	
Fluconazole[†]	Renal	15.2–30	q24hr	D	≤50	50% ↓	NI	Y (He)[ΣΣΣ] ? (P)
Flucytosine	Renal	2.5–7.4	q6hr	I	20–40	NI	q12hr	Y (He)
					10–20	NI	q24hr	? (P)
					<10	NI	q24–48hr	
Foscamet	Renal	2–4.5	Induct: q8hr Maint: q24hr	D	See package insert for adjustments for induction and maintenance.			? (He) ? (P)
Ganciclovir	Renal	2.5–3.6	Induct: q12hr IV Maint: q24hr IV PO	D,I	**Induction IV**			Y (He)[§]
					50–69	2.5 mg/kg	q12hr	N (P)
					25–49	2.5 mg/kg	q24hr	
					10–24	1.25 mg/kg	q24hr	

			OR q8hr		<10	1.25 mg/kg	3 times/wk after He	
					Maintenance IV			
					50–69	2.5 mg/kg	q24hr	
					25–49	1.25 mg/kg	q24hr	
					10–24	0.625 mg/kg	q24hr	
					<10	0.625 mg/kg	3 times/wk after He	
					Maintenance PO[†]			
					50–69	1,500 mg	q24hr	
						OR 500 mg	q8hr	
					25–49	1,000 mg	q24hr	
						OR 500 mg	q12hr	
					10–24	500 mg	q24hr	
					<10	500 mg	3 times/wk after He	
Gentamicin	Renal	0.5–5	q8–24hr	I	40–60	NI	q12hr	Y (He)
					20–40	NI	q24hr	Y (P)[¶]
					<20	NI	Monitor levels	

*Route in parentheses indicates secondary route of excretion.
[†]In adults; guidelines not established in children.
***Patients on hemodialysis administer 250 mg after each dialysis session.
[ΣΣΣ]Patients on hemodialysis: administer 100% of recommended dose after each dialysis session.
[§]For patients on hemodialysis, administer 3 times per week.
[¶]May add to peritoneal dialysate to obtain adequate serum levels.

Continued

TABLE 31-1

ANTIMICROBIALS REQUIRING ADJUSTMENT IN RENAL FAILURE (Continued)

	Pharmacokinetics			Adjustments in Renal Failure				
Drug	Route of Excretion*	Normal $t_{1/2}$ (hr)	Normal Dose Interval	Method	CrCl (mL/min)	Dose	Interval	Supplemental Dose for Dialysis
Imipenem/cilastatin	Renal	1–1.4	q6–8hr	D,I	41–70 mL/min/1.73 m^2	50% ↓ in max daily dose	q6hr	Y (He) ? (P)
					21–40 mL/min/1.73 m^2	63% ↓ in max daily dose	q8hr	
					6–20 mL/min/1.73 m^2	75% ↓ in max daily dose	q12hr	
					≤5 mL/min/1.73 m^2	Should not receive imipenem unless on He		
Isoniazid	Renal (hepatic)	2–5 (slow)[#] 0.5–1.5 (fast)	q24hr	D	<10	100%	NI	Y (He) ? (P)
Kanamycin	Renal	1.8–5	q8hr	D,I	GFR > 50 mL/min	10%–40% ↓	q12hr	Y (He) Y (P)
					GFR 10–50 mL/min	30%–70% ↓	q12–18hr	
					GFR < 10 mL/min	70%–80% ↓	q24–48hr	

Lamivudine[†,**]	Renal	1.4–7	q12hr	D,I	30–49	NI	q24hr	N (He)
					15–29	First dose 100%, then 66%	q24hr	N (P)
					5–14	First dose 100%, then 33%	q24hr	
					<5	First dose 33%, then 17%	q24hr	
Levofloxacin[†]	Renal (hepatic)	6–8	q12–24hr	D,I	**500 mg q24hr Regimen**			N (He)
					20–49	First dose 500 mg, then 250 mg	q24hr	N (P)
					10–19	First dose 250–500 mg, then 250 mg	q48hr	
					750 mg q24hr Regimen			
					20–49	750 mg	q48hr	
					10–19	500 mg	q48hr	
					250 mg q24hr Regimen			
					10–19	250 mg	q48hr	

*Route in parentheses indicates secondary route of excretion.

[†]In adults; guidelines not established in children.

[#]Rate of acetylation of isoniazid.

**GFR ≥5 mL/min: Give full dose as first dose; GFR <5 mL/min: Give 33% of full dose as first dose.

Continued

TABLE 31-1

ANTIMICROBIALS REQUIRING ADJUSTMENT IN RENAL FAILURE (Continued)

	Pharmacokinetics			Adjustments in Renal Failure				
Drug	**Route of Excretion***	**Normal $t_{1/2}$ (hr)**	**Normal Dose Interval**	**Method**	**CrCl (mL/min)**	**Dose**	**Interval**	**Supplemental Dose for Dialysis**
Loracarbef	Renal	0.78–1	q12hr	D, I	10–49	50% ↓	NI	Y (P)
					OR	NI	q24hr	? (P)
					<10	NI	q3–5 days	
Meropenem	Renal	1–1.5	q8hr	D,I	26–50	NI	q12hr	Y (He)
					10–25	50% ↓	q12hr	? (P)
					<10	50% ↓	q24hr	
Metronidazole	Hepatic (renal)	6–12	q6–8hr	D	<10	50% ↓	NI	Y (He)
								Y (P)
Norfloxacin	Hepatic (renal)	2–4	q12hr	I	10–50	NI	q12–24hr	N (He)
					<10	NI	q24hr	N (P)
Oseltamivir[†]	Renal	1–10	q12–24hr	I	**Treatment of Influenza**			? (He)
					10–30	75 mg	q24hr	? (P)
					<10	No recommended dosage regimen.		
					Prophylaxis of Influenza			
					10–30	75 mg	q48hr	
					<10	No recommended dosage regimen.		

Oxacillin	Renal (hepatic)	0.3–1.8	q4–12hr	D	<10	Use lower range of usual dose.	NI	N (He) N (P)
Penicillin G–and aqueous K^+ Na^+ (IV)	Renal (hepatic)	0.5–1.2	q4–6hr	I	10–30 <10	NI NI	q8–12hr q12–18hr	Y (He) ? (P)
Penicillin V K^+ (PO)	Renal (hepatic)	30–40 min	q6–8hr	I	<10	NI	q8hr	Y (He) ? (P)
Pentamidine	Renal	6.4–9.4	q24hr	I	10–30 <10	NI NI	q36hr q48hr	N (He) N (P)
Piperacillin	Renal (hepatic)	0.5–1	q4–6hr	I	20–40 <20	NI NI	q8hr q12hr	Y (He) ? (P)
Piperacillin/ tazobactam	Renal	Piperacillin: 0.5–1 Tazobactam: 0.7–1.6	q6–8hr	D,I	20–40 <20	30% ↓ 30% ↓	q6hr q8hr	Y (He) Y (P)
Rifabutin[†]	Renal (hepatic)	16–69	q12–24hr	D	<30	50% ↓	NI	? (He) ? (P)
Rifampin	Hepatic (renal)	3–4	q12–24hr	D	10–50 <10	NI NI	NI NI	N (He) N (P)
Streptomycin sulfate	Renal	2–10	q24hr	D,I	50–80 10–50 <10	7.5 mg/kg 7.5 mg/kg 7.5 mg/kg	q24hr q24–72hr q72–96hr	? (He) ? (P)

*Route in parentheses indicates secondary route of excretion.

[†]In adults; guidelines not established in children.

Continued

TABLE 31-1

ANTIMICROBIALS REQUIRING ADJUSTMENT IN RENAL FAILURE (Continued)

	Pharmacokinetics			Adjustments in Renal Failure				
Drug	**Route of Excretion***	**Normal $t_{1/2}$ (hr)**	**Normal Dose Interval**	**Method**	**CrCl (mL/min)**	**Dose**	**Interval**	**Supplemental Dose for Dialysis**
Sulfamethoxazole/ trimethoprim (cotrimoxazole)	Sulfamethoxazole: Hepatic (renal) Trimethoprim: Renal (hepatic)	Sulfamethoxazole: 9–12 Trimethoprim: 6–11	q12hr	D	15–30 <15	50% ↓ Not recommended	NI	? (He) ? (P)
Sulfisoxazole	Renal	4–8	q6hr	I	10–50 <10	NI NI	q8–12hr q12–24hr	Y (He) ? (P)
Tetracycline	Renal (hepatic)	6–12	q6hr	I	50–80 10–50 <10	NI NI NI	q8–12hr q12–24hr q24hr	Y (He) ? (P)
Ticarcillin[††]	Renal	0.9–1.3	q4–6hr IV q6–8hr IM	I	10–30 <10	NI NI	q8hr q12hr	Y (He) ? (P)
Ticarcillin/ clavulanate[††]	Renal	Ticarcillin: 0.9–1.3 Clavulanate: 1–1.5	q4–6hr	I	10–30 <10 <10 *AND* hepatic impairment	NI NI NI	q8hr q12hr q24hr	Y (He) ? (P)
Tobramycin[‖]	Renal	0.5–5	q6–8hr	I	Any degree of renal insufficiency	2.5 mg/kg; Subsequent doses determined by levels		Y (He) Y (P)[¶]

Valacyclovir[†]	88% as acyclovir in urine	Valacyclovir: ~30 min Acyclovir: 2–3	q12–24hr	D,I	**Herpes Zoster (Adults)**			Y (He) ? (P)
					30–49	1 g	q12hr	
					10–29	1 g	q24hr	
					<10	500 mg	q24hr	
					Genital Herpes (Adol/Adults): Initial Episode			
					10–29	1 g	q24hr	
					<10	500 mg	q24hr	
					Genital Herpes (Adol/Adults): Recurrent Episode			
					<10	500 mg	q24hr	
					Genital Herpes (Adol/Adults): Suppressive			
					<10	500 mg	q24hr (for usual dose of 1 g q24hr)	
						OR		
						500 mg	q48hr (for usual dose of 500 mg q24hr)	

*Route in parentheses indicates secondary route of excretion.
[†]In adults; guidelines not established in children.
[‖]Subsequent doses best determined by measurement of serum levels and assessment of renal insufficiency.
[¶]May add to peritoneal dialysate to obtain adequate serum levels.
[††]May inactivate aminoglycosides in patients with renal impairment.

Continued

TABLE 31-1

ANTIMICROBIALS REQUIRING ADJUSTMENT IN RENAL FAILURE (Continued)

	Pharmacokinetics			Adjustments in Renal Failure				
Drug	Route of Excretion*	Normal $t_{1/2}$ (hr)	Normal Dose Interval	Method	CrCl (mL/min)	Dose	Interval	Supplemental Dose for Dialysis
Valacyclovir—cont'd					**Herpes Labialis (Adol/Adults)**			
					30–49	1 g	q12hr × 2 doses	
					10–29	500 mg	q12hr × 2 doses	
					<10	500 mg	Single dose	
Valganciclovir (see ganciclovir)								
Vancomycin[‖]	Renal	2.2–8	q6–12hr	I	>90	Nl	q6hr	N (He)[††]
					70–89	Nl	q8hr	N (P)
					46–69	Nl	q12hr	
					30–45	Nl	q18hr	
					15–29	Nl	q24hr	
					<15	10–20 mg/kg	Subsequent doses best determined by levels.	

*Route in parentheses indicates secondary route of excretion.

‖Subsequent doses best determined by measurement of serum levels and assessment of renal insufficiency.

††May inactivate aminoglycosides in patients with renal impairment.

CrCl, Creatinine clearance; GFR, glomerular filtration rate; He, hemodialysis; Induct, induction; K^+, potassium; Maint, maintenance; Na^+, sodium; Nl, normal; P, peritoneal dialysis; $t_{1/2}$, half-life with normal renal function.

III. NONANTIMICROBIALS REQUIRING ADJUSTMENT IN RENAL FAILURE (TABLE 31-2)

TABLE 31-2

NONANTIMICROBIALS REQUIRING ADJUSTMENT IN RENAL FAILURE[1–4]

	Pharmacokinetics			Adjustments in Renal Failure				
Drug	Route of Excretion*	Normal $t_{1/2}$ (hr)	Normal Dose Interval	Method	CrCl (mL/min)	Dose	Interval	Supplemental Dose for Dialysis
Acetaminophen	Hepatic	2–4	q4–6hr	I	10–50	NI	q6hr	N (He)
					<10	NI	q8hr	N (P)
Acetazolamide	Renal	2.4–5.8	q6–24hr	I	10–50	NI	q12hr	Y (He)
					<10	Avoid use		? (P)
Allopurinol	Renal	1–3	q6–12hr	D	10–50	50% ↓	NI	? (He)
					<10	70% ↓	NI	? (P)
Aminocaproic Acid	Renal	1–2	q4–6hr	D	Oliguria/ESRD	75% ↓	NI	? (He)
								? (P)
Aspirin[†]	Hepatic (renal)	3–10	q4hr	I	10–50	NI	q4–6hr	Y (He)
					<10	Avoid use		N (P)
Atenolol	Renal (GI)	3.5–7	q24hr	D, I	15–35	1 mg/kg *OR* 50 mg	q24hr	Y (He)
					<15	1 mg/kg *OR* 50 mg	q48hr	N (P)
Azathioprine[‡]	Hepatic (renal)	0.7–3	q24hr	D	10–50	25% ↓	NI	Y (He)
					<10	50% ↓	NI	? (P)
Bismuth subsalicylate	Hepatic (renal)	Salicylate: 2–5 Bismuth: 21–72 days	q3–4hr	D	Avoid use in patients with renal failure			NA

*Route in parentheses indicates secondary route of excretion.

[†]With large doses, the $t_{1/2}$ is prolonged up to 30 hr.

[‡]Azathioprine rapidly converted to mercaptopurine ($t_{1/2}$ = 0.5–4 hr).

Continued

TABLE 31-2

NONANTIMICROBIALS REQUIRING ADJUSTMENT IN RENAL FAILURE (Continued)

	Pharmacokinetics			Adjustments in Renal Failure				
Drug	**Route of Excretion***	**Normal $t_{1/2}$ (hr)**	**Normal Dose Interval**	**Method**	**CrCl (mL/min)**	**Dose**	**Interval**	**Supplemental Dose for Dialysis**
Calcium supplements	GI	Variable	Variable		<25	May require dosage adjustment depending on calcium level		
Captopril	Renal (hepatic)	1–12.5	q6–24hr	D	10–50 <10	25% ↓ 50% ↓	NI NI	Y (He) N (P)
Carbamazepine	Hepatic (renal)	Initial: 25–65 Subsequent: 8–17	q6–24hr	D	<10	25% ↓ (monitor serum levels)	NI	? (He) ? (P)
Cetirizine	Renal (hepatic)	6.2–9	q12–24hr	D	**<6 yr with Renal Impairment** Use not recommended **6–11 yr** Any degree of Insufficiency **≥12 yr** 11–30 <11	 <2.5 mg 15 mg Use not recommended	 q24hr q24hr	? (He) ? (P)
Chloral hydrate	Renal	8–11	q6–8hr	NA	<50	Avoid use		NA
Chloroquine	Renal (hepatic)	3–5 days	q6hr–7 days	D	<10	50% ↓	NI	N (He) N (P)
Chlorothiazide	Renal	0.75–2	q12–24hr	NA	<30	May be ineffective Use not recommended		NA

Cimetidine	Renal (hepatic)	1.4–2	q6–12hr	D, I	>40	NI	q6hr	Y (He)
					20–40	NI	q8hr	? (P)
						OR 25% ↓	NI	
					<20	NI	q12hr	
						OR 50% ↓	NI	
Codeine	Hepatic (renal)	2.5–3.5	q4–6hr	D	10–50	25% ↓	NI	? (He)
					<10	50% ↓	NI	? (P)
Desloratadine	Renal (GI)	27	q24hr	I	Any degree of renal impairment	NI	q48hr	? (He) ? (P)
Digoxin[§]	Renal	18–48	q12–24hr	D, I	**Digitalizing Dose**			N (He)
					ESRD	50% ↓	NA	N (P)
					Maintenance Dose			
					10–50	25%–75% ↓	NI	
						OR NI	q36hr	
					<10	75%–90% ↓	NI	
						OR NI	q48hr	
Diphenhydramine	Hepatic	2–8	q6–8hr	I	10–50	NI	q6–8hr	? (He)
					<10	NI	q6–8hr	? (P)
Disopyramide[‖]	Renal (GI)	3.15–10	q6hr	I	30–40	NI	q8hr	? (He)
					15–30	NI	q12hr	? (P)
					<15	NI	q24hr	
EDTA calcium chloride[‖]	Renal	1.5 (IM) 0.3 (IV)	q4hr IM q12hr IV	D, I	**Serum Creatinine: IV Dose**			? (He)
					≤2 mg/dL	1 g/m^2	q24hr × 5 days	? (P)
					2–3 mg/dL	500 mg/m^2	q24hr × 5 days	
					3–4 mg/dL	500 mg/m^2	q48hr × 3 doses	
					>4 mg/dL	500 mg/m	Once weekly	

*Route in parentheses indicates secondary route of excretion.

§Decrease loading dose by 50% in end-stage renal disease because of decreased volume of distribution.

‖Guidelines in adults; guidelines not established in children.

Continued

TABLE 31-2

NONANTIMICROBIALS REQUIRING ADJUSTMENT IN RENAL FAILURE (Continued)

	Pharmacokinetics			Adjustments in Renal Failure				
Drug	**Route of Excretion***	**Normal $t_{1/2}$ (hr)**	**Normal Dose Interval**	**Method**	**CrCl (mL/min)**	**Dose**	**Interval**	**Supplemental Dose for Dialysis**
Enalapril (IV: Enalaprilat)	Renal (hepatic)	1.3–6.3 (PO)	q6–24hr	D	10–50	0%–25% ↓	NI	? (He)
		5.1–38 (IV)			<10	50% ↓	NI	N (P)
					Use not recommended in infants and children ≤16 yr with GFR <30 mL/min/1.73m^2			
Enoxaparin[‖,¶]	Renal	4.5–7	q12hr	I	<30	NI	q24hr	? (He) ? (P)
Famotidine	Renal	0.8–5	q8–12hr	D, I	10–50	50% ↓	NI	? (He)
						OR NI	q24hr	? (P)
					<10	NI	q36–48hr	
Felbamate[‖]	Renal	20–30	q6–8hr	D	Any degree of renal impairment	50% ↓	NI	? (He) ? (P)
Fentanyl	Renal (hepatic)	2–4	q30min–1hr	D	10–50	25% ↓	NI	NA
					<10	50% ↓	NI	
Fexofenadine	GI (renal)	14–18	q14–18hr	I	Any degree of renal impairment	NI	q24hr	? (He) ? (P)
Flecainide	Renal/hepatic	8–27	q8–12hr	D	<20	25%–50%↓	NI	N (He) N (P)
Furosemide	Renal (hepatic)	0.5	q6–24hr PO q6–12hr IV		Avoid use in oliguric states			N (He) N (P)
Gabapentin[‖]	Renal (hepatic)	4.7–9	q8hr	D, I	30–59	200–700 mg	q12hr	Y (He)
					15–29	200–700 mg	q24hr	N (P)
					<15	100–300 mg	q24hr	

Hydralazine[#]	Hepatic (renal)	2–8	q4–6hr (IV) q6–12hr (PO)	I	10–50	NI	q8hr(fast acetylator)	? (He)
					<10	NI	q8–16hr q12–24hr (slow acetylator)	? (P)
Insulin (regular)**	Hepatic (renal)	1.5	Variable	D	10–50	25% ↓	NI	N (He)
					<10	50%–75% ↓	NI	N (P)
Levetiracetam[‖]	Renal	5–8	q12hr	D	**Children**			Y (He)
					<50	50% ↓	NI	N (P)
					Adults			
					50–80	500–1,000 mg	NI	
					30–50	250–750 mg	NI	
					<30	250–500 mg	NI	
					ESRD on dialysis	500–1,000 mg	q24hr	
Lisinopril	Renal	11–13	q24hr	D	10–30	50% ↓	NI	Y (He)
					<10	75% ↓	NI	N (P)
					Use not recommended for children with CrCl <30 mL/min/1.73m^2			
Lithium	Renal	18–24	q6–8hr	D	10–50	25%–50% ↓	NI	Y (He)
					<10	50%–75% ↓	NI	N (P)
Loratadine	Renal/hepatic	Loratadine: 8.4 Metabolite: 28	q24hr	I	<30	NI	q48hr	? (He) ? (P)

*Route in parentheses indicates secondary route of excretion.

‖Guidelines in adults; guidelines not established in children.

¶Monitor antifactor Xa closely.

#Dose interval varies for rapid and slow acetylators with normal and impaired renal function.

**Renal failure may cause hyposensitivity or hypersensitivity to insulin; adjust to clinical response and blood glucose.

Continued

TABLE 31-2

NONANTIMICROBIALS REQUIRING ADJUSTMENT IN RENAL FAILURE (Continued)

	Pharmacokinetics			Adjustments in Renal Failure				
Drug	**Route of Excretion***	**Normal $t_{1/2}$ (hr)**	**Normal Dose Interval**	**Method**	**CrCl (mL/min)**	**Dose**	**Interval**	**Supplemental Dose for Dialysis**
Meperidine	Renal (hepatic)	2.3–4	q3–4hr	D	10–50	25% ↓	NI	? (He)
	Normeperidine: Renal				<10	50% ↓	NI	? (P)
Methadone	Hepatic (renal)	4–87	q3–12hr	D	<10	25%–50% ↓	NI	N (He)
								N (P)
Methyldopa	Hepatic (renal)	1–3	q6–12hr PO	I	>50	NI	q8hr	Y (He)
			q6–8hr IV		10–50	NI	q8–12hr	? (P)
					<10	NI	q12–24hr	
Metoclopramide	Renal	2.5–6	q6hr PO	D	40–50	25% ↓	NI	? (He)
			q6–8hr IV		10–40	50% ↓	NI	? (P)
					<10	50%–75%↓	NI	
Midazolam	Hepatic (renal)	2.2–6.8	Variable	D	10–29	25% ↓	NI	NA
					<10	50% ↓	NI	
Milrinone	Renal	1.5–3.8	Continuous infusion	D	50 mL/min/1.73 m^2		0.43 mcg/kg/min	NA
					40 mL/min/1.73 m^2		0.38 mcg/kg/min	
					30 mL/min/1.73 m^2		0.33 mcg/kg/min	
					20 mL/min/1.73 m^2		0.28 mcg/kg/min	
					10 mL/min/1.73 m^2		0.23 mcg/kg/min	
					5 mL/min/1.73m^2		0.2 mcg/kg/min	
Morphine	Hepatic (renal)	1–67.8	Variable	D	10–50	25% ↓	NI	? (He)
					<10	50% ↓	NI	? (P)
Neostigmine	Hepatic (renal)	0.5–2.1	Variable	D	10–50	50% ↓	NI	? (He)
					<10	75% ↓	NI	? (P)

Oxcarbazepine	Renal	Oxcarbazepine: 2 MHD: 9	q12hr	D	<30	50% ↓ in initial dose and slower titration	NI	? (He) ? (P)
Pancuronium bromide	Renal (hepatic)	1.8	q30–60min OR continuous infusion	D	10–50 <10	50% ↓ Avoid use	NI	? (He) ? (P)
Phenazopyridine	Renal (hepatic)	?	q8hr for2 days	I	50–80 <50	NI Avoid use	q8–16hr	NA
Phenobarbital	Hepatic (renal, 30%)	37–140	q8–12hr	I	<10	NI	q24hr	Y (He) Y (P)
Primidone	Hepatic (renal, 20%)	Primidone: 10–12 Metabolite: 16	q6–12hr	I	>50 10–50 <10	NI NI NI	q12hr q12–24hr q24hr	Y (He) ? (P)
Procainamide	Hepatic (renal)	Procainamide: 1.7–4. 7 NAPA: 6–8	q3–6hr PO q4–6hr IM	I	**Oral** 10–50 <10	 NI NI	 q6–12hr q8–24hr	Y (He) N (P)
					IV (Adult) Maintenance 10–50 <10	 33% ↓ 67% ↓	 NI NI	
					IV (Adult) Loading Dose Severe renal 12 mg/kg impairment		 NA	
Quinidine	Renal	2.5–8	q4–12hr	D	<10	25% ↓	NI	Y (He) N (P)

*Route in parentheses indicates secondary route of excretion.

Continued

TABLE 31-2

NONANTIMICROBIALS REQUIRING ADJUSTMENT IN RENAL FAILURE (Continued)

	Pharmacokinetics			Adjustments in Renal Failure				
Drug	**Route of Excretion***	**Normal $t_{1/2}$ (hr)**	**Normal Dose Interval**	**Method**	**CrCl (mL/min)**	**Dose**	**Interval**	**Supplemental Dose for Dialysis**
Ranitidine	Renal (hepatic)	1.8–2.5	q12hr PO	D	10–50	50% ↓	NI	N (He)[††]
			q6–8hr IV/IM		<10	75% ↓	NI	? (P)
Spironolactone	Renal (hepatic)	Spironolactone: ↓ 1.3–1.4	q6–24hr	I	10–50	NI	q12–24hr	NA
		Canrenone: 13–24			<10	Avoid use		
Terbutaline (IV/PO)	Renal (hepatic)	2.9–14	Variable	D	<50	NI	NI	? (He) ? (P)
Thiopental	Hepatic (renal)	3–11.5	One-time dose	D	<10	25% ↓	NI	NA
Triamterene	Hepatic (renal)	1.6–2.5	q12–24hr	I	>50	NI	q12hr	NA
					<50	Avoid use		
Verapamil	Renal (hepatic)	2–8	Variable	D	<10	NI	NI	N (He)
					Use caution and closely monitor ECG for PR prolongation, BP and other signs of overdose			N (P)
Vigabatrin (Sabril)	Renal	5–8	q12hr	D	50–80	25% ↓	NI	? (He)
					30–50	50% ↓	NI	? (P)
					10–30	75% ↓	NI	

*Route in parentheses indicates secondary route of excretion.

[††]Adjust dose schedule to administer dose at the end of dialysis.

BP, Blood pressure; CrCl, creatinine clearance; ECG, electrocardiogram; ESRD, end-stage renal disease; GFR, glomerular filtration rate; GI, gastrointestinal; He, hemodialysis; IV, intravenous; MDH, 10-monohydroxy metabolite; NA, not applicable; maint, maintenance dose; P, peritoneal dialysis; PO, per os (by mouth).

REFERENCES

1. Taketomo C, Hodding JH, Kraus DM. *Pediatric dosage handbook.* 16th ed. Hudson, OH: Lexi-Comp; 2009.
2. Aronoff GR, Bennett WM, Berns JS, et al. *Drug prescribing in renal failure: dosing guidelines for adults.* 5th ed. Philadelphia: American College of Physicians; 2007.
3. Veltri, M, Neu AM, Fivush BA, et al. Dosing during intermittent hemodialysis and continuous renal replacement therapy: special considerations in pediatric patients. *Paediatr Drugs.* 2004;6(1):45–66.
4. Micromedex Healthcare Series (electronic version). Greenwood Village, CO: Thomson Micromedex; 2010. http://www.thomsonhc.com. Accessed August 8, 2010.

Index

Page numbers followed by "f" indicate figures, "t" indicate tables, and "b" indicate boxes.
Entries in *italics* indicate color plates.

A

A-200, formulary entry for, 929
Abdomen(s)
  acute pain in, 294–295
  radiographs of, 615–617
  trauma to
    emergent treatments for, 106
    evaluation of, 103–104
    laboratory studies of, 104–113
    radiologic evaluation of, 105–106
    secondary survey of, 90t
Abelcet, with renal failure, 1014t
Abilify (aripiprazole), dosage/side effects for, 1003t
Abortive tiptans, for migraine headaches, 510t
Absent reflexes, 506–507
Absolute risk reduction, 656
Absorptive triptans, for migraines, 510t
AccuNeb
  for anaphylaxis, 10
  for asthma, 10
  formulary entry for, 687–688
Accutane
  for acne vulgaris, 218–220
  formulary entry for, 832
Acetadote, formulary entry for, 684
Acetaminophen (Tylenol, Tempra, Panadol, Feverall, Aspirin Free Anacin)
  analgesic properties of, 138
  formulary entry for, 682
  poisoning with, 684
  with renal failure, 1027t
  toxicity of, 28t
Acetaminophen and codeine, formulary entry for, 756
Acetaminophen and oxycodone (Tylox, Roxilox, Percocet, Endocet, Roxicet), formulary entry for, 895
Acetazolamide (Diamox)
  formulary entry for, 683
  with renal failure, 1027t
Acetylcysteine (Mucomyst, Mucosol, Acetadote), formulary entry for, 684
Acetylsulfisoxazole erythromycin ethylsuccinate (Pediazole), formulary entry for, 787
Achondroplasia, growth charts for, 534
Acid phophatase, reference values for, 639t
Acid-base disturbances, analysis of, 586
Acid-base/osmolar gap disturbances
  definitions for, 289
  etiology of, 289, 290f–291f
Acidosis
  anion gap metabolic, 22t
  definition of, 246
  renal tubular, 486–487
Acinetobacter spp., sensitivity profile of, 409t
Aclovate, potency ranking of, 996t
Acne vulgaris
  algorithm for, 219t
  pathogenesis of, 217
  treatment for, 217–220, 218t
Acquired aplasias, characterization of, 327
Acquired heart disease
  bacterial endocarditis prophylaxis as, 191
  endocarditis as, 191
  Kawasaki disease as, 196–198
  Lyme disease as, 199
  myocardial disease as, 191–195
  pericardial disease as, 195–196
  rheumatic heart disease as, 198–199
ACTH. *See* Corticotropin
ACTH stimulation test, 263
Acthar Gel, formulary entry for, 757
Acticin
  for scabies, 208
  formulary entry for, 906
Actigall, formulary entry for, 971
Actinomycin D (dactinomycin), toxicity of, 1007t

Actiq
characterization of, 140t
formulary entry for, 794–795
relative potency of, 151t
with renal failure, 1030t
for RSI, 6t–7t
Activase, formulary entry for, 689
Activated protein C resistance. *See* Factor V Leiden
Active movements, 504
Acular
characterization of, 139
formulary entry for, 835–836
Acute ataxia, evaluation of, 520b
Acute bacterial sinusitis, levofloxacin for, 843
Acute dialysis
indications for, 494–495
techniques for, 495
Acute kidney injury, 494
Acute liver failure (ALF), 301–304
Acute pancreatitis
conditions associated with, 306t
diagnosis of, 306
management of, 307
presentation of, 305–307
Acute phase reactants, 620–621
Acute promyelocytic leukemia (APL), isotretinoin contraindications for, 220
Acute pyelonephritis, levofloxacin for, 843
Acute renal failure. *See* Acute kidney injury
Acute tubular necrosis (ATN), 494
Acute viral bronchiolitis, sodium chloride-inhaled preparations for, 948
Acyanotic lesions
characterization of, 183
types of, 186t
Acyclovir (Zovirax)
for antimicrobial prophylaxis, 575t
formulary entry for, 685–686
for neonatal varicella, 413t
with renal failure, 1013t
Aczone
for antimicrobial prophylaxis, 575t
formulary entry for, 761–762
Adalat CC
formulary entry for, 881–882
for hypertension emergency, 105t
Adenocard
formulary entry for, 686
for resuscitation, ii
Adenosine (Adenocard)
formulary entry for, 686
for resuscitation, ii
ADHD. *See* Attention deficit/ hyperactivity disorder
Adjuncts, for RSI, 6t
Adolescent(s)
abnormalities in, summary of, 123t
acetazolamide dosage for, 479–480
captopril dosage for, 727
contraceptive use by
barrier methods, 127t
combined hormonal, 127t
DMPA, 129f
ECP, 128
follow-up recommendations, 131
long-acting progestin methods, 128
quick start method, 130–131
drug use among, 120
eating habits of, 117
education of, 117
genital development in, 119t
health maintenance for
chief complaint, 120–121
confidentiality in, 121
family history in, 121
immunizations, 121–122
laboratory tests for, 121–122
MCV4 vaccine for, 384
physical examinations, 121
review of systems, 121
household composition, 117
pain assessments for, 137
PPE for, 132–133
examination items in, 133
medical history, 133
orthopedic examination, 134f
review of systems in, 133
psychosocial development in, 119t
pubertal development, 117
pubic hair tanner staging, 118b, 118f
scoliosis in, 131–132
sexual health of
genital ulcer management, 123t

Adolescent(s) *(Continued)*
genital wart management, 123t
infections, 122
vaginal infection management, 123t
websites for, 117
Adrenal insufficiency
characterization of, 253–256
classic, 254–255
management of, 255
nonclassic, 255
tests for, 253t
Adrenalin
for anaphylaxis, 10
anesthetics use with, 139
asthma treatment with, 10–11
characterization of, 141t
formulary entry for, 782–783
for resuscitation, ii
standard concentrations for, i
Adrenergics, toxidrome of, 23t
Adriamycin (doxorubicin), toxicity of, 1008t
Adrucil (fluorouracil), toxicity of, 1007t
Advair, formulary entry for, 804–805
Advil, formulary entry for, 821–822
Aerobic bacteria, algorithm for, 406f–407f
Aerobid
daily dose recommendations for, 804t, 993t
formulary entry for, 800
Aerolizer, formulary entry for, 807–808
Aerospan MDI
daily dose recommendations for, 804t, 993t
formulary entry for, 800
AF, formulary entry for, 867
Afrin, formulary entry for, 693
Aftate, formulary entry for, 966
Age, bone, 618
Aggression, in children, 230t
Airway(s)
assessment of, 3–7
edema in, 991
imaging of
foreign bodies, 609
lateral radiographs of, 608, 608t
normal anatomy, 610f–611f
Airway(s) *(Continued)*
inflammation of, inhaled steroids for, 992–995, 993t–994t
management of, 3–7
protection, during GI decontamination, 4
Airway clearance therapy, for cystic fibrosis, 601
Akarpine, formulary entry for, 912–913
AK-Poly-Bac Ophthalmic, formulary entry for, 711
AK-Spore H.C., formulary entry for, 916
AK-Sulf, formulary entry for, 953
AKTob
formulary entry for, 965–966
with renal failure, 1024t
AK-Tracin Ophthalmic, formulary entry for, 711
Alacol, formulary entry for, 717–718
Alanine aminotransferase (ALT)
in hepatic function test, 303t
reference values for, 639t
Albuterol (Proventil, VoSpire ER, Proventil HFA, Ventolin HFA, AccuNeb)
for anaphylaxis, 10
for asthma, 10
formulary entry for, 687–688
Alclometasone dipropionate (Aclovate), potency ranking of, 996t
Alcohols, toxicity of, 30t
Aldactone
formulary entry for, 950
for hypertension, 501t
with renal failure, 1034t
Aldolase, reference values for, 639t–647t
Aldosterone, potency of, 992t
Alenaze, formulary entry for, 717–718
Aleve, formulary entry for, 877–878
Alkaline phosphatase, reference values for, 640t
Alkeran (melphalan), toxicity of, 1008t
Allegen Ear Drops, formulary entry for, 702
Allegra
formulary entry for, 796
with renal failure, 1030t

Allergic eosinophilic gastroenteritis, 356
Allergic rhinitis
  characterization of, 354–356
  montelukast for, 873
Allergy(ies)
  to cow's milk, 558t
  to eggs, 371–374
  food, 356–359
  to penicillin, 359
Allogeneic HSCT, 569–571
Alloprim
  formulary entry for, 688
  with renal failure, 1027t
  for tumor lysis syndrome, 567
  for von Willebrand disease, 346t–347t
Allopurinol (Zyloprim, Alloprim)
  formulary entry for, 688
  with renal failure, 1027t
  for tumor lysis syndrome, 567
  for von Willebrand disease, 347t
Almacone, formulary entry for, 690–691
Alocril (Nedocromil sodium ophthalmic), 1000t
Alomide (lodoxamide tromethamine ophthalmic), 1000t
Alpha adrenergic drug extravasion, phentolamine mesylate for, 908
Alpha blockers, for hypertension, 500t
Alpha–beta-blocker, for hypertensive emergency, 105t
Alpha-tocopherol
  DRIs for, 542t
  in multivitamin drops, analysis of, 545t
  in multivitamin tablets, analysis of, 546t
Alprostadil (Postaglandin E_1)
  formulary entry for, 688–689
  standard concentrations for, i
ALT (alanine aminotransferase), in hepatic function test, 303t
AltenaGEL, formulary entry for, 690
Alteplase (Activase, Cathflo, Activase, t(PA)), formulary entry for, 689
Altered states of consciousness
  differential diagnosis of, 15b
  emergency treatments for, 13–16
Aluminum hydroxide (Amphojel, Alu-Tab, Dialume, AltenaGEL), formulary entry for, 690
Aluminum hydroxide with magnesium hydroxide (Maalox, Mylanta, Almacone, Rulox Plus, Mintox), formulary entry for, 690–691
Alu-Tab, formulary entry for, 690
Alvesco, formulary entry for, 747–748
Amantadine hydrochloride (Symmetrel)
  approval for, 393
  formulary entry for, 691
  with renal failure, 1013t
Ambiguous genitalia, 262
AmBisome, with renal failure, 1014t
Amebiasis, metronidazole for, 865
Amethopterin (methotrexate), toxicity of, 1008t
Amicar, formulary entry for, 693
Amide
  formulary entry for, 928
  for tuberculosis, 447t, 928
Amifostine, as chemotherapy adjunct, 1009t
Amikacin sulfate (Amikin)
  formulary entry for, 692
  with renal failure, 1013t
Amiloride, for hypertension, 501t
Amino acid-based formulas, 552t
Aminocaproic acid (Amicar), formulary entry for, 693
Aminoglycoside(s)
  for catheter-related bloodstream infections, 423t
  gentamicin as, 812–813
  kanamycin as, 833–834
  neomycin sulfate as, 878
  for osteomyelitis, 426t
  paromomycin sulfate as, 899–900
  streptomycin sulfate as, 950–951
  tobramycin as, 965–966
Aminopenicillin(s)
  amoxicillin as, 697
  ampicillin as, 697
  ampicillin/sulbactam as, 701–702
  formulary entry as, 697
Aminophylline, formulary entry for, 693–694
5-Aminosalicylic acid, formulary entry for, 857

Aminoxin
DRIs for, 542t
formulary entry for, 930
in multivitamin drops, analysis of, 545t
in multivitamin tablets, analysis of, 546t
Amiodarone HCl (Cordarone, Pacerone)
formulary entry for, 694–695
IV infusions of, i
for resuscitations, ii
standard concentrations for, i
Amitriptyline (Elavil)
formulary entry for, 695–696
for migraines, 512t
Amlodipine (Norvasc)
formulary entry for, 696
for hypertension, 500t
Ammonia, reference values for, 640t
Ammonium chloride, formulary entry for, 696–697
Amnesteem
for acne vulgaris, 218–220
formulary entry for, 832
Amoxicillin (Amoxil, Trimox, Wymox, Polymox, DisperMox)
for bacterial infections, 422t
formulary entry for, 697
for lymphadenitis, 425t
for meningitis, 426t
for otitis media, 426t
with renal failure, 1013t
Amoxicillin-clavulanic acid (Augmentin)
formulary entry for, 701–702
with renal failure, 1013t
Amoxil
for bacterial infections, 422t
formulary entry for, 697
for lymphadenitis, 425t
for meningitis, 426t
for otitis media, 426t
with renal failure, 1013t
Amphadase, formulary entry for, 817
Amphetamines
for ADHD, 239t
toxicity of, 43b
Amphocin, with renal failure, 1014t
Amphojel, formulary entry for, 690
Amphotericin B (Fungizone, Amphocin), with renal failure, 1014t
Amphotericin B lipid complex (Abelcet), with renal failure, 1014t
Amphotericin B liposomal (AmBisome), with renal failure, 1014t
Ampicillin (Omnipen, Principen, Totacillin)
formulary entry for, 701
for gonococcal infections, 420t
for meningitis, 421t
neonatal critical care dosing of, 1010t
with renal failure, 1014t
with sulbactam, for mastoiditis, 425t
Ampicillin/sulbactam (Unasyn)
formulary entry for, 701–702
with renal failure, 1014t
Amylase, reference values for, 640t
Anacin
analgesic properties of, 139
formulary entry for, 703–704
for Kawasaki disease, 198
with renal failure, 1027t
Anaerobes, in animal bites, 96t
Anaerobic infection(s), metronidazole for, 865
Analgesia(s)
acetaminophen for, 682
amitriptyline for, 695–696
aspirin for, 703–704
codeine for, 755
codeine and acetaminophen for, 756
fentanyl for, 794–795
hydromorphone for, 820
ibuprofen for, 821–822
imipramine for, 823–824
local anesthetics for, 139–142
meperidine for, 140t
methadone for, 140t, 859
morphine for, 140t, 878
naproxen sodium as, 877
nonopioid, 137–139
opioids, 139
opium tincture for, 890–891
oxycodone for, 693
oxycodone and acetaminophen for, 895
oxycodone and aspirin for, 693
pain thresholds of, 149t
paregoric for, 899
patient-controlled, 148

Analgesia(s) *(Continued)*
PCA, 148–150
standard-risk patient and, 137–143
websites for, 137
Anaphylaxis
definitions of, 9
food allergy-induced, 356
management of, 9–10
Anaprox, formulary entry for, 877–878
Anaspaz, for palliative care, 581t
Anatomic asplenia, immunization recommendations for, 381
Ancef
for bacterial endocarditis prophylaxis, 193t
formulary entry for, 732
with renal failure, 1015t
Ancobon
formulary entry for, 798
with renal failure, 1018t
Ancylostoma caninum, mebendazole for, 855
Androstenedione, normal values for, 269t
Anemia
age-specific indices of, 323t, 325f
causes of, 322–328
chronic inflammation, 328
classification of, 326t
darbepoetin alfa dose adjustments for, 763t
epoetin alfa for, 784
gender-specific indices of, 325f
general evaluation of, 322
hematologic, 573
macrocytic, 327
sickle cell
characterization of, 328–329
complications of, 329t
immunization recommendations for, 381
maintenance of, 331t
Anesthesia. *See also* Sedation
fasting recommendations for, 143t
local
analgesic properties of, 139–142
commonly used, 141t
injectables, 142t
toxicity of, 139–142
Angiostrongylosis, thiabedazole for, 962
Angiotensin-converting enzyme (ACE) inhibitor
captopril as, 727
enalapril maleate as, 780
for hypertension, 500t
lisinopril as, 848
losartan as, 851–852
risks of, 970
Angiotensin-II receptor blocker (ARB), for hypertension, 500t
Angloedema, food allergy-induced, 356
Anion gap metabolic acidosis, due to poisoning, 22t
Ankle(s), injuries to, splints for, 87
Ankylosing spondylitis, naproxen sodium as, 877
Annuria/oliguria, mannitol for, 854
Anthelmintic
mebendazole as, 854–855
thiabedazole as, 962
Anthrax, 750
Anthrax exposure, levofloxacin for, 843
Antiarrhythmic
adenosine as, 686
amiodarone as, 694–695
digoxin as, 770
esmolol HCl as, 789–790
flecainide acetate as, 797
lidocaine as, 844–845
metoprolol as, 864
phenytoin as, 909–910
procainamide as, 922
propranolol as, 924–925
quinidine as, 931–932
Antibiotic prophylaxis
for specific cardiac conditions, 193b
for UTI evaluation, 482
Antibiotic(s)
amikacin sulfate as, 692
amoxicillin as, 697
amoxicillin-clavulanic acid as, 701–702
ampicillin/sulbactam as, 701–702
azithromycin as, 708–710
aztreonam as, 710
bacitracin as, 711
cefactor as, 731–732
cefadroxil as, 732
cefazolin as, 732
cefdinir as, 733

Antibiotic(s) *(Continued)*
cefepime as, 733
cefixime as, 734–735
cefotaxime as, 734–735
ceftriaxone as, 738–739
cephalexin as, 740
chloramphenicol as, 741
ciprofloxacin as, 749–750
clarithromycin as, 751–752
clindamycin as, 752–753
dapsone as, 761–762
dicloxacillin sodium as, 769
doxycycline as, 777
ertapenem as, 786–787
erythromycin ethylsuccinate and acetylsulfisoxazole as, 787
erythromycin preparations as, 218t
for GBS infection, 420t
gentamicin as, 812–813
imipenem and cilastin as, 823
kanamycin as, 833–834
levofloxacin as, 842–843
linezolid, 847
meropenem as, 858
metronidazole as, 865–866
minocycline as, 870
murpirocin as, 874
nafcillin as, 876
neomycin sulfate as, 878
neomycin/polymyxin B/bacitracin as, 878–879
neonatal critical care dosing of, 1010t
nitrofurantion as, 882–883
ofloxacin as, 887
paromomycin sulfate as, 899–900
penicillin as, 575t
penicillin benzathine as, 903
penicillin G, benzthine, procaine as, 903
penicillin G procaine as, 904
penicillin V potassium as, 904–905
pentamidine isethionate as, 905
piperacillin as, 913–914
piperacillin with tazobactam as, 914
quinupristin and dalfopristin as, 932
sensitivity-based selection of, 405, 408t–409t
streptomycin sulfate as, 950–951
sulfadiazine as, 953–954
ticarcillin and ciavulanate as, 964
tobramycin as, 965–966

Antibiotic(s) *(Continued)*
topical
for acne vulgaris, 217
murpirocin as, 874
neomycin/polymyxin B/bacitracin as, 878–879
polymyxin B sulfate and trimethoprim sulfate as, 916
silver sulfadiazine as, 945
trimethoprim-sulfamethoxazole as, 954
vancomycin as, 974–976
Antibody deficiency(ies), subcutaneous immune globulin for, 363
Antibody(ies), anti-CCP, 622
Antibody-deficient disorders, IVIG therapy for, 361–362
Anticholinergic(s)
for allergic rhinitis, 355–356
atropine sulfate as, 706–707
benztropine mesylate as, 714
cyclopentolate as, 758–759
cyclopentolate with phenylephrine as, 759
glycopyrrolate as, 814
ipratroplum bromide as, 827–828
oxybutynin chloride as, 894
scopolamine hydrobromide as, 942
toxicity of, 31t
toxidrome of, 23t
Anticholinesterase agent(s)
edrophonium chloride as, 779
neostigmine as, 879
toxidrome of, 24t
Anticoagulant(s)
enoxaparin as, 780–782
heparin sodium as, 816–817
for stroke, 522
warfarin as, 983–984
Anticonvulsant(s)
carbamazepine as, 727–728
diazepam, 768–769
divalproex sodium as, 773–774
felbamate as, 793–794
fosphenytoin as, 690–691
gabapentin as, 810–811
lamotrigine as, 837–840
levetiracetam, 841–842
lorazepam as, 851
for migraines, 512t
oxcarbazepine, 893–894
phenytoin as, 909–910

Anticonvulsant(s) *(Continued)*
topiramate as, 967
valproic acid as, 973–974
zonisamide as, 732
Anti-cyclic citrullinated peptide (CCP), antibodies of, 622
Antidepressant(s)
amitriptyline as, 695–696
carbamazepine as, 727–728
diazepam as, 768–769
divalproex sodium as, 773–774
felbamate as, 793–794
fluoxetine hydrochloride as, 801–802
fluvoxamine as, 805t
fosphenytoin as, 690–691
gabapentin as, 810–811
imipramine as, 823–824
for migraines, 512t
nortriptyline hydrochloride, 108t
paroxetine as, 900–901
sertraline as, 944
SSRIs as, 1004t
toxicity of, 32t
trazodone as, 968
Antidote(s)
for acetaminophen toxicity, 29t
for alcohol toxicity, 30t
for antidepressant toxicity, 32t
for antihistamine toxicity, 33t
for benzodiazepine toxicity, 34t
for beta-blockers, 35t
for calcium channel blockers, 36t
for hypoglycemics, 37t
for NSAIDs, 39t
for salicytates, 137
Antiemetic(s)
chloramphenicol as, 741
dexamethasone as, 766–767
dimenhydrinate as, 772
dolasetron as, 775
dronabinol as, 778
droperidol as, 778
granisetron as, 814
hydralazine hydrochloride as, 818
lorazepam as, 851
metoclopramide as, 863
ondansetron as, 889–890
prochlorperazine as, 922–923
promethazine as, 923–924
scopolamine hydrobromide as, 942
trimethobenzamide as, 970
Antifungal(s)
amphotericin B as, 1014t
amphotericin B lipid complex as, 1014t
amphotericin B liposomal as, 1014t
caspofungin as, 810–811
clotrimazole as, 754–755
fluconazole as, 797–798
flucytosine as, 798
griseofulvin as, 815
itraconazole as, 833
ketoconazole as, 833
micafungin sodium as, 866–867
miconazole as, 867
tolnaftate as, 966
voriconazole as, 981–982
Antihistamine(s)
for atopic dermatitis, 212
azelastine as, 708
brompheniramine with phenylephrine as, 717–718
carbinoxamine and pseudoephedrine as, 729–730
cetirizine as, 740–741
chlorpheniramine maleate as, 744
cyproheptadine as, 760–761
diphenhydramine as, 773
fexofenadine as, 796
hydralazine hydrochloride as, 818
for migraines, 512t
olopatadine as, 887–888
promethazine as, 923–924
sedating, properties of, 137
toxicity of, 33t
Antihypertensive(s)
amlodipine as, 696
captopril as, 727
clonidine as, 754
diazoxide as, 769
enalapril maleate as, 780
esmolol HCl as, 789–790
hydralazine hydrochloride as, 818
hydrochlorothiazide as, 818
labetalol as, 836
lisinopril as, 848
losartan as, 851–852
methyldopa as, 860
metoprolol as, 864
for migraines, 512t
minoxidil as, 870–871
nicardipine as, 881
nifedipine as, 881–882

Antihypertensive(s) *(Continued)*
nitroglycerin as, 882–883
phentolamine mesylate as, 908
propranolol as, 924–925
verapamil as, 978
Antihyperuricemic agent, rasburicase as, 933–934
Antihypoglycemic agent(s)
diazoxide as, 769
glucagon as, 813
Anti-inflammatory(ies)
aspirin as, 703–704
corticotropin as, 757
cortisone acetate as, 757
dexamethasone as, 766–767
hydrocortisone as, 819
mesalamine as, 857
olsalazine as, 888
prednisone as, 919–920
sulfasalazine as, 955
Antilirium
as anticholinergic antidote, 33t
formulary entry for, 911
Antimalarial(s)
chloroquine HCl/phosphate as, 742–743
hydroxychloroquine as, 820–821
mefloquine HCl as, 856
primaquine phosphate as, 920
Antimanic agent, lithium as, 849
Antimicrobial prophylaxis, 575t
Antimigraine agent(s)
ergotamine tartrate as, 786
prochlorperazine as, 922–923
propranolol as, 924–925
sumatriptan succinate as, 955–956
valproic acid as, 973–974
Antiminth, formulary entry for, 927–928
Antinuclear antibody(ies)
laboratory studies of, 621
reference values for, 640t
Antiparasitic agent(s)
metronidazole as, 865–866
pyrimethamine as, 930–931
Anti-Parkinson's agent, benztropine mesylate as, 714
Antiplatelet therapy, for stroke, 522
Antipsychotic(s), 1004t
aripirazole as, 1003t
chlorpromazine as, 745
Antipsychotic(s) *(Continued)*
clozapine as, 1003t
haloperidol as, 815–816, 1003t
olanzapine as, 1003t
quetiapine as, 1004t
risperdal as, 939–940
risperidone as, 1003t
thioridazine as, 963
ziprasidone as, 1004t
Antipyretic(s)
acetaminophen as, 682
aspirin as, 703–704
ibuprofen for, 822
Antipyrine and benzocaine (Allegen Ear Drops, Antipyrine, Antipyrine and benzocaine Otic, Autoguard Otic, Auralgan), formulary entry for, 702
ANTIROBE
for bacterial vaginosis, 422t
for cellulitis, 423t
formulary entry for, 752–753
for lymphadenitis, 425t
for mastoiditis, 425t
for osteomyelitis, 426t
for pneumonia, 428t
Antispasmodic(s), oxybutynin chloride as, 894
Antistreptolysin O titer, reference values for, 641t
Antithrombin III deficiency, characterization of, 338b
Antithyroid agent(s)
methimazole as, 856–857
potassium iodide as, 917
propylthiouracil as, 925
Antituberculous agent(s)
ethambutol HCl as, 791
isoniazid as, 831
rifampin as, 937–938
streptomycin sulfate as, 950–951
Antiviral(s)
acyclovir as, 685–686
amantadine hydrochloride as, 691
cidofovir as, 748
famciclovir as, 792
ganciclovir as, 731
lamivudine as, 837
nevirapine as, 879–880
oseltamivir phosphate as, 891–892

Antiviral(s) *(Continued)*
ribavirin as, 934–936
rimantadine as, 938
valacyclovir as, 971–972
valganciclovir as, 971–972
zidovudine as, 984
Antizol, formulary entry for, 806–807
Anxiety disorders
in childhood, 230t, 240
hydroxyzine for, 821
Anxiolytic(s)
buspirone as, 1005t
diazepam as, 768–769
hydroxyzine as, 821
lorazepam as, 851
SSRIs as, 1005t
Anzemet, formulary entry for, 775
Aorta(s), contraction of, CHD/exam findings of, 186t
Aortic stenosis (AS), CHD/exam findings of, 186t
Apex, 168
Apgar scores, neonatal, 205, 457t
APL. *See* Acute promyelocytic leukemia
Aplasias
acquired, 327
congenital, 327
Aplastic anemia, characterization of, 327
Apnea
central, bradycardia without, 465
neonatal
causes of, 466f
characterization of, 465
theophylline for, 957
Apparent-life-threatening events (ALTE), pulmonary, 591–592
Apresoline
formulary entry for, 818
for hypertension, 501t
for hypertensive crisis, 43
for hypertensive emergency, 105t, 818
for renal failure, 1031t
Aquachloral Supprettes
formulary entry for, 741
properties of, 145
with renal failure, 1031t
for sedation, 137
Aquasol A
DRIs for, 542t
in multivitamin drops, analysis of, 545t
Aquasol A *(Continued)*
in multivitamin tablets, analysis of, 546t
reference values for, 647t
Aquasol E
DRIs for, 542t
in multivitamin drops, analysis of, 545t
in multivitamin tablets, analysis of, 546t
Aquavit-E
DRIs for, 542t
in multivitamin drops, analysis of, 545t
in multivitamin tablets, analysis of, 546t
Aralen
formulary entry for, 742–743
with renal failure, 1028t
Aranesp, formulary entry for, 762–764
Arestin
for acne vulgaris, 218t
formulary entry for, 870
Arginine HCL (R-Gene), formulary entry for, 702–703
Aripiprazole (Abilify), dosage/side effects for, 1003t
Aristospan, formulary entry for, 969
Arm(s), injuries to
long arm posterior splinting for, 85
nursemaid's elbow, 87
sugar tong forearm splinting for, 86
ulnar gutter splint for, 86
Arm recoil, in newborn assessment, 457
Arrhythmia(s)
nonventricular, 175t, 176f
propranolol for, 924–925
ventricular, 178t
Arsenic poisoning, penicillamine for, 901
Arso Forte, formulary entry for, 971
Arterial blood gas (ABG), 586
Arterial gas, reference values for, 641t
Arteriole vasodilator
formulary entry for, 769
for hypertensive emergency, 105t
Artery(ies)
dorsalis pedis, puncture of, 61
femoral, puncture of, 59
radial, puncture of, 59–61
umbilical artery catheterization, vascular access for, 65–68

Arthritis
juvenile idiopathic
characterization of, 623
classical divisions of, 625t
ethancept for, 790
juvenile rheumatoid
autoantibodies associated with, 621t
characterization of, 901
PsA, 624–626
reactive, 626–627
ASA
analgesic properties of, 139
formulary entry for, 703–704
for Kawasaki disease, 198
with renal failure, 1027t
Asacol, formulary entry for, 857
Ascaris
mebendazole for, 855
pyrantel pamoate for, 928
Ascorbic acid, formulary entry for, 703
Asmanex twisthaler
daily dose recommendations for, 805t, 993t
formulary entry for, 871–872
potency ranking of, 995t
Asparaginase (L-Asp, PEG-Asp, Elspar, Erwinia), toxicity of, 1006t
Aspartate aminotransferase (AST), reference values for, 641t
Asperger disorder, 237–238
Aspergillosis
itraconazole for, 833
voriconazole for, 982
Aspiration(s)
foreign-body, 13
soft tissue, 78–80
suprapubic bladder, 78, 79f–80f
Aspirin (ASA, Anacin, Bufferin, ZORprin)
analgesic properties of, 139
formulary entry for, 703–704
for Kawasaki disease, 198
with renal failure, 1027t
Aspirin Free Anacin
analgesic properties of, 138
with renal failure, 1027t
formulary entry for, 682
poisoning with, 684
toxicity of, 28t
Aspirin and oxycodone (Percodan, Roxiprin), formulary entry for, 693
AST (aspartate aminotransferase), in hepatic function test, 302t
Astelin
drug formulary for, 708
Asthma
acetylcysteine recommendations for, 684
adenosine contraindications for, 686
cimetidine for, 748
classification of, 593f–595f
clinical manifestations of, 592
emergency treatment of, 10–11
exacerbation prevention in, 592
fluticasone propionate for, 803t
inhaled steroid dose recommendations for, 994t
ipratroplum bromide for, 10
montelukast for, 873
prednisone dosage for, 919
salmeterol for, 941
salmeterol and fluticasone propionate for, 804
stepwise management of, 596f–598f
Asymptomatic cyanosis
amiodarone induction of, 695
due to poisoning, 22t
Ataxia, due to poisoning, 21t
Atelectasis, imaging of, 609
Atenolol (Tenormin)
formulary entry for, 704–706
for hypertension, 500t
with renal failure, 1027t
Ativan
for chemotherapy-induced nausea, 574
for palliative care, 581t
ATN. *See* Acute tubular necrosis
Atomoxetine (Strattera), formulary entry for, 705
Atopic dermatitis
characterization of, 210–213
food allergy-induced, 356
Atovaquone, for antimicrobial prophylaxis, 575t
Atrial fibrillation, 175t
Atrial flutter, 175t
Atrial septal defect (ADS), CHD/exam findings of, 186t

Atrial septostomy, for CHD, 184
Atrioventricular septal defects, CHD/exam findings of, 186t
AtroPen
for resuscitation, ii
for RSI, 6t
formulary entry for, 706–707
Atropine sulfate (Sal-Tropine, AtroPen)
formulary entry for, 706–707
for pesticide toxicity, 52
for resuscitation, ii
for RSI, 6t
Atrovent
for asthma, 10
formulary entry for, 827–828
Attention deficit/hyperactivity disorder (ADHD)
characterization of, 238
lisdexamfetamine for, 848
medications for, 239t
methylphenidate dosage for, 861
screening tests for, 232t
Augmentin
formulary entry for, 701–702
with renal failure, 1013t
Auralgan, formulary entry for, 702
Autism
characterization of, 237
risperidone dosage for, 939
Autism spectrum disorders (ASD)
characterization of, 237–238
screening tests for, 232t
Auto Ear Drops, formulary entry for, 728–729
Autoantibody(ies), in SLE, 629
Autoguard Otic, formulary entry for, 702
Autoimmune marker(s), in SLE, 628t
Autoimmune-bullous lesions, characterization of, 222–223
Autologous HSCT, 571
Avastin (bevacizumab), toxicity of, 1006t
Aventyl
formulary entry for, 108t
for migraines, 512t
Avita, formulary entry for, 968
Azactam, formulary entry for, 710
Azasan
formulary entry for, 707
with renal failure, 1027t
Azasite (Azithromycin ophthalmic)
for chlamydial infections, 420t
drug formulary for, 707
for gastroenteritis, 424t
for gonorrhea, 421t
neonatal ICU dosing with, 1000t
otitis media, 426t
for pertussis, 428t
for pneumonia, 428t
Azathioprine (Imuran, Azasan)
formulary entry for, 707
with renal failure, 1027t
Azelaic acid, for acne vulgaris, 218t
Azelastine (Astelin, Optivar), drug formulary for, 708
Azithromycin (Zithromax, Zmax, Azasite)
for chlamydial infections, 429t
drug formulary for, 708–710
for gastroenteritis, 424t
for gonorrhea, 430t
neonatal ICU dosing with, 1000t
for otitis media, 426t
for pertussis, 428t
for pneumonia, 428t
Azmacort, formulary entry for, 969
Azo-Standard
formulary entry for, 906–907
with renal failure, 1033t
AZT, in utero HIV transmission prevention by, 441t
Aztreonam (Azactam)
formulary entry for, 710
with renal failure, 1014t
Azulfidine, formulary entry for, 955

B

B lymphocytes, in peripheral blood, 366t
BAC-CGH arrays, for genetic abnormalities, 316
Baciguent Topical, formulary entry for, 711
Bacitracin (AJ-Tracin Ophthalmic, Baciguent Topical), formulary entry for, 711
Bacitracin and polymyxin B (AK-Poly-Bac Ophthalmic, Polysporin Ophthalmic, Polysporin Topical), formulary entry for, 711

Bacitracin zinc, ophthalmic use of, 1000t
Back trauma, secondary survey of, 90t
Baclofen (Lioresal, Kemstro), formulary entry for, 711–712
Bacteria, aerobic, algorithm for, 406f–407f
Bacterial endocarditis prophylaxis
  ceftriaxone dosage with, 738
  characterization of, 191
  clindamycin dosage for, 753
  dental procedures and, prophylactic regimens for, 193t
  respiratory tract procedures and, prophylactic regimens for, 193t
Bacterial meningitis
  cefepime dosage with, 733
  ceftriaxone dosage with, 738
  corticosteroids for, 992
  drug therapy for, 447t
  emergency treatment of, 14
  initial management of, 426t
Bacterial vaginosis, metronidazole for, 865
Bacteremia, initial management of, 422t
Bacitracin zinc ophthalmic, 1000t
Bactocill
  for cellulitis, 423t
  formulary entry for, 892
  for lymphadenitis, 425t
  for osteomyelitis, 426t
  with renal failure, 1023t
  for septic arthritis, 429t
Bactroban, formulary entry for, 874
Bag and mask ventilation, use of, 3
BAL, formulary entry for, 772–773
Ballard scores, 456–459
Banzel, for seizures, 517t
Barbiturate(s)
  antidote for, 34t
  clonazepam as, 753
  commonly used, 147t
  diazepam as, 768–769
  lorazepam as, 851
  midazolam as, 868
  pentobarbital, 905–906
  primidone as, 920–921
Barbiturate(s) *(Continued)*
  properties of, 137
  toxicity of, 34t
Basal energy expenditure (Bee)
  calculation of, 536–537
  definition of, 535
Basal metabolic rate (BMR), definition of, 535
BCNU (carmustine), toxicity of, 1006t
Beclomethasone dipropionate, daily dose recommendations for, 993t
Bee. *See* Basal energy expenditure
Behavior
  age-appropriate, 230t
  disorders of, 238–239
Benadryl
  for chemotherapy-induced nausea, 574
  formulary entry for, 773
  for NSAIDs toxicity, 137
  for palliative care, 581t
  properties of, 137
  with renal failure, 1029t
Benazepril, for hypertension, 500t
Benign rolandic epilepsy, 515t
Benzalkonium chloride, 1000t
Benzodiazepine(s)
  for chemotherapy-induced nausea, 574
  as cocaine antidote, 44
  commonly used, 147t
  for hypertensive crisis, 43
  overdose from, 799
  properties of, 137–143
  toxicity of, 34t
Benzoyl peroxide (BPO)
  for acne vulgaris, 217
  formulary entry for, 713
Benztropine mesylate (Cogentin)
  formulary entry for, 714
  for phenothiazine toxicity, 39t
Bereavement, 582
Beriberi, thiamine for, 962
Beta-1 selective adrenergic blocker(s)
  atenolol as, 704
  esmolol as, 789–790
  metoprolol, 864

Beta-2 adrenergic agonist(s)
albuterol as, 687–688
budesonide as, 718–719
fluticasone propionate as, 802–803
formoterol as, 718–719
levalbuterol as, 841
salmeterol as, 941
terbutaline as, 959–960
Beta-arginine vasopressin, formulary entry for, 977
Beta-blocker(s)
alpha-induced hypertension from, 44
for hypertension, 500t
toxicity of, 35t
Beta-lactamase inhibitor(s)
ampicillin/sulbactam as, 701–702
piperacillin as, 913–914
ticarcillin and ciavulanate as, 964
Betamethasone
dosage recommendations for, 804t
formulary entry for, 714–715
potency of, 992t
Betamethasone base (Celestone), formulary entry for, 714
Betamethasone dipropionate (Diprolene, Diprosone, Maxivate)
formulary entry for, 714
potency ranking of, 995t
Betamethasone valerate (Beta-Val), formulary entry for, 714
Bethanechol chloride, formulary entry for, 715–716
Bevacizumab (Avastin), toxicity of, 1006t
Beta-Val, formulary entry for, 714
Bicarbonate (HCO_3^-)
intracellular/extracellular composition of, 276t
reference values for, 641t
Bicillin C-R, formulary entry for, 903
Bicillin L-A, formulary entry for, 903
Bicitra
formulary entry for, 947
for resuscitation, ii
BiCNU (carmustine), toxicity of, 1006t
Biguanide(s)
metformin as, 858
toxicity of, 28t–41t
Biliary atresia
imaging of, 617
ursodiol for, 971
Biliary obstruction, 305t
Bilious emesis differential, 470–471
Bilirubin
reference values for, 641t
in urine, 477, 478t
Bilirubin metabolism disorders, 305t
Biocef
for cellulitis, 423t
formulary entry for, 740
for influenza, 425t
for lymphadenitis, 425t
with renal failure, 1016t
Bipolar disorder, risperidone dosage for, 939
Biostatistics
commonly used tests for, 653t
for medical literature, 652–657
websites for, 651
Biotin
DRIs for, 542t
in multivitamin tablets, analysis of, 546t
Bipolar disorder, in children, 241
Birth trauma, 459
Bisacodyl (Dulcolax, Fleet Laxative, Bisacodyl, Doxidan), formulary entry for, 716
Bis-chloronitrosourea (carmustine), toxicity of, 1006t
Bismuth subsalicylate (Pepto-Bismol, Kaopectate)
formulary entry for, 716–717
with renal failure, 1027t
Bisoprolol, for hypertension, 500t–501t
Bite(s)
infections from, 422t
management of, 111–112
types of, 96t
wound considerations for, 108
Bladder irrigation, neomycin/polymyxin B/bacitracin for, 878
Blastomycosis, itraconazole for, 833
Blaxin
for bacterial endocarditis prophylaxis, 193t
formulary entry for, 751–752
with renal failure, 1017t
Bleeding disorders
common types of, 345b
differential diagnosis of, 344f
gastrointestinal, 293–294, 294t
Bleph (sulfacetamide sodium ophthalmic), 1000t

Bleph 10, formulary entry for, 953
Blood chemistry, reference values for, 639t–647t
Blood fluid sampling
chest tube placement in, 72–74, 73f
lumbar puncture for, 70–72, 71f
paracentesis for, subxiphoid approach for, 77f
pericardiocentesis for, 75
soft tissue aspiration for, 78–80
suprapubic bladder aspiration for, 78, 79f
thoracentesis for, 72–74, 74f
urinary bladder catheterization for, 77–78
Blood gas, reference values for, 641t
Blood pressure
level percentiles, 156t, 164f
mean systolic regression, 166f
measuring, 154
parameters of, 496
Blood sampling
catheterization and, 59–61
dorsalis pedis artery punctures, 61
external jugular puncture for, 58–59
femoral artery/vein punctures, 59
fingersticks for, 57–58
heelsticks for, 57–58
lead levels, 50t
posterior tibial punctures, 61
radial artery puncture for, 59–61
Blood smears, interpretation of, 352
Blood transfusions, oncologic, 573–574
Blood volume, estimation of, 348t
Blood, hyperviscosity of, 976
Blood-borne pathogens
infections from, 450–452
in UTIs, 480
Blunt thoracic trauma
emergent treatments for, 106
evaluation of, 103–104
laboratory studies of, 104–113
radiologic evaluation of, 105–106
BMI. *See* Body mass index
BMR. *See* Basal metabolic rate
Bocotra (citrate mixture), formulary entry for, 751
Body fluids
cerebrospinal, 648t
conversion formulas for, 650
exudate/transudate, 648t
synovial, in rheumatic disease, 649t
Body mass index (BMI)
for boys 2 to 20 years, 530f
definition of, 533–534
for girls 2 to 20 years, 530f
percentiles, 534
Body surface area (BSA) method, 272, 273t
Bone age, 618
Bone marrow transplants
complications of, 571–573
GVHD as, 571–572
hemorrhagic cystitis as, 573
thrombotic microangiopathy as, 572–573
veno-occlusive disease as, 572
IVIG therapy for, 362
Bones, long, trauma to, 94–96
Borrelia burgdorferi, 448
Bowel. *See also* Gastrointestinal (GI) tract
cleansing of, 915
obstructions, imaging of, 616
BPO (Benzoyl peroxide), for acne vulgaris, 217
Bradycardia
without central apnea, 465
characterization of, 175t
neonatal, 465
due to poisoning, 20t
succinylchyoline for, 952
Bradypnea, due to poisoning, 20t
Breastfeeding
drug dosage and, 664
HIV exposure from, 441–442, 451
iron supplementation and, 544
Breathing
assessment of, 7
management of, 7–8
Brethine. *See* Terbutaline (Brethine)
Brevibloc, formulary entry for, 789–790
Brisk reflexes, 506
British Anti-Lewisite, formulary entry for, 772–773
Brompheniramine with phenylephrine (Alacol, Alenaze, Dimetapp), formulary entry for, 717–718

Bronchiolitis
acute viral, sodium chloride-inhaled preparations for, 948
cefdinir for, 733
theophylline for, 961
Bronchospasm(s)
atropine sulfate for, 706
exercise-induced, montelukast for, 873
theophylline for, 961
Brown recluse, toxicity of, 53–54
Budesonide (Pulmicort, Formoterol, Rhinocort)
for allergic rhinitis, 355–356
daily dose recommendations for, 993t–994t
dosage recommendations for, 804t
formulary entry for, 718–719
for hypertension, 501t
Budesonide and formoterol (Symbicort), formulary entry for, 720
Bufferin
analgesic properties of, 139
formulary entry for, 703–704
for Kawasaki disease, 198
with renal failure, 1027t
Bullous lesions
autoimmune types of, 222–223
impetigo as, 222
Bumetanide (Bumex), formulary entry for, 720–721
Buminate, formulary entry for, 687
Bupropion (Wellbutrin), dosage/side effects for, 1005t
Burkholderia cepacia, sensitivity profile of, 408t–409t
Burns
assessment chart, 99f
bullous lesions from, 223
from cigarettes, *Trauma, Burns, and Common Critical Care Emergencies Color Plate 5*
classification of, 98t
emergent management of, 99–100
evaluation of, 97
from hot water, *Trauma, Burns, and Common Critical Care Emergencies Color Plate 1*
management of, 100–102
fluid, 101f
inpatient, 100–102
mapping of, 99
Burns *(Continued)*
prevention of, 102
thermal, 98t
Buspirone (BuSpar), dosage/side effects for, 1005t
Busulfan (Myleran), toxicity of, 1006t
Butyrophenone, toxicity of, 39t

C

CAE. *See* Criteria for atrial enlargement
Cafcit, formulary entry for, 721
Caffeine citrate (Cafcit), formulary entry for, 721
CAH. *See* Congenital adrenal hyperplasia
Calan, with renal failure, 1034t
Calciferol, formulary entry for, 785–786
Calcijex, formulary entry for, 722–723
Calcionate, formulary entry for, 724–725
Calciquid, formulary entry for, 724–725
Calcitonin-salmon (Miacalcin, Fortical Nasal Spray), formulary entry for, 721–722
Calcitriol
cyanocobalamin with, 758
DRIs for, 542t
formulary entry for, 745–746, 981
for hyperparathyroidism, 252
for hypoparathyroidism, 252
in multivitamin drops, analysis of, 545t
in multivitamin tablets, analysis of, 546t
normal values for, 266t
for rickets resistant, 785
Calcitriol (1,25-dihydroxycholecalciferol, Rocaltrol, Calcijex), formulary entry for, 722–723
Calcium
in cow's milk formulas, 548t–557t
in enteral formulas, 548t–557t
parenteral nutrition formulations, 561t
Calcium (Ca^{2+})
DRIs for, 542t
in enteral formulas, 549t–556t
in multivitamin tablets, analysis of, 546t
reference values for, 642t
serum disturbances of, 284–286
Calcium acetate (PhosLo), formulary entry for, 722–723

Calcium carbonate (Tums, Os-Cal), formulary entry for, 723
Calcium channel blocker(s)
  for hypertension, 500t
  for migraines, 512t
  toxicity of, 36t
Calcium chloride
  for calcium channel blocker toxicity of, 36t
  formulary entry for, 723–724
  for resuscitation, ii
Calcium citrate, formulary entry for, 724
Calcium disodium versenate, formulary entry for, 779
Calcium glubionate (Calcionate, Calciquid), formulary entry for, 724–725
Calcium gluconate (Cal-G), formulary entry for, 725
Calcium lactate (Cal-Lac), formulary entry for, 726
Calcium phosphate, tribasic, formulary entry for, 726
Calcium supplementation
  for hyperparathyroidism, 252
  for hypoparathyroidism, 252
  vitamin D resistant rickets with, 785
Calcium supplements
  monitoring of, 252
  with renal failure, 1028t
Cal-G, formulary entry for, 725
Calorie(s)
  calculations of, 271–272
  common modulars, 549t
  in enteral formulas, 550t
  in human milk, 548t
  increased need for, formulas for, 558t
  in infant formula, 550t
  metabolism of, 272f
Camphorated opium tincture, formulary entry for, 899
Camptosar (Irinotecan), toxicity of, 1007t
Canasa, formulary entry for, 857
Cancer
  antimicrobial prophylaxis in, 575t
  bone marrow transplants, complications of, 571–573
  darbepoetin alfa for, 689
  fever in, 570f
Cancer *(Continued)*
  hematologic care and complications in, 573–574
  HSCT for, 569–571
  nausea treatment for, 574–575
  neutropenia in, 570f
  oncologic emergencies of, 564–569
    cerebrovascular accident as, 568
    hyperleukocytosis as, 564–567
    increase intracranial pressure as, 568
    respiratory distress as, 568–569
    spinal cord compression as, 567–568
    superior vena cava syndrome as, 568–569
    tumor lysis syndrome as, 567
  patients, immunization for, 381t
  signs/symptoms of, 565t–566t
  survivors, treatment of, 575–576
  vaccines and, 381, 381t
  websites for, 564
Candidiasis
  diagnosis of, 450
  esophageal
    micafungin for, 866
    voriconazole for, 982
  invasive, 866
  oral, 451t
  prophylaxis
    micafungin for, 866
    micafungin sodium for, 866
  skin, 451t
  systemic, 798
  vaginal, 755
Cankaid, formulary entry for, 728–729
Cannabinoids, for chemotherapy-induced nausea, 574
Capex shampoo, potency ranking of, 995t
Capillary blood gas (CBG), 586
Capnography, 585
Capoten
  formulary entry for, 727
  for hypertension, 500t
  with renal failure, 1028t
Captopril (Capoten)
  formulary entry for, 727
  for hypertension, 500t
  with renal failure, 1028t
Capute scales, 229
Carafate, formulary entry for, 952–953
Carbamates, toxicity of, 52

Carbamazepine (Epitol, Tegretol, Carbatrol)
adenosine effects on, 686
formulary entry for, 727–728
with renal failure, 1028t
for seizures, 516t
toxicity of, 48
Carbamide peroxide (Debrox, Murine Ear, Auto Ear Drops, Cankaid, Gly-Oxide, Orajel Perioseptic), formulary entry for, 728–729
Carbatrol
adenosine effects on, 686
formulary entry for, 727–728
with renal failure, 1028t
for seizures, 516t
toxicity of, 48
Carbinoxamine (Palgic), formulary entry for, 729
Carbinoxamine and pseudoephedrine (Sildex, Cordron-D, Pseudo Carb Pediatric, Hydro-Tussin, CBX), formulary entry for, 729–730
Carbohydrate(s)
caloric modulars of, 549t
in cow's milk formulas, 551t
in enteral formulas, 551t
in human milk, 549t
in infant formula, 549t
intolerances of, formula's for, 558t–559t
Carbon dioxide (CO_2), reference values for, 642t
Carbon monoxide, toxicity of, 27
Carboplatin (CBOCA, Paraplatin), toxicity of, 1006t
Carboxamide (dacarbazine), toxicity of, 1007t
Cardiac arrest algorithm, see pages after Index
Cardiac arrest, sodium bicarbonate dosage and, 947
Cardiac change, as death approaches, 580
Cardiology
acquired heart disease in, 191–199
amitriptyline contraindicated for, 696
bacterial endocarditis prophylaxis as, 191
endocarditis as, 191
Kawasaki disease as, 196–198
Lyme disease as, 199
Cardiology *(Continued)*
myocardial disease as, 191–195
pericardial disease as, 195–196
rheumatic heart disease as, 198–199
cardiac cycle in, 155f
congenital heart disease in
acyanotic lesions in, 183
amitriptyline contraindicated for, 696
chest radiographs of, 185–190
cyanotic lesions in, 183
cyanotic type of, 188t
echocardiography of, 191
exercise recommendations for, 192t
imaging of, 185–191
interventions for, 184–185
lesion types of, 186t
major syndromes of, 184t
electrocardiography for
abnormalities in, 174
basic principles of, 169–173
CAE in, 174f
hexaxial reference system for, 170f
horizontal reference system for, 170f
long QT ranges in, 181–183
MI in children, 180–181, 181f
nonpathologic changes in, 173f
nonventricular arrhythmias in, 175t
nonventricular conduction disturbances, 178t
normal parameters for, 170t
normal T-wave axis for, 173t
pathologic changes in, 173f
quadrants of mean, location of, 172f
secondary findings in, 181
supraventricular arrhythmias in, 175t
ventricular arrhythmias, 178t
ventricular conduction disturbances, 180t
ventricular hypertrophy criteria for, 174b
imaging in, 185–191
lipid monitoring recommendations for, 168–169
goals for, 169
hyperlipidemia management in, 169
screening criteria for, 168–169

Cardiology *(Continued)*
physical examinations for, 154–167
blood pressure, 154, 158t, 162t, 164f–166f
heart murmurs, 167, 167t, 168b
heart sounds in, 154–164, 166b
systolic/diastolic sounds in, 164–165
websites for, 154
Cardiopulmonary resuscitation, atropine sulfate for, 706
Cardiovascular system, dysfunction, due to poisoning, 22t
Cardizem, formulary entry for, 771
Carmustine (bis-chloronitrosourea, BCNU, BiCNU), toxicity of, 1006t
Carmustine, toxicity of, 1006t
Carnitine (levocarnitine, Carnitor, L-Carnitine), formulary entry for, 730
Carnitor, formulary entry for, 730
Case-control study, 655t
Caspofungin (Cancidas), formulary entry for, 810–811
CAT (clinical adaptive test), 229
Cat bites, 96t
Catapres, formulary entry for, 754
Catch-up growth, 537–538
Catheter(s)
central line placement of, 613
central venous, placement of, 61–63
umbilical arterial, placement of, 69f
Catheterization
blood sampling and, 59–61
pelvic fractures and, 78
umbilical vein/artery, vascular access for, 65–68
urinary bladder
for blood fluid sampling, 77–78
suprapubic, aspiration for, 77–78
Catheter-related bloodstream infections, initial management of, 423t
Cathflo, formulary entry for, 689
CBOCA (carboplatin), toxicity of, 1006t
CBX, formulary entry for, 729–730
CCNU (lomustine), toxicity of, 1008t
CCP. *See* Anti-cyclic citrullinated peptide
2-CdA (cladribine), toxicity of, 1006t
CDDP (cisplatin), toxicity of, 1006t
Ceclor
formulary entry for, 731–732
with renal failure, 1014t
Cecon, formulary entry for, 703
Cedax, with renal failure, 1016t
Cefactor (Ceclor, Raniclor)
formulary entry for, 731–732
with renal failure, 1014t
Cefadroxil (Duricef)
formulary entry for, 732
with renal failure, 1014t
Cefazolin (Ancef, Zolicef)
for bacterial endocarditis prophylaxis, 193t
formulary entry for, 732
with renal failure, 1015t
Cefdinir (Omnicef)
formulary entry for, 733
for lymphadenitis, 425t
with renal failure, 1015t
Cefepime (Maxipime)
formulary entry for, 733
with renal failure, 1015t
Cefixime (Suprax)
formulary entry for, 734–735
for gonorrhea, 430t
with renal failure, 1015t
Cefoxitin (Mefoxin)
for gonorrhea, 430t
with renal failure, 1015t
Cefizox
for bacterial endocarditis prophylaxis, 422t
formulary entry for, 738
for gonorrhea, 430t
for meningitis, 426t
for PID, 432t
with renal failure, 1016t
Cefotan
formulary entry for, 735
for PID, 432t
with renal failure, 1015t
Cefotaxime (Claforan)
formulary entry for, 734–735
for gonorrhea, 430t
for meningitis, 426t
neonatal critical care dosing of, 1010t
with renal failure, 1015t
Cefotetan (Cefotan)
formulary entry for, 735
for PID, 432t
with renal failure, 1015t

Cefpodoxime proxetil (Vantin)
for gonorrhea, 431t
with renal failure, 1015t
Cefprozil (Cefzil)
formulary entry for, 736
with renal failure, 1016t
Cefprozil proxetil, formulary entry for, 736
Ceftazidime (Fortaz, Tazidime, Taxicef)
formulary entry for, 737
for osteomyelitis, 426t
for otitis media, 426t
with renal failure, 1016t
Ceftibuten (Cedax)
with renal failure, 1016t
Ceftin, formulary entry for, 739–987
Ceftizoxime (Cefizox)
for bacterial endocarditis prophylaxis, 422t
formulary entry for, 738
for gonorrhea, 430t
for meningitis, 426t
for PID, 432t
with renal failure, 1016t
Ceftriaxone (Rocephin)
for bacterial endocarditis prophylaxis, 422t
formulary entry for, 738–739
for gonorrhea, 430t
for meningitis, 426t
for meningococcus exposure, 395
Cefuroxime (Zinacef)
formulary entry for, 739–987
for lymphadenitis, 425t
for otitis media, 426t
with renal failure, 1016t
Cefuroxime axetil (Ceftin), formulary entry for, 739–987
Cefzil
formulary entry for, 736
with renal failure, 1016t
Celestone, formulary entry for, 714–715
Celexa (citalopram), dosage/side effects for, 1004t
Celiac disease, 301
CellCept, formulary entry for, 874–875
Cellulitis, initial management of, 423t
Central alpha agonists, for hypertension, 500t–501t
Central nervous system (CNS), malignancies of, signs/symptoms of, 565t–566t
Central venous catheter placement, 61–63
Cephalexin (Keflex, Biocef)
for cellulitis, 423t
formulary entry for, 740
for influenza, 425t
for lymphadenitis, 425t
with renal failure, 1016t
Cephalosporin(s)
for catheter-related bloodstream infections, 423t
cefactor as, 731–732
cefadroxil as, 732
cefdinir as, 733
cefepime as, 733
cefotaxime as, 734–735
ceftazidime as, 737
ceftizoxime as, 738
ceftriaxone as, 738–739
cefuroxime as, 739–987
cephalexin as, 740
resistance to, 411f
Cephradine (Velosef), with renal failure, 1016t
Cephulac, formulary entry for, 836–837
Cerebral edema, diabetes-associated, 246
Cerebral palsy (CP)
characterization of, 236
classification of, 238t
Cerebrospinal fluid (CSF) shunting, for hydrocephalus, 518
Cerebrospinal fluids, 648t
Cerebrovascular accidents, 568
Cerebyx
formulary entry for, 690–691
for status epilepticus, 17
toxicity of, 48
Cervical spine trauma, imaging of, 607
Cetacort
for adrenal insufficiency, 256
formulary entry for, 819
for glucocorticoid deficiency, 989
for hyperparathyroidism, 253
for hypoparathyroidism, 252
Cetirizine (Zyrtec)
for allergic rhinitis, 355–356
formulary entry for, 740–741
with pseudoephedrine, 740–741
with renal failure, 1028t

CGD. *See* Constitutional growth delay
CHARGE syndrome, 459
CHD. *See* Congenital heart disease
Chelating agent(s)
  deferoxamine as, 764–765
  dimercaprol as, 772–773
  penicillamine as, 901
  succimer as, 951
Chelation therapy, for lead poisoning, 50t
Chemet, formulary entry for, 951
Chemical burns, 98t
Chemoprophylaxis
  influenza A and B, 392–393
  postexposure, 395
Chemotherapy
  agents of, 1009t
  anemia associated, darbepoetin alfa dose adjustments for, 763t
  nausea and vomiting from
    granisetron for, 814
    serotonin ($5\text{-}HT_3$) for, 574
    systemic corticosteroids for, 991
Chest radiograph(s)
  atelectasis *versus* infiltrate on, 609
  cardiac anatomy on, 612f–613f
  central line placement in, 613
  empyema on, 610
  ETT placement in, 613
  evaluations by, 185, 190
  heat contours images from, 190f
  lung anatomy on, 612f–613f
  mediastinal masses on, 611
  parapneumonic effusions on, 610
  parenchymal findings on, 610–611
  pneumonia on, 609
Chest trauma, secondary survey of, 90t
Chest tube(s), placement of, blood fluid sampling, 72–74, 73f
Chibroxin
  formulary entry for, 884–885
  with renal failure, 1022t
Child abuse
  beatings, *Trauma, Burns, and Common Critical Care Emergencies Color Plate 2*
  bruising marks
    on face, *Trauma, Burns, and Common Critical Care Emergencies Color Plate 4*
    on legs, *Trauma, Burns, and Common Critical Care Emergencies Color Plate 6*
Child abuse *(Continued)*
    on lower back, *Trauma, Burns, and Common Critical Care Emergencies Color Plate 3*
  burns
    from cigarette, *Trauma, Burns, and Common Critical Care Emergencies Color Plate 5*
    from hot water, *Trauma, Burns, and Common Critical Care Emergencies Color Plate 1*
  emergency care for, 102
  facial slaps as, *Trauma, Burns, and Common Critical Care Emergencies Color Plate 4*
  skeletal injury in, 103t
Children
  age-appropriate behavior of, 230t–231t
  anxiety syndromes in, 230t
  behavioral disorders in, 238–239
  developmental disorders in, 236–238
  growth-plate injury to, 95t
  lead poisoning in, 50–51
  long bone fracture unique to, 95f
  mental health disorders in, 239–241
  MI in, 180–181
  pain assessments for
    developmental response to, 138t
    overview, 137
Chlamydia infections, initial treatment of, 429t
Chloral hydrate (Aquachloral Supprettes)
  formulary entry for, 741
  properties of, 145
  with renal failure, 1031t
  for sedation, 137
Chloramphenicol (Chloromycetin)
  formulary entry for, 741
  for meningitis, 426t
Chloride (Cl^-)
  intracellular/extracellular composition of, 276t
  in multivitamin tablets, analysis of, 547t
  reference values for, 642t
Chlorobutanol ophthalmic, 1002t
Chloromycetin
  formulary entry for, 741
  for meningitis, 426t

Chloroquine HCl/phosphate (Aralen)
  formulary entry for, 742–743
  with renal failure, 1028t
Chlorothiazide (Diuril, Diurigen)
  formulary entry for, 743
  with renal failure, 1028t
Chlorpheniramine maleate (Chlor-Trimeton), formulary entry for, 744
Chlorpromazine (Thorazine)
  for chemotherapy-induced nausea, 574
  formulary entry for, 745
Chlorthalidone, for hypertension, 501t
Chlor-Trimeton, formulary entry for, 744
Cholecalciferol, formulary entry for, 745–746
Cholestasis, characterization of, 301
Cholestyramine (Questran, Prevalite), formulary entry for, 746–747
Choline
  DRIs for, 542t
  in multivitamin tablets, analysis of, 547t
Choline magnesium trisalicylate
  analgesic properties of, 139
  formulary entry for, 747
Cholinergic agent(s)
  bethanechol chloride as, 715–716
  neostigmine as, 879
  physostigmine salicylate as, 911
  pilocarpine as, 912–913
  toxidrome of, 23t
Christmas disease. *See* Factor IX deficiency
Chromium
  DRIs for, 542t
  in formulas, 542t
  in multivitamin tablets, analysis of, 547t
Chromosome(s), abnormalities of, 305t
Chronic hypertension
  causes of, 498t
  classification of, 499t
  definitions of, 496
  drugs for, 500t–501t
  evaluation of, 496–498
  treatment of, 498–499, 502
Chronic inflammatory demyelinating polyneuropathy, IVIG therapy for, 362
Chronic kidney disease, 495–496
  characterization of, 495–496
  clinical manifestations of, 497t
Chronic pancreatitis, 307
Chronic renal failure. *See* Chronic kidney disease
Chronulac, formulary entry for, 836–837
Churg-Strauss syndrome, 631t
Chvostek sign
  due to hypocalcemia, 284
  due to poisoning, 21t
Ciavulanate and ticarcillin (Timentin)
  formulary entry for, 964
  with renal failure, 1024t
Ciclesonide (Alvesco Omnaris)
  formulary entry for, 747–748
  for allergic rhinitis, 355–356
Cidofovir (Vistide), formulary entry for, 748
Cigarette burns, *Trauma, Burns, and Common Critical Care Emergencies Color Plate 5*
Cilastin and imipenem (Primaxin)
  formulary entry for, 823
  with renal failure, 1020t
Ciloxan ophthalmic
  formulary entry for, 749–750
  for meningococcus exposure, 395
  with renal failure, 1016t
Cimetidine (Tagamet)
  for asthma, 748
  formulary entry for, 749
  for methemoglobinemia, 52
  with renal failure, 1029t
  for warts, 207t
Cipro
  formulary entry for, 749–750
  for meningococcus exposure, 395
  with renal failure, 1016t
Cipro HC Otic, formulary entry for, 749
Ciprodex, formulary entry for, 749
Ciprofloxacin (Cipro, Ciloxan ophthalmic)
  formulary entry for, 749–750
  for meningococcus exposure, 395
  with renal failure, 1016t
Circulation
  assessment of, 3
  changes in, as death approaches, 580
  management of, 8t

Cisplatin (*cis*-platinum, CDDP, Platinol), toxicity of, 1006t
Citalopram (Celexa), dosage/side effects for, 1004t
Citrate mixture, formulary entry for, 751
Citrobacter spp., sensitivity profile of, 408t
Cl^-. *See* Chloride
Cladribine (2-CdA, Leustatin), toxicity of, 1006t
Claforan
  formulary entry for, 734–735
  for gonorrhea, 430t
  for meningitis, 426t
  neonatal critical care dosing of, 1010t
  with renal failure, 1015t
CLAMS (clinical linguistic and auditory milestone scale), 229
Claravis
  for acne vulgaris, 218–220
  formulary entry for, 832
Clarinex, with renal failure, 1017t
Clarithromycin (Blaxin)
  for bacterial endocarditis prophylaxis, 193t
  formulary entry for, 751–752
  with renal failure, 1017t
Claritin
  formulary entry for, 850
  for renal failure, 1017t
Clavulanic acid
  for lymphadenitis, 425t
  for otitis media, 426t
Clear liquid diet formulas for, 558t
Cleocin
  for bacterial vaginosis, 422t
  for cellulitis, 423t
  formulary entry for, 752–753.
  for lymphadenitis, 425t
  for mastoiditis, 425t
  for osteomyelitis, 426t
  for pneumonia, 428t
Clindamycin (ANTIROBE, Cleocin, ClindaRobe, Clinsol)
  for acne vulgaris, 218t
  for bacterial vaginosis, 422t
  for cellulitis, 423t
  formulary entry for, 752–753
  for lymphadenitis, 425t
Clindamycin (ANTIROBE, Cleocin, ClindaRobe, Clinsol) *(Continued)*
  for mastoiditis, 425t
  for osteomyelitis, 426t
  for pneumonia, 428t
ClindaRobe
  for acne vulgaris, 218t
  for bacterial vaginosis, 422t
  for cellulitis, 423t
  formulary entry for, 752–753
  for lymphadenitis, 425t
  for mastoiditis, 425t
  for osteomyelitis, 424t
  for pneumonia, 428t
Clinical tests, 656t
Clinitest tablet, 477
Clinsol
  for acne vulgaris, 218t
  for bacterial vaginosis, 422t
  for cellulitis, 423t
  formulary entry for, 752–753
  for lymphadenitis, 425t
  for mastoiditis, 425t
  for osteomyelitis, 426t
  for pneumonia, 428t
Clobetasol propionate (Clobex, Olux foam, Temovate), potency ranking of, 995t
Clobex, potency ranking of, 995t
Clofarabine (Clolar), toxicity of, 1006t
Clolar, toxicity of, 1006t
Clonazepam (Klonopin)
  formulary entry for, 753
  for seizures, 516t
Clonidine (Catapres, Duraclon)
  formulary entry for, 754
  for hypertension, 500t
  for sedation, 151
  toxicity of, 36t
Clostridium difficile colitis, metronidazole for, 976
Clotrimazole (Lotrimin AF, Cruex, Gyne-Lotrimin, Mycelex), formulary entry for, 754–755
Clozapine (Clozaril), dosage/side effects for, 1003t
CMV. *See* Cytomegalovirus
Coagulation
  age-specific values of, 336t–337t
  cascade of, 335f
  disseminated intravascular, 345b

Coagulation *(Continued)*
hypercoagulable states in
causes of, 338b
extended workup for, 338b
presentation of, 335–343
warfarin dosing adjustments for, 340t
warfarin dosing guidelines for, 339t, 342t
tests of, 334–335
Cobalamin
DRIs for, 542t
in multivitamin drops, analysis of, 545t
in multivitamin tablets, analysis of, 546t–547t
reference values for, 647t
Cobb angle, 132f
Cocaine, toxicity of, 43b–44b
Codeine
formulary entry for, 755
with renal failure, 1029t
Codeine and acetaminophen, formulary entry for, 756
Cogentin
formulary entry for, 714
for phenothiazine toxicity, 28t–41t
Cognitive-behavioral therapy, for depression, 241
Cognitive/motor development, screening tests for, 232t
Cohort study, 655t
Colace, formulary entry for, 774–775
Cold injury burns, 98t
Colic, 230t
Colitis, *Clostridium difficile*
metronidazole for, 866
vancomycin for, 975
Colyte, formulary entry for, 915
Coma
due to poisoning, 21t
medicines for, 14
scales for, 15t
Common warts, 206
Communication disorders, 236
Compazine
formulary entry for, 922–923
for palliative care, 581t
Complement system, 622–623
Compro
formulary entry for, 922–923
for palliative care, 581t
Comvax, immunoprophylaxis for, 402
Concerta
for ADHD, 239t
formulary entry for, 860–862
Concussions, from sports-related injuries, 97–102
Congenital adrenal hyperplasia (CAH), ambiguous genitalia from, 254–255
Congenital aplasias, 327
Congenital heart disease (CHD)
acyanotic lesions in, 183, 186t
antibiotic prophylaxis for, 193b
chest radiographs of, 185–190
cyanotic lesions in, 183
cyanotic type of, 188t–189t
echocardiography of, 191
exercise recommendations for, 192t
imaging of, 185–191, 613–615
interventions for, 184–185
lesion types of, 186t
major syndromes of, 184t
Congenital infection(s)
cytomegalovirus as, 416
enterovirus as, 412t–414t
group B streptococcal (GBS) as, 416
herpes simplex virus as, 410
intrauterine as, 410–416
parvovirus as, 412t–414t
rubella as, 410, 413t, 415–416, 440t
syphilis as, 410, 412t–413t, 415, 440t
toxoplasmosis as, 408t–409t, 410, 415
varicella as, 414t, 444
Congenital syphilis, penicillin G preparations for, 902
Congenital toxoplasmosis, sulfadiazine for, 953–954
Conjugated hyperbilirubinemia, neonatal, 469
Conjunctivitis
initial management of, 420t
levofloxacin for, 843
Conotruncal anomaly face syndrome. *See* 22q11 syndrome
Constipation
definitions of, 297
MiraLax for, 915
senna/sennosides for, 943
treatment for, 298, 837
Constitutional growth delay (CGD), 257
Contact burns, 98t

Contact dermatitis, characterization of, 223–224
Contraceptive(s)
barrier methods
advantages/disadvantages for, 127t
combined hormonal
advantages/disadvantages for, 127t
contraindications for, 123–128
DMPA, 129f
ECP, 128
follow-up recommendations, 131
long-acting progestin methods
contraindications for, 128
medroxyprogesterone for, 855
Conversion formulas, 650
Coordination, examination of, 507
Copegus, formulary entry for, 934–936
Copper
DRIs for, 542t
in formulas, 542t
in multivitamin tablets, analysis of, 546t
parenteral nutrition formulations, 561t
Coraid
for adrenal insufficiency, 256
for glucocorticoid deficiency, 989
for hyperparathyroidism, 253
for hypoparathyroidism, 252
formulary entry for, 819
Cordarone
formulary entry for, 694–695
IV infusions of, i
for resuscitations, ii
standard concentrations for, i
Cordran, potency ranking of, 995t
Cordron-D, formulary entry for, 729–730
Corneal ulcer, levofloxacin for, 843
Cortef
for adrenal insufficiency, 256
for hyperparathyroidism, 253
for hypoparathyroidism, 252
formulary entry for, 819
for glucocorticoid deficiency, 989
Corticosteroid(s)
asthma treatment with, 10
for atopic dermatitis, 212
creams
for alopecia areata, 216
for atopic dermatitis, 212
Corticosteroid(s) *(Continued)*
for anaphylaxis, 10
for hemangiomas, 205
immunization recommendations for, 382, 385t
inhaled
dosage recommendations for, 804t–805t
for airway inflammation, 992–995, 993t–994t
systemic
for bacterial meningitis, 992
body surface area nomogram for, 990f
for cerebral edema, 991
for chemotherapy-induced nausea, 991
for endocrine disorders, 989
for idiopathic thrombocytic purpura, 992
pulmonary treatments with, 991
for spinal cord injury, 991–992
topical, 995–996
potency ranking of, 995t–996t
vaccines and, 382, 382t
Corticotropin (H. P. Acthar Gel), formulary entry for, 757
Cortisol
levels, measurement of, 253t, 264
potency of, 992t
Cortisone acetate
formulary entry for, 757
potency of, 992t
Cortisporin
formulary entry for, 916
with renal failure, 1000t
Co-trimoxazole, for acne vulgaris, 218t
Coumadin
dosing adjustments for, 340t
dosing guidelines for, 340t
excessive anticoagulation by, 342t
formulary entry for, 983–984
international normalized ratio for, 341t
medications influencing, 343b
toxicity of, 52–53
Covera-HS, with renal failure, 1034t
Cow's milk-based formulas
enteral nutritional components in, 549t–556t
nutritional components in, 549t–556t

Cozaar for, hypertension, 500t
C-peptide, diabetes-associated, 243
Crackles, 585t
Cradle cap. *See* Seborrheic dermatitis
Cranial nerves, examination of, 505t
Craniosynostosis, 607
C-reactive protein, reference values for, 642t
Creatine kinase, reference values for, 642t
Creatine phosphokinase, reference values for, 642t
Creatinine, reference values for, 642t
Creatinine clearance, for renal function assessment, 483–484
Criteria for atrial enlargement (CAE), 174f
Critical care emergency(ies)
  acute hypertension, 104–105
  animal bites
    management of, 111–112
    types of, 96t
    wound considerations for, 108
  burns
    assessment chart, 99f
    from cigarettes, *Trauma, Burns, and Common Critical Care Emergencies Color Plate 5*
    classification of, 98t
    emergent management of, 99–100
    evaluation of, 97
    management of, 100–102, 101f
    from hot water, *Trauma, Burns, and Common Critical Care Emergencies Color Plate 1*
  child abuse
    approach to, 102
    facial slaps, 2f
    management of, 102–104
    skeletal injury in, 103t
  increased intracranial pressure (ICP), 106–107
  respiratory failure
    characterization of, 107–112
    ventilator setting changes in, 112t
  shock, 108t
    basic treatment for, 109t
    categorization of, 108t
    physiologic response in, 109t
    types of, 107
Crohn's disease, 298–299
Crolom, formulary entry for, 757
Cromolyn (Intal, NasalCrom, Gastrocrom, Crolom, Opticrom)
  for allergic rhinitis, 355–356
  formulary entry for, 757
Cross-sectional study, 655t
Crotalids, toxicity of, 53
Croup. *See* Laryngotracheobronchitis
Cruex, formulary entry for, 754–755
Cryoprecipitates, 350
Cryptococcus neoformans, itraconazole for, 833
Cryptorchidism, signs/symptoms of, 566t
C-spine films, 607–608
CTX
  for SLE, 629
  toxicity of, 1006t
Culture-positive UTIs
  imaging studies of, 481–482
  treatment for, 480–481
Cuprimine, formulary entry for, 901
Curosurf, formulary entry for, 957–958
Cushing evaluation, 264
Cutaneous larva migraines, thiabedazole for, 962
Cutaneous leishmaniasis, pentomone isethionate for, 905
Cutivate
  for asthma, 803t
  daily dose recommendations for, 802t
  formulary entry for, 802–803
  potency ranking of, 995t
Cyanide, toxicity of, 49
Cyanocobalamin/Vitamin D, formulary entry for, 758
Cyanosis
  methemoglobinemia-induced, 51–52
  neonatal, 462
Cyanosis unresponsive to oxygen, due to poisoning, 22t
Cyanotic congenital heart disease, lesions in, 188t–189t
Cyanotic lesions, 183
Cyclomydril, 759
Cyclopentolate, formulary entry for, 758–759
Cyclopentolate with phenylephrine (Cyclomydril), formulary entry for, 759
Cyclophosphamide (CTX, Cytoxan)
  for SLE, 629
  toxicity of, 1006t

Cyclosporine (Sandimmune), formulary entry for, 759–760
Cyclosporine microemulsion (Neoral), formulary entry for, 759–760
Cyclosporine modified (Gengraf), formulary entry for, 759–760
Cyproheptadine (Periactin)
formulary entry for, 760–761
for migraines, 512t
Cystic fibrosis (CF)
azithromycin for, 709
cefepime dosage with, 733
clinical manifestations of, 601t
common complications of, 602
diagnosis of, 600–601
formulas for, 559t
meropenem for, 857
sodium chloride-inhaled preparations for, 948
therapies for, 601
ursodiol for, 971
Cystinuria, penicillamine for, 901
Cystitis
hemorrhagic, in bone marrow transplants, 573
initial treatment of, 435t
Cystospaz, for palliative care, 581t
Cytarabine (Ara-C), toxicity of, 1006t
Cytochrome P450 system
inducers/inhibitors of, 998t
paroxetine effects on, 901
Cytomegalovirus (CMV)
diagnosis of, 416
neonatal management of, 414t
valganciclovir, 972
Cytovene
for seizures, 516t–517t
formulary entry for, 731
with renal failure, 1018t
Cytoxan (cyclophosphamide)
toxicity of, 1006t
for SLE, 629

D

Dacarbazine (DIC, DTIC, imidazole, carboxamide), toxicity of, 1007t
Dacryocystitis, initial management of, 423t
Dactinomycin, toxicity of, 1007t
Dalfopristin and quinupristin, formulary entry for, 932
Dandruff, selenium sulfide for, 942
Dantrium, formulary entry for, 761
Dantrolene (Dantrium), formulary entry for, 761
Dapsone (Aczone, Diaminodiphenylsulfone)
for antimicrobial prophylaxis, 575t
formulary entry for, 761–762
Daraprim, formulary entry for, 930–931
Darbepoetin alfa (Aranesp), formulary entry for, 762–764
Daunorubicin (daunomycin), toxicity of, 1007t
Daytrana
for ADHD, 239t
formulary entry for, 860–862
DDAVP
for diabetes, 257
formulary entry for, 765–766
for von Willebrand disease, 347t
Death and dying
bereavement following, 582
body, mind and spirit changes in, 580
conceptualization of, 578t
pronouncements of, 581–582
Debrox, formulary entry for, 728–729
Decadron
for airway edema, 991
for bacterial meningitis, 447t
for chemotherapy-induced nausea, 574
formulary entry for, 766–767
for idiopathic thrombocytic purpura, 992
potency of, 992t
Decongestant(s)
brompheniramine with phenylephrine as, 717–718
carbinoxamine and pseudoephedrine as, 729–730
fexofenadine as, 796
oxymetazoline as, 693
phenylephrine as, 908–909
pseudoephedrine as, 926
Deep vein thrombosis prophylaxis
enoxaparin for, 781
heparin sodium for, 817
Deferoxamine mesylate (Desferal)
formulary entry for, 764–765
as hypoglycemic antidote, 38t
for iron toxicity, 38t

Deficit replacement, strategy for, 277–278
Deficit repletion, fluids, 274
Degenerative disorders
lysosomal, 319
peroxisomal, 319
Dehydration
clinical observations in, 274t
types of, 275f
Dehydroepiandrosterone (DHEA), normal values for, 267t
Delay, definition of, 227
Delayed puberty, 259–260, 261f
Delirium, due to poisoning, 21t
Deltasone
for asthma, 10
dose equivalence for, 992t
formulary entry for, 919–920
Demerol
for analgesia, 140t
characterization of, 140t
relative potency of, 151t
for renal failure, 1032t
toxicity of, 28t–41t
Dental abscesses, initial management of, 423t
Dental procedures, prophylactic regimens for, 193t
Denver II Developmental Assessment, 233
Deodorized tincture of opium, formulary entry for, 890–891
Depacon. *See* Valproic acid
Depakene
formulary entry for, 973–974
for seizures, 517t
toxicity of, 48
Depakote
formulary entry for, 773–774, 973–974
for migraines, 512t
for seizures, 517t
toxicity of, 48
Depen, formulary entry for, 901
Depomedroxyprogesterone acetate (DMPA), 129f
Depo-Provera, formulary entry for, 855
Depp-Sub Q Provera, formulary entry for, 855
Depression
in children, 240–241
due to poisoning, 21t
Depression *(Continued)*
ethanol and, 45
imipramine for, 823
paroxetine for, 900
screening tests for, 232t
sertraline for, 944
trazodone for, 968
Derma-Smoothe, potency ranking of, 996t
Dermatitis, contact, 223–224
Dermatologic disorders
acne vulgaris as, 217–220
alopecia areata as, 216
autoimmune-bullous lesions as, 222–223
bullous lesions as, 222–224
burns as, 223
clinical description of, 201
contact dermatitis as, 223–224
due to poisoning, 20t–22t
erythema toxicum neonatorum as, 220
evaluation of, 201
hair loss as, 214–217
hemangiomas as, 201–206
ichthyosis as, 214
impetigo as, 222
lesions as, 201
lumps as, 201–208
miliaria as, 220
molluscum contagiosum as, 207
mongolian spots as, 222
neonatal, 220–222
neonatal acne as, 220
papular urticaria as, 213
papulosquamous lesions as, 210–214
poison ivy as, 223–224
pyogenic granuloma as, 208
reactive erythema as, 208, 209f
scabies as, 208
seborrheic dermatitis as, 222
telogen effluvium as, 216
tinea capitis as, 214–216
tinea corporis as, 214
tinea versicolor as, 214
transient neonatal pustular melanosis as, 220
warts as, 206–207
websites for, 201
Dermatomes, 506f

Dermatomyositis, autoantibodies associated with, 621t
Dermatop, potency ranking of, 996t
Desferal
 formulary entry for, 764–765
 as hypoglycemic antidote, 38t
 for iron toxicity, 38t
Desloratadine (Clarinex)
 for allergic rhinitis, 355–356
 with renal failure, 1029t
Desmopressin acetate (DDAVP, Stimate)
 for diabetes, 257
 formulary entry for, 765–766
 for von Willebrand disease, 347t
Desonide (DesOwen, Verdeso foam), potency ranking of, 996t
DesOwen, potency ranking of, 996t
Desoximetasone (Topicort), potency ranking of, 995t
Desyrel, formulary entry for, 968
Development
 assessment tools for, 229–233
 characterization of, 226
 definitions in, 226
 milestones for, 228t–229t
 normal, guidelines for, 227
 screenings for, 227–233
 sexual, 259–262
Developmental disorders
 ADHD as, 238
 autism spectrum, 237–238
 cerebral palsy as, 236
 communication-associated, 236
 evaluation of, 233–236
 interventions for, 241–242
 learning associated, 236
 types of, 236–238
 websites for, 226
Developmental night walking, 230t
Developmental quotient (DQ), definition of, 227
Developmental screening(s)
 age-appropriate behavioral issues, 230t–231t
 commonly used, 229–233
  ages and stages questionnaire, 233
  Capute scales, 229
  cognitive/motor, 232t
  Denver II, 233
  by diagnosis, 232t
Developmental screening(s) *(Continued)*
  Gesell block skills, 233
  Gesell figures, 233
  Goodenough-Harris Draw-a-Person test, 233
  parent-based questionnaire, 233
 guidelines for, 227
 milestones, 228t–229t
 reach out and read milestones, 230t
Deviancy, definition of, 227
Dexamethasone (Decadron, Hexadrol, Maxidex)
 for airway edema, 991
 for bacterial meningitis, 447t
 for chemotherapy-induced nausea, 574
 formulary entry for, 766–767
 for idiopathic thrombocytic purpura, 992
 potency of, 992t
Dexamethasone and ciprofloxacin (Ciprodex), formulary entry for, 749
Dexamethasone suppression test, 264
Dexrazoxane, as chemotherapy adjunct, 1009t
Dextrose, for resuscitation, ii
DHEA. *See* Dehydroepiandrosterone
Di-5-ASA, formulary entry for, 888
Diabetes insipidus (DI), 256–257
Diabetes mellitus
 A-32 kg patient with, 246f
 characteristics at presentation of, 244t
 classification of, 243–244
 diagnostic criteria for, 243
 DKA in, 244–246, 245f
 monitoring of, 247
 type II, 247
Diabetic ketoacidosis (DKA), 244–246, 245f
Diabetic mother, infant of, 459–460
Dialume, formulary entry for, 690
Dialysis patient(s)
 drug adjustments for, 1012
 formulas for, 559t
Diaminodiphenylsulfone
 for antimicrobial prophylaxis, 575t
 formulary entry for, 761–762

Diamond-Blackfan anemia, 327
Diamox
  formulary entry for, 683
  with renal failure, 1027t
Diarrhea
  bismuth subsalicylate for, 717
  definition of, 295
  etiology of, 296
  evaluation of, 295
  loperamide for, 849
  management of, 296–297
  neomycin sulfate for, 878
Diastat
  formulary entry for, 768–769
  for palliative care, 581t
Diastat AcuDial
  formulary entry for, 768–769
  for palliative care, 581t
Diastolic heart murmurs, 167t
Diastolic opening snap, 165
Diastolic sounds, 164–165
Diazepam (Valium, Diastat, Diastat AcuDial)
  formulary entry for, 768–769
  for palliative care, 581t
Diazoxide (arteriole vasodilator)
  formulary entry for, 769
  for hypertensive emergency, 105t
DIC (dacarbazine), toxicity of, 1007t
Dicloxacillin sodium (Dycill, Pathocil)
  formulary entry for, 769
  for lymphadenitis, 425t
Dietary reference intakes (DRIs)
  fat requirements of, 539t
  for fiber, 544t
  for minerals, 542t
  protein requirements of, 539t
  values of, 538
Diethylene triamine pentaacetic acid (DTPA), for UTI evaluation, 481
Diflorasone diacetate (Popcorn, Florone), potency ranking of, 995t
Diflucan
  formulary entry for, 797–798
  with renal failure, 1018t
  for tinea capitis, 215
DiGeorge syndrome. *See* 22q11 syndrome
Digibind, formulary entry for, 771
DigiFab, formulary entry for, 771
Digitalis, ECG findings for, 181
Digitek
  formulary entry for, 770
  toxicity of, 48
Digoxin (Lanoxin, Digitek, Lanoxicaps)
  formulary entry for, 770
  with renal failure, 1029t
  toxicity of, 48
Digoxin Immune Fab (ovine) (Digibind, DigiFab), formulary entry for, 771
Dihydroxyanthracenedione dihydrochloride (Mitoxantrone), toxicity of, 1008t
1,25-Dihydroxycholecalciferol, formulary entry for, 722–723
Dilacor, formulary entry for, 771
Dilantin
  for seizures, 517t
  formulary entry for, 909–910
  toxicity of, 48
Dilated cardiomyopathy, characterization of, 191–195
Dilated funduscopic exam, for ROP, 473
Dilaudid
  characterization of, 140t
  formulary entry for, 820
  relative potency of, 151t
Diltiazem (Cardizem, Dilacor, Tiazac), formulary entry for, 771
Dimenhydrinate (Dramamine), formulary entry for, 772
Dimercaptosuccinic acid (DMSA), for UTI evaluation, 481
Dimercaprol (British Anti-Lewisite, BAL), formulary entry for, 772–773
Dimercaptosuccinic acid, formulary entry for, 951
Di-mesalazine, formulary entry for, 888
Dimetapp, formulary entry for, 717–718
Dipentum, formulary entry for, 888
Diphenhydramine (Benadryl)
  for allergic rhinitis, 355–356
  for chemotherapy-induced nausea, 574
  for palliative care, 581t
  formulary entry for, 773

Diphenhydramine (Benadryl) *(Continued)*
for NSAIDs toxicity, 137
properties of, 137
with renal failure, 1029t
Diphtheria and tetanus toxoids and acellular pertussis (DTaP) vaccine
for adolescents and young adults, 384
age-based schedule for, 372f–373f
for cancer, 381t
contraindications/precautions for, 379t
immunoprophylaxis for, 384–386
for pregnant patients, 384
Diprivan
for RSI, 6t
properties of, 145
for sedation, 145
Diprolene
formulary entry for, 715
potency ranking of, 995t
Diprolene AF, formulary entry for, 715
Dipropionate augmented (Diprolene, Diprolene AF), formulary entry for, 715
Diprosone, formulary entry for, 714
Dipyridamole
adenosine effects on, 686
for Kawasaki disease, 198
Direct Coombs test, for anemia diagnosis, 327
Disopyramide (Norpace), with renal failure, 1029t
DisperMox
for bacterial infections, 422t
formulary entry for, 697
for lymphadenitis, 425t
for meningitis, 426t
for otitis media, 426t
with renal failure, 1013t
Disseminated intravascular coagulation, 345b
Dissociation, definition of, 227
Diuretic(s)
acetazolamide as, 479
ammonium chloride as, 696–697
bumetanide as, 720–721
chlorothiazide as, 743
Diuretic(s) *(Continued)*
furosemide as, 809–810
hydrochlorothiazide as, 818
for hypertension, 501t
mannitol as, 854
spironolactone as, 950
triamterene as, 970
Diurigen
formulary entry for, 743
with renal failure, 1028t
Diuril
formulary entry for, 743
with renal failure, 1028t
Divalproex sodium (Depakote)
for migraines, 512t
formulary entry for, 773–774
toxicity of, 48
DKA. *See* Diabetic ketoacidosis
DMPA. *See* Depomedroxyprogesterone acetate
DMSA, formulary entry for, 951
DNA analysis, for genetic abnormalities, 315
DNAR. *See* Do not attempt resuscitation
DNAse, formulary entry for, 776
Do not attempt resuscitation (DNAR), 579
Dobutamine (Dobutrex), formulary entry for, 774
DOC (deoxycorticosterone) acetate, potency of, 992t
Docusate (Colace, Surfak), formulary entry for, 774–775
Dog/cat bites, infections from, 422t
Dolasetron (Anzemet), formulary entry for, 775
Dolophine
for analgesia, 140t
formulary entry for, 859
relative potency of, 151t
with renal failure, 1032t
toxicity of, 28t–41t
Dopamine (Intropin)
for IV infusions, i
formulary entry for, 775–776
Dopram, formulary entry for, 776–777
Dornase alfa (DNAse, Pulmozyme), formulary entry for, 776
Dorsalis pedis artery, blood sampling puncture of, 61

Dobutamine, standard concentrations for, i
Down syndrome, growth charts for, 534
Doxapram HCL (Dopram), formulary entry for, 776–777
Doxazosin, for hypertension, 501t
Doxorubicin (Adriamycin), toxicity of, 1008t
Doxycycline (Vibramycin, Periostat)
  for acne vulgaris, 218t
  for ehrlichiosis/anaplasmosis, 449
  formulary entry for, 777
  for Lyme disease, 448
  for Rocky Mountain spotted fever, 449
Dramamine, formulary entry for, 772
DRIs. *See* Dietary reference intakes
Drisdol, formulary entry for, 785–786
Dronabinol (tetrahydrocannabinol, THC, Marinol)
  for chemotherapy-induced nausea, 574
  formulary entry for, 778
Droperidol (Inapsine), formulary entry for, 778
Drug dosage
  adjustments for renal failure
    antimicrobials requiring, 1013t–1026t
    methods for, 1012
    nonantimicrobials requiring, 1013
  breastfeeding categories, 664
  do not use list, 662t
  pregnancy categories and, 664
  sample entry, 663
Drug toxicity
  acetaminophen, 28t
  actinomycin D, 1007t
  adriamycin, 1007t
  adrucil, 1007t
  alcohols, 30t
  alkeran, 1008t
  amphetamines, 43
  anticholinergics, 31t
  antidepressants, 32t
  antihistamines, 33t
  asparaginase, 1006t
  avastin, 1006t
  barbiturates, 34t
  benzodiazepines, 34t
  beta-blockers, 35t
  busulfan, 1006t
Drug toxicity *(Continued)*
  butyrophenone, 39t
  calcium channel blockers, 36t
  camptosar, 1007t
  carbamates, 52
  carbamazepine, 48
  carboplatin, 1006t
  carboxamide, 1007t
  carmustin, 1006t
  cisplatin, 1006t
  clofarabine, 1006t
  cytarabine, 1006t
  cytoxam, 1006t
  daunomycin, 1007t
  digoxin, 48
  dihydroxyanthracenedione dihydrochloride, 1008t
  divalproex sodium, 48
  fosphenytoin, 48
  hypoglycemics, 37t
  iron, 38t
  lomustine, 1008t
  NSAIDs, 39t
  phenothiazines, 39t
  salicylates, 40t
  6-TG (thioguanine), 1008t
  valproic acid, 48
Drugs
  administration of
    by intramuscular injection, 81
    by subcutaneous injections, 81
  chemotherapeutic, 1006t–1009t
  effecting warfarin therapy, 343b
  trade and generic names for, 664–681
DSMA. *See* Dimercaptosuccinic acid
DTaP vaccine. *See* Diphtheria and tetanus toxoids and acellular pertussis (DTaP) vaccine
DTIC (dacarbazine), toxicity of, 1007t
DTPA. *See* Diethylene triamine pentaacetic acid
Duodenal ulcer(s)
  famotidine for, 793
  lansoprazole for, 840
  omeprazole for, 889
  ranitidine for, 933
  sucralfate for, 952
Duraclon, formulary entry for, 754
Duragesic
  characterization of, 140t
  for RSI, 6t
  formulary entry for, 794–795

Duragesic *(Continued)*
relative potency of, 151t
with renal failure, 1030t
Duramist, formulary entry for, 693
Duricef
formulary entry for, 732
with renal failure, 1014t
Dycill
formulary entry for, 769
for lymphadenitis, 425t
Dynacin
for acne vulgaris, 218t
formulary entry for, 870
Dyrenium
for hypertension, 501t
for hyperthyroidism, 251t
with renal failure, 1034t
Dysmenorrhea, naproxen sodium as, 877
Dyspnea, morphine for, 581t

E
ECMO, 465
ECP. *See* Emergency contraceptive pill
Echocardiography, long QT ranges in, 181–183
Ecstasy, toxicity of, 44b
Eczema. *See* Atopic dermatitis
Edema
ehrlichiosis and, 449
hydrochlorothiazide for, 818
in renal disease, 490
Edetate (EDTA) calcium disodium (calcium disodium versenate), formulary entry for, 779
Efidac/24Pesudeophedrine
cetirizine with, 740–741
formulary entry for, 926
loratadine with, 850
Egg allergies, skin testing for, 371–374
Ehrlichia chaffeensis, 449
Ehrlichia ewingii, 449
Ehrlichiosis, 449
Eikenella corrodens, in animal bites, 96t
Ejection click, 164–165
Elavil
formulary entry for, 695–696
for migraines, 512t
Elbow(s), nursemaid's, 87
Electrical burns, 98t
Electrocardiography (ECG)
abnormalities in, 174
basic principles of, 169–173
CAE in, 174f
hexaxial reference system for, 170f
horizontal reference system for, 170f
MI in children, 181f
for nonfebrile seizures, 511
nonpathologic changes in, 173f
nonventricular arrhythmias in, 175t–176t, 176f
nonventricular conduction disturbances, 178t–179t
normal parameters for, 170t
normal T-wave axis for, 173t
pathologic changes in, 173f
quadrants of mean, location of, 172f
secondary findings in, 181
supraventricular arrhythmias in, 154
ventricular arrhythmias, 178t
ventricular conduction disturbances, 180t
ventricular hypertrophy criteria for, 174b
Electroencephalogram (EEG)
for developmental disorders, 236
for paroxysmal events, 511
Electrolyte(s)
composition in various body fluids, 281t
deficits in
in hyponatremic dehydration, 282t
replacement strategy for, 277–278
for diabetes, 245f
maintenance requirements of, 271–274
Electrolyte disturbances
hyponatremia as, 277
due to poisoning, 22t
in serum calcium, 284–286
in serum magnesium, 286–287
in serum phosphate, 288–289
in serum potassium, 283–284
in serum sodium, 281, 282t
Elevated intraocular pressure, pilocarpine for, 912
Elimite
for scabies, 208
formulary entry for, 906
Elitek, formulary entry for, 933–934
Elixophyllin
formulary entry for, 960–961
toxicity of, 20t–22t

Elocon
daily dose recommendations for, 871t, 993t
formulary entry for, 871–872
potency ranking of, 995t–996t
Elspar (Asparaginase), toxicity of, 1006t
Emergency(ies), oncologic, 564–569
cerebrovascular accident as, 568
hyperleukocytosis as, 564–567
increase intracranial pressure as, 568
respiratory distress as, 568–569
spinal cord compression as, 567–568
superior vena cava syndrome as, 568–569
tumor lysis syndrome as, 567
Emergency contraceptive pill (ECP), 128
Emergency management
for airway conditions, 3–7
for anaphylaxis, 9–10
for breathing conditions, 7–8
for circulation conditions, 8–9
for gastrointestinal conditions, 293–295
for neurologic conditions, 13–17
for respiratory conditions, 10–13
EMLA. *See* Lidocaine and Prilocaine
Emotional changes, as death approaches, 580
Empyema, imaging of, 609
E-Mycin, formulary entry for, 787–788
Enalapril maleate (Vasotec)
for hypertension, 500t
for hypertensive emergency, 105t
formulary entry for, 780
with renal failure, 1030t
Enbrel, formulary entry for, 790–791
Encephalitis, emergency treatment of, 14
Encopresis
definitions of, 297
treatment for, 298
Endocarditis
characterization of, 191
prosthetic valve, rifampin dosage for, 937
vancomycin for, 975
Endocet, formulary entry for, 895
Endocrine disorders
abnormal growth as, 257
adrenal function, 253–257
diabetes as, 243–247
parathyroid function, 247–253
pituitary function, 253–257
thyroid function, 247–253
websites for, 243
Endocrine normal values
for androstenedione, 269t
for dehydroepiandrosterone, 267t
for estradiol, 266t
for gonadotropins, 269t
for 17-hydroxyprogeterone, 267t
for insulin-like growth factor 1, 267t
for insulin-like growth factor-binding protein, 268t
for testosterone, 266t
for vitamin D, 266t
Endocrine tests and procedures
ACTH stimulation test, 263
Cushing evaluation, 264
glucagon stimulation test, 264–265
for infants, 250t
neonatal hypoglycemia, 264–265
normal values for, 265–269
DHEA, 266t
estradiol, 266t
17-hydroxyprogesterone, 267t
IGF-1, 267t
IGF-BP3, 268t
mean stretched penile length, 268t
testicular size, 269t
testosterone, 266t
vitamin D, 266t
OGTT, 262
for thyroid function, 247, 248t–249t
vasopressin test, 264
water deprivation test, 263–264
Endotracheal tube(s)
placement of, 613
size of, 457t
Engraftment, HSCT from, 571
Enlon, formulary entry for, 779
Enoxaparin (Lovenox)
formulary entry for, 780–782
with renal failure, 1030t
Enteral nutrition
for children (ages 1 to 10), 554t–555t

Enteral nutrition *(Continued)*
for children and adults, 556t–557t
components for, 549t–556t
infant formula components of, 549t–551t
overview of, 545
Enterobacter spp., sensitivity profile of, 408t–409t
Enterobius
mebendazole for, 854
pyrantel pamoate for, 928
Enterococci, sensitivity profile of, 409t
Enterocolitis, food-induced, 356
Enterovirus
diagnosis of, 416
neonatal management of, 414t
Enulose, formulary entry for, 836–837
Enzymes, serum muscle, 623
Eosinophilic enterocolitis
mebendazole for, 855
pyrantel pamoate for, 928
Eosinophilic esophagitis (EE), 300
Epidemiological Studies Depression Scale for Children, 240
Epididymitis, initial treatment of, 429t
Epiglottis, emergency-associated, 12
Epilepsy
events mimicking, 513t
intractable, formulas for, 558t
seizures of
characterization of, 511
classification of, 514b
differential diagnosis of, 513t
imaging of, 513
syndromes of, 515t
treatment for, 514–518, 516t–517t
Epinephrine HCl (Adrenalin, Epi-pen)
for anaphylaxis, 10
anesthetics use with, 139
asthma treatment with, 10–11
characterization of, 141t
formulary entry for, 782–783
for resuscitation, ii
standard concentrations for, i
Epinephrine intramuscular, for anaphylaxis, 9–10
Epinephrine, Racemic (S-2 inhalant), formulary entry for, 783
Epi-pen
for anaphylaxis, 10
anesthetics use with, 139
Epi-pen *(Continued)*
asthma treatment with, 10–11
characterization of, 141t
formulary entry for, 782–783
for resuscitation, ii
standard concentrations for, i
Epithelial cells, in urine, 478
Epitol
adenosine effects on, 686
formulary entry for, 727–728
with renal failure, 1028t
for seizures, 516t
toxicity of, 48
Epivir
formulary entry for, 837
with renal failure, 1021t
Epoetin alfa (Epogen, Procrit), formulary entry for, 784–785
Epogen, formulary entry for, 784–785
Epsom salts
asthma treatment with, 11
formulary entry for, 853–854
for resuscitation, ii
Ergocalciferol (Drisdol, Calciferol), formulary entry for, 785–786
Ergotamine tartrate (Ergomar), formulary entry for, 786
Erosive esophagitis
lansoprazole for, 840
pantoprazole for, 898
ranitidine for, 933
Ertapenem (Invanz)
formulary entry for, 786–787
with renal failure, 1017t
Erwinia (Asparaginase), toxicity of, 1006t
Ery-Ped, formulary entry for, 787–788
Erythema. *See* Reactive erythema
Erythema toxicum neonatorum, characterization of, 220
Erythrocin (Erythromycin preparations)
for acne vulgaris, 218t
for chlamydial infections, 420t
formulary entry for, 787–788
Erythrocyte sedimentation rate, 639t–647t
Erythromycin
for acne vulgaris, 218t
for cellulitis, 423t
for chlamydial infections, 420t

Erythromycin *(Continued)*
for gastroenteritis, 218t
for gonorrhea, 430t
for pneumonia, 428t
Erythromycin ethylsuccinate and acetylsulfisoxazole (Pediazole), formulary entry for, 787
Erythromycin ophthalmic (Oticin)
for cellulitis, 423t
for conjunctivitis, 423t
toxicity of, 1000t
Erythromycin preparations (Erythrocin, Pediamycin, E-Mycin, Ery-Ped)
for acne vulgaris, 218t
for chlamydial infections, 420t
formulary entry for, 787–788
Erythropoietin. *See* Epoetin alfa
Escalate treatment, abandonment of, 579
Escherichia coli, 479
Escitalopram (Lexapro), dosage/side effects for, 1004t
Eskalith
formulary entry for, 849
for renal failure, 1031t
Esmolol HCl (Brevibloc), formulary entry for, 789–790
Esomeprazole, formulary entry for, 789–790
Esophageal atresia, imaging of, 616
Esophageal candidiasis, micafungin for, 866
Esophagitis
erosive
lansoprazole for, 840
omeprazole for, 888
famotidine for, 793
Esophagus. *See also* Gastrointestinal (GI) tract
eosinophilic, 300
foreign bodies in, imaging of, 609
Estimated energy requirements (EERs)
definition of, 535
equations, 536
for healthy children, 537t
under stress conditions, 536–537
Estradiol, normal values for, 266t
Estrogen, contraindications for, 123–128
Ethambutol HCl (Myambutol)
formulary entry for, 791
with renal failure, 1017t
Ethancept (Enbrel), formulary entry for, 790–791
Ethanol
as alcohol antidote, 20t–22t
toxicity of, 45b
Ethosuximide (Zarontin)
formulary entry for, 791–792
for seizures, 516t
Etomidate, for RSI, 6t
Etoposide (VP-16, VePesid), toxicity of, 1007t
ETT (endotracheal tube), use of, 4
Evidence-based medicine
clinical studies evaluation in, 656t
framework for, 651–652
study design comparison in, 655t
Ewing's sarcoma, signs/symptoms of, 566t
Excitation, due to poisoning, 20t–22t
Exogenous surfactant therapy, for neonates, 463
Expiratory pressures, maximal, measurement of, 587–588
Extended-release nifedipine, for hypertension, 500t
External jugular puncture(s), 58–59
Extracellular fluid composition, 276t
Extracorporeal membrane oxygenation (ECMO), for PPHN, 465
Extradural fluid collections, 459f
Extrapyramidals, toxidrome of, 24t
Extremities trauma, secondary survey of, 90t
Exudate fluids, reference values for, 648t
Eye movements, tests for, 505t
Eyelids, tests for, 505t

F

Facial slaps, 2f
Factor V Leiden, characterization of, 338b
Factor VIII deficiency, characterization of, 345b
Factor IX deficiency, characterization of, 345b, 346t
Famciclovir (Famvir)
formulary entry for, 792
with renal failure, 1017t
Familial short stature (FSS), 257

Famotidine (Pepcid)
formulary entry for, 792–793
with renal failure, 83t
Famvir
formulary entry for, 792
with renal failure, 1017t
Fanconi syndrome
characterization of, 39, 327
presentation of, 327
FAS. *See* Fetal alcohol syndrome
Fat(s)
caloric modulars of, 549t
dietary requirements for, 539t
in enteral formulas, 549t–556t
in human milk, 549t–556t
in infant formulas, 549t–556t
malabsorption of, formulas for, 558t–559t
5-FC
formulary entry for, 798
with renal failure, 1018t
Feeding tubes, formulas for, 558t–559t
Felbamate (Felbatol)
formulary entry for, 793–794
with renal failure, 1030t
for seizures, 516t
Felbatol
formulary entry for, 793–794
with renal failure, 1030t
for seizures, 516t
Felodipine, for hypertension, 500t
Femoral vein(s), catheter placement in, 62, 64f
Fentanyl (Sublimate, Duragesic, Fentora, Actiq)
characterization of, 140t
formulary entry for, 794–795
relative potency of, 151t
with renal failure, 1030t
for RSI, 6t
Ferric gluconate. *See* Iron—injectable preparations
Ferric gluconate (IV), 829
Ferritin, reference values for, 642t
Ferrous sulfate. *See* Iron—oral preparations
Fetal alcohol syndrome (FAS), 184t, 460
Fetal hydantoin syndrome, 460
Fetal valproate syndrome, 460
Fever(s)
oncologic-induced, 570f
seizure associated with, 512b, 519f
Feverall
analgesic properties of, 138
formulary entry for, 682
poisoning with, 684
with renal failure, 1027t
Fexofenadine (Allegra)
for allergic rhinitis, 355–356
fexofenadine with, 796
formulary entry for, 796
with renal failure, 1030t
FFP (fresh frozen plasma), 350
Fiber Therapy, formulary entry for, 927
Fiberall, formulary entry for, 927
Fibrillation, ventricular, 178t
Filgrastim (Neupogen, G-CSF), formulary entry for, 796
Fingersticks, 57–58
First degree heart block, 178t
FISH. *See* Fluorescence in situ hybridization
Fisher's exact test, 653t
FK506, formulary entry for, 958–959
FLACC scale, 137, 138t
Flagyl
for acne vulgaris, 218t
for bacterial vaginosis, 422t
formulary entry for, 865–866
for gastroenteritis, 218t
neonatal critical care dosing of, 1010t
for PID, 432t
with renal failure, 1022t
Flame burns, 98t
Flat warts, 206
Flecainide acetate (Tambocor)
formulary entry for, 797
with renal failure, 1030t
Fleet, formulary entry for, 948–949
Fleet Babylax, formulary entry for, 813
Fleet Mineral Oil, formulary entry for, 869
Fleet Phospho-Soda, formulary entry for, 948–949
Fletcher's Castoria, formulary entry for, 943

Flonase
for asthma, 803t
daily dose recommendations for, 802t
formulary entry for, 802–803
potency ranking of, 995t
Florinef acetate
formulary entry for, 799
for mineralocorticoid deficiency, 989–991
Florone, potency ranking of, 995t
Flovent Diskus
for asthma, 803t
daily dose recommendations for, 802t
formulary entry for, 802–803
potency ranking of, 995t
Flow-volume curve, 589f
Floxin
formulary entry for, 887
for gonorrhea, 430t
Fluconazole (Diflucan)
formulary entry for, 797–798
with renal failure, 1018t
for tinea capitis, 215
Flucytosine (Ancobon, 5-FC, 5-fluorocytosine)
formulary entry for, 798
with renal failure, 1018t
Fludara (fludarabine), toxicity of, 1007t
Fludrocortisone acetate (Florinef acetate, 9-Flurohydrocortisone)
formulary entry for, 799
for mineralocorticoid deficiency, 989–991
Fluid(s)
deficits of
solute calculations, 276
volume of, 274
for diabetes, 245f
newborns' requirements for, 461t
Fluid and electrolyte management
acid-base/osmolar gap disturbances in, 289
deficit repletion in, 274–281
goals of, 271
maintenance requirements for, 271–274
ongoing losses in, 281
serum electrolyte disturbances in, 281–289
calcium, 283–284
magnesium, 286–287
Fluid and electrolyte management *(Continued)*
phosphate, 288–289
potassium, 283–284
sodium, 281
Flumadine
approval for, 393
for influenza, 425t
Flumazenil (Romazicon)
as benzodiazepine antidote, 34t
formulary entry for, 799
for sedation reversal, 146
Flunarizine, for migraines, 512t
Flunisolide (Nasarel, Aerospan, Aerobid)
for allergic rhinitis, 355–356
daily dose recommendations for, 804t, 993t
formulary entry for, 800
Fluocinolone acetonide (Synalar, Capex shampoo, Derma-Smoothe), potency ranking of, 995t
Fluocinonide (Vanos, Lidex), potency ranking of, 995t
Fluorescence in situ hybridization (FISH), for genetic abnormalities, 315
Fluoride (Luride, Fluoritab, Pediaflor)
concentration in water, 801t
DRIs for, 542t
formulary entry for, 800–801
in formulas, 542t
in multivitamin drops, 545t
in multivitamin tablets, 547t
supplementation of, 544
Fluoritab, formulary entry for, 800–801
9-α-Fluorocortisone, potency of, 992t
5-Fluorocytosine
formulary entry for, 798
with renal failure, 1018t
9-Fluorohydrocortisone
formulary entry for, 799
for mineralocorticoid deficiency, 989–991
Fluoroquinolone, for gastroenteritis, 424t
5-Fluorouracil (5-FU, Adrucil), toxicity of, 1007t

Fluoxetine hydrochloride (Prozac, Sarafem)
  dosage/side effects for, 1004t
  formulary entry for, 801–802
Flurandrenolide (Cordran), potency ranking of, 995t
Flushing, due to poisoning, 22t
Fluticasone (Flovent, Salmeterol)
  for allergic rhinitis, 355–356
  daily dose recommendations for, 993t–994t
Fluticasone furoate (Veramyst), dosage recommendations for, 802
Fluticasone propionate (Flonase HFA, Cutivate, Flovent Diskus)
  for asthma, 803t
  daily dose recommendations for, 804t–805t
  formulary entry for, 802–803
  potency ranking of, 995t–996t
Fluticasone propionate and salmeterol (Advair), formulary entry for, 804–805
Fluvoxamine (Luvox)
  dosage/side effects for, 1004t
  formulary entry for, 805t
Folate
  in multivitamin tablets, analysis of, 546t
  reference values for, 643t
Folex (Methotrexate), toxicity of, 1008t
Folic acid (Folvite), formulary entry for, 806
Follicle-stimulating hormone (FSH), delayed puberty caused by, 260
Folvite, formulary entry for, 806
Fomepizole (Antizol)
  as alcohol antidote, 30t
  formulary entry for, 806–807
Fontan procedure, for CHD, 184
Food allergies
  diagnosis of, 357–358
  epidemiology of, 356
  evaluation of, 357f
  management of, 357f
  manifestations of, 356
  natural history of, 358–359
  skin testing for, 371–374
Food-induced enterocolitis, 356
Foradil, formulary entry for, 807–808
Forced expiratory flow (FEF), 590
Forced expiratory volume (FEV), 589
Forced vital capacity (FVC), 589
Foreign bodies, airway, imaging of, 609
Foreign-body aspiration, causes of, 13
Fosinopril, for hypertension, 500t
Formoterol
  budesonide with, 720
  dose recommendations for, 804t–805t, 994t
  formulary entry for, 807–808
Formoterol (Foradil, Aerolizer, Perforomist), formulary entry for, 807–808
Formoterol fumarate and mometasone furoate (Dulera), formulary entry for, 872
Formula(s)
  amino acid-based, enteral nutritional components in, 552t–557t
  cow's milk-based
    enteral nutritional components in, 550t–555t
  iron supplementation and, 545
  oral rehydration solutions, 559t
  preparation of, 548t
  preterm, nutritional components in, 548t–549t
  for special clinical conditions, 558t–559t
    enteral nutritional components in, 549t–556t
  websites for, 524–535
Fortamet
  for diabetes, 247
  for polycystic ovarian syndrome, 259
Fortaz
  formulary entry for, 737
  for osteomyelitis, 426t
  for otitis media, 426t
  with renal failure, 1016t
Fortical Nasal Spray, formulary entry for, 721–722
Forward bending test, 132f
Foscarnet (Foscavir)
  formulary entry for, 808
  with renal failure, 1018t

Fosphenytoin (Cerebyx)
formulary entry for, 690–691
for status epilepticus, 17
toxicity of, 48
Fractures
long bone
characteristics of, 94–96
unique to children, 95f
stress, imaging of, 618
Fragile X syndrome, characterization of, 317
Free water deficit (FWD), 277
Frostbite, 98t
FSH. *See* Follicle-stimulating hormone
5-FU (fluorouracil), toxicity of, 1007t
Fulvicin
formulary entry for, 815
for tinea capitis, 214–216
Fungal infections
amphotericin B for, 1014t
amphotericin B lipid complex for, 1014t
amphotericin B liposomal for, 1014t
caspofungin for, 810–811
clotrimazole for, 754–755
common types of, 451t
diagnosis of, 450,
fluconazole for, 797–798
flucytosine for, 798
griseofulvin for, 815
itraconazole for, 833
ketoconazole for, 833
micafungin sodium for, 866–867
miconazole for, 867
tolnaftate for, 966
voriconazole for, 981–982
Fungizone, with renal failure, 1014t
Furadantin, formulary entry for, 882–883
Furosemide (Lasix)
formulary entry for, 809–810
for hypertension, 501t
for hyperthyroidism, 251t
for renal failure, 1030t

G

G6PD assay. *See* Glucose-6-phosphate dehydrogenase (G6PD) assay
Gabapentin (Neurontin, Gabarone)
formulary entry for, 810–811
for renal failure, 1030t
for seizures, 516t
Gabitril
formulary entry for, 963–964
for seizures, 517t
Galactose, reference values for, 643t
Gallstone(s), ursodiol for, 971
Galzin, formulary entry for, 985–986
Gamma benzene hexachloride, formulary entry for, 846
Gamma-glutamyl transferase (GGT), reference values for, 643t
Gamma-hydroxybutyrate (GBH), toxicity of, 45b
Ganciclovir (Cytovene)
formulary entry for
with renal failure, 1018t
Gantrisin, with renal failure, 1024t
Garamycin
formulary entry for, 812–813
for PID, 432t
with renal failure, 1019t
for septic arthritis, 421t, 429t
Gas chromatography, poison screenings by, 19
Gas exchange
evaluation of, 584–586
capnography, 585
oxyhemoglobin dissociation curve, 586f
pulse oximetry, 584–585
respiratory auscultation in, 585t
respiratory rates in, 585t
Gas mass spectroscopy, poison screenings by, 19
Gastric acid proton pump inhibitor
esomeprazole as, 789–790
lansoprazole as, 840–841
omeprazole as, 888
pantoprazole as, 898–899
Gastric ulcers
lansoprazole for, 840
omeprazole for, 889
ranitidine for, 933
Gastrocrom, formulary entry for, 757
Gastroenteritis
allergic eosinophilic, 356
initial management of, 424t

Gastroenterology
emergencies in, 293–295
acute abdominal pain, 294–295
GI bleeding, 293–294, 294t
GI tract conditions in, 295–301
bilious emesis differential, 470–471
bleeding, 293–294
celiac disease, 301
constipation, 297–298
diarrhea, 295–297
EE, 300
encopresis, 297–298
GER, 299–300
IBD, 298–299
necrotizing enterocolitis as, 470
hepatic conditions in, 301–305
pancreatitis in, 305–307
websites for, 293
Gastroesophageal reflux (GER)
metoclopramide for, 863
seizures *versus*, 513t
Gastrointestinal (GI) tract
aluminum hydroxide for, 690
bleeding in, characterization of, 293–294
changes in, as death approaches, 580
conditions of
bilious emesis differential, 470–471
celiac disease, 301
constipation, 297–298
diarrhea, 295–297
EE, 300
encopresis, 297–298
food allergy syndromes, 356
GER, 299–300
IBD, 298–299
imaging of, 615–617
necrotizing enterocolitis, 470
vomiting, 296t
poison-associated decontamination of, 22–26
Gastrointestinal reflux disease (GERD)
characterization of, 299–300
esomeprazole for, 789
famotidine for, 793
lansoprazole for, 840
metoclopramide for, 863
omeprazole for, 888
pantoprazole for, 898
ranitidine for, 933
Gas-X, formulary entry for, 945–946
GBH. *See* Gamma-hydroxybutyrate
GBL. *See* Gamma-hydroxybutyrolactone
GBS. *See* Group B streptococcal (GBS) infection
G-CSF, formulary entry for, 796
Gemcitabine (Pyrimidine analog), toxicity of, 1007t
Genetic diagnostic tests, 315–316
Genetics
common syndromes in, 316–318
22Q11 syndrome as, 317–318
fragile X syndrome a, 317
marfan syndrome as, 317
Prader-Willi syndrome as, 318
Trisomy 13 as, 318
Trisomy 18 as, 318
Trisomy 21 as, 316
Turner syndrome as, 316–317
consultation for, 320
degenerative disorders in, 318–320
lysosomal, 319
peroxisomal, 319
dysmorphology of, 315–316
inborn errors of metabolism in, 310–315
definition of, 310–315
differential diagnosis of, 310
evaluation of, 310
hypoglycemia in, 312–315, 314f
laboratory test for, 311b
management of, 311–312
presentation of, 310
sample collection for, 312t
newborn metabolic screen in, 309–310
websites for, 309
Gengraf, formulary entry for, 759–760
Genital herpes
acyclovir for, 685
famciclovir for, 792
valacyclovir for, 972
Genital ulcers, management of, 125t–126t
Genital warts, management of, 125t–126t
Genitalia, ambiguous, 262
Genitals, development of, 119t
Genitourinary tract, imaging of, 617
Genitourinary trauma, secondary survey of, 90t

Gentamicin (Garamycin)
  formulary entry for, 812–813
  for PID, 432t
  with renal failure, 1019t
  for septic arthritis, 421t, 429t
Geodon (Ziprasidone), dosage/side effects for, 1004t
GERD. *See* Gastrointestinal reflux disease
Gesell block skills, 233, 235f
Gesell figures, 233, 234f
GGT (gamma-glutamyl transpeptidase), in hepatic function test, 302t
GI tract. *See* Gastrointestinal (GI) tract
Giant cell vasculitis, 631t
Giardiasis, metronidazole for, 865
Glasgow coma scale, i
Glaucoma
  acetazolamide for, 479
  amitriptyline contraindicated for, 696
  atomoxetine contraindicated for, 705
Gleevec (Imatinib), toxicity of, 1007t
Glenn shunt, for CHD, 184
Glomerular diseases, 492–493
Glomerular function assessment
  filtration rate
    normal values of, 484t
    proportionality constant, 484t
  with nuclear medicine scans, 484
GlucaGen
  for beta-blocker toxicity, 35t
  for hypoglycemics, 37t
  formulary entry for, 813
Glucagon Emergency Kit
  for beta-blocker toxicity, 35t
  for hypoglycemics, 37t
  formulary entry for, 813
Glucagon HCl (GlucaGen, Glucagon Emergency Kit)
  for beta-blocker toxicity, 35t
  for hypoglycemics, 37t
  formulary entry for, 813
Glucagon stimulation test, 264–265
Glucocorticoid deficiency, systemic corticosteroids for, 989
Glucophage
  for diabetes, 247
  for polycystic ovarian syndrome, 259
Glucose
  in cerebrospinal fluid, 648t
  for hypoglycemic seizures, 45
Glucose *(Continued)*
  newborns' requirements for, 460
  reference values for, 643t
Glucose tolerance, impaired, formulas for, 559t
Glucose-6-phosphate dehydrogenase (G6PD) assay, for anemia diagnosis, 327
Glucosuria, 477
Glycerin (Fleet Babylax, Sani-Supp), formulary entry for, 813
Glycopyrrolate (Robinul), formulary entry for, 814
Gly-Oxide, formulary entry for, 728–729
GoLYTELY, formulary entry for, 915
Gonadotropins, normal values for, 269t
Gonorrhea
  azithromycin for, 709
  cefixime for, 430t–431t
  cefoxitin for, 430t–431t
  ceftriaxone for, 430t–431t
  initial management of, 430t–431t
  probenecid for, 430t–431t
Goodenough-Harris Draw-a-Person Test, 233
Graft-*versus*-host disease (GVHD), in cancer survivors, 576
Granisetron (Kytril), formulary entry for, 814
Granulomatous disease
  differential diagnosis of, 632–633
  sarcoidosis in, 633
Graves disease
  characterization of, 250
  methimazole for, 250
  propylthiouracil for, 250
Griseofulvin (Grifulvin V, Grisactin, Fulvicin)
  formulary entry for, 815
  for tinea capitis, 214–216
Group A streptococcal pharyngitis, penicillin V potassium for, 904
Group A streptococci, Bicillin L-A for, 903
Group B streptococcal (GBS) infection
  diagnosis of, 416
  IAP for, 417f–419f
Growth
  catch-up, 537–538, 538b
  delay of, 257, 258f

Growth *(Continued)*
evaluation of, 525–533
failure of, 537
Growth charts
BMI (boys), 532f
BMI (girls), 530f
head circumference (boys), 528f
head circumference (girls), 526f
interpretation of, 534
length and weight (girls), 525f
length-to-weight ratio (boys), 527f–528f
length-to-weight ratio (girls), 526f
for preterm infants, 533f
for special populations, 534
stature and weight (boys), 531f
stature and weight (girls), 529f
WHO, 537–538
Growth-plate injuries, Salter-Harris classification of, 95t
Guillain-Barré syndrome, IVIG therapy for, 362
GVHD. *See* Graft-*versus*-host disease
Gyne-Lotrimin, formulary entry for, 754–755

H

Haemophilus influenza B (HIB) vaccine
age-based schedule for, 374f
for cancer patients, 381t
catch-up schedule for, 374f
immunoprophylaxis for, 386–387
schedule for, 372f
Halcinonide (Halog), potency ranking of, 995t
Haldol
dosage/side effects for, 1003t
formulary entry for, 815–816
for palliative care, 581t
Hallucinogens, toxicity of, 45b–46b
Halog, potency ranking of, 995t
Haloperidol (Haldol)
dosage/side effects for, 1003t
formulary entry for, 815–816
for palliative care, 581t
Hands, injuries to, thumb spica splint for, 87
Haptoglobin
for anemia diagnosis, 327
reference values for, 644t
Hashimoto's thyroiditis, 250
HCO_3^-. *See* Bicarbonate
HCTZ (hydrochlorothiazide)
formulary entry for, 818
for hypertension, 501t
Head trauma
imaging of, 607
minor closed (CHT)
associated symptoms of, 93
imaging indications for, 92b
injury mechanism in, 92–93
management of, 93
physical examination of, 91–93
secondary survey of, 90t
sports-related, 97–102
Head(s)
circumference
for boys, 528f
for girls, 526f
control of, tests for, 505t
imaging of, 606–607
Headache(s)
acute, differential diagnosis of, 508b
chronic, differential diagnosis of, 509b
classification of, 507
evaluation of, 507–509
imaging, 509
physical, 507
warning signs of, 508b
Hearing, tests for, 505t
Heart(s)
abnormal sounds of, 166b
anatomy, imaging of, 614f–615f
chest radiography of, 185, 190f
imaging of, 613–615, 614f–615f
sounds from, 154–164
Heart block(s)
conduction, 179f
degrees of, 178t–179t
Heart murmur(s)
characteristics of, 167
common innocent, 167t
systolic/diastolic, 167t
Heelsticks, 57–58
Heel-to-ear maneuver, in newborn assessment, 457
Heiner syndrome, 356
Heinz body preparation, for anemia diagnosis, 327
Helicobacter pylori
bismuth subsalicylate for, 717
metronidazole for, 866

Hemangiomas
  clinical manifestations of, 204
  management of, 205–206
  pathogenesis of, 201
  size of, 204
Hematologic anemia, 573
Hematologic diseases
  conjugated hyperbilirubinemia as, 469
  polycythemia as, 469–470
  unconjugated hyperbilirubinemia in newborns as, 467–469
Hematologic disorder(s), in SLE, 628t
Hematology
  anemia in, 322–328
    age-specific indices of, 323t–324t, 325f
    causes of, 322–328
    classification of, 326t
    gender-specific indices of, 325f
    general evaluation of, 322
    macrocytic, 327
  bleeding disorders
    common types of, 345b
    differential diagnosis of, 344f
  blood component replacement in, 343–352
    complications of, 351
    directed donor considerations for, 351–352
    PRBC exchange transfusion, 350
    product components for, 348–350
    volume, 343
  blood smear interpretation in, 352
  coagulation in, 334–343
    age-specific values of, 336t–337t
    cascade of, 335f
    disseminated intravascular, 345b
    hypercoagulable states in, 335–343, 338b
    tests of, 334–335
  hemoglobinopathies in, 328–332
    hemoglobin electrophoresis as, 328
    sickle cell anemia as, 328–329, 329t–331t
    thalassemias as, 329–332
  neonatal Hb electrophoresis patterns, 328t
  neutropenia in, 332
  thrombocytopenia in, 332–334
Hematopoietic stem cell transplantation (HSCT)
  goal of, 569
  types of, 569–571
Hematuria
  characterization of, 487
  diagnostic strategy for, 488f
  management algorithm for, 489f
Hemiplegia, acute onset of, 521b
Hemodialysis, 1012
Hemoglobin (Hb)
  neonatal electrophoresis patterns of, 328t
  in urine, 477
Hemoglobin A, reference values for, 644t
Hemoglobin electrophoresis, 328
Hemoglobin F, reference values for, 644t
Hemoglobinopathies
  hemoglobin electrophoresis as, 328
  sickle cell anemia as, 328–329, 329t–331t
  thalassemias as, 329–332
Hemolytic anemia, characterization of, 326–327
Hemolytic disorders, 305t
Hemolytic uremic syndrome (HUS), in bone marrow transplants, 572–573
Hemolytic-uremic syndrome/thrombotic thrombocytopenic purpura (HUS/TTP), 345b
Hemophilia, factor replacement in, 348t
Hemophilia B. *See* Factor IX deficiency
Hemorrhage, categorization of, 108t
Hemorrhagic cystitis, in bone marrow transplants, 573
Henoch-Schönlein purpura (HSP), 630–632, 631t
Heparin sodium
  formulary entry for, 816–817
  protamine sulfate as antidote for, 926
Hepatitis A (HAV) vaccine
  catch-up schedule for, 374f
  contraindications/precautions for, 376t–379t
  dosages/schedule for, 388t
  immunoprophylaxis for, 387–388
  interval schedule for, 375t
  for pregnant patients, 384
  schedule for, 372f

Hepatitis B (HBV) vaccine
age considerations for, 382
catch-up schedule for, 374f
contraindications/precautions for, 376t
dosages/schedule for, 389t
immunoprophylaxis for, 388–389
interval schedule for, 375t
for pregnant patients, 384
Hepatitis A virus (HAV)
IMIG therapy for, 363
serologic markers of, 304t
Hepatitis B virus (HBV)
diagnosis of, 416
neonatal management of, 414t
serologic markers of, 304t
transmission of, 452
Hepatitis C virus (HCV)
diagnosis of, 416
neonatal management of, 414t
ribavirin dosage for, 934
serologic markers of, 304t
transmission of, 452
Hepatoblastoma, signs/symptoms of, 566t
Hepatocytes, injury to, 301
Herpes, genital
acyclovir for, 685
famciclovir for, 792
valacyclovir for, 972
Herpes labialis
acyclovir for, 685
famciclovir for, 792
valacyclovir for, 971
Herpes simplex virus (HSV)
acyclovir for, 685
immunocompetent, acyclovir dosage and, 685
immunocompromised, acyclovir dosage and, 685
neonatal management of, 413t
Herpes zoster virus
acyclovir for, 685
valacyclovir for, 972
Hexadrol
for airway edema, 991
for bacterial meningitis, 447t
for chemotherapy-induced nausea, 574
formulary entry for, 766–767
Hexadrol *(Continued)*
for idiopathic thrombocytic purpura, 992
potency of, 992t
Hexaxial reference system, 170f
HFA
for asthma, 803t
daily dose recommendations for, 804t–805t
formulary entry for, 802–803
HIB. *See* Haemophilus influenza B (HIB) vaccine
High intestinal obstruction(s), imaging of, 616
Hip(s), disorders, imaging of, 618
Histamine-1 antagonists, for chemotherapy-induced nausea, 574
Histamine-1 receptor antagonist, for anaphylaxis, 10
Histiocytic disease, signs/symptoms of, 566t
Histoplasma capsulatum, itraconazole for, 833
Histoplasmosis, nonmeningeal, itraconazole for, 833
History, medical
for adolescent health, 121
AMPLE, 89–93
for poison evaluation, 19
psoriasis, 624
urinary tract infections, 476
HIV/AIDS
classification system for, 443t
counseling and testing for, 437–438
immunizations in, 444
in utero exposure to, 439t–441t
itraconazole for, 833
IVIG therapy for, 362
management of, 443–444
mother to child transmission of, 438–442
neonatal management of, 414t
nevirapine for, 442
occupational exposure to, 391
opportunistic infections in, 442–443
perinatal, management of, 438–442
vaccine administration recommendations for, 393
vaccines and, 380–381
zidovudine, 985

HLA (human leukocyte antigen) B27, 626
Holliday-Segar method, 272, 272t, 273b
Homocystinemia, characterization of, 338b
Hookworm
mebendazole for, 855
pyrantel pamoate for, 928
Hot water burns, *Trauma, Burns, and Common Critical Care Emergencies Color Plate 1*
HPV. *See* Human papilloma virus
HSCT. *See* Hematopoietic stem cell transplantation
HSP. *See* Henoch-Schönlein purpura
HSV. *See* Herpes simplex virus
Human albumin (Buminate), formulary entry for, 687
Human bites
common organisms in, 96t
infections from, 422t
Human milk, enteral nutritional components in, 548t–549t
Human papilloma virus (HPV)
for adolescents and young adults, 389
age-based schedule for, 373f
catch-up schedule for, 374f
contraindications/precautions for, 376t–379t
immunoprophylaxis for, 389–390
interval schedule for, 375t
vaccines for, 384
Humatin, formulary entry for, 899–900
HUS. *See* Hemolytic uremic syndrome
HUS/TTP. *See* Hemolytic-uremic syndrome/thrombotic thrombocytopenic purpura
Hyaluronidase (Amphadase, Hydase, Hylenex, Vitrase), formulary entry for, 817
Hycamptin (Topotecan), toxicity of, 1009t
Hydase, formulary entry for, 817
Hydralazine hydrochloride (Apresoline)
formulary entry for, 818
for hypertension, 501t
for hypertensive crisis, 43
for hypertensive emergency, 105t, 818
for renal failure, 1031t
Hydrea (Hydroxyurea), toxicity of, 1007t
Hydrocephalus, management of, 479–480
Hydrochlorothiazide (HCTZ, Hydrodiuril)
formulary entry for, 818
for hypertension, 501t
Hydrocortisone (Colocort, Cortef, Coraid, Micor, Nutracort, Hytone, Locoid, Pandel, Synacort)
for adrenal insufficiency, 256
formulary entry for, 819
for glucocorticoid deficiency, 989
for hyperparathyroidism, 253
for hypoparathyroidism, 252
Hydrocortisone base, 819
Hydrocortisone and ciprofloxacin (Cipro HC Otic), formulary entry for, 749
Hydrocortisone valerate (Westcort), potency ranking of, 995t–996t
Hydrodiuril
formulary entry for, 818
for hypertension, 501t
Hydromorphone HCl (Dilaudid)
characterization of, 140t
formulary entry for, 820
relative potency of, 151t
Hydro-Tussin, formulary entry for, 729–730
Hydroxychloroquine (Plaquenil, Quineprox)
formulary entry for, 820–821
for SLE, 629
Hydroxyprogesterone, normal values for, 267t
7-Hydroxyprogesterone, serum, normal values for, 267t
Hydroxyurea (Hydrea), toxicity of, 1007t
Hydroxyzine (Vistaril)
formulary entry for, 821
properties of, 137
Hylenex, formulary entry for, 817
Hyoscyamine (Anaspaz, Cystospaz), for palliative care, 581t
Hyperammonemia, differential diagnosis of, 313f
Hyperandrogenism, 259
Hyperbilirubinemia
characterization of, 304–305
differential diagnosis of, 305t
Hypercalcemia, calcitonin-salmon for, 721

Hypercoagulable states
causes of, 338b
extended workup for, 338b
presentation of, 335–343
warfarin dosing guidelines for, 339t, 341t–342t
Hyperglycemia, neonatal, management of, 461t
Hyperimmune globulins, 364
Hyperkalemia
algorithm for, 285f
causes of, 284t
Hyperleukocytosis
characterization of, 564
management of, 564–567
Hyperlipidemia, management of, 169
Hypernatremia, 282t
Hypernatremic dehydration, 275f
Hyperparathyroidism, 252–253
Hyperphosphatemia
aluminum hydroxide dosage for, 690
calcium acetate for, 722
Hyperpyrexia, due to poisoning, 20t
Hypertension
chronic
causes of, 498t
classification of, 499t
definitions of, 496
drugs for, 500t–501t
evaluation of, 496–498
treatment of, 498–499, 502
hypokalemia from, 283t
methyldopa for, 853
metoprolol for, 864
nifedipine for, 882
due to poisoning, 20t
propranolol for, 924
Hypertension emergency(ies)
assessment of, 104–105
management of, 105–106
medications for, 105t
Hyperthyroidism, 248–252, 251t
Hypertrophic cardiomyopathy, for myocardial disease, 194
Hyperuricemia
probenecid for, 921
rasburicase for, 933
Hyperviscosity, blood, 976
Hypoalbuminemia, albumin for, 687
Hypocalcemia
calcium carbonate for, 723
calcium gluconate for, 725
characterization of, 284–285
Hypocalcemia *(Continued)*
etiologies of, 286b
magnesium sulfate for, 854
Hypochloremia, arginine for, 702
Hypoglycemia
diazepam for, 768
glucagon HCl for, 813
IEM associated, 312–315
neonatal
management of, 461t
tests for, 264–265
due to poisoning, 22t
Hypoglycemics, toxicity of, 37t
Hypoglycemic seizures, glucose for, 45
Hypokalemia
algorithm for, 285f
aluminum hydroxide induction of, 691
causes of, 283t
Hypomagnesemia
characterization of, 286–287
etiologies of, 287b
magnesium oxide for, 853
magnesium sulfate for, 854
Hyponatremia, 282t
Hyponatremic dehydration
excess electrolyte deficits in, 277
excess sodium in, 278
replacement schedule for, 275f
Hypoparathyroidism, ergocalciferol for, 785
Hypophosphatemia, phosphorus supplements for, 911
Hypoparathyroidism, 252
Hypotension
asthma-associated, 11
phenylephrine for, 908
due to poisoning, 20t
Hypothermia, due to poisoning, 20t
Hypoxia, due to poisoning, 20t
Hytone
for adrenal insufficiency, 256
formulary entry for, 819
for glucocorticoid deficiency, 989
for hyperparathyroidism, 253
for hypoparathyroidism, 252

I

IAP. *See* Intrapartum antimicrobial prophylaxis
IBD. *See* Inflammatory bowel disease
Ibuprofen (Motrin, Advil, NeoProfen), formulary entry for, 821–822

Ichthyosis, characterization of, 214
Idamycin (Idarubicin), toxicity of, 1007t
Idarubicin (idamycin), toxicity of, 1007t
Idiopathic thrombocytic purpura, systemic corticosteroids for, 992
IDM syndrome, dominant cardiac defect in, 184t
IEM. *See* Inborn errors of metabolism
Ifex, toxicity of, 1007t
Ifosfamide, toxicity of, 1007t
Ifotamidemide (isophosphamide, Ifex), toxicity of, 1007t
IGF-1. *See* Insulin-like growth factor-1
IGF-BP3. *See* Insulin-like growth factor-binding protein
IGRA. *See* Interferon gamma release assay
Imatinib (Gleevec), toxicity of, 1007t
Imidazole (Dacarbazine), toxicity of, 1007t
IMIG. *See* Intramuscular immune globulin
Imipenem and cilastin (Primaxin)
  formulary entry for, 823
  with renal failure, 1020t
Imipramine (Tofranil), formulary entry for, 823–824
Immune globulin
  formulary entry for, 824–825
  for HIV/AIDS patients, 362
  for Kawasaki disease, 197–198
Immune thrombocytopenic purpura, IVIG therapy for, 362
Immunization(s)
  for cancer patients, 381, 381t
  guidelines for, 371–374
  for HIV-infected children, 444
  intervals for, 375t
  by intramuscular injection, 81
  for patients on corticosteroids, 382t
  for pregnant patients, 384
  schedules for, 371
    7-year-olds to 18-year-olds, 373f
    catch-up, 374f
    infants to 6-year-olds, 372f
  by subcutaneous injection, 81
Immunodeficiency
  acyclovir dosage and, 685
  evaluation of, 360, 360t–361t
  therapies for, 361–364
Immunoglobulin(s)
  complement pathway for, 367f
  levels of, 368t
  reference values, 364
  serum levels, 364t–366t
Immunoprophylaxis
  combination vaccines, 402–403
  disease-specific recommendations, 384–403
  DTaP, 384–386
  guidelines, for special hosts, 375–384
  HAV, 387–388
  HBV, 388–389
  HIB, 386–387
  HPV, 389–390
  influenza, 390–393
  meningococcal, 395
  MMR vaccine, 393–394
  pneumococcal, 396
  poliomyelitis, 396–397
  rabies vaccines, 397–399
  rotavirus, 400–401
  RSV, 399
  varicella vaccine, 401–402
  websites for, 370
Immunosuppressant(s)
  azathioprine as, 707
  cortisone acetate as, 757
  cyclosporine as, 759–760
  hydrocortisone as, 256
  methylprednisolone as, 10
  prednisone as, 919–920
  sirolimus as, 946–947
  tacrolimus as, 946–947
  topical, pimecrolimus as, 913
Imodium, formulary entry for, 849–850
Impetigo, characterization of, 222
Imuran
  formulary entry for, 707
  with renal failure, 1027t
Inactivated poliovirus (IPV) vaccine
  for cancer patients, 381t
  catch-up schedule for, 374f
  immunoprophylaxis for, 396–397
  for inactivated poliovirus, 396–397

Inactivated poliovirus (IPV) vaccine
(Continued)
interval schedule for, 375t
for pregnant patients, 384
Inapsine, formulary entry for, 778
Inborn errors of metabolism (IEM)
definition of, 310–315
differential diagnosis of, 310
evaluation of, 310
hypoglycemia in, 312–315, 314f
laboratory test for, 311b
management of, 311–312
presentation of, 310
sample collection for, 312t
Increased intracranial pressure (ICP),
emergency care for, 106–107
Inderal
formulary entry for, 924–925
for hemangiomas, 205–206
for hypertension, 500t
for migraines, 512t
Indirect Coombs test, for anemia
diagnosis, 327
Individuals with Disabilities Education
Act (IDEA), 241
Indomethacin (Indocin)
formulary entry for, 825–826
for IVH, 467, 471
for PDA, 467
Infantile proctocolitis, 356
Infantile spasms, 515t
Infant(s)
age-appropriate behavior of,
230t–231t
common infections of, 420t–435t
dermatologic disorders in,
220–222
low birth weight
immunizations for, 355
serum IGG levels for, 365t
pain assessment for
developmental response in, 137
overview of, 140
premature
apnea in, 465
CMV in, 413t
electrolyte requirements for, 462t
exogenous caloric requirements
for, 462
glucose requirements for, 460
hyperglycemia in, 461t
hypoglycemia in, 461t
Infant(s) *(Continued)*
indomethacin for, 466
insensible water loss in, 460t
iron requirements for, 461
necrotizing enterocolitis in, 470
nonventricular arrhythmias in,
176f
PDA in, 466
periventricular leukomalacia in,
471
phototherapy for, 467–468, 468t
varicella in, 414t
thyroid tests for, 250t
ZDV treatment for, 442
Infasurf, formulary entry for, 957
Infection(s)
anaerobic, metronidazole for, 865
bacterial
amoxicillin for, 422t
MRSA, 847
Staphylococcus aureus, 937
from bites, 422t
from blood-borne pathogens,
450–452
catheter-related bloodstream, 423t
cefepime dosage with, 733
chlamydial, 429t
common pediatric
HIV/AIDS, 437–444
management of, 420t–435t
PID as, 437
congenital
cytomegalovirus as, 416
diagnosis of, 405
enterovirus as, 414t, 416
group B streptococcal (GBS) as,
416
HBC as, 416
HBV as, 416
herpes simplex virus as, 410
HSV as, 416
intrauterine as, 410–416
neonatal management of,
412t–414t
parvovirus as, 413t, 416
presentations of, 410
rubella as, 410, 413t, 415–416,
439t–440t
syphilis as, 410, 412t, 415,
439t–440t
toxoplasmosis as, 408t–409t, 410,
415

Infection(s) *(Continued)*
varicella as, 414t, 444
VZV as, 416
fever with localizing source of, 410, 411f, 436f
fungal and yeast, 450
group B streptococcal
diagnosis of, 416
IAP for, 417f–419f
hepatic, 305t
HIV/AIDS as
classification system for, 443t
counseling and testing for, 437–438
immunizations in, 444
in utero exposure to, 438–442, 439t–441t
IVIG therapy for, 362
management of, 443–444
opportunistic infections in, 442–443
perinatal, management of, 438–442
in internationally adopted children, 452
intrauterine, 410
meropenem for, 857
from mucous membrane exposure, 450
from needlesticks, 450
from PEP exposure, 450–452
perinatal viral, 405
diagnosis of, 405
neonatal management of, 412t–414t
presentations of, 410–415
from postspinal fusion, 429t
red cell aplasia and, 327
sexual, 122
sexually transmitted, 429t
skin
meropenem for, 857
uncomplicated, linezolid for, 847
tick-borne, 446–450
anaplasmosis as, 449
ehrlichiosis as, 449
Lyme disease as, 446–448
Rocky Mountain spotted fever as, 448–449
tuberculosis as
drug therapy for, 445–446, 447t
testing for, 444–445, 446b

Infection(s) *(Continued)*
urinary tract
culture-positive, 481–482
evaluation of, 479–483
imaging of, 617
initial treatment of, 420t–435t
levofloxacin for, 843
medical history of, 476
phenazopyridine for, 907
vaginal, 124t
from ventriculoperitoneal shunts, 435t
Infiltrate, 609
Inflammation
chronic, anemia of, 328
ibuprofen for, 822
indomethacin for, 825
methylprednisolone for, 862
Inflammatory bowel disease (IBD)
classification of, 298–299
metronidazole for, 866
Influenza
amantadine hydrochloride for, 691
chemoprophylaxis for, 392–393
immunoprophylaxis for, 390–393
initial management of, 425t
vaccine for, 384, 392t
Influenza A
amantadine hydrochloride for, 691
rimantadine for, 938
INH
formulary entry for, 831
with renal failure, 1020t
for tuberculosis, 447t
Inhalants, toxicity of, 47b–48b
Inhalation burns, 98t
Inhalation injuries, due to poisoning, 26
Inhaled ribavirin, formulary entry for, 936
Inspiratory pressures, maximal, measurement of, 587–588
Insulin
for diabetes, 245f
formulary entry for, 826
products of, 997t
for renal failure, 1031t
for resuscitation, ii
Insulin-like growth factor-1 (IGF-1), normal values for, 267t
Insulin-like growth factor-binding protein (IGF-Bp3), normal values for, 268t

Intal, formulary entry for, 757
Intellectual disability (ID)
characterization of, 236
classification of, 237t
Interferon gamma release assay (IGRA), 444–445
Intracellular fluid composition, 276t
Intracranial pressure, oncologic-associated, characterization of, 568
Intractable epilepsy, formulas for, 558t
Intramuscular immune globulin (IMIG), 363
Intraosseous (IO) infusion, vascular access for, 63–65, 65f
Intrapartum antimicrobial prophylaxis (IAP), 417f–418f
Intraspinal lesions, examination of, 505
Intrauterine infections, 410
Intravenous immune globulin (IVIG), 361–362
for Kawasaki disease, 197–198
for unconjugated hyperbilirubinemia in newborns, 467
Intraventricular hemorrhages (IVH), neonatal, 471
Intubation
asthma treatment with, 11
indications for, 3–7
paralysis for, with succinylcholine, 951
treatment algorithm for, 5f
Intussusception, imaging of, 616–617
Invanz
formulary entry for, 786–787
with renal failure, 1017t
Invasive aspergillosis, voriconazole for, 982
Invasive candidasis, micafungin sodium for, 866
Iodide. *See* Potassium iodide
Iodine
in formulas, 542t
in multivitamin tablets, analysis of, 546t
Iohexol (Omnipaque), formulary entry for, 826–827
Ipratropium bromide (Atrovent)
for allergic rhinitis, 355–356
for asthma, 10
formulary entry for, 827–828
IPV vaccine. *See* Inactivated poliovirus (IPV) vaccine
Iquix
formulary entry for, 842–843
for PID, 432t
with renal failure, 1021t
Irbesartan, for hypertension, 500t
Irinotecan (Camptosar, IRN), toxicity of, 1007t
IRN (irinotecan), toxicity of, 1007t
Iron (Fe)
in cow's milk formulas, 550t–555t
DRIs for, 542t
in enteral formulas, 548t–557t
in formulas, 542t
in human milk, 548t–549t
in infant formula, 548t–553t
in multivitamin drops, analysis of, 545t
in multivitamin tablets, analysis of, 546t
newborns' requirements for, 461
reference values for, 644t
supplementation, 544–545
toxicity of, 38t
Iron deficiency anemia
iron dextran for, 829
iron sucrose for, 829
iron—oral preparations for, 830
Iron dextran. *See* Iron—injectable preparations
Iron sucrose. *See* Iron—injectable preparations
Iron-deficiency anemia, 322
Iron—injectable preparations, formulary entry for, 829–830
Iron—oral preparations, formulary entry for, 830–831
Irradiated blood products, 349
Islet cell autoantibodies, diabetes-associated, 243
Isonatremic dehydration, 275f, 276
Isoniazid (INH, Nydrazid, Laniazid)
formulary entry for, 831
with renal failure, 1020t
for tuberculosis, 447t
Isophosphamide (Ifosfamide), toxicity of, 1007t
Isoproterenol (Isuprel), formulary entry for, 832
Isoptin, renal with renal failure, 1034t

Isopto Carpine, formulary entry for, 912–913
Isopto Hyoscine, formulary entry for, 942
Isotretinoin (Accutane, Amnesteem, Claravis, Sotret)
  for acne vulgaris, 218–220
  formulary entry for, 832
Isradipine, for hypertension, 500t
Itraconazole (Sporanox), formulary entry for, 833
IVH. *See* Intraventricular hemorrhages
IVIG. *See* Intravenous immune globulin

J

Jantoven
  dosing adjustments for, 340t
  dosing guidelines for, 340t
  excessive anticoagulation by, 342t
  formulary entry for, 983–984
  international normalized ratio for, 341t
  medications influencing, 343b
  toxicity of, 52–53
Jaundice
  due to poisoning, 22t
  transient neonatal, 305t
JIA. *See* Juvenile idiopathic arthritis
Joint fluid analysis
  algorithm for, 624f
  for reactive arthritis diagnosis, 626
Jugular vein(s)
  external, puncture of, 58–59
  internal, catheter placement in, 62
Juvenile dermatomyositis, 634–635
Juvenile idiopathic arthritis (JIA)
  characterization of, 623
  classical divisions of, 625t
  ethancept for, 790
Juvenile myoclonic epilepsy, 515t
Juvenile rheumatoid arthritis (JRA)
  autoantibodies associated with, 621t
  ethancept for, 790
  indomethacin for, 825
  naproxen sodium as, 877
  penicillamine for, 901
  sulfasalazine for, 955

K

K+. *See* Potassium
Kanamycin (Kantrex)
  formulary entry for, 833–834
  with renal failure, 1020t
  for tuberculosis, 447t
Kantrex
  formulary entry for, 833–834
  with renal failure, 1020t
  for tuberculosis, 447t
Kaopectate
  formulary entry for, 716–717
  with renal failure, 1027t
Karyotyping
  for genetic abnormalities, 315
  indications for, 320
Kawasaki disease
  characterization of, 196–198
  clinical features of, 631t
  IVIG therapy for, 362
  management of, 197–198
  osteomalacia in, 253
  rickets in, 253
Kayexalate, formulary entry for, 949
Keflex
  for cellulitis, 423t
  formulary entry for, 740
  for influenza, 425t
  for lymphadenitis, 425t
  with renal failure, 1016t
Kemstro, formulary entry for, 711–712
Kenalog, formulary entry for, 969
Keppra
  for seizures, 516t
  for renal failure, 1031t
Keratolytics (lactic acid, salicylic acid, tretinoin), for warts, 207t
Kerion
  characterization of, 215
Ketamine (Ketalar)
  formulary entry for, 834–835
  properties of, 145
  for RSI, 6t
  toxicity of, 46b
Ketoacidosis, in diabetes, 243
Ketoconazole (Nizoral, Nizoral A-D), formulary entry for, 834–835
Ketones, in urine, 477
Ketorolac (Toradol, Acular)
  characterization of, 139
  formulary entry for, 835–836
Ketotifen fumarate ophthalmic, 1002t
Kidney(s)
  sodium deficits and, 282t
  stones, 502
  transplants, 875

Kinrix, immunoprophylaxis for, 402
Kionex, formulary entry for, 949
Klinefelter syndrome, characterization of, 318
Klonopin
formulary entry for, 753
for seizures, 516t
Kondremul, formulary entry for, 869
Konsyl, formulary entry for, 927
K-PHOS, formulary entry for, 911
Kruskall-Wallis test, 653t
Kytril, formulary entry for, 814

L

Labetalol (Normodyne, Trandate)
formulary entry for, 836
for hypertensive emergency, 105t
Labor, ZDV treatment during, 442
Laceration repair, basic, 81–84
skin staples for, 84
suturing for, 81–84
tissue adhesives for, 84
Laceration(s), body region risks in, 82f
Lactate, reference values for, 644t
Lactate dehydrogenase (LDH)
for anemia diagnosis, 327
reference values for, 644t
Lactic acid, for warts, 207t
Lactose intolerance, formulas for, 558t
Lactulose (Cephulac, Chronulac, Enulose), formulary entry for, 836–837
LAIV. *See* Live intranasal influenza vaccine
Lamictal
formulary entry for, 837–840
for seizures, 516t
Lamisil granules, for tinea capitis, 215
Lamivudine (Epivir, 3TC)
formulary entry for, 837
with renal failure, 1021t
Lamotrigine (Lamictal)
formulary entry for, 837–840
for seizures, 516t
Laniazid
formulary entry for, 831
with renal failure, 1020t
for tuberculosis, 447t
Lanoxicaps
formulary entry for, 770
with renal failure, 1029t
toxicity of, 48
Lanoxin
formulary entry for, 770
with renal failure, 1029t
Lansoprazole (Prevacid), formulary entry for, 840–841
Lariam, formulary entry for, 856
Laryngoscope blade, use of, 4
Laryngotracheobronchitis, emergency-associated, 12–13
Lasix
formulary entry for, 809–810
for hypertension, 501t
for hyperthyroidism, 251t
for renal failure, 1030t
L-Asp (asparaginase), toxicity of, 1006t
Late syphilis, initial treatment of, 433t
Lateral recumbent position, opening pressure for, 648t
Laxative(s)
aluminum hydroxide as, 691
bisacodyl as, 716
docusate as, 774–775
glycerin as, 813
lactulose as, 691
magnesium citrate as, 852
magnesium hydroxide as, 853
mineral oil as, 869
polyethylene glycol as, 915
psyllium as, 927
senna as, 943
sodium phosphate as, 948–949
Lax-Pills, formulary entry for, 943
L-Carnitine, formulary entry for, 730
Lead, reference values for, 644t
Lead chelation therapy, 901
Lead poisoning(s)
blood testing guidelines for, 50t
characterization of, 49–51
chelation therapy for, 50t
Learning disabilities (LDs), 236
Left bundle-branch block (LBBB), 180t
Length, weight and
for boys, 527f–528f
degree conversion for, 650

Length, weight and *(Continued)*
  for girls, 525f–526f
  for preterm infants, 533f
Lennox-Gastaut syndrome, topiramate for, 967
Leucovorin, as chemotherapy adjunct, 1009t
Leukemia, signs/symptoms of, 565t
Leukocytes, age-specific differentials for, 333t
Leukocyte-poor PRBCs, 348–349
Leustatin (Cladribine), toxicity of, 1006t
Levalbuterol (Xopenex), formulary entry for, 841
Levaquin
  formulary entry for, 842–843
  for PID, 432t
  with renal failure, 1021t
Levetiracetam (Keppra)
  formulary entry for, 841–842
  for renal failure, 1031t
  for seizures, 516t
Levocarnitine, formulary entry for, 730
Levocetirizine (Xyzal), for allergic rhinitis, 355–356
Levofloxacin (Levauin, Quixin, Iquix)
  formulary entry for, 842–843
  for PID, 429t
  with renal failure, 1021t
Levophed, formulary entry for, 105t
Levothyroxine (T_4, Synthroid), formulary entry for, 843–844
Lexapro (Escitalopram), dosage/side effects for, 1004t
LH. *See* Luteinizing hormone
Lialda, formulary entry for, 857
Lidex, potency ranking of, 995t
Lidocaine (Xylocaine, L-M-X, Lidoderm)
  characterization of, 141t
  formulary entry for, 844–845
  for IV infusions, i
  for RSI, 6t
Lidocaine and prilocaine, formulary entry for, 845–846
Lidoderm
  characterization of, 141t
  formulary entry for, 844–845
  for IV infusions, i
  for RSI, 6t
Likelihood ratio, 657
Limit setting, need for, 231t
Lindane (Gamma benzene hexachloride), formulary entry for, 846
Linezolid (Zyvox), formulary entry for, 847
Lioresal, formulary entry for, 711–712
Lipase, reference values for, 644t
Lipids, reference values for, 645t
Lipid monitoring recommendations
  goals for, 169
  hyperlipidemia management in, 169
  screening criteria for, 168–169
Liquid Pred
  for asthma, 10
  dose equivalence for, 992t
  formulary entry for, 919–920
Lisdexamfetamine, formulary entry for, 847–848
Lisinopril (Prinivil, Zestril)
  formulary entry for, 848
  for hypertension, 500t, 848
  for renal failure, 1031t
Literacy milestones, 230t
Lithium (Lithobid, Eskalith)
  formulary entry for, 849
  for renal failure, 1031t
Live intranasal influenza vaccine (LAIV), interval schedule for, 375t
Liver
  acute failure of
    arginine chloride contraindicated for, 702
    characterization of, 301–304
  factor sites, 345b
  function studies of
    components of, 301
    evaluation of, 302t–303t
  hepatitis of, 304t
  hyperbilirubinemia of, 304–305, 305t
Liver cells. *See* Hepatocytes
LLSB, 168
LMA (laryngeal mask airway), indications for, 3
L-M-X
  characterization of, 141t
  formulary entry for, 844–845
  for IV infusions, i
  for RSI, 6t

Local anesthetics
  analgesic properties of, 139–142
  commonly used, 141t, 142t
  toxicity of, 139–142
Locoid
  for adrenal insufficiency, 256
  formulary entry for, 819
  for glucocorticoid deficiency, 989
  for hyperparathyroidism, 253
  for hypoparathyroidism, 252
Lodoxamide tromethamine ophthalmic (Alomide), 1000t
Loeys-Dietz, dominant cardiac defect in, 184t
Lomustine (CCNU), toxicity of, 1008t
Long arm posterior splinting, 85
Long bones, trauma to, 94–96
Loniten
  formulary entry for, 870–871
  for hypertension, 501t
  for hypertensive emergency, 105t
Loperamide (Imodium), formulary entry for, 849–850
Lopressor
  formulary entry for, 864
  for hypertension, 500t
Loracarbef (Lorabid), with renal failure, 1022t
Loratadine (Claritin)
  for allergic rhinitis, 355–356
  for renal failure, 1029t
Loratadine and pseudoephedrine (Claritin), formulary entry for, 850
Lorazepam (Ativan)
  for chemotherapy-induced nausea, 574
  formulary entry for, 851
  for palliative care, 581t
Losartan (Cozaar)
  formulary entry for, 851–852
  for hypertension, 500t, 851
Lotrimin, formulary entry for, 867
Lotrimin AF, formulary entry for, 754–755
Lovenox
  formulary entry for, 780–782
  with renal failure, 1030t
Low-molecular-weight heparin, 340. *See* Enoxaparin
Loxosceles recluse, toxicity of, 53–54
L-PAM (Melphalan), toxicity of, 1008t
LSD intoxication, 46
Lumbar puncture(s), for blood fluid sampling, 70–72, 71f
Luminal
  for conjugated hyperbilirubinemia, 469
  formulary entry for, 907
  with renal failure, 1033t
  for seizures, 516t
  for status epilepticus, 17
Lung(s)
  chest radiography of, 190
  imaging of, 614f–615f
  volume readings of, 590t
Luride, formulary entry for, 800–801
LUSB, 168
Luteinizing hormone (LH), delayed puberty caused by, 260
Luvox (fluvoxamine), dosage/side effects for, 1004t
Luxiq foam, potency ranking of, 995t
Lyme disease, 446–448
  characterization of, 199
Lymphadenitis, initial management of, 425t
Lymphoma, signs/symptoms of, 565t
Lysosomal disorders, characterization of, 319

M
Maalox, formulary entry for, 690–691
Macrobid, formulary entry for, 882–883
Macrodantin, formulary entry for, 882–883
MAG-3. *See* Mercaptoacetyl triglycine
Magnesium (Mg^{2+})
  DRIs for, 543t
  in formulas, 543t
  in multivitamin tablets, analysis of, 547t
  parenteral nutrition formulations, 561t
  reference values for, 645t
  serum disturbances of, 286–287
Magnesium citrate, formulary entry for, 852

Magnesium hydroxide
with aluminum hydroxide, formulary entry for, 690–691
formulary entry for, 852–853
Magnesium oxide, formulary entry for, 853
Magnesium sulfate (Epsom salts)
asthma treatment with, 11
formulary entry for, 853–854
for resuscitation, ii
Malar rash, in SLE, 628t
Malaria
hydroxychloroquine for, 820–821
prophylaxis
chloroquine HCl/phosphate for, 742
mefloquine for, 856
quinidine for, 931
primaquine phosphate for, 920
Manganese
DRIs for, 543t
in formulas, 543t
in multivitamin tablets, analysis of, 547t
Mannitol (Osmitrol, Resectisol), formulary entry for, 854
Mann-Whitney U test, 653t
MAOIs (monoamine oxidase inhibitors), toxicity of, 32t
Marfan syndrome
characterization of, 317
dominant cardiac defect in, 184t
Marijuana, characterization of, 46b
Marinol
for chemotherapy-induced nausea, 574
formulary entry for, 778
Mastication muscles, tests for, 505t
Mastoiditis, initial management of, 425t
Matulane (Procarbazine), toxicity of, 1008t
Maxidex
for airway edema, 991
for bacterial meningitis, 447t
for chemotherapy-induced nausea, 574
formulary entry for, 766–767
for idiopathic thrombocytic purpura, 992
potency of, 992t
Maxipime
formulary entry for, 733
with renal failure, 1015t
Maxivate, formulary entry for, 714
Maxolon
for chemotherapy-induced nausea, 574
formulary entry for, 863
with renal failure, 1032t
toxicity of, 29t
MBC. *See* Minimum bactericidal concentrations
MCNS. *See* Minimal changes nephrotic syndrome
MCV4. *See* Meningococcal conjugate vaccine
Measles prophylaxis
IMIG therapy for, 363
Measles, mumps, and rubella (MMR) vaccine
age-based schedule for, 373f
for cancer patients, 381t
catch-up schedule for, 374f
contraindications/precautions for, 378t
immunoprophylaxis for, 393–394
Mebendazole (Vermox), formulary entry for, 854–855
Mechlorethamine (nitrogen mustard, mustine, mustargen), toxicity of, 1008t
Meckel diverticulum, imaging of, 616–617
Mediastinal masses, imaging of, 611
Medical literature, biostatistics for, 652–657
Medication administration
by intramuscular injection, 81
by subcutaneous injections, 81
Medrol
for anaphylaxis, 991
for asthma, 10
formulary entry for, 862–863
Medroxyprogesterone (Depo-Provera, Provera, Depp-Sub Q Provera), formulary entry for, 855
Mefloquine HCl (Lariam), formulary entry for, 856
Mefoxin
for gonorrhea, 430t
with renal failure, 1015t

Mellaril, formulary entry for, 963
Melphalan, toxicity of, 1008t
Memory making, 578
Meningitis
ampicillin/sulbactam for, 701
cefotaxime dosage with, 1015t
cefotaxime for, 734
cefepime for, 733
ceftriaxone for, 738
meropenem for, 857
Meningococcal conjugate vaccine (MCV4)
for adolescents and young adults, 384
for cancer patients, 381t
contraindications/precautions for, 376t–379t
immunoprophylaxis, 395
interval schedule for, 375t
Men's Rogaine Extra Strength
formulary entry for, 870–871
for hypertension, 501t
for hypertensive emergency, 105t
Mental changes, as death approaches, 580
Mental health
disorders of, 239–241
screenings of, 232t
Mental status, examination of, 504
Mentzer index, 322
Meperidine HCl (Demerol)
for analgesia, 140t
characterization of, 140t
relative potency of, 151t
for renal failure, 1032t
toxicity of, 28t
Mephyton
DRIs for, 542t
formulary entry for, 912
in multivitamin drops, analysis of, 545t
in multivitamin tablets, analysis of, 546t
Mercaptoacetyl triglycine (MAG-3), for UTI evaluation, 481
Mercaptopurine (6-MP), toxicity of, 1008t
Meropenem (Merrem)
formulary entry for, 858
with renal failure, 1022t
Mesalamine (Asacol, Canasa, Lialda, Pentasa, Rowasa, FIV-ASA, 5-aminosalicylic acid, 5-ASA), formulary entry for, 857
Mesna, as chemotherapy adjunct, 1009t
Metabolism
inborn errors of, 310–315
definition of, 310–315
differential diagnosis of, 310
evaluation of, 310
hypoglycemia in, 312–315, 314f
laboratory test for, 311b
management of, 311–312
presentation of, 310
sample collection for, 312t
Metadate
for ADHD, 239t
for anaphylaxis, 991
for asthma, 10
formulary entry for, 862–863
Metamucil, formulary entry for, 927
Metformin (Glucophage, Fortamet, Riomet)
for diabetes, 247
formulary entry for, 858
for polycystic ovarian syndrome, 259
Methadone HCl (Dolophine, Methadose)
for analgesia, 140t
formulary entry for, 859
relative potency of, 151t
with renal failure, 1032t
as sedative-hypnotic antidote, 47
toxicity of, 28t
Methemoglobin, reference values for, 645t
Methemoglobinemia
methylene blue for, 860
toxicity of, 51–52
Methimazole (Tapazole)
formulary entry for, 856–857
for Graves disease, 250
Methotrexate (MTX, Amethoplerin, Folex, Mexate), toxicity of, 1008t
Methyldopa
formulary entry for, 860
with renal failure, 1032t
Methylene blue (Urolene Blue)
formulary entry for, 860
for methemoglobinemia, 51

Methylin
Methylphenidate HCl (Ritalin, Methylin, Metadate, Concerta, Daytrana)
  for ADHD, 239t
  formulary entry for, 860–862
Methylprednisolone (Medrol)
  for anaphylaxis, 10, 991
  for asthma, 10
  formulary entry for, 862–863
  potency of, 992t
  for spinal cord injury, 991–992
Methylxanthines
  adenosine with, 686
  asthma treatment with, 11
Metoclopramide (Reglan, Maxolon)
  for chemotherapy-induced nausea, 574
  formulary entry for, 863
  with renal failure, 1032t
  toxicity of, 29t
Metolazone (Zaroxolyn)
  for *C.* colitis, 976
  formulary entry for, 863–864
Metoprolol (Lopressor, Toprol-XL)
  formulary entry for, 864
  for hypertension, 500t
MetroCream, formulary entry for, 865–866
MetroGel
  for acne vulgaris, 218t
  for bacterial vaginosis, 422t
  formulary entry for, 865–866
  for gastroenteritis, 218t
  neonatal critical care dosing of, 1010t
  for PID, 432t
  with renal failure, 1022t
MetroLotion, formulary entry for, 865–866
Metronidazole (Flagyl, Protostat, MetroGel, MetroLotion, MetroCream, Noritate)
  for acne vulgaris, 218t
  for bacterial vaginosis, 422t
  formulary entry for, 865–866
  for gastroenteritis, 218t
  neonatal critical care dosing of, 1010t
  for PID, 432t
  with renal failure, 1022t
Mexate (methotrexate), toxicity of, 1008t
Mg^{2+}. *See* Magnesium
MI. *See* Myocardial infarction
Miacalcin, formulary entry for, 721–722
MIC. *See* Minimum inhibitory concentrations
Micafungin sodium (Mycamine), formulary entry, 866–867
Micatin, formulary entry for, 867
Miconazole (Monistat, Micatin, Lotrimin, AF, M-Zole, Vagistat-3), formulary entry for, 867
Micor
  for adrenal insufficiency, 256
  for glucocorticoid deficiency, 989
  for hyperparathyroidism, 253
  for hypoparathyroidism, 252
Microscopic polyangiitis, 631t
Microbiology, 405
Midazolam (Versed)
  formulary entry for, 868
  with renal failure, 1032t
  for RSI, 6t
  for sedation, 151t
Midsystolic click, 165
Migraine headache(s), 510–511
  abortive tiptans for, 510t
  absorptive triptans for, 504
  preventive therapies for, 512t
  propranolol for, 924
  valproic acid for, 975
Miliaria, characterization of, 220
Milrinone (Primacor)
  formulary entry for, 869
  with renal failure, 1032t
Mineral(s)
  DIRs for, 542t
  newborns' requirements for, 460–461
Mineral oil (Kondremul, Fleet Mineral Oil), formulary entry for, 869
Mineralocorticoid deficiency, 989–991
Minimal changes nephrotic syndrome (MCNS), 492–493
Minimum bactericidal concentrations (MBC), 405
Minimum inhibitory concentrations (MIC), 405
Minocin
  for acne vulgaris, 218t
  formulary entry for, 870
Minocycline (Minocin, Dynacin, Arestin)
  for acne vulgaris, 218t
  formulary entry for, 870

Minoxidil (Loniten, Rogaine, Men's Rogaine Extra Strength)
formulary entry for, 870–871
for hypertension, 501t
for hypertensive emergency, 105t
Mintox, formulary entry for, 690–691
Miosis, due to poisoning, 21t
MiralLax, formulary entry for, 915
Mirtazapine (Remeron), dosage/side effects for, 1005t
Mitochondrial disorders, characterization of, 319–320
Mitoxantrone (dihydroxyanthracenedione dihydrochloride, Novantrone), toxicity of, 1008t
MMR. *See* Measles, mumps, and rubella (MMR) vaccine
Mobitz type I, 178t
Mobitz type II, 179t
Molluscum contagiosum, 202f–203f, *Dermatology Color Plate 1*
morphology of, 207
treatment for, 207
Molybdenum
DRIs for, 543t
in formulas, 543t
in multivitamin tablets, analysis of, 547t
Mometasone (Asmanex twisthaler, Elocon, Nasonex)
for allergic rhinitis, 355–356
daily dose recommendations for, 804t–805t, 993t
formulary entry for, 871–872
potency ranking of, 995t
Mometasone furoate and formoterol fumarate (Dulera), formulary entry for, 872
Mongolian spots, characterization of, 222
Monistat, formulary entry for, 867
Monoclonal factor VIII, 350
Montelukast (Singulair), formulary entry for, 872–873
Morganella spp., sensitivity profile of, 408t
Morphine sulfate (Roxanol, MS Contin, Oramorph SR)
for analgesia, 140t
characterization of, 140t
Morphine sulfate (Roxanol, MS Contin, Oramorph SR) *(Continued)*
formulary entry for, 878
for palliative care, 581t
paregoric comparison to, 899
relative potency of, 151t
with renal failure, 1032t
Motor evaluation, 504
Motor neuron findings, 505t
Motrin, formulary entry for, 821–822
Mouth pharynx, tests for, 505t
Mouth-to-mouth breathing, description of, 7–8
Movement, examination of, 507
Moxifloxacin hydrochloride ophthalmic, 1002t
6-MP (mercaptopurine), toxicity of, 1008t
MRSA infection(s), linezolid for, 847
MS Contin
for analgesia, 140t
characterization of, 140t
formulary entry for, 878
for palliative care, 581t
relative potency of, 151t
with renal failure, 1032t
MTX (methotrexate), toxicity of, 1008t
Mucomyst, formulary entry for, 684
Mucosol, formulary entry for, 684
Mucous membrane exposure, infections from, 450
Multiple regression by least squares method, 653t
Multivitamin(s)
drops, analysis of, 545t
tablets, analysis of, 545t
Murine Ear, formulary entry for, 728–729
Murpirocin (Bactroban), formulary entry for, 874
Muscle bulk, examination of, 504
Musculoskeletal repair, splinting procedures for, 85–87
Musculoskeletal screening(s), for adolescents, 134f
Mustargen, toxicity of, 1008t
Mustine (mechlorethamine), toxicity of, 1008t
Mustargen (mechlorethamine), toxicity of, 1008t

Myambutol
  formulary entry for, 791
  with renal failure, 1017t
Myasthenia gravis, pyrethrins dosage for, 929
Mycamine, formulary entry, 866–867
Mycelex, formulary entry for, 754–755
Mycifradin, formulary entry for, 878
Mycobacterium avium complex
  clarithromycin for, 752
  rifabutin for, 936
  tuberculosis with, pyrazinamide for, 447t, 928
Mycobutin
  formulary entry for, 936–937
  with renal failure, 1023t
Mycophenolate mofetil (CellCept), formulary entry for, 874–875
Mycophenolate sodium (Myfortic), formulary entry for, 874–875
Mycostatin, formulary entry for, 886
Mydriasis, due to poisoning, 21t
Myfortic, formulary entry for, 874–875
Mylanta, formulary entry for, 690–691
Mylanta Gas, formulary entry for, 945–946
Myleran (busulfan), toxicity of, 1006t
Mylicon, formulary entry for, 945–946
Myocardial disease
  characterization of, 191–195
  myocarditis as, 195
Myocardial infarction (MI)
  in children, 180–181
  sequential changes during, 181f
Myocarditis, characterization of, 195
Myoglobin, in urine, 477
Mysoline
  formulary entry for, 920–921
  with renal failure, 1033t
M-Zole, formulary entry for, 867

N

Na$^+$. *See* Sodium
N-acetylcysteine (NAC), as acetaminophen antidote, 29t
Nafcillin (Unipen, Nallpen)
  formulary entry for, 876
  for osteomyelitis, 426t
  septic arthritis, 429t
Nallpen, formulary entry for, 876
Naloxone (Narcan)
  administration of, 148b
  as antidote, 37t
  coma treatment with, 14
  formulary entry for, 876–877
  for resuscitation, ii
  for sedation reversal, 146, 874
Naproxen sodium (Aleve, Anaprox, Naprelan), formulary entry for, 877–878
Narcan
  administration of, 148b
  as antidote, 37t
  coma treatment with, 14
  formulary entry for, 876–877
  for resuscitation, ii
  for sedation reversal, 146, 874
Narcotics, toxidrome of, 25t
Nasalcrom, formulary entry for, 757
Nasarel
  daily dose recommendations for, 804t–805t, 993t
  formulary entry for, 800
Nasacort, formulary entry for, 969
Nasoduodenal tube(s), placement of, 617
Nasonex
  daily dose recommendations for, 804t–805t, 993t
  formulary entry for, 871–872
  potency ranking of, 995t
Nafcillin, for dacrocystitis, 423t
Nausea and vomiting
  chemotherapy-induced
    cannabinoids for, 574
    chlorpromazine for, 574
    dexamethasone for, 574
    diphenhydramine for, 574
    dronabinol for, 574
    granisetron for, 814
    histamine-1 antagonists for, 574
    lorazepam for, 574
    metoclopramide for, 574
    promethazine for, 574
    serotonin (5-HT$_3$) for, 574
    substance P for, 575
    systemic corticosteroids for, 991
    treatments for, 574–575
  in dying patients, 581t
  postoperative
    dolasetron for, 775
    granisetron for, 775
    metoclopramide for, 863

Nausea and vomiting *(Continued)*
radiation-induced, dolasetron for, 775
zinc salts for, 986
Navelbine (vinorelbine), toxicity of, 1009t
Nebcin
formulary entry for, 965–966
with renal failure, 1024t
Nebulization
sodium chloride for, 948
terbutaline in, 959
NebuPent
for antimicrobial prophylaxis, 575t
formulary entry for, 905
with renal failure, 1023t
Neck, trauma to, 100
secondary survey of, 90t
Necrotizing enterocolitis, 470
Nedocromil sodium ophthalmic (Alocril), 1000t
Needlesticks, infections from, 450
Negative predictive value, 657
Neisseria meningitidis prophylaxis, rifampin dosage for, 937
Nembutal
formulary entry for, 905–906
for sedation, 147t
Neo-Fradin, formulary entry for, 878
Neomycin sulfate (Mycifradin, Neo-Fradin, Neo-TABs)
formulary entry for, 878
ophthalmic use of, 1000t
Neomycin/polymyxin B/bacitracin (Neosporin), formulary entry for, 878–879
Neonatal abstinence syndrome, 472
Neonatal alloimmune thrombocytopenia (NAIT), 306
Neonatal apnea
causes of, 466f
characterization of, 465
theophylline for, 957
Neonatal enterocolitis, imaging of, 615–617
Neonatal hemorrhagic disease, phytonadione for, 912
Neonatal infant pain scale (NIPS), 137
Neonatal seizures, 515t
Neonate(s)
acne in
characterization of, 220
apnea in, 465, 466f
Neonate(s) *(Continued)*
assessment of, 210
anomalies and malformations, 459–460
Apgar scores in, 205
Ballard scores in, 456–459
birth trauma, 459
vital signs in, 205–206
bradycardia in, 465
calcium gluconate dosage for, 725
cardiac diseases in, 466–467
common infections of, 420t–435t
cyanosis in, 462
electrolyte requirements of, 462t
extradural fluid collections in, 459f
GI diseases in, 470–471
glucose requirements of, 460
Hb electrophoresis patterns in, 328t
hematologic diseases in, 467–470
conjugated hyperbilirubinemia as, 469
polycythemia as, 469–470
unconjugated hyperbilirubinemia as, 467–469
hypoglycemia in, tests for, 264–265
infection management for, 412t–414t
magnesium disturbances in, 287b
mineral and vitamin requirements of, 460–461
neurologic diseases in, 471–472
nutritional requirements of, 462
rashes in, evolution of, 221f
respiratory diseases in
general considerations for, 463
PPHN as, 463–465
RDS as, 463
resuscitation of, 455, 456f
ROP in, 473–474
thrombocytopenia in, 306
transient jaundice in, 305t
water loss in, 460t
water requirements of, 461t
ZDV treatment for, 442
Neonatology websites, 455
NeoProfen, formulary entry for, 821–822
Neoral, formulary entry for, 759–760
Neosporin (Poly B sulfate, bacitracin zinc, neomycin sulfate)
formulary entry for, 878–879
ophthalmic use of, 1000t

Neostigmine (Prostigmin)
  formulary entry for, 879
  with renal failure, 1032t
Neo-Synephrine, formulary entry for, 693
Neo-TABs, formulary entry for, 878
Nephrology
  acute dialysis in, 494–495
  acute kidney in, 494
  chronic hypertension in
    causes of, 498t
    characterization of, 496–499
    classification of, 499t
    drugs for, 500t–501t
    treatment of, 502
  chronic kidney disease in, 495–496
  glomerular diseases in, 492–493
  nephrolithiasis in, 499–502
  renal disease, clinical manifestations of, 487–492
    edema as, 490
    hematuria as, 487, 488f–489f
    oliguria as, 490–492, 492t
    proteinuria as, 487–490, 491f
  renal functioning test in, 483–486
    creatinine clearance as, 483–484
    glomerular function as, 484, 484t
    tubular, 485–486, 486t, 490t
  tubular disorders in, 486–487
  urinalysis in
    dipstick method, 476–477
    microscopy for, 477–478
  urinary tract infections in
    cultures for, 480–483
    evaluation of, 479–483
    history of, 476
    laboratory studies for, 479–480
    physical examination of, 479
  websites for, 476
Nephrotic syndrome, mycophenolate for, 875
Nerve(s), impairment of, 506f
Nervous system, instability of, due to poisoning, 21t
Neupogen, formulary entry for, 796
Neuraminidase inhibitors, for influenza, 425t
Neuroblastoma, signs/symptoms of, 565t
Neuroimaging
  for developmental disorders, 236
  headache evaluation with, 509
Neurokinin-1 antagonist, for chemotherapy-induced nausea, 575
Neurologic disorder(s)
  ataxia as, 520
  headaches as, 507–511
    classification of, 507
    evaluation of, 507–509, 508b
  hydrocephalus as, 518–520
  intraventricular hemorrhages as, 471
  migraine headaches as, 510–511
  neonatal abstinence syndrome, 472
  paroxysmal events as, 511–518
  peripheral nerve injuries as, 472
  periventricular leukomalacia as, 471
  sensory associated, 504–506
  in SLE, 628t
  stroke as, 520–522
    etiology of, 520
    initial workup for, 521
    management of, 521–522
Neurologic emergency(ies)
  altered states of consciousness, 13–16
  management of, 13–17
Neurologic examination(s)
  for cerebellar function, 507b
  coordination, 507
  cranial nerves, 505t
  mental status, 504
  motor skills, 504
  movement, 507
  sensory norms, 504
  tendon reflexes, 506–507
Neurologic trauma, secondary survey of, 90t
Neurology, websites for, 504
Neuromuscular blockers, for RSI, 7t
Neuromuscular maturity, 456–457
Neurontin
  formulary entry for, 810–811
  for renal failure, 1030t
  for seizures, 516t
Neurosyphilis, initial treatment of, 433t
Neut
  formulary entry for, 947
Neutropenia
  in cancer patients, 570f, 574
  characterization of, 332
  differential diagnosis of, 332b

Nevirapine (Viramune, NVP), formulary entry for, 879–880
NGT (Nasogastric tube), use of, 4
Niacin
DRIs for, 542t
formulary entry for, 880
in multivitamin drops, analysis of, 545t
in multivitamin tablets, analysis of, 546t
Nicardipine (Cardene)
formulary entry for, 881
for hypertensive emergency, 105t
Nifedipine (Adalat CC, Nifediac CC, Procardia)
formulary entry for, 881–882
for hypertension emergency, 105t
Night terrors, 231t
Nightmares, 231t
Nipride
formulary entry for, 884
for hypertensive emergency, 43, 105t
Nitrofurantion (Furadantin, Macrodantin, Macrobid), formulary entry for, 882–883
Nitrogen mustard (mechlorethamine), toxicity of, 1008t
Nitroglycerin (Nitro-Bid, Nitrostat, Nitro-Time, Nitro-Dur, NitroMist), formulary entry for, 882–883
Nitropress, for hypertensive emergency, 43, 105t
Nitroprusside (Nitropress, Nipride)
formulary entry for, 884
for hypertensive emergency, 43, 105t
Nitrostat, formulary entry for, 882–883
Nizoral, formulary entry for, 834–835
Nonmeningeal histoplasmosis, itraconazole for, 833
Nonparametric regression, 653t
Nonsteroidal antiinflammatory drugs (NSAIDs)
analgesic properties of, 139
for SLE, 629
toxicity of, 39t
Nonventricular arrhythmias
classification of, 175t–176t
premature atrial contraction in, 176f
Nonventricular conduction disturbances, 178t–179t
Noonan syndrome, dominant cardiac defect in, 184t
Norepinephrine bitartrate (Levophed), formulary entry for, 105t
Norfloxacin (Noroxin, Chibroxin)
formulary entry for, 884–885
with renal failure, 1022t
Noritate
for acne vulgaris, 218t
for bacterial vaginosis, 422t
formulary entry for, 865–866
for gastroenteritis, 218t
neonatal critical care dosing of, 1010t
for PID, 432t
with renal failure, 1022t
Normodyne, formulary entry for, 836
Noroxin
formulary entry for, 884–885
with renal failure, 1022t
Norpace, with renal failure, 1029t
Nortriptyline hydrochloride (Pamelor, Aventyl)
formulary entry for, 108t
for migraines, 512t
Norvasc
formulary entry for, 696
for hypertension, 500t
Norwood procedure, for CHD, 185
Nostrilla, formulary entry for, 693
Novantrone (mitoxantrone), toxicity of, 1008t
NSAIDs. *See* Nonsteroidal antiinflammatory drugs
Nucleic acid amplification tests (NAATs), 122
NuLYTELY, formulary entry for, 915
Number needed to treat, 656
Nursemaid's elbow, 87
Nutracort
for adrenal insufficiency, 256
for glucocorticoid deficiency, 989
formulary entry for, 819
for hyperparathyroidism, 253
for hypoparathyroidism, 252
Nutr-E-Sol
DRIs for, 542t
in multivitamin drops, analysis of, 545t
in multivitamin tablets, analysis of, 546t

Nutrition
dietary reference intakes for, 538–539
elements of, 542t
fat requirements of, 539t
fiber of, 544t
protein requirements of, 539t
values of, 538
vitamins of, 540t
energy needs for, 535–538
enteral, 545
components for, 549t–556t
for children (ages 1 to 10), 549t–556t
for children and adults, 549t–556t
infant formula components of, 549t–556t
for malnourished infants and children, 537–538
newborns' requirements for, 462
parenteral, 560
formulation recommendations for, 561t
initiation/advancement of, 560t
monitoring schedule for, 562t
need for, 560
vitamin-mineral supplementation for, 539–545
websites for, 524
Nutritional status
elements of, 524
indicators of, 525–535
NVP, formulary entry for, 879–880
Nydrazid
formulary entry for, 831
with renal failure, 1020t
for tuberculosis, 447t
Nystatin (Mycostatin, Nilstat), formulary entry for, 886

O

Obesity
in cancer survivors, 576
endocrine etiology for, 259
management recommendations for, 534
Obsessive compulsive disorder
fluvoxamine for, 805
paroxetine for, 900
sertraline for, 944
Obstructive sleep apnea syndrome (OSAS), 602–603
Occlusive dressings, 996
OCL, formulary entry for, 915
Octreotide acetate (Sandostatin)
formulary entry for, 886
for hypoglycemic toxicity, 20t
Ocuflox (Ofloxacin)
formulary entry for, 887
for gonorrhea, 430t
ophthalmic properties of, 1001t
for PID, 432t
Ocusulf-10, formulary entry for, 953
Odd ratio, 656
Odors, from poison victims, 22t
Ofloxacin (Floxin, Ocuflox), 1001t
formulary entry for, 887
for gonorrhea, 430t
for PID, 432t
OGTT. *See* Oral glucose tolerance test
Olanzapine (Zyprexa), dosage/side effects for, 1003t
Olfactory, tests for, 505t
Oliguria
characterization of, 490–492
laboratory differentiation of, 492t
Olopatadine (Patanol)
formulary entry for, 887–888
ophthalmic properties of, 1001t
Olsalazine (Dipentum, Di-mesalazine, Di-5-ASA), formulary entry for, 888
Olux foam, potency ranking of, 995t
Omeprazole (Prilosec), formulary entry for, 888
Omnaris, formulary entry for, 747–748
Omnicef
formulary entry for, 733
for lymphadenitis, 425t
with renal failure, 1015t
Omnipaque. *See* Iohexol
Omnipen
formulary entry for, 701
for gonococcal infections, 420t
for meningitis, 421t
neonatal critical care dosing of, 1010t
with renal failure, 1014t
with sulbactam, for mastoiditis, 425t
Oncology. *See* Cancer

Oncovin (vincristine), toxicity of, 1009t
Ondansetron (Zofran)
formulary entry for, 889–890
for palliative care, 581t
One sample *t* test, 653t
Ophthalmia neonatorum, initial management of, 420t
Opiate(s)
analgesic properties of, 139
commonly used, 140t
properties of, 143–148
relative potencies of, 151t
withdrawal symptoms/signs of, 472b
Opiate intoxication, naloxone for, 876
Opiate withdrawal, paromomycin sulfate for, 899
Opioid tapering
examples of, 151b–152b
guidelines for, 150–151
indication for, 150
withdrawal from, 150
Opioids, toxicity of, 46b–47b
Opium tincture (Deodorized tincture of opium), formulary entry for, 890–891
Opticrom, formulary entry for, 757
Optivar, drug formulary for, 708
Orajel Perioseptic, formulary entry for, 728–729
Oral allergy syndrome, 356
Oral glucose tolerance test (OGTT), 262
Oral rehydration solutions, 559t
Oral rehydration therapy
composition of, 279t–280t
for diarrhea, 296–297
use of, 278–281
Oral ribavirin, formulary entry for, 935
Oral ulcers, in SLE, 628t
Oramorph SR
for analgesia, 140t
characterization of, 140t
formulary entry for, 878
for palliative care, 581t
relative potency of, 151t
with renal failure, 1032t
Orapred
for asthma, 10
formulary entry for, 919
for glucocorticoid deficiency, 989
potency of, 992t
Orasone
for asthma, 10
dose equivalence for, 992t
formulary entry for, 919–920
Orazinc, formulary entry for, 985–986
Orbital cellulitis
imaging of, 607
initial management of, 426t
Organic phosphorus compounds, toxicity of, 52
Oropharyngeal candidiasis, nystatin for, 886
OSAS. *See* Obstructive sleep apnea syndrome
Os-Cal, formulary entry for, 723
Oseltamivir phosphate (Tamiflu)
approval for, 392
formulary entry for, 891–892
for influenza, 425t
with renal failure, 1022t
Osmitrol, formulary entry for, 854
Osmolality
in enteral formulas, 549t–556t
in human milk, 548t–550t
in infant formula, 549t–556t
reference values for, 645t
OsmoPrep, formulary entry for, 948–949
Osmotic fragility test, for anemia diagnosis, 327
Osteomalacia, 253
Osteomyelitis
imaging of, 618
initial management of, 426t
Osteosarcoma, signs/symptoms of, 566t
Otic, formulary entry for, 916
Otitis media
ceftriaxone dosage with, 738
initial management of, 426t
levofloxacin for, 843
Ovarian pathology, 617
Overweight, management recommendations for, 534
Oxacillin (Bactocill)
for cellulitis, 423t
formulary entry for, 892
for lymphadenitis, 425t
for osteomyelitis, 426t
with renal failure, 1023t
for septic arthritis, 429t

Oxcarbazepine (Trileptal)
formulary entry for, 893–894
with renal failure, 1033t
for seizures, 516t
Oxybutynin chloride (Ditropan, Oxytrol), formulary entry for, 894
Oxycodone (Roxicodone, OxyContin)
characterization of, 140t
formulary entry for, 693
Oxycodone and acetaminophen (Tylox, Roxilox, Percocet, Endocet, Roxicet), formulary entry for, 895
Oxycodone and aspirin (Percodan, Roxiprin), formulary entry for, 693
OxyContin
formulary entry for, 693
Oxyhemoglobin dissociation curve, 586f
Oxymetazoline (Afrin, Duramist, Neo-Synephrine, Nostrilla, Visine), formulary entry for, 693

P

PA. *See* Physical activity coefficient
PAC. *See* Premature atrial contraction
Pacerone
for resuscitation, ii
formulary entry for, 694–695
standard concentrations for, i
Packed RBC (PRBC) transfusion, 350
Paclitaxel (Taxol), toxicity of, 1008t
Pain assessment(s)
for adolescents, 137
analgesia protocols and, 149t
developmental response to, 138t
FLACC for, 138t
for infants, 137
for preschoolers, 137
sedation protocols and, 149t
Pain management
analgesics for, 137–139
ibuprofen for, 822
morphine for, 581t
PAL. *See* Physical activity level
Palgic, formulary entry for, 729
Palivizumab (Synagis)
formulary entry for, 896–897
for RVS immunoprophylaxis, 400
Palliative care
authorization forms, examples of, 579b
death-associated changes and, 580
decision making in, 577–578
definition of, 577
intervention limitations in, 579–580
medications used in, 581t
memory making in, 578
rituals in, 579
team composition, 577
Palliative superior vena cava-to-pulmonary artery shunts, for CHD, 184
Palliative systemic-to-pulmonary artery shuts, for CHD, 184
Palmitate-A 5000
DRIs for, 542t
formulary entry for, 979–980
in multivitamin drops, analysis of, 545t
in multivitamin tablets, analysis of, 546t
reference values for, 647t
2-PAM
for pesticides toxicity, 52
formulary entry for, 918
Pamelor
formulary entry for, 108t
for migraines, 512t
Pamix, formulary entry for, 927–928
Panadol
analgesic properties of, 138
formulary entry for, 682
poisoning with, 684
with renal failure, 1027t
toxicity of, 28t
Panayiotopoulos syndrome, 515t
Pancreatic enzymes, formulary entry for, 897
Pancreatic enzyme supplement(s)
characterization of, 996
cytochrome P450 inducers/inhibitors as, 998t
insulin products of, 995–996
pancrelipase, 995–996
Pancreatitis
acute, 305–307, 306t
characterization of, 305–307
chronic, 307

Pancrelipase, products of, 997t
Pancuronium bromide
  formulary entry for, 897–898
  with renal failure, 1033t
Pandel
  for adrenal insufficiency, 256
  formulary entry for, 819
  for glucocorticoid deficiency, 989
  for hyperparathyroidism, 253
  for hypoparathyroidism, 252
Pantoprazole (Protonix), formulary entry for, 898–899
Pantothenic acid
  DRIs for, 542t
  in multivitamin tablets, analysis of, 546t
Papular urticaria
  characterization of, 213
Papulosquamous lesions
  algorithm for, 211f
  atopic dermatitis as, 210–213
Paracentesis
  procedures for, 75–77
  subxiphoid approach for, 76f–77f
Paralysis, due to poisoning, 21t
Paralytics, for RSI, 7t
Paraplatin (carboplatin), toxicity of, 1006t
Parapneumonic effusions, imaging of, 609
Parathyroid disorders
  hyperparathyroidism and, 252
  hypoparathyroidism and, 252
Parathyroid hormone (PTH), function of, 252
Pacerone. *See* Amiodarone HCl (Cordarone, Pacerone)
Paregoric (camphorated opium tincture), formulary entry for, 899
Parenteral nutrition
  formulation recommendations for, 561t
  initiation/advancement of, 560t
  monitoring schedule for, 562t
  need for, 560
Paromomycin sulfate (Humatin), formulary entry for, 899–900
Parotitis, initial management of, 427t
Paroxetine (Paxil, Pexeva), formulary entry for, 900–901
Paroxysmal events
  imaging of, 513
  seizures as
    characterization of, 511
    classification of, 514b
    febrile illness associated with, 512b
    syndromes of, 515t
    treatments for, 514–518, 516t–517t
Parvovirus
  diagnosis of, 416
  neonatal management of, 413t
Passive movements, 504
Pasteurella multocida, in animal bites, 96t
Patanol, formulary entry for, 887–888
Patanol/Pataday, 1000t
Patent ductus arteriosus (PDA)
  characterization of, 466–467
  CHD/exam findings of, 186t
  management of, 467
Pathocil
  formulary entry for, 769
  for lymphadenitis, 425t
Patient-controlled analgesia
  administration routes of, 150
  complications from, 150
  definition of, 148
  indications for, 148
  orders for, 150t
Paxil, formulary entry for, 900–901
PCA. *See* Patient-controlled analgesia
PCECV. *See* Purified chicken embryo cell vaccine
PCP intoxication, 46
PCV. *See* Pneumococcal conjugate vaccine
Peak expiratory flow rate (PEFR), 586–587, 588t
Pearson's *r*, 653t
Pediaflor, formulary entry for, 800–801
Pediamycin, formulary entry for, 787–788
Pediapred
  for asthma, 10
  formulary entry for, 919
  for glucocorticoid deficiency, 989
  potency of, 992t
Pediarix, immunoprophylaxis for, 402
Pediatric BLS healthcare providers, see pages after Index

Pediatric bradycardia algorithm, see pages after Index
Pediatric cardiac arrest algorithm, see pages after Index
Pediatric tachycardia algorithm, see pages after Index
Pediazole, formulary entry for, 787
Pediculus capitis, permethrin for, 906
PediOtic, formulary entry for, 916
PEFR. *See* Peak expiratory flow rate
PEG-Asp (asparaginase), toxicity of, 1006t
Pelvic fractures, catheterization and, 78
Pelvic inflammatory disease (PID)
  cefotetan for, 432t
  ceftizoxime for, 432t
  characterization of, 437
  garamycin for, 432t
  gentamicin for, 432t
  initial treatment of, 432t
  levofloxacin for, 432t
  ocuflox for, 432t
  ofloxacin for, 432t
Pelvis trauma, secondary survey of, 90t
Penicillamine (Cuprimine, Depen), formulary entry for, 901
Penicillin G preparations
  aqueous potassium and sodium, formulary entry for, 902
  benzathine, formulary entry for, 903
  benzathine and penicillin G procaine, formulary entry for, 903
  procaine, formulary entry for, 904
Penicillin G, with renal failure, 1023t
Penicillin V potassium (Veetids)
  characterization of, 902
  formulary entry for, 904–905
  with renal failure, 1023t
Penicillin, for antimicrobial prophylaxis, 575t
Penis, length, mean stretched, 268t
Pentacel, immunoprophylaxis for, 403
Pentamidine isethionate (Pentam 300, NebuPent)
  for antimicrobial prophylaxis, 575t
  formulary entry for, 905
  with renal failure, 1023t
Pentobarbital (Nembutal)
  formulary entry for, 905–906
  for sedation, 147t
Pentothal
  with renal failure, 1034t
  for RSI, 6t
  for sedation, 151t
PEP (postexposure prophylaxis), exposure to, 450–452
Pepcid, formulary entry for, 792–793
Peptic ulcer(s)
  aluminum hydroxide for, 690
  famotidine for, 793
  pantoprazole for, 898
Pepto-Bismol
  formulary entry for, 716–717
  with renal failure, 1027t
Percodan, formulary entry for, 693
Perdiem, formulary entry for, 927
Perforomist, formulary entry for, 807–808
Periactin
  formulary entry for, 760–761
  for migraines, 512t
Pericardial disease, characterization f, 195–196
Pericardiocentesis, procedures for, 75
Pericarditis, in SLE, 628t
Perinatal viral infections, diagnosis of, 405
Periorbital cellulitis, initial management of, 427t
Periostat
  for acne vulgaris, 218t
  for ehrlichiosis, 449
  for Lyme disease, 448
  for Rocky Mountain spotted fever, 449
Peripheral alpha antagonists, for hypertension, 501t
Peripheral intravenous placement, 61–68
Peripheral nerve injuries, 472
Peritoneal dialysis, 1012
Periventricular leukomalacia, 471
Permethrin (Elimite, Acticin, Nix)
  formulary entry for, 906
  for scabies, 208
Peroxisomal disorders, characterization of, 319
Persistent pulmonary hypertension of the newborn (PPHN), 463–465
Pertussis
  azithromycin for, 709
  exposure to, 386

Pervasive developmental disorder, 237–238
Pesticides, toxicity of, 52
Pexeva, formulary entry for, 900–901
Pfizerpen, formulary entry for, 902
pH
  arterial blood, 587f
  urine, 476
Pharyngitis
  cefdinir for, 733
  initial management of, 427t
Phazyme, formulary entry for, 945–946
Phenazopyridine HCl (Pyridium, Azo-Standard)
  formulary entry for, 906–907
  with renal failure, 1033t
Phenergan
  for chemotherapy-induced nausea, 574
  formulary entry for, 923–924
Phenobarbital (Luminal)
  for conjugated hyperbilirubinemia, 469
  formulary entry for, 907
  with renal failure, 1033t
  for seizures, 516t
  for status epilepticus, 17
Phenothiazines, toxicity of, 31t
Phentolamine mesylate (Regitine), formulary entry for, 908
Phenylalanine, reference values for, 645t
Phenylephrine HCl (Neo-Synephrine)
  brompheniramine with, 717–718
  cyclopentolate with, 759
  formulary entry for, 908–909
  standard concentrations for, i
Phenytoin (Dilantin, Phenytek)
  formulary entry for, 909–910
  for seizures, 517t
  toxicity of, 48
PhosLo, formulary entry for, 722–723
Phosphate ion (PO_4^{3-})
  intracellular/extracellular composition of, 276t
  serum disturbances of, 288–289
Phosphate supplementation, vitamin D resistant rickets with, 785
Phosphorus
  in cow's milk formulas, 549t–556t
  DRIs for, 543t
  in enteral formulas, 549t–556t
Phosphorus *(Continued)*
  in formulas, 543t
  in infant formula, 549t–556t
  in multivitamin tablets, analysis of, 542t, 546t
  parenteral nutrition formulations, 561t
  reference values for, 639t–647t
Phosphorus supplements (K-PHOS, Ur-KP-Neutral, sodium phosphate, potassium phosphate), formulary entry for, 911
Photosensitivity, in SLE, 628t
Phototherapy
  guidelines for, 468f, 468t
  for unconjugated hyperbilirubinemia in newborns, 467
Phthirus pubis, permethrin for, 906
Physical activity coefficient(s)
  definition of, 535
  levels of, 535t
Physical activity level (PAL), definition of, 535
Physical examinations
  cardiac, 154–167
  for head trauma, 91–93
  for health maintenance, 121
  nephrology, 479
  pulmonary, 584
  for UTI, 479
Physiologic anemia of infancy, characterization of, 328
Physostigmine salicylate (Antilirium)
  as anticholinergic antidote, 31t
  formulary entry for, 911
Phytonadione (Mephyton, Vitamin K)
  DRIs for, 542t
  formulary entry for, 912
  in multivitamin drops, analysis of, 545t
  in multivitamin tablets, analysis of, 546t
PID. *See* Pelvic inflammatory disease
Pilocarpine HCl (Akarpine, Isopto Carpine, Pilocar, Salagen), formulary entry for, 912–913
Pimecrolimus, formulary entry for, 913
Pin-Rid, formulary entry for, 927–928
Pinworms (Entererobius)
  mebendazole for, 854
  pyrantel pamoate for, 928

Pin-X, formulary entry for, 927–928
Piperacillin (Pipracil)
 formulary entry for, 913–914
 with renal failure, 1023t
Piperacillin with tazobactam (Zosyn)
 formulary entry for, 914
 with renal failure, 1023t
Pitressin, formulary entry for, 977
Plantar warts, 206
Plaque psoriasis, ethancept for, 790
Plaquenil
 formulary entry for, 820–821
 for SLE, 629
Platelet, smear interpretation of, 352
Platelet transfusion, 349–350
Platinol (cisplatin), toxicity of, 1006t
Pleuritis, in SLE, 628t
Plexus impairment, 506f
Plexus injuries, characterization of, 472t
Plus disease, 473
Pneumococcal conjugate vaccine
 for cancer patients, 381t
 for high-risk patients, 380t
 immunoprophylaxis for, 396
 interval schedule for, 375t
 PCV7 transition to, 397t
 schedule for, 372f
Pneumocystis jiroveci. See Pneumocytic carinii pneumonia (PCP)
Pneumocytic carinii pneumonia (PCP)
 pentamidine isethionate for, 905
 sulfamethoxazole and trimethoprim for, 955
Pneumonia
 azithromycin for, 709
 imaging of, 609
 initial management of, 428t
 levofloxacin for, 843
 linezolid for, 847
 neonatal, initial management of, 420t
 pediatric, management of, 428t
Poison ivy
 characterization of, 223–224
Poisoning(s)
 acute management of, 20–27
  ABCs for, 20
  active removal for, 27
  antidotes for, 27
Poisoning(s) *(Continued)*
  decontamination for, 20–22
  enhanced elimination for, 27
  GI decontamination for, 22–26
  inhalation injuries and, 26
 antidotes to
  for acetaminophen, 28t
  for alcohol, 30t
  for anticholinergics, 31t
  for antidepressants, 32t
  for antihistamines, 33t
  for benzodiazepines, 34t
  for beta-blockers, 35t
  for calcium channel blockers, 36t
  for hypoglycemics, 37t
  for NSAIDs, 39t
  for salicytates, 137
 carbon monoxide, 27
 cyanide, 49
 due to drug(s) of abuse, 43b–48b
  with amphetamine, 43
  with cocaine, 43–44
  with ecstasy, 44
  with ethanol, 45
  with GBH, 45
  with GBL, 45
  with hallucinogens, 45–46
  with inhalants, 47–48
  with ketamine, 46
  with marijuana, 46
  with opioids, 46–47
  with sedative-hypnotics, 47
 initial evaluation for, 19–20
  clinical diagnostic aids, 20t–22t, 42f
  history, 19
  laboratory findings, 19
  radiology, 22t
 lead
  blood testing guidelines for, 50t
  characterization of, 49–51
 due to medication ingestion of
  with acetaminophen, 28t
  with alcohols, 30t
  with anticholinergics, 31t
  with antidepressants, 32t
  with antihistamines, 33t
  with barbiturates, 34t
  with benzodiazepines, 34t
  with beta-blockers, 35t
  with butyrophenone, 39t

Poisoning(s) *(Continued)*
with calcium channel blockers, 36t
with carbamazepine, 48
with clonidine, 36t
with digoxin, 48
with hypoglycemics, 37t
with iron, 38t
with NSAIDs, 39t
with phenothiazines, 39t
with salicylates, 40t
methemoglobinemia, 51–52
due to pesticides, 52
due to rodenticides, 52–53
due to spiders, 53–54
due to superwarfarins, 52–53
toxidromes of
ABCs for, 23t–25t
adrenergics, 23t
anticholinergics, 23t
anticholinesterase, 24t
extraphyramidals, 24t
narcotics, 25t
opiods, 25t
sedative-hypnotics, 25t
sympathomimetics, 23t
withdrawal, 25t
due to venomous snakes, 53
websites for, 19
Poly B sulfate ophthalmic, 1000t–1001t
Polyarteritis nodosa, 631t
Polycitra
formulary entry for, 947
for resuscitation, ii
Polycystic ovaries, 259
Polycythemia, neonatal, 469–470
Polyethylene glycol electrolyte solution (GoLYTELY, Colyte, NuLYTELY, OCL, TriLyte, MiralLax), formulary entry for, 915
Polymox
for bacterial infections, 422t
formulary entry for, 697
for lymphadenitis, 425t
for meningitis, 426t
for otitis media, 426t
with renal failure, 1013t
Polymyositis, autoantibodies associated with, 621t
Polymyxin B sulfate, 1000t–1001t
Polymyxin B sulfate and bacitracin. *See* Bacitracin and Polymyxin B
Polymyxin B sulfate/hydrocortisone (Cortisporin, AK-Spore H. C, Otic, PediOtic), formulary entry for, 916
Polymyxin B sulfate and trimethoprim sulfate (Polytrim, Ophthalmic Solution), formulary entry for, 916
Polymyxin B sulfate ophthalmic, 1000t–1001t
Polyneuropathy, 506
Poly-Pred, 1001t
Polysporin ophthalmic, 1001t
Polysporin Ophthalmic, formulary entry for, 711
Polysporin Topical, formulary entry for, 711
Polytrim (Trimethoprim sulfate, polymyxin B sulfate, benzalkonium chloride)
characterization of, 1001t
formulary entry for, 916
Popliteal angle, in newborn assessment, 457
Poractant Alfa. *See* Surfactant, pulmonary
Porcelain, reference values for, 645t
Positive antinuclear antibody(ies), in SLE, 628t
Positive predictive value, 657
Postaglandin E_1, standard concentrations for, i
Posterior ankle splints, 87
Postoperative nausea and vomiting
dolasetron for, 775
granisetron for, 775
metoclopramide for, 863
Postspinal fusion infection, initial management of, 429t
Posture, in newborn assessment, 456
Potassium
in cow's milk formulas, 549t–556t
in enteral formulas, 549t–556t
parenteral nutrition formulations, 561t
Potassium (K^+)
dehydration-associated, 275f
in enteral formulas, 549t–556t
in human milk, 548t–549t
in infant formula, 549t–556t

Potassium (K+) *(Continued)*
- intracellular/extracellular composition of, 276t
- in multivitamin tablets, analysis of, 547t
- neonatal requirements for, 462t
- reference values for, 645t
- serum disturbances of, 283–284

Potassium chloride, ravine chloride as alternative for, 702
Potassium iodide (Iosat, Pima, SSKI, ThyroShield, ThyroSafe), formulary entry for, 917
Potassium phosphate, formulary entry for, 911
Potassium supplements, formulary entry for, 917–918
Power, examination of, 504
PPE. *See* Preparticipation physical evaluation
PPHN. *See* Persistent pulmonary hypertension of the newborn
Prader-Willi syndrome, characterization of, 318
Pralidoxime chloride (2-PAM, Protopam)
- formulary entry for, 918
- for pesticides toxicity, 52

Prazosin, for hypertension, 501t
Prealbumin, reference values for, 645t
Precocious puberty, 260–262
Pred-Forte (Prednisolone acetate), 1001t
Prednicarbate (Dermatop), potency ranking of, 996t
Prednisolone (Orapred, Prelone, Pediapred)
- for asthma, 10
- formulary entry for, 919
- for glucocorticoid deficiency, 989
- potency of, 992t

Prednisolone acetate ophthalmic, 1001t
Prednisone (Orasone, Deltasone, Liquid Pred)
- for asthma, 10
- dose equivalence for, 992t
- formulary entry for, 919–920

Pregnancy
- amantadine hydrochloride contraindications during, 691
- drug dosage and, 664
- epididymitis during, 429t

Pregnancy *(Continued)*
- HIV during, 438–442, 439t–441t
- immunization considerations for, 384
- syphilis testing during, 415
- vaccines and, 382

Prelone
- for asthma, 10
- formulary entry for, 919
- for glucocorticoid deficiency, 989
- potency of, 992t

Premature atrial contraction (PAC), 175t
Premature infants, 176f
- apnea in, 465
- CMV in, 413t
- electrolyte requirements for, 462t
- exogenous caloric requirements for, 462
- glucose requirements for, 460
- hyperglycemia in, 461t
- hypoglycemia in, 461t
- indomethacin for, 466
- insensible water loss in, 460t
- iron requirements for, 461
- necrotizing enterocolitis in, 470
- PDA in, 466
- periventricular leukomalacia in, 471
- phototherapy for, 467–468, 468t
- varicella in, 414t

Premature ventricular contraction (PVC), 178t
Prenatal counseling, indications for, 320
Preparticipation physical evaluation (PPE), for adolescents
- examination items in, 133
- medical history, 133
- orthopedic examination, 134f
- review of systems in, 133

Pressor
- for resuscitation, ii
- standard concentrations for, i

Preterm infants
- formulas for, 549t–554t
- growth charts for, 533f

Prevalite, formulary entry for, 746–747
Prilocaine, characterization of, 141t
Prilocaine and lidocaine, formulary entry for, 845–846

Prilosec, formulary entry for, 888
Primacor
formulary entry for, 869
with renal failure, 1032t
Primaquine phosphate, formulary entry for, 920
Primary acid-base disorders, determination of, 289
Primary biliary cirrhosis, penicillamine for, 901
Primary skin lesions
characterization of, 201
pattern diagnosis of, 202f–203f
Primaxin
formulary entry for, 823
with renal failure, 1020t
Primidone (Mysoline)
formulary entry for, 920–921
with renal failure, 1033t
Principen
formulary entry for, 701
for gonococcal infections, 420t
for meningitis, 421t
neonatal critical care dosing of, 1010t
with renal failure, 1014t
with sulbactam, for mastoiditis, 425t
Prinivil, formulary entry for, 848
Probability, calculating changes in, 658f
Probenecid, formulary entry for, 921
Probiotics, for diarrhea, 297
Procainamide (Pronestyl, Procanbid)
formulary entry for, 922
with renal failure, 1033t
Procarbazine (Matulane), toxicity of, 1008t
Procardia
for hypertension emergency, 105t
formulary entry for, 881–882
Procedure(s)
for basic laceration repair, 81–84
skin staples for, 84
suturing for, 81–84
tissue adhesives for, 84
for blood fluid sampling, 70–80
chest tube placement in, 72–74, 73f
lumbar puncture for, 70–72, 71f
paracentesis for, 75–77, 76f–77f
pericardiocentesis for, 75
soft tissue aspiration for, 78–80
Procedure(s) *(Continued)*
suprapubic bladder aspiration for, 78, 79f–80f
thoracentesis for, 72–74, 74f
urinary bladder catheterization for, 77–78
for blood samplings, 57–61
catheterization for, 59–61
dorsalis pedis artery puncture for, 61
external jugular puncture for, 58–59
femoral artery/vein puncture for, 59
heelstick for, 57–58
posterior tibial puncture for, 61
radial artery puncture for, 59–61
consent for, 57
general guidelines for, 57
for immunization and medication administration, 81
risks in, 57
for splinting, 85–87
basic, 85
long arm posterior, 85
posterior ankle, 87
radial head subluxation reduction, 87
sugar tong forearm, 86
thumb spica, 84
ulnar gutter, 86
volar, 87
for vascular access, 61–68
central venous catheter placement, 61–63
intraosseous infusion, 63–65, 65f
peripheral intravenous placement for, 61
umbilical artery/vein catheterization, 65–68
Prochlorperazine (Compazine, Compro)
formulary entry for, 922–923
for palliative care, 581t
Procrit, formulary entry for, 784–785
Proctitis, sucralfate for, 952
Proctocolitis, infantile, 356
Product moment correlation coefficient, 653t
Progesterone, contraindications for, 123–128
Progestin, long-acting, 128
Prograf, formulary entry for, 958–959

Prokinetic agent(s)
erythromycin preparations as, 787–788
metoclopramide as, 863
Promethazine (Phenergan)
for chemotherapy-induced nausea, 574
formulary entry for, 923–924
Pronestyl
formulary entry for, 922
with renal failure, 1033t
Pronto, formulary entry for, 929
Prophylactic therapy
curosurf for, 957
infasurf for, 957
survanta for, 956
Prophylaxis
aluminum hydroxide dosage for, 690
antibiotic
for specific cardiac conditions, 193b
for UTI evaluation, 482
antimicrobial, 575t
acyclovir for, 575t
cancer and, 575t
azithromycin for, 709
bacterial endocarditis, 191
ceftriaxone dosage with, 738
characterization of, 191
clindamycin dosage for, 753
dental procedures and, 193t
respiratory tract procedures and, 193t
candida, micafungin for, 866
CMV, valganciclovir for, 972–973
endocarditis, vancomycin for, 975
influenza A, 691
isoniazid for, 831
itraconazole for, 833
malaria
chloroquine HCL/phosphate for, 742
mefloquine for, 856
measles
IMIG therapy for, 363
migraine
propranolol for, 924
valproic acid for, 975
Mycobacterium avium complex, 936
oseltamivir for, 892
pyridoxine for, 930
Prophylaxis *(Continued)*
rheumatic fever
Bicillin L-A for, 903
penicillin V potassium for, 904
sulfadiazine for, 953–954
rubella, IMIG therapy for, 363
UTIs, 482
Propofol (Diprivan)
properties of, 145
for RSI, 6t
for sedation, 145
Propranolol (Inderal)
formulary entry for, 924–925
for Hashimoto's thyroiditis, 252
for hemangiomas, 205–206
for hypertension, 500t
for migraines, 512t
Propylthiouracil (PTU)
formulary entry for, 925
for Graves disease, 250
Proquad, immunoprophylaxis for, 403
Prostaglandin E. *See* Alprostadil
Prosthetic valve endocarditis, rifampin dosage for, 937
Prostigmin
formulary entry for, 879
with renal failure, 1032t
Protamine sulfate, formulary entry for, 926
Protein(s)
caloric modulars of, 549t
in cerebrospinal fluid, 648t
complement, levels of, 622–623
dietary requirements for, 539t
in enteral formulas, 549t–556t
in human milk, 548t–549t
in infant formulas, 549t–556t
intolerances of, formulas for, 558t–559t
intracellular/extracellular composition of, 276t
parenteral nutrition formulations, 561t
in urine, 477, 490t
Protein C deficiency, characterization of, 338b
Protein electrophoresis, reference values for, 645t
Protein S deficiency, characterization of, 338b
Proteinuria(s)
characterization of, 487–490
evaluation of, 491f
Protonix, formulary entry for, 898–899

Protopam
formulary entry for, 918
for pesticides toxicity, 52
Protopic, formulary entry for, 958–959
Protostat
for acne vulgaris, 218t
for bacterial vaginosis, 422t
formulary entry for, 865–866
for gastroenteritis, 218t
neonatal critical care dosing of, 1010t
for PID, 432t
with renal failure, 1022t
Proventil
for anaphylaxis, 10
for asthma, 10
formulary entry for, 687–688
Proventil HFA
for anaphylaxis, 10
for asthma, 10
formulary entry for, 687–688
Provera, formulary entry for, 855
Providencia spp., sensitivity profile of, 408t
Prozac (fluoxetine)
dosage/side effects for, 1004t
formulary entry for, 801–802
Pruritus, hydroxyzine for, 821
PsA. *See* Psoriatic arthritis
Pseudo Carb Pediatric, formulary entry for, 729–730
Pseudoephedrine (Sudafed, Efidac/24Pesudeophedrine)
cetirizine with, 740–741
formulary entry for, 926
loratadine with, 850
Pseudoephedrine, carbinoxamine with, 729–730
Pseudoephedrine and loratadine (Claritin), formulary entry for, 850
Pseudomonas aeruginosa
in cystic fibrosis patients, 601
sensitivity profile of, 408t
Pseudotumor cerebri, acetazolamide for, 479–480, 740–741
Psorcon, potency ranking of, 995t
Psoriasis
history of, 624
plaque, ethancept for, 790
Psoriatic arthritis (PsA), 624–626
Psychosis
aripirazole for, 1003t
chlorpromazine for, 745
Psychosis *(Continued)*
clozapine for, 1003t
haloperidol for, 815–816, 1003t
olanzapine for, 1003t
due to poisoning, 21t
quetiapine for, 1004t
risperdal for, 939–940
risperidone for, 1003t
thioridazine for, 963
ziprasidone for, 1004t
Psychosocial development, 119t
Psyllium (Metamucil, Fiberall, Serutan, Konsyl, Perdiem, Fiber Therapy), formulary entry for, 927
Puberty
delayed, 259–260, 261f
precocious, 260–262
Pubic hair Tanner staging, 118b, 118f
Pulmicort
daily dose recommendations for, 993t
dosage recommendations for, 718t–719t
formulary entry for, 718–719
for hypertension, 501t
Pulmonary function tests
compensatory response calculation for, 588t
flow-volume curve in, 589f
maximal pressure as, 587–588
PEFR as, 586–590, 588t
spirometry as, 588–590, 590t
Pulmonary hypertension, sildenafil for, 944
Pulmonary stenosis (PS), CHD/exam findings of, 186t
Pulmonary vasodilatory therapy, for PPHN, 464–465
Pulmonology
apparent-life-threatening event in, 591–592
asthma in, 590t
classification of, 593f–595f
clinical manifestations of, 592
exacerbation prevention in, 592
stepwise management of, 596f–598f
bronchiolitis in, 599
bronchopulmonary dysplasia in, 599–600
cystic fibrosis in, 600–602
clinical manifestations of, 601t
common complications of, 602

Pulmonology *(Continued)*
diagnosis of, 600–601
therapies for, 601
gas exchange evaluation in, 584–586
capnography, 585
oxyhemoglobin dissociation curve, 586f
pulse oximetry, 584–585
respiratory auscultation in, 585t
respiratory rates, 585t
OSAS in, 602–603
pulmonary function tests in, 586–590
compensatory response calculation for, 588t
flow-volume curve in, 589f
maximal pressure as, 587–588
PEFR as, 586–587, 588t
spirometry as, 588–590, 590t
respiratory physical examinations in, 584
SIDS in, 603, 603b
websites for, 584
Pulmozyme, formulary entry for, 776
Pulse oximetry, 584–585
Pulsus paradoxus, 154
Puncture(s)
external jugular, 58–59
femoral artery/vein, 59
lumbar, for blood fluid sampling, 70–72, 71f
Pupillary dilation, phenylephrine for, 909
Purified chicken embryo cell vaccine (PCECV), 397
Pyelonephritis, initial treatment of, 435t
Pyloric stenosis, imaging of, 616
Pyogenic granuloma
morphology of, 208
treatment for, 208
Pyrantel pamoate (Antiminth, Reese's Pinworm, Pamix, Pin-Rid, Pin-X), formulary entry for, 927–928
Pyrazinamide (pyrazinoic acid, amide)
formulary entry for, 928
for tuberculosis, 447t, 928
Pyrazinoic acid
formulary entry for, 928
for tuberculosis, 447t, 928
Pyrethrins (Tisit, A-200, Pyrinyl, Pronto, RID), formulary entry for, 929
Pyridium
formulary entry for, 906–907
with renal failure, 1033t
Pyridoxine (Aminoxin, vitamin B_6)
DRIs for, 542t
formulary entry for, 930
in multivitamin drops, analysis of, 545t
in multivitamin tablets, analysis of, 546t
Pyrimethamine (Daraprim), formulary entry for, 930–931
Pyrimidine analog (gemcitabine), toxicity of, 1007t
Pyrinyl, formulary entry for, 929

Q

22q11 syndrome
characterization of, 317–318
dominant cardiac defect in, 184t
QT ranges, long, diagnosis of, 181–182
Questran, formulary entry for, 746–747
Quetiapine (Seroquel), dosage/side effects for, 1004t
Quick start method, 130–131
Quinapril, for hypertension, 500t
Quineprox, formulary entry for, 820–821
Quinidine (Quinidex)
formulary entry for, 931–932
with renal failure, 1033t
Quinupristin and dalfopristin (Synercid), formulary entry for, 932
Quixin
formulary entry for, 842–843
for PID, 429t
with renal failure, 1021t

R

Rabies, IMIG therapy for, 363
Rabies vaccines
immunoprophylaxis for, 397–399
postexposure prophylaxis of, 398–399, 398t
Racemic epinephrine, for anaphylaxis, 10
Radial arteries, puncture of, 59–61
Radial head subluxation reduction, 87
Radiation, nausea and vomiting from, granisetron for, 775

Radiology
abdomen, 615–617
airway, 608–609
foreign bodies, 609
lateral radiographs of, 608, 608t
normal anatomy, 610f–611f
vascular rings of, 609
chest, 609–613
atelectasis *versus* infiltrate, 609
cardiac anatomy, 612f–613f
central line placement, 613
empyema, 610
ETT placement, 613
lung anatomy, 612f–613f
mediastinal masses, 611
parapneumonic effusions, 610
parenchymal findings, 610–611
pneumonia, 609
extremities, 618
general principles of, 606
genitourinary tract, 617
head, 606–607
heart, 613–615, 614f–615f
orbital cellulitis, 607
spine, 607–608
Raniclor
formulary entry for, 731–732
with renal failure, 1014t
Ranitidine HCl (Zantac)
formulary entry for, 933
with renal failure, 1034t
Rapamune, formulary entry for, 946–947
Rasburicase (Elitek), formulary entry for, 933–934
Rashes
neonatal, evolution of, 221f
in SLE, 628t
RDS. *See* Respiratory distress syndrome
Reactive arthritis as, 626–627
Reactive erythema, 208, 211f
Rebetol, formulary entry for, 934–936
Recombinant factor VIII, 350
Recombinant factor IX, 350
Red blood cell(s)
replacement of, 348–349
smear interpretation of, 352
in urine, 477–478
Red cell aplasia, characterization of, 327
Reese's Pinworm, formulary entry for, 927–928
Reflex(s)
rating scale for, 507b
tendons, 506–507
Refractory dermatomyositis, IVIG therapy for, 362
Refractory polymyositis, IVIG therapy for, 362
Regitine, formulary entry for, 908
Reglan
formulary entry for, 863
with renal failure, 1032t
toxicity of, 24t
Regression by least squares method, 653t
Relative risk, 656
Relative risk reduction, 656
Remeron (mirtazapine), dosage/side effects for, 1005t
Renal diseases
acute injury and, 494
chronic, 495–496, 497t
clinical manifestations of, 487–492
edema as, 490
hematuria as, 487, 488f–489f
oliguria as, 490–492, 492t
proteinuria as, 487–490, 491f
in SLE, 628t
Renal failure
dosage adjustments for
allopurinol, 688
amoxicillin, 697
antimicrobials requiring, 1013t–1026t
darbepoetin, 689
epoetin alfa, 784
methods for, 1012
nonantimicrobials requiring, 1027t–1034t
formulas for, 559t
Renal functioning test(s)
creatinine clearance as, 483–484
glomerular function as, 484, 484t
tubular, 485–486, 486t, 490t
Renal tubular acidosis, 486–487
Renova, formulary entry for, 968
Resectisol, formulary entry for, 854
Respiratory auscultation, 585t
Respiratory changes, as death approaches, 580

Respiratory diseases, neonatal
general considerations for, 463
PPHN as, 463–465
RDS as, 463
Respiratory distress, oncologic-associated, characterization of, 568–569
Respiratory distress syndrome (RDS), 463
Respiratory emergencies
asthma, 10–11
epiglottis, 12
foreign-body aspiration, 13
glycopyrrolate for, 814
laryngotracheobronchitis, 12–13
upper airway obstruction, 12–13
Respiratory failure
characterization of, 107–112
ventilator setting changes in, 112t
Respiratory rates, normal, 585t
Respiratory syncytial virus (RSV), palivizumab for, 399–400, 896
Restrictive cardiomyopathy, for myocardial disease, 194–195
Resuscitation
medications for, ii
neonatal, 455
overview of, 456f
Reticulocyte count, for anemia diagnosis, 326
Retin-A, formulary entry for, 968
Retina
examination of
age-based timing of, 473t
follow-up schedule for, 474t
zones of, 474f
Retinoblastoma, signs/symptoms of, 566t
Retinoids, for acne vulgaris, 217–220
Retinol
formulary entry for, 979–980
in multivitamin drops, analysis of, 545t
in multivitamin tablets, analysis of, 546t
reference values for, 647t
Retinopathy of prematurity (ROP), characterization of, 473–474
Retrospective study, 655t
Retrovir, in utero HIV transmission prevention by, 441t
Revatio, formulary entry for, 944–945
Reversol, formulary entry for, 779
R-Gene, formulary entry for, 702–703
Rhabdomyolysis, hydration treatment for, 44
Rheumatic disease(s)
arthritides as, 623–627
JIA as, 623–627
PsA as, 624–626
reactive arthritis as, 626–627
granulomatous disease as, 632–634
differential diagnosis of, 632–633
sarcoidosis in, 633
juvenile dermatomyositis as, 634–635
laboratory studies of, 620–623
for acute phase reactants, 620–621
for antinuclear antibodies, 621
for autoantibodies, 621–622, 621t
for complement system, 622–623
joint fluids, 623, 624f
for rheumatoid factors, 621
serum muscle enzymes, 623
urinalysis as, 623
SLE as, 627–630
classification of, 627, 628t
clinical features of, 628–629
drug-induced, 629–630
treatment of, 629
synovial fluid in, 628t
vasculitis as, 630–632
general characterization of, 630
HSP induction of, 630–632, 631t
syndromes of, 631t
websites for, 620
Rheumatic fever prophylaxis
Bicillin L-A for, 903
penicillin V potassium for, 904
sulfadiazine for, 953–954
Rheumatic heart disease
characterization of, 198–199
diagnostic guidelines for, 198b
Rheumatoid arthritis. *See* Juvenile rheumatoid arthritis
Rheumatoid factor(s)
laboratory studies of, 621
reference values for, 646t
Rhinitis medicamentosa, 355
Rhinocort
daily dose recommendations for, 993t
dosage recommendations for, 804t

Rhinocort *(Continued)*
formulary entry for, 718–719
for hypertension, 501t
Rh_o immune globulin intravenous (WinRho-SDF), formulary entry for, 934
Rhonchi, 585t
Ribavirin (Rebetol, Copegus, Ribaspheres, Virazole), formulary entry for, 934–936
Riboflavin
formulary entry for, 936
in multivitamin drops, analysis of, 545t
in multivitamin tablets, analysis of, 546t
reference values for, 647t
Rickets
Kawasaki disease-associated, 253
vitamin D resistant, 785
Rickettsia rickettsii, 448
RID, formulary entry for, 929
Rifabutin (Mycobutin)
formulary entry for, 936–937
with renal failure, 1023t
Rifampin (Rimactane, Rifadin)
formulary entry for, 937–938
with renal failure, 1023t
Right bundle-branch block (RBBB), 180t
Rimactane
formulary entry for, 937–938
with renal failure, 1023t
Rimantadine (Flumadine)
approval for, 393
formulary entry for, 938
for influenza, 425t
Riomet
for diabetes, 247
for polycystic ovarian syndrome, 259
Risperdal, formulary entry for, 939–940
Risperidone (Risperdal)
dosage/side effects for, 1003t
formulary entry for, 939–940
Ritalin
for ADHD, 239t
for anaphylaxis, 991
for asthma, 10
formulary entry for, 860–862
Rituals, 579
Robinul, formulary entry for, 814
Rocaltrol, formulary entry for, 722–723
Rocephin
for bacteremia, 422t
for gonorrhea, 430t
for meningitis, 426t
for meningococcus exposure, 395
Rocky Mountain spotted fever, 448–449
Rocuronium (Zemuron)
formulary entry for, 940–941
for RIS, 7t
Rodent bites, 96t
Rodenticides, toxicity of, 52–53
Rogaine
formulary entry for, 870–871
for hypertension, 501t
for hypertensive emergency, 105t
Romazicon
formulary entry for, 799
for sedation reversal, 146
Root impairment, 506f
ROP. *See* Retinopathy of prematurity
Rota Teq, immunoprophylaxis for, 400
Rotarix, immunoprophylaxis for, 400
Rotavirus
contraindications/precautions for, 379t
immunoprophylaxis for, 400–401
schedule for, 400
Roundworms
mebendazole for, 855
pyrantel pamoate for, 928
Rowasa, formulary entry for, 857
Roxanol
for analgesia, 140t
characterization of, 140t
formulary entry for, 878
for palliative care, 581t
relative potency of, 151t
with renal failure, 1032t
Roxicet, formulary entry for, 895
Roxicodone
characterization of, 140t
formulary entry for, 693
Roxilox, formulary entry for, 895
Roxiprin, formulary entry for, 693
RSI (Rapid sequence intubation)
medications for, 6t–7t
use of, 4
RSV. *See* Respiratory syncytial virus
Rubella, diagnosis of, 415–416

Rubella prophylaxis, IMIG therapy for, 363
Rufinamide (Banzel), for seizures, 517t
Rulox Plus, formulary entry for, 690–691
RUSB, 168

S
S-2 inhalant, formulary entry for, 783
Sabril
formulary entry for, 979
for seizures, 517t
Salagen, formulary entry for, 912–913
Salicylates, toxicity of, 40t
Salicylazosulfapyridine, formulary entry for, 955
Salicylic acid, for warts, 207t
Salmeterol (Serevent Diskus), formulary entry for, 941
Salmeterol and fluticasone propionate (Advair), formulary entry for, 804–805
Salmonella, sensitivity profile of, 408t
Salter-Harris classification, 95t
Sal-Tropine
formulary entry for, 706–707
for resuscitation, ii
for RSI, 6t
Sandimmune, formulary entry for, 759–760
Sandostatin
formulary entry for, 886
for hypoglycemic toxicity, 20t
Sani-Supp, formulary entry for, 813
Sarafem
dosage/side effects for, 1004t
formulary entry for, 801–802
Sarcoidosis, in granulomatous disease, 633
SAS, formulary entry for, 955
Scabies
characterization of, 208
permethrin for, 906
Scald burns, 98t, *Trauma, Burns, and Common Critical Care Emergencies Color Plate 1*
Scarf sign, in newborn assessment, 457
Schizophrenia
risperidone dosage for, 939
thioridazine for, 963
Scoliosis
assessment of, 131
Cobb angle for, 132f
forward bending test for, 132f
imaging of, 608
treatment of, 131–132
Scopace, formulary entry for, 942
Scopolamine hydrobromide (Transderm Scop, Isopto Hyoscine, Scopace), formulary entry for, 942
Screening(s)
for ADHD, 232t
for ASD, 232t
cognitive/motor, 232t
for depression, 232t
developmental
age-appropriate behavioral issues, 230t–231t
commonly used, 229–233
guidelines for, 227
milestones, 228t–229t
reach out and read milestones, 230t
gas chromatography, 19
gas mass spectroscopy, 19
lipid monitoring, 168–169
mental health, 232t
musculoskeletal, for adolescents, 134f
Scurvy, ascorbic acid for, 703
Seborrhea, selenium sulfide for, 942
Seborrheic dermatitis
characterization of, 222
Secondary skin lesions
characterization of, 201
pattern diagnosis of, 202f–203f
Second-degree block, 178t–179t
Secretions, in dying patients, 581t
Sedation. *See also* Anesthesia
atropine sulfate dose before, 706
complications from, 144
definitions of, 143
discharge criteria for, 146
midazolam for, 868
monitoring of, 144
opioid tapering, 150–151
pain thresholds of, 149t
pharmacologic agents for, 145–146
preparation of, 143–144
protocols for, 148, 149t
reversal of, 799
web resources for, 137

Sedative-hypnotics
common, properties of, 137
for RSI, 6t
toxicity of, 47b
toxidrome of, 25t
Sediment, in urine, 478
Seizures
acetazolamide contraindicated for, 683
acute management of, 16t
amitriptyline contraindicated for, 696
classification of, 514b
DTaP recommendations for, 385
in dying patients, 581t
febrile illness associated with, 512b, 519f
hypoglycemic, glucose for, 45
imaging of, 513
levetiracetam for, 841–842
nonepileptic causes of, 511
pyridoxine dependent, 930
syndromes of, 515t
topiramate for, 967
treatments for, 514–518, 515t–517t
vigabatrin for, 979
zonisamide for, 986
Selective norepinephrine reuptake inhibitor, for ADHD, 239t
Selective serotonin reuptake inhibitors (SSRIs)
citalopram as, 1004t
escitalopram as, 1004t
fluvoxamine as, 1004t
fluoxetine as, 1004t
sertraline as, 1004t
toxicity of, 32t
Selenium
DRIs for, 543t
in multivitamin tablets, analysis of, 547t
parenteral nutrition formulations, 561t
Selenium sulfide (Selsun), formulary entry for, 942
Senna (Senokot, Senna-Gen, Lax-Pills, Fletcher's Castoria), formulary entry for, 943
Senna-Gen, formulary entry for, 943
Sennosides, formulary entry for, 943
Senokot, formulary entry for, 943
Sensation changes, as death approaches, 580
Sensitivity tests, 656–657
Sensory evaluation, 504
Separation anxiety, 230t
Sepsis, initial management of, 421t
Septic arthritis, initial management of, 421t
Serevent Diskus, formulary entry for, 941
Seroquel (Quetiapinel), dosage/side effects for, 1004t
Serotonin (5-HT_3), for chemotherapy-induced nausea, 574
Serotonin norepinephrine reuptake inhibitor, dosage/side effects for, 1005t
Serratia spp., sensitivity profile of, 408t
Sertraline HCl (Zoloft)
dosage/side effects for, 1004t
formulary entry for, 944
Serum muscle enzymes, 623
Serum osmolar gap, due to poisoning, 22t
Serutan, formulary entry for, 927
Sex hormone binding protein (SHBG), 259
Sex hormones. *See* Estradiol; Testosterone
Sexual abuse, HIV infection from, 450–451
Sexual development
ambiguous genitalia in, 262
delayed puberty in, 259–260, 261f
precocious puberty in, 260–262
Shock
basic treatment for, 109t
categorization of, 108t
emergency care for, 107
physiologic response in, 109t
Shprintzen syndrome. *See* 22q11 syndrome
Shunt dysfunction, cause of, 518
Shunts
Glenn, 184
palliative superior vena cava-to-pulmonary artery, 184
palliative systemic-to-pulmonary artery, 184

SIADH. *See* Syndrome of inappropriate antidiuretic hormone secretion
Sibling relationships, 231t
Sickle cell anemia
  characterization of, 328–329
  complications of, 329t–330t
  immunization recommendations for, 381
  maintenance of, 331t
SIDS. *See* Sudden infant death syndrome
Sildenafil (Revatio, Viagra), formulary entry for, 944–945
Sildex, formulary entry for, 729–730
Silver sulfadiazine (Silvadene, Thermazene, SSD Cream)
  formulary entry for, 945
Simethicone (Mylicon, Phazyme, Mylanta Gas, Gas-X), formulary entry for, 945–946
Singulair, formulary entry for, 872–873
Sinusitis
  azithromycin for, 709
  cefdinir for, 733
  initial treatment of, 434t
Sinusoidal obstruction syndrome. *See* Veno-occlusive disease
Sirolimus (Rapamune), formulary entry for, 946–947
Skeletal injuries, child abuse-associated, 103t
Skeletal survey, 618
Skin
  abrasions, from child abuse, 1f–2f
  disorders of. *See* Dermatologic disorders
  primary lesions on
    characterization of, 201
    pattern diagnosis of, 202f
  secondary lesions on
    characterization of, 201
    pattern diagnosis of, 203f
  staples, for laceration repair, 84
  tests
    for egg allergies, 371–374
    for food allergies, 371–374
Skin infection(s)
  meropenem for, 857
  uncomplicated, linezolid for, 847
Skin staples, 84
Skin trauma, secondary survey of, 90t
SLE. *See* Systemic lupus erythematosus
Sleep, changes in, as death approaches, 580
Snakes. *See* Venomous snakes
SOAP (suction, oxygen, airway, supplies, pharmacology), use of, 4
Sodium (Na^+)
  in cow's milk formulas, 549t–556t
  deficits
    dehydration-associated, 275f
    replacement of, 278
  in enteral formulas, 549t–556t
  intracellular/extracellular composition of, 276t
  in multivitamin tablets, analysis of, 547t
  neonatal requirements for, 462t
  parenteral nutrition formulations, 561t
  reference values for, 646t
  serum disturbances of, 281
Sodium bicarbonate ($NaHCO_3^-$, Bicitra, Polycitra, Neut)
  formulary entry for, 947
  for resuscitation, ii
Sodium chloride, arginine chloride as alternative for, 702
Sodium chloride-inhaled preparations, formulary entry for, 948
Sodium phosphate (Fleet, Fleet Phospho-Soda, Visicol, OsmoPrep), formulary entry for, 911, 948–949
Sodium polystyrene sulfonate (Kayexalate, SPS, Kionex), formulary entry for, 949
Soft tissue(s), aspiration of, 78–80, 79f–80f
Solu-Metadate, formulary entry for, 860–862
Solute fluid deficit (SFD), 277
Sotret
  for acne vulgaris, 218–220
  formulary entry for, 832
Soy-based formulas
  enteral nutritional components in, 550t–557t
Spearman's rank correlation coefficient, 653t

Specific gravity, of urine, 476
Specificity tests, 656–657
Spiders, toxicity of, 53–54
Spinal cord(s)
  compression of, characterization of, 567–568
  examination of, 505
  imaging of, 607–608
  injury to, methylprednisolone for, 991–992
Spinal dysraphism, 608
Spirillum minus, in animal bites, 96t
Spiritual changes, as death approaches, 580
Spirometry, 588–590, 590t
Spironolactone (Aldactone)
  formulary entry for, 950
  for hypertension, 501t
  with renal failure, 1034t
Splinting
  basic, 85
  long arm posterior, 85
  posterior ankle, 87
  radial head subluxation reduction, 87
  sugar tong forearm, 86
  thumb spica, 86
  ulnar gutter, 86
  volar, 87
SPS, formulary entry for, 949
Square window, in newborn assessment, 457
SSD Cream
  formulary entry for, 945
Staphylococcus aureus, in animal bites, 96t
Staphylococcus aureus infections, rifampin dosage for, 937
Staphylococcus viridans, in dog bites, 96t
Staples, skin, 84
Stature, weight and
  for boys, 531f
  for girls, 529f
Status epilepticus
  acute management of, 17
  diazepam for, 768
  lorazepam for, 853
  phenytoin dosage for, 910
Stem cell transplants, *Candida* prophylaxis in, 866
Stenosis
  aortic, CHD/exam findings of, 186t
  pulmonary, CHD/exam findings of, 186t
Stenotrophomonas maltophilia, sensitivity profile of, 409t
Steroid hormones. *See also* Corticosteroid(s)
  biosynthetic pathway of, 254f
  for chemotherapy-induced nausea, 574
  for spinal cord compression, 568
Stimate
  formulary entry for, 765–766
  for von Willebrand disease, 347t
Stimulant(s)
  cocaine as, 43–44
  ecstasy as, 44
Stomach. *See* Gastrointestinal (GI) tract
Stomatitis, sucralfate for, 952
Stranger anxiety, 230t
Staphylococcus spp., sensitivity profile of, 408t
Strattera, formulary entry for, 705
Strength
  examination of, 504
  rating scale for, 505b
Streptobacilles moniliformis, in animal bites, 96t
Streptococcal meningitis, penicillin G preparations for, 902
Streptomycin sulfate
  formulary entry for, 950–951
  with renal failure, 1023t
Stress fractures, imaging of, 618
Stress ulcer, sucralfate for, 952
Stridor, 585t
Stroke(s)
  differential diagnosis of, 521b
  etiology, 520
  initial workup for, 521
  management of, 521–522
Structural diagnostic tests, for genetic abnormalities, 316
Subclavian vein(s), catheter placement in, 62, 63f
Subcutaneous immune globulin, 363
Subcutaneous injections, 81
Sublimaze
  characterization of, 140t
  formulary entry for, 794–795

Sublimaze *(Continued)*
relative potency of, 151t
with renal failure, 1030t
for RSI, 6t
Substance P, for chemotherapy-induced nausea, 575
Succimer (Chemet, DMSA, [dimercaptosuccinic acid]), formulary entry for, 951
Succinylcholine
formulary entry for, 951–952
for RSI, 7t
Sucralfate (Carafate), formulary entry for, 952–953
Sudafed
cetirizine with, 740–741
formulary entry for, 926
loratadine with, 850
Sudden infant death syndrome (SIDS), 603, 603b
Sugar(s), in urine, 477
Sugar tong forearm splinting, 86
Sulbactam, with ampicillin, for mastoiditis, 425t
Sulfacetamide sodium ophthalmic (AK-Sulf, Bleph 10, Ocusulf-10), formulary entry for, 953, 1000t
Sulfadiazine, formulary entry for, 953–954
Sulfamethoxazole and Trimethoprim (Co-trimoxazole)
for acne vulgaris, 218t
formulary entry for, 954
with renal failure, 1024t
Sulfasazine (salicylazosulfapyridine, SAS, Azulfidine), formulary entry for, 955
Sulfisoxazole (Gantrisin), with renal failure, 1024t
Sumatriptan succinate (Imitrex), formulary entry for, 955–956
Sumycin
for acne vulgaris, 218t
with renal failure, 1024t
Sunkist Vitamin C, formulary entry for, 703
Superior vena cava syndrome, oncologic-associated, characterization of, 568–569
Superwarfarins, toxicity of, 52–53
Supplemental oxygen, for newborns, 463
Supplementation
calcium, monitoring of, 252–253
fluoride, 544
iron, 253
vitamin D, 539
vitamin-mineral, 539–545
Supplements, pancreatic enzymes, 996
Suprapubic bladder, aspirations of, 78, 79f–80f
Supraventricular tachycardia
adenosine dosage for, 686
characterization of, 175t
Suprax
formulary entry for, 734–735
for gonorrhea, 430t
with renal failure, 1015t
Surfactant pulmonary/beractant (Survanta), formulary entry for, 956
Surfactant pulmonary/calfactant (Infasurf), formulary entry for, 957
Surfactant pulmonary/poractant ALFA (Curosurf), formulary entry for, 957–958
Surfak, formulary entry for, 774–775
Survanta, formulary entry for, 956
Suturing
guidelines for, 83t
procedures for, 82–84
techniques of, 81
vertical mattress, 82f
SVT, 175t
Symbicort, formulary entry for, 720
Symmetrel
approval for, 393
formulary entry for, 691
with renal failure, 1013t
Sympathomimetic(s)
cyclopentolate with phenylephrine as, 759
dobutamine as, 774
dopamine as, 775–776
epinephrine as, 782–783
pseudoephedrine as, 926
toxidrome of, 23t
Sympathomimetics, toxidrome of, 23t
Synacort
for adrenal insufficiency, 256
formulary entry for, 819

Synacort *(Continued)*
for glucocorticoid deficiency, 989
for hyperparathyroidism, 253
for hypoparathyroidism, 252
Synagis
formulary entry for, 896–897
for RVS immunoprophylaxis, 400
Synalar, potency ranking of, 995t
Syndrome of inappropriate antidiuretic hormone secretion (SIADH), 256
Synercid, formulary entry for, 932
Synovial fluids, in rheumatic disease, 628t
Synthroid, formulary entry for, 843–844
Syphilis
Bicillin L-A for, 903
congenital, penicillin G preparations for, 902
diagnosis of, 415
initial treatment of, 433t
Systemic corticosteroids
for endocrine disorders, 989
for pulmonary disorders, 991
Systemic lupus erythematosus (SLE)
autoantibodies associated with, 621t
classification of, 627, 628t
clinical features of, 628–629
definition of, 627–630
drug-induced, 629–630
treatment of, 629
Systolic heart murmurs, 167t
Systolic sounds, 164–165

T

T lymphocytes, in peripheral blood, 366t
T_4, formulary entry for, 843–844
Tachycardia
characterization of, 175t
due to poisoning, 20t
supraventricular, 176t
ventricular, 178t
Tachypnea, due to poisoning, 20t
Tacrolimus (Prograf, FK506, Protopic), formulary entry for, 958–959
Tagamet
for asthma, 748
formulary entry for, 749
with renal failure, 1029t
for warts, 207t
Takayasu arthritis, 631t
Tambocor
formulary entry for, 797
with renal failure, 1030t
Tamiflu
approval for, 392
formulary entry for, 891–892
for influenza, 425t
with renal failure, 1022t
Tanner stages, 269t
Tanner staging, 118b, 118f
Tapazole
formulary entry for, 856–857
for Graves disease, 250
Taxol, toxicity of, 1008t
Tazicef
formulary entry for, 737
for osteomyelitis, 426t
for otitis media, 426t
with renal failure, 1016t
Tazidime
formulary entry for, 737
for osteomyelitis, 426t
for otitis media, 426t
with renal failure, 1016t
Tazobactam, piperacillin with, formulary entry for, 914
3TC
formulary entry for, 837
with renal failure, 1021t
TCIs. *See* Topical calcineurin inhibitors
Td. *See* Tetanus and diphtheria (Td) vaccine
Tegretol
adenosine effects on, 686
formulary entry for, 727–728
with renal failure, 1028t
for seizures, 516t
toxicity of, 48
Telogen effluvium
clinical presentation of, 216
pathogenesis of, 216
Temodar (temozolomide), toxicity of, 1008t
Temovate, potency ranking of, 995t
Temozolomide (Temodar), toxicity of, 1008t
Temper tantrums, 231t
Temperature(s), conversion formulas for, 650
Temporal arthritis, 631t

Tempra
analgesic properties of, 138
formulary entry for, 682
poisoning with, 684
with renal failure, 1027t
toxicity of, 28t
Tendon(s), reflexes of, 506–507
Teniposide (VM-26), toxicity of, 1008t
Tenormin
formulary entry for, 704–706
for hypertension, 500t
with renal failure, 1027t
Tensilon, formulary entry for, 779
Tension pneumothorax
characterization of, 94
needle decompression for, 72
Terazosin, for hypertension, 501t
Terbinafine (Lamisil granules), for tinea capitis, 215
Terbutaline (Brethine)
asthma treatment with, 11
formulary entry for, 959–960
with renal failure, 1034t
standard concentrations for, i
Testicles, size, Tanner stages, 269t
Testicular tumors, signs/symptoms of, 566t
Testosterone, normal values for, 266t
Tetanus and diphtheria (Td) vaccine, for cancer patients, 381t
Tetracaine, characterization of, 141t
Tetracycline HCl (Sumycin)
for acne vulgaris, 218t
formulary entry for, 960
with renal failure, 1024t
Tetrahydrocannabinol
for chemotherapy-induced nausea, 574
formulary entry for, 778
Tetralogy spells, propranolol for, 924
6-TG (thioguanine), toxicity of, 1008t
Thalassemias, characterization of, 329–332
THC
for chemotherapy-induced nausea, 574
formulary entry for, 778
Theo-24
formulary entry for, 960–961
toxicity of, 20t–22t
TheoCap
formulary entry for, 960–961
toxicity of, 20t–22t
Theophylline (Theo-24, Theochron, Uniphyl, TheoCap, Elixophyllin)
formulary entry for, 960–961
toxicity of, 20t–22t
Thermal burns, 98t, *Trauma, Burns, and Common Critical Care Emergencies Color Plate 5*
Thermazene
formulary entry for, 945
Thermic effect of food (TEF), definition of, 535
Thiabedazole (Mintezol), formulary entry for, 962
Thiamilate
coma treatment with, 14
formulary entry for, 962
in multivitamin drops, analysis of, 545t
in multivitamin tablets, analysis of, 546t
for status epilepticus, 16t
Thiamine (vitamin B_1, Thiamilate)
coma treatment with, 14
formulary entry for, 962
in multivitamin drops, analysis of, 545t
in multivitamin tablets, analysis of, 546t
for status epilepticus, 16t
Thiamine deficiency. *See* Beriberi
Thioguanine (6-TG, 6-thioguanine), toxicity of, 1008t
Thiopental sodium (Pentothal)
with renal failure, 1034t
for RSI, 6t
for sedation, 151t
Thioridazine (Mellaril), formulary entry for, 963
Thiotepa, toxicity of, 1009t
Third degree heat block. *See* Mobitz type I
Thoracentesis, procedures for, 72–74, 74f
Thorazine
for chemotherapy-induced nausea, 574
formulary entry for, 745
Thrombocytopenia
in cancer patients, 573–574
causes of, 332–334

Thrombocytopenia *(Continued)*
characterization of, 345b
definition of, 332
Thrombocytopenic purpura (TTP), in bone marrow transplants, 572–573
Thrombolytic therapy
alteplase for, 689
characterization of, 522
Thrombosis(es)
evaluation of, 335–339
risks for, 338b, 339
treatment of, 339–343
Thrombotic microangiopathy, in bone marrow transplants, 572–573
Thumb spica splint, 84
Thyroid disorders. *See also* Parathyroid disorders
Graves diseases, 250
Hashimoto's thyroiditis, 250
hyperthyroidism as, 248–252, 251t
neonatal thyrotoxicosis as, 252
Thyroid function tests, 247, 248t, 249t
Thyrotoxicosis, propranolol for, 924
Tiagabine (Gabitril)
formulary entry for, 963–964
for seizures, 517t
Tiazac, formulary entry for, 771
Tibia(s), posterior, puncture of, 61
Ticarcillin (Ticar), with renal failure, 1024t
Ticarcillin and clavulanate (Timentin)
formulary entry for, 964
with renal failure, 1024t
Tick-borne illnesses
anaplasmosis as, 449
ehrlichiosis as, 449
Lyme disease as, 446–448
rocky mountain spotted fever as, 448–449
Tigan, formulary entry for, 970
Timentin
formulary entry for, 964
with renal failure, 1024t
Tinactin, formulary entry for, 966
Tinea capitis, characterization of, 214–216
Tinea corporis, characterization of, 214
Tinea versicolor, characterization of, 214
Tisit, formulary entry for, 929
Tissue adhesive(s), 84
TIV. *See* Trivalent influenza vaccine
TOBI
formulary entry for, 965–966
with renal failure, 1024t
Tobramycin (Nebcin, Tobrex, AKTob, TOBI)
formulary entry for, 965–966
with renal failure, 1024t
Tobramycin ophthalmic, 1002t
Tobrex
formulary entry for, 965–966
with renal failure, 1024t
Tofranil, formulary entry for, 823–824
Toilet training, 231t
Tolnaftate (Tinactin, Aftate), formulary entry for, 966
Tonic clonic seizures, topiramate for, 967
Topical antibiotics, for acne vulgaris, 217, 218t
Topical calcineurin inhibitors (TCIs), for atopic dermatitis, 212
Topicort, potency ranking of, 995t
Topiramate (Topamax)
formulary entry for, 967
for migraines, 512t
for seizures, 517t
Topotecan (Hycamptin), toxicity of, 1009t
Toprol-XL
formulary entry for, 864
for hypertension, 500t
Toradol
characterization of, 139
formulary entry for, 835–836
Totacillin
formulary entry for, 701
for gonococcal infections, 420t
for meningitis, 421t
neonatal critical care dosing of, 1010t
with renal failure, 1014t
with sulbactam, for mastoiditis, 425t
Total energy expenditure (TEE), definition of, 535
Total iron-building capacity (TIBC), reference values for, 646t
Tourette's syndrome, haloperidol for, 816

Toxicity, vancomycin, 975
Toxicology screens, types of, 19
Toxocariasis, mebendazole for, 855
Toxoplasmosis
congenital, sulfadiazine for, 953–954
diagnosis of, 415
pyrimethamine dosage for, 930
tPA, formulary entry for, 689
Tracheoesophageal fistula (TEF), imaging of, 616
Traction alopecia
clinical presentation of, 216
pathogenesis of, 216
treatment for, 216
Trained night feeding, 230t
Trandate, formulary entry for, 836
Transderm Scop, formulary entry for, 942
Transferrin, reference values for, 646t
Transfusion(s)
blood product components for, 348–350
complications of, 351
donor acceptances criteria for, 352
donor rejection criteria for, 351
PRBC exchange, 350
Transient erythroblastopenia of childhood (TEC), characterization of, 327
Transient neonatal jaundice, 305t
Transient neonatal pustular melanosis, characterization of, 220
Transplantation(s)
bone marrow, complications of, 571–573
stem cell, *Candida* prophylaxis in, 866
tacrolimus for, 958
Transthoracic echocardiography (TEE), characterization of, 191
Transudate fluids, reference values for, 648t
Trauma(s)
abdominal, 617
emergent treatments for, 106
evaluation of, 103–104
laboratory studies of, 104–113
radiologic evaluation of, 105–106
AMPLE history of, 89–93
Trauma(s) *(Continued)*
blunt thoracic
emergent treatments for, 106
evaluation of, 103–104
laboratory studies of, 104–113
radiologic evaluation of, 105–106
cervical spine, 607
to extremities, imaging of, 618
minor closed head (CHT)
associated symptoms of, 93
imaging indications for, 92b
injury mechanism in, 92–93
management of, 93
overview of, 89–91
physical examination of, 91–93
sports-related, 97–102
systemic corticosteroids for, 991
neck injury-related, 100
orthopedic/long bone, 94–96
primary survey of, 89
secondary survey of
organ systems in, 90t
procedures for, 89–96
Trazodone (Desyrel)
dosage/side effects for, 1005t
formulary entry for, 968
Tretinoin (Retin-A, Avita, Renova), formulary entry for, 968
Tretinoin (Vesanoid), for warts, 207t
Triamcinolone
for allergic rhinitis, 355–356
potency of, 992t
Triamcinolone acetonide (Azmacort, Nasacort, Kenalog, Aristospan)
formulary entry for, 969
potency ranking of, 995t
Triamterene (Dyrenium)
formulary entry for, 970
for hyperthyroidism, 251t
with renal failure, 1034t
Trichinosis, thiabedazole for, 962
Trichomoniasis, metronidazole for, 865
Trichophyton tonsurans, characterization of, 214
Trichostrongylus, pyrantel pamoate for, 928
Trichotillomania
clinical presentation of, 217
pathogenesis of, 217

Trichuris, mebendazole for, 855
Tricyclic antidepressants, toxicity of, 32t
Trifluridine ophthalmic, 1002t
Triglycerides, reference values for, 646t
TriHIBit, immunoprophylaxis for, 403
Trileptal
  formulary entry for, 893–894
  with renal failure, 1033t
  for seizures, 516t
Trilisate. *See* Choline magnesium trisalicylate
TriLyte, formulary entry for, 915
Trimethobenzamide HCl (Tigan), formulary entry for, 970
Trimethoprim sulfate
  ophthalmic, 1001t
  polymyxin B sulfate with, formulary entry for, 916
Trimethoprim-sulfamethoxazole (Co-trimoxazole)
  for acne vulgaris, 218t
  formulary entry for, 954
  with renal failure, 1024t
Trimox
  for bacterial infections, 422t
  formulary entry for, 697
  for lymphadenitis, 425t
  for meningitis, 426t
  for otitis media, 426t
  with renal failure, 1013t
Triamterene (Dyrenium), for hypertension, 501t
Trisomy 13, characterization of, 318
Trisomy 18, characterization of, 318
Trisomy 21
  characterization of, 316
  dominant cardiac defect in, 184t
Trivalent influenza vaccine (TIV)
  contraindications/precautions for, 378t
  for pregnant patients, 384
Troponin-I, reference values for, 647t
Trousseau sign, 284
  due to hypocalcemia, 284
  due to poisoning, 21t
Trypanosomiasis spp., pentomone isethionate for, 905
TTP. *See* Thrombocytopenic purpura
Tuberculosis
  drug therapy for, 445–446, 447t
  pyrazinoic acid dosage for, 928
  rifampin dosage for, 937
  testing for, 444–445, 446b
Tubular disorders, 486–487
Tumor lysis syndrome
  allopurinol dosage use and, 688
  characterization of, 567
Tums, formulary entry for, 723
Turbidity, urine, 476
Turner syndrome
  characterization of, 316–317
  dominant cardiac defect in, 184t
  growth charts for, 534
TWINRIX, immunoprophylaxis for, 403
Two sample *t* test, 653t
Two way analysis of variance, 653t
Tylenol
  analgesic properties of, 138
  formulary entry for, 682
  poisoning with, 684
  with renal failure, 1027t
  toxicity of, 28t
Tylox, formulary entry for, 895
Type 3 renal tubular acidosis, 487

U

Ulcer(s)
  duodenal
    famotidine for, 793
    lansoprazole for, 840
    omeprazole for, 889
    ranitidine for, 933
    sucralfate for, 952
  genital, 122
  omeprazole for, 888
  peptic
    aluminum hydroxide for, 690
    famotidine for, 793
    pantoprazole for, 898
  NSAID-induced, lansoprazole for, 840
  ranitidine for, 933
  SLE-associated, 628t
  stress, sucralfate for, 952
Ulcerative colitis (UC), 299
Ulnar gutter splint, 86
Umbilical artery, catheterization, vascular access for, 65–68
Umbilical cord blood, HSCT from, 571

Umbilical veins, catheterization of
catheter placement for, 69f
vascular access for, 65–68
Unasyn
formulary entry for, 701–702
with renal failure, 1014t
Unconjugated hyperbilirubinemia in newborns, neonatal, 467
Unfractionated heparin (UFH), 339–340, 339t–340t
Unipen, formulary entry for, 876
Uniphyl
formulary entry for, 960–961
toxicity of, 20t–22t
Upper airway obstruction, emergency treatment of, 12–13
Urea nitrogen, reference values for, 647t
Uric acid, reference values for, 647t
Urinalysis
dipstick method for, 476–477
microscopy for, 477–478
for rheumatic diseases, 623
for UTIs, 480t
Urinary acidification, 697
Urinary bladder(s)
catheterization, for blood fluid sampling, 77–78
suprapubic, aspiration for, 77–78
Urinary tract infections (UTIs)
culture-positive
antibiotic prophylaxis for, 481–482
imaging studies of, 481–482
treatment for, 480–481
evaluation of, 479–483
cultures for, 480–483
history in, 476
laboratory studies for, 479–480, 480t
physical examination for, 479
imaging of, 617
initial treatment of, 435t
levofloxacin for, 843
phenazopyridine for, 907
Urine
bilirubin in, 477
epithelial cells in, 478
hemoglobin in, 477
ketones in, 477
myoglobin in, 477
pH, 476
Urine *(Continued)*
proteins in, 477
red blood cells in, 477–478
sediment in, 478
specific gravity of, 476
sugars in, 477
turbidity of, 476
urobilinogen in, 477
white blood cells in, 478
Urine gram stain, purpose of, 478
Ur-KP-Neutral, formulary entry for, 911
Urobilinogen, in urine, 477, 478t
Urolene Blue
formulary entry for, 860
for methemoglobinemia, 51
Ursodiol (Actigall, Urso 250, Urso Forte), formulary entry for, 971
Urticaria, food allergy-induced, 356
Uterine pathology, 617
UTIs. *See* Urinary tract infections (UTIs)

V

Vaccine(s)
abbreviations of, 370b
administration of, 371–374
asplenia and, 381
for cancer patients, 381, 381t
combination, 402–403
corticosteroid therapy and, 382, 382t
DTaP
for adolescents and young adults, 384
age-based schedule for, 372f
for cancer, 381t
contraindications/precautions for, 376t
immunoprophylaxis for, 384–386
for pregnant patients, 384
egg allergies and, 371–374
for haemophilus influenza B
age-based schedule for, 374f
for cancer patients, 381t
catch-up schedule for, 374f
immunoprophylaxis for, 386–387
schedule for, 372f
for hepatitis A
catch-up schedule for, 374f
contraindications/precautions for, 376t
dosages/schedule for, 388t
immunoprophylaxis for, 387–388
interval schedule for, 375t

Vaccine(s) *(Continued)*
for pregnant patients, 384
schedule for, 372f
for hepatitis B
age considerations for, 382
catch-up schedule for, 374f
contraindications/precautions for, 376t
dosages/schedule for, 389t
immunoprophylaxis for, 388–389
interval schedule for, 375t
for pregnant patients, 384
for HIV/AIDS patients, 380–381
immunoprophylaxis guidelines for, 375–384
for inactivated poliovirus
for cancer patients, 381t
catch-up schedule for, 374f
interval schedule for, 375t
for pregnant patients, 384
informed consent for, 371
for MCV4
for adolescents, 384
for cancer patients, 381t
contraindications/precautions for, 379t
for adolescents and young adults, 384
immunoprophylaxis, 395
interval schedule for, 375t
minimum age/interval, 375t
for MMR
age-based schedule for, 373f
for cancer patients, 381t
catch-up schedule for, 374f
contraindications/precautions for, 378t
immunoprophylaxis for, 393–394
for PCEC, 397
for PCV
contraindications/precautions for, 376t
interval schedule for, 375t
for rabies
immunoprophylaxis for, 397–399
postexposure prophylaxis of, 398–399
for reactive arthritis patients, 388–389
rotavirus, 379t
schedules for
catch-up, 374f
infants to 6-year-olds, 372f

Vaccine(s) *(Continued)*
7-year-olds to 18-year-olds, 373f
for splenectomy patients, 381
for tetanus and diphtheria, 381t
for trivalent influenza
contraindications/precautions for, 378t
for pregnant patients, 384
for varicella zoster virus
for adolescents and young adults, 384
for cancer patients, 381t
contraindications/precautions for, 378t
immunoprophylaxis for, 401–402
schedule for, 372f
for yellow fever, 374
Vasodilators, for hypertension, 501t
Vaginal infections, diagnostic features of, 123t
Vagistat-3, formulary entry for, 867
Valganciclovir (Valcyte), formulary entry for, 972–973
Valacyclovir (Valtrex)
formulary entry for, 971–972
with renal failure, 1025t
Valcyte, formulary entry for, 971–973
Valganciclovir (Valcyte), formulary entry for, 971–972
Valium
formulary entry for, 768–769
Valproic acid (VPA, Depakote, Depakene)
formulary entry for, 973–974
for seizures, 517t
toxicity of, 48
Valtrex
formulary entry for, 971–972
with renal failure, 1025t
Vancomycin (Vancocin)
for catheter-related bloodstream infections, 423t
for cellulitis, 423t
formulary entry for, 974–976
for lymphadenitis, 425t
for meningitis, 426t
neonatal critical care dosing of, 1010t
for pneumonia, 428t
with renal failure, 1026t

Vanos, potency ranking of, 995t
Vantin
for gonorrhea, 431t
with renal failure, 1015t
Varicella-Zoster immune globulin (human), formulary entry for, 976
Varicella zoster virus (VZV)
acyclovir dosage and, 685
diagnosis of, 416
neonatal management of, 414t
vaccine for, 384
valacyclovir for, 971
Varicella zoster virus (VZV) vaccine
for adolescents and young adults, 384
for cancer patients, 381t
contraindications/precautions for, 378t
immunoprophylaxis for, 401–402
schedule for, 372f
VariZIG
immunoprophylaxis for, 401–402
for neonatal varicella, 414t
Vascular access
for central venous catheter placement, 61–63
for intraosseous infusion, 63–65, 65f
for peripheral intravenous placement, 61
for umbilical artery/vein catheterization, 65–68
Vasculitis
autoantibodies associated with, 621t
general characterization of, 630
HSP induction of, 630–632, 631t
syndromes of, 631t
Vasopressin (Pitressin, beta-arginine vasopressin)
in diabetes insipidus, 256
formulary entry for, 977
for resuscitation, ii
standard concentrations for, i
Vasopressin test, 264
Vasotec
formulary entry for, 780
for hypertension, 500t
for hypertensive emergency, 105t
with renal failure, 1030t
VATER association, 459
VATER/VACTERL syndrome, dominant cardiac defect in, 184t
VCFS syndrome, dominant cardiac defect in, 184t
VCR (vincristine), toxicity of, 1009t
VCUG. *See* Voiding cysto-urethrogram
Vecuronium, for RSI, 7t
Veetids
characterization of, 902
formulary entry for, 904–905
with renal failure, 1023t
Vein(s)
external jugular, puncture of, 58–59
femoral
catheter placement in, 62, 64f
puncture of, 59
internal jugular, catheter placement in, 62
subclavian, catheter placement in, 62, 63f
umbilical, catheterization of, vascular access for, 65–68
Velban (vinblastine), toxicity of, 1009t
Velocardiofacial syndrome. *See* 22q11 syndrome
Velosef, renal with renal failure, 1016t
Venlafaxine (Effexor), dosage/side effects for, 1005t
Venomous snakes, toxicity of, 53
Veno-occlusive disease, in bone marrow transplants, 572
Venous blood gas (VBG), 586
Venous vasodilator, for hypertensive emergency, 105t
Ventriculoperitoneal (VP) shunts
malfunction of, 607
use of, 518
Ventilation, bag and mask, 3
Ventilator, setting changes in, 112t
Ventolin HFA
for anaphylaxis, 10
for asthma, 10
formulary entry for, 687–688
Ventricular arrhythmias, 178t
Ventricular conduction disturbances, 180t
Ventricular fibrillation, 178t
Ventricular hypertrophy, criteria for, 174b
Ventricular septal defect (VSD), CHD/exam findings of, 186t
Ventricular tachycardia, 178t
Ventriculoperitoneal shunt infections, initial treatment of, 435t

VePesid (etoposide), toxicity of, 1007t
Veramyst, dosage recommendations for, 802
Verapamil (Isoptin, Calan, Verelan, Covera-HS)
  formulary entry for, 978
  with renal failure, 1034t
Verdeso foam. *See* Desonide (DesOwen, Verdeso foam)
Verdeso foam, potency ranking of, 996t
Verelan, with renal failure, 1034t
Vermox, formulary entry for, 854–855
Versed
  formulary entry for, 868
  with renal failure, 1032t
  for RSI, 6t
  for sedation, 151t
Vertical mattress suturing, 82f
Vesanoid, for warts, 207t
Vesicoureteral reflux
  antibiotic prophylaxis for, 483t
  international classification of, 478t
Vessels, imaging of, 615
VFEND, formulary entry for, 981–982
Viagra, formulary entry for, 944–945
Vibramycin
  for acne vulgaris, 218t
  for Lyme disease, 448
Vigabatrin (Sabril)
  formulary entry for, 979
  for seizures, 517t
Vigamox, 1002t
Vinblastine (VLB, vincaleukoblastine, Velban), toxicity of, 1009t
Vincaleukoblastine, toxicity of, 1009t
Vincristine (VCR, Oncovin), toxicity of, 1009t
Vinorelbine (Navelbine), toxicity of, 1009t
Viramune, formulary entry for, 879–880
Virazole, formulary entry for, 934–936
Viroptic, 1002t
Visceral larva migraines, mebendazole for, 855
Visceral leishmaniasis, pentomone isethionate for, 905
Visicol, formulary entry for, 948–949
Visine, formulary entry for, 693
Vision, tests for, 505t
Vistaril
  formulary entry for, 821
  properties of, 137
Vitamin(s)
  DRI for, 540t
  drops, analysis of, 545t
  newborns' requirements for, 460–461
Vitamin A (Aquasol A, Palmitate-A 5000)
  DRIs for, 542t
  formulary entry for, 979–980
  in multivitamin drops, analysis of, 545t
  in multivitamin tablets, analysis of, 546t
  reference values for, 647t
Vitamin B_1
  coma treatment with, 14
  DRIs for, 542t
  formulary entry for, 962
  in multivitamin drops, analysis of, 545t
  in multivitamin tablets, analysis of, 546t
  for status epilepticus, 16t
Vitamin B_2
  DRIs for, 542t
  formulary entry for, 936
  in multivitamin drops, analysis of, 545t
  in multivitamin tablets, analysis of, 546t
  reference values for, 647t
Vitamin B_3. *See* Niacin
Vitamin B_6
  DRIs for, 542t
  formulary entry for, 930
  in multivitamin drops, analysis of, 545t
  in multivitamin tablets, analysis of, 546t
Vitamin B_{12}
  DRIs for, 542t
  in multivitamin drops, analysis of, 545t
  in multivitamin tablets, analysis of, 546t
  reference values for, 647t

Vitamin C (ascorbic acid, Cecon, Sunkist Vitamin C)
DRIs for, 542t
formulary entry for, 703
in multivitamin tablets, analysis of, 546t
reference values for, 647t
Vitamin D (Calcitriol). *See also* Calcitriol
cyanocobalamin with, 758
DRIs for, 542t
for hyperparathyroidism, 252
for hypoparathyroidism, 252
formulary entry for, 745–746, 981
in multivitamin drops, analysis of, 545t
in multivitamin tablets, analysis of, 546t
normal values for, 266t
rickets resistant, 785
Vitamin D deficiency, 253t
Vitamin D supplementation
monitoring of, 252
recommend dosage for, 539
Vitamin E (Alpha-tocopherol, Aquasol E, Aquavit-E, Nutr-E-Sol)
DRIs for, 542t
in multivitamin drops, analysis of, 545t
in multivitamin tablets, analysis of, 546t
Vitamin K
deficiency, 345b
DRIs for, 542t
formulary entry for, 912
in multivitamin drops, analysis of, 545t
in multivitamin tablets, analysis of, 546t
for warfarin toxicity, 52–53
Vitamin-mineral supplementation, 539–545
Vitrase, formulary entry for, 817
VLB (vinblastine), toxicity of, 1009t
VM-26 (teniposide), toxicity of, 1008t
Voiding cysto-urethrogram (VCUG), for UTI evaluation, 481–482
Volar splints, 87
Vomiting. *See* Nausea and vomiting
von Willebrand disease
characterization of, 347t
hepatic factors in, 345b
Voriconazole (VFEND), formulary entry for, 981–982
VoSpire ER
for anaphylaxis, 10
for asthma, 10
formulary entry for, 687–688
VP-16 (etoposide), toxicity of, 1007t
VPA
for seizures, 517t
formulary entry for, 973–974
toxicity of, 48

W

Waist circumference ratio, 535
Waist-height ratio, 535
Warfarin (Coumadin, Jantoven, Warfarin)
dosing adjustments for, 340t
dosing guidelines for, 340t
excessive anticoagulation by, 342t
formulary entry for, 983–984
international normalized ratio for, 341t
medications influencing, 343b
toxicity of, 52–53
Warts
genital, 122
morphology of, 206–207
treatment for, 207t
Water
deprivation test, 263–264
newborns' loss of, 460t
Wegener granulomatosis, 631t
Weight
acetaminophen dosage and, 682
acetylcysteine dosage and, 684
kanamycin dosage and, 833t
lamotrigine dosage and, 838t
length and
degree conversion for, 650
for boys, 527f–528f
for girls, 525f–526f
for preterm infants, 533f
lidocaine and prilocaine dosage and, 846t
oseltamivir dosage and, 838t
oxcarbazepine dosage and, 893t
stature and
for boys, 531f
for girls, 529f
Wellbutrin, dosage/side effects for, 1005t
Wenckebach. *See* Mobitz type I

Wernicke's encephalopathy syndrome, thiamine for, 962
Westcort, potency ranking of, 995t
Wheezes, 585t
Whipworms, mebendazole for, 855
White blood cells
smear interpretation of, 352
in urine, 478
WHO. *See* World Health Organization
Wilcoxon matched pairs test, 653t
Williams syndrome, dominant cardiac defect in, 184t
Wilms' tumor, signs/symptoms of, 565t
Wilson's disease, penicillamine for, 901
Withdrawal, toxidrome of, 25t
Wolff-Parkinson-White (WPW), 180t
World Health Organization (WHO), growth charts of, 525–528
Wrist(s), injuries to, volar splints for, 87
Wycillin, formulary entry for, 904
Wymox
for bacterial infections, 422t
formulary entry for, 697
for lymphadenitis, 425t
for meningitis, 426t
otitis media for otitis media, 426t
with renal failure, 1013t

X

χ^2 test, 653t
Xerostomia, pilocarpine for, 913
Xopenex, formulary entry for, 841
Xylocaine
characterization of, 141t
formulary entry for, 844–845
for IV infusions, i
for RSI, 6t

Y

Yellow fever vaccine, 374

Z

Zaditor, 1002t
Zafirlukast (Accolate), formulary entry for, 984
Zanamivir
approval for, 392
for influenza, 425t
Zantac
formulary entry for, 933
with renal failure, 1034t
Zarontin
formulary entry for, 791–792
for seizures, 516t
Zaroxolyn
for *C.* colitis, 976
formulary entry for, 863–864
ZDV, in utero HIV transmission prevention by, 441t
Zemuron
formulary entry for, 940–941
for RIS, 7t
Zestril, formulary entry for, 848
Zidovudine (ZDV, AZT, Retrovir)
formulary entry for, 984
in utero HIV transmission prevention by, 441t
Zinacef
formulary entry for, 739–987
for lymphadenitis, 425t
for otitis media, 426t
with renal failure, 1016t
Zinc
dietary reference intake for, 542t
DRIs for, 542t
in formulas, 542t
in multivitamin tablets, analysis of, 547t
parenteral nutrition formulations, 561t
Zinc salts (Galzin, Orazinc, Zincate), formulary entry for, 985–986
Ziprasidone, dosage/side effects for, 1004t
Zithromax
for chlamydial infections, 420t
drug formulary for, 707
for gastroenteritis, 424t
for gonorrhea, 430t
neonatal ICU dosing with, 1000t
for otitis media, 426t
for pertussis, 428t
for pneumonia, 428t
Zmax
for chlamydial infections, 420t
drug formulary for, 707
for gastroenteritis, 424t
for gonorrhea, 430t
neonatal ICU dosing with, 1000t
for otitis media, 426t
for pertussis, 428t
for pneumonia, 428t

Zofran
  formulary entry for, 889–890
  for palliative care, 581t
Zolicef
  for bacterial endocarditis prophylaxis, 193t
  formulary entry for, 732
  with renal failure, 1015t
Zoloft, formulary entry for, 944
Zonisamide (Zonegran)
  formulary entry for, 986–987
  for seizures, 517t
ZORprin
  analgesic properties of, 139
  formulary entry for, 703–704
  for Kawasaki disease, 198
  with renal failure, 1027t
Zosyn
  formulary entry for, 914
  with renal failure, 1023t
Zovirax
  for antimicrobial prophylaxis, 575t
  formulary entry for, 685–686
  for neonatal varicella, 413t–414t
  with renal failure, 1013t
Zyloprim
  formulary entry for, 688
  with renal failure, 1027t
  for tumor lysis syndrome, 567
  for von Willebrand disease, 347t
Zymar, 1002t
Zyprexa, dosage/side effects for, 1003t
Zyrtec
  formulary entry for, 740–741
  with renal failure, 1028t

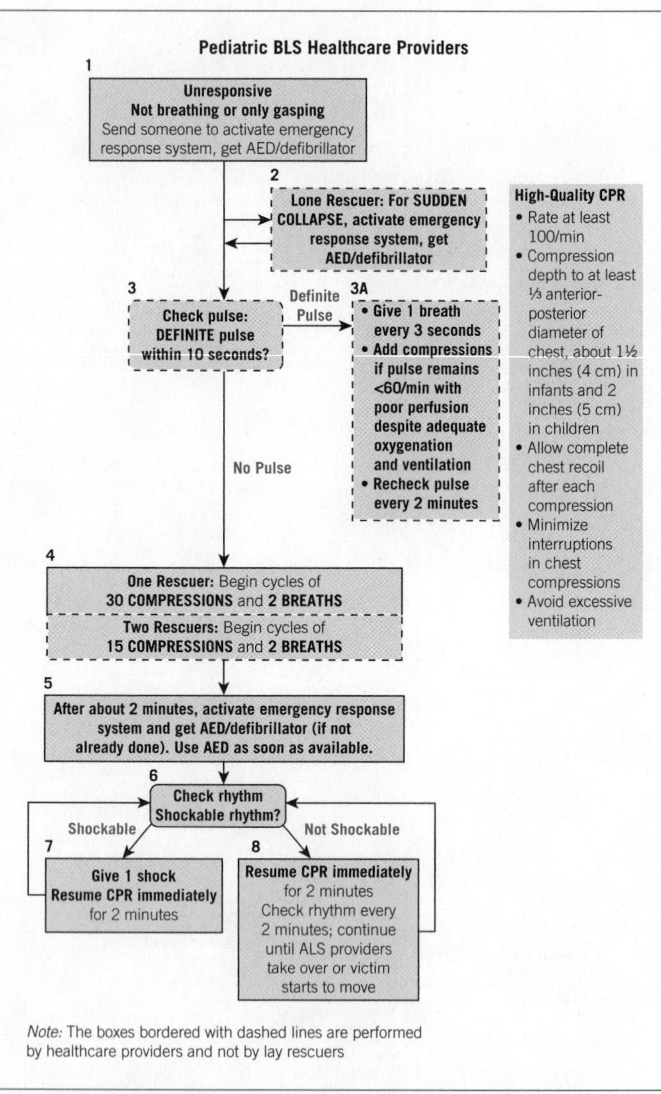

Pediatric BLS healthcare providers algorithm. *Reprinted with Permission. 2010 American Heart Association Guidelines for Cardiopulmonary Resuscitation and Emergency Cardiovascular Care. Part 13. Circulation. 2010;122:S862–S875.*

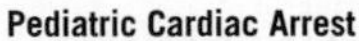

Shout for Help/Activate Emergency Response

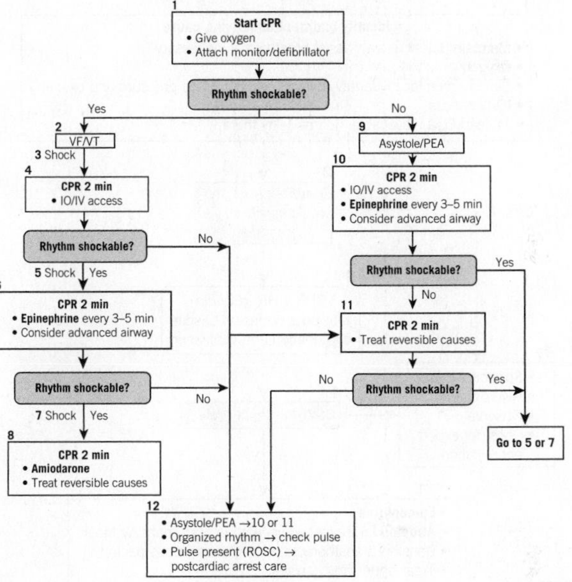

Doses/Details

CPR Quality
- Push hard (≥⅓ of anterior-posterior diameter of chest) and fast (at least 100/min) and allow complete chest recoil
- Minimize interruptions in compressions
- Avoid excessive ventilation
- Rotate compressor every 2 minutes
- If no advanced airway, 15:2 compression-ventilation ratio. If advanced airway, 8–10 breaths per minute with continuous chest compressions

Shock Energy for Defibrillation
First shock 2 J/kg, second shock 4 J/kg, subsequent shocks ≥4 J/kg, maximum 10 J/kg or adult dose.

Drug Therapy
- **Epinephrine IO/IV Dose:** 0.01 mg/kg (0.1 mL/kg of 1:10 000 concentration). Repeat every 3–5 minutes. If no IO/IV access, may give endotracheal dose: 0.1 mg/kg (0.1mL/kg of 1:1000 concentration).
- **Amiodarone IO/IV Dose:** 5 mg/kg bolus during cardiac arrest. May repeat up to 2 times for refractory VF/pulseless VT.

Advanced Airway
- Endotracheal intubation or supraglottic advanced airway
- Waveform capnography or capnometry to confirm and monitor endotracheal tube placement
- Once advanced airway in place give 1 breath every 6–8 seconds (8–10 breaths per minute)

Return of Spontaneous Circulation (ROSC)
- Pulse and blood pressure
- Spontaneous arterial pressure waves with intra-arterial monitoring

Reversible Causes
- **H**ypovolemia
- **H**ypoxia
- **H**ydrogen ion (acidosis)
- **H**ypoglycemia
- **H**ypokalemia/hyperkalemia
- **H**ypothermia
- **T**ension pneumothorax
- **T**amponade, cardiac
- **T**oxins
- **T**hrombosis, pulmonary
- **T**hrombosis, coronary

Pediatric cardiac arrest algorithm. *Reprinted with Permission. 2010 American Heart Association Guidelines for Cardiopulmonary Resuscitation and Emergency Cardiovascular Care. Part 14: Pediatric advanced life support. Circulation. 2010;122:S885.* © 2010 American Heart Association, Inc.

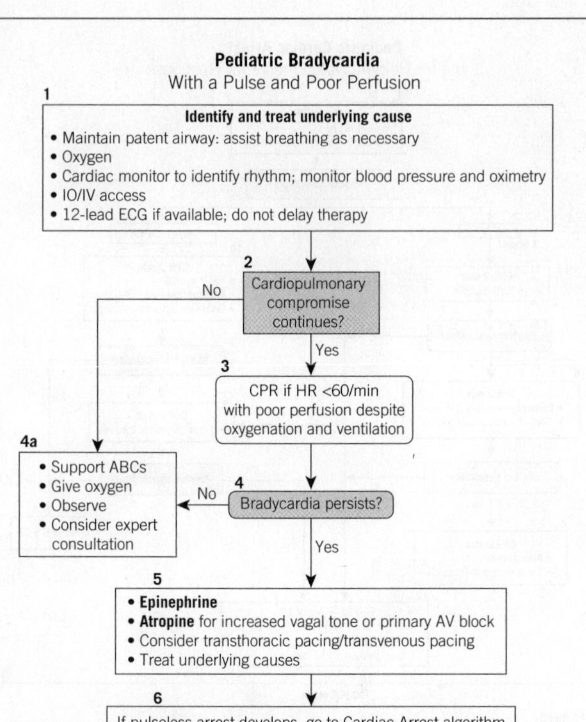

Cardiopulmonary Compromise

- Hypotension
- Acutely altered mental status
- Signs of shock

Doses/Details

Epinephrine IO/IV Dose: 0.01 mg/kg (0.1 mL/kg of 1:10 000 concentration). Repeat every 3–5 minutes. If IO/IV access not available but endotracheal (ET) tube in place, may give ET dose: 0.1 mg/kg (0.1 mLkg of 1:1000).

Atropine IO/IV Dose: 0.02 mg/kg. May repeat once. Minimum dose 0.1 mg and maximum single dose 0.5 mg.

Pediatric bradycardia algorithm. *Reprinted with Permission. 2010 American Heart Association Guidelines for Cardiopulmonary Resuscitation and Emergency Cardiovascular Care. Part 14: Pediatric advanced life support. Circulation. 2010;122:S887.*